Pharmacology and Physiology in Anesthetic Practice

PHARMACOLOGY AND PHYSIOLOGY IN ANESTHETIC PRACTICE

ROBERT K. STOELTING, M.D.

Professor and Chairman
Department of Anesthesia
Indiana University School of Medicine
Indianapolis, Indiana

J. B. LIPPINCOTT COMPANY

Philadelphia

London   Mexico City   New York   St. Louis   São Paulo   Sydney

Acquisitions Editor: Lewis Reines
Sponsoring Editor: Sanford J. Robinson
Manuscript Editor: Helen Ewan
Indexer: Barbara Littlewood
Art Director: Tracy Baldwin
Production Manager: Kathleen P. Dunn
Production Coordinator: George V. Gordon
Compositor: Progressive Typographers
Printer/Binder: R. R. Donnelley & Sons Company

6 5 4 3

Library of Congress Cataloging-in-Publication Data

Stoelting, Robert K.
  Pharmacology and physiology in anesthetic practice.

  Includes bibliographies and indexes.
    1. Anesthetics — Physiological effect. 2. Anesthesia.
3. Human physiology. 4. Pharmacology. I. Title.
[DNLM: 1. Anesthetics — pharmacodynamics. 2. Physiology.
QV 81 S872p]
RD81.S87   1987   615'.781   86-21017
ISBN 0-397-50771-2

The author and publisher have exerted every effort to
ensure that drug selection and dosage set forth in this text
are in accord with current recommendations and practice
at the time of publication. However, in view of ongoing
research, changes in government regulations, and the
constant flow of information relating to drug therapy and
drug reactions, the reader is urged to check the package
insert for each drug for any change in indications and
dosage and for added warnings and precautions. This is
particularly important when the recommended agent is a
new or infrequently employed drug.

P R E F A C E

Anesthesiology is a medical specialty that requires daily application of principles of pharmacology and physiology in the care of patients. Reference textbooks of pharmacology and physiology often serve as the repository of information that is pertinent to all medical aspects of pharmacology and physiology. Clearly, only portions of these textbooks are relevant to the clinical practice of anesthesia. In this regard, the goal of *Pharmacology and Physiology in Anesthetic Practice* is to provide students as well as practicing anesthesiologists with an in-depth but concise and current presentation of those aspects of pharmacology and physiology that are relevant either directly or indirectly to the perioperative anesthetic management of patients.

Preparation of a textbook of this scope requires unique and reliable support from others. In this regard, special accolades go to my secretary, Deanna Walker, for her skillful preparation of the many revisions that preceded the final manuscript. Ellyn Traub receives my appreciation for her skillful preparation of the original art work. Lewis Reines, president of J. B. Lippincott Company, again earned my admiration for his professionalism and constant ability to provide encouragement and resources for the evolution of this textbook. Finally, my wife and daughters deserve my special thanks for again enduring the time commitment required for another textbook.

Robert K. Stoelting, M.D.

C O N T E N T S

SECTION I

PHARMACOLOGY

CHAPTER 1

Pharmacokinetics and Pharmacodynamics of Injected and Inhaled Drugs

INTRODUCTION

Pharmacokinetics is the quantitative study of the absorption, distribution, metabolism, and excretion of injected or inhaled drugs and their metabolites (*i.e.,* what the body does to a drug) (Hug, 1978; Stanski and Watkins, 1982). Coupled with the dose of drug administered, pharmacokinetics determines the concentration of drug at its sites of action (*i.e.,* receptors) and, thus, the intensity of the drug's effects with time. Pharmacokinetics also determines variations in plasma concentrations of a drug among patients resulting from differences in its absorption, distribution, and elimination. Selection and adjustment of drug dosage schedules and interpretation of measured plasma concentrations of drugs are facilitated by an understanding of pharmacokinetic principles.

Pharmacodynamics is the study of the intrinsic sensitivity or responsiveness of receptors to a drug and the mechanisms by which these effects occur (*i.e.,* what the drug does in the body) (Hull, 1979; Maze, 1981; Stanski and Watkins, 1982). Structure activity relationships relate the actions of drugs to their chemical structure and facilitate design of drugs with more desirable pharmacologic properties. Intrinsic sensitivity of receptors is determined by measuring plasma concentrations of a drug required to evoke specific pharmacologic responses (Kauffman, 1981). Variability exists in the intrinsic sensitivity of receptors among patients. As a result, at similar plasma concentrations of drug, some patients show a therapeutic response, others show no response, and, in others, toxicity develops.

DESCRIPTION OF DRUG RESPONSE

Hyperreactive is the term used for people in whom an unusually low dose of drug produces its expected pharmacologic effects. *Hypersensitive* is the term usually reserved for people who are allergic to a drug. *Hyporeactive* describes people who require unusually large doses of drug to evoke expected pharmacologic effects. Hyporeactivity acquired from chronic exposure to a drug is better termed *tolerance*. Cross-tolerance frequently develops between drugs of different classes that produce similar pharmacologic effects (*e.g.,* alcohol and inhaled anesthetics). Tolerance that develops acutely with only a few doses of a drug, such as thiopental, is termed *tachyphylaxis*. The most important factor in the development of tolerance to drugs such as the opioids, barbiturates, and alcohol is neuronal adaptation referred to as cellular tolerance. Other mechanisms of tolerance may include enzyme induction and depletion of neurotransmitters by virtue of sustained stimulation. Immunity is present when hyporeactivity is due to formation of antibodies. Idiosyncrasy is present when an unusual effect of a drug occurs in a small percentage of patients regardless of the dose of drug. More appropriately, unusual effects of drugs should be described precisely in terms of their documented or likely mechanisms (*e.g.,* allergy, genetic difference).

An *additive effect* means that a second drug acting with the first drug will produce an effect equal to an algebraic summation. For example, the anesthetic effects of two different inhaled anesthetics are additive as reflected by MAC equivalents (Quasha *et al*, 1980) (see the section entitled Minimum Alveolar Concentration). Synergistic means two drugs interact to produce an effect that is greater than algebraic summation. Antagonism is when two drugs interact to produce an effect less than algebraic summation.

A drug that activates a receptor by binding to the receptor is called an *agonist*. An *antagonist* is a drug that binds to the receptor without activating the receptor and at the same time prevents an agonist from stimulating the receptor. Competitive antagonism is present when increasing concentrations of the antagonist progressively inhibit the response to an unchanging concentration of agonist. Noncompetitive antagonism is present when, after administration of an antagonist, even high concentrations of agonist cannot completely overcome the antagonism.

Termination of drug effect is by metabolism, excretion, or redistribution. Redistribution is a factor in terminating drug effect primarily when a highly lipid-soluble drug is administered rapidly intravenously.

PHARMACOKINETICS OF INJECTED DRUGS

Compartmental Models

Pharmacokinetics of injected drugs has been simplified by considering the body to be comprised of a number of compartments representing theoretical spaces. This approach permits a mathematical modeling of the disposition of a drug within the body based on its pharmacokinetics. In this regard, it is essential that the analytical procedures used in pharmacokinetic studies measure the parent drug and its metabolites separately.

A two-compartment model can be used to illustrate basic concepts of pharmacokinetics that also apply to more complex models (Fig. 1-1) (Stanski and Watkins, 1982). In the two-compartment model, drug is introduced by intravenous injection directly into the central compartment. Drug subsequently distributes to a peripheral compartment only to return eventually to the central compartment where clearance from the body occurs.

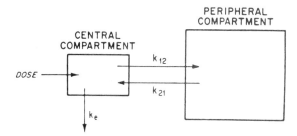

FIGURE 1-1. A two-compartment pharmacokinetic model as derived from a biexponential plasma decay curve (see Fig. 1-2). K_{12} and k_{21} are the rate constants that characterize intercompartmental transfer of drugs, and k_e is the rate constant for overall drug elimination from the body. (From Stanski DR, Watkins WD. Drug Disposition in Anesthesia. New York, Grune and Stratton, 1982. Reproduced by permission of the authors and publisher.)

The central compartment includes intravascular fluid and highly perfused tissues (*e.g.,* heart, brain, lungs, liver, kidneys) into which uptake of drug is rapid (see the section entitled Distribution). In an adult, these tissues represent about 10% of body mass but receive almost 75% of the cardiac output. This central compartment is defined only in terms of its apparent volume, which is calculated and does not necessarily correspond to actual anatomic volumes (see the section entitled Volume of Distribution). Likewise, the peripheral compartment is defined in terms of its apparent volume. A large calculated volume for the peripheral compartment suggests extensive uptake of drug by those tissues that constitute the peripheral compartment. Any residual drug present in the peripheral compartment at the time of repeat injection will diminish the effect of distributive processes on the reduction of the plasma concentration and lead to exaggerated effects of the repeat dose (*i.e.,* cumulative drug effect). The degree of cumulative drug effect can be calculated knowing the drug's volume of distribution, elimination half-time, and dosing interval.

Despite the usefulness of compartmental models to depict the pharmacokinetics of drugs, it must be appreciated that these pharmacokinetic characteristics are most often derived from healthy and ambulatory adults with a low fat-to-lean body ratio. Conversely, drugs are most likely to be administered to patients with chronic disease at various extremes of age, hydration, and nutrition.

Plasma Concentration Curves

A graphic plot of the logarithm of the plasma concentration of drug versus time following a rapid (bolus) intravenous injection characterizes the distribution and elimination half-times of that drug (Fig. 1-2) (Stanski and Watkins, 1982). Logarithms provide a convenient means for managing the large range in the plasma concentrations encountered after an intravenous injection of drug. In addition, logarithms are appropriate for depiction of the first-order kinetics characteristic of the distribution and elimination of most drugs.

Distribution and Elimination Phases

Two distinct phases (*i.e.,* biexponential) are present on the graphic plot of the decline in the plasma concentration of a drug (Fig. 1-2) (Stanski and Watkins, 1982). The first phase is designated the distribution (alpha) phase. This phase begins immediately after intravenous injection of the drug and reflects its distribution from the circulation to peripheral tissues. The second phase is designated the elimination (beta) phase. This phase is characterized by a gradual decline in the plasma concentration of the drug and reflects its

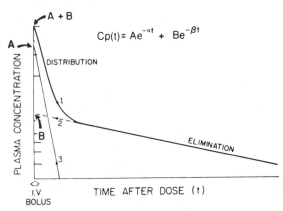

FIGURE 1-2. Schematic depiction of the decline in the plasma concentration of drug with time following rapid intravenous injection into the central compartment (see Fig. 1-1). Two distinct phases (*e.g.,* biexponential) characterize this curve, being designated the distribution and elimination phases. (From Stanski DR, Watkins WD. Drug Disposition in Anesthesia. New York, Grune and Stratton, 1982. Reproduced by permission of the authors and publisher.)

elimination from the central vascular compartment by renal and hepatic clearance mechanisms (see Fig. 1-1) (Stanski and Watkins, 1982).

ELIMINATION HALF-TIME. The rate of drug elimination can be characterized by the slope of the line representing the log plasma concentration of drug plotted against time during the elimination phase. The numerical value of the slope of the elimination phase is defined as the first-order rate constant. The concept of elimination half-time, however, is used more frequently than the rate constant. *Elimination half-time* is the time necessary for the plasma concentration of drug to decline 50% during the elimination phase. Conversely, *half-life* refers to the total amount of drug in the body and the time necessary for elimination of 50% of this total from the body. Half-time and half-life are not equal when the decline of drug concentrations in all tissues does not parallel the decline in the plasma concentration.

Elimination half-time of a first-order process can be estimated graphically by selecting any point on the straight line portion of the elimination phase and measuring the time interval to the point on the same line that represents one-half the original concentration (Fig. 1-2) (Stanski and Watkins, 1982). The elimination half-time can also be calculated as 0.63 divided by the elimination rate constant for that drug.

Elimination half-time of a drug is directly proportional to its volume of distribution and inversely proportional to its clearance. For this reason, renal or hepatic disease that alters volume of distribution and/or clearance will alter the elimination half-time.

The amount of drug remaining in the body is related to the number of elimination half-times that have elapsed. For example, if 50% of a drug is eliminated in 10 minutes, another 10 minutes will be required for elimination of one-half the remaining drug. About five elimination half-times are required for almost complete (96.9%) elimination of a drug (Table 1-1) (Hug, 1978). For this reason, drug accumulation is predictable if dosing intervals are less than this period of time. Drug accumulation continues until the rate of drug elimination equals the rate of drug administration. As with drug elimination, the time necessary for a drug to achieve a steady state plasma concentration (Cpss) with intermittent dosing is about five elimination half-times.

Table 1-1

Relationship of Half-Times to Amount of Drug Eliminated

Number of Half-Times	Fraction of Initial Amount Remaining	Percent of Initial Amount Eliminated
0	1	0
1	1/2	50
2	1/4	75
3	1/8	87.5
4	1/16	93.8
5	1/32	96.9
6	1/64	98.4

(Adapted from Hug CC. Pharmacokinetics of drugs administered intravenously. Anesth Analg 1978; 57:704–23 with permission of the author and publisher)

Route of Administration and Systemic Absorption of Drugs

The choice of route of administration for a drug should be based on an appreciation of factors that influence the systemic absorption of drugs. The rate of systemic absorption of a drug determines its intensity and duration of action. Changes in the rate of systemic absorption may necessitate an adjustment in the dose or time interval between repeated drug doses (Azarnoff and Huffman, 1976).

Systemic absorption, regardless of the route of drug administration, is dependent on drug solubility. Local conditions at the site of absorption alter solubility, particularly in the gastrointestinal tract. Circulation to the site of absorption is also important in the rapidity of absorption. For example, increased blood flow by external massage or local application of heat enhances systemic absorption, whereas decreased blood flow due to vasoconstriction impedes drug absorption. Finally, the area of absorbing surface to which a drug is exposed is an important determinant of drug absorption.

Oral Administration

Oral administration of a drug is the most convenient and economic route of administration. Disadvantages of the oral route of administration include (1) emesis because of irritation of the gastrointestinal mucosa by the drug, (2) destruction of the drug by digestive enzymes or low gas-

tric fluid *p*H, and (3) irregularities in absorption in the presence of food or other drugs. Furthermore, drugs may be metabolized by enzymes or bacteria in the gastrointestinal tract before systemic absorption can occur.

Following oral administration, the onset of drug effect is largely determined by the rate and extent of absorption from the gastrointestinal tract. The principal site of drug absorption after oral administration is from the small intestine, reflecting the large surface area of this portion of the gastrointestinal tract. Lipid solubility is necessary to facilitate drug absorption across epithelial cells lining the gastrointestinal tract. Changes in gastrointestinal *p*H that favor the lipid-soluble nonionized fraction of drug thus favor systemic absorption. Drugs, such as aspirin, which are weak acids, become more highly ionized in the alkaline environment of the small intestine, but absorption is still great because of the large surface area. Furthermore, absorption also occurs in the stomach, where gastric fluid *p*H is low.

FIRST-PASS HEPATIC EFFECT. Drugs absorbed from the gastrointestinal tract enter the portal venous blood and thus pass through the liver before entering the systemic circulation for delivery to tissue receptors (Fig. 1-3). This is known as the *first-pass hepatic effect,* and, for drugs that undergo extensive hepatic extraction and metabolism (*e.g.,* propranolol, lidocaine), this is the reason for large differences between effective oral and intravenous doses (Routledge and Shand, 1979).

Sublingual Administration

The sublingual route of administration permits rapid onset of drug effect by virtue of bypassing

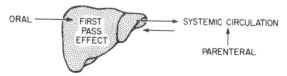

FIGURE 1-3. Drugs administered orally are absorbed from the gastrointestinal tract into the portal venous blood and pass through the liver (*e.g.,* first-pass hepatic effect) before entering the systemic circulation for distribution to receptors. Conversely, intravenously administered drugs gain rapid access to the systemic circulation without an initial impact of metabolism in the liver.

the liver and thus preventing the first-pass hepatic effect on the initial plasma concentration of drug. For example, venous drainage from the sublingual area is into the superior vena cava. Evidence of the value of bypassing the first-pass hepatic effect is the efficacy of sublingual nitroglycerin. Conversely, oral administration of nitroglycerin is ineffective because extensive first-pass hepatic metabolism prevents achievement of a therapeutic plasma concentration. Buccal administration is an alternative to sublingual placement of drug, being better tolerated and less likely to stimulate salivation. Salivation speeds solution of a tablet so that it is more easily swallowed and rendered less active (Bell *et al,* 1985).

Drugs administered rectally also bypass the liver and enter directly into the systemic circulation. Nevertheless, rectal absorption is often unpredictable, and irritation of the rectal mucosa may occur.

Transdermal Administration

Transdermal administration of drugs provides sustained therapeutic plasma concentrations of the drug with a low total dosage that results in minimal associated drug-induced side effects (Shaw and Chandrasekaran, 1978; Shaw and Urquhart, 1980). This route of administration is devoid of the complexity of continuous intravenous infusion techniques, and the low incidence of side effects owing to the minimal total dose administered contributes to high patient compliance and acceptance. Characteristics of drugs that favor predictable transdermal absorption include (1) combined water and lipid solubility, (2) molecular weight less than 1000, and (3) *p*H 5 to 9 in a saturated aqueous solution. Scopolamine, clonidine, and nitroglycerin are examples of drugs that undergo predictable transdermal absorption (see Chapters 10, 15, and 16).

The rate-limiting step in transdermal absorption of drugs is diffusion across the stratum corneum of the epidermis. Significant differences in the thickness and chemistry of the stratum corneum are reflected in the skin's permeability. For example, skin may be 10 to 20 μm thick on the back and abdomen compared with 400 to 600 μm on the palmar surfaces on the hands. Likewise, skin permeation studies have shown substantial regional differences for systemic absorption of

scopolamine (Shaw and Chandrasekaran, 1978). The postauricular zone, because of its thin epidermal layer and somewhat higher temperature, is the only area that is sufficiently permeable for predictable and sustained absorption of scopolamine. Systemic absorption is least when scopolamine is applied to the thigh and intermediate when applied to the back or chest.

It is likely that transdermal absorption of drug initially occurs along sweat ducts and hair follicles (*i.e.,* diffusion shunts). Following saturation of skin binding sites with drug, diffusion through the stratum corneum becomes the dominant pathway for absorption. The stratum corneum sloughs and regenerates at a rate such that 7 days of adhesion appears to be the duration limit for one application of a transdermal system. There is no evidence for active transport of drugs across the skin.

Parenteral Administration

Parenteral administration may be required to ensure absorption of the active form of the drug. Systemic absorption after parenteral injection is usually more rapid and more predictable than after oral administration. The effective administered dose can be more precisely determined when absorption is predictable. Parenteral administration is the only acceptable route of drug administration in an unconscious or otherwise uncooperative patient.

Systemic absorption from subcutaneous and intramuscular injection sites occurs by simple diffusion along the concentration gradient from the site of drug deposition to plasma. Rate of systemic absorption is limited by the area of the absorbing capillary membranes and by solubility of the drug in interstitial fluid. Large aqueous channels in vascular endothelium account for the unimpeded diffusion of drug molecules, regardless of their lipid solubility (see Chapter 39).

Intravenous administration avoids those factors that limit systemic absorption by other routes. As a result, the desired concentration of drug in the blood can be more rapidly and precisely acheived by this route of administration. Irritant drugs are more comfortably administered by this route because blood vessel walls are relatively insensitive and the injected drug is rapidly diluted in the blood.

Distribution of Drugs Following Systemic Absorption

Following systemic absorption of drug, the highly perfused tissues initially receive a proportionally large amount of the total dose (Table 1-2). Subsequently, as the plasma concentration of drug declines below that in the highly perfused tissues, drug leaves these tissues to be delivered to less well-perfused sites such as skeletal muscles and fat (Table 1-2).

Variation in tissue blood flow may have an important impact on distribution of drugs and, thus, the duration of their pharmacologic effects. For example, awakening after a single dose of thiopental reflects redistribution of drug from highly perfused brain to poorly perfused inactive tissues such as fat and skeletal muscles (see Chapter 4).

Uptake of a drug by tissues is determined by tissue blood flow and the tissue's capacity to accept drug (Table 1-3) (Hug, 1978). For drugs able to penetrate membranes rapidly, tissue perfusion can be the rate-limiting factor in the exchange of drug between plasma and tissues. The concentration gradient for the diffusible fraction of drug (*i.e.,* that fraction that is lipid soluble, nonionized, and unbound) determines both the rate and direction of net transfer between plasma and the tissue. For example, initially, after administration of a drug, the concentration gradient favors drug passage from plasma into tissues. At equilibrium, the concentration gradient is zero and the net exchange of drug is also zero. With continuing elimination of drug, the plasma concentration declines below that in tissues. At this time, the direction of drug movement is reversed such that drug leaves

Table 1-2
Body Tissue Compartments

	Body Mass (percent of 70-kg adult)	Blood Flow (percent of cardiac output)
Vessel-rich group	10	75
Muscle group	50	19
Fat group	20	6
Vessel-poor group	20	<1

Table 1-3
Rate and Capacity of Tissue Uptake of Drugs

Determinants of Tissue Uptake of Drug
Blood flow
Concentration gradient
Physicochemical properties of drug
 Lipid solubility
 Ionization
 Molecular size
 Protein binding
Blood–brain barrier
Membrane transport mechanisms

Determinants of Capacity of Tissue to Store Drug
Solubility
Binding to macromolecules
*p*H
Active transport
Tissue mass
Metabolism
Excretion

(Adapted from Hug CC. Pharmacokinetics of drugs administered intravenously. Anesth Analg 1978; 57:704–23; with permission of the author and the International Anesthesia Research Society.)

tissues to enter the plasma along a concentration gradient. Therefore, a tissue that preferentially accumulates drug may act as a reservoir to maintain the plasma concentration and thus prolong its duration of action. Similarly, repeated or large doses of drug may saturate inactive tissue sites, thus inhibiting the role of these tissues in providing a source of redistribution that limits the initial duration of drug action. When this occurs, the duration of action of drugs such as thiopental and fentanyl becomes dependent on metabolism rather than on redistribution.

Capacity of tissues to accept drug is largely dependent on the solubility of the drug in the tissue and the mass of the tissue (Table 1-3) (Hug, 1978). For example, a drug could exhibit limited solubility in skeletal muscles, but the large mass of this tissue (*i.e.,* about 50% of body weight) would exert a dominant role in distribution of the drug.

Central Nervous System Distribution

Distribution of drugs to the central nervous system from the circulation is restricted because of the limited permeability characteristic of brain capillaries (*i.e.,* the blood–brain barrier). In contrast to capillaries elsewhere, brain capillaries lack intracellular pores and pinocytotic vesicles (see Chapter 39). Tight junctions between capillary endothelial cells thus restrict flow of highly ionized water-soluble substances. In addition, pericapillary glial cells provide another barrier that must be traversed after drugs cross the capillary endothelium. Conversely, cerebral blood flow is the only limitation to permeation of the central nervous system by highly nonionized lipid-soluble drugs. It is important to recognize that the blood–brain barrier is subject to change and can be overcome by administration of large doses of drug. Furthermore, acute head injury and arterial hypoxemia may be associated with disruption of the blood–brain barrier.

Volume of Distribution

Volume of distribution (Vd) of a drug is a mathematical expression of the sum of the apparent volumes of the compartments that constitute the compartmental model (Fig. 1-1) (Stanski and Watkins, 1982). As such, this value depicts the distribution characteristics of a drug in the body. The Vd is calculated as the dose of drug injected intravenously divided by the resulting plasma concentration of drug before elimination starts.

The Vd is influenced by physicochemical characteristics of the drug, including (1) lipid solubility, (2) binding to plasma proteins, and (3) molecular size. Binding to plasma proteins and poor lipid solubility limit passage of drug to tissues, thus maintaining a high concentration in the plasma and a small calculated Vd. Examples of poorly lipid-soluble drugs with a Vd similar to extracellular fluid volume are the nondepolarizing neuromuscular blocking drugs. A lipid-soluble drug that is highly concentrated in tissues with a resulting low plasma concentration will have a calculated Vd that exceeds total body water. Examples of lipid-soluble drugs with Vd that exceed total body water are thiopental and diazepam.

Ionization

Most drugs are weak acids or bases that are present in solutions as both ionized and nonionized molecules (Albert, 1952). Solubility characteristics of the ionized and nonionized molecules determine the ease with which drugs may diffuse through lipid components of cell membranes. This diffusion is particularly important because drugs are often too large to pass through membrane channels.

Characteristics of Ionized and Nonionized Molecules

The nonionized drug molecule is usually lipid soluble and can diffuse across lipid cell membranes that constitute the blood–brain barrier, renal tubular epithelium, gastrointestinal epithelium, and hepatocytes (Table 1-4). As a result, this fraction of drug is pharmacologically active, undergoes reabsorption from renal tubules, is absorbed from the gastrointestinal tract, and is susceptible to hepatic metabolism. Conversely, the ionized fraction is poorly lipid soluble and cannot penetrate lipid cell membranes with ease (Table 1-4). Ionization causes the drug to be repelled from portions of cells with similar charges. A high degree of ionization thus impairs absorption of drug from the gastrointestinal tract, limits access to drug-metabolizing enzymes in the hepatocytes, and facilitates renal excretion of unchanged drug, since reabsorption across the renal tubular epithelium is unlikely. Although the degree of ionization greatly influences the rate of diffusion across parenchymal cell membranes, it has little or no effect on diffusion across vascular capillaries.

Determinants of Degree of Ionization

The degree of ionization of a drug is a function of its dissociation constant (pKa) and the pH of the surrounding fluid. When pK and pH are identical,

Table 1-4
Characteristics of Nonionized and Ionized Drug Molecules

	Nonionized	*Ionized*
Pharmacologic effect	Active	Inactive
Solubility	Lipids	Water
Cross lipid barriers (gastrointestinal tract, blood–brain barrier, placenta)	Yes	No
Renal excretion	No	Yes
Hepatic metabolism	Yes	No

50% of the drug exists in the ionized form. Small changes in pH can result in large changes in the extent of ionization, especially if the pH and pK values are similar. Acid drugs, such as barbiturates, tend to be highly ionized at an alkaline pH, whereas basic drugs, such as opioids and local anesthetics, are highly ionized at an acid pH.

Ion Trapping

A concentration difference of total drug can develop on two sides of a membrane that separates fluids with different pHs (Fig. 1-4) (Hug, 1978). As a result of this pH difference, the degree of ionization of a drug is also different on each side of the membrane. The nonionized lipid-soluble fraction of drug equilibrates across the cell membrane, but the total concentration of drug is very different on each side of the membrane because of the impact of pH on the fraction of drug that exists in the nonionized form. This is an important consideration because one fraction of the drug may be more pharmacologically active than the other fraction.

Systemic administration of a weak base, such as an opioid, can result in accumulation of ionized drug (*i.e.,* ion trapping) in the acid environment of the stomach. A similar phenomenon occurs in the transfer of basic drugs, such as local anesthetics, across the placenta from mother to fetus where the fetal pH is lower than maternal pH. The lipid-soluble nonionized fraction of local anesthetic crosses the placenta and is converted to the poorly lipid-soluble ionized fraction in the more acidic environment of the fetus. The ionized fraction in the fetus cannot easily cross the placenta back to the maternal circulation and, thus, is effectively trapped in the fetus. At the same time, conversion of the nonionized to ionized fraction maintains a gradient for continued passage of local anesthetic into the fetus. The resulting accumulation of local anesthetic in the fetus is accentuated by the acidosis that accompanies fetal distress.

Protein Binding

A variable amount of most drugs is bound to plasma proteins that include albumin, alpha-1 acid glycoprotein and lipoproteins (Wood, 1986). Most acidic drugs bind to albumin, whereas basic drugs select alpha-1 acid glycoprotein. Protein binding has an important effect on distribution of drugs, since only the free or unbound fraction is readily available to cross cell membranes and act on receptors. As a result it is the unbound fraction of drug that is pharmacologically active. Nevertheless, some protein-bound drug seems to be able to cross lipid membranes as represented by the blood–brain barrier (Wood, 1986).

Volume of distribution of drugs is inversely related to protein binding. For example, high protein binding limits passage of drugs into tissues, thus resulting in high drug plasma concentrations and a small calculated Vd (see the section entitled Volume of Distribution). Clearance of drug is also influenced by protein binding, since it is the unbound fraction in the plasma that has ready access to hepatic drug metabolizing enzymes and it is this fraction of drug that undergoes glomerular filtration.

The drug–protein complex is maintained by a weak bond (ionic, hydrogen, or van der Walls bond) and can dissociate when the plasma concentration of drug declines as a result of hepatic or renal clearance of the unbound drug fraction. In this regard, protein binding of drugs may actually facilitate elimination by acting as a transport mechanism to deliver drugs to sites of clearance.

Alterations in protein binding are usually of

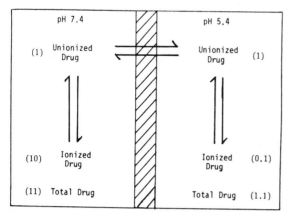

FIGURE 1-4. A concentration difference of total drug can develop on two sides of a membrane that separates fluids with different pHs. At steady state, the nonionized (unionized) drug concentration on both sides of the membrane is similar, but the concentration of ionized drug differs. (From Hug CC. Pharmacokinetics of drugs administered intravenously. Anesth Analg 1978;57: 704–23. Reproduced by permission of the author and the International Anesthesia Research Society.)

importance only for drugs that are highly protein bound such as warfarin, propranolol, phenytoin, and diazepam. For example, for a drug that is 98% protein bound, a decrease in binding to 96% will double the plasma fraction of unbound drug with potential associated increases in pharmacologic effects. Conversely, a decrease in protein binding from 70% to 68% results in only a 7% increase in the free fraction of drug in plasma.

Determinants of Protein Binding

The extent of protein binding depends largely on lipid solubility of the specific drug. In general, the degree of protein binding parallels lipid solubility. For example, pentobarbital is less highly bound to protein than is its more lipid-soluble thioanalog, thiopental. In addition to lipid solubility, the fraction of total drug in plasma that is protein bound is determined by the drug concentration and the number of available binding sites. Low plasma concentrations of drugs are likely to be more highly protein bound than are higher plasma concentrations of the same drug. Statements as to the percent of protein binding of a drug are not meaningful unless the plasma concentration of drug and availability of binding sites (*i.e.,* plasma concentration of albumin) are also known.

Binding of drugs to plasma albumin is often nonselective such that many drugs with similar physicochemical characteristics can compete with each other and with endogenous substances for the same protein binding sites. For example, sulfonamides can displace unconjugated bilirubin from binding sites on albumin, leading to the risk of bilirubin encephalopathy in the newborn.

Renal failure may decrease the percent of drug bound to protein even in the absence of changes in plasma concentrations of albumin or other proteins (Reidenberg, 1974). For example, the free fraction of phenytoin is increased in patients with renal failure such that toxic plasma concentrations are likely to occur if the total dose of drug is not decreased. This occurrence in the presence of normal plasma concentrations of albumin suggests that an alteration in protein structure or displacement of phenytoin from its protein binding sites by a metabolic factor that is normally excreted by the kidneys has occurred (Booker and Darcey, 1973). Albumin concentrations tend to be lower in elderly patients, but the impact of this change is small compared to the effect of disease states that result in renal or hepatic dysfunction.

Increases in the plasma concentration of alpha-1 acid glycoprotein occur in response to surgery, chronic pain, and acute myocardial infarction (Wood, 1986). An increase of this protein fraction in patients with rheumatoid arthritis leads to increased protein binding of lidocaine and propranolol (Piafsky *et al,* 1978). The plasma concentration of alpha-1 acid glycoprotein is reduced in neonates, resulting in decreased protein binding of several drugs, including d-tubocurarine, metocurine, diazepam, propranolol, and lidocaine (Wood and Wood, 1981).

It is important to consider protein binding when comparing maternal to fetal ratios for drugs. For example, total body concentrations of drugs may be different, but the pharmacologic effects are similar because the free concentration of drug is similar.

Clearance of Drugs from the Systemic Circulation

Clearance is the volume of plasma cleared of drug by renal excretion, metabolism in the liver or other organs or both, or a combination of these events per unit of time. Almost all drugs given in therapeutic dose ranges are cleared from plasma at a rate proportional to the amount of drug present (*i.e.,* first-order kinetics). Even at therapeutic doses, however, a few drugs will exceed the metabolic or excretory capacity of the body to clear drugs by first-order kinetics. In this situation, only a constant amount of drug is cleared per unit of time until the plasma concentration decreases below the limit of clearance saturation (*i.e.,* zero-order kinetics).

Clearance is one of the most important pharmacokinetic variables to be considered when defining a constant drug infusion regimen. To maintain an unchanging plasma concentration of drug, the intravenous infusion rate must be equal to the rate of clearance of drug by hepatic and renal mechanisms. Knowledge of the elimination half-time for a drug is crucial for achieving a constant plasma concentration of drug. Nevertheless, individual variations in Vd and clearance may alter the elimination half-time of a drug in an individual patient compared with values calculated from normal patients.

Hepatic Clearance

The hepatic clearance of a drug is the product of hepatic blood flow and the hepatic extraction ratio. If the hepatic extraction ratio is large (above 0.7), the clearance of drug will be dependent upon hepatic blood flow, whereas changes in enzyme activity have minimal influence (Fig. 1-5) (Wilkinson and Shand, 1975). Thus, a high hepatic extraction ratio results in perfusion-dependent elimination. If the hepatic extraction ratio is less than 0.3, only a small fraction of the drug delivered to the liver is removed per unit of time. As a result, an excess of drug is available for hepatic elimination mechanisms, and changes in hepatic blood flow will not greatly influence hepatic clearance. An increase in enzyme activity, however, as associated with enzyme induction or decrease in protein binding, will greatly increase hepatic clearance of a drug with a low hepatic extraction ratio. This type of hepatic elimination is termed *capacity-dependent elimination* (Wilkinson and Shand, 1975).

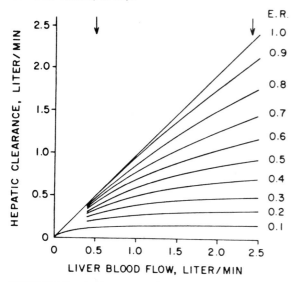

FIGURE 1-5. An increase in hepatic blood flow within the physiologic range denoted by the arrows produces minimal changes in hepatic clearance of drugs with a low extraction ratio (ER). Conversely, for drugs with a high ER, an increase in hepatic blood flow produces a nearly proportional increase in hepatic clearance. (From Wilkinson GR, Shand DG. A physiologic approach to hepatic drug clearance. Clin Pharmacol Ther 1975;18:377–90. Reproduced by permission of the authors and publisher.)

Biliary Excretion

Most of the metabolites of drugs produced in the liver are excreted in bile into the gastrointestinal tract. Often, these metabolites are reabsorbed from the gastrointestinal tract into the circulation for ultimate elimination in the urine. Organic anions such as glucuronides are actively transported into bile by carrier systems similar to those that transport these anions into renal tubules.

Renal Clearance

The kidneys are the most important organs for the elimination of unchanged drugs or their metabolites. Water-soluble compounds are excreted more efficiently by the kidneys than are compounds with high lipid solubility. This emphasizes the important role of metabolism in converting lipid-soluble drugs to water-soluble metabolites.

Renal excretion of drugs involves (1) glomerular filtration, (2) active tubular secretion, and (3) passive tubular reabsorption. The amount of drug that enters the renal tubular lumen is dependent on the fraction of drug bound to protein and the glomerular filtration rate. Renal tubular secretion involves active transport processes, which may be selective for certain drugs and metabolites, including protein-bound compounds. Reabsorption from renal tubules removes drug that has entered tubules by glomerular filtration and tubular secretion. This reabsorption is most prominent for lipid-soluble drugs that can easily cross cell membranes of renal tubular epithelial cells to enter pericapillary fluid. Indeed, a highly lipid-soluble drug, such as thiopental, is almost completely reabsorbed such that little or no unchanged drug is excreted in the urine. Conversely, production of less lipid-soluble metabolites limits renal tubule reabsorption and facilitates excretion in the urine.

The rate of reabsorption from renal tubules is influenced by factors such as *p*H and rate of renal tubular urine flow. Passive reabsorption of weak bases and acids is altered by urine *p*H, which influences the fraction of drug that exists in the ionized form. For example, weak acids are excreted more rapidly in an alkaline urine. This occurs because alkalinization of the urine results in more ionized drug that cannot easily cross renal tubular epithelial cells, resulting in less passive reabsorption.

Drug elimination by the kidneys is correlated with endogenous creatinine clearance or serum creatinine concentration. The magnitude of elevation of these indices provides an estimate of the necessary downward adjustment in drug dosage.

Metabolism of Drugs

The role of metabolism (biotransformation) is to convert pharmacologically active lipid-soluble drugs into water-soluble and often pharmacologically inactive metabolites. Increased water solubility reduces the Vd for a drug and enhances its renal excretion. A lipid-soluble parent drug is poorly excreted because of the ease of reabsorption from the lumens of renal tubules into pericapillary fluid. In the absence of metabolism, a lipid-soluble drug such as thiopental would continue to undergo reabsorption from renal tubules and have an elimination half-time of about 100 years. Metabolism to water-soluble metabolites, however, reduces its reabsorption from renal tubules and thus facilitates elimination in the urine.

It is important to recognize that metabolism does not always lead to the production of pharmacologically inactive metabolites. For example, diazepam and propranolol may be metabolized to active compounds. In some instances, an inactive parent compound (*e.g.,* cyclophosphamide) is administered and subsequently undergoes metabolism to active metabolites. These examples emphasize that metabolism is not always synonymous with deactivation or even detoxification.

Rate of Metabolism

Rate of metabolism of most drugs is determined by the concentration of drug at the site of the metabolism and by the intrinsic rate of the metabolism process. Hepatic blood flow often determines delivery and, thus, concentration of drug at the site of metabolism. The intrinsic rate of metabolism reflects factors and events that influence enzyme activity, such as genetics and enzyme induction.

FIRST-ORDER KINETICS. Most drug metabolism follows linear or first-order kinetics such that a constant fraction of available drug is metabolized in a given time period. First-order kinetics depends on the plasma concentration of drug in the sense that the absolute amount of drug eliminated per unit of time is greatest when its plasma concentration is greatest. However, the fraction of total drug that is eliminated during first-order kinetics is independent of the plasma concentration of drug.

ZERO-ORDER KINETICS. Zero-order kinetics occurs when the plasma concentration of drug exceeds the capacity of metabolizing enzymes (*i.e.,* saturation of the enzymes is present). Therefore, zero-order kinetics is nonlinear and is characterized by metabolism of a constant amount of drug per unit time. This contrasts with the constant fraction of drug metabolized during first-order kinetics. As a result, the absolute amount of drug eliminated per unit of time during zero-order kinetics is the same, regardless of its plasma concentration. The intrinsic activity of enzymes determines the constant amount of drug metabolized per unit of time. Alcohol, aspirin, and phenytoin are drugs that exhibit zero-order kinetics at even therapeutic concentrations.

Pathways of Metabolism

The four basic pathways of metabolism are (1) oxidation, (2) reduction, (3) hydrolysis, and (4) conjugation. Phase I reactions include oxidation, reduction, and hydrolysis (Drayer, 1974). Phase II reactions are when the parent drug, or a metabolite, reacts with an endogenous substrate such as a carbohydrate or amino acid to form a more water-soluble conjugate.

Hepatic microsomal enzymes are responsible for the metabolism of most drugs. Other sites of drug metabolism include plasma, lungs, kidneys, and the gastrointestinal tract. The evolutionary development of drug-metabolizing enzymes is most likely related to ingestion of toxic alkaloids in plants. In this regard, drug metabolism has evolved as a means of protection against environmental toxins.

HEPATIC MICROSOMAL ENZYMES. Hepatic microsomal enzymes, which participate in the metabolism of many drugs, are located principally in hepatic smooth endoplasmic reticulum. These microsomal enzymes are also present in the kidneys, gastrointestinal tract, and adrenal cortex. The term *microsomal enzymes* is derived from the fact that centrifugation of homogenized cells (usually hepatocytes) concentrates fragments of the disrupted smooth endoplasmic reticulum in what is designated as the microsomal fraction. The microsomal fraction also includes an iron-containing homoprotein termed *cytochrome P-450*. The designation "cytochrome P-450" emphasizes this substance's absorption peak at 450 nm when it combines with carbon monoxide. The cytochrome P-450 system is also known as the mixed function oxidase system because it involves both oxidation and reduction steps. Cytochrome P-450 functions as the terminal oxidase in the electron transport scheme. Considering the large number of different drugs metabolized by the cytochrome P-450 system, it is likely that this system is actually a large number of different protein enzymes (Coon, 1981).

Microsomal enzymes catalyze most of the oxidation, reduction, and conjugation reactions that lead to metabolism of drugs. Lipid solubility of a drug favors passage across cell membranes and thus facilitates access of drugs to microsomal enzymes in hepatocytes and other cells. Individual differences in microsomal enzyme activity are genetically determined. Indeed, rates of drug metabolism vary sixfold or more among persons as a reflection of differences in microsomal enzyme activity.

Hepatic microsomal enzyme activity is low in neonates, especially premature infants. The presence of (1) decreased metabolizing enzyme activity, (2) poorly developed blood–brain barrier, and (3) immature mechanisms for excretion of drugs often combine to make the neonate sensitive to toxic effects of drugs (Morselli, 1976).

ENZYME INDUCTION. A unique feature of hepatic microsomal enzymes is the ability of drugs or chemicals to stimulate activity of these enzymes (Conney, 1967; Gelehrter, 1976). Increased enzyme activity produced by drugs or chemicals is known as enzyme induction. Enzyme induction also occurs to a limited extent in lungs, kidneys, and the gastrointestinal tract.

Phenobarbital and polycyclic hydrocarbons are examples of substances that induce microsomal enzymes. The resulting increase in microsomal enzyme activity produced by phenobarbital is attributed to increased synthesis of cytochrome P-450 and cytochrome P-450 reductase.

NONMICROSOMAL ENZYMES. Nonmicrosomal enzymes catalyze reactions responsible for metabolism of drugs by conjugation and hydrolysis and to a lesser extent by oxidation and reduction. These nonmicrosomal enzymes are present principally in the liver but are also found in plasma and the gastrointestinal tract. All conjugation reactions except for conjugation to glucuronic acid are catalyzed by nonmicrosomal enzymes. Conjugation with acetic acid, glycine, glutathione, and sulfate are examples of nonmicrosomal enzyme reactions. Nonspecific esterases in the liver, plasma, and gastrointestinal tract are examples of nonmicrosomal enzymes responsible for hydrolysis of drugs that contain ester bonds (*e.g.*, succinylcholine, atracurium, ester local anesthetics). Hydrolysis of drugs by nonmicrosomal enzymes in the gastrointestinal tract can contribute to reduced drug effect, which is incorrectly attributed to poor oral absorption of drug.

Individual variation in activity of nonmicrosomal enzymes is similar to that present for microsomal enzymes. Nonmicrosomal enzymes such as plasma cholinesterase and acetylating enzymes do not, however, undergo enzyme induction (Stoelting and Petersen, 1975). The activity of these enzymes is genetically determined, as emphasized by patients with atypical cholinesterase enzyme and people who are classified as being rapid or slow acetylators (Uetrecht and Woosley, 1981).

OXIDATIVE METABOLISM. Hepatic microsomal enzymes, including cytochrome P-450 enzymes, are crucial for the oxidation and resulting metabolism of many drugs. These enzymes require an electron donor in the form of reduced nicotinamide adenine dinucleotide (NADPH) and molecular oxygen for their activity. The molecule of oxygen is split, with one atom of oxygen oxidizing each molecule of drug and the other oxygen atom being incorporated into a molecule of water. A loss of electrons results in oxidation, whereas a gain of electrons results in reduction.

The rate of oxidative drug metabolism is determined by the (1) concentration of cytochrome P-450 enzymes, (2) concentration of cytochrome P-450 reductase, and (3) affinities of drug for the enzymes. Rate of oxidation of drugs may also be influenced by the presence of other competing endogenous and exogenous substrates.

Epoxide intermediates in the oxidative metabolism of drugs are capable of covalent binding with macromolecules and may be responsible for drug-induced organ toxicity, such as hepatic dysfunction. Normally, these highly reactive intermediates have such a transient existence that they exert no biologic action. When enzyme induction occurs, however, large amounts of reactive intermediates may be produced, leading to organ damage. This is especially likely to occur if the antioxidant glutathione, which is in limited supply in the liver, is depleted by the reactive intermediates (Park and Breckenridge, 1981).

Examples of oxidative metabolism of drugs catalyzed by cytochrome P-450 enzymes include hydroxylation, deamination, desulfuration, dealkylation, and dehalogenation. Demethylation of morphine to normorphine is an example of oxidative dealkylation. Dehalogenation involves oxidation of a carbon–hydrogen bond to form an intermediate metabolite that is unstable and spontaneously loses a halogen atom. Halogenated volatile anesthetics are susceptible to dehalogenation, often leading to the release of bromide, chloride, and fluoride ions. Aliphatic oxidation is oxidation of a side chain. For example, oxidation of the side chain of thiopental converts the highly lipid-soluble parent drug to the more water-soluble carboxylic acid derivative. Thiopental also undergoes desulfuration to pentobarbital by an oxidative step (see Chapter 4).

REDUCTIVE METABOLISM. Reductive pathways of metabolism, like oxidative pathways, involve cytochrome P-450 enzymes. Under conditions of low oxygen partial pressures, the cytochrome P-450 enzymes transfer electrons directly to a substrate such as halothane rather than to oxygen. This electron gain imparted to the substrate occurs only when insufficient oxygen is present to compete for electrons.

HYDROLYSIS. Enzymes responsible for hydrolysis of drugs do not involve the cytochrome P-450 system (see the section entitled Nonmicrosomal Enzymes). Hydrolysis of glucuronide conjugates secreted into the bile occurs in the gastrointestinal tract and is necessary for release of drug to become available for enterohepatic recirculation.

CONJUGATION. Conjugation with glucuronic acid involves cytochrome P-450 enzymes and constitutes the major proportion of metabolites of phenols, alcohols, and carboxylic acids. When conjugated to a lipid-soluble drug or metabolite, hydrophilic glucuronic acid renders the substance (1) pharmacologically inactive, (2) more water soluble, and (3) more highly ionized at physiologic pH. As a result, glucuronide conjugates are less likely to be reabsorbed into the systemic circulation and are excreted into the bile and urine.

Conjugation can occur only when the drug contains a reactive group such as a carboxyl, primary amine, sulfhydryl, or hydroxyl, which are capable of acting as a substrate for the enzymes of conjugation. If the parent drug does not contain such groups, it becomes necessary for metabolism to occur with insertion of such a group before conjugation can take place. Glucuronic acid is always readily available from glucose. Reduced microsomal enzyme activity interferes with conjugation, leading to hyperbilirubinemia of the neonate and the risk of bilirubin encephalopathy (Morselli, 1976). This reduced microsomal enzyme activity is responsible for increased toxicity in the neonate of drugs that are normally inactivated by conjugation with glucuronic acid. Conjugation with glucuronic acid is also reduced during pregnancy, presumably because of elevated levels of progesterone.

Dose-Response Curves

Dose-response curves depict the relationship between dose of drug administered and the resulting pharmacologic effect. The hyperbolic dose-response curve demonstrates increasing drug effect with increasing doses until a maximum effect is reached, after which further increases in dose produce no additional effects. The dose that produces just a detectable effect is the threshold dose.

Dose-response curves are characterized by differences in (1) potency, (2) slope, (3) efficacy, and (4) individual responses (Fig. 1-6). Logarith-

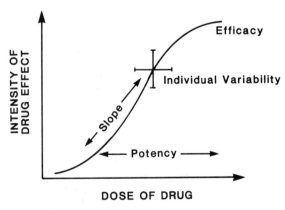

FIGURE 1-6. Dose-response curves are characterized by differences in potency, slope, efficacy, and individual responses.

mic transformation of dosage is frequently used, because it permits display of a wide range of doses.

Potency

Potency of a drug is depicted by its location along the dose axis of the dose-response curve. Factors that influence potency of a drug include (1) absorption, (2) distribution, (3) metabolism, (4) excretion, and (5) affinity for the receptor. For clinical purposes, the potency of a drug makes little difference as long as the effective dose of the drug can be administered conveniently. Low potency is a disadvantage only if the effective dose is so large that it becomes awkward to administer the required volume.

It is possible to compare potencies between two drugs only when the dose-response curves are parallel (Fig. 1-7) (Stoelting and Miller, 1984). When the dose-response curves deviate from parallelism, potency must be described individually at each level of response.

EFFECTIVE DOSES. The dose of drug required to produce a specific effect in 50% of persons is designated the median effective dose (ED50, not ED_{50}). If death is the end point, the median effective dose is termed the *median lethal dose* (LD50). Doses required to produce a specified drug effect in different percentages of the population are expressed in a similar manner (*e.g.,* ED90, LD20).

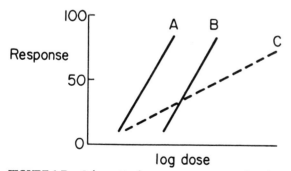

FIGURE 1-7. Schematic dose-response curves that depict parallelism *(curves A and B)* and deviation from parallelism *(curve C compared with A or B)*. A potency ratio can be derived only when the dose-response curves for two drugs are parallel. (From Stoelting RK, Miller RD, eds: Basics of Anesthesia. Churchill Livingstone Inc, New York, 1984. Reproduced by permission of the authors and publisher.)

Slope

The slope of the dose-response curves is influenced by the number of receptors that must be blocked before a drug effect occurs. For example, if a drug must occupy a majority of receptors before an effect occurs, the slope of the dose-response curve will be steep. A steep dose-response curve is characteristic of neuromuscular blocking drugs and inhaled anesthetics (*e.g.,* MAC) and means that small increases in dose evoke intense increases in drug effect. For example, a 1 MAC concentration of volatile anesthetic prevents skeletal muscle movement in response to a painful surgical skin incision in 50% of patients, whereas a modest increase to about 1.3 MAC prevents movement in at least 95% of patients. Furthermore, when the dose-response curve is steep, the difference between the concentration that is therapeutic and that which is toxic may be small. This is true for volatile anesthetics characterized by small differences between the dose that produces desirable degrees of central nervous system depression and undesirable degrees of cardiac depression.

Efficacy

The maximal effect of a drug reflects its efficacy (*i.e.,* intrinsic activity). This efficacy is reflected by the plateau in dose-response curves. It must be recognized that undesired effects (side effects) of a drug may limit dosage to below the concentration associated with maximal effect. Differences in efficacy are emphasized by pharmacologic effects of opioids versus aspirin in relieving pain. Opioids relieve pain of high intensity, whereas maximal doses of aspirin are effective only against mild discomfort. Efficacy and potency of a drug are not necessarily related.

THERAPEUTIC INDEX. Therapeutic index or margin of safety is the difference between the dose of drug required to produce a desired effect and the dose that produces undesired effects. No drug produces only a single effect. In laboratory studies, the therapeutic index is often defined as the ratio between the median lethal dose and median effective dose (LD50/ED50). Drugs have multiple therapeutic indices, depending on the therapeutic response being considered and the dose of drug necessary to evoke that response. For example, the therapeutic index for aspirin to relieve headache is greatly different from the therapeutic index to relieve pain of rheumatoid arthritis.

Individual Responses

Individual responses to a drug may vary as a reflection of differences in pharmacokinetics (*e.g.,* bioavailability, renal function, liver function, cardiac function, patient age, enzyme activity) and pharmacodynamics (*e.g.,* receptor responsiveness, drug concentration, genetics) among patients. This may even account for differences in pharmacologic effects of drugs in the same patient at different times. Drug interactions may also alter the intensity of drug effect (see the section entitled Drug Interactions).

The relative importance of the numerous factors that contribute to variations in individual responses to drugs depends, in part, on the drug itself and its usual route of excretion. Drugs that are excreted primarily unchanged by the kidneys tend to exhibit smaller differences in pharmacokinetics than do drugs that are metabolized. Of drugs that are extensively metabolized, those with slower rates of clearance tend to exhibit the greatest individual variations. In this regard, the most important determinant of the rate of metabolism is genetic. Equally important, the dynamic state of receptor concentration, as influenced by diseases and other drugs, plays an important role in the variation of drug responses observed among patients (see the section entitled Concentration of Receptors). Finally, inhaled anesthetics, by virtue of altering circulatory, hepatic, and renal function, may influence the pharmacokinetics of injected drugs.

BIOAVAILABILITY. Bioavailability describes the amount and rate of absorption of drug administered by a nonvascular route (*e.g.,* oral, intramuscular, subcutaneous). Absorption may be incomplete because of (1) physicochemical properties of the drug (*e.g.,* lipid and water solubility, molecular size), (2) the presence of food or other drugs in the gastrointestinal tract, (3) gastric emptying times, (4) *p*H in the gastrointestinal tract, and (5) characteristics of the specific pharmaceutical formulation (bioequivalence). As a result of these factors, individual variations in responses to drugs may occur.

RENAL FUNCTION. Renal function is a variable that contributes to the variation in drug response observed among patients. The magnitude of renal dysfunction is quantitated by the creatinine clearance. The dose of drug is decreased or the dosing interval is increased in proportion to the decrease in creatinine clearance. Creatinine clearance can be measured directly, or it can be estimated from the plasma concentration of creatinine (Cockroft and Gault, 1976).

LIVER FUNCTION. There is no liver function test that can quantitate the degree of liver impairment in the same way that creatinine clearance does for renal function. Factors to consider in evaluating changes in drug disposition produced by liver dysfunction include (1) altered protein binding, (2) altered drug metabolizing ability, and (3) portosystemic shunting. Chronic liver disease reduces hepatic blood flow and causes some of the portal blood to flow directly to the systemic circulation (*i.e.,* portosystemic shunting). These changes, combined with decreased hepatic enzyme activity, result in increased delivery of active drug to the systemic circulation. For example, clearance following oral administration of propranolol is halved, and systemic availability is increased in patients with cirrhosis of the liver (Wood *et al,* 1978).

Drugs with low hepatic extraction ratios are principally influenced by metabolizing activity of the hepatic enzymes. Changes, however, are unpredictable because not all pathways are equally affected by liver disease. For example, clearance of diazepam, which is oxidized by the microsomal mixed-function oxidase system, is reduced in the presence of liver disease, whereas drugs such as oxazepam and lorazepam, which are eliminated using conjugation pathways, are not affected (see Chapter 5).

CARDIAC FUNCTION. Reductions in hepatic blood flow associated with cardiac failure result in decreased hepatic clearance of lidocaine. When lidocaine is used to suppress cardiac dysrhythmias in patients with a low cardiac output, a lower than normal infusion rate should be used. The loading dose of lidocaine should also be reduced in these patients because of the smaller Vd.

PATIENT AGE. Patient age may be responsible for variations in drug response. Nonuniform organ maturation is responsible for variations in the very young, whereas nonuniform organ deterioration is responsible in the elderly.

Many metabolic mechanisms are poorly developed in premature and newborn infants, resulting in toxic plasma concentrations of drug if conventional doses are administered (Morselli, 1976). Gastric emptying is prolonged until about 6 to 12 months of age, and gastric pH does not reach adult values until about 3 years of age. Total body water, including extracellular fluid, is greater in the newborn but gradually decreases to adult values by about 12 months of age. Renal function is greatly reduced in neonates and infants but approaches adult values at 6 to 12 months of age.

In elderly patients, variations in drug response reflect (1) decreased cardiac output, (2) enlarged fat compartment, (3) reduced protein binding, and (4) a decline in renal function. Decreased cardiac output reduces hepatic blood flow and thus delivery of drug to the liver for metabolism. This decreased delivery, combined with the possibility of decreased hepatic enzyme activity may greatly prolong the duration of action of drugs such as lidocaine and fentanyl (Bentley *et al*, 1982). An enlarged fat compartment may increase the Vd and lead to the accumulation of lipid-soluble drugs such as diazepam and thiopental (Jung *et al*, 1982; Klotz *et al*, 1975). Increased total body fat content and decreased plasma protein binding of drugs accounts for the increased Vd that accompanies aging. A parallel decrease in total body water accompanies increased fat stores. The net effect of these changes is an increased vulnerability of elderly patients to cumulative drug effects. Indeed, there is an increased incidence of drowsiness following administration of diazepam to elderly patients. There is no convincing evidence that age-related changes in the responsiveness of receptors are responsible for variation of drug responses among elderly patients.

ENZYME ACTIVITY. Alterations in enzyme activity as reflected by enzyme induction may be responsible for variations in drug responses among people. For example, cigarette smoke contains polycyclic hydrocarbons that induce mixed-function hepatic oxidases leading to increased dose requirements for drugs such as theophylline and tricyclic antidepressants (Vestal and Wood, 1980). Acute alcohol ingestion can inhibit metabolism of drugs. Conversely, chronic alcohol use (greater than 200 g day^{-1}) induces microsomal enzymes that metabolize drugs (Iber, 1977). This accelerated metabolism due to enzyme induction may manifest as tolerance to drugs such as barbiturates.

GENETIC DIFFERENCES. Variations in drug responses among persons is due, in part, to genetic differences that may also affect receptor sensitivity. Pharmacogenetics describes genetically determined disease states that are initially revealed by altered responses to specific drugs (Vesell, 1979). Examples of diseases that are unmasked by drugs include (1) atypical cholinesterase enzyme revealed by prolonged neuromuscular blockade following administration of succinylcholine, (2) malignant hyperthermia triggered by succinylcholine or volatile anesthetics, (3) glucose-6-phosphate dehydrogenase deficiency, in which certain drugs cause hemolysis, and (4) intermittent porphyria, in which barbiturates evoke an acute attack.

Genetic variations in metabolic pathways may have important clinical implications. For example, acetylation may be slow or fast, depending on genetic determinants (Uetrecht and Woosley, 1981). Rapid acetylators are homozygous or heterozygous for a gene controlling an acetylating enzyme, whereas slow acetylation is a homozygous recessive trait. Isoniazid and hydralazine are examples of drugs in which pharmacologic responses are influenced by the rate of acetylation.

Drug Interactions

A drug interaction occurs when one drug alters the intensity of pharmacologic effects of another drug given concurrently (Cullen and Miller, 1979; Rawlins, 1978). The net result of a drug interaction may be enhanced or diminished effects of one or both of the drugs, leading to desired or undesired effects. Drug interactions may reflect alterations in absorption, distribution, metabolism, or clearance of one drug by another (*i.e.,* pharmacokinetic drug interactions) or alterations in interactions between agonists and antagonists at drug receptors (*i.e.,* pharmacodynamic interactions).

Beneficial Drug Interactions

An example of a beneficial drug interaction is the concurrent administration of propranolol with hydralazine so as to prevent compensatory increases in heart rate that would offset the blood-pressure – lowering effects of hydralazine. Furthermore, the concurrent use of these two drugs with different mechanisms of action permits a greater sustained reduction in blood pressure with lower doses of each drug. Use of lower doses also minimizes the likelihood of adverse side effects. Multiple drug therapy is usual in cancer chemotherapy and for the treatment of infectious diseases. Interactions between drugs are frequently used to counter the effects of agonist drugs, as reflected by the use of naloxone to antagonize opioids.

Adverse Drug Interactions

Adverse drug interactions become more likely as the number of drugs being administered to a patient increases. The mechanisms most likely responsible for adverse drug interactions involve pharmacokinetic changes. For example, one drug may interact with another to (1) impair absorption, (2) compete with the same plasma protein binding sites, (3) alter metabolism by enzyme induction or inhibition, or (4) change the rate of renal excretion. Drug interactions leading to adverse responses can also occur at receptor sites. Adverse drug interactions typically manifest as impaired therapeutic efficacy or enhanced toxicity or both.

PHARMACODYNAMICS OF INJECTED DRUGS

Mechanism of Drug Action

The most common mechanism by which drugs exert pharmacologic effects is by the interaction of the drug with a specific protein macromolecule in the cell membrane (Maze, 1981). This protein macromolecule in the cell membrane is referred to as a receptor. The drug–receptor interaction alters the function or conformation of a specific cellular component that initiates or prevents a series of changes characteristic of the pharmacologic effects of the drug. Specific receptors and subtypes of receptors are identified using radioactive-labeled drugs and hormones. Prior to the advent of these radioactive binding techniques, receptors could be considered only concepts that were useful in describing the pharmacologic effects of drugs. Radioactive binding techniques have also made it possible to demonstrate that the concentration (density) of receptors in cell membranes changes (e.g., dynamic) in response to biologically relevant stimuli. Clearly, these receptors exist for endogenous regulatory substances such as hormones and neurotransmitters. A drug ad-

ministered as an exogenous substance is an incidental "passenger" for these receptors.

Receptors for polypeptide hormones and catecholamines are present in cell membranes of responsive cells. Conversely, receptors for steroid hormones are present in the cytoplasm of cells. Receptors for thyroid hormones are present in the chromatin of target cells.

Classification of Receptors

Receptors are identified and subsequently classified primarily on the basis of effects of specific antagonists and by the relative potencies of known agonists. Such a classification serves as a practical basis for summarizing the pharmacologic effects of agonist drugs and the likely effects of antagonist drugs.

Multiple subtypes of receptors exist for many receptors. For example, there are differences in the ligand binding properties for acetylcholine at cholinergic nicotinic receptors present in ganglia of the autonomic nervous system compared with those at the neuromuscular junction. This difference is emphasized by nondepolarizing neuromuscular blocking drugs that block the nicotinic receptor at the neuromuscular junction but exert minimal or no effect at nicotinic receptors in autonomic ganglia. Likewise, ganglionic blocking drugs used to lower blood pressure do not produce skeletal muscle paralysis. Other examples of receptor subtypes include alpha-1 and alpha-2 receptors, beta-1 and beta-2 receptors, H_1 and H_2 receptors, and the various subtypes of opioid receptors.

Second Messenger

Receptors often function as a mechanism for the regulation of the intracellular concentration of adenosine $3',5'$-monophosphate (cyclic AMP). Cyclic AMP is designated the second messenger. Conceptually, a recognition site in the lipid bilayer of cell membranes facing the exterior of cells interacts with the water-soluble endogenous ligand (Maze, 1981). It is likely that this recognition site is the enzyme adenylate cyclase (i.e., first messenger). This ligand–recognition site interaction activates a subsequent interaction with catalytic sites also present in the lipid bilayer cell membranes but facing the interior of cells. Activation of this catalytic site catalyzes the conversion of adenosine triphosphate (ATP) to cyclic AMP.

Alternately, the effector may open channels in cell membranes, allowing ionic fluxes to move along concentration and electrical gradients. The importance of recognition sites facing the exterior of cell membranes is related to the poor lipid solubility of many polypeptide hormones and catecholamines, which could not otherwise penetrate the lipid barrier of cell membranes to initiate a physiologic effect.

The action of a large number of hormones appears to be mediated by cyclic AMP, which functions as a second messenger by activating protein kinases that phosphorylate proteins. These proteins are usually enzymes; thus, phosphorylation changes their activity. For example, binding of epinephrine to beta-adrenergic receptors in membranes of cells involved in synthesis of glycogen results in generation of cyclic AMP and phosphorylation of the enzyme glycogen synthetase. Phosphorylated glycogen synthetase has decreased enzyme activity, so that synthesis of glycogen from glucose is inhibited. At the same time, however, the breakdown of glycogen to glucose is enhanced.

Steroids, which are more lipid soluble than polypeptide hormones and catecholamines, are exceptions to the general concept that regulation of intracellular cyclic AMP concentrations is the determinant of physiologic responses. The lipid solubility of steroids allows these hormones to pass through cell membranes and enter the cytoplasm, where they bind to receptors. This intracellular receptor–steroid combination in some way regulates the concentration of specific messenger ribonucleic acid (RNA). Because the rate of synthesis of proteins is determined by RNA, steroids are able to alter this rate of synthesis in organs such as the liver.

Concentration of Receptors

The concentration of receptors in the lipid portion of cell membranes is dynamic, either increasing (up-regulation) or decreasing (down-regulation) in response to specific stimuli. For example, an excess of endogenous ligand, as present in a patient with a pheochromocytoma, results in a decrease in the concentration of beta-adrenergic receptors in cell membranes (e.g., down-regulation) in an attempt to reduce the magnitude of stimulation. Likewise, prolonged treatment of asthma with a beta agonist results in tachyphylaxis associated with a decrease in the concentration of

receptors (Galant et al, 1978). Conversely, chronic interference with activity of receptors as produced by a beta antagonist may result in increased numbers of receptors in cell membranes (i.e., up-regulation) such that an exaggerated response (i.e., hypersensitivity) occurs if the blockade is abruptly reversed such as by the sudden discontinuation of propranolol (Fraser et al, 1981).

Disease states may reflect inappropriate regulation of the concentration of receptors in cell membranes. For example, antibodies against beta-adrenergic receptors may occur in asthmatics, leading to a predominance of bronchoconstrictor activity. Patients with myasthenia gravis often manifest antibodies to acetylcholine receptors. The number of beta-adrenergic receptors may be reduced in the elderly. Indeed, more isoproterenol is necessary to increase heart rate in the elderly compared with younger people (Vestal et al, 1979).

Changing concentrations of receptors in the lipid bilayer of cell membranes emphasizes that receptors determine that pharmacologic responses to drugs are not static components of the cell but rather are in a dynamic state. This dynamic state is modulated by a variety of exogenous and endogenous factors that may influence the pharmacologic response to drugs in different people or the same person at different times. Keeping this concept in mind, variable pharmacologic responses often evoked by drugs become more predictable.

Characteristics of Drug – Receptor Interaction

A drug or endogenous substance (ligand) is an agonist if the drug–receptor interaction elicits a pharmacologic effect by virtue of an alteration in the functional properties of receptors. A drug is an antagonist when it interacts with receptors but does not alter the functional properties of receptors and, at the same time, prevents response of receptors to an agonist. If inhibition can be overcome by increasing the concentration of agonist, the antagonist drug is said to produce competitive blockade. This type of antagonism is produced by neuromuscular blocking drugs and beta-adrenergic antagonists that act reversibly at receptors. An agonist drug that binds only weakly to receptors may produce minimal pharmacologic effects even though a maximal concentration is present. Such a drug is known as a *partial agonist*. Examples of partial agonists are the opioid agonist–antagonist drugs.

INTRINSIC ACTIVITY. Intrinsic activity (*e.g.,* agonist, partial agonist, antagonist) reflects the different intensity of effects of drugs of the same chemical class that bind to the same receptors. Efficacy, which is the same as intrinsic activity, ultimately determines the maximal pharmacologic responses produced by drugs. Affinity of a drug for specific receptors determines the position of the dose-response curve and, thus, the relative potency of that drug. For example, increased affinity of a drug for its receptor moves the dose-response curve to the left.

The affinity of drugs for a specific receptor in cell membranes and the intrinsic activity are closely related to chemical structure. For example, minor modifications in the structure of a drug molecule, especially changes in stereoisomerism, can result in dramatic changes in the drug's pharmacologic properties. This knowledge may be used to design more precise agonist and antagonist drugs with minimal side effects.

RECEPTOR OCCUPANCY THEORY. It is traditionally assumed that the intensity of effect produced by binding of drugs to receptors is proportional to the fraction of receptors occupied by the drug. Conceptually, maximal drug effects occur when all the receptors are occupied. This receptor occupancy theory, however, does not explain differences in intrinsic activity between drugs that occupy the same number of receptors producing responses ranging from full stimulation to antagonism.

STATE OF RECEPTOR ACTIVATION. A modification of the receptor occupancy theory that is consistent with differences in intrinsic activity of drugs is the concept of activated and nonactivated states for receptors (Papadimetriou and Worcel, 1974). In this theory, when an agonist binds to receptors, it converts the receptors from a nonactivated to an activated state. Full agonists are able to convert most of the receptors they occupy to the activated state, partial agonists convert only a fraction of the receptors they occupy to the activated state, and antagonists do not activate any of the receptors they occupy to the activated state. Increasing doses of a partial agonist in the presence of a maximal effect produced by an agonist results in competitive antagonism of the effect of the agonist. Conversely, addition of a partial agonist in the presence of less than a maximal effect produced by the agonist will result in additional drug action to the maximal effect of the partial agonist.

DRUG RECEPTOR BOND. The action of drugs on receptors requires binding to occur between drugs and receptors by a physicochemical force. Bonds between the drug and receptor may be covalent, ionic, hydrogen, and van der Walls. It is likely that multiple types of bonds between drugs and receptors occur involving reactive groups on drugs and complimentary regions of receptors.

A covalent bond is formed by sharing a pair of electrons between atoms. This is a strong bond, and, because of its high stability, it plays little role in the reversible binding of drugs to receptors. Covalent bonding is involved in the inactivation of cholinesterase enzyme by organophosphates (*e.g.,* insecticides) and prolonged alpha-adrenergic blockade as produced by phenoxybenzamine.

Ionic bonds arise from electrostatic forces existing between groups of opposite charge. Acidic or basic drugs that are ionized at plasma pH can readily combine with available charged groups on proteins.

Hydrogen bonds occur between hydroxyl groups or amino groups and an electronegative carbonyl oxygen group. Van der Walls forces are weak bonds between two atoms or groups of atoms of different molecules. When the configuration between drug and receptor is sterically similar, these bonds can form readily.

Nonreceptor Drug Action

Several drugs act by mechanisms other than combination with receptors in cell membranes. For example, chelating agents are capable of forming strong bonds with metallic cations that may be bound normally or abnormally in the body. Antacids neutralize gastric acid by a direct action.

Plasma Drug Concentrations

Plasma drug concentrations are a reliable monitor of therapy only when interpreted in parallel with the clinical course of the patient (Koch-Weser, 1972). Furthermore, serial measurements of plasma drug concentrations at selected intervals are more informative than isolated determinations. It is misleading to measure the plasma concentrations of drugs during the rapidly changing distribution phase. Likewise, at a later time, when the gradient is reversed, drug concentrations at receptors are probably higher than that existing in plasma. In this regard, individual kinetic characteristics of each drug must be considered to determine an optimal time during the elimination phase for measurement of a steady state plasma concentration of drug. Finally, it is important to know whether the analytical technique used measures both free and protein-bound drug. Most often, the technique for determining the plasma concentration of a drug measures the total concentration of drug and does not discriminate between protein-bound or free drug. Nevertheless, pharmacologic effects usually reflect only the free fraction of drug in the plasma. Indeed, drug toxicity from phenytoin and diazepam are more frequent in patients with associated hypoalbuminemia, suggesting that measurement of the free fraction of these drugs would permit better prediction of drug toxicity.

Relationship of Plasma and Receptor Drug Concentration

Typically, there is a direct relationship between the (1) dose of drug administered, (2) resulting plasma concentration, and (3) intensity of drug effect. This emphasizes the relationship between the concentration of drug at its site of action (receptors) and the plasma concentration. In patients, the plasma concentration of drug is the most practical measurement for monitoring the receptor concentration. The plasma concentration should be proportional, if not equal, to the receptor concentration. Furthermore, factors influencing the concentration of drug in plasma (*e.g.,* tissue uptake, renal excretion, hepatic metabolism) will also affect the drug's concentration at receptors. During acute drug therapy, the number of receptors is constant and the formation, therefore, of the drug–receptor complex and resulting pharmacologic effect depends on only the plasma concentration of drug. Likewise, the onset and duration of drug effects are related to the rise and decline of the drug concentration at responsive receptors as reflected by corresponding changes in the plasma concentration.

Appropriateness of Initial and Maintenance Doses

Measurement of plasma concentrations of drugs along with clinical observations serves to verify the appropriateness of the initial loading and maintenance doses. A knowledge of plasma concentrations of drugs is particularly useful for guiding initial and maintenance doses in patients with renal or hepatic disease and in patients at the extremes of age when the risk of drug accumulation and toxicity is increased.

The initial loading dose is necessary to promptly establish a therapeutic plasma concentration of drug. This initial dose will be larger than the subsequent maintenance dose. Changes in the Vd will influence the size of the initial dose. For example, in the presence of an increased Vd, the drug is diluted in a large volume, and, thus, a larger initial dose is required to produce the same plasma concentration of drug that would be obtained with a smaller dose and a normal Vd. The maintenance dose of a drug must be adjusted downward in the presence of renal or hepatic dysfunction so as to prevent drug accumulation due to a prolonged elimination half-time. This adjustment can be achieved by reducing the maintenance dose or increasing the time interval between doses.

PHARMACOKINETICS OF INHALED ANESTHETICS

Pharmacokinetics of inhaled anesthetics describes their (1) absorption (uptake) from alveoli into pulmonary capillary blood, (2) distribution in the body, and (3) eventual elimination by way of the lungs. A series of partial pressure gradients beginning at the anesthetic machine serve to drive the inhaled anesthetic across various barriers (*e.g.,* alveoli, capillaries, cell membranes) to the sites of action in the brain. The principal objective of inhalation anesthesia is to achieve a constant and optimal brain partial pressure of the inhaled anesthetic.

The brain and all other tissues equilibrate with the partial pressures of inhaled anesthetics delivered to them by arterial blood (Pa) (Fig. 1-8) (Stoelting and Miller, 1984). Likewise, arterial blood equilibrates with alveolar partial pressures (PA) of anesthetics. This emphasizes that the PA of

$$\textsf{P}_{\textsf{A}} \rightleftarrows \textsf{P}_{\textsf{a}} \rightleftarrows \textsf{P}_{\textsf{br}}$$

FIGURE 1-8. The alveolar partial pressure (PA) of an inhaled anesthetic is in equilibrium with the arterial blood (Pa) and brain (Pbr). As a result, the PA is an indirect measurement of anesthetic partial pressure at the brain. (From Stoelting RK, Miller RD, eds: Basics of Anesthesia. Churchill Livingstone Inc, New York, 1984. Reproduced by permission of the authors and the publisher.)

inhaled anesthetics mirrors the brain partial pressure (Pbr). This is the reason that PA is used as an index of depth of anesthesia and recovery from anesthesia and measure of anesthetic equal potency (*e.g.,* minimum alveolar concentration, MAC). Understanding those factors that determine the PA and thus the Pbr permits control of the doses of inhaled anesthetics delivered to the brain.

Determinants of the Alveolar Partial Pressure

The PA and ultimately the Pbr of inhaled anesthetics is determined by input (delivery) into the alveoli minus uptake (loss) of the drug from alveoli into arterial blood (Table 1-5) (Stoelting and Miller, 1984). Input of inhaled anesthetics depends on the (1) inhaled partial pressures, (2) alveolar ventilation (VA), and (3) characteristics of the anesthetic breathing system. Uptake of inhaled anesthetics from alveoli depends on (1) lipid solubility, (2) cardiac output (CO), and (3) alveolar-to-venous partial pressure difference (A-vD). Percutaneous loss of inhaled anesthetics occurs but is too small to influence the rate of rise in the PA (Stoelting and Eger, 1969a). For example, the greatest loss occurs during administration of nitrous oxide when the estimated percutaneous loss is 5 to 10 ml min^{-1} with an alveolar concentration of 70%. With the possible exception of methoxyflurane, the magnitude of metabolism of other inhaled anesthetics is too small to influence the rate of increase of the PA (Berman *et al,* 1973). This lack of effect reflects the large excess of anesthetic molecules administered and the saturation, by anesthetic concentrations of inhaled drugs, of enzymes responsible for anesthetic metabolism (Halsey *et al,* 1971; Sawyer *et al,* 1971).

Table 1-5
Factors Determining Partial Pressure Gradients Necessary for Establishment of Anesthesia

Transfer of Inhaled Anesthetic from Anesthetic Machine to Alveoli
  Inspired partial pressure
  Alveolar ventilation
  Characteristics of anesthetic breathing system
Transfer of Inhaled Anesthetic from Alveoli to Arterial Blood
  Blood: gas partition coefficient
  Cardiac output
  Alveolar-to-venous partial pressure difference
Transfer of Inhaled Anesthetic from Arterial Blood to Brain
  Brain: blood partition coefficient
  Cerebral blood flow
  Arterial-to-venous partial pressure difference

(Adapted from Stoelting RK, Miller RD, eds: Basics of Anesthesia. Churchill Livingstone Inc., New York, 1984; by permission.)

Inhaled Partial Pressure

A high inhaled partial pressure (PI) delivered from the anesthetic machine is required during initial administration of the inhaled anesthetic. High initial input offsets the impact of uptake and thus accelerates induction of anesthesia as reflected by the rate of rise in the PA and thus Pbr. With time, as uptake into the blood decreases, the PI is decreased to match the reduced anesthetic uptake and thus maintain a constant and optimal Pbr. If the PI is maintained constant with time, the PA and the Pbr will increase progressively as uptake diminishes.

CONCENTRATION EFFECT. The impact of PI on the rate of rise of the PA of an inhaled anesthetic is known as the *concentration effect* (Fig. 1-9) (Eger, 1963). The concentration effect states that the greater the PI, the more rapidly the PA approaches the PI. The greater PI provides input to offset uptake and thus speeds the rate at which the PA rises.

The concentration effect results from (1) a concentrating effect and (2) an augmentation of tracheal inflow (Stoelting and Eger, 1969b). The concentrating effect reflects concentration of the inhaled anesthetic in a smaller lung volume due to uptake of all gases in the lung. At the same time, anesthetic input (*i.e.,* tracheal inflow) is in-

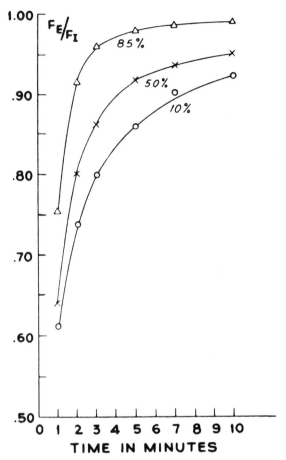

of the second gas reflects increased tracheal inflow of all the inhaled gases (first and second gases) and concentration of the second gas in a smaller lung volume (*i.e.*, concentrating effect) due to the high volume uptake of the first gas (Fig. 1-11) (Stoelting and Eger, 1969b).

Alveolar Ventilation

Increased VA, like PI, promotes input of anesthetics to offset uptake. The net effect is a more rapid rate of rise in the PA and induction of anesthesia. Decreased VA has the opposite effect, acting to decrease input and thus slow the establish-

FIGURE 1-9. The impact of the inhaled concentration of an anesthetic on the rate at which the alveolar concentration approaches the inspired (FE/FI) is known as the concentration effect. (From Eger EI. Effect of inspired anesthetic concentration on the rate of rise of alveolar concentration. Anesthesiology 1963;24:153–7. Reproduced by permission of the author and publisher.)

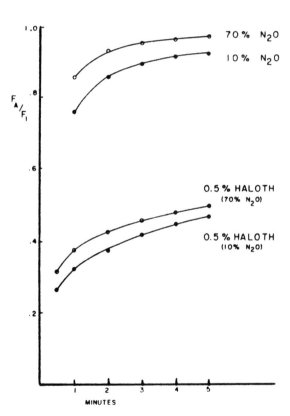

creased to fill the space (*i.e.*, void) produced by uptake of gases.

SECOND GAS EFFECT. The second gas effect reflects the ability of high volume uptake of one gas (first gas) to accelerate the rate of rise of the PA of a concurrently administered companion gas (second gas) (Fig. 1-10) (Epstein *et al,* 1964). For example, the initial large volume uptake of nitrous oxide accelerates the uptake of companion gases such as a volatile anesthetic. This increased uptake

FIGURE 1-10. The second gas effect is the accelerated rise in the alveolar concentration of a second gas, halothane (HALOTH), toward the inspired (FA/FI) in the presence of a high inhaled concentration of the first gas (nitrous oxide). (From Epstein RM, Rackow H, Salanitre E, Wolf G. Influence of the concentration effect on the uptake of anesthetic mixtures: The second gas effect. Anesthesiology 1964;25:364–71. Reproduced by permission of the authors and publisher.)

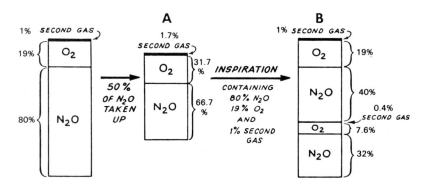

FIGURE 1-11. The second gas effect results from a concentrating effect *(A)* and an augmentation of tracheal inflow *(B)*. (From Stoelting RK, Eger EI. An additional explanation for the second gas effect: A concentrating effect. Anesthesiology 1969;30:273–7. Reproduced by permission of the authors and publisher.)

ment of a PA and Pbr necessary for the induction of anesthesia.

In addition to increased input, the decreased $PaCO_2$ produced by hyperventilation of the lungs acts to decrease cerebral blood flow. Conceivably, the impact of increased input on the rate of rise of the PA would be offset by decreased delivery of anesthetic to the brain.

The impact of changes in VA on the rate of rise in the PA depends on the solubility of the anesthetic. For example, changes in VA influence the rate of rise of the PA of a soluble anesthetic more than a poorly soluble anesthetic. Indeed, the rate of rise in the PA of a poorly soluble anesthetic, such as nitrous oxide, is rapid regardless of the VA. This occurs because uptake of nitrous oxide is limited because of its poor solubility. Conversely, uptake of a soluble drug is great, and increasing VA provides more drug input to offset loss by way of uptake. As a result, increases in VA greatly accelerate the rate at which the PA of a soluble anesthetic approaches the PI. This emphasizes that switching from spontaneous to controlled ventilation of the lungs, which is likely also to be associated with increased VA, will probably increase the depth of anesthesia (*i.e.,* PA) produced by a soluble anesthetic.

Inhaled anesthetics influence their own uptake by virtue of depressant effects on VA. Increasing concentrations of volatile anesthetics reduce VA and thus input. This, in effect, is a negative feedback mechanism that prevents establishment of an excessive depth of anesthesia when high PI is administered. This protective mechanism is lost when mechanical ventilation of the lungs replaces spontaneous ventilation.

Anesthetic Breathing System

Characteristics of the anesthetic breathing system that influence the rate of rise of the PA are the (1) volume of the external breathing system, (2) the solubility of inhaled anesthetics in the rubber or plastic components of the breathing system, and (3) gas inflow from the anesthetic machine. The volume of the anesthetic breathing system acts as a buffer to slow achievement of the PA. High gas inflow rates (5–10 L min^{-1}) from the anesthetic machine negate this buffer effect. Solubility of inhaled anesthetics in the components of the anesthetic breathing system initially slows the rate at which the PA increases. At the conclusion of the administration of an anesthetic, however, reversal of the partial pressure gradient in the anesthetic breathing system results in elution of the anesthetic, which slows the rate at which the PA decreases.

Solubility

Solubility of inhaled anesthetics in blood and tissues is denoted by the partition coefficient (Table 1-6). A partition coefficient is a distribution ratio describing how the inhaled anesthetic distributes itself between two phases at equilibrium (*i.e.,* when the partial pressures are identical). For example, a blood:gas partition coefficient of 1.4 means that the concentration of inhaled anesthetic is 1.4 in the blood and 1 in alveolar gas when the partial pressures of that anesthetic in these two phases are identical. The partition coefficient may also be thought of as reflecting the relative capacity of each phase to accept anesthetic.

Table 1-6
Comparative Solubilities of Inhaled Anesthetics

	Blood:Gas Partition Coefficient	Brain:Blood Partition Coefficient	Muscle:Blood Partition Coefficient	Fat:Blood Partition Coefficient	Oil:Gas Partition Coefficient
Soluble					
Methoxyflurane	12	2	1.3	49	970
Intermediate Solubility					
Halothane	2.4	2.6	3.5	60	224
Enflurane	1.9	2.6	1.7	36	98
Isoflurane	1.4	3.7	4.0	45	98
Poorly Soluble					
Nitrous oxide	0.47	1.1	1.2	2.3	1.4

Partition coefficients are temperature dependent. For example, the solubility of a gas in a liquid is increased when the temperature of the liquid decreases.

BLOOD:GAS PARTITION COEFFICIENTS. Based on their blood:gas partition coefficients, inhaled anesthetics are traditionally categorized as (1) soluble (methoxyflurane), (2) having intermediate solubility (halothane, enflurane, isoflurane), and (3) poorly soluble (nitrous oxide) (Table 1-6). Blood can be considered a pharmacologically inactive reservoir, the size of which is determined by the solubility of the anesthetic in blood. When the blood:gas partition coefficient is high, a large amount of anesthetic must be dissolved in the blood before the Pa equilibrates with the PA. For example, the high solubility of methoxyflurane slows the rate at which the PA and Pbr rise; thus, induction of anesthesia is slow (Fig. 1-12). The impact of high blood solubility on the rate of rise of the PA can be offset, to some extent, by increasing the PI. When blood solubility is low, as with nitrous oxide, minimal amounts of inhaled anesthetic must be dissolved before equilibrium is reached; thus, the rate of rise of PA and Pa and, thus, the induction of anesthesia is rapid (Fig. 1-12).

The greater solubility of volatile anesthetics in blood than can be accounted for by their solubility in lipids and water most likely reflects protein binding of these drugs. Blood:gas partition coefficients are altered by individual variations in water, lipid and protein content, and hematocrit of

whole blood (Laasberg and Hedley-White, 1970). For example, blood:gas partition coefficients are about 20% less in blood with an hematocrit of 21% compared with blood with an hematocrit of 43% (Ellis and Stoelting, 1975). Presumably, this decreased solubility reflects the reduction in lipid-dissolving sites normally presented by erythrocytes. Conceivably, reduced solubility of volatile anesthetics in anemic blood would manifest as an

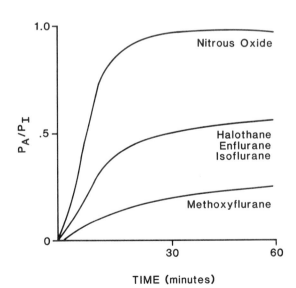

FIGURE 1-12. The rate at which the alveolar partial pressure (PA) approaches the inspired partial pressure (PI) is principally determined by solubility of the anesthetic in blood.

increased rate of rise in the PA and a more rapid induction of anesthesia. Not all investigators, however, have reported reductions in solubility of volatile anesthetics with decreases in hematocrit (Lerman *et al*, 1984). Ingestion of a fatty meal alters the composition of blood, resulting in about a 20% increase in the solubility of volatile anesthetics in blood (Munson *et al*, 1978).

TISSUE : BLOOD PARTITION COEFFICIENTS. Tissue : blood partition coefficients determine the time necessary for equilibration of tissues with the Pa. This time can be predicted by calculating a time constant (amount of inhaled anesthetic that can be dissolved in the tissue divided by tissue blood flow) for each tissue. One time constant on an exponential curve represents 63% equilibration. Three time constants are equivalent to about 95% equilibration.

Brain : blood partition coefficients for volatile anesthetics are about 2.5, resulting in a time constant of about 5 minutes (*i.e.*, 2.5 times 100 divided by 50 ml min^{-1} of blood flow to every 100 g of brain tissue) (Table 1-6). Therefore, complete equilibration between partial pressures in the arterial blood and brain requires about 15 minutes (*i.e.*, three time constants). Three time constants for nitrous oxide is about 6 minutes, reflecting the low brain : blood partition of about 1 (Table 1-6). Tissue : blood partition coefficients of inhaled anesthetics for most lean tissues are almost 1, emphasizing that different lean tissues do not have greatly different capacities for anesthetics (Table 1-6). The exception is fat, which has a large capacity to hold anesthetic, as reflected by high fat : blood partition coefficients (Table 1-6). The resulting large capacity of fat to store anesthetic and the low blood flow to this tissue serves to prolong the time required to narrow anesthetic partial pressure differences between arterial blood and fat.

Fasting before elective operations or associated with disease processes results in transport of fat to the liver. In animals, liver : blood partition coefficients for volatile anesthetics increase 15% to 20% after 6 hours of starvation and 35% to 42% after 24 hours (Fassoulaki and Eger, 1986). Brain : gas and blood : gas partition coefficients are not altered by starvation for these same periods of time. It is possible that increased anesthetic uptake by the liver would modestly slow the rate of increase in the concentration of volatile drug during induction of anesthesia.

OIL : GAS PARTITION COEFFICIENTS. Oil : gas partition coefficients parallel anesthetic requirements. For example, MAC can be calculated as 150 divided by the oil : gas partition coefficient. Using this calculation, the predicted MAC for enflurane is about 1.5% (*i.e.*, 150 divided by the oil : gas partition coefficient of 98) (Table 1-6). The constant, 150, is the average value of the product of oil : gas solubility and MAC for numerous inhaled drugs with widely divergent lipid solubilities.

NITROUS OXIDE TRANSFER TO CLOSED GAS SPACES. The blood : gas partition coefficient of nitrous oxide (0.47) is 34 times greater than nitrogen (0.014). This differential solubility means that nitrous oxide can leave the blood to enter an air-filled cavity 34 times more easily (*i.e.*, rapidly) than nitrogen can leave the cavity to enter blood (Eger and Saidman, 1965). As a result of this preferential transfer of nitrous oxide, the volume or pressure of the air-filled cavity increases. Passage of nitrous oxide into an air-filled cavity surrounded by a compliant wall (*e.g.*, intestinal gases, pneumothorax, pulmonary blebs, air bubbles) causes the gas space to expand. Conversely, passage of nitrous oxide into an air-filled cavity surrounded by a noncompliant wall (*e.g.*, middle ear, cerebral ventricles, supratentorial space) causes an increase in intracavitary pressure.

The magnitude of volume or pressure increase is influenced by the (1) partial pressure of nitrous oxide, (2) blood flow to the air-filled cavity, and (3) duration of nitrous oxide administration. In an animal model, the inhalation of 75% nitrous oxide doubles the volume of a pneumothorax in 10 minutes, emphasizing the high blood flow to this area (Fig. 1-13) (Eger and Saidman, 1965). Likewise, air bubbles (*e.g.*, emboli) expand rapidly when exposed to nitrous oxide (Fig. 1-14) (Munson and Merrick, 1966). In contrast to the rapid expansion of a pneumothorax, the increase in bowel gas volume produced by nitrous oxide is slow.

The middle ear is an air-filled cavity that passively vents by way of the eustachian tube when pressures reach 20 to 30 cmH$_2$O. Nitrous oxide diffuses into the middle ear more rapidly than nitrogen leaves, and middle ear pressures may become excessive if eustachian tube function is compromised by inflammation or edema. Indeed, tympanic membrane rupture has been attributed to this mechanism following administration of nitrous oxide. Negative middle ear pressures may

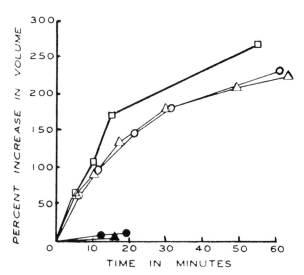

FIGURE 1-13. Inhalation of 75% nitrous oxide rapidly increases the volume of a pneumothorax *(open symbols)*. Inhalation of oxygen *(solid symbols)* does not alter the volume of a pneumothorax. (From Eger EI, Saidman LJ. Hazards of nitrous oxide anesthesia in bowel obstruction and pneumothorax. Anesthesiology 1965;26:61–66. Reproduced by permission of the authors and publisher.)

develop after discontinuation of nitrous oxide, leading to serous otitis. Nausea and vomiting that follows anesthesia may be due to multiple mechanisms, but the possible role of altered middle ear pressures as a result of nitrous oxide should be considered.

Cardiac Output

The CO influences uptake and, therefore, PA by carrying away more or less anesthetic from alveoli. A high CO results in more rapid uptake, so that the rate of rise in the PA, and thus the induction of anesthesia, is slowed. A low CO speeds the rate of rise of the PA, because there is less uptake to oppose input.

The effect of CO on the rate of increase in the PA may seem paradoxical. For example, the uptake of more drug by an increased CO should speed the rate of rise of partial pressure in tissues and thus narrow the A-vD for anesthetics. Indeed, an increase in CO does hasten the equilibration of tissue anesthetic partial pressure with the Pa. Nevertheless, the Pa is lower than it would be if CO were normal. Conceptually, a change in CO is an-

alagous to the effect of a change in solubility. For example, doubling CO increases the capacity of blood to hold anesthetic, just as solubility increases the capacity of the same volume of blood.

As with VA, changes in CO most influence the rate of rise of PA of a soluble anesthetic. Conversely, the rate of rise of the PA of a poorly soluble anesthetic, such as nitrous oxide, is rapid regardless of CO. As a result, changes in CO exert little influence on the rate of rise of the PA of nitrous oxide. In contrast, doubling the CO will greatly increase the uptake of soluble anesthetic from alveoli, thus slowing the rate of rise of the PA. This effect of solubility suggests that a low CO, as with shock, could produce an unexpectedly high PA of a soluble anesthetic. This is potentially dangerous because soluble volatile anesthetics in high doses may produce cardiovascular depression.

Volatile anesthetics that depress CO can exert a positive feedback response that contrasts with

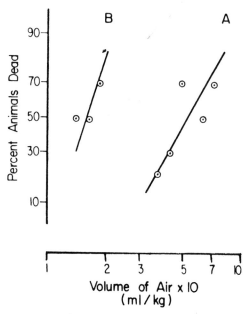

FIGURE 1-14. Nitrous oxide rapidly expands air bubbles as reflected by the volume of injected air necessary to produce 50% mortality in animals breathing nitrous oxide (0.16 ml kg⁻¹) *(A)* compared with animals breathing oxygen (0.55 ml kg⁻¹) *(B)*. (From Munson ES, Merrick HC. Effect of nitrous oxide on venous air embolism. Anesthesiology 1966;27:783–7. Reproduced by permission of the authors and publisher.)

the negative feedback response on spontaneous ventilation exerted by these drugs. For example, depression of CO due to an excessive dose of volatile anesthetic results in an increase in the PA, which further increases anesthetic depth and thus cardiac depression. The administration of a volatile anesthetic that depresses cardiac output plus controlled ventilation of the lungs results in a situation characterized by unopposed input of anesthetic (*e.g.,* VA) combined with decreased uptake (*e.g.,* CO). The net effect of this combination of events can be an unexpected rapid rise in PA and an excessive depth of anesthesia.

Distribution of CO will influence the rate of rise in the PA of an anesthetic. For example, increases in CO are not necessarily accompanied by proportional increases in blood flow to all tissues. Preferential perfusion of vessel-rich group tissues when the CO increases results in a more rapid rise in the PA of anesthetic than would occur if the increased CO was distributed equally to all tissues. Indeed, infants have a relatively greater perfusion of vessel-rich group tissues than do adults and, consequently, show a faster rate of rise of the PA toward the PI (Salanitre and Rackow, 1969).

IMPACT OF SHUNT. In the absence of an intracardiac or intrapulmonary right-to-left shunt, it is valid to assume that the PA and Pa of inhaled anesthetics are essentially identical. The presence of a shunt, however, serves to increase the PA and decrease the Pa such that a partial pressure gradient develops between these two phases.

A right-to-left intracardiac or intrapulmonary shunt slows the rate of induction of anesthesia. This slowing reflects dilutional effects of shunted blood containing no anesthetic on the partial pressure of anesthetic in blood coming from ventilated alveoli. A similar mechanism is responsible for a reduction in the PaO_2 in the presence of an intracardiac or intrapulmonary shunt.

The relative impact of a right-to-left shunt on the rate of rise in the Pa depends on the solubility of the anesthetic. For example, shunt slows the rate of rise of the Pa of a poorly soluble anesthetic more than that of a soluble anesthetic (Fig. 1-15) (Stoelting and Longnecker, 1972). This occurs because uptake of a soluble anesthetic offsets dilutional effects of shunted blood on the Pa. Uptake of a poorly soluble drug is minimal, and dilutional effects on Pa are relatively unopposed. This impact of solubility in the presence of shunt is opposite to that observed with changes in CO and VA.

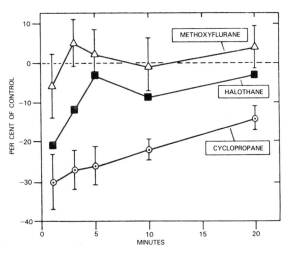

FIGURE 1-15. A right-to-left intrapulmonary shunt slows the rate of rise of the arterial concentration of a poorly soluble anesthetic (cyclopropane) more than an anesthetic (methoxyflurane) that is highly soluble in blood. (From Stoelting RK, Longnecker DE. Effect of right-to-left shunt on rate of increase in arterial anesthetic concentration. Anesthesiology 1972;36:352–6. Reproduced by permission of the authors and publisher.)

Left-to-right tissue shunts (*e.g.,* arteriovenous fistulas) result in delivery of blood to the lungs containing a higher Pv of inhaled anesthetic than that present in blood that has passed through tissues. As a result, left-to-right tissue shunts offset the decrease in Pa of inhaled anesthetic produced by a right-to-left intrapulmonary shunt (Eger, 1974). In this regard, it is unlikely that left-to-right tissue shunts will influence uptake of inhaled anesthetics in the absence of an intrapulmonary shunt. Nevertheless, inhaled anesthetics may normally produce some degree of left-to-right tissue shunting by increasing cutaneous blood flow. Indeed, the increase in cutaneous blood flow associated with administration of volatile anesthetics is often sufficient to arterialize peripheral venous blood (France *et al,* 1974; Williamson and Munson, 1982).

Alveolar-to-Venous Partial Pressure Difference

The A-vD reflects tissue uptake of the inhaled anesthetic. Factors that determine the fraction of anesthetic removed from blood traversing a tissue parallel those factors that determine uptake at the lungs (*e.g.,* tissue solubility, tissue blood flow, and arterial-to-tissue partial pressure difference).

Highly perfused tissues (*e.g.,* brain, heart, kidneys) account for less than 10% of body mass but receive about 75% of the CO (Table 1-2). As a result of the small mass and high blood flow, these tissues, known as the vessel-rich group, equilibrate rapidly with the Pa. Indeed, after about three time constants, approximately 75% of the returning venous blood is at the same partial pressure as the PA. Therefore, uptake of a volatile anesthetic is greatly decreased after about 15 minutes, as reflected by a narrowing of the inspired-to-alveolar partial pressure difference.

Skeletal muscles and fat represent about 70% of the body mass but receive only about 25% of the CO (Table 1-2). As a result of the large tissue mass, sustained tissue uptake of the inhaled anesthetics continues, and the effluent venous blood is at a lower partial pressure than the PA. For this reason, the alveolar-to-arterial difference for anesthetic is maintained, and uptake from the lungs continues, even after several hours of continuous administration.

Recovery from Anesthesia

Recovery from anesthesia is depicted by the rate of decline in the PA (*e.g.,* Pbr) of the anesthetic. Although similarities exist between the rate of induction and recovery, as reflected by changes in the PA of the inhaled anesthetic, there are important differences between the two events. For ex-

ample, failure of certain tissues to reach equilibrium with the PA of the inhaled anesthetic means that the rate of decline of the PA during recovery from anesthesia will be more rapid than the rate of increase of the PA during induction of anesthesia. Indeed, even after a prolonged anesthetic, it is unlikely that skeletal muscles and, almost certain, that fat will not have equilibrated with the PA of the inhaled anesthetic. Thus, when the PI of an anesthetic is abruptly reduced to zero at the conclusion of an anesthetic, these tissues initially cannot contribute to the transfer of drug back into blood for delivery to the lungs and exhalation. As long as a gradient exists between the Pa and that in tissues, the tissues will continue to take up anesthetic. Thus, during recovery from anesthesia, the continued passage of anesthetic from blood to tissues, such as fat, acts to speed the rate of decline in the PA of that anesthetic.

The difference between the rate of change in the PA during recovery from anesthesia and induction of anesthesia depends on the solubility of the inhaled anesthetic and the duration of anesthesia (Fig. 1-16) (Stoelting and Eger, 1969c). The rate of decline of the PA of a poorly soluble drug, such as nitrous oxide, is rapid, regardless of the duration of anesthesia. The potential impact of lack of tissue equilibration and subsequent continued tissue uptake that speeds the rate of decline in the PA during recovery becomes more important with soluble anesthetics. With soluble anesthetics, however, this impact of continued tissue uptake is lessened with prolonged administration of the inhaled anesthetic. For example, prolonged administration of a soluble anesthetic can result in suffi-

FIGURE 1-16. The rate at which the alveolar concentration declines from the concentration present when the anesthetic is discontinued (FE/FO) is determined by the solubility of the anesthetic in the blood (lambda) and the duration of anesthesia. (From Stoelting RK, Eger EI. The effects of ventilation and anesthetic solubility on recovery from anesthesia: An *in vivo* and analog analysis before and after equilibration. Anesthesiology 1969;30:290–6. Reproduced by permission of the authors and publisher.)

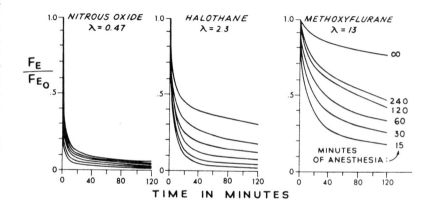

cient storage for tissues to act as a reservoir to maintain the PA when the PI is reduced to zero.

Saturation of enzymes responsible for metabolism of inhaled anesthetics prevents any significant impact on the rate of rise of the PA during induction of anesthesia. During recovery from anesthesia, the PA is greatly reduced, and enzyme saturation may not be present. As a result, metabolism of inhaled anesthetics could theoretically speed the rate of decline of the PA. Indeed, the rate of decline of the PA of halothane is more rapid than that of enflurane (Munson *et al,* 1978). This observation is consistent with the greater magnitude of metabolism of halothane (15% – 20%) compared with enflurane (2% – 3%) (see Chapter 2).

Anesthetic that has been absorbed into the components of the anesthetic breathing system will pass from the components back into the gases of the breathing circuit at the conclusion of anesthesia. This anesthetic, if not washed out of the system by high gas flows, can be delivered to the patient and retard the rate of decline in the PA of the anesthetic. Likewise, exhaled gases of the patient contain anesthetic that will be rebreathed in the absence of high fresh gas flows into the anesthetic breathing circuit. For these reasons, fresh gas flow rates of at least 5 L min^{-1} of oxygen are commonly used at the conclusion of anesthesia.

Diffusion Hypoxia

Diffusion hypoxia occurs when inhalation of nitrous oxide is abruptly discontinued, leading to a reversal of partial pressure gradients such that the nitrous oxide leaves the blood to enter alveoli (Fink, 1955). This initial high-volume outpouring of nitrous oxide from the blood into the alveoli can so dilute the PAO_2 that the PaO_2 decreases (Sheffer *et al,* 1972). In addition to dilution of the PAO_2 by nitrous oxide, there is also a dilution of carbon dioxide in the lungs, which reduces the stimulus to ventilation. This decreased stimulus to breath exaggerates the impact on PaO_2 of the outpouring of nitrous oxide into the alveoli. Outpouring of nitrous oxide into alveoli is greatest during the first 1 to 5 minutes following its discontinuation at the conclusion of anesthesia. For this reason, it is common practice to fill the lungs with oxygen at the end of anesthesia to ensure that arterial hypoxemia will not occur as a result of dilution of the PAO_2 by nitrous oxide.

PHARMACODYNAMICS OF INHALED ANESTHETICS

Minimum Alveolar Concentration

Minimum alveolar concentration (MAC) of an inhaled anesthetic at 1 atmosphere, which prevents skeletal muscle movement in response to a noxious stimulus (*e.g.,* surgical skin incision) in 50% of patients, is the standard by which inhaled anesthetics are compared (Table 1-7) (Merkel and Eger, 1963). The fact that the alveolar concentration reflects the partial pressure at the site of anesthetic action (*e.g.,* brain) has made MAC the most useful index of anesthetic equal potency. The use of equal potent doses (*i.e.,* comparable MAC concentrations) of inhaled anesthetics is mandatory for comparing effects of these drugs or organ function (see Chapter 2).

Similar MAC concentrations of inhaled anesthetics produce equivalent depression of the central nervous system. Conversely, similar MAC concentrations may produce different effects on blood pressure, CO, and ventilation (see Chapter 2). For example, 1 MAC enflurane (1.68%) depresses CO more than a 1 MAC concentration of isoflurane (1.15%). This emphasizes that MAC represents only one point on the dose-response curve of effects produced by inhaled anesthetics and that these dose-response curves for various inhaled anesthetics are not parallel.

MAC values for inhaled anesthetics are additive. For example, 0.5 MAC nitrous oxide plus 0.5 MAC isoflurane has the same effect at the brain as does a 1 MAC concentration of either anesthetic alone. The fact that 1 MAC for nitrous oxide ex-

Table 1-7
Comparative Potencies of Inhaled Anesthetics

	Minimum Alveolar Concentration (MAC) (30– 55 yr old, 37° C, P_B 760 mm Hg)
Nitrous oxide	104%*
Halothane	0.74%
Enflurane	1.68%
Isoflurane	1.15%
Methoxyflurane	0.16%

* Determined in a hyperbaric chamber in males 21 to 35 years old.

ceeds 100% means that this anesthetic cannot be used alone at 1 atmosphere and still provide an acceptable inhaled concentration of oxygen.

Dose-response curves for inhaled anesthetics, although not parallel, are all steep. This is emphasized by the fact that a 1 MAC dose prevents skeletal muscle movement in response to a painful surgical skin incision in 50% of patients, whereas a modest increase to about 1.3 MAC prevents movement in at least 95% of patients.

Use of MAC allows a quantitative analysis of the effect of various pharmacologic and physiologic factors on anesthetic requirements (Table 1-8) (Quasha *et al*, 1980; Stoelting and Miller,

---

Table 1-8

Impact of Physiologic and Pharmacologic Factors on Minimum Alveolar Concentration (MAC)

Increase in MAC
  Hyperthermia
  Hypernatremia
  Drug-induced elevations in CNS catecholamine stores
  Chronic alcohol abuse
Decrease in MAC
  Hypothermia
  Hyponatremia
  Pregnancy
  Lithium
  Pancuronium
  Magnesium
  Lidocaine
  PaO_2 below 38 mmHg
  Blood pressure below 40 mmHg
  Increasing age
  Preoperative medication
  Drug-induced decreases in CNS catecholamine stores
  Acute alcohol abuse
No Change in MAC
  Duration of anesthesia
  Hyperkalemia
  Hypokalemia
  Anesthetic metabolism
  Thyroid gland dysfunction
  Male or female
  $PaCO_2$ 15–95 mmHg
  $PaCO_2$ above 38 mmHg
  Blood pressure above 40 mmHg

(By permission, Stoelting RK, Miller RD, eds: Basics of Anesthesia. Churchill Livingstone Inc., New York, 1984)

1984). Likewise, factors that do not alter MAC can be defined (Table 1-8).

Mechanism of Anesthesia

The mechanism by which inhaled anesthetics produce progressive and occasionally selective depression of the central nervous system (*i.e.*, anesthesia) is not known. Most evidence is consistent with inhibition of synaptic transmission in the central nervous system produced by an action of inhaled anesthetics at hydrophobic (*e.g.*, lipophilic) sites in biologic membranes. A single theory, however, to explain the mechanism of anesthesia, seems unlikely.

Meyer–Overton Theory (Critical Volume Hypothesis)

Correlation between lipid solubility of inhaled anesthetics (*i.e.*, oil:gas partition coefficient) and anesthetic potency (*i.e.*, MAC) suggests that anesthesia occurs when a sufficient number of anesthetic molecules dissolve (*i.e.*, critical concentration) in crucial hydrophobic sites such as lipid cell membranes. This critical concentration is approximately 20 mM at 1.3 MAC (Lowe and Ernst, 1981). Conceptually, expansion of cell membranes by dissolved anesthetic molecules could exert pressure on channels necessary for sodium flux and the subsequent development of action potentials necessary for synaptic transmission. Evidence supporting this theory is the observation that high pressures (40–100 atmospheres) partially antagonize the action of inhaled anesthetics (*i.e.*, pressure reversal) presumably by returning (compressing) lipid membranes to their "awake" contour (Halsey and Smith, 1975). Nevertheless, not all lipid-soluble drugs are anesthetics and, in fact, some may be convulsants.

Protein Receptor Hypothesis

Existence of protein receptors in the central nervous system as a site and mechanism of action of inhaled anesthetics is suggested by the steep dose-response curve for inhaled anesthetics. Indeed, a crucial degree of receptor occupancy is characteristic of a steep dose-response curve. Receptor specificity is also suggested by conversion of an anesthetic to a nonanesthetic by increasing the molecular weight despite corresponding increases in lipid solubility.

Recognition that there is an endogenous pain suppression system has led to the speculation that inhaled anesthetics could act by evoking the release of endorphins that attach to specific receptors (see Chapter 3). Based on current evidence, it is likely that inhaled anesthetics may produce some degree of analgesia by stimulating the release of endorphins. Nevertheless, it is unlikely that inhaled anesthetics produce unconsciousness characteristic of general anesthesia by the release of endorphins.

Alteration in Neurotransmitter Availability

In vitro studies have demonstrated the ability of both inhaled and injected anesthetics to inhibit metabolic breakdown of the inhibitory neurotransmitter, gamma-aminobutyric acid (GABA). This inhibition leads to increased brain concentrations of GABA and the speculation that anesthesia may arise from enhanced synaptic inhibition resulting from accumulation of this inhibitory neurotransmitter. Inhibition of GABA breakdown is greatest with halothane, followed by enflurane, thiopental, and ketamine (Cheng and Brunner, 1981). Morphine does not influence the breakdown of GABA.

REFERENCES

Albert A. Ionization, *p*H and biological activity. Pharmacol Rev 1952;4:136–67.

Azarnoff DL, Huffman DH. Therapeutic implications of bioavailability. Annu Rev Pharmacol Toxicol 1976;16:53–66.

Bell MDD, Murray GR, Mishra P, Calvey TN, Weldon BD, Williams NE. Buccal morphine —a new route for analgesia. Lancet 1985;1:71–3.

Bentley JB, Borel JD, Nad RE, Gillespie TJ. Age and fentanyl pharmacokinetics. Anesth Analg 1982;61:968–71.

Berman ML, Lowe HJ, Bochantin J, Hagler K. Uptake and elimination of methoxyflurane as influenced by enzyme induction in the rat. Anesthesiology 1973;38:352–7.

Booker HE, Darcey B. Serum concentrations of free diphenylhydantoin and their relationship to clinical intoxication. Epilepsia 1973;14:177–84.

Cheng S-C, Brunner EA. Effects of anesthetic agents on synaptosomal GABA disposal. Anesthesiology 1981;55:34–40.

Cockcroft DW, Gault MH. Prediction of creatinine clearance from serum creatinine. Nephron 1976;16:31–41.

Conney AH. Pharmacological implications of microsomal enzyme induction. Pharmacol Rev 1967;19:317–66.

Coon MJ. Drug metabolism by cytochrome P-450: Progress and perspectives. Drug Metab Dispos 1981;9:1–4.

Cullen BF, Miller MG. Drug interactions and anesthesia: A review. Anesth Analg 1979;58:413–23.

Drayer DE. Pathways of drug metabolism in man. Individualization of drug therapy. Med Clin North Am 1974;58:927–44.

Eger EI. Effect of inspired anesthetic concentration on the rate of rise of alveolar concentration. Anesthesiology 1963;24:153–7.

Eger EI. Anesthetic Uptake and Action. Baltimore, Williams and Wilkins. 1974:146.

Eger EI, Saidman LJ. Hazards of nitrous oxide anesthesia in bowel obstruction and pneumothorax. Anesthesiology 1965;26:61–6.

Ellis DE, Stoelting RK. Individual variations in fluroxene, halothane and methoxyflurane blood–gas partition coefficients, and the effect of anemia. Anesthesiology 1975;42:748–50.

Epstein RM, Rackow H, Salanitre E, Wolf G. Influence of the concentration effect on the uptake of anesthetic mixtures: The second gas effect. Anesthesiology 1964;25:364–71.

Fassoulaki A, Eger EI. Starvation increases the solubility of volatile anaesthetics in rat liver. Br J Anaesth 1986;58:327–9.

Fink BR. Diffusion anoxia. Anesthesiology 1955;16:511–9.

France CJ, Eger EI, Bendixen HH. The use of peripheral venous blood for *p*H and carbon dioxide tension determinations during general anesthesia. Anesthesiology 1974;40:311–4.

Fraser J, Nadeau J, Robertson D, Wood AJJ. Regulation of human beta receptors by endogenous catecholamines. Relationship of leukocyte beta–receptor density to the cardiac sensitivity to isoproterenol. J Clin Invest 1981;67:1777–84.

Galant SP, Duriseti L, Underwood S, Insel PA. Decreased beta-adrenergic receptors on polymorphonuclear leukocytes after adrenergic therapy. N Engl J Med 1978;299:933–6.

Gelehrter TD. Enzyme induction. N Engl J Med 1976;294:522–6, 589–95, 646–51.

Halsey MJ, Sawyer DC, Eger EI, Bahlman SH, Impelman DMK. Hepatic metabolism of halothane, methoxyflurane, cyclopropane, Ethrane and Forane in miniature swine. Anesthesiology 1971;35:43–7.

Halsey MJ, Smith B. Pressure reversal of narcosis produced by anesthetics, narcotics and tranquilizers. Nature 1975;257:811–3.

Hug CC. Pharmacokinetics of drugs administered intravenously. Anesth Analg 1978;57:704 – 23.

Hull CJ. Pharmacokinetics and pharmacodynamics. Br J Anaesth 1979;51:579 – 94.

Iber FL. Drug metabolism in heavy consumers of ethyl alcohol. Clin Pharmacol Ther 1977;22:735 – 42.

Jung D, Mayersohn M, Perrier D, Calkins J, Saunders R. Thiopental disposition as a function of age in female patients undergoing surgery. Anesthesiology 1982;56:263 – 8.

Kauffman RE. Clinical interpretation and application of drug concentration data. Pediatr Clin North Am 1981;28:35 – 45.

Klotz U, Avant GR, Hoyuma RJ, Schenker S, Wilkinson GR. The effects of age and liver disease on the disposition and elimination of diazepam in adult man. J Clin Invest 1975;55:347 – 57.

Koch-Weser J, Sellers EM. Binding of drugs to serum albumin. N Engl J Med 1976;294:311 – 6; 526 – 31.

Laasberg HL, Hedley-White J. Halothane solubility in blood and solutions of plasma proteins: Effects of temperature, protein composition and hemoglobin concentration. Anesthesiology 1970;32:351 – 6.

Lerman J, Gregory GA, Eger EI. Hematocrit and the solubility of volatile anesthetics in blood. Anesth Analg 1984;63:911 – 4.

Lowe HJ, Ernst EA. The Quantitative Practice of Anesthesia: Use of the Closed Circuit. Baltimore, Williams and Wilkins, 1981:38.

Maze M. Clinical implications of membrane receptor function in anesthesia. Anesthesiology 1981;55:160 – 71.

Merkel G, Eger EI. A comparative study of halothane and halopropane anesthesia. Including method for determining equipotency. Anesthesiology 1963;24:346 – 57.

Morselli PL. Clinical pharmacokinetics in neonates. Clin Pharmacokinet 1976;1:81 – 98.

Munson ES, Eger EI, Tham MK, Embro WJ. Increase in anesthetic uptake, excretion and blood solubility in man after eating. Anesth Analg 1978;57:224 – 31.

Munson ES, Merrick HC. Effect of nitrous oxide on venous air embolism. Anesthesiology 1966;27:783 – 7.

Papadimitriou A. Worcel M. Dose – response curves for angiotensin II and synthetic analogues in three types of smooth muscle. Existence of different forms of receptor sites for angiotensin II. Br J Pharmacol 1974;50:291 – 7.

Park BK, Breckenridge AM. Clinical implications of enzyme induction and enzyme inhibition. Clin Pharmacokinet 1981;6:1 – 24.

Piafsky KM, Borga O, Odar-Cederlof I, Johansson C, Sjoqvist F. Increased plasma protein binding of propranolol and chlorpromazine mediated by disease-induced elevations of plasma $alpha_1$-acid glycoprotein. N Engl J Med 1978;299:1435 – 9.

Quasha AL, Eger EI, Tinker JH. Determination and application of MAC. Anesthesiology 1980;53:315 – 34.

Rawlins MD. Drug interactions and anaesthesia. Br J Anaesth 1978;50:689 – 93.

Reidenberg MM. Effect of disease states on plasma protein binding of drugs. Med Clin North Am 1974;58:1103 – 9.

Routledge PA, Shand DG. Presystemic drug elimination. Annu Rev Pharmacol Toxicol 1979;19:447 – 68.

Sawyer DC, Eger EI, Bahlman SH, Cullen BF, Impelman D. Concentration dependence of hepatic halothane metabolism. Anesthesiology 1971;34:230 – 4.

Shaw JE, Chandrasekaran SK. Controlled topical delivery of drugs for systemic action. Drug Metab Rev 1978;8:223 – 33.

Shaw J, Urquhart J. Programmed, systemic drug delivery by the transdermal route. Trends Pharmacol Sci 1980;1:208 – 11.

Sheffer L, Steffenson JL, Birch AA. Nitrous oxide – induced diffusion hypoxia in patients breathing spontaneously. Anesthesiology 1972;37:436 – 9.

Stanski DR, Watkins WD. Drug disposition in anesthesia. New York, Grune and Stratton, 1982.

Stoelting RK, Eger EI. Percutaneous loss of nitrous oxide, cyclopropane, ether and halothane in man. Anesthesiology 1969a;30:278 – 83.

Stoelting RK, Eger EI. An additional explanation for the second gas effect: a concentrating effect. Anesthesiology 1969b;30:273 – 7.

Stoelting RK, Eger EI. The effects of ventilation and anesthetic solubility on recovery from anesthesia: An *in vivo* and analog analysis before and after equilibration. Anesthesiology 1969c;30:290 – 6.

Stoelting RK, Longnecker DE. Effect of right-to-left shunt on rate of increase in arterial anesthetic concentration. Anesthesiology 1972;36:352 – 6.

Stoelting RK, Miller RD. Basics of Anesthesia. New York, Churchill Livingstone, 1984:11.

Stoelting RK, Peterson C. Phenobarbital or diazepam therapy and plasma cholinesterase activity. Anesthesiology 1975;42:356 – 7.

Uetrecht JP, Woosley RL. Acetylator phenotype and lupus erythematosus. Clin Pharmacokinet 1981; 6:118 – 34.

Vesell ES. Pharmacogenetics — multiple interactions between gases and environment as determinants of drug response. Am J Med 1979;66:183 – 7.

Vestal RE, Wood AJJ. Influence of age and smoking on drug kinetics in man. Studies using model compounds. Clin Pharmacokinet 1980;5:309 – 19.

Vestal RE, Wood AJJ, Shand DG. Reduced beta-adrenoceptor sensitivity in the elderly. Clin Pharmacol Ther 1979;26:181 – 6.

Wilkinson GR, Shand DG. A physiologic approach to hepatic drug clearance. Clin Pharmacol Ther 1975;18:377 – 90.

Williamson DC, Munson ES. Correlation of peripheral venous and arterial blood gas values during general anesthesia. Anesth Analg 1982;61:950–2.

Wood AJJ, Kornhauser DM, Wilkinson GR, Shand DG, Branch RA. The influence of cirrhosis on steady state blood concentrations of unbound propranolol after oral administration. Clin Pharmacokinet 1978;3:478–87.

Wood M. Plasma drug binding. Implications for anesthesiologists. Anesth Analg 1986;65:786–804.

Wood M, Wood AJJ. Changes in plasma drug binding and alpha$_1$ acid glycoprotein in mother and newborn infant. Clin Pharmacol Ther 1981;29:522–6.

C H A P T E R 2

Inhaled Anesthetics

INTRODUCTION

The discovery of the anesthetic properties of nitrous oxide, diethyl ether, and chloroform in the 1840s was followed by a hiatus of about 80 years before other inhaled anesthetics were introduced (Fig. 2-1) (Eger, 1984a). In 1950, all available inhaled anesthetics were either flammable or potentially toxic to the liver. Recognition that combining carbon with fluorine decreased flammability led to the introduction, in 1951, of the first halogenated hydrocarbon anesthetic, fluroxene. Fluroxene was used clinically for several years before its voluntary withdrawal from the market because of potential flammability and increasing concern that this drug could cause organ toxicity (Johnston *et al,* 1973).

Halothane was synthesized in 1951 and introduced for clinical use in 1956. The propensity for alkane derivatives, such as halothane, however, to enhance the arrhythmogenic effects of epinephrine led to the search for new inhaled anesthetics derived from ethers. Methoxyflurane, a methyl ethyl ether, was the first such derivative and was introduced for clinical use in 1960. Although this drug does not enhance the arrhythmogenic effects of epinephrine, its extreme solubility in blood and lipids results in a prolonged induction and slow recovery from anesthesia. More important, however, is the extensive hepatic metabolism of methoxyflurane (up to 50% of an absorbed dose), leading to the production of fluoride in amounts sufficient to produce nephrotoxicity, especially if

the duration of administration exceeds 2.5 MAC hours. Enflurane was the next methyl ethyl ether derivative introduced for clinical use in 1973. This drug does not enhance the arrhythmogenicity of epinephrine and, unlike halothane and methoxyflurane, is resistant to metabolism, thus minimizing the likelihood of hepatotoxicity or nephrotoxicity. Isoflurane, the isomer of enflurane, was introduced for clinical use in 1981. This drug is the most resistant of all the inhaled anesthetics to metabolism, emphasizing the unlikely occurrence of organ toxicity following its administration.

Commonly administered inhaled anesthetics are currently limited to the inorganic gas, nitrous oxide, and the volatile liquids, halothane, enflurane, and isoflurane (Fig. 2-2). Available but rarely administered inhaled anesthetics include the cyclic hydrocarbon gas, cyclopropane, and the volatile liquids, diethyl ether and methoxyflurane (Fig. 2-2). Volatile liquids are administered as vapors following their evaporation in devices known as vaporizers.

Nitrous Oxide

Nitrous oxide is a low molecular weight, odorless to sweet smelling nonflammable gas of low potency and poor blood solubility that is most commonly administered in combination with opioids or volatile anesthetics to produce general anesthesia (Table 2-1). Although nitrous oxide is nonflam-

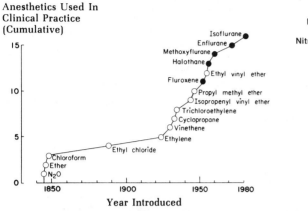

Anesthetics Used In Clinical Practice (Cumulative)

Year Introduced

FIGURE 2-1. Inhaled anesthetics introduced into clinical practice. Solid circles are drugs that contain fluorine. (From Eger EI. Isoflurane [Forane]. A compendium and reference. Madison, Wisconsin, Ohio Medical Products, 1984:1–110. Reproduced by permission of the author and publisher.)

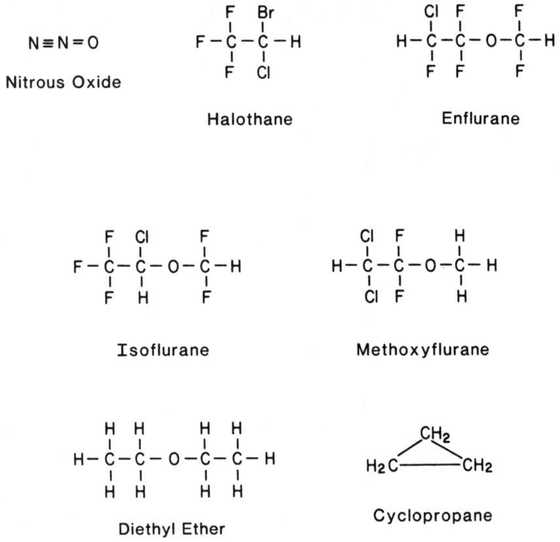

FIGURE 2-2. Inhaled anesthetics.

Table 2-1
Physical and Chemical Properties of Inhaled Anesthetics

	Nitrous Oxide	Halothane	Enflurane	Isoflurane
Molecular weight	44	197	184	184
Specific gravity (25°C)		1.86	1.52	1.50
Boiling point (°C)		50.2	56.5	48.5
Vapor pressure (mmHg; 20°C)	Gas	244	172	240
Odor	Sweet	Organic solvent	Ethereal	Ethereal
Pungency	None	None	Moderate	Moderate
Preservative necessary	No	Yes	No	No
Stability				
Soda lime	Yes	No	Yes	Yes
Sunlight	Yes	No	Yes	Yes
Reacts with metal	No	Yes	No	No

mable, it will support combustion. The poor blood solubility of nitrous oxide permits rapid achievement of an alveolar and brain partial pressure of the drug. For example, inhalation of 60% to 70% nitrous oxide results in nearly 90% equilibration in about 15 minutes. During this time, about 10 L of nitrous oxide will have been absorbed from the alveolar gas into the body. This high volume absorption of nitrous oxide is responsible for several unique effects of nitrous oxide when administered in the presence of volatile anesthetics or air-containing cavities (see Chapter 1). Analgesic effects of nitrous oxide are prominent, but skeletal muscle relaxation is minimal. Increasing awareness of the possible adverse effects related to the high volume absorption of this drug and appreciation of potential toxic effects on organ function may lead to a decline in the use of nitrous oxide in future years (Eger, 1985a).

Halothane

Halothane is a clear nonflammable volatile liquid at room temperature with a sweet nonpungent odor (Table 2-l). An intermediate solubility in blood combined with a high potency permits rapid onset and recovery from anesthesia using halothane alone or in combination with nitrous oxide or injected drugs such as opioids (Table 2-1).

Halothane was developed on the basis of predictions that its halogenated structure would provide nonflammability, intermediate blood solubility, anesthetic potency, and molecular stability. Specifically, carbon-fluorine decreases flammability, and the trifluorocarbon contributes to molecular stability. The presence of a carbon-chlorine bond and carbon-bromine bond plus the retention of a hydrogen atom ensures anesthetic potency. Despite its chemical stability, halothane is susceptible to decomposition to hydrochloric acid, hydrobromic acid, chloride, bromide, and phosgene. For this reason, halothane is stored in amber-colored bottles, and thymol is added as a preservative to prevent spontaneous oxidative decomposition. Thymol that remains in vaporizers following vaporization of halothane can cause vaporizer turnstiles or temperature compensating devices to malfunction.

Enflurane

Enflurane is a clear nonflammable volatile liquid at room temperature with a pungent ethereal odor (Table 2-1). Its intermediate solubility in blood combined with a high potency permits rapid onset and recovery from anesthesia using enflurane alone or in combination with nitrous oxide or injected drugs such as opioids (Table 2-1). Enflurane does not require the presence of a preservative such as thymol.

Isoflurane

Isoflurane is a clear nonflammable volatile liquid at room temperature with a pungent ethereal odor (Table 2-1). Its intermediate solubility combined with a high potency permits rapid onset and recovery from anesthesia using isoflurane alone or in combination with nitrous oxide or injected drugs such as opioids (Table 2-1). Isoflurane is characterized by extreme physical stability, undergoing no detectable deterioration during 5 years of storage or on exposure to soda lime or sunlight. The stability of isoflurane negates the need to add preservatives such as thymol to the commercial preparation.

Although isoflurane is an isomer of enflurane, the manufacturing processes are not similar. For example, the compounds used at the start of manufacturing are different with 2,2,2-trifluoroethanol, the starting compound for isoflurane and chlorotrifluorethylene for enflurane. The subsequent purification of isoflurane by distillation is complex and expensive.

Sevoflurane

Sevoflurane is a fluorinated methyl ethyl ether with a low blood : gas (0.6) and oil : gas (55) partition coefficient (Holaday and Smith, 1981). It has a vapor pressure of 160 mmHg at 20 Celsius and a predicted MAC in adult patients of 2.6%. Solubility characteristics and potency of sevoflurane facilitate rapid induction of anesthesia and subsequent emergence when the drug is discontinued. Inhalation of sevoflurane is not irritating to the airways, and there is a high degree of patient acceptance. Cardiopulmonary effects of sevoflurane appear to be similar to those of other volatile anesthetics. Plasma fluoride concentrations average 22.1 μmol L^{-1} after 1 hour of administration. This peak level declines rapidly, often declining to near normal values in less than 1 hour, reflecting the poor lipid solubility of the drug.

Sevoflurane was withdrawn from clinical investigation in 1980, principally because of its metabolism to fluoride. Nevertheless, its solubility characteristics and potency could make sevoflurane a useful volatile anesthetic for surgical procedures when rapid onset and awakening are desired, as for outpatients.

COMPARATIVE PHARMACOLOGY

Inhaled anesthetics often evoke differing pharmacologic effects at comparable MAC concentrations. Measurements obtained from normothermic volunteers exposed to equal potent concentrations of inhaled anesthetics during controlled ventilation of the lungs to maintain normocarbia have provided the basis of comparison for pharmacologic effects of these drugs on various organ systems (Eger, 1984a). In this regard, it is important to recognize that the surgically stimulated patient with other confounding variables may respond differently than the healthy volunteer (Table 2-2).

CENTRAL NERVOUS SYSTEM EFFECTS

Inhaled anesthetics produce characteristic alterations on the electroencephalogram (EEG). Furthermore, these drugs evoke changes in cerebral blood flow that may increase intracranial pressure in patients with space-occupying intracranial lesions. Cerebral metabolic oxygen requirements are reduced in parallel with drug-induced declines in cerebral activity. Volatile anesthetics do not cause retrograde amnesia or prolonged impairment of intellectual function. Sleepiness may last longer following prolonged administration of halothane than other inhaled anesthetics because of its metabolism to bromide.

Mental impairment is not detectable in volunteers breathing 1600 ppm nitrous oxide (0.16%) or 16 ppm halothane (0.0016%) (Frankhuizen et al, 1978). It is, therefore, unlikely that impairment of mental function results from inhalation of trace concentrations of anesthetics by those who work

Table 2-2
Variables That Influence Pharmacologic Effects of Inhaled Anesthetics

Anesthetic concentration
Spontaneous versus controlled ventilation of the lungs
Variations from normocapnia
Surgical stimulation
Patient age
Co-existing disease
Concomitant drug therapy
Intravascular fluid volume
Preoperative medication
Injected drugs used to establish and maintain anesthesia and produce skeletal muscle relaxation
Alterations in body temperature

in the operating room. Reaction times do not increase significantly until 10% to 20% nitrous oxide is inhaled (Garfield et al, 1975).

Electroencephalogram

Volatile anesthetics in concentrations below 0.4 MAC similarly increase the frequency and voltage of the EEG (see Chapter 41). At about 0.4 MAC, there is an abrupt shift of high voltage activity from posterior to anterior portions of the brain (Tinker et al, 1977). Cerebral metabolic oxygen requirements also begin to decline abruptly at about 0.4 MAC. It is likely that these changes reflect a transition from wakefulness to unconsciousness. Furthermore, amnesia probably occurs at this dose of volatile anesthetic. As the dose of volatile anesthetic approaches 1 MAC, the frequency on the EEG decreases and maximum voltage occurs. During administration of isoflurane burst, suppression appears on the EEG at about 1.5 MAC, and, at 2 MAC, electrical silence predominates (Eger et al, 1971). Electrical silence does not occur with enflurane, and only unacceptably high concentrations (greater than 3.5 MAC) of halothane produce this effect.

The effects of nitrous oxide on the EEG are similar to those produced by volatile anesthetics. Slower frequency and higher voltage develops on the EEG as the dose of nitrous oxide is increased or when nitrous oxide is added to a volatile anesthetic to provide a greater total MAC concentration.

Seizure Activity

Enflurane can produce fast-frequency and high-voltage activity on the EEG that often progresses to spike-wave activity, which is indistinguishable from changes that accompany a seizure (Neigh *et al,* 1971). This EEG activity may be accompanied by tonic-clonic twitching of the skeletal muscles of the face and extremities. The likelihood of enflurane-evoked seizure activity is increased when the concentration of enflurane exceeds 2 MAC or when hyperventilation of the lungs lowers the $PaCO_2$ below 30 mmHg. Repetitive auditory stimuli can also initiate seizure activity during the administration of enflurane. There is no evidence of anaerobic metabolism in the brain during seizure activity produced by enflurane. Furthermore, in an animal model, enflurane does not enhance pre-existing epileptic foci—the possible exception being certain types of myoclonic epilepsy and photosensitive epilepsy (Oshima *et al,* 1985).

Isoflurane does not evoke seizure activity on the EEG, even in the presence of deep levels of anesthesia, hypocapnia, or repetitive auditory stimulation. Indeed, isoflurane possesses anticonvulsant properties, being able to suppress seizure activity produced by flurothyl (Koblin *et al,* 1980). An intriguing but undocumented speculation is that the greater MAC value for enflurane compared with its isomer, isoflurane, reflects the need for a higher concentration to suppress the central nervous system-stimulating effects of enflurane.

Animals picked up by the tail experience seizures in the first 15 to 90 minutes following discontinuation of nitrous oxide but not of volatile anesthetics (Smith *et al,* 1979). It is speculated that these withdrawal seizures reflect acute drug dependence. In patients, delerium or excitement during recovery from anesthesia that included nitrous oxide could reflect this phenomenon.

Evoked Potentials

Volatile anesthetics cause dose-related depression in the amplitude and an increase in the latency of the cortical component of median nerve somatosensory evoked potentials. This depression is least with halothane, intermediate with isoflurane, and greatest with enflurane (Peterson *et al,* 1986). For example, in neurologically intact patients a monitorable cortical wave form is reliably maintained in the presence of 60% nitrous oxide plus 1 MAC halothane but not isoflurane or enflurane. Even nitrous oxide may decrease the amplitude of cortical somatosensory evoked potentials (McPherson *et al,* 1985) (see Chapter 41).

Cerebral Blood Flow

Volatile anesthetics administered during normocapnia in concentrations above 0.6 MAC produce dose-dependent increases in cerebral blood flow (Fig. 2-3) (Eger, 1984a). This drug-induced increase in cerebral blood flow occurs despite concomitant reductions in cerebral metabolic oxygen requirements) (see the section entitled Cerebral Metabolic Oxygen Requirements). The greatest increase in cerebral blood flow occurs with halothane, is intermediate with enflurane, and is least with isoflurane. For example, at 1.1 MAC, cerebral blood flow increases almost 200% during administration of halothane, 30% to 50% with enflurane, and is unchanged with isoflurane. In patients with intracranial space-occupying lesions, the administration of halothane–nitrous oxide in concentrations equivalent to about 1.5 MAC increases regional cerebral blood flow 166% compared with 35% during enflurane and no change with isoflurane (Eintrei *et al,* 1985). Nitrous oxide also in-

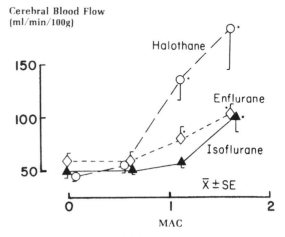

FIGURE 2-3. Cerebral blood flow measured in the presence of normocapnia and absence of surgical stimulation. *P < 0.05. (From Eger EI. Isoflurane [Forane]. A compendium and reference. Madison, Wisconsin, Ohio Medical Products, 1984:1–110. Reproduced by permission of the author and publisher.)

creases cerebral blood flow, but its restriction to concentrations less than 1 MAC limits the magnitude of this change.

Anesthetic-induced increases in cerebral blood flow occur within minutes of initiating administration of the inhaled drug and occur whether blood pressure is unchanged or decreased, emphasizing the action of inhaled anesthetics as cerebral vasodilators. Isoflurane may produce less direct cerebral vascular vasodilation than halothane because of a lesser increase in cyclic AMP relative to adenosine triphosphate (Sprague *et al*, 1974).

Animals exposed to halothane demonstrate a time-dependent decrease in the previously elevated cerebral blood flow beginning after about 30 minutes and reaching predrug levels after 150 minutes (Albrecht *et al*, 1983). This normalization of cerebral blood flow reflects a concomitant increase in cerebral vascular resistance that is not altered by alpha- or beta-adrenergic blockade or as a result of changes in cerebrospinal fluid *p*H (Albrecht *et al*, 1983; Warner *et al*, 1985).

In animals, autoregulation of cerebral blood flow in response to changes in blood pressure is retained during administration of 1 MAC isoflurane but not halothane (Fig. 2-4) (Drummond *et al*, 1982; Eger, 1984b). Indeed, increases in blood pressure produce smaller increases in brain protrusion during administration of isoflurane (and enflurane) compared with halothane (Drummond *et al*, 1982). It is speculated that loss of autoregulation during administration of halothane is responsible for the greater brain swelling seen in animals anesthetized with this drug. Inhaled anesthetics do not alter the responsiveness of the cerebral circulation to changes in $PaCO_2$.

Cerebral Metabolic Oxygen Requirements

Inhaled anesthetics produce dose-dependent reductions in cerebral metabolic oxygen requirements (Theye and Michenfelder, 1968). Isoflurane produces reductions in cerebral metabolic oxygen requirements that exceed those produced by an equivalent MAC concentration of halothane (Todd and Drummond, 1984). Above 2 MAC isoflurane, the EEG becomes isoelectric and additional increases in the concentration of anesthetic do not produce further decreases in cerebral metabolic oxygen requirements (Newberg *et al*, 1983). Unchanged cerebral blood flow and decreased cerebral metabolic oxygen requirements during isoflurane-induced controlled hypotension for clipping of cerebral aneurysms indicate that global cerebral oxygen supply–demand balance is favorably altered in patients anesthetized with this anesthetic (Newman *et al*, 1986).

The greater decrease in cerebral metabolic oxygen requirements produced by isoflurane may explain why cerebral blood flow is not increased by this anesthetic at concentrations below 1.1 MAC. For example, decreased cerebral metabolism means that less carbon dioxide is produced, which thus opposes any increase in cerebral blood flow. Isoflurane-induced reductions in cerebral metabolic oxygen requirements may account for the ability of this anesthetic to protect the brain from ischemic damage produced by profound hypotension (Newberg and Michenfelder, 1983).

Intracranial Pressure

Inhaled anesthetics produce elevations in intracranial pressure that parallel increases in cerebral blood flow produced by these drugs. Patients with space-occupying intracranial lesions are most vulnerable to these drug-induced elevations in intracranial pressure. Hyperventilation of the lungs sufficient to lower the $PaCO_2$ to about 30 mmHg opposes the tendency for inhaled anesthetics to increase intracranial pressure (Adams *et al*, 1981).

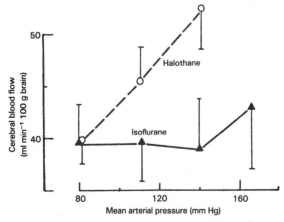

FIGURE 2-4. Autoregulation of cerebral blood flow as measured in animals. Mean ± SE. (From Eger EI. Pharmacology of isoflurane. Br J Anaesth 1984; 56:71S – 99S. Reproduced by permission of the author and publisher.)

In this regard, isoflurane differs from halothane in that hyperventilation can be established simultaneously with initiation of administration rather than before introducing the anesthetic. With enflurane, it must be remembered that hyperventilation of the lungs increases the risk of seizure activity, which could lead to an elevation in cerebral metabolic oxygen requirements and carbon dioxide production. These enflurane-induced changes will tend to increase cerebral blood flow, which could further increase intracranial pressure. The ability of nitrous oxide to elevate intracranial pressure is probably less than that of volatile anesthetics, reflecting the restriction of the dose of this drug to less than 1 MAC.

Cerebrospinal Fluid Production

Enflurane increases both the rate of production and resistance to reabsorption of cerebrospinal fluid, which may contribute to sustained increases in intracranial pressure associated with administration of this drug (Artru, 1984a). Conversely, isoflurane does not alter production of cerebrospinal fluid and, at the same time, decreases resistance to its reabsorption (Artru, 1984b). These observations are consistent with minimal increases in intracranial pressure observed during administration of isoflurane. Increases in intracranial pressure associated with administration of nitrous oxide presumably reflect elevations in cerebral blood flow, since enhanced production of cerebral spinal fluid does not occur in the presence of this anesthetic (Artru, 1982).

CIRCULATORY EFFECTS

Inhaled anesthetics produce dose-dependent and drug-specific circulatory effects (Eger, 1984a). These effects manifest on blood pressure, heart rate, cardiac output, stroke volume, right atrial pressure, peripheral vascular resistance, cardiac rhythm, and coronary blood flow. Circulatory effects of inhaled anesthetics may be different in the presence of (1) controlled ventilation of the lungs compared with spontaneous breathing, (2) preexisting cardiac disease, or (3) drugs that act directly or indirectly on the heart. Mechanisms of circulatory effects are diverse but often reflect effects of inhaled anesthetics on (1) myocardial contractility, (2) peripheral vascular smooth mus-

cle tone, and (3) autonomic nervous system activity.

Blood Pressure

Volatile anesthetics produce dose-dependent reductions in blood pressure, with enflurane and isoflurane producing somewhat greater decreases than halothane (Fig. 2-5) (Calverley *et al*, 1978b; Eger *et al*, 1970; Eger, 1984a; Stevens *et al*, 1971). In contrast with volatile anesthetics, nitrous oxide produces either no change or modest increases in blood pressure (Fig. 2-5) (Eger, 1984a; Hornbein *et al*, 1982). Substitution of nitrous oxide for a portion of the volatile anesthetic reduces the magnitude of blood pressure depression produced by the same MAC concentration of the volatile anesthetic alone (Fig. 2-6) (Dolan *et al*, 1974; Eger, 1984a). Surgical stimulation also reduces the magnitude of blood pressure reduction produced by volatile anesthetics. The decrease in blood pressure produced by enflurane and halothane is,

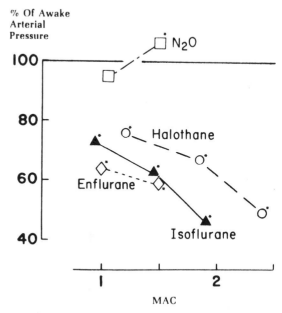

FIGURE 2-5. Impact of inhaled anesthetics on blood pressure in the presence of normocapnia and absence of surgical stimulation. *P < 0.05. (From Eger EI. Isoflurane [Forane]. A compendium and reference. Madison, Wisconsin, Ohio Medical Products, 1984:1–110. Reproduced by permission of the author and publisher.)

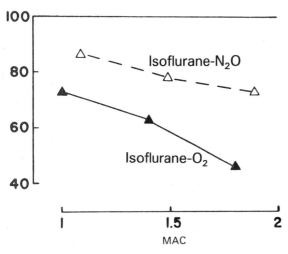

FIGURE 2-6. The substitution of nitrous oxide for a portion of isoflurane produces less depression of blood pressure than the same dose of volatile anesthetic alone. (From Eger EI. Isoflurane [Forane]. A compendium and reference. Madison, Wisconsin, Ohio Medical Products, 1984:1–110. Reproduced by permission of the author and publisher.)

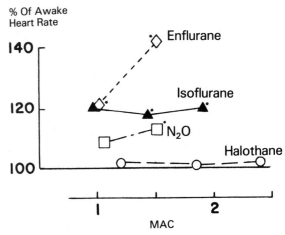

FIGURE 2-7. Impact of inhaled anesthetics on heart rate in the presence of normocapnia and in the absence of surgical stimulation. *$P < 0.05$. (From Eger EI. Isoflurane [Forane]. A compendium and reference. Madison, Wisconsin, Ohio Medical Products, 1984:1–110. Reproduced by permission of the author and publisher.)

in part or whole, a consequence of decreases in myocardial contractility and cardiac output, whereas with isoflurane, the decrease in blood pressure results almost entirely from a decrease in peripheral vascular resistance (see the section entitled Mechanism of Circulatory Effects).

Heart Rate

Heart rate is not substantially altered during the administration of nitrous oxide or halothane (Fig. 2-7) (Eger, 1984a). Enflurane produces dose-dependent elevations in heart rate, whereas isoflurane elevates heart rate similar amounts independent of the dose above 1 MAC (Fig. 2-7) (Eger, 1984a).

The presence of an intact carotid sinus baroreceptor reflex response during administration of enflurane and isoflurane is suggested by increases in heart rate during drug-induced reductions in blood pressure. Indeed, in humans, isoflurane produces less depression of the carotid sinus reflex–mediated heart rate response to changes in blood pressure than do enflurane and halothane (Fig. 2-8) (Kotrly *et al*, 1984). Evidence of carotid

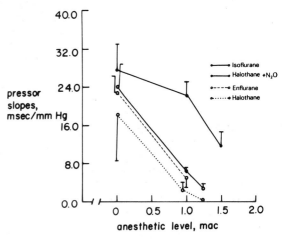

FIGURE 2-8. Pressor slopes, as a reflection of carotid sinus baroreceptor reflex activity, are best maintained during administration of isoflurane. (From Kotrly KJ, Ebert TJ, Vucins E, Igler FO, Barney JA, Kampine JP. Baroreceptor reflex control of heart rate during isoflurane anesthesia in humans. Anesthesiology 1984;60:173–9. Reproduced by permission of the authors and publisher.)

sinus depression by halothane is the absence of heart rate changes despite drug-induced reductions in blood pressure. Halothane may also slow the rate of sinus node depolarization and delay conduction of cardiac impulses through the atrioventricular node and His–Purkinje system (see the section entitled Cardiac Dysrhythmias). Nitrous oxide also depresses the carotid sinus, but quantitating this effect is difficult because of the limited potency of nitrous oxide and its frequent administration with other anesthetics.

In addition to less depression of the carotid sinus, isoflurane may increase heart rate by virtue of modest beta-agonist stimulation characterized by greater drug-induced depression of the parasympathetic than sympathetic nervous system (Skovsted and Sapthavichaikul, 1977). Indeed, isoflurane-induced increases in heart rate are more likely to occur in younger patients and may be accentuated by the presence of other drugs (atropine, meperidine, pancuronium) that accelerate heart rate. Administration of an opioid appears to minimize the likelihood of isoflurane-induced increases in heart rate (Cahalan *et al,* 1983). Heart rate increases during the administration of isoflurane also seem to be blunted in elderly patients (Linde *et al,* 1975; Mallow *et al,* 1976).

The effects of volatile anesthetics on heart rate and blood pressure may be influenced by the awake level of autonomic nervous system activity. For example, increased sympathetic nervous system activity, as accompanies apprehension, may artificially elevate awake heart rate and blood pressure and alter the magnitude of the pharmacologic effects of volatile anesthetics. Likewise, excess awake parasympathetic nervous system activity may result in unexpected increases in heart rate when anesthesia is established.

Cardiac Output and Stroke Volume

Administration of isoflurane during controlled ventilation of the lungs to maintain normocapnia does not alter cardiac output from awake levels (Fig. 2-9) (Eger, 1984a). In contrast, halothane and enflurane produce dose-dependent reductions in cardiac output that principally reflect reductions in stroke volume (*e.g.,* myocardial contractility) (Fig. 2-9) (Eger, 1984a). Isoflurane also decreases stroke volume, but this is offset by an increase in heart rate such that cardiac output is

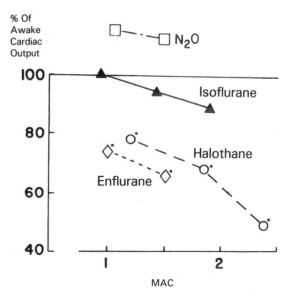

FIGURE 2-9. Impact of inhaled anesthetics on cardiac output in the presence of normocapnia and absence of surgical stimulation. *P < 0.05. (From Eger EI. Isoflurane [Forane]. A compendium and reference. Madison, Wisconsin, Ohio Medical Products, 1984:1–110. Reproduced by permission of the author and publisher.)

unchanged. The increase in heart rate associated with administration of enflurane is insufficient to offset decreases in stroke volume, and cardiac output is decreased. Cardiac output is modestly increased by nitrous oxide, possibly reflecting mild sympathomimetic effects of this drug (see the section entitled Mechanism of Circulatory Effects).

Failure of isoflurane to alter cardiac output may reflect activation of homeostatic mechanisms that obscure direct cardiac depressant effects (see the section entitled Mechanism of Circulatory Effects). Indeed, volatile anesthetics, including isoflurane, produce similar dose-dependent depression of myocardial contractility when studied *in vitro* using isolated papillary muscle preparations (Kemmotsu *et al,* 1973). *In vitro* depression of myocardial contractility produced by nitrous oxide is about one-half that produced by comparable concentrations of volatile anesthetics. Direct myocardial depressant effects *in vivo* are most likely offset by sympathomimetic effects of nitrous oxide.

Another possible explanation for the lesser impact of isoflurane on myocardial contractility may be a greater anesthetic potency of isoflurane relative to halothane and enflurane (Eger, 1984b). For example, the multiple of MAC times the oil : gas partition coefficient for halothane, enflurane, and isoflurane is 168, 163, and 105, respectively. The implication is that isoflurane may more readily depress the brain and, thus, at a given MAC value, appear to spare the heart. Indeed, in animals, the lesser myocardial depression associated with administration of isoflurane manifests as a greater margin of safety between the dose that produces anesthesia and that which produces cardiovascular collapse (Wolfson *et al,* 1978).

Right Atrial Pressure

Inhaled anesthetics produce dose-dependent increases in right atrial pressure, presumably reflecting direct myocardial depression and drug effects on the peripheral vasculature (Fig. 2-10) (Eger, 1984a). Consistent with minimal *in vivo* depression of myocardial contractility during administration of isoflurane is failure of the right

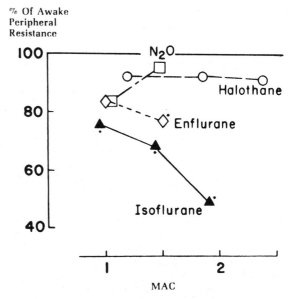

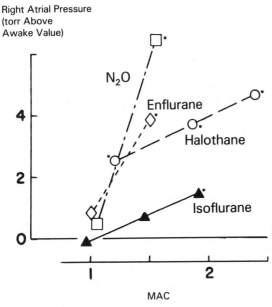

FIGURE 2-10. Impact of inhaled anesthetics on right atrial pressure in the presence of normocapnia and absence of surgical stimulation. *P < 0.05. (From Eger EI. Isoflurane [Forane]. A compendium and reference. Madison, Wisconsin, Ohio Medical Products, 1984:1–110. Reproduced by permission of the author and publisher.)

FIGURE 2-11. Impact of inhaled anesthetics on peripheral vascular resistance in the presence of normocapnia and absence of surgical stimulation. *P < 0.05. (From Eger EI. Isoflurane [Forane]. A compendium and reference. Madison, Wisconsin, Ohio Medical Products, 1984:1–110. Reproduced by permission of the author and publisher.)

atrial pressure to increase compared with other inhaled anesthetics. Peripheral vasodilating effects of isoflurane, and to a lesser extent of enflurane, would also minimize effects of direct myocardial depression produced by these drugs on right atrial pressure. Elevated right atrial pressure during administration of nitrous oxide most likely reflects increased pulmonary vascular resistance owing to sympathomimetic effects of this drug (Smith *et al,* 1970).

Peripheral Vascular Resistance

Isoflurane produces a dose-dependent decrease in peripheral vascular resistance that exceeds that produced by enflurane (Fig. 2-11) (Eger, 1984a). Peripheral vascular resistance does not change during administration of halothane or nitrous oxide (Fig. 2-11) (Eger, 1984a). Substitution of nitrous oxide for a portion of the isoflurane dose reduces the magnitude of decrease in peripheral vascular resistance produced by administration of isoflurane.

The effect of isoflurane on peripheral vascular resistance is predictable considering this drug's known effects on blood pressure and cardiac output (see Fig. 44-7). Likewise, the absence of a change in peripheral vascular resistance during administration of halothane emphasizes that reductions in blood pressure produced by this drug parallel decreases in myocardial contractility and cardiac output.

The decrease in peripheral vascular resistance during administration of isoflurane principally reflects a substantial (up to fourfold) increase in skeletal muscle blood flow (Stevens *et al*, 1971). Cutaneous blood flow is also increased by isoflurane. Implications of these alterations in blood flow may include (1) excess (wasted) perfusion relative to oxygen needs, (2) loss of body heat due to increased cutaneous blood flow, and (3) enhanced delivery of drugs, such as neuromuscular blocking drugs to the neuromuscular junction. A beta-agonist effect due to isoflurane is consistent with vascular smooth muscle relaxation in skeletal muscle but does not explain vasodilation in the brain.

Failure of peripheral vascular resistance to decline during administration of halothane does not mean that this drug lacks vasodilating effects on certain organ systems. Clearly, halothane is a potent cerebral vasodilator, and cutaneous vasodilation is prominent (see the section entitled Cerebral Effects). These vasodilating effects of halothane, however, are offset by absent changes or vasoconstriction in other vascular beds such that the overall effect is an unchanged calculated peripheral vascular resistance.

The increase in cutaneous blood flow produced by all volatile anesthetics is likely to reflect a central inhibitory action of these anesthetics on temperature-regulating mechanisms. Conversely, administration of 40% nitrous oxide produces constriction of cutaneous blood vessels, whereas the combination with halothane results in no change or in an increase in cutaneous blood flow (Eisele and Smith, 1972). Cutaneous blood flow does not change when nitrous oxide is administered in the presence of enflurane (Smith *et al*, 1978). Skeletal muscle blood flow increases when nitrous oxide is administered in the presence of halothane but not enflurane or isoflurane (Dolan *et al*, 1974; Smith *et al*, 1978).

Pulmonary Vascular Resistance

Volatile anesthetics appear to exert little or no predictable effect on pulmonary vascular smooth muscle. Conversely, nitrous oxide may produce increases in pulmonary vascular resistance that are exaggerated in patients with preexisting pulmonary hypertension (Hilgenberg *et al*, 1980; Schulte-Sasse *et al*, 1982). The newborn with or without preexisting pulmonary hypertension may also be uniquely vulnerable to pulmonary vascular vasoconstricting effects of nitrous oxide (Eisele *et al*, 1986). In patients with congenital heart disease, these increases in pulmonary vascular resistance may increase the magnitude of right-to-left intracardiac shunting of blood and further jeopardize arterial oxygenation.

Duration of Administration

Administration of a volatile anesthetic for 5 hours or longer is accompanied by recovery from the depressant circulatory effects of these drugs. For example, compared with measurements at 1 hour, the same MAC concentration after 5 to 6 hours is associated with a return of cardiac output toward predrug levels (Figs. 2-12 and 2-13) (Bahlman *et al*, 1972; Calverley *et al*, 1978b). After 5 hours, heart rate is also increased, but blood pressure is unchanged as the increase in cardiac output is offset by a decline in peripheral vascular resistance. Evidence of recovery with time is most apparent during administration of halothane, is intermediate with enflurane, and is minimal during inhalation of isoflurane. Minimal evidence of recovery during administration of isoflurane is predictable, because this drug does not substantially alter cardiac output even at 1 hour.

The return of cardiac output toward predrug levels with time in association with increases in heart rate and peripheral vasodilation resembles a beta-adrenergic agonist response. Indeed, pretreatment with propranolol prevents evidence of recovery with time from the circulatory effects of volatile anesthetics (Price *et al*, 1970).

Cardiac Dysrthythmias

The ability of volatile anesthetics to reduce the dose of epinephrine necessary to evoke ventricu-

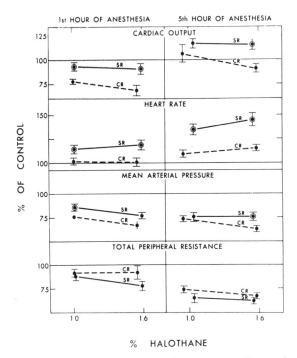

FIGURE 2-12. Comparison of circulatory effects of halothane during spontaneous breathing (SR) and controlled ventilation (CR) of the lungs after 1 hr and 5 hr of administration of halothane. (From Bahlman SH, Eger EI, Halsey MJ, *et al*. The cardiovascular effects of halothane in man during spontaneous ventilation. Anesthesiology 1972;36:494–502. Reproduced by permission of the authors and publisher.)

lar cardiac dysrhythmias is greatest with halothane, intermediate with enflurane, and least with isoflurane. For example, the dose of submucosally injected epinephrine necessary to produce ventricular cardiac dysrhythmias in 50% of patients anesthetized with a 1.25 MAC concentration of a volatile anesthetic is 2.1, 3.4, and 6.7 μg kg^{-1} during administration of halothane, enflurane, and isoflurane, respectively (Fig. 2-14) (Johnston *et al*, 1976). This order of arrhythmogenic potential is consistent with the alkane structure of halothane compared with ether derivatives such as enflurane and isoflurane. In contrast to adults, children tolerate higher doses of subcutaneous epinephrine (7.8–10 μg kg^{-1}) injected with or without lidocaine during halothane anesthesia (Karl *et al*, 1983; Ueda *et al*, 1983). Mechanical stimulation associated with injection of epineph-

rine for repair of cleft palate has been associated with cardiac dysrhythmias (Ueda *et al*, 1983).

Inclusion of lidocaine, 0.5% in the epinephrine solution that is injected submucosally nearly doubles the dose of epinephrine necessary to provoke ventricular cardiac dyshythmias (Fig. 2-14) (Johnston *et al*, 1976). A similar response occurs when lidocaine is combined with epinephrine injected submucosally during administration of enflurane (Horrigan *et al*, 1978). Despite this apparent protective effect of lidocaine, the systemic concentrations of the local anesthetic remain below 1μg ml^{-1} following its subcutaneous injection with epinephrine (Stoelting, 1978).

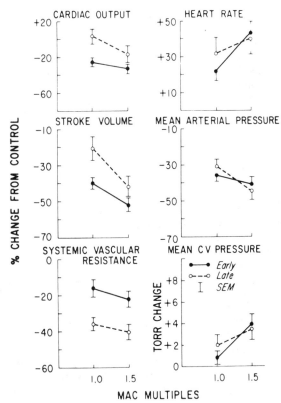

FIGURE 2-13. Comparison of circulatory effects of enflurane after 1 hr *(solid line)* and 6 hr *(broken line)* of administration during controlled ventilation of the lungs to maintain normocapnia. (From Calverley RK, Smith NT, Prys–Roberts C, Eger EI, Jones CW. Cardiovascular effects of enflurane anesthesia during controlled ventilation in man. Anesth Analg 1978;57:619–28. Reproduced by permission of the authors and the International Anesthesia Research Society.)

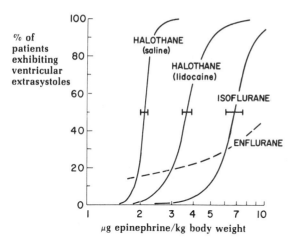

FIGURE 2-14. Percent of patients developing ventricular cardiac dysrhythmias (three or more premature ventricular contractions considered a positive response) with increasing doses of submucosal epinephrine injected during administration of 1.25 MAC concentrations of the volatile anesthetic. (From Johnston RR, Eger EI, Wilson C. A comparative interaction of epinephrine with enflurane, isoflurane, and halothane in man. Anesth Analg 1976;55:709–12. Reproduced by permission of the authors and the International Anesthesia Research Society.)

In animals, enhancement of the arrhythmogenic potential of epinephrine is independent of the dose of halothane between alveolar concentrations of 0.5% and 2% (Metz and Maze, 1985). If true in patients, it is likely that cardiac dysrhythmias owing to epinephrine will persist until the halothane concentration declines to below 0.5%. For this reason, therapeutic interventions other than decreasing the inhaled concentration of halothane will be required to promptly treat cardiac dysrhythmias owing to epinephrine.

The mechanism for the difference between volatile anesthetics and the arrthythmogenic potential of epinephrine may reflect the effects of these drugs on the rate of transmission of cardiac impulses through the heart. For example, both isoflurane and halothane slow conduction of cardiac impulses through the atrioventricular node, but only halothane also slows conduction through the His–Purkinje system (Atlee and Alexander, 1977; Blitt *et al*, 1979). Slow conduction of cardiac impulses through the His–Purkinje system during administration of halothane would increase the likelihood of cardiac dysrhythmias due to a reentry mechanism (see Chapter 48). A role of

alpha- and beta-adrenergic receptors in the heart is suggested by the increased dose of epinephrine required to produce cardiac dysrhythmias in dogs anesthetized with halothane and pretreated with droperidol, prazosin, or metoprolol (Fig. 2-15) (Maze and Smith, 1983; Maze *et al*, 1985).

Junctional rhythm leading to reductions in blood pressure is common during administration of halothane. The appearance of this cardiac rhythm disturbance most likely reflects suppression of sinus node activity by halothane.

Coronary Blood Flow

Isoflurane is a more potent coronary artery vasodilator than halothane or enflurane in animals and patients with coronary artery disease (Gelman *et al*, 1984a; Reiz *et al*, 1983; Rydvall *et al*, 1984). Conceivably, isoflurane-induced coronary artery vasodilation combined with an associated reduction in perfusion pressure could result in diver-

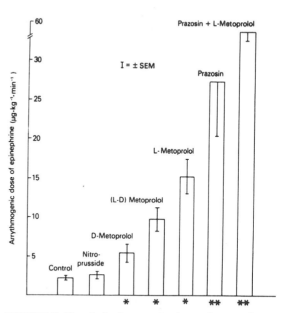

FIGURE 2-15. Arrhythmogenic dose of epinephrine during halothane anesthesia (1.2 MAC) in the dog following different treatments. *P < 0.05. **P < 0.01. (From Maze M, and Smith CM. Identification of receptor mechanism mediating epinephrine-induced arrhythmias during halothane anesthesia in the dog. Anesthesiology 1983;59:322–6. Reproduced by permission of the authors and publisher.)

sion of blood flow from diseased areas of myocardium to areas with normally responsive coronary arteries (*e.g.,* coronary steal syndrome) (Reiz and Ostman, 1985). Indeed, evidence of myocardial ischemia (ST changes on the electrocardiogram and decreased lactate extraction) has been observed in patients with coronary artery disease who have been anesthetized with nitrous oxide – isoflurane but not nitrous oxide – opioids (Reiz *et al,* 1983). Nitrous oxide may enhance the vasodilating properties of isoflurane (Reiz, 1983). Nevertheless, most patients do not develop myocardial ischemia during administration of isoflurane, emphasizing the importance of avoiding drug-induced events that (1) may reduce myocardial oxygen delivery (*e.g.,* decreased perfusion pressure, increased left ventricular end-diastolic pressure) or (2) increase myocardial oxygen requirements (*e.g.,* tachycardia) (Eger, 1984b; Moffitt *et al,* 1984). In this regard, inclusion of an opioid or prior treatment with a beta-adrenergic antagonist may minimize the occurrence of events that alter the balance between myocardial oxygen requirements and delivery. Furthermore, a low concentration of isoflurane (about 0.4 MAC) plus 50% nitrous oxide administered to patients with coronary artery disease produces only a modest decline in mean arterial pressure and improves tolerance to pacing-induced myocardial ischemia (Tarnow *et al,* 1986).

In another study, halothane and enflurane were observed to produce modest increases in myocardial vascular resistance (Merin and Basch, 1981). Despite the potential for this response to reduce coronary blood flow, there is no evidence of myocardial ischemia based on lactate extraction. Furthermore, autoregulation of coronary artery blood flow seems to remain intact during administration of these anesthetics.

In an animal model, collateral coronary artery circulation is maintained during administration of halothane in the presence of a normal heart rate (Sivarajan and Bashein, 1985). Tachycardia, however, severely limits blood flow to the collateralized subendocardium.

Spontaneous Breathing

The circulatory effects of volatile anesthetics during spontaneous breathing are different from those observed during normocapnia and controlled ventilation of the lungs. The difference reflects the impact of sympathetic nervous system stimulation due to accumulation of carbon dioxide (*i.e.,* respiratory acidosis) and improved venous return during spontaneous breathing. In addition, carbon dioxide may have a direct relaxing effect on peripheral smooth muscle. Indeed, cardiac output and blood pressure are depressed less, heart rate is elevated, and peripheral vascular resistance is decreased during spontaneous breathing compared with measurements during administration of volatile anesthetics in the presence of controlled ventilation of the lungs to maintain normocapnia (Fig. 2-12) (Bahlman *et al,* 1972; Calverley *et al,* 1978a; Cromwell *et al,* 1971).

Preexisting Diseases and Drug Therapy

Preexisting cardiac disease may influence the significance of circulatory effects produced by inhaled anesthetics. For example, volatile anesthetics decrease myocardial contractility of normal and failing cardiac muscle similar amounts, but the significance is greater in diseased cardiac muscle because contractility is impaired before drug administration (Shimosato *et al,* 1973). In patients with coronary artery disease, administration of 40% nitrous oxide produces evidence of myocardial depression that does not occur in patients without heart disease (Eisele and Smith, 1972). Valvular heart disease may influence the significance of anesthetic-induced circulatory effects. In this regard, peripheral vasodilation produced by isoflurane is undesirable in patients with aortic stenosis but may be beneficial in those with mitral or aortic regurgitation.

Arterial hypoxemia may enhance cardiac depressant effects of volatile anesthetics (Cullen and Eger, 1970). Conversely, anemia does not alter anesthetic-induced circulatory effects compared with measurements from normal animals (Loarie *et al,* 1979).

Prior drug therapy that alters sympathetic nervous system activity (*e.g.,* antihypertensives, beta-adrenergic antagonists) may influence the magnitude of circulatory effects produced by volatile anesthetics (see Chapters 14 and 15). Calcium entry blockers decrease myocardial contractility and thus render the heart more vulnerable to direct depressant effects of inhaled anesthetics. In animals, depressant effects of verapamil on cardiac output are greater during administration of enflurane than isoflurane (see Chapter 18).

Mechanism of Circulatory Effects

Volatile Anesthetics

There is no single mechanism that explains depressant circulatory effects of volatile anesthetics in all situations. Proposed mechanisms include (1) direct myocardial depression, (2) inhibition of central nervous system sympathetic outflow, (3) peripheral autonomic ganglion blockade, (4) attenuated carotid sinus baroreceptor activity, (5) decreased formation of cyclic AMP, (6) decreased release of catecholamines from the adrenal medulla, and (7) decreased influx of calcium through slow channels. Indeed, the negative inotropic effect of 1% halothane may be due, in part, to decreased calcium ion influx through slow channels (Lynch *et al*, 1981). Absence of this effect at 0.5% halothane, however, suggests that additional mechanisms, not involving slow calcium channels, also participate in the negative inotropic effect of this drug. Plasma catecholamine concentrations typically do not increase during administration of volatile anesthetics, as evidence that these drugs do not activate and may even depress activity of the central and peripheral sympathetic nervous system.

Isoflurane may be unique among the volatile anesthetics in possessing mild beta-adrenergic agonist properties and producing less inhibition of the carotid sinus baroreceptor. These effects are consistent with the maintenance of cardiac output, increased heart rate, elevated skeletal muscle blood flow, coronary artery vasodilation, and decreased peripheral vascular resistance that may accompany the administration of isoflurane (Stevens *et al*, 1971). A beta-agonist effect of isoflurane, however, is not supported by animal data failing to demonstrate a difference between volatile anesthetics with or without beta-adrenergic blockade (Philbin and Lowenstein, 1976).

Nitrous Oxide

Nitrous oxide administered alone or added to an unchanged concentration of volatile anesthetic produces signs of mild sympathomimetic stimulation characterized by elevations in plasma concentrations of catecholamines, mydriasis, increases in body temperature, diaphoresis, increases in right atrial pressure, and evidence of vasoconstriction in the systemic and pulmonary circulations. Evidence of this sympathomimetic effect is more prominent when nitrous oxide is administered in the presence of halothane than enflurane or isoflurane (Smith *et al*, 1970). It is presumed that this mild sympathomimetic effect masks any direct depressant effects of nitrous oxide on the heart.

Nitrous oxide-induced increases in sympathetic nervous system activity may reflect activation of brain nuclei that control beta-adrenergic outflow from the central nervous system (Fukunaga and Epstein, 1973). Sympathetic nervous system stimulation may also result because nitrous oxide can inhibit uptake of norepinephrine by the lungs, thus making more neurotransmitter available to receptors (Naito and Gillis, 1973).

In contrast to sympathomimetic effects observed with nitrous oxide alone or added to volatile anesthetics, the administration of nitrous oxide in the presence of opioids results in evidence of profound circulatory depression characterized by decreases in blood pressure and cardiac output and elevations of left ventricular end-diastolic pressure and peripheral vascular resistance (Lappas *et al*, 1975; McDermott and Stanley, 1974; Stoelting and Gibbs, 1973). It is possible that opioids block centrally mediated sympathomimetic effects of nitrous oxide, thus unmasking its direct depressant effects on the heart (Flaim *et al*, 1978).

VENTILATION EFFECTS

Inhaled anesthetics produce dose-dependent and drug-specific effects on the (1) pattern of breathing, (2) ventilatory response to carbon dioxide, (3) ventilatory response to hypoxemia, and (4) airway resistance. The PaO_2 predictably declines during administration of inhaled anesthetics in the absence of supplemental oxygen. Drug-induced inhibition of hypoxic pulmonary vasoconstriction as a mechanism for this decrease in oxygenation has not been confirmed during one-lung ventilation in patients inhaling halothane or isoflurane (see Fig. 46-3). Changes in intraoperative PaO_2 and the incidence of postoperative pulmonary complications are not different in patients anesthetized with halothane, enflurane, or isoflurane (Gold *et al*, 1983).

Pattern of Breathing

Inhaled anesthetics, except for isoflurane, produce dose-dependent increases in the rate of

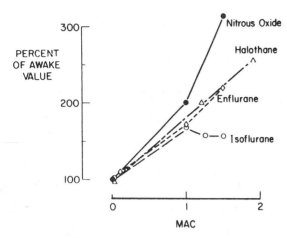

FIGURE 2-16. Impact of inhaled anesthetics on rate of breathing in the absence of surgical stimulation. (From Eger EI. Respiratory effects of nitrous oxide. In Nitrous Oxide. New York, Elsevier, 1985:109. Reprinted by permission of the author and publisher from Eger, Nitrous Oxide. Copyright 1985 by Elsevier Science Publishing Co., Inc.)

breathing (Fig. 2-16) (Eger, 1985b). Isoflurane increases the rate of breathing similar to other inhaled anesthetics up to a dose of 1 MAC. Above a 1 MAC concentration, however, isoflurane does not produce a further increase in the rate of breathing. Nitrous oxide increases the rate of breathing more than other inhaled anesthetics at concentrations above 1 MAC. The effect of inhaled anesthetics on the rate of breathing presumably reflects central nervous system stimulation. Activation of pulmonary stretch receptors by inhaled anesthetics has not been demonstrated. The exception may be nitrous oxide, which at anesthetic concentrations that exceed 1 MAC may also stimulate pulmonary stretch receptors (Eger, 1985b).

Tidal volume is decreased in association with anesthetic-induced increases in the rate of breathing. The net effect of these changes is a rapid and shallow pattern of breathing during general anesthesia. The increase in rate of breathing is insufficient to offset the reduction in tidal volume, leading to a decline in minute ventilation and elevation of $PaCO_2$. The pattern of breathing during general anesthesia is also characterized as regular and rhythmic in contrast to the awake pattern of intermittent deep breaths separated by varying intervals.

Ventilatory Response to Carbon Dioxide

Volatile anesthetics produce dose-dependent depression of ventilation characterized by a decreased ventilatory response to carbon dioxide and an increase in $PaCO_2$. In the absence of surgical stimulation or other drugs and at comparable MAC concentrations, enflurane produces the greatest elevation in $PaCO_2$, followed by isoflurane and then halothane (Fig. 2-17) (Bahlman *et al*, 1972; Calverley *et al*, 1978a; Cromwell *et al*, 1971; Eger, 1984a). The presence of chronic obstructive airways disease, however, may accentuate the magnitude of increase in $PaCO_2$ produced by volatile anesthetics (Pietak *et al*, 1975). Nitrous oxide does not increase the $PaCO_2$, suggesting that substitution of this anesthetic for a portion of the volatile anesthetic would result in less depression of ventilation. Indeed, nitrous oxide combined with a volatile anesthetic produces less depression of ventilation and elevation in $PaCO_2$ than does the same MAC concentration of the volatile drug alone (France *et al*, 1974; Lam *et al*, 1982). This ventilatory depressant-sparing effect of nitrous oxide is detectable with all three volatile anesthetics, but the greatest impact occurs

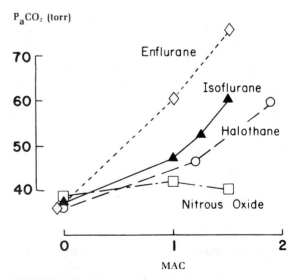

FIGURE 2-17. Impact of inhaled anesthetics on the resting $PaCO_2$ (mmHg) in the absence of surgical stimulation. (From Eger EI. Isoflurane [Forane]. A compendium and reference. Madison, Wisconsin, Ohio Medical Products. 1984:1–110. Reproduced by permission of the author and publisher.)

when nitrous oxide is used to replace an equivalent amount of enflurane (Lam *et al,* 1982).

Despite the apparent benign effect of nitrous oxide on ventilation, the slope of the carbon dioxide response curve is depressed similarly and shifted rightward by anesthetic concentrations of all inhaled anesthetics (Fig. 2-18) (Eger, 1984a; Fourcade *et al,* 1971; Knill *et al,* 1979). Subanesthetic concentrations (0.1 MAC) of inhaled anesthetics, however, do not alter the ventilatory response to carbon dioxide.

In addition to nitrous oxide, surgical (*i.e.,* painful) stimulation and duration of drug administration influence the magnitude of increase in $PaCO_2$ produced by volatile anesthetics.

Surgical Stimulation

Surgical stimulation elevates minute ventilation about 40% by virtue of increases in tidal volume and rate of breathing. The $PaCO_2$, however, declines only about 10% (*e.g.,* 4 – 6 mmHg) despite this large increase in minute ventilation (Fig. 2-19) (Eger, 1984a; France *et al,* 1974). The reason for this discrepancy is speculated to be an increased production of carbon dioxide resulting

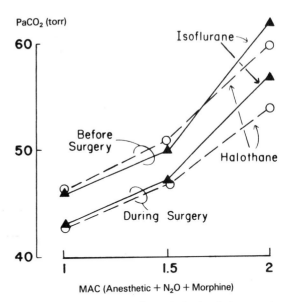

FIGURE 2-19. Impact of surgical stimulation on the resting $PaCO_2$ (mmHg) during administration of isoflurane or halothane. (From Eger EI. Isoflurane [Forane]. A compendium and reference. Madison, Wisconsin, Ohio Medical Products. 1984:1–110. Reproduced by permission of the author and publisher.)

from activation of the sympathetic nervous system in response to surgical stimulation. Increased production of carbon dioxide is presumed to offset the impact of increased minute ventilation on the $PaCO_2$.

Duration of Administration

After about 5 hours of administration, the elevation in $PaCO_2$ produced by a volatile anesthetic is less than that present during administration of the same dose of anesthetic for 1 hour (Table 2-3) (Calverley *et al,* 1978a). Likewise, the slope and position of the carbon dioxide response curve returns toward normal after about 5 hours of administration of the volatile anesthetics (Lam *et al,* 1982). The reason for this apparent recovery from the ventilatory depressant effects of inhaled anesthetics with time is not known.

Mechanism of Depression

Anesthetic-induced depression of ventilation (*e.g.,* elevated $PaCO_2$) most likely reflects direct depressant effects of these drugs on the medullary ventilatory center. An additional mechanism may

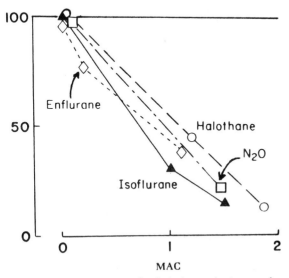

FIGURE 2-18. Impact of inhaled anesthetics on the slope of the line depicting the ventilatory response to carbon dioxide. (From Eger EI. Isoflurane [Forane]. A compendium and reference. Madison, Wisconsin, Ohio Medical Products. 1984:1–110. Reproduced by permission of the author and publisher.)

Table 2-3
*Evidence for Recovery from the Ventilatory
Depressant Effects of Volatile Anesthetics*

Enflurane (MAC)	Arterial PCO_2	
	One Hour of Administration	Five Hours of Administration
1	61 mmHg	46 mmHg
2	Apnea	67 mmHg

(Data from Calverley RK, Smith NT, Jones CW, Prys-Roberts C, Eger EI. Ventilatory and cardiovascular effects of enflurane anesthesia during spontaneous ventilation in man. Anesth Analg 1978; 57:610–8.)

be the ability of halothane and possibly other inhaled anesthetics to selectively interfere with intercostal muscle function, contributing to loss of chest stabilization during spontaneous breathing (Tusiewicz *et al,* 1977). This loss of chest stabilization could interfere with expansion of the chest in response to chemical stimulation of ventilation as normally produced by elevations of the $PaCO_2$ or arterial hypoxemia. Furthermore, this loss of chest stabilization means that descent of the diaphragm tends to cause the chest to collapse inward during inspiration, contributing to reductions in lung volumes, particularly the functional residual capacity. It is thus likely that halothane-induced depression of ventilation reflects both a central and peripheral effect of the drug.

Management of Depression

The predictable ventilatory depressant effects of volatile anesthetics are most often managed by institution of mechanical (*i.e.,* controlled) ventilation of the lungs. In this regard, the inherent ventilatory depressant effects of volatile anesthetics facilitate the initiation of controlled ventilation of the lungs.

Assisted ventilation of the lungs is a questionably effective method for offsetting the ventilatory depressant effects of volatile anesthetics. For example, the apneic threshold (*i.e.,* maximal $PaCO_2$, which does not initiate spontaneous ventilation) is only 3 to 5 mmHg lower than the $PaCO_2$ present during spontaneous ventilation (Ravin

lowered to 47 to 45 mmHg by assisted ventilation of the lungs before apnea occurs.

Ventilatory Response to Hypoxemia

All inhaled anesthetics, including nitrous oxide, profoundly depress the ventilatory response to arterial hypoxemia that is normally mediated by the carotid bodies. For example, 0.1 MAC produces 50% to 70% depression and 1.1 MAC, 100% depression of this response (Knill *et al,* 1982; Yacoub *et al,* 1976). This contrasts with the absence of significant depression of the ventilatory response to carbon dioxide during administration of 0.1 MAC concentrations of volatile anesthetics. Inhaled anesthetics also attenuate the usual synergistic effect of arterial hypoxemia and hypercapnia on stimulation of ventilation.

Airway Resistance

Volatile anesthetics produce dose-dependent and similar reductions in airway resistance following antigen-induced bronchoconstriction in an animal model (Fig. 2-20) (Hirshman *et al,* 1982). Despite these observations, there is lack of evidence that bronchodilating effects of volatile anesthetics, specifically halothane, are an effective method for treating status asthmaticus that is unresponsive to more conventional treatments. Likewise, data demonstrating decreases in airway resistance in asthmatic patients during administration of a volatile anesthetic are not available. Furthermore, in the absence of bronchoconstriction, the bronchodilating effects of volatile anesthetics are difficult to demonstrate, because normal bronchomotor tone is low and only minimal additional relaxation of bronchial smooth muscle is possible.

Halothane and enflurane reverse the bronchoconstricting effects of hypocapnia, with halothane being more efficacious at lower doses. This effect is not prevented by beta-adrenergic blockade, suggesting a direct bronchodilating effect of volatile anesthetics. In addition, volatile anesthetics probably contribute to bronchial smooth muscle relaxation by virtue of drug-induced reductions in afferent (vagal) nerve traffic from the central nervous system.

Like other inhaled anesthetics, nitrous oxide

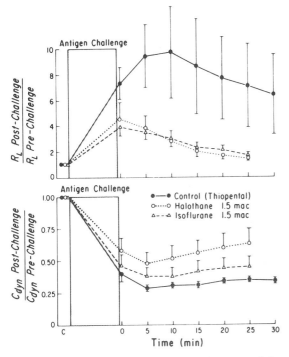

FIGURE 2-20. Increases in airway resistance and decrease in pulmonary compliance follow Ascaris antigen challenge during anesthesia in dogs. These changes are similarly attenuated by halothane and isoflurane. Mean ± SD. (From Hirshman CA, Edelstein G, Peetz S, Wayne S, Downes H. Mechanism of action of inhalational anesthesia on airways. Anesthesiology 56:1982;107–11. Reproduced by permission of the authors and publisher.)

muscle rigidity. Inhaled anesthetics are not irritating to the airways; thus, increased secretions or elevations in airway resistance by this mechanism are unlikely.

HEPATIC EFFECTS

Hepatic Blood Flow

Portal vein blood flow decreases during administration of 1 MAC halothane or isoflurane to animals (Gelman *et al.,* 1984b). At the same time, hepatic artery blood flow increases during administration of isoflurane and remains unchanged during administration of halothane despite associated reductions in blood pressure and cardiac

output. These data suggest that hepatic oxygen supply is maintained better during isoflurane than during halothane anesthesia.

In other reports, halothane has been shown to reduce hepatic blood flow in parallel with decreases in blood pressure and cardiac output (Cooperman, 1972). If the $PaCO_2$ increases during administration of halothane, there is a reduction in splanchnic vascular resistance and hepatic blood flow may increase (Epstein *et al,* 1966). Selective hepatic artery vasoconstriction has been reported in otherwise healthy patients during the administration of halothane (Benumof *et al,* 1976). Hepatic blood flow is reduced during administration of nitrous oxide in the presence of skeletal muscle paralysis and mechanical ventilation of the lungs, most likely reflecting transmission of positive airway pressure to the venous circulation (Cooperman, 1972).

Ideally, anesthetic-induced reductions in hepatic blood flow would be accompanied by similar reductions in hepatic oxygen consumption. Hepatic blood flow during anesthesia, however, decreases more than splanchnic oxygen consumption. Conceivably, this could result in anaerobic metabolism reflected by excess lactate production. Nevertheless, increased splanchnic lactate production has not been observed during anesthesia (Epstein *et al,* 1966). Therefore, it seems unlikely that reductions in hepatic blood flow produced by anesthetic drugs or techniques jeopardize hepatocyte viability.

Drug Clearance

Volatile anesthetics may interfere with clearance of drugs from the plasma by virtue of reductions in hepatic blood flow or inhibition of drug-metabolizing enzymes. Despite reductions in hepatic blood flow, decreases in drug clearance during administration of halothane seem to be principally due to inhibition of hepatic drug-metabolizing enzymes (Reilly *et al,* 1985).

Liver Function Tests

Halothane, but not isoflurane or enflurane, is associated with a transient elevation of bromsulphalein retention following prolonged administration (8.8 to11.6 MAC hr) in the absence of surgical stimulation (Eger *et al,* 1976; Stevens *et al.,*

1973). Transient elevations of liver transaminase enzymes follow prolonged administration of enflurane but not halothane or isoflurane. These changes following prolonged administration of halothane and enflurane are statistically significant but not clinically important. In the presence of surgical stimulation, bromsulphalein retention and elevations of liver transaminase enzymes transiently follow the administration of even isoflurane, suggesting that changes in hepatic blood flow evoked by painful stimulation can adversely alter hepatic function independent of the volatile anesthetic.

Hepatotoxicity

All anesthetics studied in the hypoxic rat model that includes enzyme induction may produce centrilobular necrosis, but the incidence is greatest with halothane, followed by fentanyl and then nitrous oxide (Fassoulaki *et al,* 1984). Enflurane and isoflurane are the least likely inhaled anesthetics to produce centrilobular necrosis in the hypoxic rat model. The combination of nitrous oxide with halothane accentuates hepatic injury produced by halothane in this animal model (Ross *et al,* 1984). In the liver, nitrous oxide inactivates methionine synthetase. The role of this inhibition in the production of liver disease, if any, is not known.

Small changes in the inhaled hypoxic concentration of oxygen may influence the likelihood of centrilobular necrosis following the administration of an anesthetic. For example, hepatic damage may occur in the rat model following administration of any anesthetic when the inhaled concentration of oxygen is 10% (Fig. 2-21) (Shingu *et al,* 1983b). Conversely, hepatic damage occurs following administration of halothane, but not enflurane or isoflurane, when the inhaled concentration of oxygen is 12% or 14% (Fig. 2-21) (Shingu *et al,* 1983b).

Mechanism

It is speculated that arterial hypoxemia with subsequent inadequate hepatocyte oxygenation is the principal mechanism responsible for centrilobular necrosis that occurs in the hypoxic rat model. Indeed, hypoxia in the absence of anesthetic drugs can produce hepatic damage in the rat model (Shingu *et al,* 1982). Any anesthetic drug

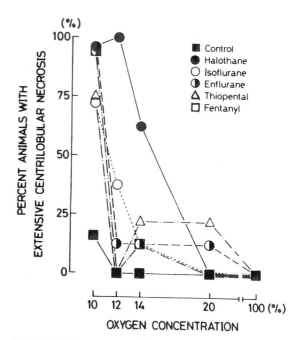

FIGURE 2-21. Hepatic damage may occur in the rat model following administration of inhaled or injected drugs when the inhaled oxygen concentration is 10%. Conversely, hepatic damage occurs following administration of halothane, but not enflurane or isoflurane, when the inhaled concentration of oxygen is 12% or 14%. (From Shingu K, Eger EI, Johnson BH, VanDyke RA, Lurz FW, Cheng A. Effect of oxygen concentration, hyperthermia, and choice of vendor on anesthetic-induced hepatic injury in rats. Anesth Analg 1983;62:146–50. Reproduced by permission of the authors and the International Anesthesia Research Society.)

that decreases alveolar ventilation or reduces hepatic blood flow could exaggerate preexisting arterial hypoxemia, thus contributing to hepatocyte damage. Preexisting hepatic disease, such as cirrhosis, may be associated with marginal hepatocyte oxygenation, which would be further jeopardized by depressant effects of anesthetics on hepatic blood flow or alveolar ventilation or both. For example, anesthetics could enhance the hepatotoxic effects of arterial hypoxemia by preventing the liver's capacity to use the decreased amount of available oxygen (Shingu *et al,* 1983b). Despite the theoretical adverse effects of preexisting liver disease, it has been demonstrated that postanesthetic hepatic dysfunction is minimal and similar in cirrhotic and noncirrhotic rats (Baden *et al,* 1985).

Hepatic hypoxia may be greater with halothane than isoflurane anesthesia because of greater reductions in hepatic blood flow produced by halothane (Gelman *et al,* 1984b). Evidence of an hepatotoxic role of reductive intermediary metabolites of halothane is not supported by occurrence of similar hepatic damage following administration of other anesthetics that do not undergo significant metabolism or metabolism by pathways other than reductive routes (Fassoulaki *et al,* 1984; Shingu *et al,* 1983a; VanDyke, 1981) (see the section entitled Metabolism).

Further evidence for the role of hepatocyte hypoxia in the production of hepatic damage is the observation that reduction in body temperature to 32°C prevents centrilobular necrosis in the hypoxic rat model following administration of enflurane and isoflurane but not halothane (Shingu *et al,* 1983b). The protective effect of hypothermia presumably reflects decreased hepatic oxygen requirements.

Halothane-Associated Hepatic Dysfunction

Halothane-associated hepatic dysfunction most commonly manifests as elevated body temperature and increased plasma concentrations of liver transaminase enzymes in the first 7 days postoperatively. Jaundice may or may not develop. Typically, the patient is a middle-aged obese female. An allergic reaction is suggested by eosinophilia and occurrence of hepatic dysfunction after repeated exposures to halothane, often at intervals separated by less than 4 weeks. Further support for an allergic reaction is the observation that plasma from some patients recovering from halothane-associated hepatic dysfunction contains antibodies that bind to the surfaces of specially prepared hepatocytes that have been exposed to halothane (Vergani *et al,* 1980). The possibility of a genetic susceptibility factor is suggested by (1) case reports of halothane hepatitis in closely related females, (2) strain differences in the susceptibility of rats to halothane-induced hepatic necrosis, and (3) demonstration of damage to lymphocytes from patients with suspected halothane-associated hepatic dysfunction when exposed to electrophilic metabolites (Farrell *et al,* 1985; Gourlay *et al,* 1981).

It is estimated that severe and occasionally fatal liver damage occurs in about every 30,000 administrations of halothane (Summary of the National Halothane Study, 1977). In contrast, a similar cause-and-effect relationship cannot be documented following the administration of enflurane or isoflurane (Eger *et al,* 1986; Stoelting *et al,* 1987). Indeed, the diagnosis of anesthetic-associated hepatic dysfunction is often a diagnosis of exclusion. In this regard, inhaled anesthetics may be incriminated as the cause of hepatic dysfunction when a more detailed evaluation of the patient and additional laboratory measurements would possibly establish a mechanism of hepatotoxicity unrelated to the anesthetic.

Mesenteric Blood Flow

Volatile anesthetics are associated with reductions in mesenteric blood flow principally due to indirect effects of these drugs by virtue of decreases in blood pressure and cardiac output. A role for circulating catecholamines is suggested by return of mesenteric blood flow to normal during general anesthesia following administration of phentolamine (Tverskoy *et al,* 1985).

RENAL EFFECTS

Volatile anesthetics produce similar dose-related reductions in renal blood flow, glomerular filtration rate, and urine output (Cousins *et al,* 1976; Mazze *et al,* 1974). These changes are not a result of release of antidiuretic hormone but rather most likely reflect effects of volatile anesthetics on blood pressure and cardiac output. Preoperative hydration attenuates or abolishes effects of volatile anesthetics on renal function. Halothane does not alter autoregulation of renal blood flow (see Chapter 53). Renal function following kidney transplantation is not influenced by the volatile anesthetic administered (Cronnelly *et al,* 1984).

Nephrotoxicity

Fluoride-induced nephrotoxicity is a potential hazard following metabolism of volatile anesthetics, principally enflurane (see the section entitled Metabolism). Peak plasma fluoride concentrations following a 2.5 MAC hour exposure to enflurane are about 20 μM L^{-1}, which is approximately one-third the level considered to be potentially nephrotoxic. Minimal metabolism of halothane and isoflurane to inorganic fluoride is insufficient to introduce even a theoretical risk of fluoride-induced nephrotoxicity. Indeed, the ability to concentrate urine remains unaltered following short-term (less than 4.9 MAC hours) administration of volatile anesthetics, including enflurane (Fig. 2-22) (Cousins *et al*, 1976). Conversely, prolonged administration (9.6 MAC hours or longer) of enflurane, but not halothane, is associated with detectable decreases in urine concentrating ability despite plasma fluoride concentrations averaging 15 μM L^{-1} (Fig. 2-23) (Mazze *et al*, 1977). This observation that even low plasma fluoride concentrations may transiently interfere with renal tubular function suggests that administration of enflurane to patients with preexisting renal disease might be harmful. Nevertheless, there is no detectable reduction in renal function in patients with chronic renal disease who un-

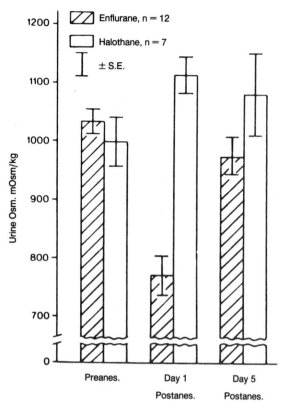

FIGURE 2-23. Prolonged administration (9.6 MAC hours) of enflurane, but not halothane, is associated with transient impairment of the ability of the renal tubules to concentrate urine. (From Mazze RI, Calverley RK, Smith NT. Inorganic fluoride nephrotoxicity: Prolonged enflurane and halothane anesthesia in volunteers. Anesthesiology 1977;46:265 – 71. Reproduced by permission of the authors and publisher.)

dergo elective operations and receive halothane or enflurane (Mazze *et al*, 1984). In fact, plasma creatinine declines and creatinine clearance increases following anesthesia with either anesthetic.

SKELETAL MUSCLE EFFECTS

Enflurane and isoflurane produce skeletal muscle relaxation that is about twofold greater than that associated with a comparable dose of halothane. Nitrous oxide does not relax skeletal muscles, and, in doses that exceed 1 MAC, it may produce skeletal muscle rigidity.

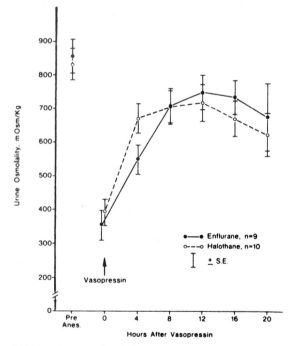

FIGURE 2-22. The ability to concentrate urine in response to administration of vasopressin remains unaltered following short-term administration of halothane (4.9 MAC hr) or enflurane (2.7 MAC hours). (From Cousins MJ, Greenstein LR, Hitt BA, Mazze RI. Metabolism and renal effects of enflurane in man. Anesthesiology 1976;44:44 – 53. Reproduced by permission of the authors and publisher.)

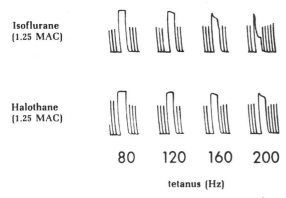

Isoflurane
(1.25 MAC)

Halothane
(1.25 MAC)

80   120   160   200

tetanus (Hz)

FIGURE 2-24. The thenar response to continuous (tetanus) stimulation at increasing frequency (Hz) is less likely to be sustained during administration of isoflurane compared with halothane. (From Miller RD, Eger EI, Way WL, Stevens WC, Dolan WM. Comparative neuromuscular effects of Forane and halothane alone and in combination with d-tubocurarine in man. Anesthesiology 1971;35:38–42. Reproduced by permission of the authors and publisher.)

The ability of skeletal muscles to sustain contractions in response to high-frequency (greater than 120 Hz) continuous stimulation is often impaired in the presence of 1.25 MAC enflurane or isoflurane, but not halothane or nitrous oxide (Fig. 2-24) (Miller *et al*, 1971). Increased doses of enflurane and isoflurane further impair the ability of skeletal muscles to sustain a contraction in response to high frequency stimulation.

Volatile anesthetics produce dose-dependent enhancement of the effects of neuromuscular blocking drugs with the effects of enflurane and isoflurane being similar and greater than halothane (see Chapter 8). Nitrous oxide does not significantly potentiate the effects of neuromuscular blocking drugs.

In vitro isoflurane and halothane produce similar potentiation of the effects of neuromuscular blocking drugs (Vitez *et al*, 1974). This discrepancy with *in vivo* observations cannot be entirely explained by differences in skeletal muscle blood flow associated with these two drugs. Another explanation may be that human skeletal muscle is more readily depressed *in vivo* by isoflurane than halothane, whereas these differences do not exist for skeletal muscles from animals used for *in vitro* experiments.

chamber) to produce skeletal muscle rigidity appear to be unique to this inhaled anesthetic (Hornbein *et al*, 1982). This effect is consistent with enhancement of skeletal muscle rigidity produced by opioids when low concentrations of nitrous oxide are administered.

Malignant Hyperthermia

Volatile anesthetics can trigger malignant hyperthermia, but enflurane and isoflurane are less potent in this regard than is halothane. Nitrous oxide compared with volatile anesthetics is a weak trigger for malignant hyperthermia. For example, augmentation of caffeine-induced contracture of frog sartorius muscle by nitrous oxide is 1.3 times, whereas that for isoflurane is 3 times, enflurane 4 times, and halothane 11 times (Reed and Strobel, 1978). Even considering its lower potency, nitrous oxide still exerts a lesser effect than volatile anesthetics.

OBSTETRIC EFFECTS

Volatile anesthetics produce similar and dose-dependent reductions in uterine smooth muscle contractility and blood flow (Fig. 2-25) (Eger,

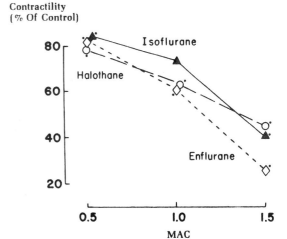

Contractility
(% Of Control)

80

Isoflurane

Halothane

60

40

Enflurane

20

0.5   1.0   1.5

MAC

FIGURE 2-25. Impact of volatile anesthetics on contractility of uterine smooth muscle strips studies *in vitro*. *P < 0.05. (From Eger EI. Isoflurane [Forane]. A compendium and reference. Madison, Wisconsin, Ohio

1984a; Munson and Embro, 1977; Palahniuk and Shnider, 1974). These changes are modest at 0.5 MAC (*e.g.,* analgesic concentrations) but become substantial at concentrations above 1 MAC. Nitrous oxide does not alter uterine contractility in doses used to provide analgesia during vaginal delivery.

Anesthetic-induced uterine relaxation may be desirable to facilitate removal of retained placenta. Conversely, uterine relaxation produced by volatile anesthetics may contribute to blood loss due to uterine atony. Indeed, blood loss during therapeutic abortion is greater in patients anesthetized with a volatile anesthetic compared with that in patients receiving a nitrous oxide – barbiturate – opioid anesthetic (Cullen *et al,* 1970; Dolan *et al,* 1972).

In animals, evidence of fetal distress does not accompany anesthetic-induced reductions in maternal uterine blood flow as long as the anesthetic concentration does not exceed 1.5 MAC (Biehl *et al,* 1983). Furthermore, volatile anesthetics at about 0.5 MAC concentrations combined with 50% nitrous oxide ensure amnesia during cesarean section and do not produce detectable effects on the newborn (Warren *et al,* 1983). Inhaled anesthetics rapidly cross the placenta to enter the fetus, but these drugs are likewise rapidly exhaled by the newborn infant. Nitrous oxide analgesia for vaginal delivery develops more rapidly than with volatile anesthetics, but, after about 10 minutes, all inhaled drugs provide comparable analgesia.

RESISTANCE TO INFECTION

Inhaled anesthetics, particularly nitrous oxide, produce dose-dependent inhibition of polymorphonuclear leukocytes and their subsequent migration (*i.e.,* chemotaxis) for phagocytosis, which is necessary for the inflammatory response to infection (Duncan and Cullen, 1976). Nevertheless, decreased resistance to bacterial infection owing to inhaled anesthetics seems unlikely, considering the duration and dose of these drugs that are administered. Furthermore, when leukocytes reach the site of infection, their ability to phagocytize bacteria appears to be normal.

Inhaled anesthetics do not have bacteriostatic effects at clinically useful concentrations. Conversely, the liquid volatile anesthetic may be bactericidal (Johnson and Eger, 1979). All volatile anesthetics (doses as low as 0.2 MAC) produce

dose-dependent inhibition of measles virus replication and reduce mortality in mice receiving intranasal influenza virus (Knight *et al,* 1983). This inhibition may reflect anesthetic-induced decreases in deoxyribonucleic acid (DNA) synthesis.

GENETIC EFFECTS

The Ames test, which identifies chemicals that act as mutagens and carcinogens, is negative for enflurane, isoflurane, and nitrous oxide, including their known metabolites (Baden *et al,* 1977; Waskell, 1978). Halothane also results in a negative Ames test, but potential metabolites may be positive (Sachder *et al,* 1980). In animals, inhaled anesthetics administered during vulnerable periods of gestation may act as teratogens, producing skeletal anomalies (Bussard *et al,* 1974; Lane *et al,* 1980; Pope and Persaud, 1978). Learning function may be impaired in newborn animals exposed *in utero* to inhaled anesthetics (Chalon *et al,* 1982; Mazze *et al,* 1984b).

The increased incidence of spontaneous abortions in operating room personnel may reflect a teratogenic effect from chronic exposure to trace concentrations of inhaled anesthetics, especially nitrous oxide (Cohen *et al,* 1971; Lane *et al,* 1980; Rosenberg and Kirves, 1973). Nitrous oxide irreversibly oxidizes the cobalt atom of vitamin B_{12} such that the activity of vitamin B_{12}-dependent enzymes (*e.g.,* methionine synthetase, thymidylate synthetase) is reduced. Indeed, in mice, inactivation of methionine synthetase is produced after administration of as little as 0.1% (*i.e.,* 1000 ppm) nitrous oxide for 4 hours (Fig. 2-26) (Koblin *et al,* 1981). Higher inhaled concentrations of nitrous oxide are associated with more rapid enzyme inhibition, as evidenced by a decrease in methionine synthetase activity of more than 50% within 30 minutes of exposure of animals to about 80% nitrous oxide. In contrast to animals, the onset of nitrous oxide-induced inhibition of vitamin B_{12}-dependent enzymes in humans may be slow. For example, patients inhaling 60% to 70% nitrous oxide for less than 4 hours do not manifest evidence of enzyme inhibition up to 2 hours postoperatively (Nunn *et al,* 1986). Conversely, exposure of patients to nitrous oxide for 8 hours is associated with reductions in the plasma concentration of methionine and abnormal thymidine synthesis (Amess *et al,* 1978; Skacel *et al,* 1983).

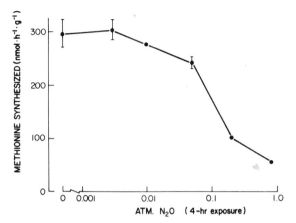

FIGURE 2-26. Nitrous oxide administered to mice for 4 hours irreversibly oxidizes the cobalt atom of vitamin B_{12} such that activity of vitamin B_{12}-dependent enzymes, including methionine synthetase, are reduced. (From Koblin DD, Watson JE, Deady JE, Stokstad ELR, Eger EI. Inactivation of methionine synthetase by nitrous oxide in mice. Anesthesiology 1981;54:318–24. Reproduced by permission of the authors and publisher.)

Volatile anesthetics do not alter activity of vitamin B_{12}-dependent enzymes.

Methionine synthetase converts homocysteine to methionine, which is necessary for formation of myelin. Thymidylate synthetase is important in the conversion of deoxyrubinine to thymidine and the subsequent formation of DNA. Interference with myelin formation and DNA synthesis could have significant effects on the rapidly growing fetus, manifesting as spontaneous abortions or congenital anomalies. Inhibition of these enzymes could also manifest as depression of bone marrow function and neurologic disturbances (see the sections entitled Bone Marrow Function and Peripheral Neuropathy). The speculated, but undocumented, role of trace concentrations of nitrous oxide in the production of spontaneous abortions has led to the use of scavenging systems designed to remove anesthetic gases, including nitrous oxide, from the operating room atmosphere. Nevertheless, animal studies using intermittent exposure to trace concentrations of nitrous oxide, halothane, enflurane, and isoflurane have not revealed harmful reproductive effects (Mazze, 1985). Conversely, exposure of pregnant rats to 75% nitrous oxide for 6 hours daily on 3 consecutive days is associated with increased

fetal resorptions (*i.e.,* abortions) (Mazze *et al,* 1986).

BONE MARROW FUNCTION

Human bone marrow appears to be particularly sensitive to nitrous oxide, with mild megaloblastic depression being detectable following administration of 50% nitrous oxide for 12 to 24 hours (Amess *et al,* 1978; O'Sullivan *et al,* 1981). These bone marrow effects occur as a result of nitrous oxide–induced interference with activity of vitamin B_{12}-dependent enzymes, which are necessary for synthesis of DNA and the subsequent formation of erythrocytes (see the section entitled Genetic Effects). Bone marrow activity recovers within 12 hours when nitrous oxide is withdrawn.

PERIPHERAL NEUROPATHY

Animals exposed to 15% nitrous oxide for up to 15 days develop ataxia and exhibit evidence of spinal cord and peripheral nerve degeneration. People who chronically inhale nitrous oxide for nonmedical purposes may develop a neuropathy characterized by a sensorimotor polyneuropathy that is often combined with signs of posterior and lateral spinal cord degeneration resembling pernicious anemia (Layzer *et al,* 1978). The speculated mechanism of this neuropathy is the ability of nitrous oxide to irreversibly oxidize the cobalt atom of vitamin B_{12} such that activity of vitamin B_{12}-dependent enzymes, including methionine synthetase, is reduced (see the section entitled Genetic Effects).

TOTAL BODY OXYGEN REQUIREMENTS

Total body oxygen requirements are reduced similar amounts by volatile anesthetics. Oxygen requirements of the heart decrease more than those of other organs, reflecting drug-induced reductions in cardiac work associated with declines in blood pressure and myocardial contractility. Theoretically, reduced oxygen requirements would protect tissues from ischemia that might result from decreased oxygen delivery associated with drug-induced reductions in perfusion pressure. Reductions in total body oxygen requirements probably reflect metabolic depressant ef-

Table 2-4
Metabolism of Inhaled Anesthetics

	Percent of Absorbed Anesthetic Recovered as Metabolites
Nitrous oxide	0.004%
Halothane	20%
Enflurane	2.4%
Isoflurane	0.17%

fects as well as reduced functional needs in the presence of anesthetic-produced depression of organ function.

METABOLISM

Inhaled anesthetics undergo varying degrees of metabolism in the liver, and, to a lesser extent, in the lungs, kidneys, and gastrointestinal tract (Table 2-4). The importance of this metabolism relates to the potential toxic effects of intermediary metabolites or end-metabolites on the kidneys, liver, and reproductive organs. Metabolism does not influence the rate of induction of anesthesia or the inhaled concentration of anesthetic necessary for maintenance of anesthesia, since the inhaled anesthetics are administered in great excess of the amount metabolized.

Determinants of Metabolism

The magnitude of metabolism of inhaled anesthetics is determined by (1) the chemical structure of the anesthetic, (2) hepatic enzyme activity, (3) blood concentration of the anesthetic, and (4) genetic factors. Overall, genetic factors appear to be the most important determinant of drug-metabolizing enzyme activity. In this regard, humans are active metabolizers of drugs compared with lower animal species such as the rat.

Chemical Structure

The ether bond and carbon halogen bond are the sites in the anesthetic molecule most susceptible to oxidative metabolism. Oxidation of the ether bond is less likely when hydrogen atoms on the carbons surrounding the oxygen atom of this bond are replaced with halogen atoms. Two halogen atoms on a terminal carbon represent the optimal arrangement for dehalogenation, whereas a terminal carbon with three fluorine atoms is very resistant to oxidative metabolism. The bond energy for carbon-fluorine is twice that for carbon-bromine or carbon-chlorine. The absence of ester bonds in inhaled anesthetics negates any role of metabolism by hydrolysis.

Hepatic Enzyme Activity

The activity of hepatic cytochrome P-450 enzymes responsible for metabolism of volatile anesthetics may be increased by a variety of drugs, including the anesthetics themselves. For example, volatile anesthetics may induce hepatic microsomal enzymes responsible for their own metabolism (Linde and Berman, 1971). Phenobarbital, phenytoin, and isoniazid may increase defluorination of volatile anesthetics, especially enflurane. Prolonged enflurane anesthesia in the absence of surgery and chronic exposure to trace concentrations of halothane increase hepatic microsomal enzyme activity.

There is evidence in patients that short (1 hour) surgical stimulation increases hepatic microsomal enzyme activity independent of the anesthetic drug (halothane or isoflurane) or technique (spinal) used (Loft *et al,* 1985). Conversely, surgery lasting longer than 4 hours can lead to depressed microsomal enzyme activity (Pessayre *et al,* 1978).

Blood Concentration

The fraction of anesthetic that undergoes metabolism on passing through the liver is influenced by the blood concentration of the anesthetic (Fig. 2-27) (Sawyer *et al,* 1971; White *et al,* 1979). For example, a 1 MAC concentration saturates hepatic enzymes and reduces the fraction of anesthetic that is removed (*e.g.,* metabolized) during a single passage through the liver. Conversely, subanesthetic concentrations (0.1 MAC or less) undergo extensive metabolism on passage through the liver.

Inhaled anesthetics that are not highly soluble in blood and tissues (nitrous oxide, enflurane, isoflurane) tend to be rapidly exhaled by the lungs at the conclusion of an anesthetic. As a result, less drug is available to continually pass through the liver at low blood concentrations conducive to metabolism. This is reflected in the magnitude of metabolism of these drugs (Table 2-4). Halothane

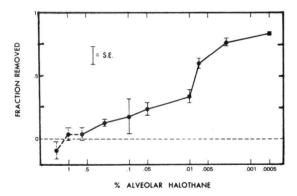

FIGURE 2-27. Fraction of halothane removed during passage through the liver at progressively decreasing alveolar concentrations. (From Sawyer DC, Eger EI, Bahlman SH, Cullen BF, Impelman D. Concentration dependence of hepatic halothane metabolism. Anesthesiology 1971;34:230–5. Reproduced by permission of the authors and publisher.)

and methoxyflurane are more soluble in blood and lipids and thus likely to be stored in tissues that act as a reservoir to maintain subanesthetic concentrations for prolonged periods of time following discontinuation of their administration.

Disease states such as cirrhosis of the liver or cardiac failure could theoretically alter metabolism by reducing hepatic blood flow and drug delivery or decreasing the amount of viable liver and thus enzyme activity. Obesity, for reasons that are not known, predictably increases defluorination of halothane and enflurane (Bentley *et al*, 1979; Young *et al*, 1975).

Nitrous Oxide

An estimated 0.004% of an absorbed dose of nitrous oxide undergoes reductive metabolism to nitrogen in the gastrointestinal tract (Hong *et al*, 1980a; Trudell, 1985). Anaerobic bacteria, such as pseudomonas, are responsible for this reductive metabolism. Reductive products of some nitrogen compounds include free radicals that could produce toxic effects on cells. The potential toxic role of these metabolites, however, remains undocumented.

Oxygen concentrations above 10% in the gastrointestinal tract and antibiotics inhibit metabolism of nitrous oxide by anaerobic bacteria. There is no evidence that nitrous oxide undergoes oxidative metabolism in the liver (Hong *et al*, 1980b).

Halothane

Halothane undergoes oxidative and, to a lesser extent, reductive metabolism, with about 20% of an absorbed dose appearing in the urine as metabolites (Rehder *et al*, 1967).

Oxidative Metabolism

The principal oxidative metabolite of halothane is trifluoroacetic acid, which has no known toxic effects. Chloride and bromide are also oxidative metabolites of halothane. The energy bond for carbon-fluorine is strong, accounting for the absence of detectable amounts of fluoride as oxidative metabolites of halothane.

It is estimated the plasma concentrations of bromide increase 0.5 mEq L^{-1} MAC hr^{-1} of halothane administration (Fig. 2-28) (Johnstone *et al*, 1975). Because signs of bromide toxicity such as somnolence and confusion do not occur until

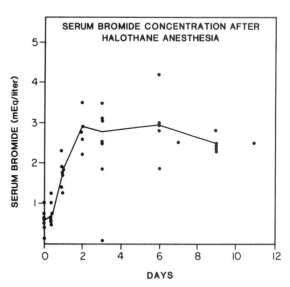

FIGURE 2-28. Serum bromide concentrations in volunteers following prolonged (about 7 hours) exposure to halothane (From Johnstone RE, Kennell EM, Behar MG, Brummund W, Ebersole RC, Shaw LM. Increased serum bromide concentration after halothane anesthesia in man. Anesthesiology 1975;42:598–60. Redrawn by permission of the authors and publisher.)

plasma concentrations of bromide exceed about 6 mEq L^{-1}, the likelihood of symptoms from metabolism of halothane seems remote. Nevertheless, prolonged halothane anesthesia may more likely be associated with intellectual impairment than a similar dose of an anesthetic that is not metabolized to bromide.

Reductive Metabolism

Reductive metabolism, which among the volatile anesthetics has only been documented to occur during breakdown of halothane, is most likely to occur in the presence of hepatocyte hypoxia and enzyme induction. Volatile reductive metabolites of halothane include 2-chloro-1, 1,1-trifluoroethane and 2-chloro-1, 1-difluoroethylene. The volatile metabolite, 2 bromo-2-chloro-1, 1-difluoroethylene is due to reaction of halothane with soda lime within the anesthetic circuit. Fluoride and bromide are also reductive metabolites of halothane.

Hepatotoxicity of halothane may reflect the ability of reductive metabolites to bind covalently with tissue macromolecules and initiate events that end in cell death (deGroot and Noll, 1983). In this regard, detection of an increased plasma concentration of fluoride following administration of halothane implies that reductive metabolism has occurred. Indeed, plasma fluoride concentrations correlate with hepatotoxicity in the hypoxic rat model for halothane hepatotoxicity. Nevertheless, increased plasma concentrations of fluoride following administration of halothane to morbidly obese patients is not associated with changes in liver transaminase enzymes (Nawaf and Stoelting, 1979). Furthermore, peak plasma concentrations of fluoride (about 10 μM L^{-1}) are far below the nephrotoxic concentration of about 50 μM L^{-1} (see the section entitled Renal Effects).

Deuterium substitution in the halothane molecule is less reactive than the carbon-halogen bond. In animals, deuterated halothane undergoes less oxidative metabolism, but activity by way of the reductive pathway is not altered since scisson of the carbon-halogen bond is not involved in this pathway (Sipes *et al*, 1981).

Enflurane

Enflurane undergoes oxidative metabolism with about 2.4% of an absorbed dose appearing in the urine as metabolites (Chase *et al*, 1971). This minimal metabolism of enflurane reflects its chemical stability and low solubility in tissues such that the drug is exhaled unchanged rather than repeatedly passing through the liver at low plasma concentrations conducive to metabolism.

The principal oxidative metabolites of enflurane are inorganic fluoride and organic fluoride compounds. Fluoride results from dehalogenation of the terminal carbon atom. Oxidation of the ether bond and release of additional fluoride does not occur, reflecting the chemical stability imparted to this bond by the surrounding halogens. As with isoflurane, the methyl portion of the molecule seems to be resistant to oxidation, and reductive metabolism does not occur (Burke *et al*, 1981).

Enzyme induction with phenobarbital or phenytoin increases the liberation of fluoride from enflurane *in vitro* but not *in vivo* (Mazze *et al*, 1982). This observation is most likely due to low tissue solubility of enflurane such that, *in vivo*, the availability of substrate (*e.g.*, enflurane) becomes the rate-limiting factor, whereas *in vitro*, the substrate concentration is controlled and the effect of enzyme induction manifests as increased metabolism of enflurane to fluoride (Greenstein *et al*, 1975). For these reasons, it seems unlikely that the nephrotoxic potential of enflurane would be increased by enzyme induction. An exception may be patients who are being treated with isoniazid, because this drug can increase defluorination of enflurane in genetically susceptible patients (*e.g.*, rapid acetylators) (see Chapter 28).

Isoflurane

Isoflurane undergoes oxidative metabolism with about 0.17% of an absorbed dose appearing in the urine as metabolites (Holaday *et al*, 1975). This minimal metabolism of isoflurane reflects its chemical stability and low solubility in tissues such that the drug is exhaled unchanged rather than repeatedly passing through the liver at low plasma concentrations conducive to metabolism. Chemical stability of isoflurane is ensured by the trifluorocarbon and the presence of halogen atoms on three sides of the ether bond.

Metabolism of isoflurane begins with oxidation of the carbon-halogen link of the alpha carbon atom, leading to an unstable compound that subsequently decomposes to difluoromethanol and trifluoroacetic acid. Difluoromethanol breaks down to formic acid and, in the process, releases two fluoride ions. Trifluoroacetic acid is the principal organic fluoride metabolite of isoflurane (Hitt *et al,* 1974). As with enflurane, the methyl portion of the molecule seems to be resistant to oxidation, and reductive metabolism does not occur (Burke *et al,* 1981). The minimal changes in plasma concentrations of fluoride resulting from metabolism of isoflurane (peak less than 5 μM L^{-1}) plus the absence of reductive metabolism render nephrotoxicity or hepatotoxicity following administration of isoflurane unlikely.

Enzyme induction with phenobarbital or phenytoin increases the liberation of fluoride from isoflurane *in vitro* but not *in vivo* (Mazze *et al,* 1982). Even in the presence of enzyme induction, however, the metabolism of isoflurane and resulting plasma concentrations of fluoride remain much less than with enflurane. Likewise, isoniazid, which dramatically increases metabolism of enflurane in susceptible patients, fails to significantly alter metabolism of isoflurane (see Chapter 28).

REFERENCES

Adams RW, Cucchiari RF, Gronert GA, Messick JM, Michenfelder JD. Isoflurane and cerebrospinal fluid pressure in neurosurgical patients. Anesthesiology 1981;54:97–9.

Albrecht RF, Miletich DJ, Madala LR. Normalization of cerebral blood flow during prolonged anesthesia. Anesthesiology 1983;58:26–31.

Amess JAL, Burman JF, Rees GM, Nancekievill DG, Mollin DL. Megaloblastic hemopoiesis in patients receiving nitrous oxide. Lancet 1978;2:339–41.

Artru AA. Anesthetics produce prolonged alterations of CSF dynamics. Anesthesiology 1982;57:A356.

Artru AA. Effects of halothane, enflurane, isoflurane and fentanyl on resistance to reabsorption of cerebrospinal fluid. Anesth Analg 1984a;63:180.

Artru AA. Isoflurane does not increase the rate of CSF production in the dog. Anesthesiology 1984b;60:193–7.

Atlee JL, Alexander SC. Halothane effects on conductivity of the AV node and His–Purkinje system in the dog. Anesth Analg 1977;56:378–86.

Baden JM, Kelley M, Wharton RS, Hitt BA, Simmon VF, Mazze RI. Mutagenicity of halogenated ether anesthetics. Anesthesiology 1977;46:346–50.

Baden JM, Kundomal YR, Luttropp ME, Maze M, Kosek JC. Effects of volatile anesthetics or fentanyl on hepatic function in cirrhotic rats. Anesth Analg 1985;64:1183–8.

Bahlman SH, Eger EI, Halsey MJ, *et al.* The cardiovascular effects of halothane in man during spontaneous ventilation. Anesthesiology 1972;36:494–502.

Bentley JB, Vaughn RW, Miller MS, Calkins JM, Gandolfi AJ. Serum inorganic fluoride levels in obese patients during and after enflurane anesthesia. Anesth Analg 1979;58:409–12.

Benumof JL, Bookstein JJ, Saidman LJ, Harris R. Diminished hepatic arterial flow during halothane administration. Anesthesiology 1976;45:545–51.

Biehl DR, Yarnell R, Wade JG, Sitar D. The uptake of isoflurane by the foetal lamb in utero: effect on regional blood flow. Can Anaesth Soc J 1983;30:581–6.

Blitt CD, Raessler KL, Wightman MA, Groves BM, Wall CL, Geha DG. Atrioventricular conduction in dogs during anesthesia with isoflurane. Anesthesiology 1979;50:210–2.

Burke TR, Branchflower RV, Lees DE, Pohl LR. Mechanism of defluorination of enflurane. Identification of an organic metabolite in rat and man. Drug Metab Dispos 1981;9:19–24.

Bussard DA, Stoelting RK, Peterson C, Ishaq M. Fetal changes in hamsters anesthetized with nitrous oxide and halothane. Anesthesiology 1974;41:275–8.

Cahalan MK, Lurz FW, Beaupre PM, Schwartz LA, Eger EI. Narcotics alter the heart rate and blood pressure response to inhalational anesthetics. Anesthesiology 1983;59:A26.

Calverley RK, Smith NT, Jones CW, Prys-Roberts C, Eger EI. Ventilatory and cardiovascular effects of enflurane anesthesia during spontaneous ventilation in man. Anesth Analg 1978a;57:610–8.

Calverley RK, Smith NT, Prys-Roberts C, Eger EI, Jones CW. Cardiovascular effects of enflurane anesthesia during controlled ventilation in man. Anesth Analg 1978b;57:619–28.

Chalon J, Ramanathan S, Turndorf H. Exposure to isoflurane affects learning function of murine progeny. Anesthesiology 1982;57:A360.

Chase RE, Holaday DA, Fiserova-Bergerova V, Saidman LJ, Mack FE. The biotransformation of Ethrane in man. Anesthesiology 1971;35:262–7.

Cohen EN, Bellville JW, Brown BW. Anesthesia, pregnancy and miscarriage: A study of operating room nurses and anesthetists. Anesthesiology 1971;35:343–7.

Cooperman LH. Effects of anaesthetics on the splanchnic circulation. Br J Anaesth 1972;44:967–70.

Cousins MJ, Greenstein LR, Hitt BA, Mazze RI. Metabolism and renal effects of enflurane in man. Anesthesiology 1976;44:44–53.

Cromwell TH, Stevens WC, Eger EI, et al. The cardiovascular effects of compound 469 (Forane) during spontaneous ventilation and CO$_2$ challenge in man. Anesthesiology 1971;35:17–25.

Cronnelly R, Salvatierra O, Feduska NJ. Renal allograft

function following halothane, enflurane, or isoflurane anesthesia. Anesth Analg 1984;63:202.

Cullen DJ, Eger EI. The effects of halothane on respiratory and cardiovascular responses to hypoxia in dogs: A dose response study. Anesthesiology 1970;33:487–96

Cullen BF, Margolis AJ, Eger EI. The effects of anesthesia and pulmonary ventilation on blood loss during elective therapeutic abortion. Anesthesiology 1970;32:108–13.

deGroot H, Noll T. Halothane hepatotoxicity: relation between metabolic activation, hypoxia, covalent binding, lipid peroxidation, and liver cell damage. Hepatology 1983;3:601–6.

Dolan WM, Eger EI, Margolis AJ. Forane increases bleeding in therapeutic suction abortion. Anesthesiology 1972;36:96–7.

Dolan WM, Stevens WC, Eger EI, *et al*. The cardiovascular and respiratory effects of isoflurane-nitrous oxide anesthesia. Can Anaesth Soc J 1974;21:557–68.

Drummond JC, Todd MM, Shapiro HM. CO_2 responsiveness of the cerebral circulation during isoflurane anesthesia and N_2O sedation in cats. Anesthesiology 1982;57:A333.

Duncan PG, Cullen BF. Anesthesia and immunology. Anesthesiology 1976;45:222-38.

Eger EI. Isoflurane (Forane). A compendium and reference. Madison, Wisconsin, Ohio Medical Products, 1984a:1–110.

Eger EI. Pharmacology of isoflurane. Br J Anaesth 1984b;56:71S–99S.

Eger EI. Nitrous Oxide. New York: Elsevier, 1985a.

Eger EI. Respiratory effects of nitrous oxide. In: Eger EI, ed. Nitrous oxide, New York: Elsevier, 1985b:109.

Eger EI, Calverley RK, Smith NT. Changes in blood chemistries following prolonged enflurane anesthesia. Anesth Analg 1976;55:547–9.

Eger EI, Smith NT, Stoelting RK, Cullen DJ, Kadis LB, Whitcher CE. Cardiovascular effects of halothane in man. Anesthesiology 1970;32:396–409.

Eger EI, Smuckler EA, Ferrell LD, Goldsmith CH, Johnson BH. Is enflurane hepatotoxic? Anesth Analg 1986;65:21–30.

Eger EI, Stevens WC, Cromwell TH. The electroencephalogram in man anesthetized with Forane. Anesthesiology 1971;35:504–8.

Eintrei C, Leszniewski W, Carlsson C. Local application of ^{133}Xenon for measurement of regional cerebral blood flow (rCBF) during halothane, enflurane, and isoflurane anesthesia in humans. Anesthesiology 1985;63:391–4.

Eisele JH, Milstein JM, Goetzman BW. Pulmonary vascular responses to nitrous oxide in newborn lambs. Anesth Analg 1986;65:62–4.

Eisele JH, Smith NT. Cardiovascular effects of 40 percent nitrous oxide in man. Anesth Analg 1972;51:956–63.

Epstein RM, Deutsch S, Cooperman LH, Clement AJ, Price HL. Splanchnic circulation during halothane anesthesia and hypercapnia in normal man. Anesthesiology 1966;27:654–61.

Farrell G, Prendergast D, Murray M. Halothane hepatitis: Detection of a constitutional susceptibility factor. N Engl J Med 1985;313:1310–4.

Fassoulaki A, Eger EI, Johnson BH, *et al*. Nitrous oxide, too, is hepatotoxic in rats. Anesth Analg 1984;63:1076–80.

Flaim SF, Zelis R, Eisele JH. Differential effects of morphine on forearm blood flow: Attenuation of sympathetic control of the cutaneous circulation. Clin Pharmacol Ther 1978;23:542–6.

Fourcade HE, Stevens WC, Larson CP. The ventilatory effects of Forane, a new inhaled anesthetic. Anesthesiology 1971;35:26–31.

France CJ, Plumer MH, Eger EI, Wahrenbrock EA. Ventilatory effects of isoflurane (Forane) or halothane when combined with morphine, nitrous oxide and surgery. Br J Anaesth 1974;46:117–20.

Frankhuizen JL, Vlek CAJ, Burm AGL, Rejger V. Failure to replicate negative effects of trace anesthetics on mental performance. Br J Anaesth 1978;50:229–34.

Fukunaga AF, Epstein RM. Sympathetic excitation during nitrous oxide–halothane anesthesia in the cat. Anesthesiology 1973;39:23–36.

Garfield JM, Garfield FB, Sampson J. Effects of nitrous oxide on decision-strategy and sustained attention. Psychopharmacologia 1975;42:5–10.

Gelman S, Fowler KC, Smith LR. Regional blood flow during isoflurane and halothane anesthesia. Anesth Analg 1984a;63:557–65.

Gelman S, Fowler KC, Smith LR. Liver circulation and function during isoflurane and halothane anesthesia. Anesthesiology 1984b;61:726–30.

Gold MI, Schwam SJ, Goldberg M. Chronic obstructive pulmonary disease and respiratory complications. Anesth Analg 1983;62:975–81.

Gourlay GK, Adams JF, Cousins MJ, Hall P. Genetic differences in reductive metabolism and hepatotoxicity of halothane in three rat strains. Anesthesiology 1981;55:96–103.

Greenstein LR, Hitt BA, Mazze RI. Metabolism *in vitro* of enflurane, isoflurane, and methoxyflurane. Anesthesiology 1975;42:420–4.

Hilgenberg JC, McCammon RL, Stoelting RK. Pulmonary and systemic vascular responses to nitrous oxide in patients with mitral stenosis and pulmonary hypertension. Anesth Analg 1980;59:323–6.

Hirshman CA, Edelstein G, Peetz S, Wayne R, Downes H. Mechanism of action of inhalational anesthesia on airways. Anesthesiology 1982;56:107–11.

Hitt B, Mazze RI, Cousins MJ, Edmunds HN, Barr GA, Trudell JR. Metabolism of isoflurane in Fischer 344 rats and man. Anesthesiology 1974;40:62–7.

Holaday DA, Fiserova-Bergerova V, Latto IP, Zumbiel

MA. Resistance of isoflurane to biotransformation in man. Anesthesiology 1975;43:325–32.

Holaday DA, Smith FR. Clinical charcteristics and biotransformation of sevoflurane in healthy human volunteers. Anesthesiology 1981;54:100–6.

Hong K, Trudell JR, O'Neil JR, Cohen EN. Metabolism of nitrous oxide by human and rat intestinal contents. Anesthesiology 1980a;52:16–9.

Hong K, Trudell JR, O'Neil JR, Cohen EN. Biotransformation of nitrous oxide. Anesthesiology 1980b;53:354–55.

Hornbein TF, Eger EI, Winter PM, Smith C, Wetstone D, Smith KH. The minimum alveolar concentration of nitrous oxide in man. Anesth Analg 1982;61:553–6.

Horrigan RW, Eger EI, Wilson EI, Wilson C. Epinephrine-induced arrhythmias during enflurane anesthesia in man—a non-linear dose-response relationship and dose-dependent protection from lidocaine. Anesth Analg 1978;57:547–50.

Johnson BH, Eger EI. Bactericidal effects of anesthetics. Anesth Analg 1979;58:136–8.

Johnston RR, Cromwell TH, Eger EI, Cullen D, Stevens WC, Joas T. The toxicity of fluroxene in animals and man. Anesthesiology 1973;38:313–9.

Johnston RR, Eger EI, Wilson C. A comparative interaction of epinephrine with enflurane, isoflurane and halothane in man. Anesth Analg 1976;55:709–12.

Johnstone RE, Kennell EM, Behar MG, Brummund W, Ebersole RC, Shaw LM. Increased serum bromide concentration after halothane anesthesia in man. Anesthesiology 1975;42:598–601.

Karl HW, Swedlow DB, Lee KW, Downes JJ. Epinephrine–halothane interactions in children. Anesthesiology 1983;58:142–5.

Kemmotsu O, Hashimoto Y, Shimosato S. Inotropic effects of isoflurane on mechanics of contraction in isolated cat papillary muscles from normal and failing hearts. Anesthesiology 1973;39:470–7.

Knight PR, Bedows E, Nahrwold ML, Maassab HF, Smitka CW, Busch MT. Alterations in influenza virus pulmonary pathology induced by diethyl ether, halothane, enflurane and pentobarbital in mice. Anesthesiology 1983;58:209–15.

Knill RL, Clement JL. Variable effects of anaesthetics on the ventilatory response to hypoxaemia in man. Can Anaesth Soc J 1982;29:93–9.

Knill RL, Manninen PH, Clement JL. Ventilation and chemoreflexes during enflurane sedation and anaesthesia in man. Can Anaesth Soc J 1979;26:353–60.

Koblin DD, Eger EI, Johnson BH, Collins P, Terrell RC, Spears L. Are convulsant gases also anesthetics? Anesthesiology 1980;53:S47.

Koblin DD, Watson JE, Deady JE, Stokstad ELR, Eger EI. Inactivation of methionine synthetase by nitrous oxide in mice. Anesthesiology 1981;54:318–24.

Kotrly KJ, Ebert TJ, Vucins E, Igler FO, Barney JA, Kam-

pine JP. Baroreceptor reflex control of heart rate during isoflurane anesthesia in humans. Anesthesiology 1984;60:173–9.

Lam AM, Clement JL, Chung DC, Knill RL. Respiratory effects of nitrous oxide during enflurane anesthesia in humans. Anesthesiology 1982;56:298–303.

Lane GA, Nahrwold ML, Tait AR. Anesthetics as teratogens: nitrous oxide is fetotoxic, xenon is not. Science 1980;210;899–901.

Lappas DG, Buckley MJ, Laver MB, Daggett WM, Lowenstein E. Left ventricular performance and pulmonary circulation following addition of nitrous oxide to morphine during coronary-artery surgery. Anesthesiology 1975;43:61–9.

Layzer RB, Fishman RA, Schafer JA. Neuropathy following abuse of nitrous oxide. Neurology 1978;28:504–6.

Linde HW, Berman ML. Nonspecific stimulation of drug-metabolizing enzymes by inhalation anesthetic agents. Anesth Analg 1971;50:656–65.

Linde HW, Oh SO, Homi J, Joshi C. Cardiovascular effects of isoflurane and halothane during controlled ventilation in older patients. Anesth Analg 1975;54:701–4.

Loarie DJ, Wilkinson P, Tyberg J, White A. The hemodynamic effects of halothane in anemic dogs. Anesth Analg 1979;58:195–200.

Loft S, Boel J, Kyst A, Rasmussen B, Hansen SH, Dossing M. Increased hepatic microsomal enzyme activity after surgery under halothane or spinal anesthesia. Anesthesiology 1985;62:11–6.

Lynch C, Vogel S, Sperelakis N. Halothane depression of myocardial slow action potentials. Anesthesiology 1981;55:360–8.

Mallow JE, White RD, Cucchiara RF, Tarhan S. Hemodynamic effects of isoflurane and halothane in patients with coronary artery disease. Anesth Analg 1976;55:135–8.

Maze M, Hayward E, Gaba DM. Alpha-adrenergic blockade raises epinephrine-arrhythmia threshold in halothane-anesthetized dogs in a dose-dependent fashion. Anesthesiology 1985;63:611–5.

Maze M, Smith CM. Identification of receptor mechanism mediating epinephrine-induced arrhythmias during halothane anesthesia in the dog. Anesthesiology 1983;59:322–6.

Mazze RI. RI. Fertility, reproduction, and postnatal survival in mice chronically exposed to isoflurane. Anesthesiology 1985;63:663–7.

Mazze RI, Calverley RK, Smith NT. Inorganic fluoride nephrotoxicity: Prolonged enflurane and halothane anesthesia in volunteers. Anesthesiology 1977;46:265–71.

Mazze RI, Cousins MJ, Barr GA. Renal effects and metabolism of isoflurane in man. Anesthesiology 1974;40:536–40.

Mazze RI, Fujinaga M, Rice SA, Harris SB, Baden JM. Reproductive and teratogenic effects of nitrous oxide, halothane, isoflurane and enflurane in Sprague–Dawley rats. Anesthesiology 1986; 64:339–44.

Mazze RI, Sievenpiper TS, Stevenson J. Renal effects of isoflurane in patients with abnormal renal function. Anesthesiology 1984a;60:161–3.

Mazze RI, Wilson AI, Rice SA, Baden JM. Effects of isoflurane on reproduction and fetal development in mice. Anesth Analg 1984b;63:249.

Mazze RI, Woodruff RE, Heerdt MD. Isoniazid-induced enflurane defluorination in humans. Anesthesiology 1982;57:5–8.

McDermott RW, Stanley TH. The cardiovascular effects of low concentrations of nitrous oxide during morphine anesthesia. Anesthesiology 1974;41:89–91.

McPherson RW, Mahla M, Johnson R, Traystman RJ. Effects of enflurane, isoflurane, and nitrous oxide on somatosensory evoked potentials during fentanyl anesthesia. Anesthesiology 1985;62:626–33.

Merin RG, Basch S. Are the myocardial function and metabolic effects of isoflurane really different from those of halothane and enflurane? Anesthesiology 1981;55:398–408.

Metz S, Maze M. Halothane concentration does not alter the threshold for epinephrine-induced arrhythmias in dogs. Anesthesiology 1985;62:470–4.

Miller RD, Eger EI, Way WL, Stevens WC, Dolan WM. Comparative neuromuscular effects of Forane and halothane alone and in combination with d-tubocurarine in man. Anesthesiology 1971;35:38–42.

Moffitt EA, Barker RA, Glenn JJ, et al. Myocardial metabolism and hemodynamic responses with isoflurane anesthesia for coronary artery surgery. Anesth Analg 1984;63:252.

Munson ES, Embro WJ. Enflurane, isoflurane and halothane and isolated human uterine muscle. Anesthesiology 1977;46:11–4.

Naito H, Gillis CN. Effects of halothane and nitrous oxide on removal of norepinephrine from the pulmonary circulation. Anesthesiology 1973;39:575–80.

Nawaf K, Stoelting RK. SGOT values following evidence of reductive biotransformation of halothane in man. Anesthesiology 1979;51:185–6.

Neigh JL, Garman JK, Harp JR. The electroencephalographic pattern during anesthesia with Ethrane: effects of depth of anesthesia, $PaCO_2$ and nitrous oxide. Anesthesiology 1971;35:482–7.

Newberg LA, Michenfelder JD. Cerebral protection by isoflurane during hypoxemia or ischemia. Anesthesiology 1983;59:29–35.

Newberg LA, Milde JH, Michenfelder JD. The cerebral metabolic effects of isoflurane at and above concentrations that suppress cortical electrical activity. Anesthesiology 1983;59:23–8.

Newman B, Gelb AW, Lam AM. The effect of isoflurane-induced hypotension on cerebral blood flow and cerebral metabolic rate for oxygen in humans. Anesthesiology 1986;64:307–10.

Nunn JF, Sharer NM, Bottiglieri T, Rossiter J. Effect of short-term administration of nitrous oxide on plasma concentrations of methionine, tryptophan, plenylalanine and S-adenosyl methionine in man. Br J Anesth 1986;58:1–10.

Oshima E, Urabe N, Shingu K, Mori K. Anticonvulsant actions of enflurane on epilepsy models in cats. Anesthesiology 1985;63:29–40.

O'Sullivan H, Jennings F, Ward K, McCann S, Scott JM, Weir DG. Human bone marrow biochemical function and megaloblastic hematopoiesis after nitrous oxide anesthesia. Anesthesiology 1981;55:645–9.

Palahniuk RJ, Shnider SM. Maternal and fetal cardiovascular and acid base changes during halothane and isoflurane anesthesia in the pregnant ewe. Anesthesiology 1974;41:462–72.

Pessayre D, Allemand H, Benoist C, Afifi F, Francois M, Henhamon JP. Effect of surgery under general anesthesia on antipyrine metabolism. Br J Clin Pharmacol 1978;6:505–13.

Peterson DO, Drummond JC, Todd MM. Effects of halothane, enflurane, isoflurane, and nitrous oxide on somatosensory evoked potentials in humans. Anesthesiology 1986;65:35–40.

Philbin DM, Lowenstein E. Lack of beta-adrenergic activity of isoflurane in the dog: a comparison of circulatory effects of halothane and isoflurane after propranolol administration. Br J Anaesth 1976;48:1165–70.

Pietak S, Weenig CS, Hickey RF, Fairley HB. Anesthetic effects of ventilation in patients with chronic obstructive pulmonary disease. Anesthesiology 1975;42:160–6.

Pope WDB, Persaud TVN. Foetal growth retardation in the rat following chronic exposure to the inhalation anaesthetic enflurane. Experientia 1978;34:1332–3.

Price HL, Skovsted P, Pauca AW, Cooperman L. Evidence for B-receptor activation produced by halothane in normal man. Anesthesiology 1970;32:389–95.

Ravin MB, Olsen MB. Apneic thresholds in anesthetized subjects with chronic obstructive pulmonary disease. Anesthesiology 1972;37:450–4.

Reed SB, Strobel GE. An *in vitro* model of malignant hyperthermia: Differential effects of inhalation anesthetics on caffeine-induced muscle contractures. Anesthesiology 1978;48:254–9.

Rehder K, Forbes J, Alter H, Hessler O, Stier A. Halothane biotransformation in man: A quantitative study. Anesthesiology 1967;28:711–5.

Reilly CS, Wood AJJ, Koshakji RP, Wood M. The effect of halothane on drug disposition in intrinsic drug metabolizing capacity and hepatic blood flow. Anesthesiology 1985;63:70–6.

Reiz S. Nitrous oxide augments the systemic and coronary haemodynamic effects of isoflurane in patients with ischaemic heart disease. Acta Anaesthesiol Scand 1983;27:464–9.

Reiz S, Balfors E, Sorensen MD, Ariola S, Friedman A, Truedsson H. Isoflurane — a powerful coronary vasodilator in patients with ischemic heart disease. Anesthesiology 1983;59:91–7.

Reiz S, Ostman M. Regional coronary hemodynamics during isoflurane–nitrous oxide anesthesia in patients with ischemic heart disease. Anesth Analg 1985;64:570–6.

Rosenberg P, Kirves A. Miscarriages among operating theatre staff. Acta Anesthesiol Scand 1973;53:37–42.

Ross JAS, Monk SJ, Duffy SW. Effect of nitrous oxide on halothane-induced hepatotoxicity in hypoxic, enzyme-induced rats. Br J Anaesth 1984;56:527–33.

Rydvall A, Haggmark S, Nyhman H, Reiz S. Effects of enflurane on coronary haemodynamics in patients with ischaemic heart disease. Acta Anaesthesiol Scand 1984;28:690–5.

Sachder K, Cohen EN, Simmou VF. Genotoxic and mutagenic assays of halothane metabolites in *Bacillus subtilis* and *Salmonella typhimurium*. Anesthesiology 1980;53:31–9.

Sawyer DC, Eger EI, Bahlman SH, Cullen BF, Impelman D. Concentration dependence of hepatic halothane metabolism. Anesthesiology 1971;34:230–5.

Schulte-Sasse U, Hess W, Tarnow J. Pulmonary vascular responses to nitrous oxide in patients with normal and high pulmonary vascular resistance. Anesthesiology 1982;57:9–13.

Shimosato S, Yasuda I, Kemmotsu O, Shanks C, Gamble C. Effect of halothane on altered contractility of isolated heart muscle obtained from cats with experimentally produced ventricular hypertrophy and failure. Br J Anaesth 1973;45:2–9.

Shingu K, Eger EI, Johnson BH. Hypoxia per se can produce hepatic damage without death in rats. Anesth Analg 1982;61:820–3.

Shingu K, Eger EI, Johnson BH, *et al.* Hepatic injury induced by anesthetic agents in rats. Anesth Analg 1983a;62:140–5.

Shingu K, Eger EI, Johnson BH, VanDyke RA, Lurz FW, Cheng A. Effect of oxygen concentration, hyperthermia, and choice of vendor on anesthetic-induced hepatic injury in rats. Anesth Analg 1983b;62:146–50.

Sipes IG, Gandolfi AJ, Pohl LR, Krishna G, Brown BR. Comparison of the biotransformation and hepatotoxicity of halothane and deuterated halothane. J Pharmacol Exp Ther 1980;214:716–20.

Sivarajan M, Bashein G. Effect of halothane on coronary collateral circulation. Anesthesiology 1985;62:588–96.

Skacel PO, Hewlett AM, Lewis JD, Lumb M, Nunn JF, Chanarin I. Studies on the haemopoietic toxicity of nitrous oxide in man. Br J Haematol 1983;53:189–94.

Skovsted P, Sapthavichaikul S. The effects of isoflurane on arterial pressure, pulse rate, autonomic nervous system activity and barostatic reflexes. Can Anaesth Soc J 1977;24:304–14.

Smith NT, Calverley RK, Prys-Roberts C, Eger EI, Jones CW. Impact of nitrous oxide on the circulation during enflurane anesthesia in man. Anesthesiology 1978;48:345–9.

Smith NT, Eger EI, Stoelting RK, Whayne TF, Cullen D, Kadis LB. The cardiovascular and sympathomimetic responses to the addition of nitrous oxide to halothane in man. Anesthesiology 1970;32:410–21.

Smith RA, Winter PM, Smith M, Eger EI. Convulsions in mice after anesthesia. Anesthesiology 1979;50:501–4.

Sprague DH, Yang JC, Ngai SH. Effects of isoflurane and halothane on contractility and the cyclic 3′,5′-adenosine monophosphate system in the rat aorta. Anesthesiology 1974;40:162–7.

Stevens WC, Cromwell TH, Halsey MJ, Eger EI, Shakespeare TF, Bahlman SH. The cardiovascular effects of a new inhalation anesthetic, Forane, in human volunteers at constant arterial carbon dioxide tension. Anesthesiology 1971;35:8–16.

Stevens WC, Eger EI, Joas TA, Cromwell TH, White A. Dolan WM. Comparative toxicity of isoflurane, halothane, fluroxene and diethyl ether in human volunteers. Can Anaesth Soc J 1973;20:357–68.

Stoelting RK. Plasma lidocaine concentrations following subcutaneous or submucosal epinephrine–lidocaine injection. Anesth Analg 1978;57:724–6.

Stoelting RK, Blitt CD, Cohen PJ, Merin RG. Hepatic dysfunction after isoflurane anesthesia. Anesth Analg (in press).

Stoelting RK, Gibbs PS. Hemodynamic effects of morphine and morphine–nitrous oxide in valvular heart disease and coronary-artery disease. Anesthesiology 1973;38:45–52.

Summary of the National Halothane Study: Possible association between halothane anesthesia and postoperative hepatic necrosis. JAMA 1977;197:775–88.

Tarnow J, Markschies-Hornung A, Schulte-Sasse U. Isoflurane improves the tolerance to pacing-induced myocardial ischemia. Anesthesiology 1986;64:147–56.

Theye RA, Michenfelder JD. The effect of halothane on canine cerebral metabolism. Anesthesiology 1968;29:1113–8.

Tinker JH, Sharbrough FW, Michenfelder JD: Anterior shift of the dominant EEG rhythm during anesthesia in the Java monkey: correlation with anesthetic potency. Anesthesiology 1977;46:252–9.

Todd MM, Drummond JC. A comparison of the cerebro-vascular and metabolic effects of halothane and iso-flurane in the cat. Anesthesiology 1984;60:276–82.

Trudell JR. Metabolism of nitrous oxide. In Eger EI, ed. Nitrous Oxide. New York, Elsevier, 1985;203.

Tusiewicz K, Bryan AC, Froese AB. Contributions of changing rib cage – diaphragm interactions to the ventilatory depression of halothane anesthesia. Anesthesiology 1977;47:327–37.

Tverskoy M, Gelman S, Fowler KC, Bradley EL. Intes-tinal circulation during inhalation anesthesia. Anesthesiology 1985;62:462–71.

Ueda W, Hirakawa M, Mae O. Appraisal of epinephrine administration to patients under halothane anes-thesia for closure of cleft palate. Anesthesiology 1983;58:574–6.

Van Dyke RA. Effect of fasting on anesthetic-associated liver toxicity. Anesthesiology 1981;55:A181.

Vergani D, Vergani G, Alberti A, *et al.* Antibodies to the surface of halothane altered rabbit hepatocytes in patients with severe halothane-associated hepatitis. N Engl J Med 1980;303:66–71.

Vitez TS, Miller RD, Eger EI, VanNyhuis LS, Way WL. Comparison *in vitro* of isoflurane and halothane potentiation of d-tubocurarine and succinylcholine neuromuscular blockades. Anesthesiology 1974; 41:53–6.

Warner DS, Boarini DJ, Kassell NF. Cerebrovascular ad-aptation to prolonged halothane anesthesia is not related to cerebrovascular fluid pH. Anesthesiology 1985;63:243–8.

Warren TM, Datta S, Ostheimer GW, Naulty JS, Weiss JB, Morrison JA. Comparison of the maternal and neo-natal effects of halothane, enflurane and isoflurane for cesarean delivery. Anesth Analg. 1983;62:516–20.

Waskell L. A study of the mutagenicity of anesthetics and their metabolites. Mutat Res 1978;57:141–53.

White AE, Stevens WC, Eger EI, Mazze RI, Hitt BA. En-flurane and methoxyflurane metabolism at anes-thetic and subanesthetic concentrations. Anesth Analg 1979;58:221–4.

Wolfson B, Hetrick WD, Lake CL, Siker ES. Anesthetic indices — further data. Anesthesiology 1978; 48:187–90.

Yacoub O, Doell D, Kryger MH, Anthonisen NR. De-pression of hypoxic ventilatory response by nitrous oxide. Anesthesiology 1976;45:385–9.

Young SR, Stoelting RK, Peterson C, Madura JA. Anes-thetic biotransformation and renal function in obese patients during and after methoxyflurane or halothane anesthesia. Anesthesiology 1975; 42:451–7.

CHAPTER 3

Opioid Agonists and Antagonists

INTRODUCTION

The word *opium* is derived from the Greek word for juice; the juice of the poppy is the source of 20 distinct alkaloids of opium. *Opiate* is the term used to designate drugs derived from opium. Morphine was isolated in 1803, followed by codeine in 1832 and papaverine in 1848. Morphine can be synthesized, but it is more easily derived from opium. The term *narcotic* is derived from the Greek word for stupor and traditionally has been used to refer to potent morphine-like analgesics with the potential to produce physical dependence. The development of synthetic drugs with morphine-like properties has led to use of the term *opioid* to refer to all exogenous substances, natural and synthetic, that bind specifically to any of several subpopulations of opioid receptors and produce at least some agonist (*i.e.,* morphine-like) effects. A convenient classification of opioids includes opioid agonists, opioid agonist–antagonists, and opioid antagonists (Table 3-1)

STRUCTURE ACTIVITY RELATIONSHIPS

The alkaloids in opium can be divided into two distinct chemical classes: phenanthrenes and benzylisoquinolines. The principal phenanthrene alkaloids present in opium are morphine, codeine, and thebaine (Fig. 3-1). The principal benzylisoquinoline alkaloids present in opium, which lack opioid activity, are papaverine and noscapine (Fig. 3-2).

The three rings of the phenanthrene nucleus are composed of 14 carbon atoms (Fig. 3-1). The fourth piperidine ring includes a tertiary amine nitrogen and is present in most opioid agonists. At pH 7.4, the tertiary amine nitrogen is highly ionized, making the molecule water soluble. A close relationship exists between stereochemical structure and potency of opioids, with levorotatory isomers often being the most active (Beckett and Casey, 1954).

Semisynthetic Opioids

Semisynthetic opioids result from relatively simple modification of the morphine molecule (Fig. 3-1). For example, substitution of a methyl for the hydroxyl group on carbon 3 results in codeine (methylmorphine). Substitution of acetyl groups on carbons 3 and 6 (*e.g.,* diacetylmorphine) is heroin. Thebaine has insignificant analgesic activity but serves as the precursor for etorphine (analgesc potency more than 1000 times morphine) and the opioid antagonist naloxone.

Synthetic Opioids

Synthetic opioids contain the phenanthrene nucleus of morphine but are manufactured by synthesis rather than chemical modification of morphine. Morphinan derivatives (levorphanol), methadone derivatives, benzomorphan derivatives (pentazocine), and phenylpiperidine derivatives (meperidine, fentanyl) are examples of groups of synthetic opioids. There are similarities in the molecular weight (236–336) and *p*Ka (7.7–8.5) between amide local anesthetics and phenylpiperidine derivatives (Cousins and Mather, 1984).

Table 3-1
Classification of Opioid Agonists and Antagonists

Opioid Agonists	Opioid Agonists–Antagonists
Morphine	
Meperidine	Pentazocine
Fentanyl	Butorphanol
Sufentanil	Nalbuphine
Alfentanil	Buprenorphine
Phenoperidine	Nalorphine
Codeine	Bremazocine
Dextromethorphan	Dezocine
Hydromorphone	**Opioid Antagonists**
Oxymorphone	Naloxone
Methadone	Naltrexone
Heroin	

MECHANISM OF ACTION

Opioids act as agonists at stereospecific opioid receptors in the central nervous system and other tissues (see the section entitled Opioid Receptors) (Goldstein, 1974; Leysen *et al*, 1977; Snyder, 1977). The same opioid receptors normally are activated by endogenous ligands known as *endorphins* (see the section entitled Endorphins). Only levorotatory forms of the opioid exhibit agonist activity. The affinity of most opioid agonists for receptors correlates well with their analgesic potency. It is assumed that increasing opioid receptor occupancy parallels opioid effects.

Existence of the opioid in the ionized state appears to be necessary for strong binding at the anionic opioid receptor site. Binding of an exogenous opioid agonist or endogenous ligand produces inhibition of adenylate cyclase activity (Simon and Hiller, 1978). In addition, opioids may interfere with transmembrane transport of calcium ions and act presynaptically to interfere with the release of other neurotransmitters, including acetylcholine, dopamine, norepinephrine, and substance P (Beaumont and Hughes, 1979; Snyder, 1977). Depression of cholinergic transmission in the central nervous system by virtue of opioid-induced inhibition of release of ace-

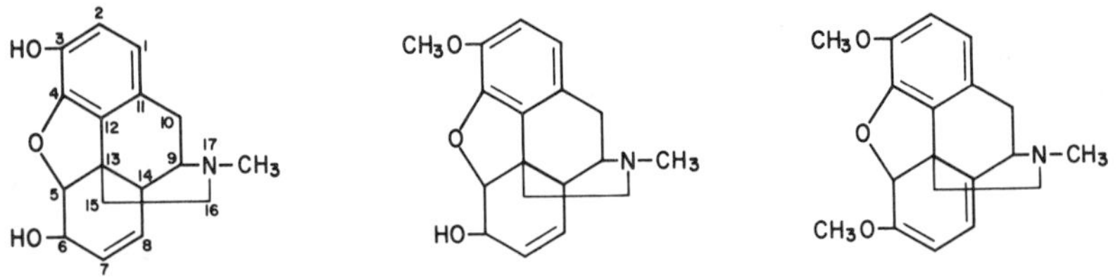

FIGURE 3-1. Phenanthrene alkaloids.

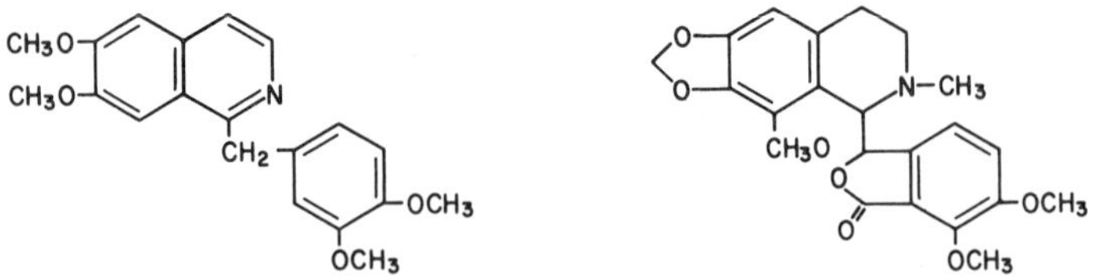

Morphine

Codeine

Thebaine

FIGURE 3-2. Benzylisoquinoline alkaloids.

Papaverine

Noscapine

tylcholine from nerve endings may play a prominent role in the analgesic and other side-effects of opioid agonists. Opioids do not alter responsiveness of afferent nerve endings to noxious stimulation, nor do they impair conduction of nerve impulses along peripheral nerves.

OPIOID RECEPTORS

There are many types of opioid receptors, each mediating a spectrum of pharmacologic effects in response to activation by an opioid with agonist activity (Table 3-2) (Martin, 1979; Maze, 1981; Vaught *et al,* 1982). Even subpopulations of opioid receptors are likely. An ideal opioid agonist would have a high specificity for receptors producing desirable responses (*e.g.,* analgesia) and little or no specificity for receptors associated with side-effects (*e.g.,* depression of ventilation, nausea, dysphoria, physical dependence).

Mu or morphine-preferring receptors are principally responsible for supraspinal analgesia. Activation of a subpopulation of mu receptors (mu-1) is speculated to result in analgesia, whereas mu-2 receptors are responsible for depression of ventilation, bradycardia, and physical dependence. Beta-endorphin is the endogenous ligand, whereas exogenous mu receptor agonists include morphine, meperidine, fentanyl, sufentanil, and alfentanil. Naloxone is a specific mu receptor antagonist attaching to but not activating the receptor.

The role of delta receptors is to modulate the activity of mu receptors. Leu-enkephalin is an endogenous agonist at the delta receptor.

Analgesia and sedation with little or no depression of ventilation are related to activation of kappa receptors. Opioid agonist–antagonists often act principally on kappa receptors. Kappa receptors are located primarily in the cerebral cortex, whereas mu receptors are located predominantly in the brain stem.

Activation of sigma receptors results in excita-

Table 3-2
Classification of Opioid Receptors

	Effect	Agonist	Antagonist
Mu-1	Supraspinal analgesia	Beta-endorphin Morphine	Naloxone Pentazocine
Mu-2	Depression of ventilation Decreased heart rate Physical dependence Euphoria	Meperidine Fentanyl Sufentanil Alfentanil	Nalbuphine
Delta	Modulate mu receptor activity	Leu-enkephalin	Naloxone Met-enkephalin
Kappa	Analgesia Sedation Depression of ventilation (?) Miosis	Dynorphin Pentazocine Butorphanol Nalbuphine Buprenorphine Nalorphine	Naloxone
Sigma	Dysphoria Hypertonia Tachycardia Tachypnea	Pentazocine (?) Ketamine (?)	Naloxone

tory symptoms such as dysphoria, hypertonia, tachycardia, and tachypnea.

Endorphins

The discovery of highly specific opioid receptors in the central nervous system led to the search and subsequent isolation of endogenous ligands that interacted with these receptors (Hughes *et al*, 1975). The first two endogenous ligands that were discovered that possessed opioid activity were the pentapeptides, leu-enkephalin, and met-enkephalin. The leucine and methionine terminal amino acids of each of these pentapeptides is emphasized by the leu and met designation. Subsequently, other endogenous opioids, including alpha, beta, gamma, and delta endorphin have been isolated.

Endorphin is a combination of the words endogenous and morphine and is applied to all endogenous peptides with opioid activity. In this regard, leu-enkephalin and met-enkephalin are specific peptides classified as endorphins. Endorphins, with the exception of beta-endorphin, are about as active as morphine (Guillemin, 1977). In contrast, beta-endorphin is 5 to 10 times more potent than morphine.

Beta-lipotropin is a 91-chain amino acid that is present in the anterior pituitary. This amino acid lacks analgesic activity but contains within its structure many of the identified endorphins. For example, amino acids 61 to 91 in beta-lipotropin is beta-endorphin, and met-enkephalin is amino acids 61 to 65. For this reason, beta-lipotropin has been speculated to function as a prohormone, with hydrolysis of various portions giving rise to endorphins. Despite this speculated role as a prohormone, there must also be other sources of endorphins, because beta-lipotropin does not contain leu-enkephalin.

Dynorphin, like beta-lipotropin, is a peptide present in the anterior pituitary. This peptide is more potent than beta-endorphin and contains, within its amino acid sequence, the pentapeptide leu-enkephalin. It is thus speculated that leu-enkephalin may be a cleavage product to dynorphin.

Endogenous Pain-Suppression System

The obvious role of opioid receptors and endor-

phins is to function as an endogenous pain-suppression system (see Chapter 43). Opioid receptors are located in areas of the brain (periaqueductal gray matter of the brain stem, amygdala, corpus striatum, and hypothalamus) and spinal cord (substantia gelatinosa) that are involved with pain perception, integration of pain impulses, and responses to pain. Modulation of pain is likely to occur at supraspinal and spinal cord sites. Spinal cord actions of endorphins are presumed to be directly on opioid receptors in the substantia gelatinosa. This spinal cord site is the first site in the central nervous system for integration of sensory information. Conceptually, painful stimuli travel by way of afferent excitatory fibers to the thalamus, followed by activation of a complex multisynaptic descending pain-suppression system (see Chapter 43).

Analgesia induced by electrical stimulation of specific sites in the brain or mechanical stimulation of peripheral areas (*e.g.,* acupuncture) most likely reflects release of endorphins (Pomeranz and Chiu, 1976). Even the analgesic response to a placebo may also involve the release of endorphins.

Intraspinal Opioids

The identification of opioid receptors in the substantia gelatinosa of the spinal cord has led to new concepts in the treatment of acute and chronic pain (Cousins and Mather, 1984). For example, intrathecal injection in adults of a low dose of morphine (0.5–1 mg) may produce analgesia lasting an average of 20 hours. Slightly higher doses of morphine (2–8 mg) placed in the epidural space produce similar intense and long-lasting analgesia, presumably by diffusion into the lumbar spinal fluid and attachment to spinal cord opioid receptors. Analgesia is dose related and specific for visceral rather than somatic (*e.g.,* cannot use for anesthesia) pain. Relief of postoperative pain is predictable, but relief of pain during labor is unreliable, especially with epidural placement of the opioid. Analgesia produced in this manner, in contrast to administration of intravenous opioids or regional analgesia with local anesthetics, is not associated with sympathetic nervous system denervation, skeletal muscle weakness, or loss of proprioception. Therefore, postoperative patients receiving intrathecal or extradural opioids are able to ambulate pain-free without the occurrence of orthostatic hypotension or skeletal muscle weakness.

Side-effects associated with intrathecal or epidural placement of opioids include (1) pruritus, (2) urinary retention, (3) nausea and vomiting, (4) sedation, and (5) early and delayed depression of ventilation or circulation or both. Early depression of ventilation reflects systemic absorption of opioid, whereas delayed depression (6–24 hr after injection) is due to cephalad spread of the opioid in spinal fluid to medullary centers in the area of the fourth cerebral ventrical. Opioids with high lipid solubility, such as fentanyl or meperidine, attach to lipid components in the spinal cord; thus, minimal drug is available to diffuse cephalad, making delayed depression of ventilation less likely than after injection of relatively poorly lipid-soluble morphine.

OPIOID AGONISTS

Opioid agonists include but are not limited to morphine, meperidine, fentanyl, sufentanil, and alfentanil (Table 3-1). These are the opioids most likely to be used with inhaled anesthetics during general anesthesia. Indeed, high doses of morphine, fentanyl, and sufentanil have been used as the sole anesthetic in critically ill patients (see the section entitled Anesthetic Requirements).

Morphine

Morphine is the prototype opioid agonist to which all other opioids are compared (Fig. 3-1). In man, morphine produces analgesia with sedation. The ability to concentrate is diminished. Normal fears and apprehension are diminished, giving rise to euphoria, especially in the presence of pain. Other sensations include nausea, a feeling of body warmth, heaviness of the extremities, dryness of the mouth, diaphoresis, and pruritus, especially around the nose. The effect on the cerebellum is mainly depressant, causing an ataxic gait by inhibiting motor coordination. In the absence of pain, morphine may produce excessive sedation and dysphoria rather than euphoria.

The cause of pain persists, but even low doses of morphine raise the threshold to pain and modify the perception of the noxious stimulus such that it is no longer experienced as pain. Analgesia

is most prominent when morphine is administered before the painful stimulus occurs. This is a pertinent consideration in administering an opioid to patients prior to the actual surgical stimulus. Continuous dull pain is relieved by morphine more effectively than is sharp intermittent pain. In contrast to the nonopioid analgesics, morphine is effective against pain arising from viscera as well as from skeletal muscles, joints, and integumental structures (see Chapter 11).

Pharmacokinetics

Morphine is well-absorbed following intramuscular administration, with onset of effect in 15 to 30 minutes and a peak effect in 45 to 90 minutes. The duration of action is about 4 hours. Absorption of morphine from the gastrointestinal tract is not reliable. Morphine is usually administered intravenously in the perioperative period, thus eliminating the unpredictable influence of drug absorption. The peak analgesic effect of morphine administered intravenously occurs about 20 minutes after injection.

Plasma morphine concentrations following rapid intravenous injection do not correlate closely with the opioid's pharmacologic activity (Aitkenhead *et al,* 1984; Hug *et al,* 1981). Presumably, this discrepancy reflects a delay in penetration of morphine across the blood–brain barrier. Cerebrospinal fluid concentrations of morphine peak 15 to 30 minutes after intravenous injection and decay more slowly than plasma concentrations (Fig. 3-3) (Hug and Murphy, 1981). As a result, the analgesic and ventilatory depressant effects of morphine may not be evident during the initial high plasma concentrations following intravenous administration of the opioid. Likewise, these same drug effects persist despite declining plasma concentrations of morphine. Moderate analgesia probably requires maintenance of plasma morphine concentrations of at least 0.05 μg ml^{-1} (Fig. 3-4) (Berkowitz *et al,* 1975). Patient-controlled demand delivery systems usually provide good postoperative analgesia, with total doses of morphine ranging from 1.3 to 2.7 mg hr^{-1} (White, 1985).

Only a small amount of administered morphine gains access to the central nervous system. For example, it is estimated that less than 0.1% of intravenously administered morphine has entered the central nervous system at the time of peak plasma concentrations (Mule, 1971). Reasons for poor penetration of morphine into the central nervous system include (1) relatively poor lipid solubility, (2) high degree of ionization (90%) at physiologic pH, (3) protein binding, and rapid metabolism to morphine glucuronide. Since morphine has a pKa or 8.5, alkalinization of the blood,

as produced by hyperventilation of the lungs, will increase the nonionized fraction of morphine and thus facilitate its passage into the central nervous system. Nevertheless, respiratory acidosis, which decreases the nonionized fraction of morphine, results in higher brain and plasma concentrations of morphine than are present during normocarbia (Fig. 3-5) (Finck *et al*, 1977). This suggests that pH-induced increases in cerebral blood flow and facilitated delivery of morphine to the brain are more important than the fraction of drug that exists in either the ionized or nonionized fraction. In contrast to the central nervous system, morphine accumulates rapidly in kidney, liver, lung, and skeletal muscle, with the kidney having the greatest ability to concentrate (Way and Adler, 1960).

METABOLISM. The principal pathway of metabolism of morphine is conjugation with glucuronic acid in hepatic and extrahepatic sites, especially the kidneys (Way and Adler, 1960). Indeed, the major inactive metabolite of morphine is morphine-3-glucuronide. Approximately 55% of intravenously administered morphine is conjugated in adults; this may increase to 80% in physically dependent patients. Morphine-3-glucuronide is detectable in the plasma within 1 minute following intravenous injection, and its concentration exceeds that of unchanged drug by almost tenfold within 90 minutes (Fig. 3-6) (Murphy and Hug, 1981). Formation of the glucuronide conjugate is inhibited by monoamine oxidase inhibitors (Yeh and Mitchell, 1972). This is consistent with exaggerated effects of morphine when administered to

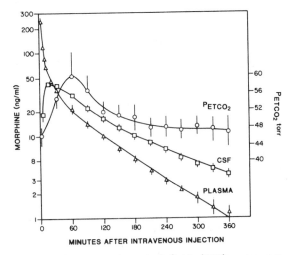

FIGURE 3-3. Cerebrospinal fluid (CSF) concentrations following intravenous administration decay more slowly than plasma concentrations. The end-tidal carbon dioxide concentration ($PETCO_2$) remains elevated despite a declining plasma concentration of morphine. Mean ± SE. (From Hug CC, Murphy MR, Rigel EP, Olson WA. Pharmacokinetics of morphine injected intravenously into the anesthetized dog. Anesthesiology 1981;54:38–47. Redrawn by permission of the authors and publisher.)

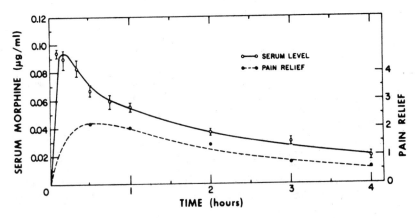

FIGURE 3-4. Moderate analgesia probably requires maintenance of a plasma (serum) concentration of morphine of at least 0.05 μg ml^{-1}. Mean ± SE. (From Berkowitz BA, Ngai SH, Yang JC, Hemstead J, Spector S. The disposition of morphine in surgical patients. Clin Pharmacol Ther 1975;17:629–35. Reproduced by permission of the authors and publisher.)

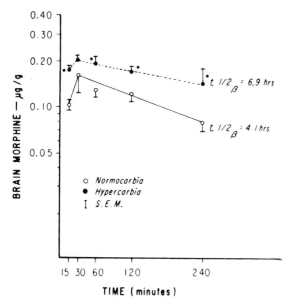

FIGURE 3-5. Hypercarbia, which decreases the nonionized fraction of morphine, results in a higher brain concentration and longer elimination half-life ($t1/2_B$) than occurs in the presence of normocarbia. $*P < 0.05$ (From Finck AD, Berkowitz BA, Hemstead J, Ngai S. Pharmacokinetics of morphine: Effects of hypercarbia on serum and brain morphine concentrations in the dog. Anesthesiology 1977;47:407–410. Reproduced by permission of the authors and publisher.)

patients being treated with these drugs (see Chapter 19).

An estimated 5% of morphine is demethylated to normorphine (Brunk *et al,* 1974). A small amount of codeine may also be formed.

Metabolites of morphine are eliminated principally in the urine, with only 7% to 10% undergoing biliary excretion. Morphine-3-glucuronide is detectable in the urine for up to 72 hours after administration of morphine. Less than 10% of morphine is excreted unchanged in the urine.

ELIMINATION HALF-TIME. Following intravenous administration, the elimination half-time of morphine is 114 minutes, and 173 minutes for morphine-3-glucuronide (Table 3-3 and Fig. 3-6) (Murphy and Hug, 1981; Stanski *et al,* 1977). The decline in the plasma concentration of morphine following initial distribution of the drug is principally due to metabolism, because only a small amount of unchanged opioid is excreted by the

kidneys. Plasma morphine concentrations are greater in elderly than in young adults, possibly reflecting age-related reductions in cardiac output (Fig. 3-7) (Berkowitz *et al,* 1975). Conversely, anesthesia appears to exert no significant effect on the elimination half-time of morphine.

Patients with renal failure exhibit higher plasma concentrations of morphine than do normal patients, which could result in increased sensitivity to the effects of the drug (Fig. 3-8) (Aitkenhead *et al,* 1984). This greater plasma concentration reflects a smaller volume of distribution in renal failure patients, as the elimination of un-

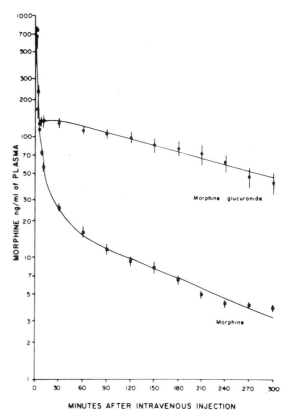

FIGURE 3-6. Morphine glucuronide is detectable in the plasma within 1 minute following intravenous injection and its concentration exceeds that of unchanged morphine by almost tenfold within 90 minutes. Mean ± SE. (From Murphy HR, Hug CC. Pharmacokinetics of intravenous morphine in patients anesthetized with enflurane-nitrous oxide. Anesthesiology 1981;54:187–92. Reproduced by permission of the authors and publisher.)

Table 3-3
Pharmacokinetics of Opioid Agonists and Antagonists

	pKa	Protein Binding (%)	Volume of Distribution (L kg⁻¹)	Clearance (ml kg⁻¹ min⁻¹)	Elimination Half-Time (min)
Morphine	7.93	30	3.2	14.7	114
Meperidine	8.50	60	3.8	15.1	180–264
Fentanyl	7.34	84	4.1	11.6	185–219
Sufentanil		92.5	1.7	12.7	148–164
Alfentanil		92	0.86	6.4	70–98
Naloxone			1.8	30.1	64

changed morphine is not changed compared with that in normal patients. Indeed, prolonged depression of ventilation (up to 7 days) has been observed in patients in renal failure following administration of morphine (Don *et al,* 1975). Plasma morphine concentrations following renal transplantation parallel postoperative creatinine clearance (Sear *et al,* 1985).

Side Effects

Side-effects described for morphine are also characteristic for other opioid agonists with rare exceptions in either incidence or magnitude.

CARDIOVASCULAR SYSTEM. Intravenous administration of morphine, even in high doses (1 mg kg⁻¹), to supine and normovolemic patients is unlikely to cause significant changes in myocardial contractility or reductions in blood pressure (Lowenstein *et al,* 1969). The same patients changing from the supine to standing position, however, may manifest orthostatic hypotension and syncope, presumably reflecting morphine-induced impairment of compensatory sympathetic nervous system responses. For example, morphine reduces sympathetic nervous system tone to

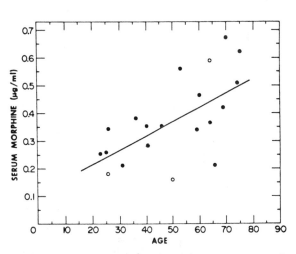

FIGURE 3-7. The plasma (serum) concentration of morphine increases progressively with advancing age. (From Berkowitz BA, Ngai SH, Yang JC, Hemstead J, Spector S. The disposition of morphine in surgical pa-

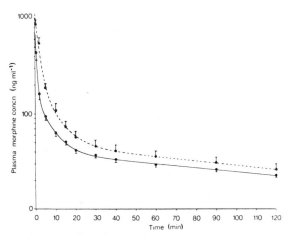

FIGURE 3-8. Patients with renal failure *(broken line)* have higher plasma concentrations of morphine than do normal patients. Mean ± SE. (From Aitkenhead AR, Vater M, Acholas K, Cooper CMS, Smith G. Pharmacokinetics of single-dose IV morphine in normal volunteers and patients with end-stage renal failure. Br J Anaesth

peripheral veins, probably by an action within the central nervous system or a direct alpha-adrenergic blocking effect on vascular smooth muscle (Lowenstein *et al,* 1972; Zelis *et al,* 1974). In addition to orthostatic hypotension, the venodilating effects of large doses of morphine may be responsible for increased intravenous fluid and whole blood replacement requirements intraoperatively (Stanley *et al,* 1974a). Morphine can also evoke reductions in blood pressure by virtue of drug-induced bradycardia or histamine release.

Morphine-induced bradycardia results from increased activity over the vagal nerves, which probably reflects stimulation of the vagal nucleus in the medulla. This opioid may also exert a direct depressant effect on the sinoatrial node and slow conduction of the cardiac impulse through the atrioventricular node. Bradycardia is not a constant finding, probably because other extraneous factors present in the patient, such as pain or anxiety, offset any heart rate – slowing effect of the drug.

Histamine release and associated hypotension are variable in both incidence and degree. The magnitude of morphine-induced histamine release and subsequent reduction in blood pressure can be minimized by (1) limiting the rate of intravenous morphine infusion to 5 mg min^{-1}, (2) keeping the patient supine to slight head-down position, and (3) optimizing intravascular fluid volume. Conversely, intravenous administration of morphine 1 mg kg^{-1} over a 10-minute period produces substantial increases in plasma concentrations of histamine that are paralleled by significant reductions in mean arterial pressure and peripheral vascular resistance (Figs. 3-9 and 3-10) (Rosow *et al,* 1982). It is important to recognize, however, that not all patients respond to this rate of morphine infusion with the release of histamine, emphasizing the individual variability associated with the administration of this drug (Fig. 3-9) (Rosow *et al,* 1982). In contrast to morphine, the intravenous infusion of fentanyl, 50 μg kg^{-1} over a 10-minute period, does not evoke release of histamine in any patient (Fig. 3-9) (Rosow *et al,* 1982). Pretreatment of patients with H$_1$ and H$_2$ receptor antagonists does not alter release of histamine evoked by morphine but does prevent changes in blood pressure and peripheral vascular resistance (Philbin *et al,* 1981) (see Chapter 21).

The release of histamine by morphine, but not equimolar concentrations of fentanyl or oxymorphone, confirms that drug-induced histamine re-

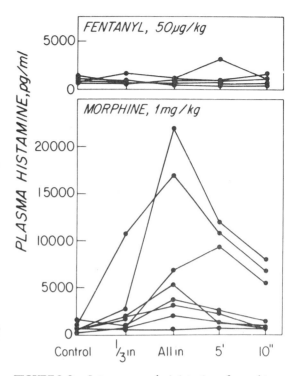

FIGURE 3-9. Intravenous administration of morphine, but not fentanyl, is associated with an unpredictable rise in the plasma concentration of histamine. (From Rosow CE, Moss J, Philbin DM, Savarese JJ. Histamine release during morphine and fentanyl anesthesia. Anesthesiology, 1982;56:93 – 6. Reproduced by permission of the authors and publisher.)

lease is not characteristic of high plasma concentrations of all opioids (Hermens *et al,* 1985). Furthermore, failure of naloxone to inhibit morphine-induced histamine release suggests that this release is not dependent on opioid receptor binding or activation.

Morphine does not sensitize the heart to catecholamines or otherwise predispose to cardiac dysrhythmias as long as hypercarbia or arterial hypoxemia does not result from ventilatory depressant effects of the opioid. Tachycardia and hypertension that occur during anesthesia with morphine are not pharmacologic effects of the opioid, but, rather are responses to noxious surgical stimulation that are not suppressed by morphine. Both the sympathetic nervous system and the renin – angiotensin mechanism contribute to these cardiovascular responses (Bailey *et al,*

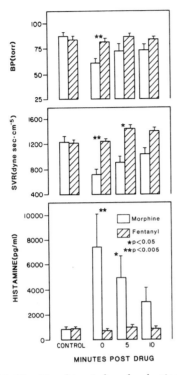

FIGURE 3-10. Morphine-induced reductions in blood pressure (BP) and peripheral (systemic) vascular resistance (SVR) are accompanied by elevations in the plasma concentration of histamine. Similar changes do not accompany the administration of fentanyl. Mean ± SE. (From Rosow CE, Moss J, Philbin DM, Savarese JJ. Histamine release during morphine and fentanyl anesthesia. Anesthesiology 1982;56:93–6. Redrawn by permission of the authors and publisher.)

1975). This emphasizes that morphine does not impair the release or peripheral effects of hormones and neurotransmitters. To the extent that morphine reduces pain, however, it may modulate the release of these substances. Very large doses of morphine, or other opioid agonists, may reduce the likelihood that tachycardia and hypertension will occur in response to noxious stimulation, but once the response has occurred, administration of additional opioid is unlikely to be effective.

During anesthesia, opioid agonists are frequently administered with inhaled anesthetics to ensure complete amnesia for the noxious surgical stimulus. The combination of an opioid agonist, such as morphine or fentanyl, with nitrous oxide results in cardiovascular depression (decreased cardiac output and blood pressure plus elevated filling pressures), which does not occur when either drug is administered alone (McDermott and Stanley, 1974; Stoelting and Gibbs, 1973). Furthermore, unexpected cardiovascular depression may occur when other intravenous drugs, such as thiamylal or diazepam, precede or are administered in the presence of an opioid agonist (Stanley *et al*, 1976; Stoelting, 1977).

VENTILATION. All opioid agonists produce dose-dependent depression of ventilation, primarily through a direct depressant effect on brain stem ventilation centers (see Chapter 49). This depression of ventilation is characterized by reduced responsiveness of these ventilation centers to carbon dioxide as reflected by an increase in the resting $PaCO_2$ and displacement of the carbon dioxide response curve to the right. Opioid agonists also interfere with pontine and medullary ventilatory centers that regulate rhythm of breathing, leading to prolonged pauses between breaths, delayed exhalation, and periodic breathing.

It is possible that opioid agonists diminish sensitivity to carbon dioxide by reducing the release of acetylcholine from neurons in the area of the medullary ventilatory center in response to hypercarbia. In this regard, it is intriguing that physostigmine, which elevates central nervous system levels of acetylcholine, may antagonize depression of ventilation, but not analgesia, produced by morphine (see Chapter 9). Depression of ventilation produced by opioid agonists is rapid and persists for several hours, as demonstrated by ventilatory responses to exogenous challenges to carbon dioxide.

Clinically, depression of ventilation produced by opioid agonists manifests as a decreased rate of breathing that is often accompanied by a compensatory increase in tidal volume. The incompleteness of this compensatory increase in tidal volume is evidenced by predictable elevations of the $PaCO_2$. High doses of opioid agonists may result in apnea, but the patient remains conscious and able to initiate a breath if so requested. Death from an opioid overdose is almost invariably attributable to depression of ventilation.

Many factors influence the magnitude and duration of depression of ventilation produced by opioid agonists. For example, elderly patients and patients who are sleeping are usually more sensitive to ventilatory depressant effects of opioids. Conversely, pain from surgical stimulation counteracts depression of ventilation produced by opioids (Eckenhoff and Oech, 1960). Likewise, the analgesic effect of opioids improves breathing that has been rapid and shallow due to pain.

Opioids produce dose-dependent depression of ciliary activity in the bronchioles. Increases in airway resistance following administration of an opioid are probably due to a direct effect on bronchial smooth muscle and an indirect action owing to release of histamine.

NERVOUS SYSTEM. Opioids, in the absence of hypoventilation, decrease cerebral blood flow and reduce intracranial pressure (Larson *et al*, 1974). These drugs must be used with caution in patients with head injury because of their (1) associated effects on wakefulness, (2) production of miosis, and (3) depression of ventilation with associated increases in intracranial pressure if the PaCO$_2$ becomes elevated. Furthermore, head injury may reduce the integrity of the blood–brain barrier, with resultant increased sensitivity to opioids.

The effect of morphine on the electroencephalogram (EEG) resembles changes associated with sleep. For example, there is replacement of rapid alpha waves by slower delta waves.

Miosis is due to an excitatory action of opioids on the autonomic nervous system component of the Edinger–Westphal nucleus of the oculomotor nerve. Tolerance to the miotic effect of morphine is not prominent. Miosis can be antagonized by atropine, and profound arterial hypoxemia can still result in mydriasis.

Opioid agonists do not alter the response to neuromuscular blocking drugs. Skeletal muscle rigidity, especially of the thoracic and abdominal muscles, is common when high doses of opioid agonists are administered rapidly intravenously and this response is enhanced by nitrous oxide (Sokoll *et al*, 1972). Central nervous system effects of opioids may be responsible for this skeletal muscle rigidity (Freund *et al*, 1973). Decreased thoracic compliance associated with skeletal muscle rigidity may interfere with adequate ventilation of the lungs and lead to impairment of venous return because of the high mechanical inflation pressures necessary to ventilate the lungs.

Analgesic responses to opioids remain relatively constant throughout adulthood. After about 60 years of age, however, there is both a decrease in sensitivity to pain and an increased analgesic response to opioids (Bellville *et al*, 1971). As a result, doses of opioids administered to elderly patients to produce analgesia are often reduced.

BILIARY TRACT. Opioids can cause spasm of biliary smooth muscle, resulting in increases in intrabiliary pressure that may be associated with epigastric distress or biliary colic. This pain may be confused with angina pectoris. Naloxone will relieve pain caused by biliary spasm but not myocardial ischemia. Conversely, nitroglycerin will relieve pain due to biliary spasm or myocardial ischemia.

Equal analgesic doses of fentanyl, morphine, meperidine, and pentazocine increase common bile duct pressure 99%, 53%, 61%, and 15% above predrug levels, respectively (Economou and Ward-McQuaid, 1971; Radnay *et al*, 1980). During surgery, opioid-induced spasm of the sphincter of Oddi may appear radiologically as a sharp constriction at the distal end of the common bile duct and be misinterpreted as a common bile duct stone (McCammon *et al*, 1978). It may be necessary to reverse biliary smooth muscle spasm with naloxone so as to correctly interpret the cholangiogram (Lang and Pilon, 1980; McCammon *et al*, 1978). Glucagon, 2 mg administered intravenously, also reverses opioid-induced biliary smooth muscle spasm and, unlike naloxone, does not antagonize analgesic effects of the opioid (Jones *et al*, 1980). Nevertheless, biliary smooth muscle spasm does not occur in most patients who receive opioids. Indeed, the incidence of spasm of the sphincter of Oddi is about 3% in patients receiving fentanyl as a supplement to inhaled anesthetics (Jones *et al*, 1981).

Contraction of the smooth muscles of the pancreatic ducts is probably responsible for elevations in plasma amylase and lipase that may be present following the administration of morphine. Such elevations may confuse the diagnosis when acute pancreatitis is a possibility.

GASTROINTESTINAL TRACT. The use of opium for treatment of diarrhea preceded its use for analgesia. Morphine reduces the propulsive peristaltic contractions of the small and large intestine and enhances the tone of the pyloric sphincter, ileocecal valve, and anal sphincter. The delay of passage of intestinal contents through the colon allows increased absorption of water to take place. As a result, constipation often accompanies therapy with opioids. Minimal tolerance to the constipating effects of opioids occurs.

NAUSEA AND VOMITING. Opioid-induced nausea and vomiting is a manifestation of direct stimulation of the chemoreceptor trigger zone in the floor of the fourth ventricle of the medulla oblongata (see Chapter 41). This may reflect the role of opioid agonists as partial dopamine agonists at dopamine receptors in the chemoreceptor trigger zone. Indeed, apomorphine is a profound emetic and is also the most potent of the opioids at dopamine receptors. Stimulation of dopamine receptors as a mechanism for opioid-induced nausea and vomiting is consistent with the antiemetic efficacy of butyrophenones (see Chapter 19).

Morphine may also cause nausea and vomiting by delaying passage of intestinal contents through the gastrointestinal tract. In addition, nausea and vomiting following administration of morphine can also reflect an increased volume of gastrointestinal secretions.

Morphine depresses the vomiting center in the medulla. As a result, the intravenous administration of morphine produces less nausea and vomiting than the administration of subcutaneous morphine, presumably because intravenously administered opioid reaches the vomiting center as rapidly as it reaches the chemoreceptor trigger zone. Nausea and vomiting are relatively uncommon in recumbent patients given morphine. This suggests that a vestibular component may be contributing to opioid-induced nausea and vomiting.

GENITOURINARY. Morphine can increase the tone and peristaltic activity of the ureter. In contrast to similar effects on the biliary tract smooth muscle, the same opioid-induced effects on the ureter can be reversed by an anticholinergic drug (see Chapter 10). Urinary urgency is produced by opioid-induced augmentation of detrusor muscle tone, but, at the same time, the tone of the vesical sphincter is enhanced, making urination difficult.

Antidiuresis that accompanies administration of morphine to animals has been attributed to opioid-induced release of antidiuretic hormone (Papper and Papper, 1964). In man, however, morphine in the absence of painful stimulation, does not evoke release of antidiuretic hormone (Philbin et al, 1976). Finally, administration of morphine to patients whose bladders are not catheterized may cause a decrease in urine output by an increase in vesical sphincter tone, resulting in retention of urine in the bladder. Indeed, when morphine is administered in the presence of an adequate intravascular fluid volume, there is no change in glomerular filtration rate or urine output (Stanley et al, 1974b).

There is evidence that epidural morphine, as administered to provide postoperative analgesia, causes an increase in the plasma concentration of antidiuretic hormones (Korinek et al, 1985). This response may reflect cephalad migration of the opioid.

CUTANEOUS CHANGES. Morphine causes cutaneous blood vessels to dilate. The skin of the face, neck, and upper thorax frequently becomes flushed and warm. These changes in cutaneous circulation are, in part, caused by the release of histamine. Histamine release probably accounts for urticaria and erythema commonly seen at the site of injection of morphine. In addition, morphine-induced histamine release probably accounts for conjunctival erythema and pruritus.

Localized cutaneous evidence of histamine release, especially along the vein into which morphine is injected, does not represent an allergic reaction. It is indeed rare that morphine evokes sufficient histamine release to result in an allergic reaction (Birt and Nickerson, 1959; Fahmy, 1981). Overall, the incidence of true allergy to opioids is extremely low (Levy and Rockoff, 1982). More often, predictable side-effects of opioids such as localized histamine release, orthostatic hypotension, and nausea and vomiting are misinterpreted as an allergic reaction.

PLACENTA. The placenta offers no real barrier to transfer of opioids from mother to fetus. Therefore, depression of the newborn can occur as a consequence of administration of opioids to the mother during labor. In this regard, maternal morphine may produce greater neonatal depression than meperidine (Way et al, 1965). This may reflect immaturity of the newborn's blood–brain barrier and a lesser dependence of meperidine on this barrier for gaining access to the central nervous system. Chronic maternal use of an opioid can result in the development of physical dependence (e.g., intrauterine addiction) in the fetus. Subsequent administration of naloxone to the newborn can precipitate a life-threatening neonatal abstinence syndrome.

DRUG INTERACTIONS. Ventilatory depressant effects of some opioids may be exaggerated by amphetamines, phenothiazines, monoamine oxidase inhibitors, and tricyclic antidepressants. For example, patients receiving monoamine oxidase inhibitors may experience exaggerated depression of ventilation and hyperpyrexia following administration of an opioid agonist, especially meperidine (see Chapter 19). This exaggerated response may reflect alterations in the rate or pathway of metabolism of the opioids or both. Sympathomimetic drugs appear to enhance analgesia produced by opioids. The cholinergic nervous system seems to be a positive modulator of opioid-induced analgesia in that physostigmine enhances and atropine antagonizes analgesia.

TOLERANCE AND PHYSICAL DEPENDENCE. Tolerance and physical dependence with repeated opioid administration is a characteristic feature of all opioid agonists and is one of the major limitations to their clinical use. Cross-tolerance develops between all the opioids. Tolerance can occur without physical dependence, but the reverse does not seem to occur.

Tolerance is the development of the need to increase the dose of opioid agonist to achieve the same analgesic effect previously achieved with a lower dose. Such acquired tolerance usually takes 2 to 3 weeks to develop with analgesic doses of morphine. The miotic and constipating actions of morphine persist while tolerance to depression of ventilation develops.

The potential for physical dependence (*e.g.,* addiction) is an agonist effect of opioids (Table 3-2). Indeed, physical dependence does not occur to opioid antagonists and is much less likely with opioid agonist–antagonists than with opioid agonists. When opioid agonist actions predominate, there often develops, with repeated use, a compulsive desire and continuous need (*e.g.,* psychological and physiologic) for the drug.

Physical dependence on morphine usually requires about 25 days to develop but may occur sooner in emotionally unstable persons. Some degree of physical dependence, however, occurs after only 48 hours of continuous medication. When physical dependence is established, discontinuation of the opioid agonist produces a typical withdrawal (abstinence) syndrome within 15

drawal include yawning, diaphoresis, lacrimation, or coryza. Insomnia and restlessness are prominent. Abdominal cramps, nausea, vomiting, and diarrhea reach their peak in 72 hours and then decline over the next 7 to 10 days. During withdrawal, tolerance to morphine is rapidly lost, and the syndrome can be terminated by a modest dose of opioid agonist. The longer the period of abstinence, the smaller the dose of opioid agonist that will be required.

Mechanisms responsible for development of tolerance or physical dependence to opioid agonists have not been conclusively determined. In many respects, symptoms of opioid withdrawal resemble a denervation hypersensitivity that might reflect an increase (*e.g.,* up-regulation) in the number of responding opioid receptors in the brain. This increase in opioid receptors could reflect chronic opioid-induced inhibition of acetylcholine release. Opioid agonists are also known to inhibit adenylate cyclase activity and cyclic AMP production (Sharma *et al,* 1976). Abrupt withdrawal of opioids leads to a marked increase in both the level of cyclic AMP and brain sympathetic nervous system activity. Indeed, clonidine, a centrally acting α_2-adrenergic agonist that diminishes transmission in central nervous system sympathetic pathways, is considered the drug of choice in suppressing withdrawal signs in persons who are physically dependent upon opioids (Devenyi *et al,* 1982, Gold *et al,* 1980). Tolerance and physical dependence are often attributed to cellular adaptation, but the proof for this premise is lacking. Tolerance is not due to enzyme induction, because no increase in the rate of metabolism of opioid agonists occurs.

OVERDOSE. The principal manifestation of opioid overdose is depression of ventilation, manifesting as a slow rate of breathing that may progress to apnea. Pupils are symmetrical and miotic unless severe arterial hypoxemia is present, which results in mydriasis. Skeletal muscles are flaccid, and upper airway obstruction may occur. Pulmonary edema commonly develops, but the mechanism for this is not known. Hypotension and seizures occur if arterial hypoxemia persists. The triad of miosis, hypoventilation, and coma should suggest overdose with an opioid. Treatment of opioid overdose is mechanical ventilation of the

Opioid Antagonists). Administration of naloxone to treat an opioid overdose in a physically dependent patient may precipitate acute withdrawal.

Meperidine

Meperidine is a synthetic opioid agonist derived from phenylpiperidine (Fig. 3-11). There are several analogs of meperidine, including fentanyl, sufentanil, alfentanil, and phenoperidine (Fig. 3-11). Structurally, meperidine is similar to atropine, and it possesses a mild atropine-like antispasmodic effect. Nevertheless, the principal pharmacologic effects of meperidine resemble morphine.

Pharmacokinetics

Meperidine is about one tenth as potent as morphine, with 80 to 100 mg administered intramuscularly being equivalent to about 10 mg of morphine. The duration of action of meperidine is 2 to 4 hours, making it a shorter-acting opioid agonist than morphine. In equal analgesic doses, meperidine produces as much sedation, euphoria, nausea, vomiting, and depression of ventilation as does morphine. Unlike morphine, meperidine is well absorbed from the gastrointestinal tract, but it nevertheless is only about one-half as effective orally as when administered intramuscularly.

METABOLISM. Metabolism of meperidine in the liver is extensive, with about 90% of the drug initially undergoing demethylation to normeperidine and hydrolysis to meperidinic acid (Burns *et al,* 1974). Normeperidine may subsequently be hydrolyzed to normeperidinic acid. Acidic metabolites are inactive and often undergo conjugation prior to their elimination in the urine. Very little meperidine (usually less than 5%) is excreted unchanged in the urine. Urinary excretion of meperidine is *p*H dependent. For example, if the urinary *p*H is reduced below 5, as much as 25% of the opioid is excreted unchanged. Indeed, acidification of the urine can be considered in an attempt to speed elimination of meperidine. Normeperidine has an elimination half-time of 15 to 40 hours and can be detected in the urine for as long as 3 days following administration of meperidine. This metabolite, in addition to having central nervous system stimulant effects, is about one-half as active as the parent compound of an analgesic. Normeperidine toxicity manifesting as myoclonus and seizures is most likely during prolonged adminis-

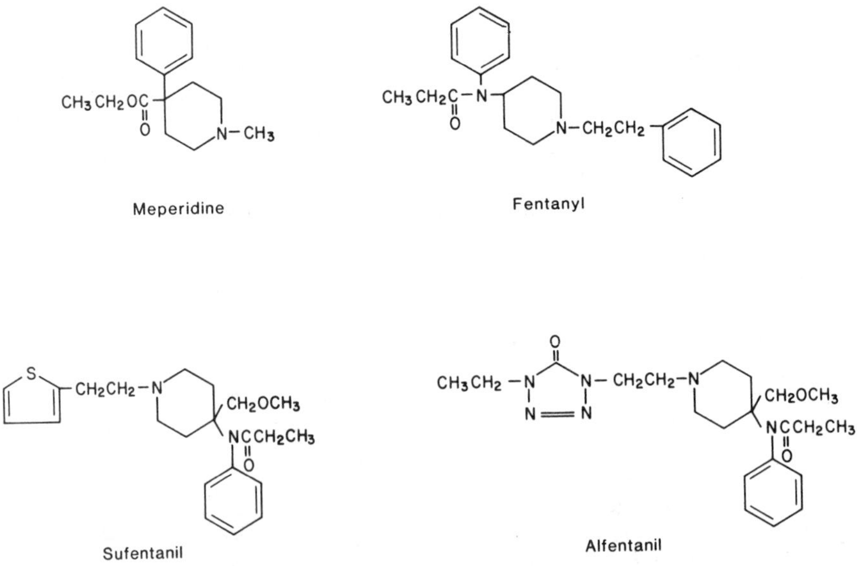

Meperidine

Fentanyl

Sufentanil

Alfentanil

FIGURE 3-11. Synthetic opioid agonists.

tration of meperidine, especially to patients with impaired renal function (Armstrong and Bersten, 1986).

ELIMINATION HALF-TIME. The elimination half-time of meperidine is 3 to 4.4 hours (Koska *et al*, 1981). Since clearance of meperidine is primarily dependent upon hepatic metabolism, it is possible that high doses of opioid would saturate enzyme systems and result in prolonged elimination half-times. Nevertheless, elimination half-time is not altered by doses of meperidine up to 5 mg kg^{-1} (Koska *et al*, 1981). About 60% of meperidine is bound to plasma proteins. Elderly patients manifest decreased plasma protein binding of meperidine, resulting in increased plasma concentrations of free drug and an apparent increased sensitivity to the opioid (Mather *et al*, 1975). Increased tolerance of alcoholics to meperidine and other opioids presumably reflects an increased volume of distribution, resulting in lower plasma concentrations of meperidine (Klotz *et al*, 1974).

Clinical Uses

The principal use of meperidine is for analgesia during labor and delivery and following surgery. Intramuscular injection of meperidine to provide postoperative analgesia results in peak plasma concentrations that vary three- to fivefold as well as times required to achieve peak concentrations that vary three- to sevenfold between patients (Austin *et al*, 1980a). The minimum analgesic plasma concentration of meperidine is highly variable among patients, yet, in the same patient, differences in concentration as small as 0.05 μg ml^{-1} can represent the margin between no relief and complete analgesia. A plasma meperidine concentration of 0.7 μg ml^{-1} would be expected to provide postoperative analgesia in about 95% of patients (Austin *et al*, 1980b). Patient-controlled demand delivery systems usually provide good postoperative analgesia, with total doses of meperidine ranging from 12 to 36 mg hr^{-1} (White, 1985).

Oral absorption may make meperidine more useful than morphine for the treatment of many forms of pain. Unlike morphine, meperidine is not useful for the treatment of diarrhea and is not an effective antitussive. During bronchoscopy, the relative lack of antitussive activity of meperidine makes it less useful. Meperidine is not used in

high doses for anesthesia because of significant negative inotropic effects (Freye, 1974; Priano and Vatner, 1981; Strauer, 1972).

Side Effects (see also the section entitled Morphine, Side Effects)

In therapeutic doses, meperidine is associated with orthostatic hypotension. In fact, hypotension after meperidine injection is more frequent and more profound than after comparable doses of morphine. Orthostatic hypotension suggests that meperidine, like morphine, interferes with compensatory sympathetic nervous system reflexes. Meperidine, in contrast to morphine, rarely causes bradycardia but instead may increase heart rate, reflecting its modest atropine-like qualities. Large doses of meperidine result in reductions in myocardial contractility, stroke volume, and elevations in cardiac filling pressures (Freye, 1974; Priano and Vatner, 1981; Strauer, 1972). This direct myocardial depressant effect is not present with other opioids, rendering meperidine unique in this respect.

Large doses of meperidine (3 – 4 g) as used by addicts may cause cerebral irritation and seizures. These effects presumably reflect accumulation of the metabolite normeperidine, which has central nervous system – stimulant effects. Normeperidine may accumulate in patients with renal disease.

Meperidine readily impairs ventilation and may even be more of a ventilatory depressant than morphine (Foldes and Tarda, 1965). Meperidine readily crosses the placenta, and concentrations of the opioid in umbilical cord blood at birth may exceed maternal plasma concentrations (Morgan *et al*, 1978). Nevertheless, meperidine produces less depression of ventilation in the newborn than does morphine (Way *et al*, 1965).

Meperidine may produce less constipation and urinary retention than morphine. After equal analgesic doses, biliary tract spasm is less after meperidine injection than after morphine injection but greater than that caused by codeine (Radnay *et al*, 1980). Meperidine does not cause miosis, but rather tends to cause mydriasis, reflecting its modest atropine-like actions. A dry mouth and an increase in heart rate is further evidence of an atropine-like effect of meperidine.

The pattern of withdrawal symptoms after abrupt discontinuation of meperidine differs from that of morphine in that there are few autonomic nervous system effects. In addition, symptoms of withdrawal develop more rapidly and are of a shorter duration compared with those of morphine.

Fentanyl

Fentanyl is a synthetic opioid agonist related to the phenylpiperidines. As an analgesic, fentanyl is 75 to 125 times more potent than morphine.

Pharmacokinetics

A single dose of fentanyl administered intravenously has a more rapid onset (within 30 seconds) and shorter duration of action than morphine. The greater potency and more rapid onset of action reflects the greater lipid solubility of fentanyl compared with that of morphine, which facilitates its passage across the blood–brain barrier. Likewise, the short duration of action of a single dose of fentanyl reflects its rapid redistribution to inactive tissue sites such as fat and skeletal muscle, with an associated decline in the plasma concentration of the drug (Fig. 3-12) (Hug and Murphy, 1981). The lungs also serve as a large inactive storage site for fentanyl. When multiple doses of fentanyl are administered or when there is continuous infusion of the drug, there is progressive saturation of these inactive tissue sites. As a result, the plasma concentration of fentanyl does not decline rapidly, and the duration of analgesia, as well as depression of ventilation, is prolonged (Murphy et al, 1979).

METABOLISM. Fentanyl is extensively metabolized by dealkylation, hydroxylation, and amide hydrolysis to inactive metabolites, including norfentanyl and desproprionylnorfentanyl, that are excreted in the bile and urine (McClain and Hug, 1980). For example, 85% of an injected dose of fentanyl appears in the urine and feces over 72 hours as metabolites, whereas less than 8% is recovered as unchanged drug in the urine. A high degree of metabolism to more polar and inactive metabolites is predictable for a highly lipid-soluble drug such as fentanyl.

ELIMINATION HALF-TIME. Despite the clinical impression that fentanyl has a short duration of action, its elimination half-time of 185 to 219 min-

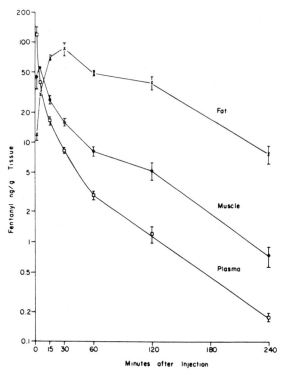

FIGURE 3-12. The short duration of action of a single dose of fentanyl reflects its rapid redistribution to inactive tissue sites such as fat and skeletal muscles with an associated decline in the plasma concentration of drug. Mean ± SE. (From Hug CC, Murphy MR. Tissue redistribution of fentanyl and termination of its effects in rats. Anesthesiology 1981;55:369–75. Reproduced by permission of the authors and publisher.)

utes is greater than that for morphine (Table 3-3). This greater elimination half-time reflects a larger volume of distribution of fentanyl, since clearance of both opioids are similar (Table 3-3). The greater volume of distribution of fentanyl is due to its higher lipid solubility and thus more rapid passage into tissues compared with the less lipid-soluble morphine. Plasma concentrations of fentanyl are maintained by its slow reuptake from inactive tissue sites, which accounts for persistent drug effects that parallel the slow elimination half-time.

In animals, the elimination half-time, volume of distribution, and clearance of fentanyl are independent of the dose of opioid between 6.4 to 640 μg kg^{-1} (Murphy et al, 1983). This suggests that saturation of clearance or tissue uptake mechanisms does not occur, even with very large doses of fentanyl.

A prolonged elimination half-time for fentanyl in elderly patients (945 minutes) is due to decreased clearance of the opioid, because volume of distribution is not changed in comparison with younger adults (Bentley *et al,* 1982). This change may reflect age-related reductions in hepatic blood flow, microsomal enzyme activity, or albumin production, as fentanyl is highly bound (84%) to protein. For these reasons, it is likely that a given dose of fentanyl will be effective for a longer period of time in elderly patients than in younger patients. A prolonged elimination half-time of fentanyl has also been observed in patients undergoing abdominal aortic surgery requiring intrarenal aortic cross-clamping (Hudson *et al,* 1986). Somewhat surprising, however, is the failure of cirrhosis of the liver to significantly prolong the elimination half-time of fentanyl (Haberer *et al,* 1982).

Clinical Uses

Fentanyl is used clinically in a wide range of doses. For example, low doses of fentanyl, 1 to 2 μg kg^{-1}, are administered intravenously to provide analgesia. Fentanyl, 2 to 10 μg kg^{-1}, may be administered as an adjuvant to inhaled anesthetics in an attempt to blunt circulatory responses (1) to direct laryngoscopy for intubation of the trachea or (2) to blunt sudden changes in the level of surgical stimulation (Sprigge *et al,* 1982). Large intravenous doses of fentanyl, 50 to 150 μg kg^{-1}, have been used alone to produce general anesthesia. High doses of fentanyl as the sole anesthetic have the advantage of stable hemodynamics owing principally to the (1) lack of direct myocardial depressant effects, (2) absence of histamine release, and (3) suppression of the stress responses to surgery (Stanley and Webster, 1978). Disadvantages of using fentanyl as the sole anesthetic include (1) failure to prevent responses to painful stimulation at any dose, especially in patients with good left ventricular function, (2) patient awareness, and (3) postoperative depression of ventilation (Hilgenberg, 1981; Sprigge *et al,* 1982; Waller *et al,* 1981; Wynands *et al,* 1983). Fentanyl combined with droperidol is used to produce neuroleptanalgesia (see Chapter 19).

In dogs, maximal analgesic, ventilatory, and cardiovascular effects are present when the plasma concentration of fentanyl is about 30 ng

ml^{-1} (Arndt *et al,* 1984). This confirms that analgesic actions of fentanyl cannot be separated from its effects on ventilation, cardiac output, and heart rate. The fact that all receptor-mediated effects are similar at the same plasma concentration of fentanyl suggests saturation of the opioid receptors.

Side Effects (see also the section entitled Morphine, Side Effects)

Persistent or recurrent depression of ventilation owing to fentanyl is a potential postoperative problem (Fig. 3-13) (Becker *et al,* 1976). Secondary peaks in plasma concentrations of fentanyl and morphine have been attributed to sequestration of fentanyl in acidic gastric fluid (*i.e.,* ion trapping). Sequestered fentanyl could then be reabsorbed from the more alkaline small intestine back into the circulation to cause an elevation of the plasma concentration of opioid and a recurrence of depression of ventilation (Stoeckel *et al,* 1979). This, however, may not be the mechanism for the secondary peak of fentanyl, because any of the absorbed opioid from the gastrointestinal tract or

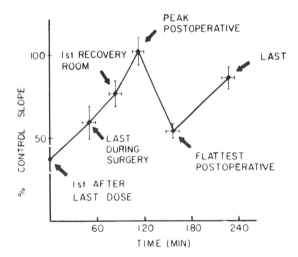

FIGURE 3-13. Recurrent fentanyl-induced depression of ventilation is evidenced by changes in the slope of the carbon dioxide ventilatory response curve. Mean ± SE. (From Becker LD, Paulson BA, Miller RD, Severinghaus JW, Eger EI. Biphasic respiratory depression after fentanyl-droperidol or fentanyl alone used to supplement nitrous oxide anesthesia. Anesthesiology 1976;44:291–6. Reproduced by permission of the authors and publisher.)

skeletal muscle as evoked by movement associated with transfer to the recovery room would be subject to extensive first-pass hepatic metabolism (Bentley *et al*, 1982). An alternative explanation for the secondary peak of fentanyl is washout of the opioid from the lung as ventilation to perfusion relationships are reestablished in the postoperative period.

In comparison with morphine, fentanyl, even in large doses (50 μg kg^{-1}), does not evoke the release of histamine (Fig. 3-9) (Rosow *et al*, 1982). As a result, dilatation of venous capacitance vessels leading to hypotension and the need for increased amounts of intravenous fluids is less likely. Bradycardia is more prominent with fentanyl than with morphine and may lead to occasional decreases in blood pressure and cardiac output (Bennett and Stanley, 1979). An anaphylactic reaction during anesthesia associated with a positive intradermal skin test to fentanyl has been reported (Bennett *et al*, 1986).

High doses of fentanyl, like other opioid agonists, can result in skeletal muscle rigidity, especially in truncal areas. This skeletal muscle spasm may be so severe that adequate ventilation of the lungs is not possible.

Fentanyl causes a progressive slowing of the EEG. High doses of fentanyl have been alleged to produce central nervous system stimulation, but a cause-and-effect relationship has not been established (Rao *et al*, 1982; Safwat and Daniel, 1983). Indeed, plasma concentrations of fentanyl as high as 1750 ng ml^{-1} following bolus administration of 150 μg kg^{-1} do not produce EEG evidence of seizure activity (Murkin *et al*, 1984). Previous reports may have misinterpreted nonpurposeful skeletal muscle movement produced by rapid infusion of fentanyl as seizure activity rather than as a variant of opioid-induced skeletal muscle rigidity.

Sufentanil

Sufentanil is a thiamyl analog of fentanyl. The analgesic potency of sufentanil is 5 to 10 times that of fentanyl, which parallels the greater affinity of sufentanil for opioid receptors compared with that of fentanyl (Stahl *et al*, 1977). An important distinction from fentanyl is the 1000-fold difference between the analgesic dose of sufentanil and the dose that produces seizures in animals (deCastro

et al, 1979). This difference is 160-fold for fentanyl and may be important when large doses of opioid agonists are used to produce anesthesia. Indeed, sufentanil may be capable of achieving a greater depth of anesthesia than other opioid agonists (see the section entitled Anesthetic Requirements).

Theoretically, the greater potency and more rapid onset of action of sufentanil compared with fentanyl will intensify specific opioid effects and reduce the likelihood or magnitude of side-effects. Indeed, the incidence of tachycardia and hypertension in response to sternotomy may be less in the presence of sufentanil than with other opioids, including fentanyl (deLange *et al*, 1982); Flacke *et al*, 1985). This, however, has not been a consistent observation (Rolly *et al*, 1979; Sebel and Bovill, 1982). Bradycardia produced by sufentanil may be sufficient to decrease cardiac output (Sebel and Bovill, 1982). As observed with other opioids, sufentanil causes a decrease in cerebral metabolic requirements for oxygen, and cerebral blood flow is reduced (Keykhah *et al*, 1985).

Supplementation of nitrous oxide with sufentanil, but not fentanyl or morphine, is associated with plasma concentrations of norepinephrine that remain below awake levels. Although sufentanil prevents the endocrine and metabolic responses to surgery before cardiopulmonary bypass, even large doses (20 μg kg^{-1}) of this opioid do not prevent these responses during or after cardiopulmonary bypass (Bovill *et al*, 1983). As observed with fentanyl, delayed depression of ventilation has also been described following the administration of sufentanil (Chang and Fish, 1985).

Pharmacokinetics

The elimination half-time of sufentanil (148 – 164 minutes) is intermediate between that of fentanyl (185 – 219 minutes) and alfentanil (70 – 98 minutes) (Table 3-3) (Bovill *et al*, 1984). A high tissue affinity is consistent with the lipophilic nature of sufentanil, which has a partition coefficient of 1754 compared with 816 for fentanyl. This high lipid solubility of sufentanil permits rapid penetrance of the blood – brain barrier and onset of central nervous system effects. A rapid redistribution to inactive tissue sites terminates the effect of small doses, but a cumulative drug effect can accompany a large dose or repeated doses of sufentanil.

Extensive protein binding of sufentanil (92.5%) compared with fentanyl (84%) contributes to a smaller volume of distribution characteristic of sufentanil. Binding to α_1-acid glycoprotein constitutes a principal proportion of the total plasma protein binding of sufentanil. Levels of alpha-1 acid glycoprotein vary over a threefold range in healthy volunteers and are increased after surgery, which would result in a decrease in the plasma free fraction of sufentanil (Fremstad *et al*, 1976; Piafsky and Borga, 1977).

In elderly patients, the clearance of sufentanil is decreased, but elimination half-time is not prolonged, reflecting a reduced volume of distribution (*e.g.*, total volume to be cleared is less) (Matteo *et al*, 1986). Nevertheless, a prolonged effect of sufentanil in elderly patients occurs, suggesting that the initial concentration gradient between the plasma and brain may be important in determining the duration of action of this opioid in persons in this age-group.

METABOLISM. Sufentanil is rapidly metabolized in animals by N-dealkylation at the piperidine nitrogen and by O-demethylation (Weldon *et al*, 1985). The products of N-dealkylation are pharmacologically inactive, whereas desmethyl sufentanil from O-demethylation has about 10% of the activity of sufentanil. Less than 1% of an administered dose of sufentanil appears unchanged in the urine. Indeed, high lipid solubility of sufentanil results in maximal renal tubular reabsorption of free drug as well as its enhanced access to hepatic microsomal enzymes. Extensive hepatic extraction means that clearance of sufentanil will be sensitive to changes in hepatic blood flow but not to alterations in the drug-metabolizing capacity of the liver.

Sufentanil metabolites are excreted almost equally in urine and feces, with 30% appearing as conjugates, presumably conjugates of desmethyl sufentanil. The production of a possibly active metabolite and the substantial amount of conjugated metabolite formation imply the possible importance of normal renal function necessary for the clearance of sufentanil. Indeed, prolonged depression of ventilation in association with an abnormally elevated plasma concentration of sufentanil has been observed in a patient with chronic renal failure (Waggum *et al*, 1985).

Alfentanil

Alfentanil is an analog of fentanyl that is less potent ($1/5 – 1/10$) and has one-third the duration of action of the parent opioid (Bovill *et al*, 1982). The onset of action of alfentanil after intravenous administration is 1 to 2 minutes in contrast to 5 to 6 minutes for fentanyl. This rapid onset of action is a result of the low pKa of alfentanil, such that nearly 90% of the drug exists in the nonionized form at physiologic pH. It is the nonionized fraction that readily crosses the blood – brain barrier. The short duration of action of alfentanil is a result of both redistribution to inactive tissue sites and hepatic metabolism by pathways identical to those described for sufentanil (see the section entitled Sufentanil). This termination of effect by redistribution of alfentanil is similar to the redistribution responsible for lowering the plasma concentrations of fentanyl and thiopental. Unlike thiopental or fentanyl, however, continuous infusion or repeated doses of alfentanil do not result in a significant cumulative drug effect.

Pharmacokinetics

The volume of distribution of alfentanil is four times smaller than that of fentanyl (Table 3-3) (Camu *et al*, 1982; Stanski and Hug, 1982). This reduced tissue accumulation of alfentanil (*e.g.*, smaller volume of distribution) compared with fentanyl reflects lower lipid solubility and greater plasma protein binding (alfentanil 92% and fentanyl 84%). Despite this lesser lipid solubility, penetration of the blood – brain barrier by alfentanil is rapid because of its high degree of nonionization at physiologic pH.

The elimination half-time of alfentanil is 70 to 98 minutes compared with 185 to 219 minutes for fentanyl (Table 3-3)(Camu *et al*, 1982). Metabolism of alfentanil in the liver to inactive metabolites is extensive, as evidenced by recovery of less than 1% of the drug unchanged in the urine. Efficiency of hepatic metabolism is emphasized by elimination of about 96% of alfentanil from the plasma within 60 minutes following its injection.

The elimination half-time of alfentanil is increased to 219 minutes in patients with cirrhosis of the liver (Ferrier *et al*, 1985). In addition, the plasma free fraction of alfentanil is increased in patients with cirrhosis of the liver. Since alfentanil is principally bound to alpha-1 acid glycoprotein and the plasma concentration of this protein is not altered by liver disease, it is presumed that the increased free fraction of alfentanil reflects an alteration of binding sites on this protein in patients with severe liver dysfunction. The combination of prolonged elimination half-time and an increased plasma free fraction of alfentanil could theoretically result in a sustained or exaggerated effect of this opioid in patients with cirrhosis of the liver.

Clinical Uses

The pharmacologic effects of alfentanil and fentanyl appear to parallel their plasma concentrations more closely than do the effects of morphine and meperidine. This, plus the rapid onset and short duration of action, makes alfentanil acceptable for producing induction of anesthesia (Nauta *et al,* 1982). For example, alfentanil 150 to 300 μg kg^{-1} administered rapidly intravenously produces unconsciousness in about 45 seconds. Furthermore, this induction of anesthesia can be followed by a continuous intravenous infusion of alfentanil, 25 to 150 μg kg^{-1}hr^{-1}, combined with an inhaled drug for maintenance of anesthesia, even for prolonged surgical procedures without a significant cumulative drug effect (Ausems *et al,* 1983). Unlike other opioids, supplemental doses of alfentanil seem to be more likely to reduce blood pressure that is elevated following painful stimulation. Alfentanil elevates biliary tract pressures similarly to fentanyl, but the duration of this increase is shorter than that produced by fentanyl (Hynynen *et al,* 1986).

Phenoperidine

Phenoperidine is chemically related to meperidine, being about 100 times more potent as an analgesic. Its side effects, including nausea, vomiting, and depression of ventilation, resemble meperidine. About 50% of an administered dose of phenoperidine appears unchanged in the urine. The remainder is metabolized to meperidine and then to meperidinic acid, which appears in the urine.

Codeine

Codeine is the result of the substitution of a methyl group for the hydroxyl group on carbon 3 of morphine (Fig. 3-1). The presence of this methyl group limits first-pass hepatic metabolism and accounts for the efficacy of codeine when administered orally.

Pharmacokinetics

The elimination half-time of codeine following oral or intramuscular administration is 3 to 3.5 hours. About 10% of administered codeine is demethylated in the liver to morphine. Indeed, codeine has a low affinity for opioid receptors and its analgesic effect may be caused by its conversion to morphine. The remaining codeine is demethylated to inactive norcodeine, conjugated or excreted unchanged by the kidneys. The plasma concentration of codeine has not been correlated with its analgesic effect.

Clinical Uses

Codeine is an effective antitussive at oral doses of 15 mg. Maximal analgesia, equivalent to that produced by 650 mg of aspirin, occurs with 60 mg of codeine. When administered intramuscularly, codeine, 120 mg, is equivalent in analgesic effect to 10 mg of morphine. Most often, codeine is included in medications as an antitussive or is combined with nonopioid analgesics for the treatment of mild to moderate pain.

Side Effects

Codeine produces minimal sedation, nausea, vomiting, and constipation. Dizziness may occur in ambulatory patients. Codeine, even in large doses, is unlikely to produce apnea. Depression of ventilation that does accompany administration of codeine is readily antagonized by naloxone. Intravenous administration of codeine is not recommended, because histamine-induced hypotension can occur. The histamine-releasing potency of codeine appears to be even greater than that of morphine. Physical dependence liability of codeine appears to be less than that of morphine and occurs only rarely after oral analgesic use.

Dextromethorphan

Dextromethorphan is equal in potency to codeine as an antitussive but lacks analgesic or physical dependency properties. Unlike codeine, this drug rarely produces drowsiness or gastrointestinal disturbances.

Hydromorphone

Hydromorphone is a derivative of morphine that is about eight times as potent as morphine but has a slightly shorter duration of action. This opioid produces somewhat more sedation and evokes less euphoria than morphine. Administered orally, the analgesic potency of hydromorphone is about one-fifth that observed after intramuscular injection. The uses and side effects of hydromorphone are the same as those of morphine.

Oxymorphone

Oxymorphone is the result of the addition of an hydroxyl group to hydromorphone. It is about 10 times as potent as morphine and seems to cause more nausea and vomiting. Physical dependence liability is great.

Methadone

Methadone is a synthetic opioid agonist that produces anlagesia and is highly effective by the oral route (Fig. 3-14). In terms of total analgesic activity, methadone administered orally is about 50% as effective as the same dose administered intramuscularly.

Pharmacokinetics

Methadone is highly bound to plasma and tissue proteins, including the brain. Gradual release from these sites serves to maintain plasma concentrations of methadone. Indeed, the elimination half-time of methadone is about 35 hours (Gourlay *et al,* 1982). Methadone is metabolized in the liver to inactive substances that are excreted in the urine and bile with small amounts of unchanged drug.

Clinical Uses

The efficient oral absorption and prolonged duration of action of methadone render this an attractive drug for suppression of withdrawal symptoms in physically dependent persons such as heroin addicts. Methadone can substitute for morphine in addicts at about one-fourth the dosage. Controlled withdrawal using methadone is milder and less acute than that from morphine. Administered intravenously, methadone, 20 mg, produces postoperative analgesia lasting more than 24 hours (Gourlay *et al,* 1982).

Side Effects

In equal analgesic doses, the pattern and incidence of side effects produced by methadone and morphine are similar. For example, methadone produces depression of ventilation, miosis, antitussive effects, decreased peristaltic activity, and biliary tract spasm. Its sedative actions and euphoric effects seem to be less than those produced by morphine. Methadone-induced miosis is less prominent than that caused by morphine, and the addict develops complete tolerance to this action.

Propoxyphene

Propoxyphene is structurally similar to methadone and binds to opioid receptors. Doses of 90 to 120 mg of propoxyphene produce analgesia and central nervous system effects similar to those produced by 60 mg of codeine and 600 mg of aspirin (Fig. 3-15). Indeed, naloxone antagonizes the pharmacologic effects of propoxyphene. The only clinical use of propoxyphene is treatment of mild to moderate pain that is not adequately relieved by aspirin. Propoxyphene does not possess antipyretic or anti-inflammatory effects, and antitussive activity is not significant.

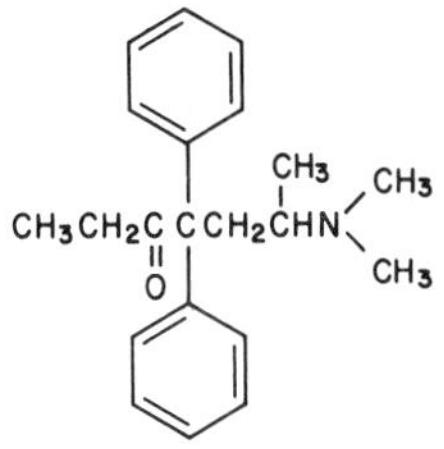

FIGURE 3-14. Methadone.

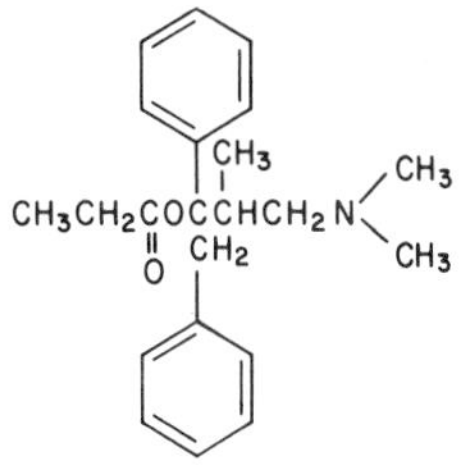

FIGURE 3-15. Propoxyphene.

Pharmacokinetics

Propoxyphene is completely absorbed after oral administration, but because of extensive first-pass hepatic metabolism (30%–70% of the absorbed drug), the systemic availability is greatly reduced. Metabolism of propoyxphene is by demethylation to yield norpropoxyphene, which is slowly excreted in the urine. The elimination half-time of propoxyphene following oral administration is about 14.6 hours (Gram *et al*, 1979).

Side Effects

The most common side effects following propoxyphene administration are vertigo, sedation, nausea, and vomiting. Propoxyphene is about one third as potent as codeine in depressing ventilation (Bellville and Seed, 1968). Overdose is complicated by seizures and depression of ventilation.

Abrupt discontinuation of chronically administered propoxyphene results in a mild withdrawal syndrome. The incidence of abuse of propoxyphene is similar to that of codeine. Intravenous administration of propoxyphene produces severe damage to veins, which limits abuse by this route. Administration of propoxyphene in combination with alcohol and other central nervous system depressants is responsible for excessive drug depression.

Heroin

Heroin is an synthetic opioid produced by acetylation of morphine (*e.g.*, diacetylmorphine). When administered parenterally, heroin acts markedly different from morphine. For example, there is rapid penetration of heroin into the brain where it is hydrolyzed to the active metabolites monoacetylmorphine and morphine. This unique rapid entrance into the central nervous system is most likely caused by the lipid solubility and chemical structure of heroin. Compared with morphine, parenteral heroin has (1) a more rapid onset, (2) lack of nausea, and (3) greater potential for physical dependency. This high physical dependency liability is the reason that heroin is not available in the United States (Angell, 1984; Mondzac, 1984).

OPIOID AGONIST–ANTAGONISTS

Opioid agonist–antagonists include pentazocaine, butorphanol, nalbuphine, buprenorphine, nalorphine, bremazocine, and dezocine (Fig. 3-16). These drugs lack the efficacy of pure agonists that is required for use during anesthesia. Antagonist properties of these drugs can attenuate the efficacy of subsequently administered opioid agonists. Side-effects are similar to those of pure agonists, and, in addition, these drugs may cause

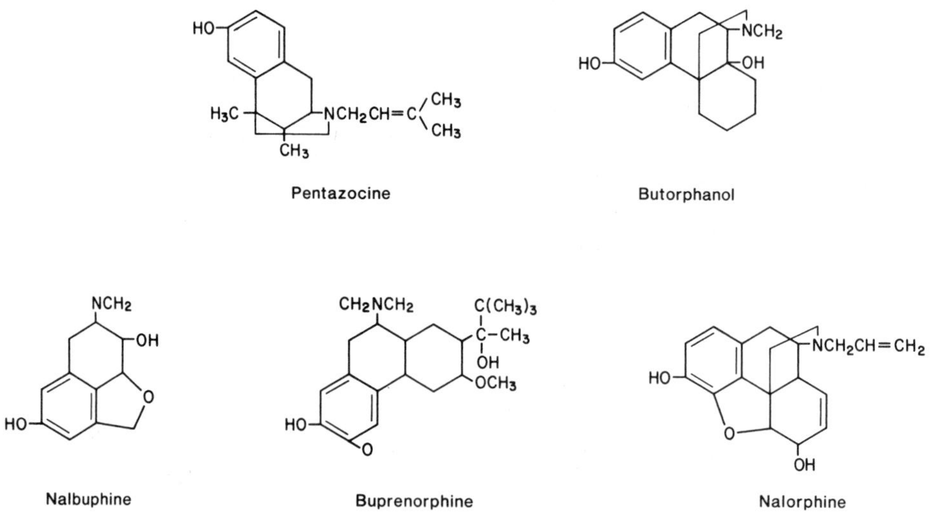

Pentazocine

Butorphanol

Nalbuphine

Buprenorphine

Nalorphine

FIGURE 3-16. Opioid agonists–antagonists.

dysphoric reactions. Advantages of opioid agonist–antagonists are the ability to produce analgesia with limited depression of ventilation and a low potential to produce physical dependence. Furthermore, these drugs have a ceiling-effect such that increasing doses do not produce additional responses. This ceiling-effect on depression of ventilation, however, is often accompanied by an equally low ceiling-effect for analgesia and ability to reduce anesthetic requirements (see the section entitled Anesthetic Requirements).

Pentazocine

Pentazocine is a benzomorphan derivative that possesses opioid agonist actions as well as weak antagonist actions. It is presumed to exert its agonist effects at delta and kappa receptors. Concomitant opioid antagonist activity is weak, being only about one-fifth as potent as nalorphine. Nevertheless, antagonist effects of pentazocine are sufficient to precipitate withdrawal symptoms when administered to patients who have been receiving opioids on a regular basis (Beaver et al, 1966). The agonist effects of pentazocine are antagonized by naloxone. Indeed, physical dependence to pentazocine can be demonstrated by abrupt withdrawal precipitated by naloxone.

Pharmacokinetics

Pentazocine is well absorbed after oral or parenteral administration. First-pass hepatic metabolism is extensive, with only about 20% of an oral dose entering the circulation (Ehrnebo et al, 1977). Metabolism of pentazocine occurs by oxidation of terminal methyl groups, and resulting inactive glucuronide conjugates are excreted in the urine. An estimated 5% to 25% of an administered dose of pentazocine is excreted unchanged in the urine, and less than 2% undergoes biliary excretion. The elimination half-time is 2 to 3 hours (Berkowitz et al, 1969).

Clinical Uses

Pentazocine, 10 to 30 mg intramuscularly or 50 mg orally, is used most often for the relief of moderate pain. An oral dose of 50 mg is equivalent in analgesic potency to 60 mg of codeine. Pentazocine is useful for treatment of chronic pain when there is a high risk of physical dependence.

Lipid solubility of pentazocine makes it a useful drug for epidural administration to produce analgesia (Kalia et al, 1983). Indeed, the onset of analgesia after epidural placement of pentazocine, 0.3 mg kg^{-1}, is rapid (3 min) compared with that of morphine, but the duration of action is shorter (10.6 hr).

Side Effects

The most common side effect of pentazocine is sedation, followed by diaphoresis and dizziness. Sedation is prominent following epidural placement of pentazocine, presumably reflecting activation of kappa receptors. Nausea and vomiting are less common than with morphine. Dysphoria, including fear of impending death, is associated with high doses of pentazocine. This tendency to dysphoria limits the physical dependence liability of pentazocine. Pentazocine produces a rise in plasma concentrations of catecholamines, which may account for increases in heart rate, systemic blood pressure, pulmonary artery blood pressure, and left ventricular end-diastolic pressure that accompany administration of this drug (Lee et al, 1976). An intramuscular pentazocine dose of 20 to 30 mg produces analgesia, sedation, and depression of ventilation similar to 10 mg of morphine. Increasing the intramuscular dose above 30 mg does not produce proportionate increases in these responses (Engineer and Jennett, 1972). Elevation of biliary tract pressure is less than that produced by equal analgesic doses of morphine, meperidine, or fentanyl (Economou and Ward-McQuaid, 1971; Radnay et al, 1980). Pentazocine crosses the placenta and may cause fetal depression. In contrast to morphine, miosis does not occur after administration of pentazocine.

Butorphanol

Butorphanol is an agonist–antagonist opioid that resembles pentazocine. Compared with pentazocine, the agonist effects of butorphanol are about 20 times greater, whereas antagonist actions are 10 to 30 times greater. It is speculated that butorphanol has a (1) low affinity for the mu receptor to produce antagonism, (2) moderate affinity for the kappa receptor to produce analgesia, and (3) minimal affinity for the sigma receptor, so the incidence of dysphoria is low (Houde, 1979).

Butorphanol is rapidly and almost completely

absorbed after intramuscular injection. In postoperative patients, an intramuscular dose of 2 to 3 mg produces analgesia and depression of ventilation similar to 10 mg of morphine. Since butorphanol is available only in the parenteral form, it is better suited for the relief of acute rather than chronic pain. The intraoperative use of butorphanol, like pentazocine, seems to be limited. The elimination half-time of butorphanol is 2.5 to 3.5 hours. Metabolism is principally to inactive hydroxybutorphanol, which is eliminated largely in the bile and to a lesser extent in the urine.

Side Effects

Common side effects of butorphanol include sedation, nausea, and diaphoresis. Dysphoria, reported frequently with other opioid agonist–antagonists, is infrequent following administration of butorphanol. Depression of ventilation is similar to that produced by similar doses of morphine. Like pentazocine, analgesic doses of butorphanol increase systemic blood pressure, pulmonary artery blood pressure, and cardiac output (Lee et al, 1976; Popio et al, 1978). Also, similar to pentazocine, the effects of butorphanol on the biliary and gastrointestinal tract seem to be milder than those produced by morphine. Finally, it may be difficult to use an opioid agonist effectively as an analgesic in the presence of butorphanol. This must be remembered when considering the use of butorphanol, or any other opioid agonist–antagonist, for preoperative medication. Withdrawal symptoms do occur after acute discontinuation of chronic therapy with butorphanol, but symptoms are mild.

Nalbuphine

Nalbuphine is an agonist–antagonist opioid that is related chemically to oxymorphone and naloxone. It is equal in potency as an analgesic to morphine, and it is about one-fourth as potent as nalorphine as an antagonist. Nalbuphine is metabolized in the liver and has an elimination half-time of 3 to 6 hours (Lake et al, 1982). Naloxone reverses the agonist effects of nalbuphine.

Nalbuphine, 10 mg administered intramuscularly, produces analgesia with an onset of effect and duration of action similar to those of morphine. Depression of ventilation is similar to that of morphine until 30 mg of nalbuphine (e.g., about 0.45 mg kg^{-1}) is exceeded, after which no further depression of ventilation occurs (e.g., a ceiling-effect) (Gal et al, 1982). A ceiling-effect for analgesia also accompanies that which occurs for depression of ventilation.

Side Effects

Sedation is the most common side effect, occurring in about one third of patients treated with nalbuphine. The incidence of dysphoria is lower than that with pentazocine or butorphanol but is qualitatively similar and increases in frequency as the dose of nalbuphine is increased. In contrast to pentazocine and butorphanol, nalbuphine does not increase systemic blood pressure, pulmonary artery blood pressure, heart rate, or atrial filling pressures (Lee et al, 1976). For this reason, nalbuphine may be useful to provide sedation with analgesia in patients with heart disease and during cardiac catheterization.

The antagonist effects of nalbuphine are speculated to occur at mu receptors (Jasinski, 1979). As a result, the subsequent use of morphine-like drugs for anesthesia after preoperative medication with nalbuphine may not provide adequate analgesia. Likewise, the efficacy of opioid agonists to provide analgesia may be compromised by nalbuphine, which has previously been administered and found to be inadequate in controlling postoperative pain. Conversely, antagonist effects of nalbuphine at mu receptors could be used to advantage in the postoperative period to reverse lingering ventilatory depressant effects of opioid agonists while still maintaining analgesia. Indeed, intravenous administration of nalbuphine, 20 mg, reverses postoperative depression of ventilation caused by fentanyl but maintains analgesia (Latasch et al, 1984). In another report, nalbuphine, 15 µg kg^{-1} antagonized the postoperative depression of ventilation associated with large doses of fentanyl (average dose 97–120 µg kg^{-1}) administered during cardiac surgery (Moldenhauer et al, 1985). Evidence of renarcotization often occurred in these patients 2 to 3 hours following administration of nalbuphine.

Abrupt withdrawal of nalbuphine after chronic administration produces withdrawal symptoms that are milder than those of morphine and more severe than those of pentazocine. The abuse potential of nalbuphine is low.

Buprenorphine

Buprenorphine is an agonist–antagonist opioid derived from the opium alkaloid thebaine. Its analgesic potency is great, with 0.3 mg administered intramuscularly being equivalent to 10 mg of morphine. Following intramuscular administration, the onset of buprenorphine effect occurs in about 30 minutes, and the duration of action is at least 8 hours, with some effects persisting 24 hours. The prolonged duration of action of buprenorphine may be due to slow dissociation from mu receptors. Antagonist effects of buprenorphine reflect the ability of this drug to displace opioid agonists from the mu receptor. It is estimated that the affinity of buprenorphine for mu receptors is 50 times greater than that of morphine (Rance, 1979). Buprenorphine is effective in relieving moderate to severe pain, such as that present in the postoperative period and that associated with cancer, renal colic, or myocardial infarction (Albert, 1982). Administered intravenously, however, buprenorphine is not adequate for performance of surgery. The high lipid solubility (5 times morphine) and affinity for opioid receptors render this an attractive drug for placement in the epidural space to produce analgesia (Lanz et al, 1984). High lipid solubility limits cephalad spread and the likelihood of delayed depression of ventilation.

There appears to be no direct relationship between plasma concentrations of buprenorphine and its pharmacologic effects. About 96% of the drug is bound to proteins. After intramuscular administration, nearly two thirds of the drug appears unchanged in the bile. The remaining buprenorphine is excreted in the urine as inactive conjugated and dealkylated metabolites (Bullingham et al, 1980).

Side Effects

Side effects of buprenorphine resemble those of other opioid analgesics, with drowsiness occurring in almost 50% of patients. The incidence of nausea and vomiting is 10% to 20%. Buprenorphine produces depression of ventilation similar to morphine, but the duration of this depression may be prolonged and resistant to antagonism with naloxone. In this regard, doxapram may be considered as a pharmacologic method to maintain adequate ventilation of the lungs and preserve analgesia in patients treated with buprenorphine.

The cardiovascular effects of buprenorphine are similar to those produced by morphine. In contrast to many other agonist–antagonist opioids, dysphoria is unlikely to occur in association with administration of this drug. Because of its antagonist properties, buprenorphine can precipitate withdrawal in patients who are physically dependent on morphine. Conversely, withdrawal symptoms in patients who are physically dependent on buprenorphine develop slowly and are of a lesser intensity than those associated with morphine. In this respect, buprenorphine resembles withdrawal from other agonist–antagonist opioids, and the risk of abuse is low.

Nalorphine

Nalorphine is equally potent to morphine as an analgesic but is not clinically useful because of a high incidence of dysphoria. The high incidence of dysphoria may reflect activity of this drug at sigma receptors. Antagonist actions of nalorphine reflect its ability to displace opioid agonists from mu receptors.

Bremazocine

Bremazocine is a benzomorphan derivative that is twice as potent as morphine as an analgesic but in animals does not produce depression of ventilation or evidence of physical dependence (Freye et al, 1983). It is speculated that bremazocine interacts selectively with kappa receptors. Failure of naloxone to reverse sedation produced by bremazocine is further evidence that this opioid is acting at other than mu receptors.

Dezocine

Dezocine is an opioid agonist–antagonist with a greater analgesic potency than morphine. Like other opioid agonist–antagonists, dezocine exhibits a ceiling-effect for depression of ventilation that parallels its analgesic activity (Gal and DiFazio, 1984). The observation that the combination of morphine and dezocine increases analgesic effects may reflect interaction of dezocine at mu and delta receptors (Rowlingson et al, 1983). The interaction at delta receptors serves to facilitate the effect of agonist activity at mu receptors (Vaught *et al*, 1982). The incidence of dysphoria is minimal after administration of dezocine.

OPIOID ANTAGONISTS

Minor changes in the structure of an opioid agonist can convert the drug into an opioid antagonist at one or more opioid receptors. The most common change is substitution of an allyl group for the methyl group on an opioid agonist. For example, naloxone is the N-allyl derivative of oxymorphone (Fig. 3-17).

Naloxone and naltrexone are pure opioid antagonists with no agonist activity that have replaced nalorphine and levorphanol, each of which possesses opioid agonist as well as antagonist activity. Both naloxone and naltrexone have a high affinity for mu and to a lesser extent delta and kappa receptors and can displace opioid agonists from these receptors. Following this displacement, the binding of naloxone or naltrexone does not activate opioid receptors, and antagonism occurs.

Naloxone

Naloxone is selectively used to (1) treat opioid-induced depression of ventilation as may be present in the postoperative period, (2) treat opioid-induced depression of ventilation in the newborn due to maternal administration of drug, (3) facilitate treatment of deliberate opioid overdose, and (4) detect suspected physical dependence.

Naloxone, 1 to 4 μg kg^{-1}, administered intravenously promptly reverses opioid-induced analgesia and depression of ventilation. The short duration of action of naloxone (30–45 min) is presumed to be due to its rapid removal from the brain (Ngai *et al*, 1976). This emphasizes that sup-

plemental doses of naloxone will likely be necessary for sustained antagonism of opioid agonists. Intramuscular supplements of about twice the initial intravenous dose provide sustained plasma concentrations of naloxone (Heisterkamp and Cohen, 1974; Longnecker *et al*, 1973). Likewise, a continuous intravenous infusion of naloxone, 5 μg kg hr^{-1}, prevents depression of ventilation without altering analgesia produced by morphine, 4 mg, placed in the epidural space (Rawal *et al*, 1986).

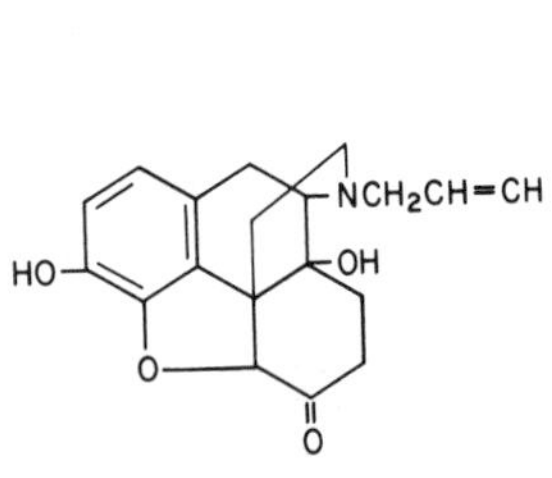

Naloxone is metabolized primarily in the liver by conjugation with glucuronic acid. The elimination half-time is 64 minutes (Table 3-3) (Berkowitz, 1976). Naloxone is absorbed orally, but metabolism during its first-passage through the liver renders it only one-fifth as potent as when administered parenterally.

Side Effects

Antagonism of opioid-induced depression of ventilation is accompanied by an inevitable reversal of analgesia.It may be possible, however, to titrate the dose of naloxone such that depression of ventilation is partially but acceptably antagonized so as to also maintain partial analgesia. Nevertheless, nausea and vomiting and cardiovascular stimulation may accompany even partial reversal of analgesia.

Nausea and vomiting appear to be closely related to the dose and speed of injection of naloxone (Kripke *et al*, 1976; Longnecker *et al*, 1973). Administering naloxone slowly over 2 to 3 minutes rather than as a bolus seems to reduce the incidence of nausea and vomiting. Fortunately, arousal occurs either before or simultaneously with vomiting, which ensures that the patient's protective reflexes have returned and the likelihood of aspiration is minimized.

Cardiovascular stimulation following administration of naloxone manifests as increased sympathetic nervous system activity, presumably reflecting the abrupt reversal of analgesia and the sudden perception of pain. Evidence of this increased sympathetic nervous system activity is tachycardia, hypertension, pulmonary edema, and cardiac dysrhythmias (Flacke *et al*, 1977; Michaelis *et al*, 1974; Tanaka, 1974). Even ventricular fibrillation has occurred following the administration of naloxone and the associated sudden

FIGURE 3-17. Naloxone.

increase in sympathetic nervous system activity (Andree, 1980; Azar and Turndorf, 1979).

Naloxone can easily cross the placenta. For this reason, administration of naloxone to an opioid-dependent parturient may produce acute withdrawal in the newborn.

Role in Treatment of Shock

Stress-induced release of endorphins may contribute to the hypotension and cardiac depression characteristic of shock. Indeed, naloxone produces a dose-related improvement in myocardial contractility and survival in animals subjected to hypovolemic shock and to a lesser extent in those subjected to septic shock (Faden, 1984). The beneficial effects of naloxone in the treatment of shock occur only with doses above 1 mg kg^{-1}. The high doses of naloxone required to produce a therapeutic response in experimental shock suggest that the effects of naloxone are not opioid-receptor mediated or, alternatively, are mediated by opioid receptors other than mu receptors, possibly delta and kappa receptors. Indeed, a selective delta receptor antagonist reverses experimental shock. In addition, high doses of naloxone may exert effects other than antagonism of opioid receptors such as alterations in calcium flux, lipid peroxidation, and inhibition of gamma-aminobutyric acid (Kraynack and Gintautas, 1982).

The site and mechanism of action of naloxone in shock remains unproven. Support for a principal effect in the central nervous system to reverse brain-mediated effects of endogenous opioids is the observation that naloxone at doses that are ineffective systemically reverses shock when administered directly into the ventricular spinal fluid. High doses of corticosteroids may mask the beneficial effects of naloxone because they inhibit the release of beta-endorphin as well as adrenocorticotrophic hormone from the anterior pituitary.

Thyrotropin-releasing hormone, like naloxone, can antagonize the effects of endorphins and, when injected into the ventricular spinal fluid, reverse experimental hypovolemic and septic shock in animals (Holaday *et al*, 1981). Combined with naloxone, the beneficial effects of thyrotropin-releasing hormone in the management of experimental shock in animals is at least additive, and possibly synergistic (Faden, 1984).

Antagonism of General Anesthesia

Reports that high doses of naloxone can partially reverse the effects of inhaled anesthetics suggest a role of endorphins in the production of general anesthesia (Arndt and Freye, 1979; Finck *et al*, 1977) (see Chapter 1). Conversely, even high doses of naloxone do not alter anesthetic requirements in animals (Harper *et al*, 1978). The occasional observation that high doses of naloxone seem to antagonize the depressant effects of inhaled anesthetics may represent drug-induced activation of the cholinergic arousal system in the brain, independent of any interaction with opioid receptors (Kraynack and Gintautas, 1982).

Naltrexone

Naltrexone, like naloxone, is a relatively pure mu receptor antagonist (Martin *et al*, 1973). In contrast to naloxone, naltrexone is highly effective orally, producing sustained antagonism of the effects of opioid agonists for as long as 24 hours. Structurally, naltrexone has a cyclopropylmethyl substitution on the tertiary nitrogen.

Cholecystokinin

Cholecystokinin is an octapeptide secreted by the mucosa of the jejunum that increases the contractility of the gallbladder (see Chapter 54). In addition, this hormone is a central nervous system neurotransmitter that can selectively antagonize analgesic effects produced by morphine when administered systemically or intrathecally (Faris *et al*, 1983). On this basis, it is speculated that cholecystokinin may act as an endogenous opioid antagonist. Indeed, proglumide, a cholecystokinin antagonist, potentiates analgesia produced in animals by morphine and endorphins (Price *et al*, 1985).

ANESTHETIC REQUIREMENTS

The contribution of opioids to total anesthetic requirements can be quantitated by determining the reduction in MAC of a volatile anesthetic in the presence of opioids. Maximal reductions in enflurane MAC of 65% are produced by morphine 5 mg kg^{-1} or a dose of fentanyl that produces a plasma concentration of 30 ng ml^{-1} (Murphy and Hug, 1982a; Murphy and Hug, 1982b). Further increases in the dose of morphine or fentanyl do not produce additional reductions in enflurane MAC, emphasizing a ceiling-effect for these opioids. This casts doubt on the ability of these opioids to reliably provide total amnesia in every patient, even with high doses. Indeed, occasional patients, especially those with minimal underlying disease, are vulnerable to recall of intraoperative events when fentanyl is used as the sole anesthetic (Hilgenberg, 1981). In contrast to morphine and fentanyl, maximal reductions in halothane MAC of greater than 90% are possible when high doses of sufentanil (0.1 μg kg^{-1} min^{-1}) are administered to rats (Fig. 3-18) (Hecker *et al*, 1983). Sufentanil may contribute to an analgesic component of general anesthesia by modulating nociception by way of the release of serotonin (Althaus *et al*, 1985).

Butorphanol and nalbuphine maximally reduce MAC 11% and 8%, respectively, even when the dose of opioid is increased 40-fold (Murphy and Hug, 1982b). Pentazocine reduces anesthetic requirements a maximal 20% (Hoffman and DiFazio, 1970). The ceiling-effect for anesthetic requirements parallels the ceiling-effect for depression of ventilation and is consistent with the clinical impression that even large doses of opioid agonist–antagonists do not produce unconsciousness or prevent patient movement in response to painful stimulation. For this reason, the use of large doses of opioid agonist–antagonists for anesthesia does not seem logical. The exception among the opioid agonist–antagonists may be dezocine, which in high doses (6 mg kg^{-1}) reduces MAC in animals by 50% (Rowlingson *et al*, 1983).

REFERENCES

Aitkenhead AR, Vater M, Acholas K, Cooper CMS, Smith G. Pharmacokinetics of single-dose I.V. morphine in normal volunteers and patients with end-stage renal failure. Br J Anaesth 1984;56:813–8.

Albert LH. Newer potent analgesics. Buprenorphine. Ration Drug Ther 1982;16:4–5.

Althaus JS, Miller ED, Moscicki JC, Hecker BR, DiFazio CA. Analgetic contribution of sufentanil during halothane anesthesia: A mechanism involving serotonin. Anesth Analg 1985;64:857–63.

Andree RA. Sudden death following naloxone administration. Anesth Analg 1980;59:782–4.

Angell M. Should heroin be legalized for the treatment of pain? N Engl J Med 1984;311:529–30.

Armstrong PJ, Berston A. Normeperidine toxicity. Anesth Analg 1986;65:536–8.

Arndt JO, Freye E. Perfusion of naloxone through the fourth cerebral ventricle reverses the circulatory and hypnotic effects of halothane in dogs. Anesthesiology 1979;51:58–63.

Arndt JO, Mikat M, Parasher C. Fentanyl's analgesic, respiratory, and cardiovascular actions in relation to dose and plasma concentration in unanesthetized dogs. Anesthesiology 1984;61:355–61.

Ausems ME, Hug CC, deLange S. Variable rate infusion of alfentanil as a supplement to nitrous oxide anesthesia for general surgery. Anesth Analg 1983;62:982–6.

Austin KL. Stapleton JV, Mather LE. Multiple intramuscular injections — A major source of variability in analgesic response to meperidine. Pain 1980a;8:47–62.

Austin KL, Stapleton JV, Mather LE. Relationship between blood meperidine concentrations and analgesic response. Anesthesiology 1980b;53:460–6.

Azar I, Turndorf H. Severe hypertension and multiple atrial premature contractions following naloxone administration. Anesth Analg 1979;58:524–5.

Bailey DR, Miller ED, Kaplan JA, Rogers PW. The renin–angiotensin–aldosterone system during cardiac surgery with morphine–nitrous oxide anesthesia. Anesthesiology 1975;42:538–44.

Beaumont A, Hughes J. Biology of opioid peptides. Annu Rev Pharmacol Toxicol 1979;19:245–67.

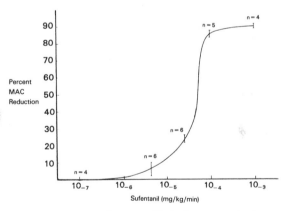

FIGURE 3-18. Reduction of halothane anesthetic requirements (MAC) in animals receiving increasing doses of sufentanil. Mean ± SE. (From Hecker BR, Lake CL, DiFazio CA, Moscicki JC. The decrease of the minimum alveolar anesthetic concentration produced by sufentanil in rats. Anesth Analg 1983;62:987–90. Reproduced by permission of the authors and the International Anesthesia Research Society.)

Beaver WT, Wallenstein SL, Houde RW, Rogers A. A comparison of the analgesia effects of pentazocine and morphine in patients with cancer. Clin Pharmacol Ther 1966;7:740–51.

Becker LD, Paulson BA, Miller RD, Severinghaus JW, Eger EI.Biphasic respiratory depression after fentanyl-droperidol or fentanyl alone used to supplement nitrous oxide anesthesia. Anesthesiology 1976;44:291–6.

Beckett AH, Casey AF. Synthetic analgesics, sterochemical considerations. J Pharm Pharmacol 1954;6:986–1001.

Bellville JW, Forrest WH, Miller E, Brown BW. Influence of age on pain relief from analgesics. JAMA 1971;217:1835–41.

Bellville JW, Seed JC. A comparison of the respiratory depressant effects of dextropropoxyphene and codeine in man. Clin Pharmacol Ther 1968;9:428–34.

Bennett MJ, Anderson LK, McMillan JC, Ebertz JM, Hanifin JM, Hirshman CA. Anaphylactic reaction during anaesthesia associated with positive intradermal skin test to fentanyl. Can Anaesth Soc J 1986;33:75–8.

Bennett GM, Stanley TH. Comparison of the cardiovascular effects of morphine-N_2O and fentanyl-N_2O balanced anesthesia in man. Anesthesiology 1979;51:S102.

Bentley JB, Borel JD, Nenad RE, Gillespie TJ. Age and fentanyl pharmacokinetics. Anesth Analg 1982;61:968–71.

Berkowitz BA. Research review. The relationship of pharmacokinetics to pharmacological activity: Morphine, methadone and naloxone. Clin Pharmacokin 1976;1:219–30.

Berkowitz BA, Asling JH, Shnider SM, Way EL. Relationship of pentazocine plasma levels to pharmacologic activity in man. Clin Pharmacol Ther 1969;10:320–8.

Berkowitz BA, Ngai SH, Yang JC, Hempstead J, Spector S. The disposition of morphine in surgical patients. Clin Pharmacol Ther 1975;17:629–35.

Birt AR, Nickerson M. Generalized flushing of the skin with urticaria pigmentosa. Arch Dermatol 1959;80:311–7.

Bovill JG, Sebel PS, Blackburn CL, Heykants J. The pharmacokinetics of alfentanil (R39209): A new opioid analgesic. Anesthesiology 1982;57:439–43.

Bovill JG, Sebel PS, Blackburn CL, Oei-Lim V, Heykants JJ. The pharmacokinetics of sufentanil in surgical patients. Anesthesiology 1984;61:502–6.

Bovill JG, Sebel PS, Fiolet JWT, Touber JL, Kok K, Philbin DM. The influence of sufentanil on endocrine and metabolic responses to cardiac surgery. Anesth Analg 1983;62:391–7.

Brunk SF, Dell M, Wilson WR. Morphine metabolism in man: Effect of aspirin. Clin Pharmacol Ther 1974;15:283–90.

Bullingham RES, McQuay HJ, Moore A, Bennett MRD. Buprenorphine kinetics. Clin Pharmacol Ther 1980;28:667–72.

Burns JJ, Berger BL, Lief PA, Wollack A, Papper EM, Brodie BB. The physiological disposition and fate of meperidine (Demerol) in man and a method for its estimation in plasma. J Pharmacol Exp Ther 1974;16:667–75.

Camu F, Gepts E, Rucquoi M, Heykants J. Pharmacokinetics of alfentanil in man. Anesth Analg 1982;61:657–61.

Chang J, Fish KJ. Acute respiratory arrest and rigidity after anesthesia with sufentanil: A case report. Anesthesiology 1985;63:710–1.

Cousins MJ, Mather LE. Intrathecal and epidural administration of opioids. Anesthesiology 1984;61:276–310.

deCastro J, van de Water A, Wouters L, Xhonneux R, Reneman R, Kay B. Comparative study of cardiovascular, neurological and metabolic side effects of eight narcotics in dogs. Acta Anaesthesiol Belg 1979;30:5–99.

deLange S, Boscoe MJ, Stanley TH. Comparison of sufentanil-O_2 and fentanyl-O_2 for coronary artery surgery. Anesthesiology 1982;56:112-8.

Devenyi P, Mitwalli A, Graham W. Clonidine therapy for narcotic withdrawal. Can Med Assoc J 1982;127:1009–11.

Don HF, Dieppa RD, Taylor P. Narcotic analgesics in anuric patients. Anesthesiology 1975;42:745–7.

Eckenhoff JE, Oech R. The effects of narcotics and antagonists upon respiration and circulation in man. Clin Pharmacol Ther 1960;1:483–524.

Economou G, Ward-McQuaid JN. A cross-over comparison of the effect of morphine, pethidine, pentazocine on biliary pressure. Gut 1971;12:218–21.

Ehrnebo M, Boreus L, Lonroth U. Bioavailability and first-pass metabolism of oral pentazocine in man. Clin Pharmacol Ther 1977;22:888–92.

Engineer S, Jennett S. Respiratory depression following single and repeated doses of pentazocine and pethidine. Br J Anaesth 1972;44:795–801.

Faden AI. Opiate antagonists and thyrotropin-releasing hormone. I. Potential role in the treatment of shock. JAMA 1984;252:1177–80.

Fahmy JH. Hemodynamics, plasma histamine, and catecholamine concentrations during an anaphylactoid reaction to morphine. Anesthesiology 1981;55:329–31.

Faris PL, Komisaruk BR, Watkins LR, Mayer DJ. Evidence for the neuropeptide cholecystokinin as an antagonist of opiate analgesia. Science 1983;219:310–2.

Ferrier C, Marty J, Bouffard Y, Haberer JP, Levron JC, Duvaldestin P. Alfentanil pharmacokinetics in patients with cirrhosis. Anesthesiology 1985;62:480–4.

Fink AD, Berkowitz BA, Hemstead J, Ngai S. Pharmacokinetics of morphine: Effects of hypercarbia on serum and brain morphine concentrations in the dog. Anesthesiology 1977;47:407–10.

Finck AD, Ngai SH, Berkowitz BA. Antagonism of general anesthesia by naloxone in the rat. Anesthesiology 1977;46:241–5.

Flacke JW, Bloor BC, Kripke BJ, et al. Comparison of morphine, meperidine, fentanyl, and sufentanil in balanced anesthesia: A double-blind study. Anesth Analg 1985;64:897–910.

Flacke JW, Flacke WE, Williams GD. Acute pulmonary edema following naloxone reversal of high-dose morphine anesthesia. Anesthesiology 1977;47:376–8.

Foldes FF, Tarda TAG. Comparative studies with narcotics and narcotic antagonists in man. Acta Anaesthesiol Scand 1965;9:121–38.

Fremstad D, Bergerud K, Haffner JW, Lunde PKN. Increased plasma binding of quinidine after surgery. A preliminary report. Eur J Clin Pharmacol 1976;10:441–4.

Freund FG, Martin WE, Wong KC, Hornbein TF. Abdominal-muscle rigidity induced by morphine and nitrous oxide. Anesthesiology 1973;38:358–62.

Freye E. Cardiovascular effects of high dosages of fentanyl, meperidine and naloxone in dogs. Anesth Analg 1974;53:40-7.

Freye E, Hartung E, Schenk GK. Bremazocine: An opiate that induces sedation and analgesia without respiratory depression. Anesth Analg 1983;62:483–8.

Gal TJ, DiFazio CA. Ventilatory and analgesic effects of dezocine in humans. Anesthesiology 1984;61:716–22.

Gal TJ, DiFazio CA, Moscicki J. Analgesic and respiratory depressant activity of nalbuphine: A comparison with morphine. Anesthesiology 1982;57:367–74.

Gold MS, Pottash AC, Sweeney DR, Kleber HD. Opiate withdrawal using clonidine. A safe, effective and rapid non-opiate treatment. JAMA 1980;243:343–6.

Goldstein A. Opiate receptors. Life Sci 1974;14:615–23.

Gourlay GK, Wilson PR, Glynn CJ. Pharmacodynamics and pharmacokinetics of methadone during the perioperative period. Anesthesiology 1982;57:458–67.

Gram LF, Schou J, Way WL, Helberg J, Bobin ND. d-Propoxyphene kinetics after single oral and intravenous doses in man. Clin Pharmacol Ther 1979;26:473–82.

Guillemin R. Endorphins, brain peptides that act like opiates. N Engl J Med 1977;296:116–8.

Haberer JP, Schoeffler P, Couderc E, Duvaldestin P. Fentanyl pharmacokinetics in anaesthetized patients with cirrhosis. Br J Anaesth 1982;54:1267–70.

Harper MH, Winter PM, Johnson BH, Eger EI. Naloxone does not antagonize general anesthesia in the rat. Anesthesiology 1978;49:3–5.

Hecker BR, Lake CL, DiFazio CA, Moscicki JC, Engle JS. The decrease of the minimum alveolar anesthetic concentration produced by sufentanil in rats. Anesth Analg 1983;62:987–90.

Heisterkamp DV, Cohen PJ. The use of naloxone to antagonize large doses of opiates administered during nitrous oxide anesthesia. Anesth Analg 1974;53:12–8.

Hermens JM, Ebertz JM, Hanifin JM, Hirshman CA. Comparison of histamine release in human skin mast cells induced by morphine, fentanyl and oxymorphone. Anesthesiology 1985;62:124–9.

Hilgenberg JC. Intraoperative awareness during high-dose fentanyl-oxygen anesthesia. Anesthesiology 1981;54:341–3.

Hoffman JC, DiFazio CA. The anesthesia-sparing effect of pentazocine, meperidine, and morphine. Arch Int Pharmacodyn 1970;186:261–8.

Holaday JW, D'Amato R, Faden AI. Thyrotropin-releasing hormone improves cardiovascular function in experimental endotoxic and hemorrhagic shock. Science 1981;213:216–8.

Houde RW. Analgesic effectiveness of the narcotic agonist-antagonists. Br J Clin Pharmacol 1979;7:297S–308S.

Hudson RJ, Thomson IR, Cannon JE, Friesen RM, Meatherall RC. Pharmacokinetics of fentanyl in patients undergoing abdominal aortic surgery. Anesthesiology 1986;64:334–8.

Hug CC, Murphy MR. Tissue redistribution of fentanyl and termination of its effects in rats. Anesthesiology 1981;55:369–75.

Hug CC, Murphy MR, Rigel EP, Olson WA. Pharmacokinetics of morphine injected intravenously into the anesthetized dog. Anesthesiology 1981;54:38–47.

Hughes J, Smith TW, Kosterlitz HW, Fothergill L, Morgan B, Morris H. Identification of two related pentapeptides from the brain with potent opiate agonist activity. Nature 1975;258:577–9.

Hynyen MJ, Turunen MT, Korttila KT. Effects of alfentanil and fentanyl on common bile duct pressure. Anesth Analg 1986;65:370–2.

Jasinski DR. Human pharmacology of narcotic antagonists. Br J Clin Pharmacol 1979;7:287S–90S.

Jones RM, Detmer M, Hill AB, Bjoraker DG, Pandit U. Incidence of choledochoduodenal sphincter spasm during fentanyl-supplemented anesthesia. Anesth Analg 1981;60:638–40.

Jones RM, Fiddian-Green R, Knight PR. Narcotic-induced choledochoduodenal sphincter spasm reversed by glucagon. Anesth Analg 1980;59:946–7.

Kalia PK, Madan R, Saksema R, Batra RK, Gode GR. Epidural pentazocine for postoperative pain relief. Anesth Analg 1983;62:949–50.

Keykhah MM, Smith DS, Carlsson C, Safo Y, Englebach I, Harp JR. Influence of sufentanil on cerebral metabolism and circulation in the rat. Anesthesiology 1985;63:274–7.

Klotz U, McHorse TS, Wilkinson GR. Schenker S. The effects of cirrhosis on the disposition and elimination of meperidine in man. Clin Pharmacol Ther 1974;16:667–75.

Korinek AM, Languille M, Bonnet F, *et al*. Effect of postoperative extradural morphine on ADH secretion. Br J Anaesth 1985;57:407–11.

Koska AJ, Kramer WG, Romagnoli A, Keats AS, Sabawala PB. Pharmacokinetics of high-dose meperidine in surgical patients. Anesth Analg 1981;60:8-11.

Kraynack BJ, Gintautas JG. Naloxone: analeptic action unrelated to opiate receptor antagonism? Anesthesiology 1982;56:251–3.

Kripke BJ, Finck AJ, Shah N, Snow JC. Naloxone antagonism after narcotic supplemented-anesthesia. Anesth Analg 1976;55:800–5.

Lake CL, DiFazio CA, Duckworth EN, Moscicki JC, Engle JS, Durbin CG. High performance liquid chromatographic analysis of plasma levels of nalbuphine in cardiac surgical patients. J Chromatogr 1982; 233:410–6.

Lang DW, Pilon RN. Naloxone reversal of morphine-induced biliary colic. Anesth Analg 1980;59:619–20.

Lanz E, Simko G, Theiss D, Glocke MH. Epidural buprenorphine—a double-blind study of postoperative analgesia and side effects. Anesth Analg 1984;63:593–8.

Larson CP, Mazze RI, Cooperman LH, Wollman H. Effects of anesthetics on cerebral, renal, and splanchnic circulations: Recent developments. Anesthesiology 1974;41:169–81.

Latasch L, Probst S, Dudziak R. Reversal by nalbuphine of respiratory depression caused by fentanyl. Anesth Analg 1984;63:814–6.

Lee G, DeMaria A, Amsterdam EA, *et al*. Comparative effects of morphine, meperidine and pentazocine on cardiocirculatory dynamics in patients with acute myocardial infarction. Am J Med 1976; 60:949–55.

Levy JH, Rockoff MA. Anaphylaxis to meperidine. Anesth Analg 1982;61:301–3.

Leysen JE, Tollenaere JP, Koch MHJ, Laduron P. Differentiation of opiate and neurolept receptor binding in rat brain. Eur J Pharmacol 1977;43:253–67.

Longnecker DE, Grazis PA, Eggers GWN. Naloxone for antagonism of morphine induced respiratory depression. Anesth Analg 1973;52:447–53.

Lowenstein E, Hollowell P, Levine FH, Daggett WM, Austen WG, Laver MB. Cardiovascular responses to large doses of intravenous morphine in man. N Engl J Med 1969;281:1389–93.

Lowenstein E, Whiting RB, Bittar DA, Sanders CA, Powell WJ. Locally and neurally mediated effects of morphine on skeletal muscle vascular resistance. J Pharmacol Exp Ther 1972;180:359–67.

Martin WR. History and development of mixed opioid agonists, partial agonists and antagonists. Br J Clin Pharmacol 1979;7:273S–9S.

Martin WR, Jasinski DR, Mansky PA. Naltrexone, an antagonist for the treatment of heroin dependence. Arch Gen Psychiatry 1973;28:748–91.

Mather LE, Tucker GT, Pflug AE, Lindop MJ, Wilkerson C. Meperidine kinetics in man. Clin Pharmacol Ther 1975;17:21–30.

Matteo RS, Ornstein E, Young WL, Schwartz AE, Port M, Chang WJ. Pharmacokinetics of sufentanil in the elderly. Anesth Analg 1986;65:S94.

Maze M. Clinical implications of membrane receptor function in anesthesia. Anesthesiology 1981;51:160-71.

McCammon RL, Viegas OJ, Stoelting RK, Dryden GE. Naloxone reversal of choledochoduodenal sphincter spasm associated with narcotic administration. Anesthesiology 1978;48:437.

McClain DA, Hug CC. Intravenous fentanyl kinetics. Clin Pharmacol Ther 1980;22:106–14.

McDermott R, Stanley TH. The cardiovascular effects of low concentrations of nitrous oxide during anesthesia. Anesthesiology 1974;41:89–91.

Michaelis LL, Hickey PR, Clark TA, Dixon WM. Ventricular irritability associated with the use of naloxone. Ann Thorac Surg 1974;18:608–14.

Moldenhauer CC, Roach GW, Finlayson DC, *et al*. Nalbuphine antagonism of ventilatory depression following high-dose fentanyl anesthesia. Anesthesiology 1985;62:647–50.

Mondzac AM. Compassionate pain relief: Is heroin the answer? N Engl J Med 1984;311:530–5.

Morgan D, Moore G, Thomas J, Triggs E. Disposition of meperidine in pregnancy. Clin Pharmacol Ther 1978;23:288–95.

Mule SJ. Physiological dispositions of narcotic agonists and antagonists. In: Clouet DH. Narcotic drugs: Biochemical pharmacology. New York. Plenum Press, 1971.

Murkin JM, Moldenhauer CC, Hug CC, Epstein CM. Absence of seizures during induction of anesthesia with high dose fentanyl. Anesth Analg 1984;63:489–94.

Murphy MR, Hug CC. Pharmacokinetics of intravenous morphine in patients anesthetized with enflurane-nitrous oxide. Anesthesiology 1981;54:187–92.

Murphy MR, Hug CC. The anesthetic potency of fentanyl in terms of its reduction of enflurane MAC. Anesthesiology 1982a;57:485–8.

Murphy MR, Hug CC. The enflurane sparing effect of morphine, butorphanol, and nalbuphine. Anesthesiology 1982b;57:489–92.

Murphy MR, Hug CC, McClain DD. Dose-dependent pharmacokinetics of fentanyl. Anesthesiology 1983;59:537–40.

Murphy MR, Olson WA, Hug CC. Pharmacokinetics of ^{3}H-fentanyl in the dog anesthetized with enflurane. Anesthesiology 1979;50:13–9.

Nauta J, deLange S, Koopman D, Spierdijk J, vanKleff J, Stanley TH. Anesthetic induction with alfentanil: a new short-acting narcotic analgesic. Anesth Analg 1982;61:267–72.

Ngai SH, Berkowitz BA, Yang YC, Hempstead J, Spector S. Pharmacokinetics of naloxone in rats and man. Basis for its potency and short duration of action. Anesthesiology 1976;44:398–401.

Papper S, Papper EM. The effects of pre-anesthetic, anesthetic, and post-operative drugs on renal function. Clin Pharmacol Ther 1964;5:205–15.

Philbin DM, Moss J, Akins CW, et al. The use of H_1 and H_2 histamine antagonists with morphine anesthesia: a double blind study. Anesthesiology 1981; 55:292–6.

Philbin DM, Wilson NE, Sokoloshi I, Coggins C. Radioimmunoassay of antidiuretic hormone during morphine anesthesia. Can Anaesth Soc J 1976;23: 290–5.

Piafsky KM, Borga O. Plasma protein binding of basic drugs. II. Importance of alpha₁-acid glycoprotein for interindividual variation. Clin Pharmacol Ther 1977;22:545–9.

Pomeranz B, Chiu D. Naloxone blockade of acupuncture analgesia: endorphin implicated. Life Sci 1976;19:1757–62.

Popio KA, Jackson DH, Ross AM, Schreiner BF, Yu PN. Hemodynamic and respiratory effects of morphine and butorphanol. Clin Pharmacol Ther 1978;23:281–7.

Priano LL, Vatner SF. Generalized cardiovascular and regional hemodynamic effects of meperidine in conscious dogs. Anesth Analg 1981;60:649–54.

Price DD, von der Gruen A, Miller J, Rafii A, Price C. Potentiation of systemic morphine analgesia in humans by proglumide, a cholecystokinin antagonist. Anesth Analg 1985;64:801–6.

Radnay PA, Brodman E, Mankikar D, Duncalf D. The effect of equi-analgesic doses of fentanyl, morphine, meperidine, and pentazocine on common bile duct pressure. Anaesthetist 1980;29:26–9.

Rance MJ. Animal and molecular pharmacology of mixed agonist-antagonist analgesic drugs. Br J Clin Pharmacol 1979;7:281S–6S.

Rao TLK, Mummaneni N, El-Etr AA. Convulsions: an unusual response to intravenous fentanyl administration. Anesth Analg 1982;61:1020–1.

Rawal N, Schott U, Dahlstrom B et al. Influence of naloxone infusion on analgesia and respiratory depression following epidural morphine. Anesthesiology 1986;64:194–201.

Rolly G, Kay B, Cockx F. A double blind comparison of high doses of fentanyl and sufentanil in man: influence on cardiovascular, respiratory and metabolic parameters. Acta Anaesthesiol Belg 1979;30:247–54.

Rosow CE, Moss J, Philbin DM, Savarese JJ. Histamine release during morphine and fentanyl anesthesia. Anesthesiology 1982;56:93–6.

Rowlinson JC, Moscicki JC, DiFazio CA. Anesthetic potency of dezocine and its interaction with morphine in rats. Anesth Analg 1983;62:899–902.

Safwat AM, Daniel D. Grand mal seizure after fentanyl administration. Anesthesiology 1983;59:78.

Sear J, Moore A, Hunniset A, et al. Morphine kinetics and kidney transplantation: morphine removal is influenced by renal ischemia. Anesth Analg 1985;64:1065–70.

Sebel PS, Bovill JG. Cardiovascular effects of sufentanil anesthesia. Anesth Analg 1982;61:115–9.

Sharma SK, Klee WA, Nirenberg M. Dual regulation of adenylate cyclase for narcotic dependence and tolerance. Proc Natl Acad Sci USA 1976;72:3092–6.

Simon EJ, Hiller JM. The opiate receptors. Annu Rev Pharmacol Toxicol 1978;18:371–94.

Snyder SH. Opiate receptors in the brain. N Engl J Med 1977;296:266–71.

Sokoll MD, Hoyt JL, Gergis SD. Studies in muscle rigidity, nitrous oxide, and narcotic analgesic agents. Anesth Analg 1972;51:16–20.

Sprigge JS, Wynands JE, Whalley DG, et al. Fentanyl infusion anesthesia for aortocoronary bypass surgery: plasma levels and hemodynamic response. Anesth Analg 1982;61:972–8.

Stahl KD, vanBever W, Janssen P, Simon EJ. Receptor affinity and pharmacological potency of a series of narcotic analgesic, anti-diarrheal and neuroleptic drugs. Eur J Pharmacol 1977;46:199–205.

Stanley TH, Bennett GM, Loeser EA, Kawamura R, Sentker CR. Cardiovascular effects of diazepam and droperidol during morphine anesthesia. Anesthesiology 1976;44:255–8.

Stanley TH, Gray NH, Isren-Amaral JH, Patton C. Comparison of blood requirements during morphine and halothane anesthesia for open-heart surgery. Anesthesiology 1974a;41:34–8.

Stanley TH, Gray NH, Bidwai AV, Lordon R. The effects of high dose morphine and morphine plus nitrous oxide on urinary output in man. Can Anaesth Soc J 1974b;21:379–84.

Stanley TH, Webster L. Anesthetic requirements and cardiovascular effects of fentanyl–oxygen and fentanyl–diazepam–oxygen anesthesia in man. Anesth Analg 1978;57:411–6.

Stanski DR, Greenblatt DJ, Lappas DG, Koch-Weser J, Lowenstein E. Kinetics of high dose intravenous morphine in cardiac surgery patients. Clin Pharmacol Ther 1977;19:752–6.

Stanski DR, Hug CC. Alfentanil—a kinetically predictable narcotic analgesic. Anesthesiology 1982; 57:435–8.

Stoeckel H, Hengstmann JH, Schuttler J. Pharmacokinetics of fentanyl as a possible explanation for recurrence of respiratory depression. Br J Anaesth 1979;51:741–5.

Stoelting RK. Influence of barbiturate anesthetic induction on circulatory responses to morphine. Anesth Analg 1977;56:615 – 7.

Stoelting RK, Gibbs PS. Hemodynamic effects of morphine and morphine-nitrous oxide in valvular heart disease and coronary artery disease. Anesthesiology 1973;38:45 – 52.

Strauer BE. Contractile responses to morphine, piritramide, meperidine, and fentanyl: a comparative study of effects on isolated ventricular myocardium. Anesthesiology 1972;37:304 – 10.

Tanaka GY. Hypertensive reaction to naloxone. JAMA 1974;228:25 – 6.

Vaught JL, Rothman RB, Westfall TC. Mu and delta receptors: Their role in analgesia and in the differential effects of opioid peptides on analgesia. Life Sci 1982;30:1443 – 55.

Waggum DC, Cork RC, Weldon ST, Gandolfi AJ, Perry DS. Postoperative respiratory depression and elevated sufentanil levels in a patient in chronic renal failure. Anesthesiology 1985;63:708 – 10.

Waller JL, Hug CC, Nagle DM, Craver JM. Hemodynamic changes during fentanyl oxygen anesthesia for aortocoronary bypass operation. Anesthesiology 1981;55:212 – 7.

Way EL, Adler TK. The pharmacologic implications of the fate of morphine and its surrogates. Pharmacol Rev 1960;12:383 – 446.

Way WL, Costley EC, Way EL. Respiratory sensitivity of the newborn infant to meperidine and morphine. Clin Pharmacol Ther 1965;6:454 – 61.

Weldon ST, Perry DF, Cork RC, Gandolfi AJ. Detection of picogram levels of sufentanil by capillary gas chromatography. Anesthesiology 1985;63:684 – 7.

White PF. Patient-controlled analgesia: A new approach to the management of postoperative pain. Semin Anes 1985;4:255 – 66.

Wynands JE, Wong P, Whalley DG, Sprigge JS, Townsend GE, Patel Y. Oxygen – fentanyl anesthesia in patients with poor left ventricular function: Hemodynamics and plasma fentanyl concentrations. Anesth Analg 1983;62:476 – 82.

Yeh SY, Mitchell CL. Effect of monoamine oxidase inhibitors on formation of morphine glucuronide. Biochem Pharmacol 1972;21:571 – 8.

Zelis R, Mansour EJ, Capone RJ, Mason DT. The cardiovascular effects of morphine: The peripheral capacitance and resistance vessels in human subjects. J Clin Invest 1974;54:1247 – 58.

Barbiturates

INTRODUCTION

In the past, it was common to classify barbiturates as long-, intermediate-, short-, and ultrashort-acting, depending on the perceived duration of action of these drugs. This classsification is no longer recommended, because it becomes misleading if the implication is that the action of these drugs ends abruptly after specified time intervals. This is clearly not the case for barbiturates; residual plasma concentrations and drug effects persist for several hours, even following administration of drugs ("ultrashort-acting") for induction of anesthesia.

COMMERCIAL PREPARATIONS

Barbiturates are prepared commercially as sodium salts that are readily soluble in water or saline to form highly alkaline solutions. For example, the pH of a 2.5% solution of thiopental is 10.5. These highly alkaline solutions are incompatible for mixture with drugs such as opioids, catecholamines, and neuromuscular blocking drugs, which are acidic in solution. The bacteriostatic properties of commercial solutions of barbiturates are due to their highly alkaline pH. Commercial preparations of barbiturates often contain a mixture of 6 parts anhydrous sodium carbonate to prevent precipitation of the insoluble free acid form of the barbiturate by atmospheric carbon dioxide.

Thiopental and thiamylal are usually prepared for clinical use in a 2.5% solution. A 5% solution is not recommended. Methohexital is used most often as a 1% solution. Solutions of barbiturates remain stable at room temperature for up to 2 weeks.

STRUCTURE ACTIVITY RELATIONSHIPS

Barbiturates are any drugs derived from barbituric acid. Barbituric acid, which lacks central nervous system activity, is a cyclic compound obtained by the combination of urea and malonic acid (Fig. 4-1). Barbiturates with sedative – hypnotic properties result from substitutions at the number 2 and 5 carbon atoms of barbituric acid (Fig. 4-2). A barbiturate with a branched chain substitution on the number 5 carbon atom usually has greater hypnotic activity than the corresponding drug with a straight chain. Drugs with a phenyl group in the number 5 carbon position, such as phenobarbital, have enhanced anticonvulsant activity. Sedative and anticonvulsant activities are separate effects of barbiturates (MacDonald and Barker, 1978). A methyl radical on the number 5 carbon atom, as is present with methohexital, confers convulsive activity manifesting as involuntary skeletal muscle movement and hypertonicity.

Barbiturates retaining an oxygen atom on the number 5 carbon of the barbituric acid ring are designated oxybarbiturates. Replacement of this oxygen atom with a sulfur atom results in thiobarbiturates, which are more lipid soluble than oxy-

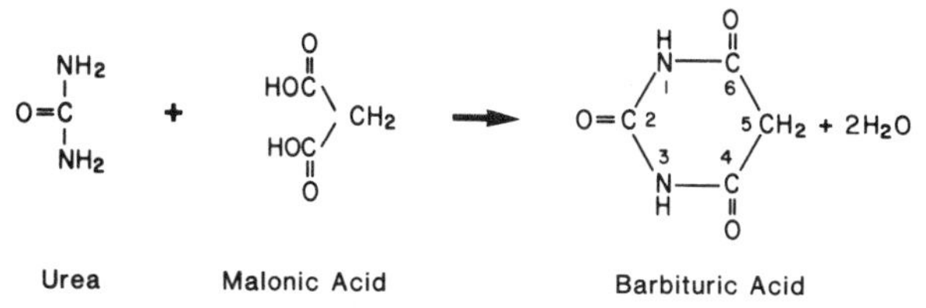

FIGURE 4-1. Barbituric acid is formed by the combination of urea and malonic acid.

barbiturates. In general, a structural change such as sulfuration that increases lipid solubility is associated with greater hypnotic potency and a more rapid onset but shorter duration of action. For example, thiopental has a more rapid onset and a shorter duration of action than its oxygen analog pentobarbital. Thiamylal is the thioanalog of the oxybarbiturate secobarbital. Addition of a methyl group to the nitrogen atom of the barbituric acid ring, as with methohexital, results in a compound that is of short duration.

MECHANISM OF ACTION

Barbiturates depress polysynaptic responses in the central nervous system, probably by means of presynaptic effects, to decrease release of neurotransmitters such as acetylcholine (Richter and Waller, 1977). In addition, barbiturates exert postsynaptic inhibition at membranes upon which gamma-aminobutyric acid (GABA) has an inhibitory action (Fragen and Avram, 1986; Ransom and Barker, 1976). GABA causes an increase in chloride conductance through ion channels resulting in hyperpolarization and, consequently, inhibition of the postsynaptic neuron. Barbiturates may decrease the rate of dissociation of GABA from its receptors and thus increase the duration of GABA-activated ion channel opening. The action of barbiturates at GABA receptor sites suggests similarities with the mechanism of action of benzodiazepines (see Chapter 5). In contrast to benzodiazepines, however, the margin of selectivity of barbiturates at these sites is small, with only slight increases in the barbiturate dose producing nonselective depression in addition to selective synaptic depression. Regardless of the mechanism, barbiturates seem to be uniquely capable of depressing the reticular activating system, which is presumed to be important in the maintenance of wakefulness. Furthermore, brain sensitivity to depressant effects of thiopental does not change in elderly patients compared with that in younger adults (Fig. 4-3) (Homer and Stanski, 1985).

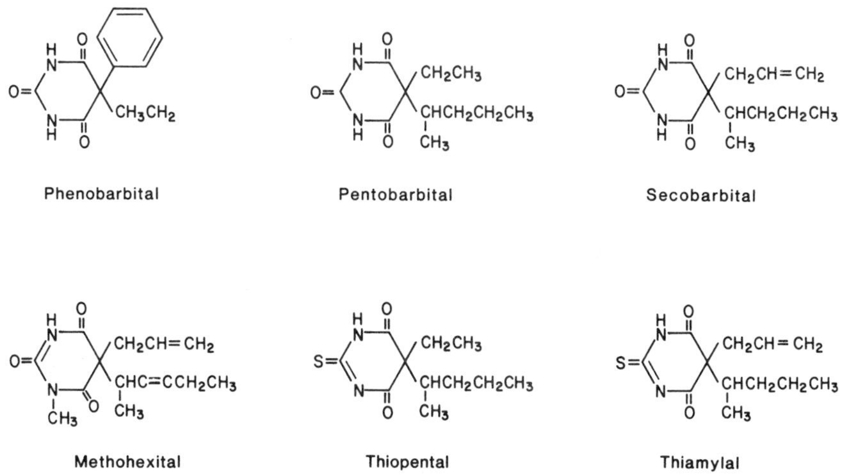

FIGURE 4-2. Barbiturates with sedative–hypnotic properties result from substitutions at the number 2 and 5 carbon atoms of barbituric acid (see Fig. 4-1).

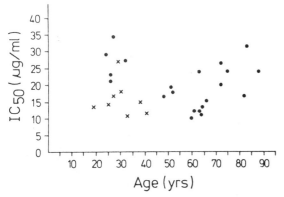

FIGURE 4-3. The plasma concentration of thiopental needed to slow activity on the electroencephalogram 50% (IC_{50}) is independent of age. Blood sampling was either arterial (X) or venous (•). (From Homer TD, Stanski DR. The effect of increasing age on the thiopental disposition and anesthetic requirement. Anesthesiology 1985;62:714–24. Reproduced by permission of the authors and publisher.)

Barbiturates selectively depress transmission in sympathetic nervous system ganglia in concentrations that have no detectable effect on nerve conduction. This effect may contribute to decreases in blood pressure that can accompany intravenous injection of barbiturates or that occur in association with a barbiturate overdose. At the neuromuscular junction, high doses of barbiturates reduce sensitivity of postsynaptic membranes to the depolarizing action of acetylcholine.

PHARMACOKINETICS

Prompt awakening following intravenous administration of thiopental, thiamylal, and methohexital reflects redistribution of these drugs from the brain to inactive tissues (Fig. 4-4) (Brodie *et al,* 1950; Price *et al,* 1960). Ultimately, however, elimination from the body depends almost entirely on metabolism, since less than 1% of these drugs are recovered unchanged in the urine (Breimer, 1976; Ghoneim and Korttila, 1977; Ghoneim and Van Hamme, 1978; Saidman and Eger, 1966).

Protein Binding

Protein binding of barbiturates parallels lipid solubility, and binding to tissues parallels binding to plasma proteins. Thiopental, as a highly lipid-soluble barbiturate, is the most avidly bound to plasma proteins, with binding to albumin ranging from 72% to 86% (Ghoneim *et al,* 1976). The higher percentage of protein binding occurs at lower plasma concentrations of thiopental. Changes in *p*H between 7.35 and 7.5 do not alter the degree of protein binding. Reduced protein binding of thiopental due to displacement from binding sites by other drugs, such as aspirin and phenylbutazone, can lead to enhanced drug effects (Chaplin *et al,* 1973). Decreased protein binding of thiopental may explain, in part, increased drug sensitivity demonstrated by patients with uremia or cirrhosis of the liver (Ghoneim and Pandya, 1975). Decreased protein binding in patients with uremia may be partially due to competitive binding inhibitors such as nitrogenous waste products. Hypoalbuminemia may account for decreased protein binding of barbiturates in patients with cirrhosis of the liver.

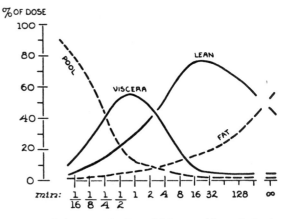

FIGURE 4-4. Distribution of thiopental from the brain to inactive tissue sites (viscera, fat, lean) following a single intravenous injection (pool) is responsible for rapid awakening. (From Price HL, Kovnat PJ, Safer JN, Conner EA, Price AB. The uptake of thiopental by body tissues and its relation to the duration of narcosis. Clin Pharmacol Ther 1960;1:16–22. Reproduced by permission of the authors and publisher.)

Distribution

Distribution of barbiturates in the body is determined by their lipid solubility, protein binding, and degree of ionization (Breimer, 1976; Ghoneim and Korttila, 1977; Ghoneim and Van Hamme, 1978). Of the factors that influence distribution of thiopental, thiamylal, and methohexital, it is lipid solubility that is most important. In addition, the initial volume of distribution of thiopental decreases exponentially with age (Fig. 4-5) (Homer and Stanski, 1985).

Thiopental, thiamylal, and methohexital undergo maximal brain uptake within 30 seconds, accounting for the rapid onset of central nervous system depression. The brain receives about 10% of the total dose in the first 30 to 40 seconds. This maximal brain concentration is followed by a decline over the next 5 minutes to one-half the initial peak concentration, owing to redistribution of drug from brain to other tissues. Indeed, redistribution is the principal mechanism accounting for early awakening following a single dose of these drugs. After about 30 minutes, the barbiturate has been further redistributed and as little as 10% remains in the vascular areas of the brain (*i.e.,* gray matter). Redistribution occurs promptly because initial high uptake of lipid-soluble drug into the brain and other highly perfused tissues causes the plasma concentration of barbiturate to decline, resulting in a reversal of the concentration gradient for the movement of drug between blood and tissues. Redistribution is much less important in determining the duration of action of less lipid-soluble barbiturates that are administered as oral hypnotics.

Skeletal muscle is the tissue into which initial redistribution of highly lipid-soluble barbiturates, such as thiopental, is most prominent (Fig. 4-4) (Price *et al,* 1960). Indeed, the initial decline in the plasma concentration of thiopental is principally due to uptake of drug into skeletal muscles, with only a modest contribution from metabolism. Equilibrium with skeletal muscles is reached in about 15 minutes following intravenous injection of thiopental.

Fat is the only compartment in which thiopental content continues to rise 30 minutes after injection (Fig. 4-4) (Price *et al,* 1960). With a fat : blood partition coefficient of about 11, thiopental will move from blood to fat as long as the concentration in fat is less than 11 times that in blood. Despite this affinity for fat, the initial uptake of drug into adipose tissue is slow, emphasizing the role of poor fat blood flow in limiting delivery of barbiturate to this tissue. Indeed, redistribution of drug to fat will not significantly affect early awakening from a single intravenous dose of barbiturate. Maximal deposition of thiopental in fat is present after about 2.5 hours, and this tissue becomes a potential reservoir for maintaining plasma concentrations of the drug. Indeed, large or repeated doses of lipid-soluble barbiturates produce a cumulative drug effect because of the storage capacity of fat. When this occurs, the usual rapid awakening, characteristic of these drugs, is absent. For this reason, the dose of thiopental is best calculated according to lean body mass so as to avoid overdose (Gilles *et al,* 1976). Furthermore, in the presence of hypovolemia, skeletal muscle blood flow is reduced and thiopental plasma concentrations are increased because of less dilution. This can result in greater initial plasma concentrations of barbiturate in blood delivered to highly perfused organs leading to exaggerated cerebral and cardiac depression.

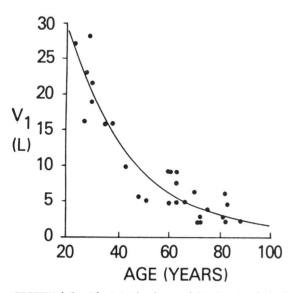

FIGURE 4-5. The initial volume of distribution (V_1) of thiopental decreases with increasing age. (From Homer TD, Stanski DR. The effect of increasing age on thiopental disposition and anesthetic requirement. Anesthesiology 1985;62:714–24. Reproduced by permission of the authors and publisher.)

The distribution of thiopental from blood to tissues will be modified by the state of ionization of the drug and its binding to plasma proteins. Since the *p*Ka of thiopental is near blood *p*H (*p*Ka 7.6), acidosis will favor the nonionized fraction of drug, whereas alkalosis has the opposite effect. The nonionized form of drug has greater access to the central nervous system by virtue of its greater lipid solubility. Acidosis will thus deepen and alkalosis will lighten barbiturate anesthesia. Evidence of increased brain penetration of barbiturate is the decrease in plasma concentration of thiopental associated with an acute reduction in blood *p*H (Brodie *et al,* 1950).

Metabolic-induced alterations in *p*H produce more pronounced effects on drug distribution than do respiratory alterations. For example, in the presence of metabolic changes, the intracellular *p*H in the brain may remain relatively unchanged, reflecting the inability of hydrogen ions to easily cross lipid barriers. As a result, movement of drug across the blood–brain barrier is favored. In contrast, respiratory-induced changes in *p*H are associated with rapid diffusion of carbon dioxide and similar changes in intracellular and extracelluar *p*H resulting in less net movement of drug.

Metabolism

Oxybarbiturates are metabolized only in hepatocytes, whereas thiobarbiturates also undergo breakdown to a small extent in extrahepatic sites, such as the kidneys, and possibly the central nervous system. Metabolites are usually inactive and always more water soluble than the parent compound, thus facilitating renal excretion.

Side chain oxidation at the number 5 carbon atom of the benzene ring to yield carboxylic acid is the most important initial step in the termination of pharmacologic activity of barbiturates by metabolism. This oxidation occurs primarily in the endoplasmic reticulum of hepatocytes. The reserve capacity of the liver to carry out oxidation of barbiturates is large, and hepatic dysfunction must be extreme before a prolonged duration of action of barbiturates owing to reduced metabolism occurs.

Thiopental

Metabolism of thiopental is almost complete (99%), but this breakdown occurs at a slow rate,

with 10% to 24% of a single dose of the drug being metabolized by the liver each hour (Mark *et al,* 1965). Clearly, the rate of metabolism of thiopental is too slow to explain the prompt recovery from central nervous system depression, emphasizing that redistribution of drug from brain to inactive tissue sites is responsible for early awakening. It is estimated that as much as 30% of the original injected dose may remain after 24 hours, emphasizing the predictability of a cumulative drug effect if repeated doses of thiopental are administered. The principal sites of metabolism of thiopental are oxidation of substituents on the number 5 carbon atom, desulfuration on the number 2 carbon atom, and hydrolytic opening of the barbituric acid ring. The majority of metabolism of thiopental occurs in the liver; a small amount may also be metabolized in the kidney and brain.

Hepatic clearance of thiopental is characterized by a low hepatic extraction ratio and capacity-dependent elimination that is influenced by hepatic enzyme activity but not hepatic blood flow. Nevertheless, enzyme induction or inhibition does not modify the duration of action of thiopental observed in animals. In patients with cirrhosis of the liver, clearance of thiopental from the plasma is not different from that in normal patients (Pandele *et al,* 1983). Therefore, it appears unlikely that a prolonged effect of a single dose of thiopental will occur in patients with cirrhosis of the liver.

Methohexital

Methohexital is metabolized to a greater extent than thiopental, reflecting its lesser lipid solubility; thus, more methohexital remains in the plasma to become available to the liver for metabolism (Whitwam, 1976). Side chain oxidation of methohexital results in the formation of an inactive metabolite, hydroxymethohexital. Overall, the hepatic clearance of methohexital is three to four times that of thiopental. Despite this greater hepatic clearance, early awakening from a single dose of methohexital, as from thiopental, depends upon redistribution to inactive tissue sites (Hudson *et al,* 1983). Nevertheless, metabolism will exert a greater role in terminating the effect of methohexital than for thiopental. For example, metabolism may be an important determinant of the time required for complete psychomotor recovery. Indeed, many psychomotor functions recover more quickly after administration of methohexital compared with thiopental (Korttila *et al*, 1975). Recovery from methohexital is predictably more rapid than that from thiopental when repeated doses of drug are administered, reflecting the greater role of metabolism in the clearance of methohexital from the plasma. The hepatic clearance of methohexital is more dependent upon changes in cardiac output and hepatic blood flow than is thiopental.

Renal Clearance

All barbiturates are filtered by the renal glomeruli, but the high degree of protein binding limits the magnitude of filtration, whereas high lipid solubility favors reabsorption of any filtered drug back into the circulation. Indeed, less than 1% of administered thiopental, thiamylal, or methohexital are recovered unchanged in the urine. Among the barbiturates, phenobarbital is the only one that undergoes significant renal excretion in the unchanged form, reflecting the lesser protein binding and lipid solubility of this barbiturate compared with that of thiopental. Renal excretion of phenobarbital can be significantly increased by osmotic diuresis. Alkalinization of the urine also hastens renal excretion of phenobarbital because of the shift toward the ionized state caused by this *p*H change.

Elimination Half-Time

Distribution half-times and volumes of distribution of thiopental and methohexital are similar (Table 4-1) (Hudson *et al*, 1983). Conversely, elimination half-times and clearances of these two drugs differ (Table 4-1) (Fig. 4-6) (Hudson *et al*, 1983). The shorter elimination half-time of methohexital compared with that of thiopental results entirely from the greater hepatic clearance of methohexital.

Elimination half-time of thiopental is increased in obese patients compared with nonobese patients, reflecting an increased volume of distribution resulting from excess fat stores (Jung *et al*, 1982). In elderly patients, a smaller initial volume of distribution results in higher plasma concentrations (*i.e.,* less dilution) and an enhanced pharmacologic effect following a single dose of thiopental (Fig. 4-5) (Homer and Stanski, 1985). Elimination half-times may be increased

Table 4-1
Comparative Pharmacokinetics

	Thiopental	*Methohexital*
Rapid distribution half-time (minutes)	8.5	5.6
Slow distribution half-time (minutes)	62.7	58.3
Elimination half-time (hours)	11.6	3.9*
Clearance (ml kg^{-1} min^{-1})	3.4	10.9*
Volume of distribution (L kg^{-1})	2.5	2.2

* Significantly different from thiopental.
(Data from Hudson RJ, Stanski DR, Burch PG. Pharmacokinetics of methohexital and thiopental in surgical patients. Anesthesiology 1983; 59:215–9.)

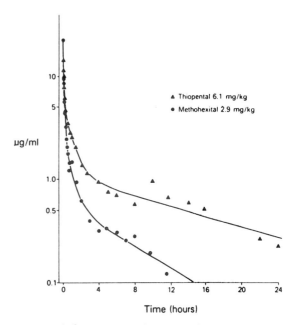

FIGURE 4-6. The rate of decline of the plasma concentration and thus elimination half-time is shorter following the intravenous administration of methohexital than following thiopental. (From Hudson RJ, Stanski DR, Burch PG. Pharmacokinetics of methohexital and thiopental in surgical patients. Anesthesiology 1983;59:215–29. Reproduced by permission of the authors and publisher.)

during pregnancy, partially because of increased binding to plasma proteins.

In pediatric patients, elimination half-times of thiopental are significantly shorter than in adults (Sorbo *et al,* 1984). These shorter elimination half-times are due to more rapid hepatic clearance of thiopental by pediatric patients. Therefore, recovery after large or repeated doses of thiopental may be more rapid for infants and children than for adults. Volume of distribution and protein binding of thiopental are not different in pediatric and adult patients.

CLINICAL USES

The principal clinical uses of barbiturates are for (1) induction of anesthesia and (2) treatment of elevated intracranial pressure. Use of phenobarbital to treat hyperbilirubinemia and kernicterus reflects barbiturate-induced increases in hepatic glucuronyl transferase enzyme activity. Other clinical uses of barbiturates are declining because these drugs (1) lack specificity of effect in the central nervous system, (2) have a lower therapeutic index than do benzodiazepines, (3) result in tolerance more frequently than do benzodiazepines, (4) have greater liability for abuse, and (5) have a high risk for drug interactions. In addition, barbiturates have other undesirable features. For example, these drugs may cause paradoxical excitement instead of sedation, especially in elderly patients or in the presence of pain. Barbiturate-induced paradoxical excitement suggests depression of central nervous system inhibitory centers as the mechanism. Small doses of barbiturates seem to lower the pain threshold, accounting for the perception that these drugs are antianalgesic. Therefore, barbiturates cannot be relied upon to produce sedation in the presence of pain. Skeletal muscle relaxation does not occur, and there is no clinically significant effect of barbiturates on the neuromuscular junction. Drowsiness may last for only a short time after a sedative – hypnotic dose of a barbiturate administered orally, but residual central nervous system effects characterized as "hangover" may persist for several hours. Barbiturates are being replaced by benzodiazepines for preanesthetic medication. The rapid onset of action of barbiturates renders these drugs useful for treatment of grand mal seizures, but, again, benzodiazepines are probably superior, providing a more specific site of action in the central nervous system.

Induction of Anesthesia

The supremacy of the barbiturates for intravenous induction of anesthesia has remained virtually unchallenged. Thiopental was introduced by Lundy in 1934 and is by far the most popular barbiturate for the intravenous induction of anesthesia. Thiamylal, however, is indistinguishable from thiopental as used for induction of anesthesia. The oxybarbiturate methohexital is the only barbiturate with actions sufficiently different so as to offer an alternative to thiopental for intravenous induction of anesthesia. The most important advantage of methohexital compared with thiopental is a more rapid recovery of consciousness, making it useful for outpatient procedures (see the section entitled Pharmacokinetics). The principal disadvantage of methohexital is the increased incidence of excitatory phenomena, such as involuntary skeletal muscle movements, including hiccough (Barron, 1968). The incidence of these excitatory phenomena is dose-dependent and may be reduced by inclusion of opioids in the preoperative medication and by use of optimum doses of methohexital (1 – 1.5 mg kg^{-1}). Indeed, high doses of methohexital, as administered in a continuous infusion for neuroanesthesia, are associated with postoperative seizures in about one third of patients (Todd *et al,* 1984).

The relative potency of barbiturates used for intravenous induction of anesthesia, assuming that thiopental is 1, is thiamylal, 1.1, and methohexital, 2.5. At a blood *p*H of 7.4, methohexital is 76% nonionized compared with 61% for thiopental, which is consistent with the greater potency of methohexital. The central nervous system is exquisitely sensitive to intravenous doses of these barbiturates that produce minimal to no effect on skeletal, cardiac, or smooth muscle. For example, intravenous thiopental, 3 to 5 mg kg^{-1}, rapidly enters the central nervous system and produces unconsciousness within 30 seconds. The dose of thiopental required to induce anesthesia decreases with age, reflecting a smaller initial volume of distribution in elderly patients, such that a given dose is diluted less and thus produces a higher plasma concentration of barbiturate compared with that in younger adults (Fig. 4-5) (Homer and Stanski, 1985). Conversely, thiopental requirements seem to be increased in children more than 1 year after thermal injury (Cote and Petkau, 1985). The reason for this apparent resistance to the effects of thiopental is not known.

Rectal administration of barbiturates, especially methohexital, 20 to 30 mg kg^{-1}, has been used to induce anesthesia in uncooperative or young patients. Loss of consciousness after rectal administration of methohexital correlates with a plasma concentration above 2 μg ml^{-1} (Liu *et al,* 1985).

Other Anesthetic Uses of Intravenous Barbiturates

Occasionally, intravenous barbiturates are used as supplements to inhaled anesthetics or as the sole anesthetic for short and usually pain-free procedures such as cardioversion or electroshock therapy. Methohexital, but not thiopental, is effective in inducing seizure activity in patients with psychomotor epilepsy undergoing cortical resection of seizure-producing areas (Ford *et al,* 1982; Musella *et al,* 1971; Rockoff and Goudsouzian, 1981).

Treatment of Elevated Intracranial Pressure

Barbiturates are administered to reduce intracranial pressure that remains elevated despite deliberate hyperventilation of the lungs and drug-induced diuresis (Shapiro *et al,* 1973). Barbiturates reduce intracranial pressure by decreasing cerebral blood volume by drug-induced cerebral vascular vasoconstriction and an associated decrease in cerebral blood flow. An isoelectric electroencephalogram (EEG) confirms the presence of maximal barbiturate-induced depression of cerebral metabolic oxygen requirements (see the section entitled Electroencephalogram). Improved outcome following head trauma has not, however, been demonstrated in patients treated with barbiturates despite the ability of these drugs to decrease and control intracranial pressure (Ward *et al,* 1985).

A hazard of high-dose barbiturate therapy as used to lower intracranial pressure is hypotension, which can jeopardize the maintenance of an adequate cerebral perfusion pressure. Doses of thiopental sufficient to suppress EEG activity in animals are more likely than those of pentobarbital to lead to hypotension and ventricular fibrillation (Roesch *et al,* 1983). In patients, doses of thiopental (37.5 mg kg^{-1}) and methohexital sufficient to produce an isoelectric EEG produce pe-

ripheral vasodilation and myocardial depression (Todd *et al,* 1984; Todd *et al,* 1985). Nevertheless, these cardiovascular effects are smaller in magnitude than those produced by the dose of isoflurane (2 MAC) required to produce an equivalent degree of depression of the EEG. This suggests that barbiturates may be hemodynamically preferable to isoflurane if profound EEG depression is desired.

The ability of barbiturate therapy to improve brain survival following global cerebral ischemia due to cardiac arrest is unlikely, since these drugs are effective only when the electroencephalogram remains active and metabolic suppression is possible (Michenfelder, 1986). During cardiac arrest, the EEG becomes flat in 20 to 30 seconds, and barbiturates would not be expected to improve outcome. Indeed, administration of thiopental, 30 mg kg^{-1}, as a single intravenous injection to comatose survivors of cardiac arrest does not increase survival or improve neurologic outcome (Brain Resuscitation Clinical Trial Study Group, 1986). Conversely, animal studies consistently show improved outcome with barbiturate therapy of incomplete cerebral ischemia that permits drug-induced metabolic suppression (Todd *et al,* 1982). Consistent with these animal data is the observation that neuropsychiatric complications following cardiopulmonary bypass that are presumably due to embolism clear more rapidly in patients treated prospectively with thiopental (average dose, 39.5 mg kg^{-1}) to maintain electroencephalographic silence (Nussmeier *et al,* 1986). This beneficial effect is accompanied by an increased need for inotropic support at the conclusion of cardiopulmonary bypass and a delayed awakening. Other patients at risk for incomplete cerebral ischemia who might benefit from prior production of electroencephalographic silence (*e.g.,* metabolic suppression) with barbiturates include those scheduled for carotid endarterectomy, thoracic aneurysm resection, and profound controlled hypotension.

Barbiturate-induced decreases in cerebral oxygen consumption appear to be greater than corresponding decreases in cerebral blood flow. Such changes in cerebral metabolism may be protective to poorly perfused areas of brain. The reduction in cerebral blood flow and increase in the perfusion to metabolism ratio render thiopental an attractive drug for induction of anesthesia in patients with increased intracranial pressure (Fig. 4-7) (Bedford *et al,* 1980).

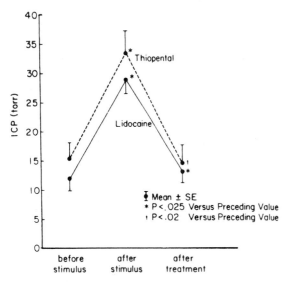

FIGURE 4-7. The intravenous administration of thiopental 3 mg kg^{-1} is as effective as lidocaine 1.5 mg kg^{-1} in lowering intracranial pressure (ICP) following surgical stimulation in patients with brain tumors. (From Bedford RF, Persing JA, Pobereskin L, Butler A. Lidocaine or thiopental for rapid control of intracranial hypertension. Anesth Analg, 1980;59:435–7. Reproduced by permission of the authors and the International Anesthesia Research Society.)

Electroencephalogram

Small intravenous doses of barbiturates increase low voltage fast activity (1–5 cycles sec^{-1}) on the EEG. This activation of the EEG is accompanied by clouding of consciousness. As the dose of barbiturate is increased, large amplitude slow waves (less than 4 cycles sec^{-1}) similar to physiologic sleep appear on the EEG and consciousness is lost, although arousal may accompany strong, painful stimuli. A further increase in dose of barbiturate causes the frequency to decrease to 1 to 3 Hz, followed by electrial silence on the EEG if the plasma concentration of barbiturate continues to increase. A continuous intravenous infusion of thiopental, 4 mg kg^{-1} hr^{-1}, produces an isoelectric EEG that is consistent with near-maximal reduction in cerebral metabolic oxygen requirements (Turcant *et al.,* 1985). Alternatively, pentobarbital administered as a continuous infusion to maintain the plasma concentration between 3 to 6 mg dl^{-1} is associated with an isoelectric EEG (Rockoff *et al,* 1979). Barbiturate-induced depression in cerebral oxygen requirements when the EEG is isoelectric is about 50% reflecting a decrease in neuronal, but not metabolic, needs for oxygen. Hypothermia is the only reliable method for decreasing the basal cellular requirements for oxygen.

Somatosensory Evoked Responses

Thiopental produces dose-dependent changes in median nerve somatosensory evoked responses and brain stem auditory evoked responses. Nevertheless, even doses of thiopental sufficient to produce an isoelectric EEG fail to render any component of these responses unobtainable (Drummond *et al,* 1985). Therefore, thiopental is an acceptable drug to administer when the ability to monitor somatosensory evoked potentials is desirable.

SIDE EFFECTS

Barbiturates are administered almost exclusively to produce depressant effects on the central nervous system. Side-effects manifesting on other organ systems include (1) development of tolerance and physical dependence, (2) allergic reactions, and (3) adverse responses associated with inadvertent intra-arterial injection.

Cardiovascular System

Oral sedative doses of barbiturates do not produce cardiovascular effects different from the slight decrease in blood pressure and heart rate that accompany normal sleep. Hemodynamic effects of equivalent doses of methohexital, thiamylal, and thiopental, as used for induction of anesthesia, are similar (Todd *et al,* 1984). In normovolemic subjects, thiopental, 5 mg kg^{-1}, administered intravenously produces a transient 10 to 20 mmHg reduction in blood pressure that is offset by a compensatory 15 to 20 beat min^{-1} increase in heart rate (Fig. 4-8) (Filner and Karliner, 1976). This dose of thiopental produces minimal to no evidence of myocardial depression. When reductions in myocardial contractility are demonstrated after induction of anesthesia with barbiturates, the magnitude of this decrease is far less than that produced by volatile anesthetics (Becker and Tonnesen, 1978; Kaplan *et al,* 1976). Cardiac dysrhythmias following induction of anesthesia with

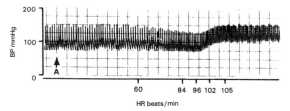

FIGURE 4-8. In normovolemic patients, the rapid intravenous administration of thiopental 5 mg kg^{-1} (A) is followed by a modest decline in blood pressure, which is subsequently offset by a compensatory increase in heart rate (HR). (From Filner BF, Karliner JS. Alterations of normal left ventricular performance by general anesthesia. Anesthesiology 1976;45:610–20. Reproduced by permission of the authors and publisher.)

barbiturates are unlikely in the presence of adequate ventilation and oxygenation.

The most likely explanation for compensatory tachycardia and unchanged myocardial contractility associated with intravenous administration of thiopental is a baroreceptor-mediated increase in peripheral sympathetic nervous system activity. In the absence of compensatory increases in peripheral sympathetic nervous system activity, as in isolated heart preparations, a negative inotropic effect of barbiturates is readily demonstrated. Direct myocardial depression may also accompany overdoses of barbiturates or the large doses of barbiturates used to lower intracranial pressure (see the section entitled Clinical Uses).

The mild and transient reduction in blood pressure that accompanies induction of anesthesia with barbiturates is principally due to peripheral vasodilatation reflecting depression of the medullary vasomotor center and decreased sympathetic nervous system outflow from the central nervous system. The resulting dilatation of peripheral capacitance vessels leads to pooling of blood, decreased venous return, and the potential for decreases in cardiac output and blood pressure (Yamamura *et al*, 1983). Histamine release can occur, but it is rarely of clinical significance (see the section entitled Allergic Reactions). Vasodilatation of cutaneous and skeletal muscle blood vessels may also contribute to heat loss and reductions in body temperature. The fact that blood pressure and cardiac output are minimally altered by induction of anesthesia with barbiturates reflects the ability of baroreceptor reflex responses to offset the effects of peripheral vasodilatation. In

the absence of compensatory baroreceptor-mediated increases in peripheral sympathetic nervous system activity, peripheral pooling of blood can result in sustained reductions in venous return, cardiac output, and blood pressure. Indeed, hypovolemic patients, who are less able to compensate for peripheral vasodilating effects of barbiturates, are highly vulnerable to marked reductions in blood pressure when these drugs are administered rapidly for induction of anesthesia. Treatment with beta-adrenergic antagonists or centrally acting antihypertensive drugs may also accentuate blood pressure reductions evoked by barbiturates by impairing the activity of compensatory baroreceptor responses.

Conceptually, the slow intravenous infusion of thiopental should be more likely to permit compensatory reflex responses and thus minimize blood pressure reductions compared with rapid intravenous injection. This would be most important in the presence of hypovolemia. Nevertheless, rapid or slow intravenous administration of thiopental to normovolemic patients produces similar reductions in blood pressure and increases in heart rate (Table 4-2) (Seltzer *et al*, 1980). Furthermore, the dose administered slowly in 50-mg increments so as to produce loss of the lash reflex was more than the single dose administered intravenously (Table 4-2) (Seltzer *et al*, 1980).

Table 4-2
Incremental vs. Rapid Injection of Thiopental

	Incremental (50 mg every 15 seconds until loss of lash reflex)	Rapid
Total dose (mg kg^{-1})	5.58	4
Systolic blood pressure decrease (mmHg)	14	16
Diastolic blood pressure decrease (mmHg)	6	9
Heart rate increase (beats min^{-1})	12	16
Measure of myocardial contractility (% decrease)	17.5	22.5

(Data from Seltzer JL, Gerson JJ, Allen FB. Comparison of the cardiovascular effects of bolus vs. incremental administration of thiopentone. Br J Anaesth 1980; 52:527–9.)

Ventilation

Barbiturates, as administered intravenously for the induction of anesthesia, produce dose-dependent depression of medullary and pontine ventilatory centers. For example, thiopental depresses the sensitivity of the medullary ventilatory center to stimulation by carbon dioxide. Apnea is especially likely in the presence of other depressant drugs as used for preoperative medication. Resumption of spontaneous ventilation following a single intravenous induction dose of barbiturate is characterized by a slow rate of breathing and reduced tidal volume. Laryngeal reflexes and the cough reflex are not depressed until large doses of barbiturates have been administered (Harrison, 1962). Stimulation of the upper airway as by laryngoscopy, intubation of the trachea, or secretions in the presence of inadequate depression of laryngeal reflexes by barbiturates may result in laryngospasm or bronchospasm. Increased irritability of the larynx because of a parasympathomimetic action of thiopental is an unlikely explanation for laryngospasm or bronchospasm. Indeed, thiopental is not likely to selectively alter parasympathetic nervous system activity, although depression of sympathetic nervous system outflow from the central nervous system could theoretically result in a predominance of vagal tone.

Liver

Thiopental, in the absence of other drugs, produces only modest reductions in hepatic blood flow. Induction doses of thiopental do not alter postoperative liver function tests (Dundee, 1955). Continuous infusion of methohexital for up to 4 hours does not produce laboratory evidence of hepatocellular damage (Prys–Roberts *et al,* 1983). In the hypoxic rat model, thiopental has a detectable, but minimal, potential to produce hepatocellular damage (Shingu *et al,* 1983).

Enzyme Induction

Barbiturates stimulate an increase in liver microsomal protein content (*e.g.,* enzyme induction) after 2 to 7 days of sustained drug administration (Conney, 1967). Phenobarbital is the most potent of the barbiturates for producing enzyme induction, leading to a 20% to 40% increase in the protein content of hepatic microsomal enzymes

(Remmer and Merker, 1963). At maximal induction of enzyme activity, rates of metabolism are approximately doubled. After discontinuation of a barbiturate, enzyme induction may persist for up to 30 days.

Altered drug responses and drug interactions may reflect barbiturate-induced enzyme induction, resulting in accelerated metabolism of (1) other drugs, such as oral anticoagulants, phenytoin, and tricyclic antidepressants; or (2) endogenous substances, including corticosteroids, bile salts, and vitamin K. Indeed, glucuronyl transferase activity is increased by barbiturates. Barbiturates also stimulate the activity of a mitochondrial enzyme (in contrast to microsomal enzyme) known as d-aminoevulinic acid synthetase. As a result, the production of heme is accelerated, and acute intermittent porphyria may be exacerbated in susceptible patients. Barbiturates can also enhance their own metabolism, which contributes to tolerance (see the section entitled Tolerance and Physical Dependence).

Kidneys

Renal effects of thiopental may include modest reductions in renal blood flow and glomerular filtration rate. The most likely explanation is drug-induced reductions in blood pressure and cardiac output. Histologic evidence of renal damage is not detectable after use of barbiturates for induction of anesthesia.

Placental Transfer

Barbiturates used for the induction of anesthesia readily cross the placenta, as evidenced by peak umbilical vein concentrations 1 minute after administration. Nevertheless, plasma fetal concentrations of barbiturates are substantially less than those in maternal plasma (Christensen *et al,* 1981; Kosaka *et al,* 1969; Mark and Poppers, 1982). Clearance by the fetal liver and dilution by blood from the viscera and extremities results in the fetal brain being exposed to lower barbiturate concentrations than are measured in the umbilical vein. Indeed, maternal doses of thiopental up to 4 mg kg^{-1} probably do not result in excessive concentrations of the barbiturate in the fetal brain (Kosaka *et al,* 1969).

Neonatal elimination half-time of thiopental following maternal administration at cesarean section is 11 to 42.7 hours (Christensen *et al,* 1981). Nevertheless, these residual drug concentrations seem to be innocuous, as evidenced by unchanged neurobehavioral scores measured 48 hours after delivery (Hodgkinson *et al,* 1978).

Tolerance and Physical Dependence

Pharmacodynamic tolerance to barbiturates occurs rapidly. For example, plasma concentrations of thiopental present on awakening are greater following a single large sleep dose than those after a single small sleep dose (Brodie *et al,* 1951). Nevertheless, this observation may be an artifact of rapid intravenous injection, resulting in a transient distortion of drug distribution between the brain and peripheral circulation.

Acute tolerance occurs earlier than does barbiturate-induced induction of microsomal enzymes. When barbiturate tolerance becomes maximal, the required effective dose of barbiturate may be increased sixfold. This magnitude of increase is at least double that which could be accounted for by increased metabolism resulting from enzyme induction.

Tolerance to sedative effects of barbiturates occurs sooner and is greater than that which occurs for the anticonvulsant and lethal effects. Thus, as tolerance to barbiturate-induced sedation increases, the therapeutic index decreases. Acute tolerance also applies to the effect of barbiturates on metabolic oxygen consumption, with supplemental doses of thiopental having less of an effect than the initial dose. The development of tolerance may be less for barbiturates that produce short-term depression.

Tolerance and physical dependence on barbiturates are closely related. The severity of the withdrawal syndrome relates to the degree of tolerance and rate of elimination of the barbiturate. Slow elimination of the barbiturate allows time for the central nervous system to diminish its compensatory excitatory responses more nearly in phase with the diminution in barbiturate-induced central nervous system depression. For example, persons who are physiologically dependent on barbiturates may be withdrawn more safely if long-acting phenobarbital is substituted for the shorter-acting barbiturate on which the patient is dependent. Nevertheless, abrupt discontinuation

of phenobarbital in patients being treated for epilepsy may result in status epilepticus, even when the patient has been taking relatively small doses of the drug.

Intra-Arterial Injection

Intra-arterial injection of thiopental usually results in intense vasoconstriction and excruciating pain (Stone and Donnelly, 1961). Vasoconstriction may obscure distal arterial pulses, and blanching of the extremity is followed by cyanosis. Gangrene and permanent nerve damage may occur. The mechanism of these changes is not fully understood. Possible explanations include (1) formation of thiopental crystals in the artery that evoke intense vasoconstriction or are carried distally to occlude end-arterioles, (2) hemolysis of erythrocytes and aggregation of platelets that occlude distal arterioles, and (3) local release of norepinephrine (Brown *et al,* 1968; Burn, 1960; Burn and Hobbs, 1959). The adverse response is not due to the alkalinity of the solution. Instead, the formation of thiopental crystals may occur because the *p*H becomes too low for the barbiturate to remain in solution (Brown *et al,* 1968; Waters, 1966). In this regard, crystal-forming ability is less likely to occur with dilute solutions of thiopental (*e.g.,* 2.5% rather than 5%). Nevertheless, inadvertent intra-arterial injection of 2.5% concentrations of thiopental or thiamylal can still cause vascular insufficiency (Dohi and Naito, 1983). Likewise, methohexital can result in changes similar to those produced by thiopental. Ultimately, the damage produced by intra-arterial injection of a barbiturate is related to the dose and concentration of drug injected. All vessels examined pathologically demonstrate a severe endoarteritis.

Treatment of an inadvertent intra-arterial injection of a barbiturate is immediate administration, through the needle that still remains in the artery, of saline to dilute the drug or a drug such as lidocaine, papaverine, or phenoxygenzamine to produce vasodilatation (Guerra, 1980). If the needle has been removed from the artery prior to recognition of the intra-arterial injection, the injection of the vasodilator drug should be made into the subclavian artery, because the affected artery will be in spasm. Direct injection of heparin into the artery may be considered (O'Donnell *et al,* 1969). Sympathectomy of the upper extremity produced by a stellate ganglion block or brachial plexus block may relieve vasoconstriction (Guerra, 1980). Despite aggressive treatment, gangrene may still occur.

Venous Thrombosis

Venous thrombosis following intravenous administration of a barbiturate for induction of anesthesia presumably reflects deposition of barbiturate crystals in the vessel. Crystal formation in veins, however, is less hazardous than in arteries because of the ever-increasing diameter of the veins. The importance of administering a dilute solution of barbiturate for induction of anesthesia is suggested by the reduced incidence of venous thrombosis after use of 2.5% thiopental and 1% methohexital, compared with 5% and 2% solutions, respectively (O'Donnell *et al,* 1969).

Allergic Reactions

Allergic reactions in association with intravenous administration of barbiturates for induction of anesthesia most likely represent anaphylaxis (*e.g,* an antigen–antibody interaction) (Watkins, 1979). Nevertheless, thiopental can also produce signs of an allergic reaction in the absence of a prior exposure, suggesting an anaphylactoid response (Hirshman *et al,* 1982). The incidence of allergic reactions to thiopental is estimated to be 1 per 30,000 patients (Clarke, 1981). The majority of reported cases are in patients with a history of chronic atopy, who often have received thiopental previously without adverse responses (Etter *et al,* 1980; Hirshman *et al,* 1982; Lilly and Hoy, 1980). Treatment of an allergic reaction following intravenous administration of thiopental, thiamylal, or methohexital must be aggressive, including epinephrine and massive intravascular fluid replacement. Mortality seems unusually high following an allergic response to thiopental (Stoelting, 1983).

Thiamylal and thiopental evoke histamine release from human skin mast cell preparations, whereas methohexital and pentobarbital are devoid of this effect (Fig. 4-9) (Hirshman *et al,* 1985). Although demonstration of *in vitro* histamine release is not confirmation that clinical symptoms of an allergic reaction are causally related to this chemical mediator, methohexital may be perferable as an induction drug in asthmatic

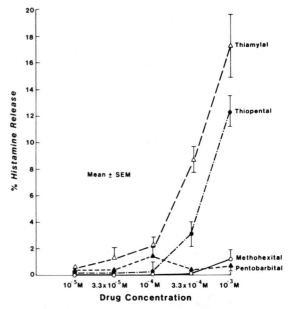

FIGURE 4-9. Thiamylal and thiopental produce dose-dependent release of histamine from human skin mast cell preparations, whereas methohexital and pentobarbital are devoid of this effect. Histamine release evoked by thiamylal is greater than thiopental at doses above 3×10^{-5} (P < 0.05). (From Hirshman CA, Edelstein RA, Ebertz JM, Hanifen JM. Thiobarbiturate-induced histamine release in human skin mast cells. Anesthesiology 1985;63:353–6. Reproduced by permission of the authors and publisher.)

patients or in those patients with a strong history of allergies.

REFERENCES

Barron DW. Effect of rate of injection on incidence of side-effects with thiopental and methohexital. Anesth Analg 1968;47:171–3.

Becker KE, Tonnesen AS. Cardiovascular effects of plasma levels of thiopental necessary for anesthesia. Anesthesiology 1978;49:197–208.

Bedord RF, Persing JA, Pobereskin L, Butler A. Lidocaine or thiopental for rapid control of intracranial hypertension. Anesth Analg 1980;59:435–7.

Brain Resuscitation Clinical Trial I Study Group. Randomized clinical study of thiopental loading in comatose survivors of cardiac arrest. N Engl J Med 1986;314:397–403.

Breimer DD. Pharmacokinetics of methohexitone following intravenous infusion in humans. Br J Anaesth 1976;48:743 – 8.

Brodie BB, Mark LC, Lief PA, Bernstein E, Papper EM. Acute tolerance to thiopental. J Pharmacol Exp Ther 1951;102:215 – 8.

Brodie BB, Mark LC, Papper EM, Bernstein E, Papper EM. The fate of thiopental in man and a method for its estimation in biological material. J Pharmacol Exp Ther 1950;98:85 – 96.

Brown SS, Lyons SM, Dundee JW. Intra-arterial barbiturates: A study of some factors leading to intravascular thrombosis. Br J Anaesth 1968;40:13 – 9.

Burn JH. Why thiopentone injected into an artery may cause gangrene. Br Med J 1960;2:414 – 6.

Burn JH, Hobbs R. Mechanism of arterial spasm following intra-arterial injection of thiopentone. Lancet 1959;1:1112 – 5.

Chaplin MD, Roszkowski AP, Richard RK. Displacement of thiopental from plasma proteins by nonsteroidal anti-inflammatory agents. Proc Soc Exp Biol Med 1973;143:667 – 71.

Christensen JH, Andreasen F, Jansen JA. Pharmacokinetics of thiopental in cesarean section. Acta Anaesthesiol Scand 1981;25:174 – 9.

Clarke RSJ. Adverse effects of intravenously administered drugs in anaesthetic practice. Drugs 1981; 22:26 – 41.

Conney AH. Pharmacological implications of microsomal enzyme induction. Pharmacol Rev 1967;19:317 – 66.

Cote CJ, Petkau AJ. Thiopental requirements may be increased in children reanesthetized at least one year after recovery from extensive thermal injury. Anesth Analg 1985;64:1156 – 60.

Dohi S, Naito H. Intra-arterial injection of 2.5% thiamylal does cause gangrene (letter). Anesthesiology 1983;59:154.

Drummond JC, Todd MM, U HS. The effect of high-dose sodium thiopental on brain stem auditory and median nerve somatosensory evoked responses in humans. Anesthesiology 1985;63:249 – 54.

Dundee JW. Thiopentone as a factor in the production of liver dysfunction. Br J Anaesth 1955;27:14 – 23.

Etter MS, Helrich M, Mackenzie CF. Immunoglobulin E fluctuation in thiopental anaphylaxis. Anesthesiology 1980;52:181 – 3.

Filner BF, Karliner JS. Alterations of normal left ventricular performance by general anesthesia. Anesthesiology 1976;45:610 – 20.

Ford EW, Morrell F, Whisler WW. Methohexital anesthesia in the surgical treatment of uncontrollable epilepsy. Anesth Analg 1982;61:997 – 1001.

Fragen RJ, Avram MF. Comparative pharmacology of drugs used for the induction of anesthesia. In Stoelting RK, Barash PG, Gallagher TJ, eds. Advances in Anesthesia. Chicago, Year Book Medical Publishers. 1986:103 – 32.

Ghoneim MM, Korttila K. Pharmacokinetics of intravenous anaesthetics: Implications for clinical use. Clin Pharmacokinet 1977;2:344 – 72.

Ghoneim MM, Pandya H. Plasma protein binding of thiopental in patients with impaired renal or hepatic function. Anesthesiology 1975;42:545 – 9.

Ghoneim MM, Pandya HB, Kelly SE, Fischer LJ, Corry RJ. Binding of thiopental to plasma proteins. Effects of distribution in the brain and heart. Anesthesiology 1976;45:635 – 9.

Ghoneim MM, VanHamme MJ. Pharmacokinetics of thiopentone: Effect of enflurane and nitrous oxide anaesthesia and surgery. Br J Anaesth 1978;50:143 – 5.

Gilles PP, DeAngelis RJ, Wynn RL. Nonlinear pharmacokinetic model of intravenous anesthesia. J Pharm Sci 1976;65:1001 – 6.

Guerra F. Thiopental forever after. In Aldrete JA, Stanley TH, eds. Trends in Intravenous Anesthesia. Chicago. Year Book Medical Publishers 1980;143.

Harrison GA. The influence of difference anesthetic agents on the response to respiratory tract irritation. Br J Anaesth 1962;34:804 – 11.

Hirshman CA, Peters J, Cartwright-Lee I. Leukocyte histamine release to thiopental. Anesthesiology 1982; 56:64 – 7.

Hirshman CA, Edelstein RA, Ebertz JM, Hanifin JM. Thiobarbiturate-induced histamine release in human skin mast cells. Anesthesiology 1985;63: 353 – 6.

Hodgkinson R, Bhatt M, Kim SS, Grewal G, Marx GF. Neonatal neurobehavioral tests following cesarean section under general and spinal anesthesia. AM J Obstet Gynecol 1978;132:670 – 4.

Homer TD, Stanski DR. The effect of increasing age on thiopental disposition and anesthetic requirement. Anesthesiology 1985;62:714 – 24.

Hudson RJ, Stanski DR, Burch PG. Pharmacokinetics of methohexital and thiopental in surgical patients. Anesthesiology 1983;59:215 – 9.

Jung D, Mayersohn M, Perrier D, Calkins J, Saunders R. Thiopental disposition in lean and obese patients undergoing surgery. Anesthesiology 1982;56:269 – 74.

Kaplan JA, Miller ED, Bailey DR. A comparative study of enflurane and halothane using systolic time intervals. Anesth Analg 1976;55:263 – 8.

Korttila K, Linnoila M, Ertama P, Hakknien S. Recovery and simulated driving after intravenous anesthesia with thiopental, methohexital, propanidid or alphadione. Anesthesiology 1975;43:291 – 9.

Kosaka Y, Takahashi T, Mark LC. Intravenous thiobarbiturate anesthesia for cesarean section. Anesthesiology 1969;31:489 – 506.

Lilly JK, Hoy RH. Thiopental anaphylaxis and reagin involvement. Anesthesiology 1980;53:335 – 7.

Liu LMP, Gaudreault P, Friedman PA, Goudsouzian NG,

Liu PL. Methohexital plasma concentrations in children following rectal administration. Anesthesiology 1985;62:567–70.

MacDonald RL, Barker JL. Different actions of anticonvulsant and anesthetic barbiturates revealed by use of cultured mammalian nerves. Science 1978; 200:775–7.

Mark LC, Poppers PJ. The dilemma of general anesthesia for cesarean section: Adequate fetal oxygenation vs. maternal awareness during operation. Anesthesiology 1982;56:405–6.

Mark LC, Brand L, Kamvyssi S, Britton RC. Thiopental metabolism by human liver in vivo and in vitro. Nature 1965;206:1117–9.

Michenfelder JD. A valid demonstration of barbiturate-induced brain protection in man — at last. Anesthesiology 1986;64:140–2.

Musella L, Wilder BJ, Schmidt RP. Electroencephalographic activation with intravenous methohexital in psychomotor epilepsy. Neurology 1971;21:594–602.

Nussmeier NA, Arlund C, Slogoff S. Neuropsychiatric complications after cardiopulmonary bypass: Cerebral protection by a barbiturate. Anesthesiology 1986;64:165–70.

O'Donnell JF, Hewitt JC, Dundee JW. Clinical studies of induction agents. XXVIII: A further comparison of venous complications following thiopentone, methohexitone and propanidid. Br J Anaesth 1969;41:681–3.

Pandele G, Chaux F, Salvadori C, Farinotti M. Duvaldestin P. Thiopental pharmacokinetics in patients with cirrhosis. Anesthesiology 1983;59:123–6.

Price HL, Kovnat PJ, Safer JN, Conner EA, Price AB. The uptake of thiopental by body tissues and its relation to the duration of narcosis. Clin Pharmacol Ther 1960;1:16–22.

Prys–Roberts C, Sear JW, Low JM, Phillips KC, Dagnino J. Hemodynamic and hepatic effects of methohexital infusion during nitrous oxide anesthesia in humans. Anesth Analg 1983;62:317–23.

Ransom BR, Barker J. Pentobarbital selectively enhances GABA-mediated postsynaptic inhibition in tissue cultured mouse spinal neurons. Brain Res 1976;114:530–35.

Remmer H, Merker HJ. Drug-induced changes in the liver endoplasmic reticulum. Association with drug metabolizing enzymes. Science 1963;142:1657–8.

Richter J, Waller MB. Effects of pentobarbital on the regulation of acetylcholine content and release in different regions of rat brain. Biochem Pharmacol 1977;26:609–15.

Rockoff MA, Goudsouzian NG. Seizures induced by methohexital. Anesthesiology 1981;54:333–5.

Rockoff MA, Marshall LF, Shapiro HM. High dose barbiturate therapy in humans: A clinical review of 60 patients. Ann Neurol 1979;6:194–9.

Roesch C, Haselby KA, Paradise RP et al. Comparison of cardiovascular effects of thiopental and pentobarbital at equivalent levels of CNS depression. Anesth Analg 1983;62:749–53.

Saidman LJ, Eger EI. The effect of thiopental metabolism on duration of anesthesia. Anesthesiology 1966;27:118–26.

Seltzer JL, Gerson JI, Allen FB. Comparison of the cardiovascular effects of bolus vs. incremental administration of thiopentone. Br J Anaesth 1980; 52:527–9.

Shapiro HR, Galindo A, Whyte JR, et al. Rapid intraoperative reduction in intracranial pressure with thiopentone. Br J Anaesth 1973;45:1057–62.

Shingu K, Eger EI, Johnson BH, et al. Hepatic injury induced by anesthetic agents in rats. Anesth Analg 1983;62:140–5.

Sorbo S, Hudson RJ, Loomis JC. The pharmacokinetics of thiopental in pediatric surgical patients. Anesthesiology 1984;61:666–70.

Stoelting RK. Allergic reactions during anesthesia. Anesth Analg 1983;62:341–56.

Stone HH, Donnelly CC. The accidental intra-arterial injection of thiopental. Anesthesiology 1961; 22:995–1006.

Todd MM, Chadwick HS, Shapiro HM, Dunlop BJ, Marshall LF, Dueck R. The neurologic effects of thiopental therapy following experimental cardiac arrest in cats. Anesthesiology 1982;57:76–86.

Todd MM, Drummond JC, Sang H. The hemodynamic consequences of high-dose methohexital anesthesia in humans. Anesthesiology 1984;61:495–501.

Todd MM, Drummond JC, Sang H. The hemodynamic consequences of high-dose thiopental anesthesia. Anesth Analg 1985;64:681–7.

Turcant A, Delhumeau A, Premel–Cabic A, et al. Thiopental pharmacokinetics under conditions of long-term infusion. Anesthesiology 1985;63:50–4.

Ward JD, Becker DP, Miller DJ et al. Failure of prophylactic barbiturate coma in the treatment of severe head trauma. J Neurosurg 1985;62:383–8.

Waters DJ. Intra-arterial thiopentone. A physico-chemical phenomenon. Anaesthesia 1966;21:346–56.

Watkins J. Anaphylactoid reactions to IV substances. Br J Anaesth 1979;51:51–60.

Whitwam JG. Methohexitone. Br J Anaesth 1976; 48:617–9.

Yamamura T, Kimura T, Furukawa K. Effects of halothane, thiamylal, and ketamine on central sympathetic and vagal tone. Anesth Analg 1983;62:129–34.

Benzodiazepines

INTRODUCTION

Benzodiazepines were initially observed to exert taming effects in animals; this led to the subsequent evaluation of these drugs in humans. In many situations, benzodiazepines have replaced barbiturates because of their favorable pharmacologic characteristics. Favorable pharmacologic characteristics of benzodiazepines include (1) production of amnesia, (2) minimal depression of ventilation or of the cardiovascular system, (3) specific site of action as anticonvulsants, (4) relative safety if taken in overdose, and (5) rarity of development of significant tolerance or physical dependence. Like barbiturates, benzodiazepines have a rapid onset and short duration of action and lack analgesic effects. Among the many benzodiazepines available, there are both similarities and differences in potency and selectivity for producing specific effects. Nevertheless, diazepam is the drug with which all other benzodiazepines are compared.

STRUCTURE ACTIVITY RELATIONSHIPS

Structurally, benzodiazepines are similar and share many active metabolites (Fig. 5-1). All important central nervous system depressant benzodiazepines contain a 5-aryl or 5-cyclohexenyl substituent on the 1,4-benzodiazepine structure. Other than this substituent, the structure activity relationship is not stringent (Greenblatt, 1974).

MECHANISM OF ACTION

Benzodiazepines are presumed to exert their antianxiety effects and skeletal muscle relaxing effects by increasing the availability of glycine inhibitory neurotransmitter, whereas the sedative action reflects the ability of benzodiazepines to facilitate actions of the inhibitory neurotransmitter, gamma-aminobutyric acid (GABA) (Fig. 5-2) (Richter, 1981). The site of action for production of amnesia by benzodiazepines has not been confirmed.

Conceptually, there are separate benzodiazepine and GABA receptors coupled to a common chloride channel (Gallagher, 1982). Chloride ions normally pass through these channels and inhibit conduction of nerve impulses. In this scheme, benzodiazepine receptors are a regulatory mechanism for the activity of GABA receptors. When benzodiazepine receptors are occupied by an endogenous inhibitor, the affinity of GABA receptors for their inhibitory neurotransmitter (e.g., GABA) is reduced. Conversely, occupation of benzodiazepine receptors by diazepam enhances the affinity of GABA for its receptors, with resulting inhibition of nerve conduction that manifests as a sedative effect.

Benzodiazepine receptors occur almost exclusively on postsynaptic nerve endings in the central nervous system. This anatomic distribution of receptors is consistent with the minimal effects of these drugs outside the central nervous system (e.g., minimal circulatory effects). The

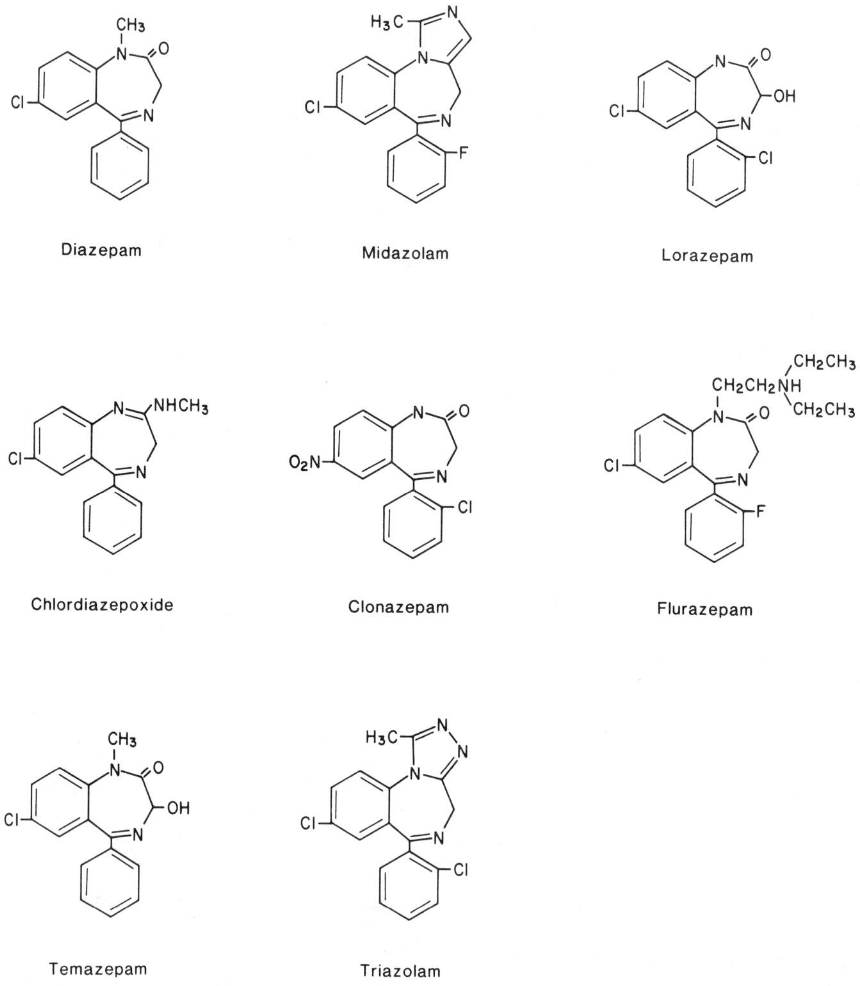

FIGURE 5-1. Benzodiazepines.

highest density of benzodiazepine receptors is in the cerebral cortex, followed in decreasing order by the hypothalamus, cerebellum, midbrain, hippocampus, medulla, and spinal cord (Mohler and Okada, 1977).

Electroencephalogram

The effects of benzodiazepines that appear on the electroencephalogram (EEG) resemble those of barbiturates in that alpha activity is decreased and low-voltage rapid beta activity is increased. This shift from alpha to beta activity occurs more in the frontal and rolandic areas with the benzodiazepines and, unlike the barbiturates, posterior spread does not occur. In common with the barbiturates, however, tolerance to the effects of benzodiazepines on the EEG does occur.

The effects of benzodiazepines on the reticular activating system are of special interest because of the importance of this region for the maintenance of wakefulness. In man, cortical somatosensory evoked potentials, thought to be modulated by the reticular activating system, are diminished in amplitude by diazepam addition,

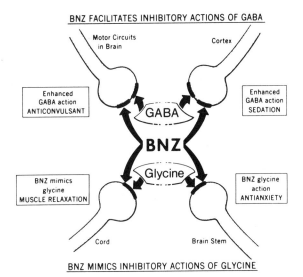

BNZ FACILITATES INHIBITORY ACTIONS OF GABA

Motor Circuits in Brain

Cortex

Enhanced GABA action ANTICONVULSANT

Enhanced GABA action SEDATION

GABA

BNZ

Glycine

BNZ mimics glycine MUSCLE RELAXATION

BNZ glycine action ANTIANXIETY

Cord

Brain Stem

BNZ MIMICS INHIBITORY ACTIONS OF GLYCINE

FIGURE 5-2. Benzodiazepines (BNZ) are presumed to exert their antianxiety effects and skeletal muscle relaxing effects by increasing the availability of glycine inhibitory neurotransmitter, whereas the sedative action reflects the ability of BNZ to facilitate actions of the inhibitory neurotransmitter, gamma-aminobutyric acid (GABA). (From Richter JJ. Current theories about the mechanisms of benzodiazepines and neuroleptic drugs. Anesthesiology 1981;54:66–72. Reproduced by permission of the author and publisher.)

the latency of the early potential is shortened, and that of the late peak is prolonged (Saletu *et al,* 1972).

Antagonist

The central nervous system actions of benzodiazepines can be antagonized within 2 minutes following the intravenous administration of a specific benzodiazepine antagonist (Fig. 5-3) (Lauven *et al,* 1985; O'Boyle *et al,* 1983). This implies a role for benzodiazepine receptors in the amnesic actions of benzodiazepines and introduces the possibility that an endogenous ligand may be involved in the memory process.

Antagonism of benzodiazepine-induced central nervous system effects with physostigmine is both nonspecific and inconsistent (Caldwell and Gross, 1982). Aminophylline, 1 mg kg⁻¹ administered intravenously, may also antagonize benzodiazepine-induced sedation (Meyer *et al,* 1984;

Wangler and Kilpatrick, 1985). Presumably, aminophylline acts by antagonizing the sedative effects of adenosine that accumulate in the central nervous system in response to administration of benzodiazepines (Phillis *et al,* 1979).

DIAZEPAM

Diazepam is the standard with which all benzodiazepines are compared. This benzodiazepine has been found to be particularly useful for (1) preoperative medication (2) induction of anesthesia and (3) treatment of seizures.

Commercial Preparation

Diazepam is dissolved in organic solvents (propylene glycol, sodium benzoate), because it is insoluble in water. The solution is viscid with a *p*H of 6.6 to 6.9. Dilution with water or saline causes cloudiness but does not alter the potency of the drug. Intramuscular or intravenous injection is often painful.

Pharmacokinetics

Diazepam is rapidly absorbed from the gastrointestinal tract after oral administration, reaching peak concentrations in about 1 hour in adults but as quickly as 15 to 30 minutes in children (Table 5-1). There is rapid uptake of diazepam into the brain followed by redistribution to inactive tissue sites, especially fat, as this benzodiazepine is highly lipid soluble. Volume of distribution of diazepam is large, reflecting extensive tissue uptake of this lipid-soluble drug. Females, with a greater body content of fat, have a larger volume of distribution for diazepam than do males (Divoll *et al,* 1983). Diazepam rapidly crosses the placenta,

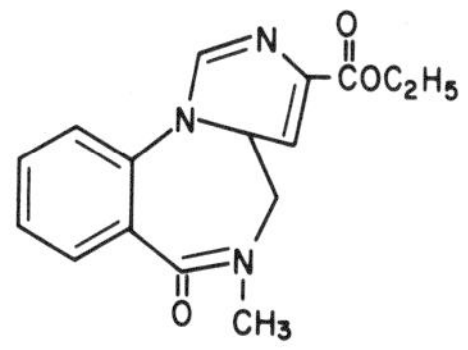

FIGURE 5-3. Benzodiazepine antagonist.

Table 5-1
Comparative Pharmacology of Benzodiazepines

	Equivalent Dose (mg kg^{-1})	Volume of Distribution (L kg^{-1})	Protein Binding (%)	Clearance (ml kg^{-1} min^{-1})	Elimination Half-Time (hr)
Diazepam	0.3–0.5	1–1.5	96–98	0.2–0.5	21–37
Midazolam	0.15–0.3	1–1.5	96–98	6–8	1–4
Lorazepam	0.05	0.8–1.3	96–98	0.7–1	10–20

achieving fetal concentrations equal to and sometimes greater than those present in the maternal circulation (Dawes, 1973). Again, the speed and ease of diazepam transfer across the placenta into the fetus is probably related to its high lipid solubility.

Protein Binding

Protein binding of benzodiazepines parallels their lipid solubility. As such, highly lipid-soluble diazepam is extensively bound, presumably to albumin (Table 5-1) (Thiessen et al, 1976). Cirrhosis of the liver or renal insufficiency with associated reductions in plasma concentrations of albumin may manifest as decreased protein binding of diazepam and an increased incidence of drug-related side effects (Greenblatt and Koch-Weser, 1974). The high degree of protein binding limits the efficacy of hemodialysis in the treatment of diazepam overdose.

Metabolism

Diazepam is principally metabolized by hepatic microsomal enzymes using an oxidative pathway of N-demethylation. The two principal metabolites of diazepam are desmethyldiazepam and oxazepam (Fig. 5-4) (Schwartz et al, 1965). Desmethyldiazepam is metabolized more slowly and is only slightly less potent than diazepam. Therefore, it is likely that this metabolite contributes to the return of drowsiness that manifests 6 to 8 hours after administration of diazepam as well as sustained effects usually attributed to the parent drug (van der Kleijn et al, 1971). Alternatively, enterohepatic recirculation may contribute to the recurrence of sedation (Eustace et al, 1975; Mahon et al, 1976). The plasma concentration of oxazepam after a single injection of diazepam is clinically

insignificant and probably reflects its rapid removal as a conjugate of glucuronic acid. Ultimately, desmethyldiazepam is excreted in the urine in the form of oxidized and glucuronide conjugated metabolites. Unchanged diazepam is not appreciably excreted in the urine.

Diazepam may induce the activity of microsomal enzymes responsible for its metabolism (Kanto and Isalo, 1973). The rate of oxidative demethylation of diazepam is slowed in the presence of cirrhosis of the liver and in elderly patients (see the following section).

Elimination Half-Time

Elimination half-time of diazepam is prolonged ranging from 21 to 37 hours in healthy volunteers (Table 5-1) (Kaplan et al, 1973). Cirrhosis of the liver is accompanied by up to fivefold increases in the elimination half-time of diazepam (Klotz et al, 1975). Likewise, the elimination half-time of diazepam increases progressively with increasing age, explaining the increased sensitivity of these patients to the drug's sedative effects (Fig. 5-5) (Klotz et al, 1975). Prolongation of the elimination half-time of diazepam in the presence of cirrhosis of the liver is due to decreased protein binding of the benzodiazepine, leading to an increased volume of distribution. In addition, hepatic clearance of diazepam is likely to be reduced, reflecting decreased hepatic blood flow. The explanation for prolonged elimination half-time of diazepam in elderly patients is also an increased volume of distribution. Presumably, increased total body fat content that accompanies aging results in an increased volume of distribution of a highly lipid-soluble drug, such as diazepam. Hepatic clearance of diazepam is not changed by aging.

Desmethyldiazepam, the principal metabo-

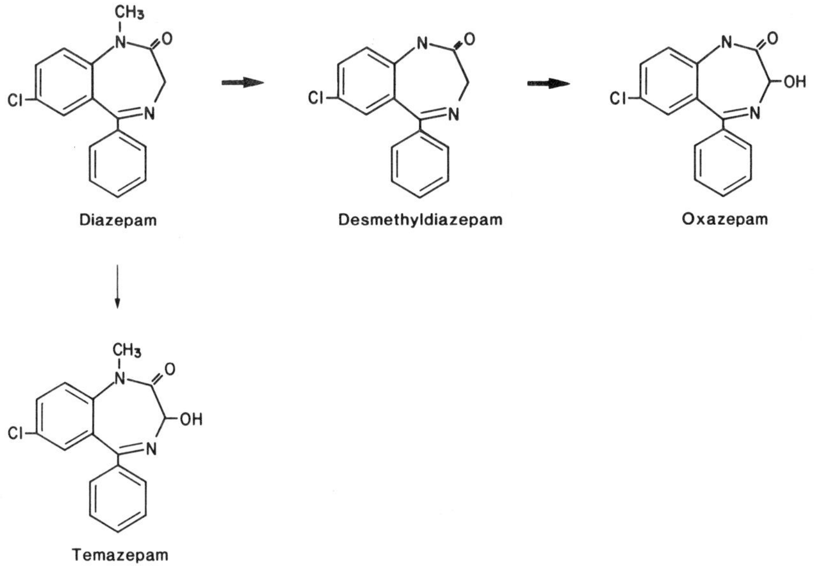

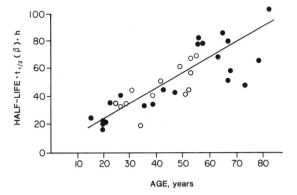

Diazepam

Desmethyldiazepam

Oxazepam

Temazepam

FIGURE 5-4. The principal metabolites of diazepam are desmethyldiazepam and oxazepam. A lesser amount of diazepam is metabolized to temazepam.

lite of diazepam, has an elimination half-time of 48 to 96 hours. As such, the elimination half-time of the metabolite may exceed that of the parent drug. Indeed, plasma concentrations of diazepam often decline more rapidly than plasma concentrations of desmethyldiazepam. This pharmacologically active metabolite can accumulate in plasma and tissues during chronic use of diaze-

pam (van der Kleijn *et al,* 1971). Prolonged somnolence associated with high doses of diazepam is likely to be due to sequestration of the parent drug and its active metabolite, desmethyldiazepam, in tissues, presumably fat, for subsequent release back into the circulation. A week or more is often required for elimination of these compounds from plasma following discontinuation of chronic diazepam therapy.

Effects on Organ Systems

Benzodiazepines, as represented by diazepam, produce minimal depressant effects on ventilation and circulation. Hepatic and renal function are not noticeably depressed. Diazepam does not increase the incidence of nausea and vomiting. There is no change in the circulating concentrations of stress-responding hormones (*e.g.,* catecholamines, antidiuretic hormone, cortisol).

Ventilation

Diazepam produces minimal depressant effects on ventilation, with detectable increases in $PaCO_2$, typically not occurring until 0.2 mg kg^{-1} intravenously is administered (Rao *et al,* 1973). The slight rise in $PaCO_2$ is due primarily to a decrease in tidal volume. Nevertheless, rarely, small doses of intravenous diazepam (<10 mg) have

FIGURE 5-5. The elimination half-time of diazepam increases progressively with increasing age. (From Klotz U, Avant GR, Hoyumpa A, Schenker S, Wilkinson GR. The effects of age and liver disease on the disposition and elimination of diazepam in adult man. J Clin Invest 1975;55:347–59 by permission of the authors and copyright permission of the American Society for Clinical Investigation.)

produced apnea (Braunstein, 1979). Combination of diazepam with other central nervous system depressants (*e.g.,* opioids, alcohol) or administration of this drug to patients with chronic obstructive airways disease may result in exaggerated or prolonged depression of ventilation (Greenblatt *et al,* 1977).

The slope of the line depicting the ventilatory response to carbon dioxide is decreased nearly 50% within 3 minutes following the intravenous administration of diazepam, 0.4 mg kg^{-1} (Fig 5-6) (Gross *et al,* 1982). This depression of the slope persists for about 25 minutes and parallels the level of consciousness. Despite the reduction in slope, the carbon dioxide response curve is not shifted to the right as observed with depression of ventilation produced by opioids. These depressant effects on ventilation seem to be a central nervous system effect, because the mechanics of

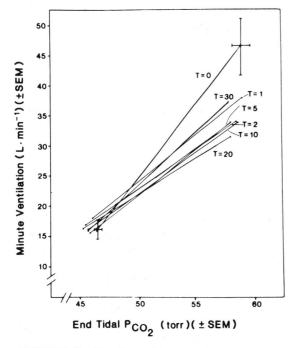

FIGURE 5-6. The slope of the line depicting the ventilatory response to carbon dioxide is depressed following (T = minutes) intravenous administration of diazepam, 0.4 mg kg^{-1}. (From Gross JB, Smith L, Smith TC. Time course of ventilatory response to carbon dioxide after intravenous diazepam. Anesthesiology 1982;57: 18–21. Reproduced by permission of the authors and publisher.)

respiratory muscles are unchanged. The ventilatory depression of benzodiazepines is reversed by surgical stimulation but not by naloxone.

Cardiovascular System

Diazepam in doses of 0.5 to 1 mg kg^{-1} administered intravenously for induction of anesthesia typically produces mild reductions in blood pressure, cardiac output, and peripheral vascular resistance that are similar in magnitude to those observed during natural sleep (*e.g.,* 10%–20% reductions) (Table 5-2) (McCammon *et al,* 1980; Rao *et al.,* 1973). There is transient depression of baroreceptor-mediated heart rate responses that is less than that evoked by volatile anesthetics but that could, in hypovolemic patients, interfere with optimal compensatory changes (Marty *et al,* 1986). Increased coronary blood flow has been observed following the administration of diazepam (Ikran *et al,* 1973.) The significance, if any, of this effect on coronary blood flow is questionable, because it is unknown whether the increased flow is diverted to ischemic areas of the myocardium. In patients with elevated left ventricular end-diastolic pressures, a small dose of diazepam significantly reduces this pressure. Diazepam appears to have no direct action on the sympathetic nervous system, and it does not cause orthostatic hypotension.

The incidence and magnitude of blood pressure reductions produced by diazepam seem to be less than those associated with barbiturates as used for induction of anesthesia (Knapp and Dubow, 1970). Nevertheless, occasionally a patient may unpredictably experience hypotension with even small doses of diazepam (Falk *et al,* 1978).

The addition of nitrous oxide following induction of anesthesia with diazepam is not associated with adverse cardiac changes (Table 5-2) (McCammon *et al,* 1980). Therefore, nitrous oxide can be added to diazepam to ensure adequate anesthesia. This contrasts with direct myocardial depression and reductions in blood pressure that occur when nitrous oxide is administered in the presence of opioids (see Chapter 3).

Skeletal Muscle

Skeletal muscle relaxant effects reflect actions of diazepam on spinal internuncial neurons and not

Table 5-2
Cardiovascular Effects of Diazepam (0.5 mg kg⁻¹)
and Diazepam – Nitrous Oxide (50%)

	Awake	Diazepam	Diazepam – Nitrous Oxide
Systolic blood pressure (mmHg)	144	125*	121*
Diastolic blood pressure (mmHg)	81	74	75
Mean arterial pressure (mmHg)	102	91*	91*
Heart rate	66	68	65
Pulmonary artery pressure (mmHg)	18.4	16.3	17.2
Pulmonary artery occluded pressure (mmHg)	11.5	10.6	11.9
Cardiac output (L min⁻¹)	5.3	5.1	4.8*
Systemic vascular resistance (dynes sec cm⁻⁵)	1391	1344	1377

* $P < 0.05$ compared with awake value.
(Data from McCammon RL, Hilgenberg JC, Stoelting RK. Hemodynamic effects of diazepam and diazepam-nitrous oxide in patients with coronary artery disease. Anesth Analg 1980; 59:438–41.)

actions at the neuromuscular junction (Dretchen *et al,* 1971). Presumably, diazepam diminishes the tonic facilitory influence on spinal gamma neurons, and, thus, skeletal muscle tone is reduced. Benzodiazepines do not produce adaquate relaxation for surgical procedures, nor does their use influence the requirements for neuromuscular blocking drugs. Tolerance occurs to the skeletal muscle relaxant effects of benzodiazepines.

Overdose

Central nervous system intoxication can be expected at diazepam concentrations that exceed 1000 ng ml⁻¹. Despite massive overdoses of diazepam (up to 700 mg), serious sequelae are unlikely to occur if cardiac and pulmonary function are supported and other drugs such as alcohol are not present (Greenblatt *el al,* 1977).

Drug Interactions

Cimetidine delays the hepatic clearance and thus prolongs the elimination half-time of both diazepam and desmethyldiazepam (Fig. 5-7) (Greenblatt *el al,* 1984a). Indeed, sedation is increased when diazepam is administered with cimetidine compared with that when diazepam is adminis-

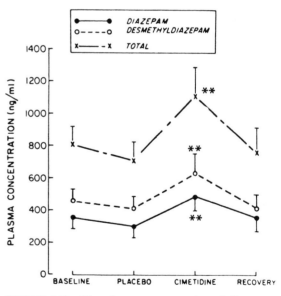

FIGURE 5-7. The plasma concentration of diazepam and its active metabolite, desmethyldiazepam, are greater when the parent drug is administered in the presence of cimetidine therapy. Mean ± SE. (From Greenblatt DJ, Abernathy DR, Morse DS, Harmatz JS, Shader RI. Clinical importance of the interaction of diazepam and cimetidine. N Engl J Med 1984;310:1639–43. Reprinted by permission of the New England Journal Medicine 1984;310:1639–43.)

tered alone. Presumably, this delayed clearance reflects cimetidine-induced inhibition of microsomal enzymes necessary for the oxidation of diazepam and desmethyldiazepam.

Interaction of alcohol with dizaepam may be particularly prominent, because alcohol increases the systemic absorption and central nervous system depressant effects of benzodiazepines. Opioids given concurrently with benzodiazepines potentiate the sedative effects of benzodiazepines. The dose of thiopental required for induction of anesthesia is reduced by diazepam (Gyermek, 1975). Diazepam, 0.2 mg kg^{-1}, reduces anesthetic requirements for halothane from 0.73% to 0.475% and doubling the dose of diazepam produces only minimal additional reductions (*e.g.*, a ceiling-effect) (Fig. 5-8) (Perisho *el al,* 1971). Halothane anesthesia reduces the rate of disappearance of diazepam from the plasma but has no significant effect on plasma concentrations of metabolites (Kanto and Isalo, 1973).

Tolerance and Physical Dependence

Tolerance to diazepam confers cross-tolerance to some extent. Habituation to diazepam can occur because of the prolonged elimination half-time and conversion to pharmacologically active metabolites (Alquander, 1978).

With abrupt discontinuation of diazepam, there is usually no evidence of withdrawal symptoms. Administration of high doses, however, for prolonged periods of time may occasionally result in withdrawal symptoms following abrupt discontinuation. Symptoms of withdrawal include anxiety, restlessness, insomnia, and, in extreme cases, seizures. Withdrawal symptoms may not appear for as long as 7 days following abrupt discontinuation.

Clinical Uses

Clinical uses of diazepam include (1) preoperative medication, (2) induction of anesthesia, (3) intravenous sedation, (4) anticonvulsant activity, (5) provision of complete anesthesia for short procedures such as cardioversion requiring minimal analgesia, (6) treatment of delerium tremens, and (7) production of skeletal muscle relaxation, which is important in the management of lumbar disc disease and rare diseases such as tetanus.

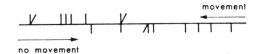

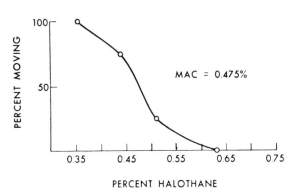

FIGURE 5-8. Diazepam, 0.2 mg kg^{-1}, reduces anesthetic requirements for halothane in patients from 0.73% to 0.475%. (From Perisho JA, Buechel DR, Miller RD. The effect of diazepam [Valium] on minimum alveolar anaesthetic requirement (MAC) in man. Can Anaesth Soc J 1971;18:536 – 40. Reproduced by permission of the authors and publisher.)

Preoperative Medication

The amnesic, calming, and sedative effects of benzodiazepines are the basis for the use of these drugs, especially diazepam, in preoperative medication. Preoperative medication with diazepam is better accomplished with oral administration than with intramuscular injection. Intramuscular injection of diazepam is painful because of the vehicle in which the drug is dissolved. Furthermore, absorption after intramuscular injection of diazepam, although usually complete, may, in some patients be unpredictable (Divoll *et al,* 1983).

Diazepam, 0.1 o 0.2 mg kg^{-1}, administered orally with 30 to 60 ml of water is rapidly absorbed from the gastrointestinal tract. Peak plasma concentrations of diazepam occur after about 55 minutes, with the estimated systemic absorption of the orally administered dose being 94%. The anterograde amnesic effect of diazepam is modest but is greatly increased when intramuscular scopolamine is administered concomitantly (Frumin *et al,* 1976). Nevertheless, anterograde amnesia, even after intravenous administration of diazepam, is transient. In contrast, lorazepam is a much more potent drug for producing amnesia.

Induction of Anesthesia

The popularity of diazepam for intravenous induction of anesthesia is related to its minimal depressant effects on ventilation and the cardiovascular system. Nevertheless, in most patients, diazepam has not represented a serious challenge to thiopental, because diazepam is slow to produce an effect while recovery is prolonged compared with the effects of barbiturates (Kanto and Isalo, 1973). Furthermore, thrombophelebitis may follow the intravenous administration of diazepam.

The potential for diazepam to produce recurrent sedation must be appreciated, especially when dealing with outpatients. Patients should not be allowed to drive for up to 24 hours after large doses of diazepam have been administered; after even small doses, patients should probably avoid alcohol for 24 hours.

Anticonvulsant Activity

The prior administration of intramuscular diazepam, 0.25 mg kg^{-1}, to monkeys protects against the occurrence of systemic toxicity produced by lidocaine. Evidence for this protection is an increased convulsant dose of lidocaine in benzodiazepine-pretreated animals (Fig. 5-9) (deJong and Heavner, 1974). Diazepam, 0.1 mg kg^{-1}, ad-

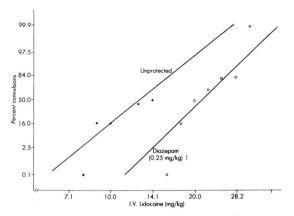

FIGURE 5-9. Prior administration of diazepam increases the intravenous dose of lidocaine required to produce convulsions compared with untreated (unprotected) animals. (From deJong RH, Heavner JE. Diazepam prevents and aborts lidocaine convulsions in monkeys. Anesthesiology 1974;41:226–30. Reproduced by permission of the authors and publisher.)

ministered intravenously, is effective in abolishing seizure activity produced by lidocaine, alcohol withdrawal (e.g., delerium tremens), and status epilepticus.

The efficacy of diazepam as an anticonvulsant may reflect its ability to facilitate the inhibitory neurotransmitter function of GABA. In contrast with nonspecific barbiturates, dizaepam selectively inhibits activity in the limbic system, particularly the hippocampus. The duration of anticonvulsant activity exceeds the elimination half-time of diazepam, suggesting a role for the pharmacologically active metabolite desmethyldiazepam.

MIDAZOLAM

Midazolam is a water-soluble benzodiazepine with an imidazole ring in its structure that accounts for stability in aqueous solutions and rapid metabolism (see Fig. 5-1) (Reves et al, 1985). Like other benzodiazepines, midazolam possesses antianxiety, sedative, amnesic, anticonvulsant, and skeletal muscle relaxant effects (see the section entitled Clinical Uses). The anticonvulsant activity of midazolam is similar to that of diazepam. Neuromuscular transmission is not affected, and the action of neuromuscular blocking drugs is not altered.

Compared with diazepam, midazolam is two to three times as potent. Indeed, midazolam has an affinity for the benzodiazepine receptor that is approximately twice that of diazepam (Mohler and Okada, 1977). Like diazepam, the central nervous system effects of midazolam are rapidly reversed by administration of a specific benzodiazepine antagonist (Lauven et al, 1985).

Commercial Preparation

The pKa of midazolam is 6.15, which permits the preparation of salts that are water soluble. The parenteral solution of midazolam used clinically is buffered to an acidic pH of 3.5. This is important because midazolam is characterized by a pH-dependent ring opening phenomenon in which the ring remains open at pH values below 4, thus maintaining water solubility of the drug. The ring closes above pH values of 4 (i.e., when exposed to physiologic pH), converting midazolam to a highly lipid-soluble drug.

Water solubility of midazolam obviates the need for a solubilizing agent such as propylene glycol that can produce venoirritation or interfere with absorption after intramuscular injection. Indeed, midazolam causes minimal to no local irritation after intravenous or intramuscular injection. Midazolam is compatible with lactated Ringer's solution and can be mixed with the acidic salts of other drugs, including opioids and anticholinergics.

Pharmacokinetics

Midazolam undergoes rapid absorption from the gastrointestinal tract and prompt passage across the blood–brain barrier (Greenblatt *et al*, 1983). Only about 50% of an orally administered dose of midazolam reaches the circulation, reflecting a substantial hepatic first-pass effect. Similar to most benzodiazepines, midazolam is bound extensively to plasma proteins; this binding is independent of the plasma concentration of midazolam (Table 5-1) (Greenblatt *et al*, 1984b). The short duration of action of a single dose of midazolam is due to its lipid solubility, leading to rapid redistribution from the brain to inactive tissue sites as well as rapid hepatic clearance.

There are important pharmacokinetic differences between midazolam and diazepam (Table 5-1) (Reves *et al*, 1985). For example, the elimination half-time of midazolam is 1 to 4 hours, which is much shorter than that of diazepam. Elimination half-time may be doubled in elderly patients, reflecting age-related reductions in hepatic blood flow and enzyme activity (Greenblatt *et al*, 1982). Volumes of distribution of midazolam and diazepam are similar, probably reflecting their similar lipid solubility and high degree of protein binding. Elderly patients and morbidly obese patients have an increased volume of distribution of midazolam resulting from enhanced distribution of the drug into peripheral adipose tissues. Clearance of midazolam is more rapid than that of diazepam. As a result of these differences, the central nervous system effects of midazolam would be expected to be shorter than those of diazepam. Indeed, tests of mental function return to normal within 4 hours after the administration of midazolam (Reves *et al*, 1985).

Metabolism

Midazolam undergoes hydroxylation by hepatic microsomal oxidative mechanisms to 1-hydroxymidazolam (Fig. 5-10) (Reves *et al*, 1985). Smaller amounts of 4-hydroxymidazolam are formed in parallel. These metabolites are excreted in the urine as glucuronide conjugates. Very little unchanged midazolam is excreted by the kidneys. The 1- and 4-hydroxy metabolites of midazolam have pharmacologic activity, although this is less than that of the parent compound (Ziegler *et al*, 1983). Neither the contribution of these metabolites to the overall clinical effects of midazolam, nor their potency or duration of action, have been established (Reves *et al*, 1985). In contrast to diazepam, H_2 receptor antagonists do not interfere with the metabolism of midazolam (Greenblatt *et al*, 1986.)

Renal Clearance

The elimination half-time, volume of distribution, and clearance of midazolam are not altered by renal failure (Vinik *et al*, 1983). This is consistent with the almost total metabolism of midazolam (see the section entitled Metabolism).

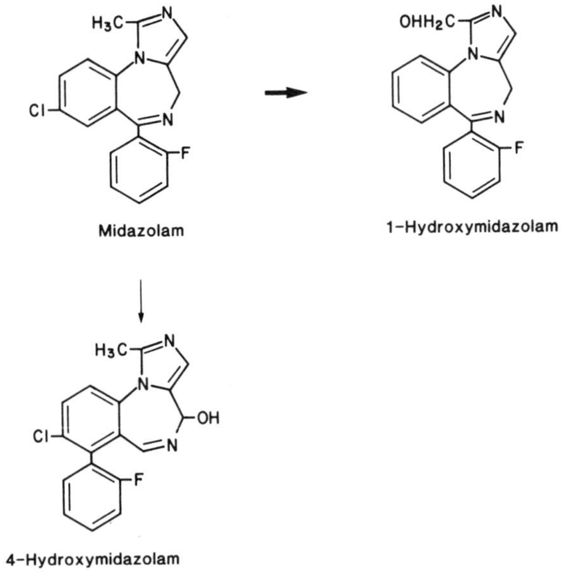

Midazolam

1-Hydroxymidazolam

4-Hydroxymidazolam

FIGURE 5-10. The principal metabolite of midazolam is 1-hydroxymidazolam. A lesser amount of midazolam is metabolized to 4-hydroxymidazolam.

Effects on Organ Systems

Cerebral Blood Flow

Midazolam produces dose-related reductions in cerebral blood flow and cerebral oxygen utilization. For example, intravenous administration of midazolam, 0.15 mg kg^{-1}, induces sleep, reduces cerebral blood flow 39%, and increases cerebral vascular resistance 52% (Forster *et al,* 1982). Patients with decreased intracranial compliance show little or no change in intracranial compliance when given midazolam in intravenous doses of 0.15 to 0.27 mg kg^{-1}. Thus, midazolam is an acceptable alternative to barbiturates for induction of anesthesia in patients with intracranial pathology. Furthermore, midazolam may protect the brain more than diazepam, but less than thiopental, against adverse effects of ischemia (Nugent *et al,* 1982). Similar to thiopental, induction of anesthesia with midazolam does not prevent increases in intracranial pressure associated with direct laryngoscopy for intubation of the trachea (Giffin *et al,* 1984).

Ventilation

Midazolam, 0.15 mg kg^{-1}, administered intravenously, depresses ventilation similar to diazepam, 0.3 mg kg^{-1} (Forster *et al,* 1980). Patients with chronic obstructive airways disease experience even greater midazolam-induced depression of ventilation. Depression of ventilation produced by midazolam is slower in onset and more prolonged than that produced by thiopental, 3.5 mg kg^{-1} (Gross *et al,* 1983). Transient apnea may occur following rapid administration of high doses (greater than 0.15 mg kg^{-1}) of midazolam, especially in the presence of preoperative medication that includes opioids (Kanto *et al,* 1982).

Cardiovascular System

Midazolam, 0.2 mg kg^{-1}, administered intravenously, for induction of anesthesia produces a greater increase in heart rate and decrease in blood pressure than does diazepam 0.5 mg kg^{-1} (Samuelson *et al,* 1981). These midazolam-induced hemodynamic changes are similar to changes produced by thiopental, 3 to 4 mg kg^{-1} (Lebowitz *et al,* 1982) (see Chapter 4). Cardiac output is not altered by midazolam. Mida-

zolam, like diazepam, produces transient depression of baroreceptor-mediated heart rate responses following intravenous administration in doses appropriate for induction of anesthesia (Marty *et al,* 1986). In the presence of hypovolemia, administration of midazolam results in enhanced blood pressure–lowering effects similar in magnitude to those produced by other intravenous induction drugs (Adams *et al,* 1985). Midazolam does not prevent blood pressure and heart rate responses evoked by intubation of the trachea.

Clinical Uses

Clinical uses of midazolam are similar to those for diazepam and include preoperative medication, induction of anesthesia, and intravenous sedation (see the section entitled Diazepam, Clinical Uses).

Preoperative Medication

Midazolam, like diazepam, is useful for preoperative medication because of its amnesic, antianxiety, and sedative effects. Onset of these effects is rapid after either oral (0.05 – 0.1 mg kg^{-1}) or intramuscular (0.5 – 0.1 mg kg^{-1}) administration. Scopolamine administered concurrently with midzaolam enhances its antianxiety and amnesic effects. Anterograde amnesia produced by midazolam, as by the other benzodiazepines, is dose related and often parallels the degree of sedation. The amnesic effect of an intravenous dose of midazolam, 5 mg, ranges from 20 to 32 minutes and may be even longer with intramuscular injection (Fragen *et al,* 1983). Prolonged amnesia could interfere with recall of oral instructions provided to outpatients, but, in this regard, midazolam is no different than thiopental (Kothary *et al,* 1981).

Intravenous Sedation

Midazolam in intravenous doses of 1 to 2.5 mg (up to 0.1 mg kg^{-1}) is effective as intravenous sedation for therapeutic procedures as well as during regional anesthesia. This drug, like diazepam, may have value for short procedures not requiring analgesia such as cardioversion and electroconvulsive therapy. Compared with diazepam, midazolam produces a more rapid onset with greater amnesia and less postoperative sedation, but the time to complete recovery is no shorter (McClure et al, 1983). Pain on injection and subsequent venous thrombosis are less likely with midazolam than with diazepam.

Induction of Anesthesia

Induction of anesthesia can be produced by intravenous administration of midazolam over 30 to 60 seconds in doses of 0.2 to 0.3 mg kg^{-1}(White, 1982). Nevertheless, thiopental usually produces induction of anesthesia 50% to 100% faster than midazolam (Fig. 5-11) (Sarnquist et al, 1980). Analgesia does not accompany induction of anesthesia with midazolam.

The dose of midazolam required for induction of anesthesia is less when preoperative medication with an opioid is included. Elderly patients require less midazolam for induction of anesthesia than do young patients (Gamble et al, 1981).

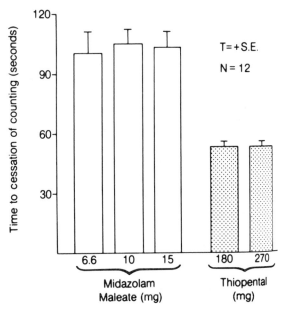

FIGURE 5-11. Induction of anesthesia as depicted by time to cessation of counting occurs in about 110 seconds following the intravenous administration of midazolam compared with about 50 seconds following thiopental injection. (From Sarnquist FH, Mathers WD, Brock–Utne J, Carr B, Canup C, Brown CR. A bioassay of a water-soluble benzodiazepine against sodium thiopental. Anesthesiology 1980;52:149–53. Reproduced by permission of the authors and publisher.)

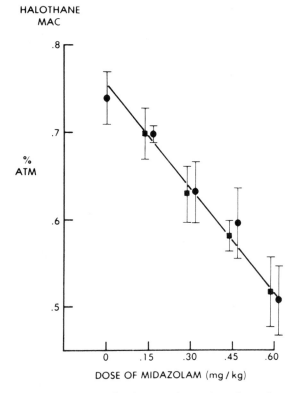

FIGURE 5-12. Midazolam produces dose-dependent reductions in anesthetic requirements (MAC) for halothane in patients. Mean ± SE. (From Melvin MA, Johnson BH, Quasha AL, Eger EI. Induction of anesthesia with midazolam decreases halothane MAC in humans. Anesthesiology 1982;57:238–41. Reproduced by permission of the authors and publisher.)

The explanation for this is not clear, because a prolonged elimination half-time should not alter the acute hypnotic effect of a single intravenous dose of midazolam. A possible explanation is increased central nervous system sensitivity to the effects of midazolam with increasing age (Greenblatt et al, 1982).

Midazolam may be used to supplement opioids or inhaled anesthetics during maintenance of anesthesia. Anesthetic requirements for halothane are reduced about 30% by midazolam, 0.6 mg kg^{-1}(Fig. 5-12) (Melvin et al, 1982). Awakening following general anesthesia that included induction of anesthesia with midazolam is one to two and one-half times longer than that observed when thiopental is used for induction of anesthesia (Jensen *et al,* 1982). Gradual awakening in patients who receive midazolam is rarely associated with nausea, vomiting, or emergence excitement. One hour after surgery, patients are equally alert with either midazolam or thiopental, and discharge time from an outpatient recovery room is similar with both anesthetics (Crawford *et al,* 1984).

LORAZEPAM

Lorazepam resembles oxazepam, differing only in the presence of an extra chlorine atom on the ortho position of the 5-phenyl moiety (see Figs. 5-1 and 5-4). It is five to ten times as potent as diazepam. Lorazepam, like diazepam, is devoid of analgesic properties but produces profound anterograde amnesia. The effects of lorazepam on the cardiovascular system, ventilation, and skeletal muscles resemble those of diazepam.

Clinical Uses

Lorazepam undergoes reliable absorption after oral and intramuscular injection, which contrasts with diazepam. Following oral administration, maximal plasma concentrations of lorazepam occur in 2 to 4 hours and persist at therapeutic levels for up to 24 to 48 hours. The recommended dose of lorazepam for preoperative medication is 50 μg kg^{-1}, not to exceed 4 mg (Fragen and Caldwell, 1976; Heisterkamp and Cohen, 1975). With this dose, maximal anterograde amnesia lasting up to 6 hours occurs, and sedation is not excessive. Larger oral doses produce additional sedation without increasing amnesia. The prolonged duration of action of lorazepam limits its usefulness for preoperative medication when rapid awakening at the end of surgery is desirable (George and Dundee, 1977).

A slow onset of effect limits the usefulness of lorazepam for (1) intravenous induction of anesthesia (2) sedation during regional anesthesia or (3) use as an anticonvulsant. Like diazepam, lorazepam is effective in limiting the incidence of emergence reactions following administration of ketamine. Although insoluble in water and thus requiring use of solvents such as polyethylene glycol or propylene glycol, lorazepam is alleged to be less painful on injection and to produce less venous thrombosis than diazepam (Hegarty and Dundee, 1977).

Pharmacokinetics

Lorazepam is conjugated with glucuronic acid to form pharmacologically inactive metabolites (Greenblatt *et al,* 1979). This contrasts with the formation of pharmacologically active metabolites following the metabolism of diazepam. The elimination half-time is 10 to 20 hours, with urinary excretion of lorazepam glucuronide accounting for more than 80% of the injected dose (see Table 5-1). This shorter elimination half-time compared with diazepam probably reflects lesser lipid solubility of lorazepam. Nevertheless, clinical effects of diazepam may be shorter because it dissociates more rapidly than lorazepam from benzodiazepine receptors, thus permitting its more rapid redistribution to inactive tissue sites. Since formation of glucuronide metabolites of lorazepam is not entirely dependent on hepatic microsomal enzymes, the metabolism of lorazepam is less likely than diazepam to be influenced by alterations in hepatic function, increasing age, or drugs such as cimetidine (see the section entitled Drug Interactions). Indeed, elimination half-time of lorazepam is not prolonged in elderly patients or in those patients treated with cimetidine.

OXAZEPAM

Oxazepam, which is a pharmacologically active metabolite of diazepam, is commercially available (see Fig. 5-4). Its duration of action is slightly shorter than that of diazepam because oxazepam is converted to pharmacologically inactive metabolites by conjugation with glucuronic acid. Indeed, the elimination half-time is relatively short, being 5 to 15 hours. Like lorazepam, the duration of action of oxazepam is unlikely to be influenced by hepatic dysfunction of administration of cimetidine (see the section entitled Drug Interactions).

Oral absorption of oxazepam is relatively slow. As a result, this drug may not be useful for the treatment of insomnia characterized by difficulty in falling asleep. Conversely, oxazepam may be useful for the treatment of insomnia characterized by nightly awakenings or shortened total sleep time.

CHLORDIAZEPOXIDE

Chlordiazepoxide was the first benzodiazepine introduced into clinical practice (see Fig. 5-1). It is not as potent as diazepam for relieving anxiety and is less active as an anticonvulsant and skeletal muscle relaxant. An active metabolite, desmethylchlordiazepoxide, has an elimination half-time of 24 to 96 hours. Physical dependence and withdrawal symptoms may occur upon discontinuation of chronic therapy.

CLONAZEPAM

Clonazepam is a highly lipid-soluble benzodiazepine that is well absorbed after oral administration (Browne, 1978). Metabolism of clonazepam is to inactive conjugated and unconjugated metabolites that appear in the urine. The elimination half-time is 24 to 48 hours. Clonazepam is particularly effective in the control and prevention of seizures, especially myoclonic and infantile spasms (see Chapter 30).

FLURAZEPAM

Flurazepam is chemically and pharmacologically similar to other benzodiazepines but is used clinically to treat insomnia (see Fig. 5-1). Following oral administration of 15 to 30 mg to adults, an hypnotic effect occurs in 15 to 25 minutes and lasts 7 to 8 hours. The percentage of rapid eye movement sleep is reduced by this drug.

The principal metabolite of flurazepam is desalkylflurazepam. This metabolite is pharmacologically active and has a long elimination half-time, which may manifest as daytime sedation (*e.g.*, hangover). Furthermore, slow elimination of this same metabolite on termination of flurazepam therapy probably accounts for rebound insomnia.

TEMAZEPAM

Temazepam is an orally active benzodiazepine used exclusively for the treatment of insomnia (see Fig. 5-1). Oral absorption is complete, but peak plasma concentrations do not reliably occur until about 2.5 hours after administration. Metabolism in the liver results in weakly active to inactive

metabolites that are conjugated with glucuronic acid. The elimination half-time of temazepam is about 15 hours.

Temazepam, 15 to 30 mg, administered to adults does not alter the proportion of rapid eye movement sleep to total sleep. Despite the relatively long elimination half-time, temazepam, as used to treat insomnia, is unlikely to be accompanied by residual drowsiness the following morning. Tolerance or signs of withdrawal do not occur, even after nightly administration for 30 consecutive days.

TRIAZOLAM

Triazolam is an orally absorbed benzodiazepine that is effective in the treatment of insomnia (see Fig. 5-1). Peak plasma concentrations following oral administration to adults of 0.25 to 0.5 mg occur in about 1 hour. The elimination half-time is 1.7 to 5.2 hours, rendering triazolam one of the shortest-acting benzodiazepines. The two principal metabolites of triazolam have little if any hypnotic activity, and their elimination half-times are less than 4 hours. Cumulative effects or tolerance to the hypnotic effects of triazolam does not seem to occur.

Triazolam does not change the proportion of rapid eye movement sleep to total sleep time. Rebound insomnia, however, may occur when this drug is discontinued.

CLORAZEPATE

Clorazepate resembles diazepam in relieving anxiety. Following oral administration, the drug is almost totally converted to desmethyldiazepam in the stomach before absorption into the systemic circulation occurs. As such, the parent drug is considered a prodrug.

HALAZEPAM

Halazepam is metabolized to the active compound desmethyldiazepam. As such, the parent drug is considered a prodrug. The principal indication for this drug is the treatment of primary anxiety disorders. The most common side-effect is drowsiness.

PRAZEPAM

Prazepam is converted to desmethyldiazepam, which is responsible for the anxiety-relieving effects of this drug. As such, the parent drug is considered a prodrug. Conversion to desmethyldiazepam in the liver occurs slowly, with peak plasma concentrations occurring about 6 hours after oral administration.

REFERENCES

Adams P, Gelman S, Reves JG, Greenblatt DJ, Alvis JM, Bradley E. Midazolam pharmacodynamics and pharmacokinetics during acute hypovolemia. Anesthesiology 1985;63:140 – 6.

Alquander C. Dependence on sedative and hypnotic drugs. Acta Psychiatr Scand 1978;270;1 – 120.

Braunstein MC. Apnea with maintenance of consciousness following intravenous diazepam. Anesth Analg 1979;58:52 – 3.

Browne TR. Clonazepam. N Engl J Med 1978;299:812 – 6.

Caldwell CB, Gross JB. Physostigmine reversal of midazolam-induced sedation. Anesthesiology 1982; 57:125 – 7.

Crawford ME, Carl P, Andersen RS, Mikkelsen BO. Comparison between midazolam and thiopentone-based balanced anaesthesia for day-care surgery. Br J Anaesth 1984;56:165 – 9.

Dawes GS. The distribution and action of drugs on the fetus *in utero*. Br J Anaesth 1973;45:766 – 9.

deJong RH, Heavner JE. Diazepam prevents and aborts lidocaine convulsions in monkeys. Anesthesiology 1974;41:226 – 30.

Divoll M, Greenblatt DJ, Ochs HR, Shader RI. Absolute bioavailability of oral and intramuscular diazepam: Effects of age and sex. Anesth Analg 1983;62:1 – 8.

Dretchen K, Ghoneim MM, Long JP. The interaction of diazepam with myoneural blocking agents. Anesthesiology 1971;34:463 – 8.

Eustace PW, Hailey DM, Cox AG, Baired ES. Biliary excretion of diazepam in man. Br J Anaesth 1975;47:983 – 5.

Falk RB, Denlinger JK, Nahrwold ML, Todd RA. Acute vasodilation following induction of anesthesia with intravenous diazepam and nitrous oxide. Anesthesiology 1978;49:149 – 50.

Forster A, Gardaz J-P, Suter PM, Gemperele M. Respiratory depression of midazolam and diazepam. Anesthesiology 1980;53:494 – 9.

Forster A, Juge O, Morel D. Effects of midazolam on cerebral blood flow in human volunteers. Anesthesiology 1982;56:453 – 5.

Fragen RJ, Caldwell N. Lorazepam premedication; Lack of recall and relief of anxiety. Anesth Analg 1976;55:792 – 6.

Fragen RJ, Funk DI, Avram MJ, Costello C, DeBruine K. Midazolam versus hydroxyzine as intramuscular premedicants. Can Anaesth Soc J 1983;30:136 – 41.

Frumin MJ, Herekar VR, Jarvik ME. Amnesic actions of diazepam and scopolamine in man. Anesthesiology 1976;45:406 – 12.

Gallager DW. Benzodiazepines and gamma-aminobutyric acid. Sleep 1982;5:S3 – S11.

Gamble JAS, Kawar P, Dundee JW, Moore J, Briggs LP. Evaluation of midazolam as an intravenous induction agent. Anaesthesia 1981;36:868 – 73.

George KA, Dundee JW. Relative amnesic actions of diazepam, flunitrazepam, and lorazepam in man. Br J Clin Pharmacol 1977;4:45 – 51.

Griffin JP, Cottrell JE, Shwiry B, Hartung J, Epstein J, Lim K. Intracranial pressure, mean arterial pressure, and heart rate following midazolam or thiopental in humans with brain tumors. Anesthesiology 1984;60:491 – 4.

Greenblatt DJ. Benzodiazepines. N Engl J Med 1974;291:1011 – 15;1239 – 43.

Greenblatt DJ, Abernathy DR, Morse DS, Harmatz JS, Shader RI. Clinical importance of the interaction of diazepam and cimetidine. N Engl J Med 1984a;310:1639 – 43.

Greenblatt DJ, Abernathy DR, Locniskar A, Harmatz JS, Limjuco RA, Shader RI. Effect of age, gender, and obesity on midazolam kinetics. Anesthesiology 1984b;61:27 – 35.

Greenblatt DJ, Allen MD, Locniskar A, Harmatz JS, Shader RI. Lorazepam kinetics in the elderly. Clin Pharmacol Ther 1979;26:103 – 13.

Greenblatt DJ, Allen MD, Noel BJ, Shader RI. Acute overdosage with benzodiazepine derivatives. Clin Pharmacol Ther 1977;4:497 – 514.

Greenblatt DJ, Arendt RM, Abernathy DR, Giles HG, Sellers EM, Shader RI. In vitro quantitation of benzodiazepine lipophilicity: Relation to in vivo distribution. Br J Anaesth 1983;55:985 – 9.

Greenblatt DJ, Koch-Weser J. Clinical toxicity of chlordiazepoxide and diazepam in relation to serum albumin concentration: A report from the Boston Collaborative Drug Surveillance Program. Eur J Clin Pharmacol 1974;7:259 – 62.

Greenblatt DJ, Locniskar A, Scavone JM *et al.* Absence of interaction of cimetidine and ranitidine with intravenous and oral midazolam. Anesth Analg 1986; 65:176 – 80.

Greenblatt DJ, Sellers EM, Shader RI. Drug Disposition in old age. N Engl J Med 1982;306:1081 – 8.

Gross JB, Smith L, Smith TC. Time course of ventilatory response to carbon dioxide after intravenous diazepam. Anesthesiology 1982;57:18 – 21.

Gross JB, Zebrowski ME, Carel WD, Gardner S, Smith TC. Time course of ventilatory depression after thiopental and midazolam in normal subjects and in patients with chronic obstructive pulmonary disease. Anesthesiology 1983;58:540–4.

Gyermek L. Clinical effects of diazepam prior to and during general anesthesia. Curr Ther Res 1975; 17:175–88.

Hegarty JE, Dundee JW. Sequelae after the intravenous injection of three benzodiazepines — diazepam, lorazepam and flunitrozepam. Br Med J 1977; 2:1384–5.

Heisterkamp DV, Cohen PJ. The effect of intravenous premedication with lorazepam (Ativan), pentobarbital or diazepam on recall. Br J Anaesth 1975;47:79–81.

Ikran H, Rubin AP, Jewkes RF. Effect of diazepam on myocardial blood flow of patients with and without coronary artery disease. Br Heart J 1973;35:626–30.

Jensen S, Schou-Olesen A, Huttel MS. Use of midazolam as an induction agent: Comparison with thiopentone. Br J Anaesth 1982;54:605–7.

Kanto J, Isalo EUM. Diazepam as an inductive agent in two kinds of combination anaesthesia: The disappearance of diazepam and its metabolites from the plasma. Ann Chir Gynaecol Fenn 1973;62:251–5.

Kanto J, Sjovall S, Vuori A. Effect of different kinds of premedication on the induction properties of midazolam. Br J Anaesth 1982;54:507–11.

Kaplan SA, Jack ML, Alexander, Weinfeld RE. Pharmacokinetic profile of diazepam in man following single intravenous and chronic oral administration. J Pharm Sci 1973;62:1789–96.

Knapp RB, Dubow H. Comparison of diazepam with thiopental as an induction agent in cardiopulmonary disease. Anesth Analg 1970;49:722–6.

Klotz U, Avant GR, Hoyumpa A, Schenker S, Wilkinson GR. The effects of age and liver disease on the disposition and elimination of diazepam in adult man. J Clin Invest 1975;55:347–59.

Kothary SP, Brown ACD, Pandit UA, Samra SK. Time course of antirecall effect of diazepam and lorazepam following oral administration. Anesthesiology 1981;55:641–4.

Lauven PM, Schwilden H. Stoeckel H, Greenblatt DJ. The effects of a benzodiazepine antagonist Ro 15-1788 in the presence of stable concentrations of midazolam. Anesthesiology 1985;63:61–4.

Lebowitz PW, Cote ME, Daniels AL, et al. Comparative cardiovascular effects of midazolam and thiopental in healthy patients. Anesth Analg 1982;61: 661–5.

Mahon WA, Inaba T, Umeda T, Tsutsumi E, Stone R. Biliary elimination of diazepam in man. Clin Pharmacol Ther 1976;19:443–50.

Marty J, Gauzit R, Lefevre P et al. Effects of diazepam and midazolam on baroreflex control of heart rate and on sympathetic activity in humans. Anesth Analg 1986;65:113–9.

McCammon RL, Hilgenberg JC, Stoelting RK. Hemody-

namic effects of diazepam and diazepam-nitrous oxide in patients with coronary artery disease. Anesth Analg 1980;59:438–41.

McClure JH, Brown DT, Wildsmith JAW. Comparison of the I.V. administration of midazolam and diazepam as sedation during spinal anaesthesia. Br J Anaesth 1983;55:1089–93.

Melvin MA, Johnson BH, Quasha AL, Eger EI. Induction of anesthesia with midazolam decreases halothane MAC in humans. Anesthesiology 1982;57:238–41.

Meyer BH, Weis OF, Muller FO. Antagonism of diazepam by aminophylline in healthy volunteers. Anesth Analg 1984;63:900–2.

Mohler H, Okada T. Benzodiazepine receptor: demonstration in the central nervous system. Science 1977;198:849–51.

Nugent M, Artru AA, Michenfelder JD. Cerebral metabolic, vascular, and protective effects of midazolam maleate: Comparison to diazepam. Anesthesiology 1982;56:172–6.

O'Boyle Co, Lambe R, Darragh A, Taffe W, Brick I, Kenny M. RO 15-1788 antagonizes the effects of diazepam in man without affecting its bioavailability. Br J Anaesth 1983;55:349–55.

Perisho JA, Buechel DR, Miller RD. The effect of diazepam (Valium) on minimum alveolar anaesthetic requirement (MAC) in man. Can Anaesth Soc J 1971;18:536–40.

Phillis JW, Edstrom JP, Ellis SW, Kirkpatrick JR. Theophylline antagonizes flurazepam-induced depression of cerebral cortical neurons. Can J Physiol Pharmacol 1979;57:917–20.

Rao S, Sherbaniuk RW, Prasad K, Lee SJK, Sproule BJ. Cardiopulmonary effects of diazepam. Clin Pharmacol 1973;14:182–9.

Reves JG, Fragen RJ, Vinik HR, Greenblatt DJ. Midazolam: Pharmacology and uses. Anesthesiology 1985;62:310–24.

Richter JJ. Current theories about the mechanisms of benzodiazepines and neuroleptic drugs. Anesthesiology 1981;54:66–72.

Saletu B, Saletu M, Ital T. Effect of minor and major tranquilizers on somatosensory evoked potentials. Psychopharmacologia 1972;24:347–58.

Samuelson PN, Reves JG, Kouchoukos NT, Smith LR, Dole KM. Hemodynamic responses to anesthetic induction with midazolam or diazepam in patients with ischemic heart disease. Anesth Analg 1981;60:802–9.

Sarnquist FH, Mathers WD, Brock-Utne J, Carr B, Canup C, Brown CR. A bioassay of a water -soluble benzodiazepine against sodium thiopental. Anesthesiology 1980;52:149–53.

Schwartz MA, Koechlin BA, Postma E, Palmer S, Krol G. Metabolism of diazepam in rat, dog, and man. J Pharmacol Exp Ther 1965;149:423–35.

Thiessen JJ, Sellers EM, Denbeigh P, Dolman L. Plasma protein binding of diazepam and tolbutamide in chronic alcoholics. J Clin Pharmacol 1976;16: 345 – 51.

vanderKleijn E, vanRossum JM, Muskens ATJM, Rijntjes NVM. Pharmacokinetics of diazepam in dogs, mice, and humans. Acta Pharmacol Toxicol 1971;29: 109 – 29.

Vinik HR, Reves JG, Greenblatt DJ, Abernathy DR, Smith LR. The pharmacokinetics of midazolam in chronic renal failure patients. Anesthesiology 1983;59: 390 – 4.

Wangler MA, Kilpatrick DS. Aminophylline is an antagonist of lorazepam. Anesth Analg 1985;64:834 – 6.

White PF. Comparative evaluation of intravenous agents for rapid sequence induction — thiopental, ketamine, and midazolam. Anesthesiology 1982;57: 279 – 84.

Ziegler WH, Schalch E, Leishman B, Eckert M. Comparison of the effects of intravenously administered midazolam, triazolam and their hydroxymetabolites. Br J Clin Pharmacol 1983;16:63s – 69s.

CHAPTER 6

Nonbarbiturate Induction Drugs

KETAMINE

Ketamine is a phencyclidine derivative that produces "dissociative anesthesia" characterized by electroencephalographic evidence of dissociation between the thalamus and limbic system (Corssen *et al*, 1968). Dissociative anesthesia resembles a cataleptic state in which the eyes remain open with a slow nystagmic gaze. The patient is noncommunicative although wakefulness may appear to be present. Varying degrees of hypertonus and purposeful skeletal muscle movements often occur independently of surgical stimulation. The patient is amnesic, and analgesia is intense. Cardiovascular stimulation and a high incidence of emergence delirium limit the clinical usefulness of ketamine.

Structure Activity Relationships

Ketamine is a water-soluble molecule that structurally resembles phencyclidine (Fig. 6-1). The presence of an asymmetric carbon atom results in the existence of two optical isomers of ketamine (White *et al*, 1982). Only the racemic mixture containing equal amounts of the two ketamine isomers is available for clinical use. When studied separately, the positive isomer is a more potent analgesic and is less likely to cause emergence reactions than the negative isomer (White *et al*, 1980). Both the positive and negative isomers of ketamine appear capable of inhibiting uptake of catecholamines back into postganglionic sympathetic nerve endings (*i.e.*, cocaine-like effect), whereas only the positive isomer prevents extraneuronal uptake of catecholamines (Lundy *et al*, 1986). The fact that individual optical isomers of ketamine differ in their pharmacologic properties suggests that this drug interacts with specific receptors.

Mechanism of Action

A number of explanations have been proposed for the intense analgesia produced by ketamine even at subanesthetic doses (Bovill and Dundee, 1971). For example, ketamine produces selective depression of the medial thalamic nuclei. Analgesia may be explained in part by lamina-specific suppression of spinal cord activity necessary for transmission of pain to higher brain centers (Kitahata *et al*, 1973). Ketamine may even bind stereospecifically to opioid receptors (Smith *et al*, 1980).

Ketamine affects central nervous system neurotransmitters, including interactions with muscarinic cholinergic receptors (Vincent *et al*, 1978). In animals, acetylcholine turnover rates are decreased by ketamine. It is of interest that physostigmine may reverse actions of ketamine (Toro-Matos *et al*, 1980) (see Chapter 9). The mechanism of analgesia produced by ketamine also appears to be related to interference with the transmission of the affective – emotional component of pain from the spinal cord to higher brain centers.

Pharmacokinetics

The pharmacokinetics of ketamine resemble thiopental in terms of rapid onset of action, relatively short duration of action, and high lipid solubility (Table 6-1). Ketamine has a pKa of 7.5 at physiologic pH 7.4 (White *et al,* 1982). Peak plasma concentrations of ketamine occur within 1 minute following intravenous administration and within 5 minutes following intramuscular injection (Cohen *et al,* 1973). Ketamine is not significantly bound to plasma proteins and leaves the blood rapidly to be distributed into tissues. Initially, ketamine is distributed to highly perfused tissues such as the brain where the peak concentration may be four to five times that present in plasma. The extreme lipid solubility of ketamine (5 – 10 times that of thiopental) ensures its rapid transfer across the blood – brain barrier (Cohen and Trevor, 1974). Furthermore, ketamine-induced increases in cerebral blood flow contribute to the delivery of drug and thus rapid achievement of high brain concentrations. Subsequently, ketamine is redistributed from the brain and other highly perfused organs to less well-perfused tissues. The elimination half-time of ketamine is 1 to 2 hours (Zsigmond and Domino, 1980).

Failure of renal function or enzyme induction to alter the duration of action of a single dose of ketamine suggests that redistribution of drug from the brain to other inactive tissue sites is primarily responsible for termination of unconsciousness. Hepatic metabolism, as with thiopental, is important for ultimate clearance of ketamine from the body. Ketamine stored in tissues may contribute to cumulative drug effects with repeated or continuous administration.

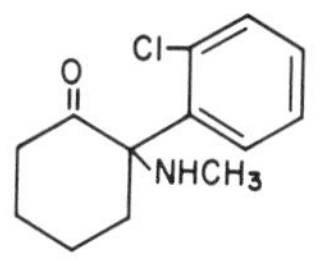

Metabolism

Ketamine is metabolized extensively by hepatic microsomal enzymes. A major pathway of metabolism is demethylation of ketamine by cytochrome P-450 enzymes to form norketamine (Fig. 6-2; White *et al,* 1982). In animals, norketamine is one-fifth to one-third as potent as ketamine. This active metabolite may contribute to prolonged effects of ketamine. Norketamine is eventually hydroxylated and then conjugated to more water-soluble and inactive glucuronide metabolites. Following intravenous administration, less than 4% of a dose of ketamine can be recovered from the urine as unchanged drug. Fecal excretion accounts for less than 5% of an injected dose of ketamine. Halothane or diazepam slow the metabolism of ketamine and prolong the drug's effects (Borondy and Glazko, 1977; White *et al,* 1976).

Chronic administration of ketamine results in stimulation of the activity of enzymes responsible for its metabolism (Marietta *et al,* 1976). Accelerated metabolism of ketamine by virtue of enzyme induction could explain, in part, the observation of tolerance to the analgesic effects of ketamine that occur in patients receiving repeated doses of ketamine. Indeed, tolerance is observed in burn patients receiving more than two short-interval exposures to ketamine (Demling *et al,* 1978). Development of tolerance is also consistent with reports of ketamine dependence (White *et al,* 1982).

FIGURE 6-1. Ketamine.

Table 6-1
Comparative Characteristics of Nonbarbiturate Induction Drugs

	Elimination Half-Time (hours)	Volume of Distribution (L kg^{-1})	Clearance (ml kg^{-1} min^{-1})	Blood Pressure	Heart Rate
Ketamine	1 – 2	2.5 – 3.5	16 – 18	Increased	Increased
Etomidate	2 – 5	2.2 – 4.5	10 – 20	No change	No change
Propofol	0.5 – 1.5	3.5 – 4.5	30 – 60	Decreased	Increased

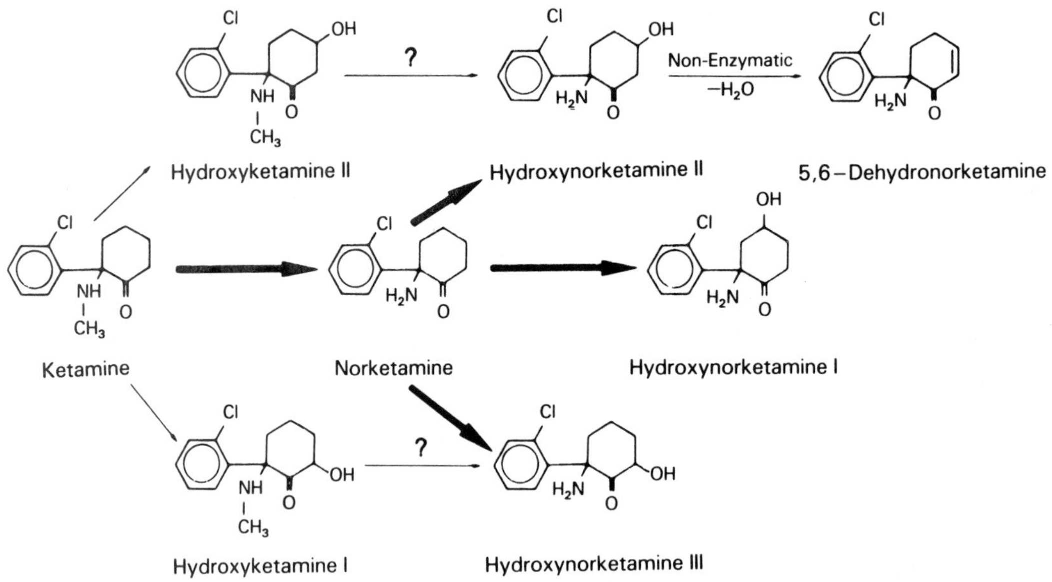

FIGURE 6-2. Metabolism of ketamine. (From White PF, Way WL, Trevor AJ. Ketamine — its pharmacology and therapeutic uses. Anesthesiology 1982;56:119-36. Reproduced by permission of the authors and publisher.)

Clinical Uses

Ketamine is unique in being effective for induction of anesthesia when given by both the intravenous (1-2 mg kg^{-1}) and intramuscular (5-10 mg kg^{-1}) routes. Intravenous injection of ketamine does not produce pain or venous irritation. The need for a higher intramuscular dose reflects a significant hepatic first-pass effect for ketamine. Consciousness is lost in 30 to 60 seconds after intravenous administration and in 2 to 4 minutes after intramuscular injection. Unconsciousness is associated with maintenance of normal or slightly depressed pharyngeal and laryngeal reflexes. Return of consciousness occurs in about 10 to 15 minutes after the usual intravenous induction dose of ketamine, but complete recovery is delayed.

A feature of ketamine administration is the subsequent development of intense analgesia. Analgesia may precede the onset of anesthesia and persist after the return of consciousness. Analgesia is alleged to be greater for somatic than for visceral pain and can be achieved with small intravenous doses of ketamine (0.2-0.5 mg kg^{-1}) that do not necessarily produce unconsciousness (Sadove *et al,* 1971). Amnesia persists for about 1 hour after apparent recovery of consciousness, but ketamine does not cause retrograde amnesia.

Because of its rapid onset of action, ketamine has been used as an intramuscular induction drug in children and in difficult-to-manage mentally retarded patients regardless of age. Ketamine has been used extensively in burn units for dressing changes, débridements, and skin-grafting procedures. The intense analgesia and ability to maintain spontaneous ventilation in what may otherwise be an airway altered by burn scar contractures are important advantages of ketamine in these patients. Tolerance may develop, however, in burn patients undergoing repeated anesthetics with ketamine (see the section entitled Metabolism). Induction of anesthesia in acutely hypovolemic patients is often accomplished with ketamine, taking advantage of the drug's cardiovascular-stimulating effects (see the section entitled Cardiovascular Effects). Beneficial effects of ketamine on airway resistance make this a potentially useful drug for rapid induction of anesthesia in patients with asthma (Corssen *et al,* 1972; Hirshman *et al,*

1979) (see the section entitled Drug Interactions).

Analgesic doses of ketamine (0.2–0.5 mg kg^{-1}) administered during labor do not depress the newborn (Akamatsu *et al*, 1974; Janeczko *et al*, 1974). Neonatal neurobehavioral scores of infants born by vaginal delivery with ketamine analgesia are lower than those born with epidural block but greater than infants delivered with thiopental–nitrous oxide (Hodgkinson *et al*, 1977). Ketamine has been used successfully for outpatient procedures when minimal intravenous doses for induction of anesthesia (0.5–1.5 mg kg^{-1}) are followed by a continuous infusion of 10 to 20 μg kg^{-1} min^{-1} (Hatano *et al*, 1976). Extensive experience with ketamine for pediatric cardiac catheterization has shown it to be highly effective. Ketamine placed in the epidural space has been reported to provide postoperative analgesia without associated depression of ventilation or cardiovascular stimulation (Islas *et al*, 1985).

Ketamine has been used safely in patients with myopathies and malignant hyperthermia (Wadhwa and Tantisira, 1974). This drug has also been used in a patient with acute intermittent porphyria, but caution is recommended because ketamine can increase ALA synthetase activity in animals (Kostrzewski and Gregor, 1978).

The use of ketamine in patients with coronary artery disease has been questioned because of increased myocardial oxygen requirements that accompany this drug's sympathomimetic effects on the heart (Reves *et al*, 1978) (see the section entitled Cardiovascular System). Nevertheless, induction of anesthesia with intravenous diazepam, 0.5 mg kg^{-1}, and ketamine, 1 to 2 mg kg^{-1}, followed by maintenance with a continuous infusion of ketamine, 15 to 30 μg kg^{-1} min^{-1}, has been proposed as an alternative to opioids and nitrous oxide for anesthesia in patients with coronary artery disease (White *et al*, 1982). Ketamine should probably be avoided in patients with severe hypertension and those with increased intracranial pressure (see the sections entitled Cardiovascular System and Central Nervous System). Nystagmus associated with administration of ketamine may be undesirable in operations or examinations of the eye performed under anesthesia.

Inclusion of an antisialagogue in the preoperative medication is recommended to avoid coughing and laryngospasm due to ketamine-induced salivary secretions. Glycopyrrolate may be a better choice because atropine or scopolamine could theoretically increase the incidence of emergence delirium (see the section entitled Emergence Delirium).

Effects Other Than Central Nervous System Depression

Central Nervous System

Ketamine is a potent cerebral vasodilator capable of increasing cerebral blood flow 60% in the presence of normocapnia (Takeshita *et al*, 1972). As a result, patients with intracranial pathology may be vulnerable to sustained elevations in intracranial pressure following administration of ketamine. The increase in cerebral blood flow and subsequent elevation in intracranial pressure produced by ketamine is blunted by prior administration of thiopental or diazepam (Dawson *et al*, 1971; Thorsen and Gran, 1980). Nevertheless, this protection is not sufficiently reliable to justify use of ketamine in patients with space-occupying intracranial lesions.

Ketamine's effects on the electroencephalogram (EEG) are characterized by abolition of alpha rhythm and a dominance of theta activity. Onset of delta activity coincides with loss of consciousness. There is depression of the auditory and visual evoked responses. Ketamine-induced excitatory activity occurs in both the thalamus and limbic system without evidence of subsequent spread of seizure activity to cortical areas (Ferrer-Allado *et al*, 1973). As such, ketamine would be unlikely to precipitate generalized convulsions in patients with seizure disorders. Indeed, ketamine does not alter the seizure threshold in epileptic patients (Celesia *et al*, 1975).

Ventilation and Airway

Ketamine does not produce significant depression of ventilation. The ventilatory response to carbon dioxide is maintained during ketamine anesthesia, and the PaCO$_2$ is unlikely to increase more than 3 mmHg (Soliman *et al*, 1975). Respiratory rate typically decreases for 2 to 3 minutes following administration of ketamine. Apnea, however, can occur if the drug is given rapidly or an opioid is administered with the preoperative medication.

Upper airway skeletal muscle tone is well-maintained, and upper airway reflexes remain relatively intact (Taylor and Towey, 1971). Despite continued presence of upper airway reflexes, ketamine anesthesia does not negate the need for protection of the lungs against aspiration by placement of a cuffed tube in the trachea. Salivary and tracheobronchial mucous gland secretions are increased by intramuscular or intravenous ketamine, necessitating use of an antisialagogue in the preoperative medication.

Ketamine is as effective as halothane or enflurane in preventing experimentally induced bronchospasm in dogs (Hirshman *et al,* 1979). This bronchodilating action of ketamine is related to its sympathomimetic properties. For these reasons, ketamine has been recommended as a desirable drug for management of patients with asthma (Corssen *et al,* 1972).

Cardiovascular System

Ketamine produces cardiovascular effects that resemble sympathetic nervous system stimulation. Systemic and pulmonary arterial blood pressure, heart rate, cardiac output, cardiac work, and myocardial oxygen requirements increase (Table 6-2) (Tweed *et al,* 1972). The rise in systolic blood pressure in adults receiving clinical doses of ketamine is 20 to 40 mmHg with a slightly smaller increase in diastolic blood pressure. Typically, blood pressure increases progressively during the

first 3 to 5 minutes following intravenous injection of ketamine and then declines to normal limits over the next 10 to 20 minutes. In contrast, ketamine administered to mildly sedated infants fails to produce hemodynamic changes in either the systemic or pulmonary circulations (Hickey *et al,* 1985).

The mechanisms for ketamine-induced cardiovascular effects are complex. Direct stimulation of the central nervous system leading to increased sympathetic nervous system outflow seems to be the most important mechanism (Wong and Jenkins, 1974). Evidence for this mechanism is the ability of inhaled anesthetics, ganglionic blockade, cervical epidural block, and spinal cord transection to prevent ketamine-induced increases in blood pressure and heart rate (Stanley, 1973; Traber *et al,* 1970) (see the section entitled Drug Interactions). Furthermore, increases in plasma concentrations of epinephrine and norepinephrine occur as early as 2 minutes following intravenous administration of ketamine and return to control levels 15 minutes later (Baraka *et al,* 1973). *In vitro,* ketamine produces direct myocardial depression, emphasizing the importance of an intact sympathetic nervous system for the cardiac stimulating effects of this drug (Schwartz and Horwitz, 1975).

The possible role of ketamine's ability to inhibit the uptake of norepinephrine back into postganglionic sympathetic nerve endings in the car-

---

Table 6-2
Circulatory Effects of Ketamine

	Control	Ketamine (2 mg kg⁻1, intravenously)	Percent Change
Heart rate (beats min⁻¹)	74	98	+33
Mean arterial pressure (mmHg)	93	119	+28
Cardiac index (L min⁻¹ m⁻²)	3.0	3.8	+29
Stroke volume index (ml m⁻²)	43	44	
Systemic vascular resistance (pru)	16.2	15.9	
Right atrial pressure (mmHg)	7	8.9	
Left ventricular end-diastolic pressure (mmHg)	13	13.1	
Pulmonary artery pressure (mmHg)	17	24.5	+44
Minute work index (kg-m m⁻²)	5.4	8.9	+40
Tension-time index (mmHg-sec)	2700	4640	+68

(Data from Tweed WA, Minuck MS, Mymin D. Circulatory responses to ketamine anesthesia. Anesthesiology 1972;37:613–9.)

diac-stimulating effects of this drug or the associated elevations of plasma catecholamine concentrations are not known (Koehntop *et al,* 1977). Depression of baroreceptor reflex activity leading to activation of the sympathetic nervous system has not been confirmed to be the mechanism responsible for ketamine's cardiovascular effects.

In shocked animals, ketamine is associated with a greater survival rate than animals anesthetized with halothane (Longnecker and Sturgill, 1976). Blood pressure may be better maintained in hemorrhaged animals anesthetized with ketamine, but greater increases in arterial lactate concentrations occur than in animals with lower arterial blood pressures anesthetized with a volatile anesthetic (Weiskopf *et al,* 1981). This suggests inadequate tissue perfusion despite maintenance of blood pressure by ketamine. Presumably, ketamine-induced vasoconstriction maintains blood pressure at the expense of tissue perfusion. Critically ill patients occasionally respond to ketamine with unexpected reductions in blood pressure and cardiac output, which may reflect depletion of catecholamine stores and exhaustion of sympathetic nervous system compensating mechanisms leading to an unmasking of ketamine's direct myocardial-depressant effects.

The effect of ketamine on cardiac rhythm is inconclusive. There is evidence that ketamine enhances the arrhythmogenicity of epinephrine (Koehntop *et al,* 1977). Conversely, ketamine may abolish epinephrine-induced cardiac dysrhythmias.

Hepatic or Renal Function

Ketamine does not significantly alter laboratory tests that reflect hepatic or renal function.

Allergic Reactions

Ketamine does not evoke the release of histamine and rarely, if ever, causes allergic reactions.

Drug Interactions

The importance of an intact and normally functioning central nervous system in determining the cardiovascular effects of ketamine is emphasized by hemodynamic depression rather than stimulation that occurs when ketamine is administered in the presence of inhaled anesthetics. For example,

depression of central nervous system sympathetic outflow by inhaled anesthetics prevents the typical increases in blood pressure and heart rate that occur when ketamine is administered alone (Stanley, 1973). Ketamine administered in the presence of halothane may result in hypotension (Bidwai *et al,* 1975). Presumably, halothane, by depressing sympathetic nervous system outflow from the central nervous system, unmasks direct cardiac-depressant effects of ketamine. Furthermore, halothane, by reducing endogenous release of norepinephrine could allow direct depressant effects of ketamine on the heart to manifest. Diazepam, 0.3 to 0.5 mg kg^{-1} administered intravenously, is also effective in preventing cardiac-stimulating effects of ketamine. In the presence of verapamil, the blood-pressure – elevating effects of ketamine may be attenuated, while drug-induced elevations in heart rate are enhanced (Fragen and Avram, 1986).

In animals, ketamine causes a dose-dependent decrease in halothane anesthetic requirements (Fig. 6-3) (White *et al,* 1975). This reduction in anesthetic requirement persists for several hours. Halothane, and presumably other volatile anesthetics, prolongs the duration of action of ketamine by delaying both its redistribution to inactive tissue sites and its metabolism (White *et al,* 1976).

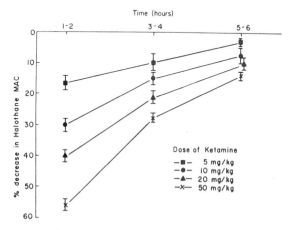

FIGURE 6-3. Ketamine produces dose-dependent decreases in halothane anesthetic requirements (MAC) in animals. Mean ± SE. (From White PF, Johnston RR, Rudwill CR. Interaction of ketamine and halothane in rats. Anesthesiology 1975;42:179 – 86. Reproduced by permission of the authors and publisher.)

Ketamine-induced enhancement of nondepolarizing neuromuscular blocking drugs may reflect interference by ketamine with calcium binding or its transport (Johnston *et al,* 1974). Alternatively, ketamine may decrease sensitivity of postjunctional membranes to ketamine. The duration of apnea following administration of succinylcholine is prolonged, possibly reflecting inhibition of plasma cholinesterase activity by ketamine. Pancuronium may enhance the cardiac-stimulating effects of ketamine.

Seizures have been observed in asthmatic patients receiving aminophylline followed by ketamine (Hirshman *et al,* 1982). Furthermore, in animals, ketamine or aminophylline alone do not alter the seizure threshold, but the combination of these two drugs reduces the seizure threshold (Hirshman *et al,* 1982).

Emergence Delirium

Emergence from ketamine anesthesia in the postoperative period may be associated with visual, auditory, proprioceptive, and confusional illusions, which may progress to delirium (White *et al,* 1980). Cortical blindness may be transiently present. Dreams and hallucinations can occur up to 24 hours after administration of ketamine. The dreams frequently have a morbid content and are often experienced in vivid technicolor. Dreams and hallucinations usually disappear within a few hours.

Mechanisms

Emergence delirium probably occurs secondary to ketamine-induced depression of the inferior colliculus and medial geniculate nucleus, leading to misinterpretation of auditory and visual stimuli (White *et al,* 1982). Furthermore, the loss of skin and musculoskeletal sensations results in decreased ability to perceive gravity, thereby producing a sensation of bodily detachment or floating in space (Collier, 1972).

Incidence

The reported incidence of emergence delirium following ketamine ranges from 5% to 30% (White *et al,* 1980). Factors associated with an increased incidence of emergence delirium include (1) age greater than 16 years, (2) female sex, (3) doses of ketamine greater than 2 mg kg^{-1}, and (4) a history of personality problems or frequent dreaming (White *et al,* 1982). It is possible that the incidence of dreaming is similar in children, but this age-group is often unable to communicate their occurrence. Indeed, there are reports of recurrent hallucinations in children as well as in adults receiving ketamine (Fine and Finestone, 1973; Meyers and Charles, 1978). Nevertheless, psychological changes in children following anesthesia with ketamine or inhaled drugs are not different (Modvig and Nielsen, 1977). Likewise, no significant long-term personality differences are present in adults receiving ketamine compared with thiopental (Moretti *et al,* 1984).

Emergence delirium occurs less frequently when ketamine is used repeatedly. For example, it is rare for emergence delirium to occur after the third or more anesthetics with ketamine. Finally, inhaled anesthetics can also produce auditory, visual, proprioceptive, and confusional illusions, but the incidence of such phenomena, especially unpleasant experiences, is indeed greater following anesthesia that includes administration of ketamine.

Prevention

A variety of drugs used in preoperative medication or as adjuvants during maintenance of anesthesia have been evaluated in attempts to prevent emergence delirium following administration of ketamine. For example, benzodiazepines, including diazepam (0.15–0.3 mg kg^{-1}) or lorazepam (25–50 μg kg^{-1}), administered intravenously 5 minutes prior to administration of ketamine for induction of anesthesia appear to be effective in preventing delirium but not in totally preventing dreaming and floating sensations during recovery (Lilburn *et al,* 1978; Mattila *et al,* 1979). Inclusion of thiopental or inhaled anesthetics may decrease the incidence of emergence delirium attributed to ketamine. Conversely, the inclusion of atropine or droperidol in the preoperative medication may increase the incidence of emergence delirium (Erbguth *et al,* 1972).

Despite contrary statements, there is no evidence that permitting patients to awaken from ketamine anesthesia in a quiet area alters the incidence of emergence delirium (Hejja and Galloon, 1975). Prospective discussion with the patient of the common side effects of ketamine (*e.g.,* dreams, floating sensations, blurred vision) is likely to reduce the incidence of emergence delirium as much as any other approach (White *et al,* 1982).

ETOMIDATE

Etomidate is a carboxylated imidazole-containing compound that is chemically unrelated to any other drug used for the induction of anesthesia (Fig. 6-4). The imidazole nucleus renders etomidate, like midazolam, water soluble at an acidic *p*H and lipid soluble at physiologic *p*H. Following an intravenous induction dose of 0.3 mg kg^{-1}, the onset of unconsciousness occurs within one arm-to-brain circulation time (Morgan *et al,* 1975). As with thiopental, an age-related decrease in the initial volume of distribution and not an alteration in brain responsiveness is the most likely explanation for the reduction in dose requirements for etomidate observed in elderly patients (Arden *et al,* 1986). Central nervous system depression may reflect a gamma-aminobutyric acid-like action of etomidate (Evans and Hill, 1978). Awakening (3 – 12 minutes) following a single intravenous dose is more rapid than after barbiturates, and there is little or no evidence of a hangover or cumulative effect. Recovery of psychomotor function after administration of etomidate is intermittent between methohexital and thiopental. Duration of action is prolonged by increasing the dose of etomidate or administering the drug as a continuous intravenous infusion. As with barbiturates, analgesia is not produced by etomidate. For this reason, administration of an opioid prior to induction of anesthesia with etomidate may be useful so as to blunt the hemodynamic responses evoked by direct laryngoscopy and intubation of the trachea.

Etomidate may be an alternative to barbiturates for intravenous induction of anesthesia in the presence of an unstable cardiovascular system or decreased intravascular fluid volume. Another use for etomidate is induction of anesthesia for brief outpatient surgical procedures. Continuous intravenous infusion of etomidate with intermittent injections of an opioid can be used for longer surgical procedures. Etomidate, like thiopental, does not trigger malignant hyperthermia in susceptible animals (Suresh and Nelson, 1985).

The use of etomidate for induction of anesthesia is associated with a greater incidence of postoperative nausea and vomiting than occurs following thiopental (Holdcroft *et al,* 1976). The incidence of this unpleasant side effect can be decreased by the prophylactic administration of intravenous droperidol. Allergic reactions seem to be infrequent following administration of etomidate. Etomidate does not evoke the release of histamine.

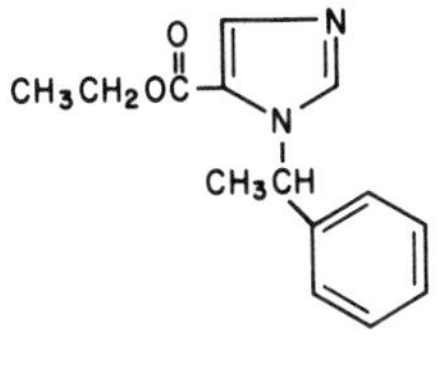

Pharmacokinetics

The volume of distribution of etomidate is larger than body weight, suggesting considerable tissue uptake (Table 6-1). Distribution of etomidate throughout body water is favored by its moderate lipid solubility and existence as a weak base (*p*Ka 4.2). Etomidate penetrates the brain rapidly, reaching peak levels within 1 minute after intravenous injection. About 76% of etomidate is bound to albumin independent of the plasma concentration of drug (Meuldermans and Heykants, 1976). Reductions in plasma albumin concentration, however, result in dramatic increases in the free plasma concentration of etomidate. Prompt awakening after a single intravenous dose of etomidate reflects principally redistribution of the drug from brain to inactive tissue sites. Rapid metabolism is also likely to contribute to prompt recovery (see the section entitled Metabolism).

Metabolism

Etomidate is rapidly metabolized by hydrolysis of the ethyl ester side chain to its carboxylic acid ester, resulting in a pharmacologically inactive compound. Hepatic microsomal enzymes and plasma esterases are responsible for this hydrolysis. Hydrolysis is nearly complete, as evidenced by recovery of less than 3% of an administered dose of etomidate as unchanged drug in the urine. About 85% of a single intravenous dose of etomidate can be accounted for as a carboxylic acid ester metabolite in the urine, while another 10% to 13% is present as this metabolite in the bile. Overall,

FIGURE 6-4.   Etomidate.

the clearance rate for etomidate is five times that of thiopental, and this is reflected in a shorter elimination half-time of 2 to 5 hours.

Effects Other Than Central Nervous System Depression

Cerebral Blood Flow

Etomidate is a potent direct cerebral vasoconstrictor that decreases cerebral blood flow and cerebral metabolic oxygen requirements 35% to 45% (Milde *et al,* 1985; Renou *et al,* 1978). As a result, previously elevated intracranial pressure is lowered by etomidate. These changes are similar to those changes produced by similar doses of thiopental (see Chapter 4).

Etomidate, like methohexital, may activate seizure foci manifesting as fast activity on the EEG (Ebrahim *et al,* 1986). For this reason, etomidate should be used with caution in patients with focal epilepsy. Conversely, this characteristic of etomidate may be used to facilitate location of seizure foci in patients undergoing cortical resection of epileptogenic tissue.

Cardiovascular System

Cardiovascular stability is characteristic of patients receiving etomidate (Patschke *et al,* 1977). An intravenous injection of etomidate, 0.3 mg kg^{-1}, evokes minimal changes in heart rate, stroke volume, or cardiac output, whereas mean arterial pressure may decline up to 15% because of decreases in peripheral vascular resistance. In animals, etomidate depresses myocardial contractility less than equally potent doses of thiopental (Kissin *et al,* 1983). Etomidate does not result in detrimental effects when injected intra-arterially. In contrast to other intravenous and volatile anesthetics, etomidate does not decrease renal blood flow. Hepatic and renal function tests are not altered by etomidate. Intraocular pressure is lowered by etomidate to a similar degree as by thiopental.

Ventilation

The depressant effects of etomidate on ventilation seem to be less than thiopental although apnea may occasionally accompany a rapid intravenous injection of the drug. In the majority of patients, etomidate-induced reductions in tidal volume (about 25%) are offset by a compensatory increase in the rate of breathing. These effects on ventilation are transient lasting only 3 to 5 minutes. Etomidate may stimulate ventilation independent of the medullary centers that normally respond to carbon dioxide (Choi *et al,* 1985). For this reason, etomidate may be useful when maintenance of spontaneous ventilation is desirable. Depression of ventilation may be exaggerated when etomidate is combined with inhaled anesthetics or opioids during continuous infusion techniques.

Pain on Injection

Pain occurring during intravenous injection of etomidate is frequent, manifesting in up to 80% of patients (Holdcroft *et al,* 1976). Pain is most likely to occur when injections of etomidate are into small veins. Preparation of etomidate without the addition of propylene glycol reduces the incidence of pain, as does inclusion of an opioid in the preoperative medication and injection of etomidate into a large vein.

Myoclonus

Involuntary muscle movements characterized as myoclonus occur in about one third of patients during induction of anesthesia with etomidate (Fragen *et al,* 1976). These involuntary skeletal muscle movements associated with etomidate occur with a greater frequency than with methohexital, whereas the incidence of hiccough is similar for both drugs. Prior intravenous administration of an opioid (fentanyl, $2-10$ μg kg^{-1}) or a benzodiazepine may reduce the incidence of myoclonus associated with administration of etomidate.

Although myoclonus may resemble seizures, it is not considered hazardous and is not associated with epileptiform discharges on the electroencephalogram. The mechanism of etomidate-induced myoclonus appears to be disinhibition of subcortical structures that normally suppress extrapyramidal motor activity (Kugler *et al,* 1977). It is possible that myoclonus could occur on awakening if the extrapyramidal system emerged more quickly than the cortex that inhibits it (Laughlin and Newberg, 1985).

Adrenocortical Suppression

Etomidate produces adrenocortical suppression as evidenced by decreased plasma concentrations of cortisol and aldosterone in the early postoperative period and by the failure of adrenocorticotropic hormone (ACTH) to evoke an increase in the concentrations of either cortisol or aldosterone (Fig. 6-5) (Fragen *et al,* 1984; Wagner *et al,* 1984).

Evidence of adrenocortical suppression was originally observed in critically ill patients receiving continuous intravenous infusions of etomidate but may also occur after a single induction dose (Wagner and White, 1984). The mechanism of adrenocortical suppression appears to be an etomidate-induced inhibition of 11-beta-hydroxylase activity, as evidenced by the accumulation of 11-deoxycorticosterone (Owen and Spence, 1984). This enzyme inhibition lasts 4 to 8 hours after an induction dose of etomidate. Despite several reports of adrenocortical suppression associated with administration of etomidate, at least one report fails to demonstrate a difference in the plasma concentrations of cortisol, corticosterone, or ACTH in patients receiving a single dose of etomidate or thiopental (Duthie *et al,* 1985). This suggests that inhibition of 11-beta-hydroxylase activity by a single dose of etomidate is incomplete, allowing the adrenal glands to respond to stimulation from ACTH.

Suppression of adrenocortical function by etomidate may be considered desirable from the standpoint of "stress-free" anesthesia. Conversely, this drug-induced suppression is considered undesirable if it prevents necessary protective responses against stresses that accompany the perioperative period (Longnecker, 1984).

PROPOFOL

Propofol is a substituted isopropylphenol that is a rapid-acting intravenous anesthetic (Fig. 6-6) (Major *et al,* 1981; Prys-Roberts *et al,* 1983). The drug is virtually insoluble in aqueous solutions, making it necessary for it to be solubilized in lecithin-containing formulations. High lipid solubility contributes to a rapid onset (less than 60 seconds) of unconsciousness following intravenous administration of 1.5 to 3 mg kg^{-1}. Awakening occurs in 4 to 8 minutes, and in contrast to barbiturates, there seems to be less postoperative sedation (*e.g.,* hangover) with this drug.

Clearance of propofol (30–60 ml kg^{-1} min^{-1}) from the plasma exceeds hepatic blood flow (Table 6-1). Hepatic metabolism clearly contributes to clearance of propofol, but tissue uptake is also important. Elimination half-time is 30 to 90 minutes. There are no known active metabolites.

Dose-dependent cardiovascular depression and ventilatory depression produced by propofol are similar to that produced by thiopental. Propofol does not seem to possess analgesic properties. Side effects are rare and include (1) pain on injection, especially when propofol is injected in a small vein, (2) involuntary skeletal muscle movements, (3) coughing, and (4) hiccoughs. Nausea and vomiting are unlikely following the administration of propofol.

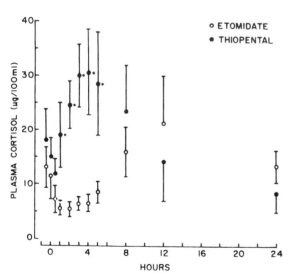

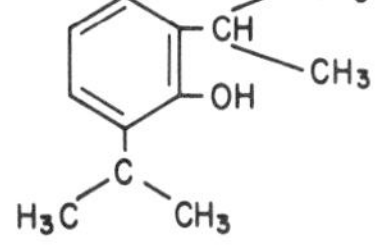

FIGURE 6-5. Etomidate, but not thiopental, is associated with a decrease in the plasma concentration of cortisol. *P<0.05 compared with thiopental. Mean ± SD. (From Fragen RJ, Shanks CA, Molteni A, Abrams MJ.: Effects of etomidate on hormonal responses to surgical stress. Anesthesiology 1984;61:652–6. Reproduced by permission of the authors and publisher.)

FIGURE 6-6. Propofol.

ALPHADIONE

Alphadione is a poorly water-soluble steroid anesthetic consisting of a three-to-one mixture of two steroids, alphaxalone, 9 mg ml^{-1} and alphadolone, 3 mg ml^{-1} (Clarke *et al,* 1972; Gyermek and Soyka, 1975). These steroids are dissolved in cremorphor EL, a nonionic surface-active solution of polyoxyethylated castor oil. Alphaxalone is the more potent of the two steroids, whereas alphadolone provides water solubility. The solution is highly viscous, making rapid intravenous injection difficult, particularly through a small needle. The *p*H of the commercial solution is about 7.

Because of its complex formulation, it is acceptable to describe dosage in terms of μl kg^{-1}. Induction of anesthesia is within one arm-to-brain circulation time following the administration of 50 to 150 μl kg^{-1} of alphadione. Analgesia is not produced, and duration of action is 5 to 10 minutes longer than with thiopental. Awakening is often associated with restlessness and sometimes agitation (Korttila *et al,* 1975).

Redistribution is the principal mechanism responsible for the rapid return of consciousness following administration of alphadione. Eventually, metabolism by hepatic microsomal enzymes, especially glucuronyl transferase, is nearly 100%. Inactive metabolites are excreted in the urine.

Cerebral blood flow, cerebral metabolic oxygen consumption, and intracranial pressure are decreased following induction of anesthesia with alphadione. Blood pressure is reduced, but the magnitude is often less than that produced by thiopental. Alphadione does not alter hepatic function. Despite similar structure, there is no apparent interaction between alphadione and the steroid neuromuscular blocking drug, pancuronium.

The incidence of alphadione-induced allergic reactions is estimated to be 1 in every 900 patients (Whitwam, 1978). These reactions may consist of erythema associated with hypotension and tachycardia and occasionally bronchospasm. Allergic reactions usually involve activation of the complement system, leading to excessive release of histamine in the absence of an antigen–antibody interaction. This relatively high incidence of severe anaphylactoid reactions will probably prevent the release of alphadione for commercial use in the United States and has resulted in its removal from clinical use in Europe.

PROPANIDID

Propanidid is a eugenol derivative that is poorly soluble in water, necessitating its preparation in a solubilizing agent such as cremophor EL or polyoxylated castor oil (Fig. 6-7). It is approximately equal in potency to thiopental, with 4 to 6 mg kg^{-1} producing rapid loss of consciousness. Recovery from the effects of propanidid is more rapid than after any other drug, reflecting its prompt hydrolysis by plasma cholinesterase (Korttila *et al,* 1975). The EEG is normal, and there is no detectable alteration of psychomotor function 30 to 60 minutes after administration of propanidid. In contrast to barbiturates, propanidid does not have an antianalgesia action. Intra-arterial injection is not followed by vascular complications.

Rapid hydrolysis by plasma cholinesterase prevents a cumulative drug effect from intermittent or continuous injections. Patients with low plasma cholinesterase activity experience a prolonged duration of anesthesia from propanidid. The duration of action of succinylcholine is slightly prolonged, presumably reflecting competition for plasma cholinesterase by propanidid.

Propanidid reduces blood pressure somewhat more than thiopental, reflecting primarily peripheral vasodilation (Bernhoff *et al,* 1972). Indeed, propanidid is likely to evoke the release of significant amounts of histamine (Lorenz *et al,* 1972). There is a biphasic effect on ventilation characterized by an initial stimulation followed by depression that may progress to apnea.

The usefulness of propanidid is greatly limited by the potential for this drug to evoke life-threatening allergic reactions (Thornton, 1971). These are anaphylactoid responses, which may be difficult to recognize because a reduction in blood pressure is a normal response to propanidid. The possibility of allergic reactions will probably prevent the commercial introduction of this drug in the United States and has resulted in its removal from clinical use in Europe. Furthermore, invol-

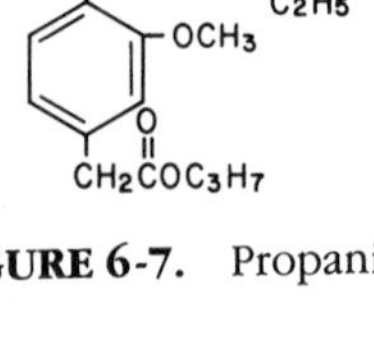

FIGURE 6-7. Propanidid.

untary skeletal muscle movements occur in about 10% of patients receiving propanidid, 4 mg kg^{-1}, and the incidence of nausea and vomiting is high.

REFERENCES

Akamatsu TJ, Bonica JJ, Rehmet R. Experiences with the use of ketamine for parturition. 1. Primary anesthetic for vaginal delivery. Anesth Analg 1974;53:284–7.

Arden JR, Holley FO, Stanski DR. Increased sensitivity to etomidate in the elderly: Initial distribution versus altered brain response. Anesthesiology 1986;65:19–27.

Baraka A, Harrison T, Kachachi T. Catecholamine levels after ketamine anesthesia in man. Anesth Analg 1973;52:198–200.

Bernhoff A, Eklund B, Kaijser L. Cardiovascular effects of short-term anaesthesia with methohexitone and propanidid in normal subjects. Br J Anaesth 1972;44:2–7.

Bidwai AV, Stanley TH, Graves CL, Kawamura R, Sentker CR. The effects of ketamine on cardiovascular dynamics during halothane and enflurane anesthesia. Anesth Analg 1975;54:588–92.

Borondy PE, Glazko AJ. Inhibition of ketamine metabolism by diazepam. Fed Proc 1977;36:938.

Bovill JG, Dundee JW. Alterations in response to somatic pain associated with anesthesia-ketamine. Br J Anaesth 1971;43:496–9.

Celesia GG, Chen R-C, Bamforth BJ. Effects of ketamine in epilepsy. Neurology 1975;25:169–72.

Choi SD, Spaulding BC, Gross JB, Apfelbaum JL. Comparison of the ventilatory effects of etomidate and methohexital. Anesthesiology 1985;62:442–7.

Clarke RSJ, Dundee JW, Carson IW, Arora MV, McCaughey W. Clinical studies with induction agents. XL. Althesin. Br J Anaesth 1972;44:845–8.

Cohen ML, Chan SL, Way WL, Trevor AJ. Distribution in the brain and metabolism of ketamine in the rat after intravenous administration. Anesthesiology 1973;39:370–6.

Cohen ML, Trevor AJ. On the cerebral accumulation of ketamine and the relationship between metabolism of the drug and its pharmacological effects. J Pharmacol Exp Ther 1974;189:351–8.

Collier BB. Ketamine and the conscious mind. Anaesthesia 1972;27:120–34.

Corssen G, Gutierrez J, Reves JC, Huber FC. Ketamine in the anesthetic management of asthmatic patients. Anesth Analg 1972;51:588–96.

Corssen G, Miyasaka M, Domino EF. Changing concepts in pain control during surgery: Dissociative anesthesia with CI-581. A progress report. Anesth Analg 1968;47:746–59.

Dawson B, Michenfelder JD, Theye RA. Effects of keta-

mine on canine cerebral blood flow and metabolism. Modification by prior administration of thiopental. Anesth Analg 1971;50:443–7.

Demling RH, Ellerbee S, Jarrett F. Ketamine anesthesia for tangential excision of burn eschar: A burn unit procedure. J Trauma 1978;18:269–70.

Duthie DJR, Fraser R, Nimmo WS. Effect of induction of anaesthesia with etomidate on corticosteroid synthesis in man. Br J Anaesth 1985;57:156–9.

Ebrahim ZY, DeBoer GE, Luders H, Hahn JF, Lesser RP. Effect of etomidate on the electroencephalogram of patients with epilepsy. Anesth Analg 1986;65:1004–6.

Erbguth PH, Reiman B, Klein RL. The influence of chlorpromazine, diazepam and droperidol on emergence from ketamine. Anesth Analg 1972;51:693–700.

Evans RH, Hill RG. GABA-mimetic action of etomidate. Experientia 1978;34:1325–7.

Ferrer-Allado T, Brechner VL, Diamond A, Cozen H, Crandall P. Ketamine-induced electroconvulsive phenomena in the human limbic and thalamic regions. Anesthesiology 1973;38:333–44.

Fine J, Finestone SC. Sensory disturbances following ketamine anesthesia — Recurrent hallucinations. Anesth Analg 1973;52:428–30.

Fragen RJ, Avram MJ. Comparative pharmacology of drugs used for the induction of anesthesia. In Stoelting RK, Barash PG, Gallagher TJ (eds): Advances in Anesthesia. Chicago, Year Book Medical Publishers, 1986:103–32.

Fragen RJ, Caldwell N, Brunner EA. Clinical use of etomidate for anesthesia induction: A preliminary report. Anesth Analg 1976;55:730–3.

Fragen RJ, Shanks CA, Molteni A, Abram MJ. Effects of etomidate on hormonal responses to surgical stress. Anesthesiology 1984;61:652–6.

Gyermek L, Soyka LF. Steroid anesthetics. Anesthesiology 1975;42:331–44.

Hatano S, Keane DM, Boggs RE, El-Naggar MA, Sadove MS. Diazepam-ketamine anesthesia for open heart surgery — a micro-mini drip administration technique. Can Anaesth Soc J 1976;23:648–56.

Hejja P, Galloon S. A consideration of ketamine dreams. Can Anaesth Soc J 1975;22:100–5.

Hickey PR, Hansen DD, Cramolini GM, Vincent RN, Lang P. Pulmonary and systemic hemodynamic responses to ketamine in infants with normal and elevated pulmonary vascular resistance. Anesthesiology 1985;62:287–93.

Hirshman CA, Downes H, Farbood A, Bergman NA. Ketamtamine block of bronchospasm in experimental canine asthma. Br J Anaesth 1979;51:713–8.

Hirshman CA, Krieger W, Littlejohn G, Lee R, Julien R. Ketamine-aminophylline-induced decrease in seizure threshold. Anesthesiology 1982;56:464–7.

Hodgkinson K, Marx GF, Kim SS, Miclat NM. Neonatal

neurobehavioral tests following vaginal delivery under ketamine, thiopental, and extradural anesthesia. Anesth Analg 1977;56:548–53.

Holdcroft A, Morgan M, Whitwam JG, Lumley J. Effect of dose and premedication on induction complications with etomidate. Br J Anaesth 1976;48:199–205.

Islas J-A, Astorga, J, Laredo M. Epidural ketamine for control of postoperative pain. Anesth Analg 1985;64:1161–2.

Janeczko GF, El-Etr AA, Younes S. Low-dose ketamine anesthesia for obstetrical delivery. Anesth Analg 1974;53:828–31.

Johnston RR, Miller RD, Way WL. The interaction of ketamine with d-tubocurarine, pancuronium, and succinylcholine in man. Anesth Analg 1974; 53:496–501.

Kissin I, Motomura S, Aultman BS, Reves JG. Inotropic and anesthetic potencies of etomidate and thiopental in dogs. Anesth Analg 1983;62:961–5.

Kitahata LM, Taub A, Kosaka Y. Lamina-specific suppression of dorsal-horn unit activity by ketamine hydrochloride. Anesthesiology 1973;38:4–11.

Koehntop DE, Liao J-C, Van Bergen FH. Effects of pharmacologic alterations of adrenergic mechanisms by cocaine, tropolene, aminophylline and ketamine on epinephrine-induced arrhythmias during halothane-nitrous oxide anesthesia. Anesthesiology 1977;46:83–93.

Korttila K, Linnoila M, Ertama P, Hakkinen S. Recovery and simulated driving after intravenous anesthesia with thiopental, methohexital, propanidid, or alphadione. Anesthesiology 1975;43:291–9.

Kostrzewski E, Gregor A. Ketamine in acute intermittent porphyria—dangerous or safe? Anesthesiology 1978;49:376–7.

Kugler J, Doenicka A, Laub M. The EEG after etomidate. Anesth Resuscitation 1977;106:31–48.

Laughlin TP, Newberg LA. Prolonged myoclonus after etomidate anesthesia. Anesth Analg 1985;64:80–2.

Lilburn JK, Dundee JW, Nair SG, Fee JPH, Johnston HML. Ketamine sequelae: Evaluation of the ability of various premedicants to attenuate its psychic actions. Anaesthesia 1978;33:307–11.

Longnecker DE. Stress free: To be or not to be? Anesthesiology 1984;61:643–4.

Longnecker DE, Sturgill BC. Influence of anesthetic agents on survival following hemorrhage. Anesthesiology 1976;45:516–21.

Lorenz W, Doenicke A, Meyer R, et al. Histamine release in man by propanidid and thiopentone: Pharmacological effects and clinical consequences. Br J Anaesth 1972;44:355–69.

Lundy PM, Lockwood PA, Thompson G, Frew R. Differential effects of ketamine isomers on neuronal and extraneuronal catecholamine uptake mechanisms. Anesthesiology 1986;64:359–63.

Major E, Verniquet AJW, Waddell TK, Savage TM, Hoffler DE, Aveling W. A study of three doses of ICI 35 868 for induction and maintenance of anaesthesia. Br J Anaesth 1981;53:267–72.

Marietta MP, White PF, Pudwill CR, Way WL, Trevor J. Biodisposition of ketamine in the rat: Self induction of metabolism. J Pharmacol Exp Ther 1976;196:536–44.

Mattila MAK, Larni HM, Nummi SE, Pekkola PD. Effect of diazepam on emergence from ketamine anaesthesia: A double-blind study. Anaesthetist 1979;28:20–3.

Meuldermans WEG, Heykants JJP. The plasma protein binding and distribution of etomidate in dog, rat and human blood. Arch Inter Pharmacodyn Ther 1976:221:150–62.

Meyers EF, Charles P. Prolonged adverse reactions to ketamine in children. Anesthesiology 1978;49:39–40.

Milde LN, Milde JH, Michenfelder JD. Cerebral functional, metabolic, and hemodynamic effects of etomidate in dogs. Anesthesiology 1985;63:371–7.

Modvig KM, Nielsen SF. Psychological changes in children after anesthesia: A comparison between halothane and ketamine. Acta Anaesth Scand 1977;21:541–4.

Moretti RJ, Hassan SZ, Goodman LI, Meltzer HY. Comparison of ketamine and thiopental in healthy volunteers: Effects on mental status, mood, and personality. Anesth Analg 1984;63:1087–96.

Morgan M, Lumley J, Whitwam JG. Etomidate, a new water-soluble non-barbiturate intravenous induction agent. Lancet 1975;1:95–6.

Owen H, Spence AA. Etomidate. Br J Anaesth 1984;56:555–7.

Patschke D, Bruckner JB, Eberlein JH, Hess W, Tarnow J, Weymar A. Effects of althesin, etomidate and fentanyl on haemodynamics and myocardial oxygen consumption in man. Can Anaesth Soc J 1977;24:57–69.

Prys-Roberts C, Davies JR, Calverley RK, Goodman NW. Haemodynamic effects of infusions of diisopropyl phenol (ICI 35 868) during nitrous oxide anaesthesia in man. Br J Anaesth 1983;55:105–11.

Renou AM, Vernheit J, Macrez P, et al. Cerebral blood flow and metabolism during etomidate anaesthesia in man. Br J Anaesth 1978;50:1047–51.

Reves JG, Lell WA, McCracken LE, Kravetz RA, Prough DS. Comparison of morphine and ketamine. Anesthetic techniques for coronary surgery: A randomized study. South Med J 1978;71:33–6.

Sadove MS, Shulman M, Hatano S, Fevold N. Analgesic effects of ketamine administration in subdissociative doses. Anesth Analg 1971;50:452–5.

Schwartz DA, Horwitz LD. Effects of ketamine on left ventricular performance. J Pharmacol Exp Ther 1975;194:410–4.

Smith DJ, Westfall DP, Adams JD. Ketamine interacts with opiate receptors as an agonist. Anesthesiology 1980;53:S5.

Soliman MG, Brinale GF, Kuster G. Response to hypercapnia under ketamine anesthesia. Can Anaesth Soc J 1975;22:486–94.

Stanley TH. Blood pressure and pulse rate responses to ketamine during general anesthesia. Anesthesiology 1973;39:648–9.

Suresh MS, Nelson TE. Malignant hyperthermia: Is etomidate safe? Anesth Analg 1985;64:420–4.

Takeshita H, Okuda Y, Sari A. The effects of ketamine on cerebral circulation and metabolism in man. Anesthesiology 1972;36:69–75.

Taylor PA, Towey RM. Depression of laryngeal reflexes during ketamine anesthesia. Br Med J 1971;2:688–9.

Thornton HL. Apparent anaphylactic reaction to propanidid. Anaesthesia 1971;26:490–3.

Thorsen T, Gran L. Ketamine/diazepam infusion anesthesia with special attention to the effect on cerebral spinal fluid pressure and arterial blood pressure. Acta Anaesth Scand 1980;24:1–4.

Toro-Matos A, Rendon-Platas AM, Avila-Valdez E, Villarrel-Guzman RA. Physostigmine antagonizes ketamine. Anesth Analg 1980;59:764–7.

Traber DL, Wilson RD, Priano LL. Blockade of the hypertensive response to ketamine. Anesth Analg 1970;49:420–6.

Tweed WA, Minuck MS, Mymin D. Circulatory response to ketamine anesthesia. Anesthesiology 1972;37:613–9.

Vincent JP, Corey D, Kamenka JM, Geneste P, Lazdunski M. Interaction of phencyclidines with the muscarinic and opiate receptors in the central nervous system. Brain Res 1978;152:176–82.

Wadhwa RK, Tantisira B. Parotidectomy in a patient with a family history of malignant hyperthermia. Anesthesiology 1974;40:191–4.

Wagner RL, White PF. Etomidate inhibits adrenocortical function in surgical patients. Anesthesiology 1984;61:647–51.

Wagner RL, White PF, Kan PB, Rosenthal MH, Feldman D. Inhibition of adrenal steroidogenesis by the anesthetic etomidate. N Engl J Med 1984;310:1415–21.

Weiskopf RB, Townsley MI, Riordan KK, Baysinger M, Mahoney E. Comparison of cardiopulmonary responses to graded hemorrhage during enflurane, halothane, isoflurane and ketamine anesthesia. Anesth Analg 1981;60:481–92.

White PF, Ham J, Way WL, Trevor AJ. Pharmacology of ketamine isomers in surgical patients. Anesthesiology 1980;52:231–9.

White PF, Johnston RR, Rudwill CR. Interaction of ketamine and halothane in rats. Anesthesiology 1975;42:179–86.

White PF, Marietta MP, Pudwill CR, Way WL, Trevor AJ. Effects of halothane anesthesia on the biodisposition of ketamine in rats. J Pharmacol Exp Ther 1976;196:545–55.

White PF, Way WL, Trevor AJ. Ketamine — its pharmacology and therapeutic uses. Anesthesiology 1982;56:119–36.

Whitwam JG. Adverse reactions to IV induction agents. Br J Anaesth 1978;50:677–87.

Wong DHW, Jenkins LC. An experimental study of the mechanism of action of ketamine on the central nervous system. Can Anaesth Soc J 1974;21:57–67.

Zsigmond EK, Domino EF. Ketamine — clinical pharmacology, pharmacokinetics, and current uses. Anesth Rev 1980;7:13–33.

C H A P T E R 7

Local Anesthetics

INTRODUCTION

Local anesthetics are drugs that produce reversible blockade of conduction of nerve impulses. With progressive increases in concentrations of local anesthetics, the transmission of autonomic, somatic sensory, and somatic motor impulses are interrupted producing autonomic nervous system blockade, anesthesia, and skeletal muscle paralysis in the area innervated by the affected nerve. Subsequent recovery of nerve conduction occurs spontaneously and is complete with no evidence of structural damage to nerve fibers as a result of exposure to the local anesthetic.

The first local anesthetic discovered was cocaine. Cocaine is an ester of benzoic acid that is present in large amounts in the leaves of *Erythroxylon coca,* a tree growing in the Andes mountains. Cocaine was introduced in 1884 by Koller as a topical anesthetic for use in ophthalamology. Halsted recognized the ability of injected cocaine to interrupt nerve conduction leading to the introduction of peripheral nerve block and subarachnoid block (spinal) anesthesia. Cocaine is unique in its ability to stimulate the cerebral cortex and produce psychologic, but probably not physiologic dependence. Another unique feature of cocaine is its ability to block the uptake of norepinephrine by postganglionic nerve endings. Evidence for this latter characteristic is vasoconstriction in the area exposed to cocaine. The topical anesthetic and vasoconstrictive effects of cocaine are used to advantage when it is desirable to both anesthetize and shrink the nasal mucosa prior to nasotracheal intubation. The abuse potential of cocaine, however, limits its use even for this purpose. Irritant properties of cocaine preclude its use for topical anesthesia of the cornea or any form of injection to produce anesthesia.

The first synthetic local anesthetic was the ester derivation, procaine, introduced by Einhorn in 1905. Lidocaine was synthesized as an amide local anesthetic by Lofgren in 1943. It produces more rapid, intense, and long-lasting conduction blockade than procaine. Unlike procaine, lidocaine is effective topically and is a highly efficacious cardiac antidysrhythmic drug. For these reasons, lidocaine is the standard to which all other local anesthetics are compared.

COMMERCIAL PREPARATIONS

Local anesthetics are poorly soluble in water and are, therefore, marketed most often as water-soluble hydrochloride salts. These hydrochloride salt solutions are acidic (pH 6) which contributes to the stability of the local anesthetic. An acidic pH is also important if epinephrine is present in the local anesthetic solution, as this catecholamine is not stable at an alkaline pH. Sodium bisulfite, which is strongly acidic, is often added to commercially prepared local anesthetic-epinephrine solutions (pH 4) to prevent oxidative decomposition of epinephrine.

Carbonated local anesthetic solutions (pH

6.5) are an alternative to hydrochloride preparations. Clinically, carbonated lidocaine has a 20% to 40% more rapid onset of action and a greater intensity of blockade than hydrochloride solutions (Bromage *et al,* 1967). Presumably, carbon dioxide diffuses rapidly into tissues so as to reduce *p*H and create a more favorable distribution of local anesthetic. Carbon dioxide more readily converts the local anesthetic amide to the more active ammonium ion by lowering the *p*H inside the membrane. This effect of carbon dioxide is opposite to that produced by tissue acidosis from infection or an epinephrine-containing local anesthetic solution with sodium bisulfite, both of which increase extracellular buffer needs (see the section entitled Pharmacokinetics).

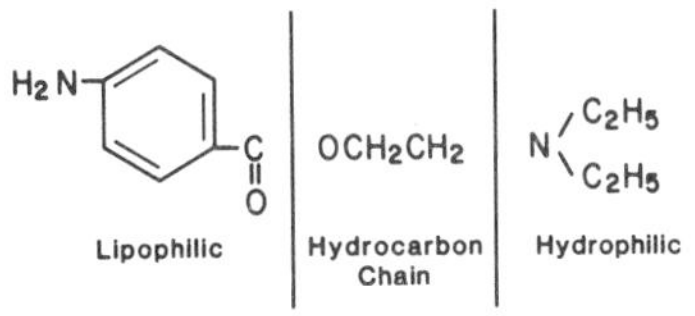

FIGURE 7-1. Local anesthetics consist of a lipophilic and hydrophilic portion separated by a connecting hydrocarbon chain.

STRUCTURE ACTIVITY RELATIONSHIPS

Local anesthetics consist of a lipophilic and hydrophilic portion separated by a hydrocarbon-connecting chain (Fig. 7-1). The hydrophilic group is usually a tertiary amine, such as diethylamine, while the lipophilic portion is usually an unsaturated aromatic ring such as para-aminobenzoic acid. The lipophilic portion is essential for anesthetic activity and therapeutically useful local anesthetics require a delicate balance between lipid solubility and water solubility. In almost all instances, the linkage of the hydrocarbon chain to the lipophilic aromatic ring is an ester (– CO –) or amide (– NHC –) bond. The nature of this bond is the basis for classifying drugs which produce conduction blockade of nerve impulses as ester local anesthetics or amide local anesthetics (Fig. 7-2). The important differences between ester and amide local anesthetics relate to the site of metabolism and the potential to produce allergic reactions (see the sections entitled Pharmacokinetics and Side Effects).

Modification of the chemical structure of a local anesthetic alters its pharmacologic effects. For example, lengthening the connecting hydrocarbon chain or increasing the number of carbon

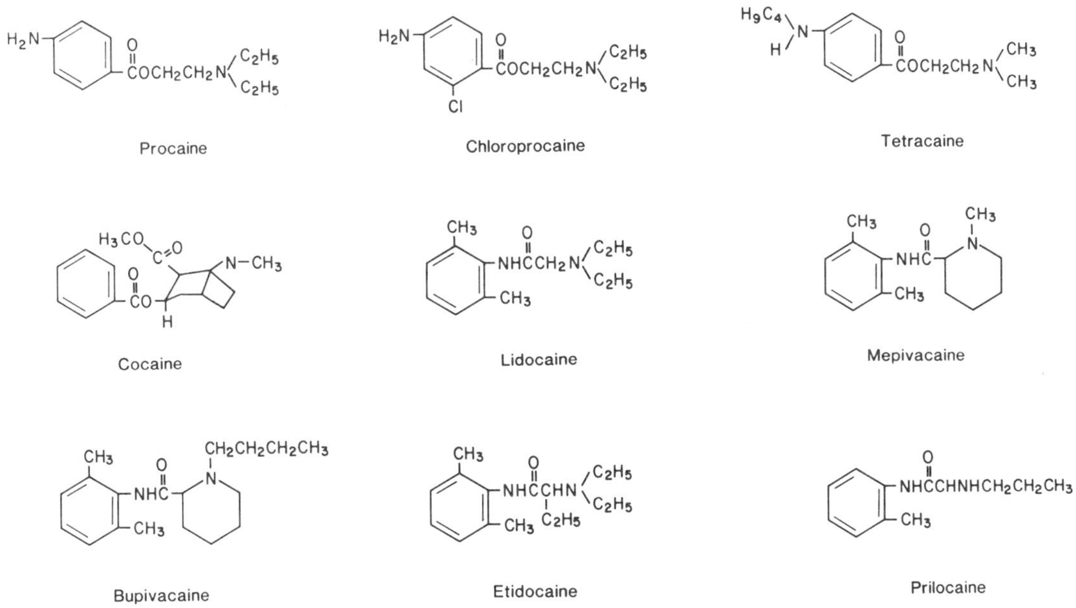

FIGURE 7-2. Ester and amide local anesthetics.

atoms on the tertiary amine or aromatic ring often results in a drug with a different lipid solubility, potency, rate of metabolism, and duration of action (Table 7-1; Fig. 7-1). Indeed, the addition of a butyl group in place of the amino group on the benzene ring of procaine results in tetracaine. Compared with procaine, tetracaine is more lipid-soluble, is ten times more potent, and has a longer duration of action corresponding to a four- to five-fold reduction in the rate of metabolism. Halogenation of procaine to chloroprocaine results in a three- to fourfold increase in the rate of hydrolysis of chloroprocaine by plasma cholinesterase. This rapid rate of hydrolysis of chloroprocaine limits the duration of action and systemic toxicity of this local anesthetic. Addition of a butyl group to the amine end of mepivacaine results in bupivacaine which is 35 times more lipid-soluble and has a potency and duration of action three to four times that of mepivacaine. Etidocaine resembles lidocaine, but a propyl group in place of an ethyl group at the amine end and addition of an ethyl group on the alpha carbon of the hydrocarbon-connecting chain produces a 50-fold increase in lipid solubility and a two- to threefold increase in the duration of action.

PHARMACOKINETICS

Local anesthetics are weak bases that have pKa values somewhat above physiologic pH (Table 7-1) (Covino and Vassallo, 1976; Tucker and Mather, 1979). As a result, less than one half the local anesthetic exists in a lipid-soluble nonionized form at physiologic pH 7.4 (Table 7-1). For example, at pH 7.4, only 5% of tetracaine exists in a nonionized form. Acidosis in the environment into which the local anesthetic is injected (*e.g.*, as present with tissue infection) further increases the ionized fraction of drug. This is consistent with the poor quality of local anesthesia that often results when a local anesthetic is injected into an acidotic infected area.

The pharmacologic profile of a local anesthetic is determined by several factors (Table 7-1). Lipid solubility seems to be the primary determinant of intrinsic local anesthetic potency. This is consistent with the fact that 90% of the nerve membrane is lipid. Protein binding influences the duration of action of local anesthesia presumably reflecting attachment to protein components of the nerve membrane. Protein binding parallels

lipid solubility with bupivacaine being more highly protein bound and potent than less lipid-soluble mepivacaine. Binding of local anesthetics to plasma proteins is reduced by systemic acidosis (Burney *et al*, 1978).

Onset of local anesthetic action reflects diffusion of the nonionized lipid-soluble form of the local anesthetic across nerve membranes (see the section entitled Mechanism of Action). Indeed, local anesthetics with pKa's nearest physiologic pH have the most rapid onset of action reflecting the presence of an optimal ratio of ionized to nonionized fraction. Intrinsic vasodilator activity will also influence apparent potency and duration of action. For example, the enhanced vasodilator action of lidocaine compared with mepivacaine results in greater vascular absorption and shorter duration of action of lidocaine. Bupivacaine and etidocaine produce similar vasodilatation but plasma concentrations of bupivacaine after epidural placement exceed etidocaine. Presumably, greater lipid solubility of etidocaine results in tissue sequestration and less drug being available for systemic absorption. Occasional prolonged sensory blockade following injection of etidocaine has been attributed to tissue sequestration.

Absorption and Distribution

Absorption of local anesthetic from its site of injection into the systemic circulation is influenced by (1) the site of injection and dosage, (2) use of epinephrine, and (3) pharmacologic characteristics of the drug (Fig. 7-3) (Covino and Vassallo, 1976) (see the section entitled Systemic Toxicity). The ultimate plasma concentration of local anesthetic is determined by the rate of tissue distribution and the rate of clearance of the drug (Table 7-1). This tissue distribution is in proportion to the tissue:blood partition coefficient of the local anesthetic and the mass and perfusion of the tissue. Patient-related factors, such as age, cardiovascular status, and hepatic function will also influence the absorption and resultant plasma concentrations of the local anesthetics. Amide local anesthetics are more widely distributed in tissues than ester local anesthetics following systemic absorption.

Lung Extraction

The lung is capable of extracting local anesthetics, such as lidocaine, bupivacaine, and prilocaine

Table 7-1
Comparative Pharmacology of Local Anesthetics

Classification	Potency	Onset	Duration After Infiltration (minutes)	Maximum Single Dose for Infiltration (adult, mg)*	Toxic Plasma Concentration (µg ml⁻¹)	pKa	Fraction Nonionized (%) pH 7.2	pH 7.4	pH 7.6	Protein Binding (%)	Lipid Solubility	Volume of Distribution (L)	Clearance (L min⁻¹)	Elimination Half Time (minutes)
Esters														
Procaine	1†	Slow	45–60	500		8.9	2	3	5	6	0.6			
Chloroprocaine	4	Rapid	30–45	600		8.7	3	5	7					
Tetracaine	16	Slow	60–180	100 (Topical)		8.5	5	7	11	76	80			
Amides														
Lidocaine	1‡	Rapid	60–120	300	>5	7.9	17	25	33	70	2.9	91	0.95	96
Mepivacaine	1	Slow	90–180	300	>5	7.6	28	39	50	77	1.0	84	0.78	114
Bupivacaine	4	Slow	240–480	175	About 1.5	8.1	11	15	24	95	28	73	0.47	210
Etidocaine	4	Slow	240–480	300	About 2	7.7	24	33	44	94	141	133	1.22	156
Prilocaine	1	Slow	60–120	400	>5	7.9	17	24	33	55	0.9			

* Increased if solution contains epinephrine
† Standard of comparison for esters
‡ Standard of comparison for amides
(Data from Covino BG, Vassallo HL: Local Anesthetics: Mechanisms of Action and Clinical Use. New York, Grune and Stratton, 1976; Tucker GT, Mather LE: Clinical pharmacokinetics of local anesthetics. Clin Pharmacokinet 1979;4:241–8.)

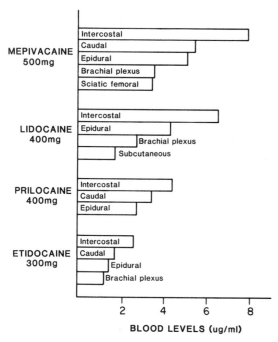

FIGURE 7-3. Peak plasma concentrations of local anesthetic are influenced by the site of injection for accomplishment of regional anesthesia. (From Covino BG, Vassallo HL. Local Anesthetics: Mechanisms of Action and Clinical Use. New York, Grune and Stratton, 1976. Reproduced by permission of the authors and publisher, 1976.)

from the circulation (Jorfeldt *et al*, 1980). Following rapid entry of local anesthetics into the venous circulation, this pulmonary extraction will limit the concentration of drug that reaches the systemic circulation for distribution to the coronary and cerebral circulations. For bupivacaine, this first-pass pulmonary extraction is dose dependent, suggesting that the uptake process becomes saturated rapidly (Rothstein *et al*, 1984). Furthermore, propranolol impairs bupivacaine extraction by the lung perhaps reflecting a common receptor site for the two drugs (Geddes *et al*, 1979; Rothstein and Pitt, 1983).

Placental Transfer

A tissue distribution of local anesthetics of clinical significance involves the placental transfer of local anesthetics. Plasma protein binding influences the rate and degree of diffusion of local an-

esthetics across the placenta (Table 7-1). Bupivacaine, which is highly protein bound (about 95%) has an umbilical vein/maternal arterial ratio of 0.14% to 0.44% compared with lidocaine which is less bound to protein (about 70%) and has a ratio of 0.52% to 0.71% (Thomas *et al*, 1976). Prilocaine, which is the least protein bound (about 55%), has a ratio of 1% to 1.18%. Ester local anesthetics, because of their rapid hydrolysis, are not available to cross the placenta in significant amounts. Acidosis in the fetus as occurs during prolonged labor can result in accumulation of local anesthetic in the fetus (*e.g.,* ion trapping) (Fig. 7-4) (Biehl *et al*, 1978).

Clearance

Clearance values and elimination half-times for amide local anesthetics probably represent mainly hepatic metabolism since renal excretion of unchanged drug is minimal (Table 7-1). Pharmacokinetic studies of ester local anesthetics are limited because of short elimination half-times due to their rapid hydrolysis in the plasma and liver.

Metabolism of Amide Local Anesthetics

Amide local anesthetics undergo varying rates of metabolism by microsomal enzymes located pri-

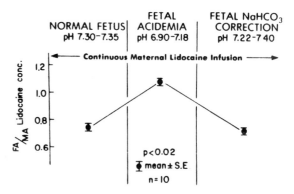

FIGURE 7-4. Fetal–maternal arterial (FA/MA) lidocaine ratios are greater during fetal acidemia compared with a normal *p*H. Mean ±SE. (From Biehl D, Shnider SM, Levinson G, Callender K. Placental transfer of lidocaine: Effects of fetal acidosis. Anesthesiology 1978;48:409–12. Reproduced by permission of the authors and publisher.)

marily in the liver. Prilocaine undergoes the most rapid metabolism, lidocaine and mepivacaine are intermediate, while the rate of breakdown of bupivacaine and etidocaine is the slowest among the amide local anesthetics (Covino and Vassallo, 1976). The initial step is conversion of the amide base to aminocarboxylic acid and a cyclic aniline derivative. Complete metabolism usually involves additional steps, such as hydroxylation of the aniline moiety and N-dealkylation of the aminocarboxylic acid.

Compared with ester local anesthetics, the metabolism of amide local anesthetics is more complex and slower. This slower metabolism means that sustained elevations of the plasma concentrations of amide local anesthetics, and thus systemic toxicity, are more likely than with ester local anesthetics. Furthermore, cumulative drug effects of amide local anesthetics are more likely than with ester local anesthetics.

LIDOCAINE. The metabolism of lidocaine is extensive such that clearance of this local anesthetic from the plasma parallels hepatic blood flow. Hepatic disease or reductions in hepatic blood flow, as occur during anesthesia, can reduce the rate of metabolism of lidocaine.

The principal pathway of metabolism of lidocaine is oxidative dealkylation in the liver to monoethylglycinexylidide followed by hydrolysis of this metabolite to xylidide (Fig. 7-5). Monoethylglycinexylidide has about 80% of the activity of lidocaine for protecting against cardiac dysrhythmias in an animal model (Burney et al, 1974). This metabolite may continue to be effective in controlling cardiac dysrhythmias after the infusion of lidocaine is discontinued. Xylidide has only about 10% of the cardiac antidysrhythmic activity of lidocaine. In humans, about 75% of xylidide is excreted in the urine as 4-hydroxy-2, 6-dimethylaniline (Covino and Vassallo, 1976). Accumulation of metabolites of lidocaine is predictable in the presence of renal failure.

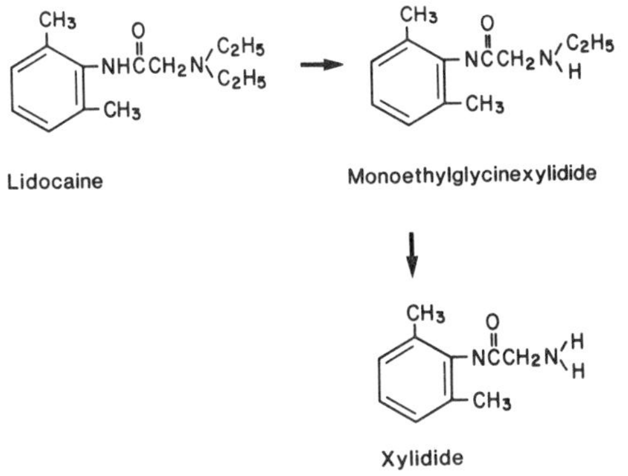

Metabolism and volume of distribution of lidocaine are decreased in patients with cardiac failure and cirrhosis of the liver (Prescott et al, 1976; Thomas et al, 1973). In these patients, the plasma concentration of lidocaine produced by a continuous intravenous infusion, as used to suppress cardiac dysrhythmias, may be unexpectedly elevated introducing an increased risk of systemic toxicity. Presumably, reductions in hepatic blood flow that accompany cardiac failure or cirrhosis of the liver are responsible for decreased metabolism and subsequent increased plasma levels of lidocaine. For example, the elimination half-time of lidocaine is increased more than fivefold in patients with liver dysfunction compared to normal patients. Decreased hepatic metabolism of lidocaine should also be anticipated when patients are anesthetized with volatile anesthetics (Fig. 7-6) (Adejepon-Yamoah et al, 1973). Likewise, drugs such as propranolol and norepinephrine, may decrease hepatic blood flow and subsequent metabolism of lidocaine (Branch et al, 1973). In patients with cardiac failure, plasma concentrations of monoethylglycinexylidide may equal the plasma concentrations of lidocaine indicating a failure of plasma clearance of lidocaine (Thomson et al, 1973). Maternal clearance of lidocaine is prolonged in toxemia of pregnancy and repeated administration of lidocaine can result in higher plasma concentrations than in normotensive parturients (Ramanathan et al, 1986).

MEPIVACAINE. Mepivacaine resembles the structure and pharmacologic properties of lidocaine (Table 7-1). The duration of action of mepivacaine is somewhat longer than lidocaine. In contrast to lidocaine, mepivacaine lacks vasodilator activity. As such, mepivacaine is an alternate selection when addition of epinephrine to the local anesthetic solution is not recommended.

BUPIVACAINE. Debutylation of bupivacaine results in the production of a xylidide metabolite (Reynolds, 1971). This metabolite undergoes further breakdown.

FIGURE 7-5. Metabolism of lidocaine.

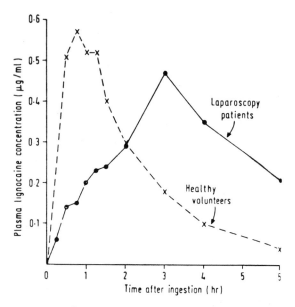

FIGURE 7-6. Plasma lidocaine (lignocaine) concentrations are greater during general anesthesia (laparoscopy patients) than in the absence of general anesthesia (healthy volunteers). (From Adejepon-Yamoah KK, Scott DB, Prescott LF. Impaired absorption and metabolism of oral lignocaine in patients undergoing laparoscopy. Br J Anaesth 1973;45:143–7. Reproduced by permission of the authors and publisher.)

ETIDOCAINE. Less than 1% of etidocaine is excreted unchanged in the urine. Despite its structural similarity to lidocaine, the metabolites of etidocaine differ from those of lidocaine.

PRILOCAINE. Prilocaine is an amide local anesthetic that is metabolized to ortho-toludine. Ortho-toludine is an oxidizing compound capable of converting hemoglobin to methemoglobin. When the dose of prilocaine exceeds 600 mg, there may be sufficient methemoglobin present ($3–5$ g dl^{-1}) to cause the patient to appear cyanotic and oxygen-carrying capacity is reduced. Methemoglobinemia is readily reversed by the intravenous administration of methylene blue 1 to 2 mg kg^{-1}, injected over 5 minutes. This therapeutic effect, however, is short-lived because methylene blue may be cleared before conversion of all the methemoglobin to hemoglobin. The unique ability of prilocaine to cause dose-related methemoglobinemia limits the clinical usefulness of this local anesthetic with the exception being intrave-

nous block anesthesia (see the section entitled Regional Anesthesia).

DIBUCAINE. Dibucaine is a quinoline derivative with an amide bond in the hydrocarbon connecting chain. This local anesthetic is metabolized in the liver and is the most slowly eliminated of all the amide derivatives.

Metabolism of Ester Local Anesthetics

Ester local anesthetics undergo hydrolysis by cholinesterase enzyme principally in the plasma and to a lesser extent in the liver. The rate of hydrolysis varies with chloroprocaine being most rapid, procaine intermediate and tetracaine the slowest (Foldes et al, 1965). The resulting metabolites are pharmacologically inactive although para-aminobenzoic acid may be an antigen responsible for subsequent allergic reactions. The exception to hydrolysis of ester local anesthetics in the plasma is cocaine which undergoes significant metabolism in the liver. Metabolites of cocaine may be responsible for sustained central nervous system effects (Miska et al, 1976).

Systemic toxicity is inversely proportional to the rate of hydrolysis emphasizing that tetracaine is more likely than chloroprocaine to result in excessive plasma concentrations. Since cerebrospinal fluid contains little or no cholinesterase, anesthesia produced by subarachnoid injection of tetracaine will persist until the drug has been absorbed into the circulation. Plasma cholinesterase activity and the rate of hydrolysis of ester local anesthetics are slowed in the presence of liver disease or an elevated blood urea nitrogen concentration (Reidenberg et al, 1972). Plasma cholinesterase activity may be reduced in parturients and in patients being treated with certain chemotherapeutic drugs (Finster, 1976; Kaniaris et al, 1979). Patients with atypical plasma chloinesterase are at increased risk for developing excess systemic concentrations of an ester local anesthetic due to absent or limited plasma hydrolysis.

PROCAINE. Procaine is hydrolyzed to para-aminobenzoic acid which is excreted unchanged in the urine and diethylaminoethanol, which is further metabolized since only 30% is recovered in the urine. Less than 5% of procaine is excreted unchanged in the urine. Increased plasma concentrations of para-aminobenzoic acid do not produce symptoms of systemic toxicity.

CHLOROPROCAINE. Addition of a chlorine atom to the benzene ring of procaine to form chloroprocaine speeds by three and one half times the rate of hydrolysis of this local anesthetic by plasma cholinesterase as compared with procaine. Resulting pharmacologically inactive metabolites of chloroprocaine are 2-chloroaminobenzoic acid and 2-diethylaminoethanol. Maternal and neonatal plasma cholinesterase activity may be decreased up to 40% at term but minimal placental passage of chloroprocaine confirms even this decreased activity is adequate to hydrolyze most of the chloroprocaine absorbed from the maternal epidural space (Kuhnert *et al*, 1980). The maternal elimination half-time of chloroprocaine following epidural administration is 1.5 to 6.4 minutes (Kuhnert *et al*, 1986a).

TETRACAINE. Tetracaine undergoes hydrolysis by plasma cholinesterase but the rate is slower than for procaine.

Renal Elimination

Poor water solubility of local anesthetics limits renal excretion of unchanged drug to usually less than 5% of the injected dose (Tucker and Mather, 1979). The exception is cocaine where 10% to 12% of unchanged drug can be recovered in the urine. Acidification of the urine facilitates renal elimination of the nonionized local anesthetic fraction by converting it to the more water-soluble ionized fraction. Water-soluble metabolites of local anesthetics, such as para-aminobenzoic acid resulting from metabolism of ester local anesthetics, are readily excreted in the urine.

Use of Vasoconstrictors

The duration of action of a local anesthetic is proportional to the time the drug is in contact with nerve fibers. For this reason, epinephrine (1 : 200,000, 5 μg ml^{-1}) or phenylephrine (1 : 20,000) is often added to local anesthetic solutions to produce vasoconstriction which limits systemic absorption and maintains the drug concentration at the nerve fiber. Indeed, addition of epinephrine to a lidocaine solution prolongs the duration of conduction blockade of nerve impulses about 50% and reduces systemic absorp-

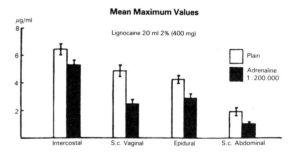

FIGURE 7-7. Addition of epinephrine (adrenaline) to the solution containing lidocaine (lignocaine) or prilocaine reduces systemic absorption of the local anesthetic by about one third. (From Scott DB, Jebson PJR, Braid B, Ortengren B, Frisch P. Factors affecting plasma levels of lignocaine and prilocaine. Br J Anaesth 1972;44:1040–9. Reproduced by permission of the authors and publisher.)

tion of local anesthetic by about one-third (Fig. 7-7) (Scott *et al*, 1972). The impact of epinephrine, however, in prolonging the duration of action and reducing systemic absorption of bupivacaine and etidocaine is less presumably because the high lipid solubility of these drugs causes them to avidly bind to tissues. In addition to reducing systemic absorption, epinephrine may enhance the intensity of conduction blockade by increasing neuronal uptake of the local anesthetic shortly after its injection.

Decreased systemic absorption of local anesthetic due to vasoconstriction produced by epinephrine increases the likelihood that the rate of metabolism will match absorption thus reducing the possibility of systemic toxicity (see the section entitled Systemic Toxicity). Whenever local anesthetic solutions containing epinephrine are administered in the presence of inhaled anesthetics, the possibility of enhanced cardiac irritability should be considered. Systemic absorption of epinephrine may accentuate hypertension in vulnerable patients. The addition of epinephrine to local anesthetic solutions, has little, if any effect on the rate of onset of local anesthesia.

Low molecular weight dextran added to local anesthetic solutions, as used for peripheral nerve blocks, prolongs the duration of action of the anesthetic. Presumably, dextran decreases the rate of systemic absorption of the local anesthetic (Kaplan *et al*, 1975).

Combinations of Local Anesthetics

Local anesthetics may be combined in an effort to produce a rapid onset (chloroprocaine) and prolonged duration (bupivacaine) of action. Local anesthetic toxicity of these mixtures is additive (Munson *et al,* 1977). Nevertheless, hydrolysis of chloroprocaine may be slowed by amide local anesthetics (Lalka *et al,* 1978). Amide ester local anesthetic mixtures containing chloroprocaine also may reduce the nonionized fraction of amide drug available reflecting the low *p*H (3.5) of chloroprocaine (Brodsky and Brock-Utne, 1978). Furthermore, tachyphylaxis to the local anesthetic mixture presumably reflects local tissue acidosis due to continued presence of a low *p*H solution.

MECHANISM OF ACTION

Local anesthetics inhibit transmission of nerve impulses(*e.g.,* conduction blockade) by preventing increases in permeability of nerve membranes to sodium ions (Ritchie and Greengard, 1966). Failure of permeability to sodium ions to increase slows the rate of depolarization such that threshold potential is not reached and thus, an action potential is not propagated (Fig. 7-8). Local anesthetics do not alter the resting transmembrane potential or threshold potential.

Sodium Channels

Sodium channels exist in (1) activated-open, (2) inactivated-closed, and (3) rested-closed states during various phases of the action potential (Hille, 1977; Kendig, 1981). During each action potential, sodium channels cycle from rested-closed to activated-open to inactivated-closed states. Before inactivated-closed sodium channels can open again, they must first pass through the rested-closed state. In the resting nerve membrane, sodium channels are distributed in equilibrium between the rested-closed and inactivated-closed states. Sodium channels in the rested-closed state have low affinity for local anesthetics while the inactivated-closed configuration has a higher affinity. By selectively binding to sodium channels in inactivated-closed states, local anesthetic molecules stabilize these channels in this configuration and prevent their change to the rested-closed and activated-open states in response to nerve impulses. Sodium channels in the inactivated-closed state are not permeable to sodium ions and thus conduction of nerve impulses in the form of propagated action potentials cannot occur.

Local Anesthetic Receptors

It is speculated that local anesthetics stabilize and maintain sodium channels in inactivated-closed states by binding to specific receptors located in the inner portion of sodium channels corresponding to the channel's internal or ''H'' gate (Hille, 1977). It is also postulated that some local anesthetic molecules may obstruct sodium channels near their external openings.

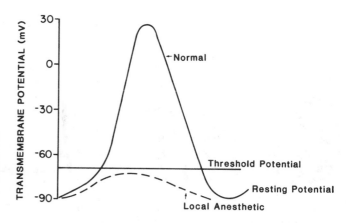

FIGURE 7-8. Local anesthetics slow the rate of depolarization of the nerve action potential such that threshold potential is not reached. As a result, an action potential cannot be propagated in the presence of local anesthetic, and conduction blockade results.

Frequency-Dependent Blockade

Sodium channels tend to recover from local anesthetic-induced conduction blockade between action potentials and develop additional conduction blockade each time sodium channels open during an action potential (*e.g.,* frequency-dependent blockade). This emphasizes that local anesthetic molecules can gain access to receptors only when sodium channels are in activated-open states. For this reason, selective conduction blockade of nerve fibers by local anesthetics may be related to the nerve's characteristic frequencies of activity as well as its anatomical properties (*e.g.,* diameter). Indeed, a resting nerve is less sensitive to local anesthetic-induced conduction blockade than is a nerve that has been repetitively stimulated. Etidocaine characteristically blocks somatic nerves before somatic sensory fibers because of frequency-dependent blockade (Bromage *et al,* 1974). In addition to local anesthetics, the pharmacologic effects of other drugs, including anticonvulsants and barbiturates, may reflect frequency-dependent blockade (Kendig, 1981).

MINIMUM CONCENTRATION

The minimum concentration of local anesthetic necessary to produce conduction blockade of nerve impulses is termed the Cm. The Cm is analogous to the minimum alveolar concentration (MAC) for inhaled anesthetics. Nerve fiber diameter influences Cm with larger nerve fibers requiring higher concentrations of local anesthetic for production of conduction blockade. An increased *p*H or a high frequency of nerve stimulation decreases Cm.

Each local anesthetic has a unique Cm reflecting differing potencies for each drug. The Cm of motor fibers is about twice that for sensory fibers emphasizing that sensory anesthesia may not be accompanied by skeletal muscle paralysis. Despite an unchanged Cm, less local anesthetic is needed for a subarachnoid block than an epidural block. This reflects greater access of drugs to unprotected nerves in the subarachnoid space.

Peripheral nerves are made up of myelinated A and B fibers and unmyelinated C fibers (see Chapter 41). There is a minimal length of myelinated nerve fiber which must be exposed to an adequate concentration of local anesthetic for conduction blockade of nerve impulses to occur. For example, if only one node of Ranvier is blocked (*e.g.,* site of changes in sodium permeability), the nerve impulse can jump (skip) across this node and conduction blockade does not occur. For conduction blockade to occur in an A fiber, it is necessary to expose at least two and preferably three successive nodes of Ranvier (about 1 cm) to an adequate concentration of local anesthetic (Franz and Perry, 1974). Both types of pain-conducting fibers (*i.e.,* myelinated A-delta and nonmyelinated C fibers) are blocked by similar concentrations of local anesthetics despite the fact that diameters of these fibers are different (see Chapter 41). Preganglionic B fibers are more readily blocked by local anesthetics than any fiber even though these fibers are myelinated.

Differential Conduction Blockade

Differential conduction blockade is illustrated by selective blockade of preganglionic sympathetic nervous system B fibers with low concentrations of local anesthetics. Slightly higher concentrations of local anesthetics interrupt conduction in small C fibers and small- and medium-sized A fibers with loss of sensation for pain and temperature. Nevertheless, touch, proprioception, and motor function are still present such that the patient will sense pressure but not pain with surgical stimulation. In an anxious patient, however, any sensation may be misinterpreted as failure of the local anesthetic.

Changes During Pregnancy

Increased sensitivity (*e.g,* more rapid onset of conduction blockade) may be present during pregnancy (Datta *et al,* 1983). Alterations in the serum protein-binding characteristics of bupivacaine may result in increased concentrations of pharmacologically active unbound drug in the plasma of parturients (Denson *et al,* 1984a). Nevertheless, progesterone which binds to the same alpha-1 acid glycoprotein as bupivacaine, does not influence protein binding of this local anesthetic (Denson *et al,* 1984b). This suggests that bupivacaine and progesterone bind to discrete but separate sites on protein molecules.

SIDE EFFECTS

The principal side effects related to the use of local anesthetics to produce local anesthesia are (1) allergic reactions and (2) systemic toxicity.

Allergic Reactions

Allergic reactions to local anesthetics are rare despite the frequent use of these drugs. It is estimated that less than 1% of all adverse reactions to local anesthetics are due to an allergic mechanism (Brown *et al,* 1981). This emphasizes that the overwhelming majority of adverse responses that are often attributed to an allergic reaction are, instead, manifestations of excess plasma concentrations of the local anesthetic (see the section entitled Systemic Toxicity).

Ester local anesthetics that produce metabolites related to para-aminobenzoic acid are more likely than amide local anesthetics, which are not metabolized to para-aminobenzoic acid, to evoke an allergic reaction. An allergic reaction following the use of a local anesthetic may be due to methylparaben or similar substances used as preservatives in commercial preparations of ester and amide local anesthetics. These preservatives are structurally similar to para-aminobenzoic acid. As a result, an allergic reaction may reflect prior stimulation of antibody production by the preservative and not the local anesthetic.

Cross-Sensitivity

Cross-sensitivity between ester local anesthetics reflects the common metabolite, para-aminobenzoic acid. A similar cross-sensitivity, however, does not exist between classes of local anesthetics. Therefore, a patient with a known allergy to an ester local anesthetic can receive an amide local anesthetic without an increased risk of experiencing an allergic reaction. Likewise, an ester local anesthetic can be administered to a patient with a known allergy to an amide local anesthetic. It is important that the "safe" local anesthetic be preservative-free.

Documentation of Allergy

Documentation of allergy to a local anesthetic is based on the clinical history and, perhaps use of intradermal testing (Incaudo *et al,* 1978). The occurrence of rash, urticaria, and laryngeal edema, with or without hypotension and bronchospasm, is highly suggestive of a local anesthetic-evoked allergic reaction. Conversely, hypotension associated with syncope or tachycardia when an epinephrine-containing local anesthetic solution is used is more suggestive of an inadvertent intravascular injection of drug (see the section entitled Systemic Toxicity). Utilization of an intradermal test requires injection of preservative-free preparations of local anesthetics to eliminate the possibility that the allergic reaction was caused by a substance other than the local anesthetic.

Systemic Toxicity

Systemic toxicity of local anesthetics is due to an excess plasma concentration of the drugs. Plasma concentrations of local anesthetics are determined by the rate of drug entrance into the circulation relative to its redistribution to inactive tissue sites and clearance by metabolism. Inadvertent direct intravascular injection of local anesthetic solutions during performance of a peripheral nerve block or epidural block is the most common mechanism for production of excess plasma concentrations of local anesthetics. Less often, excess plasma concentrations of local anesthetics result from absorption of the local anesthetic from the injection site. The magnitude of this systemic absorption depends upon the (1) dose administered into the tissues, (2) vascularity of the injection site, (3) presence of epinephrine in the solution, and (4) physiochemical properties of the drug (Table 7-1). For example, systemic absorption of local anesthetics is greatest following injection for an intercostal nerve block, intermediate for an epidural block and least for a brachial plexus block (Fig. 7-3) (Covino and Vassallo, 1976). Addition of 5 µg of epinephrine to every ml of local anesthetic solution (*i.e.* 1:200,000 dilution) reduces systemic absorption of local anesthetics by about one third (Scott *et al,* 1972) (see the section entitled Use of Vasoconstrictors).

Systemic toxicity of local anesthetics involves the central nervous system and cardiovascular system.

Central Nervous System

Low plasma concentrations of local anesthetics are likely to produce numbness of the tongue and circumoral tissues presumably reflecting delivery of drug to these highly vascular areas. As the plasma concentrations continue to rise, local anesthetics readily cross the blood–brain barrier and produce a predictable pattern of central nervous system changes. Restlessness, vertigo, tinnitus, and difficulty in focusing occur initially. Further increases in the central nervous system concentration of local anesthetic result in slurred speech and skeletal muscle twitching. This skeletal muscle twitching is often first evident in the face and extremities and signals the imminence of tonic-clonic seizures. Lidocaine and other amide local anesthetics may cause drowsiness before the onset of seizures. Seizures are classically followed by central nervous system depression which may also be accompanied by hypotension and apnea.

The onset of seizures may reflect selective depression of inhibitory cortical neurons by local anesthetics leaving excitatory pathways unopposed (see Chapter 41). An alternative explanation for seizures is local anesthetic-induced inhibition of the release of neurotransmitters, particularly gamma-aminobutyric acid. The exact site of local anesthetic-induced seizures is not known although it appears to be in the temporal lobe or the amygdala.

Plasma concentrations of local anesthetics producing signs of central nervous system toxicity depend upon the specific drug involved. Lidocaine, mepivacaine, and prilocaine demonstrate central nervous system effects at plasma concentrations of 5 to 10 μg ml^{-1}, while bupivacaine and etidocaine show central nervous system effects at venous plasma concentrations of 1.5 μg ml^{-1}. Furthermore, the active metabolite of lidocaine, monoethylglycinexylidide, may exert an additive effect in causing systemic toxicity following epidural lidocaine. For this reason, it has been recommended that the plasma concentration of lidocaine be monitored when the cumulative epidural dose of lidocaine exceeds 900 mg (Inoue *et al*, 1985). The seizure threshold for lidocaine may be related to central nervous system levels of 5-hydroxytryptophan. For example, accumulation of 5-hydroxytryptophan decreases the seizure threshold of lidocaine and prolongs the duration of seizure activity.

There is an inverse relationship between the PaCO$_2$ and seizure thresholds of local anesthetics presumably reflecting variations in cerebral blood flow and resultant delivery of drugs to the brain (deOliveira *et al*, 1974). For unknown reasons,

gallamine elevates the seizure threshold for lidocaine in animals (see Chapter 8).

Increases in the serum potassium concentration can facilitate depolarization and thus markedly increase local anesthetic toxicity. Conversely, hypokalemia, by creating hyperpolarization, can greatly decrease local anesthetic toxicity.

Cocaine in high doses (greater than 1.5 mg kg^{-1}) produces tremors, seizures, techycardia, vasoconstriction, and elevation of body temperature. The pyrogenic nature of cocaine probably reflects a direct action on heat-regulating centers in the central nervous system.

TREATMENT. Treatment of local anesthetic-induced seizures includes ventilation of the lungs with oxygen as arterial hypoxemia and metabolic acidosis occur within seconds (Moore *et al*, 1980). Equally important is the delivery of supplemental oxygen at the earliest sign of local anesthetic toxicity. Hyperventilation of the lungs seems logical in an attempt to reduce the amount of local anesthetic delivered to the brain. Conversely, this maneuver could theoretically slow removal of local anesthetic from the brain. Diazepam is effective in suppressing local anesthetic-induced seizures (see Chapter 5). Treatment of cocaine overdose includes administration of alpha- and beta-adrenergic antagonists to blunt symptoms of excess sympathetic nervous system activity.

Cardiovascular System

The cardiovascular system is more resistant to the toxic effects of high plasma concentrations of local anesthetics than is the central nervous system. For example, lidocaine in therapeutic plasma concentrations below 5 μg ml^{-1} is devoid of adverse cardiac effects producing only a decrease in the rate of spontaneous phase 4 depolarization (*e.g.*, automaticity) (see Chapter 17). Nevertheless, plasma lidocaine concentrations above 5 to 10 μg ml^{-1} and similar plasma elevations of other local anesthetics may produce profound hypotension due to relaxation of arteriolar vascular smooth muscle and direct myocardial depression. As a result, hypotension reflects both decreased peripheral vascular resistance and cardiac output.

Part of the cardiac toxicity that results from high plasma concentrations of local anesthetics results from the fact that these drugs also block cardiac sodium channels. At low concentrations of local anesthetics this effect on sodium channels probably contributes to cardiac antidysrhythmic properties of these drugs. When the plasma concentrations of local anesthetics, however, are excessive, too many cardiac sodium channels become blocked so conduction and automaticity become adversely depressed. For example, excessive plasma concentrations of lidocaine may slow conduction of the cardiac impulse through the heart manifesting as prolongation of the P–R interval and QRS complex on the electrocardiogram. Effects of local anesthetics on calcium and potassium channels may also contribute to cardiac toxicity (Arnsdorf and Bigger, 1975).

SELECTIVE CARDIAC TOXICITY. Inadvertent intravenous injection of bupivacaine may result in precipitous hypotension, cardiac dysrhythmias and atrioventricular heart block (Albright, 1979). Indeed, intravenous injection of bupivacaine or lidocaine to awake animals produces serious cardiac dysrhythmias only in animals receiving bupivacaine (Table 7-2) (Kotelko *et al,*1984). Furthermore, pregnancy may increase sensitivity to cardiotoxic effects as emphasized by occurrence of cardiopulmonary collapse with a smaller dose of bupivacaine in pregnant compared with nonpregnant animals (Fig. 7-9) (Morishima *et al,*1985). Likewise, cardiac toxicity of bupivacaine in animals is enhanced by preexisting arterial hypoxemia, acidosis, or hypercarbia.

In isolated papillary muscle preparations, V_{max}, an index of sodium current, is depressed more by bupivacaine than by lidocaine (Fig. 7-10) (Clarkson and Hondeghem, 1985). Dissociation of highly lipid-soluble bupivacaine from sodium channels is slow accounting for its persistent depressant effect on V_{max} and subsequent cardiac toxicity. In contrast, less lipid-soluble lidocaine leaves cardiac sodium channels rapidly as the channel state changes and cardiac toxicity is low. Tachycardia can enhance frequency-dependent blockade of cardiac sodium channels by bupivacaine further contributing to its selective cardiac toxicity (Kendig, 1985). Conversely, a low degree of frequency-dependent blockade may contribute to the antidysrhythmic properties of lidocaine. In anesthetized dogs, bretylium, 20 mg kg^{-1} reverses bupivacaine-induced cardiac depression and elevates the threshold for ventricular tachycardia (Kasten and Martin, 1985).

In an effort to minimize the potential for cardiotoxicity should inadvertent intravascular injection occur, the maximum recommended concentration of bupivacaine to be used for epidural block is 0.5%.

Ventilatory Response to Hypoxia

Lidocaine in clinically useful plasma concentrations depresses the ventilatory response to hypoxia (Gross *et al,* 1984). In this regard, patients with carbon dioxide retention whose resting ventilation depends on hypoxic drive may be at risk of ventilatory failure when lidocaine is administered for treatment of ventricular dysrhythmias. Con-

---

Table 7-2
Animals Manifesting Adverse Cardiac Changes Following Administration of Bupivacaine or Lidocaine

	Bupivacaine (% of animals)	Lidocaine (% of animals)
Sinus tachycardia	0	100
Supraventricular tachycardia	60	0
Atrioventricular heart block	60	0
Ventricular tachycardia	80	0
Premature ventricular contractions	100	0
Wide QRS complexes	100	0
ST–T wave changes	60	40

(Data from Kotelko DM, Shnider SM, Dailey PA, et al. Bupivacaine-induced cardiac arrhythmias in sheep. Anesthesiology 1984;60:10–8.)

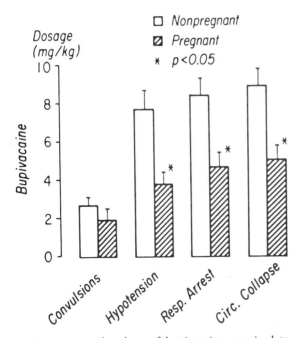

FIGURE 7-9. The dose of bupivacaine required to elicit toxic effects is less in pregnant than in nonpregnant ewes. Mean ± SE. (From Morishima HO, Pederson H, Finster M *et al.* Bupivacaine toxicity in pregnant and nonpregnant ewes. Anesthesiology 1985;63:134–9. Reproduced by permission of the authors and publisher.)

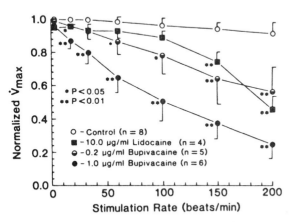

FIGURE 7-10. In an isolated papillary muscle preparation, V_{max} is depressed by bupivacaine. (From Clarkson CW, Hondeghem LM. Mechanism for bupivacaine depression of cardiac conduction: Fast block of sodium channels during the action potential with slow recovery from block during diastole. Anesthesiology 1985;62:396–405. Reproduced by permission of the authors and publisher.)

versely, systemic absorption of bupivacaine, as follows a brachial plexus block, stimulates the ventilatory response to carbon dioxide (Negre *et al*, 1985).

USES OF LOCAL ANESTHETICS

Local anesthetics are most often used to produce (1) regional anesthesia, (2) suppress grand mal seizures, (3) prevent or treat increases in intracranial pressure, (4) provide analgesia, and (5) prevent or treat cardiac dysrhythmias (see Chapter 17).

Regional Anesthesia

Regional anesthesia is classified according to the site of placement of the local anesthetic as (1) topical or surface anesthesia, (2) local infiltration, (3) peripheral nerve block, (4) intravenous block, (5) epidural block, and (6) subarachnoid or spinal block (Table 7-3).

Topical Anesthesia

Local anesthetics are used to produce topical anesthesia by placement on the mucous membrane of the nose, mouth, tracheobronchial tree, esophagus, or genitourinary tract. Cocaine (4%–10%), tetracaine (1%–2%) and lidocaine (2%–4%) are most often used. Procaine and chloroprocaine penetrate mucous membranes poorly and are not effective for topical anesthesia. Cocaine has the unique advantage of producing topical anesthesia and vasoconstriction. The latter effect decreases operative bleeding while improving surgical visualization.

Pramoxine is applied topically to skin or mucous membranes to relieve pain caused by minor burns or pruritus due to dermatoses or hemorrhoids. It may also be used to facilitate sigmoidoscopic examinations and to anesthetize the upper airway prior to direct laryngoscopy. This local anesthetic should not be injected or applied to nasal or tracheal mucosa as it may produce irritation. Structurally, pramoxine is unrelated to ester or amide local anesthetics which minimizes the danger of cross-sensitivity with other local anesthetics (Fig. 7-11).

Dyclonine is active topically being used to provide anesthesia of mucous membranes, for ex-

Table 7-3
Uses of Local Anesthetics to Produce Regional Anesthesia

	Topical Anesthesia	Local Infiltration	Peripheral Nerve Block	Intravenous Block	Epidural Block	Subarachnoid Block
Procaine	No	Yes	Yes	No	No	Yes
Chloroprocaine	No	Yes	Yes	No	Yes	No
Tetracaine	Yes	No	No	No	No	Yes
Lidocaine	Yes	Yes	Yes	Yes	Yes	Yes
Mepivacaine	No	Yes	Yes	No	Yes	No
Bupivacaine	No	Yes	Yes	Yes	Yes	Yes
Etidocaine	No	Yes	Yes	No	Yes	No
Prilocaine	No	Yes	Yes	Yes	Yes	No
Pramoxine	Yes	No	No	No	No	No
Dyclonine	Yes	No	No	No	No	No
Hexylcaine	Yes	No	No	No	No	No
Piperocaine	Yes	No	No	No	No	No

ample, prior to direct laryngoscopy (Fig. 7-11). The potency of dyclonine is similar to cocaine with an onset of action after about 10 minutes that lasts up to 1 hour.

Hexylcaine is active topically being used to provide anesthesia of mucous membranes, for example, prior to direct laryngoscopy (Fig. 7-11). Onset of anesthesia is within 5 minutes and lasts about 30 minutes. This local anesthetic is not injected because it produces tissue irritation.

Piperocaine is a benzoic acid ester used almost exclusively for topical anesthesia (Fig. 7-11). It has a more rapid onset and longer duration of action than procaine.

Topical anesthesia inhibits ciliary activity which may impair removal of secretions. Local anesthetics are absorbed into the systemic circulation following topical application to mucous membranes. Systemic absorption of tetracaine, and to a lesser extent lidocaine, following placement on the tracheobronchial mucosa produces plasma concentrations similar to those present after intravenous injection of the local anesthetic. For example, plasma lidocaine concentrations 15 minutes following laryngotracheal spray of the local anesthetic prior to intubation of the trachea were similar to those concentrations present at the same time after an intravenous injection of lidocaine (Viegas and Stoelting, 1975). This systemic absorption reflects the high vascularity of the tracheobronchial tree and the injection of the local anesthetic as a spray which spreads the solution over a wide surface area.

Local Infiltration

Local infiltration anesthesia is extravascular placement of local anesthetic in the area to be anesthetized. Subcutaneous injection of the local anesthetic in the area to be traversed for placement of an intravascular cannula is an example of infiltration anesthesia. Lidocaine is the local anesthetic most frequently used for infiltration anesthesia.

The duration of infiltration anesthesia can be approximately doubled by addition of 1 : 200,000 epinephrine to the injected local anesthetic solution. Epinephrine-containing solutions, however, should not be injected intracutaneously or into tissues supplied by end-arteries (fingers, ears, nose) because resulting vasoconstriction can produce ischemia and even gangrene.

Peripheral Nerve Block

Peripheral nerve block anesthesia is achieved by injection of local anesthetic in the vicinity of individual peripheral nerves or nerve plexuses such as the brachial plexus. When local anesthetic is deposited around a peripheral nerve, it diffuses from the outer surface. (*i.e.*, mantle) toward the center (*i.e.*, core) of the nerve along a concentration gradient (Winnie *et al*, 1977b). Consequently, nerve fibers located in the mantle of the mixed nerve are blocked first. These mantle fibers are usually distributed to more proximal anatomical structures in contrast to distal structures innervated by nerve fibers near the core of the nerve. This explains the

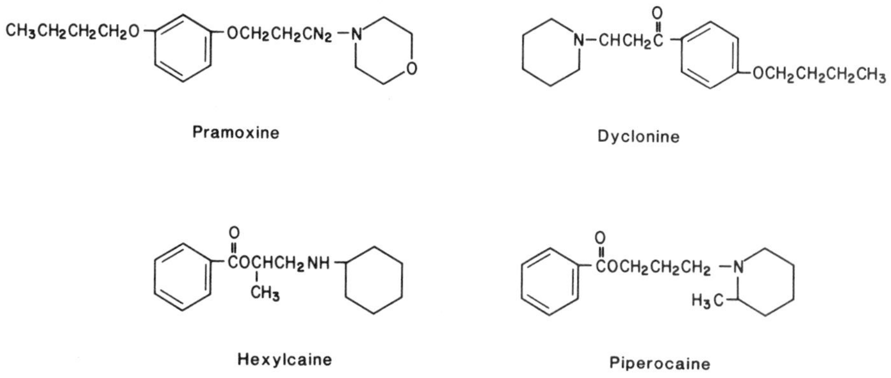

FIGURE 7-11. Local anesthetics used to produce topical anesthesia.

initial development of analgesia proximally with subsequent distal spread as local anesthetic diffuses to reach more central core nerve fibers. Conversely, recovery of sensation occurs in a reverse direction with nerve fibers in the mantle exposed to extraneural fluid being the first to lose local anesthetic such that sensation returns first to the proximal and last to the distal parts of the limb.

Skeletal muscle paralysis may precede the onset of sensory blockade if motor nerve fibers are distributed peripheral to sensory fibers in the mixed peripheral nerve (Winnie *et al*, 1977a). Indeed, the sequence of onset and recovery from blockade of sympathetic, sensory, and motor nerve fibers in a mixed peripheral nerve depend as much on the anatomical location of the nerve fibers within the mixed nerve as upon their sensitivity to local anesthetics. This differs from *in vitro* studies on single nerve fibers where diffusion distance does not play a role. In an *in vitro* model, nerve fiber size is most important, with the onset of conduction blockade being inversely proportional to fiber size. For example, the smallest sensory and autonomic nervous system fibers are blocked first, followed by larger motor and proprioceptive axons.

The rapidity of onset of sensory anesthesia following injection of a local anesthetic around a peripheral nerve depends on the *p*Ka of the drug. The *p*Ka determines the amount of local anesthetic that exists in the nonionized form at the *p*H of the tissue (Table 7-1). For example, the onset of action of lidocaine occurs in about 3 minutes while onset after bupivacaine requires about 15 minutes reflecting the greater fraction of lidocaine that exists in the lipid-soluble nonionized form.

Tetracaine, with a slow onset of anesthesia and a high potential to cause systemic toxicity, is not recommended for local infiltration or peripheral nerve block.

Duration of peripheral nerve block anesthesia depends on the dose of local anesthetic, its lipid solubility, degree of protein binding, and concomitant use of a vasoconstrictor such as epinephrine. The duration of action is more safely prolonged by epinephrine than by increasing the dose of local anesthetic which also increases the chances of systemic toxicity. Bupivacaine combined with epinephrine may produce peripheral nerve blocks lasting up to 24 hours.

Intravenous Block

Intravenous injection of a local anesthetic into an extremity isolated from the rest of the circulation by a tourniquet produces a rapid onset of anesthesia and skeletal muscle relaxation. The duration of the block is independent of the specific local anesthetic being determined by the time which the tourniquet is kept inflated. Normal sensation and skeletal muscle tone return promptly on release of the tourniquet which allows blood flow to dilute the concentration of local anesthetic.

Ester and amide local anesthetics produce satisfactory effects when used for intravenous block. Lidocaine and prilocaine are the most frequently used amide local anesthetics for intravenous block. The low incidence of thrombophlebitis and rapid metabolism of prilocaine following tourniquet deflation make this a useful local anesthetic for intravenous block. Indeed, evidence of central nervous system effects following tourniquet release was more frequent in patients receiving an intravenous block with lidocaine than with prilocaine (Kerr, 1967). The dose of prilocaine necessary for intravenous block (about 200 mg) is well below the amount likely to produce significant methemoglobinemia (600 mg). Chloroprocaine is not used for intravenous block because of a high incidence of thrombophlebitis (Harris, 1969). The mechanism by which local anesthetics produce intravenous block anesthesia is not known but probably reflects action of the drug on nerve endings as well as nerve trunks (Atkinson, 1969).

Epidural Block

Local anesthetic placed in the lumbar epidural or sacral caudal space produces epidural block by two presumed mechanisms. First local anesthetic diffuses across the dura to act on nerve roots and the spinal cord as it does when injected directly into the lumbar subarachnoid space to produce a subarachnoid block. Second, local anesthetic also diffuses into the paravertebral area through the intervertebral foramina, producing multiple paravertebral nerve blocks. These diffusion processes are slow accounting for the 15- to 30-minute delay in onset of sensory anesthesia following placement of local anesthetics in the epidural space. Lidocaine is commonly used for epidural block because of its good diffusion capabilities through tissues. Bupivacaine is often selected when prolonged epidural block is desired, as during labor. Chloroprocaine is acceptable when a rapid onset and short duration of sensory anesthesia are appropriate.

In contrast to subarachnoid block, during epidural block, there is not a zone of differential sympathetic nervous system blockade and the zone of differential motor blockade averages four and not two segments below the sensory level. Another difference from subarachnoid block is the larger dose required to produce epidural block leading to substantial systemic absorption of local anesthetic. For example, peak plasma concentrations of lidocaine are 3 to 4 μg ml^{-1} following placement of 400 mg into the epidural space. Peak plasma concentrations of bupivacaine following epidural injection of 150 mg average 1 μg ml^{-1}. Addition of 1:200,000 epinephrine to the lidocaine solution decreases systemic absorption of the local anesthetic by about one third. Systemic absorption of epinephrine produces beta-adrenergic stimulation characterized by peripheral va-

sodilation with resultant reductions in blood pressure even though cardiac output is increased by the inotropic and chronotropic effects of epinephrine.

Elevated plasma concentrations of local anesthetics following epidural block are of special importance when this technique is used to provide anesthesia to the parturient in labor. Local anesthetics cross the placenta and may produce detectable, although not necessarily adverse effects on the fetus for 24 to 48 hours. The fetus is less able to metabolize amide local anesthetics. Use of a more lipid-soluble and protein-bound local anesthetic, such as bupivacaine, limits passage across the placenta to the fetus. Even low doses of lidocaine as used for subarachnoid block during labor result in some systemic absorption as reflected by the presence of lidocaine and its metabolites in neonatal urine for longer than 36 hours (Kuhnert *et al*, 1986b).

Subarachnoid Block

Subarachnoid block is produced by injection of a local anesthetic into the lumbar subarachnoid space. Local anesthetics placed in the lumbar cerebrospinal fluid act on superficial layers of the spinal cord, but the primary site of action is the preganglionic fibers as they leave the spinal cord in the anterior rami. Because the concentration of local anesthetics in cerebrospinal fluid decreases as a function of distance from the site of injection and because different types of nerve fibers differ in their sensitivity to effects of local anesthetics, zones of differential anesthesia develop. Because preganglionic sympathetic fibers are blocked by concentrations of local anesthetics that are inadequate to affect somatic sensory or motor fibers, the level of sympathetic denervation during hyperbaric spinal anesthesia extends about two spinal segments cephalad to the level of sensory anesthesia. For the same reasons, the level of motor blockade averages two segments below sensory blockade.

Dosages of local anesthesia used for subarachnoid block vary according to the (1) height of the patient, which determines the volume of the subarachnoid space, (2) segmental level of anesthesia desired, and (3) duration of anesthesia required. Tetracaine and lidocaine are the local anesthetics most frequently used for subarachnoid block. Dibucaine is one and one half to two times as potent as tetracaine when used for subarachnoid block.

Chloroprocaine is not placed in the subarachnoid space because of potential neurotoxicity (Covino *et al,* 1980; Ravindran *et al,* 1980; Reisner *et al,* 1980).

Specific gravity of local anesthetic solutions injected into the lumbar cerebrospinal fluid is important in determining spread of the drugs. Addition of glucose to local anesthetic solutions increases specific gravity of the solutions above that of cerebrospinal fluid (hyperbaric). Addition of distilled water lowers the specific gravity of local anesthetic solutions below that of cerebrospinal fluid (hypobaric). Cerebrospinal fluid does not contain significant amounts of cholinesterase enzyme so the duration of action of ester local anesthetics as well as amides placed in the subarachnoid space is dependent on vascular absorption of the drug. Duration of anesthesia can be extended up to 100% by addition of epinephrine to the solution (maximum 0.2 mg) which presumably acts by delaying vascular absorption of the local anesthetic.

PHYSIOLOGIC EFFECTS. The goal of a subarachnoid block is to provide sensory anesthesia and skeletal muscle relaxation. It is the accompanying level of sympathetic nervous system blockade, however, that produces physiologic alterations. Plasma concentrations of local anesthetics following subarachnoid injection are too low to produce physiologic changes.

Sympathetic nervous system blockade results in arteriolar dilatation, but blood pressure does not decline proportionally because of compensatory vasoconstriction in areas with intact sympathetic nervous system innervation. Compensatory vasoconstriction occurs principally in the upper extremities and does not involve the cerebral vasculature. Even with total sympathetic nervous system blockade produced by subarachnoid block the decrease in peripheral vascular resistance is less than 15%. This change is minimal because smooth muscles of arterioles retain intrinsic tone and do not dilate maximally (see Chapter 44).

The most important cardiovascular responses produced by subarachnoid block are those that result from changes in the venous circulation. Unlike arterioles denervated by sympathetic nervous system blockade, venules do not maintain intrinsic tone and thus dilate maximally during subarachnoid block. The resulting increased vascular capacitance reduces venous return to the heart leading to reductions in cardiac output and blood pressure. This physiologic effect of subarachnoid block on venous return emphasizes the risk of extreme hypotension if this technique is used in a hypovolemic patient.

Blockade of the preganglionic cardiac accelerator fibers (T1 to T4) results in heart rate slowing particularly if decreased venous return and central venous pressure reduce stimulation of intrinsic stretch receptors in the right atrium. For example, heart rate will increase with a head-down position that increases venous return and elevates central venous pressure to stimulate stretch receptors. During a subarachnoid block, myocardial oxygen requirements are reduced as a result of decreased heart rate, venous return, and blood pressure.

Respiratory arrest that occurs with an excessive level of subarachnoid block reflects ischemic paralysis of the medullary ventilatory centers due to profound hypotension and associated reductions in cerebral blood flow. Concentrations of local anesthetic in ventricular cerebrospinal fluid are usually too low to produce pharmacologic effects on the ventilatory centers. Rarely is the cause of apnea due to phrenic nerve paralysis.

Suppression of Grand Mal Seizures

Suppression of grand mal seizures has been produced with intravenous doses of lidocaine not associated with seizure activity (Bernhard *et al,* 1955). Similar responses have been observed with mepivacaine (Berry *et al,* 1961). Presumably, these and perhaps other local anesthetics when present at low plasma concentrations are effective in suppression of seizures by virtue of initial depression of hyperexcitable cortical neurons. Nevertheless, inhibitory neurons are usually more sensitive to the depressant actions of local anesthetics than are excitatory neurons and excitatory phenomena predominate.

Prevention or Treatment of Increases in Intracranial Pressure

Intravenous lidocaine, 1.5 mg kg^{-1}, is as effective as thiopental in preventing increases in intracranial pressure evoked by intubation of the trachea in patients with decreased intracranial compliance (Bedford *et al,* 1980) (see Chapter 4). The antitussive effect of lidocaine may account, in part, for this effect. More likely, however, is the ability of lidocaine, like barbiturates, to reduce cerebral blood flow by increases in cerebral vascular resistance (Sakabe *et al*, 1974). Presumably, intracranial pressure declines in response to reductions in cerebral blood volume associated with decreases in cerebral blood flow. An advantage of using lidocaine rather than barbiturates, to lower intracranial pressure is a lesser likelihood of associated hypotension.

Intravenous lidocaine, 1.5 mg kg^{-1}, as used to prevent increases in intractranial pressure, is also effective in attenuating blood pressure but not heart rate responses associated with direct laryngoscopy for intubation of the trachea (Stoelting, 1977). Reflex-induced bronchospasm may be attenuated by intravenous lidocaine.

Analgesia

Lidocaine and procaine have been demonstrated to produce intense analgesia when injected intravenously. Use of local anesthetics for this purpose, however, is limited by the small margin of safety between intravenous analgesic doses and that which produces systemic toxicity. Nevertheless, continuous low dose infusion of lidocaine to maintain a plasma concentration of 1 to 2 μg ml^{-1} decreases the severity of postoperative pain and reduces requirements for opioids without producing systemic toxicity (Cassuto *et al*, 1985). Intravenous lidocaine also reduces anesthetic requirements for inhaled drugs. For example, halothane MAC in rats is decreased 40% by lidocaine sufficient to produce a plasma concentration of 1 μg ml^{-1} (Fig. 7-12) (DiFazio *et al*, 1976). A ceiling effect occurs above this plasma concentration as reflected by the absence of a further reduction in MAC despite more than fivefold increases in the lidocaine concentration. Intravenous lidocaine may also be administered in the perioperative period as a cough suppressant. In this regard, the cough reflex during intubation of the trachea is suppressed by plasma concentrations of lidocaine in excess of 3 μg ml^{-1} (Yukioka *et al*, 1985).

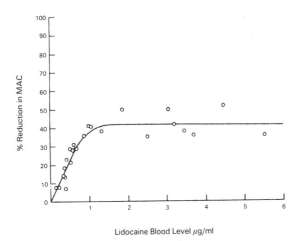

FIGURE 7-12. Halothane anesthetic requirements (MAC) are reduced in animals by about 40% when the plasma lidocaine concentration is 1 μg ml^{-1}. Further increases in the plasma lidocaine concentration do not decrease MAC an additional amount. (From DiFazio CA, Niederlehner JR, Burney RG. The anesthetic potency of lidocaine in the rat. Anesth Analg 1976;55:818–21. Reproduced by permission of the authors and the International Anesthesia Research Society.)

REFERENCES

Adejepon-Yamoah KK, Scott DB, Prescott LF. Impaired absorption and metabolism of oral lignocaine in patients undergoing laparoscopy. Br J Anaesth 1973;45:143-7.

Albright GA. Cardiac arrest following regional anesthesia with etidocaine or bupivacaine (editorial). Anesthesiology 1979;51:285-7.

Arnsdorf MF, Bigger JT. The effect of lidocaine on components of excitability in long mammalian cardiac purkinje fibers. J Pharmacol Exp Ther 1975; 195:206-15.

Atkinson DI. The mode of action of intravenous regional anaesthetics. Acta Anaesthesiol Scand 1969;36: 131-4.

Bedford RF, Persing JA, Robereskin L, Butler A. Lidocaine or thiopental for rapid control of intracranial hypertension. Anesth Analg 1980;59:435-7.

Bernhard CG, Bohm E, Hojeberg S. A new treatment of status epilepticus. Arch Neurol Psychiat 1955;74:208-14.

Berry CA, Sanner JH, Keasling HH. A comparison of the anticonvulsant activity of mepivacaine and lidocaine. J Pharmacol Exp Ther 1961;133:357-63.

Biehl D, Shnider SM, Levinson G, Callender K. Placental transfer of lidocaine: Effects of fetal acidosis. Anesthesiology 1978;48:409-12.

Branch RA, Shand DS, Wilkinson GR, Nies AS. The reduction of lidocaine clearance by dl-propranolol:

An example of hemodynamic drug interaction. J Pharmacol Exp Ther 1973;184:515-9.

Brodsky JB, Brocke-Utne JG. Mixing local anaesthetics (correspondence). Br J Anaesth 1978;50:1269.

Bromage PR, Burford MF, Crowell DE, Traunt AP. Quality of epidural blockade, III. Carbonated local anaesthetic solutions. Br J Anaesth 1967;39:197-209.

Bromage PR, Datta S, Dunford LA. Etidocaine: An evaluation in epidural analgesia for obstetrics. Can Anaesth Soc J 1974;21:535-45.

Brown DT, Beamish D, Wildsmith JAW. Allergic reaction to an amide local anaesthetic. Br J Anaesth 1981;53:435-7.

Burney RG, DiFazio CA, Foster J. Effects of pH on protein binding of lidocaine. Anesth Analg 1978;57:478-80.

Burney RG, DiFazio CA, Peach MJ, Petrie KA, Silvester MJ. Anti-arrhythmic effects of lidocaine metabolites. Am Heart J 1974;88:765-9.

Cassuto J, Wallin G, Hogstrom S, Faxen A, Rimback G. Inhibition of postoperative pain by continuous low-dose intravenous infusion of lidocaine. Anesth Analg 1985;64:971-4.

Clarkson CW, Hondeghem LM: Mechanism for bupivacaine depression of cardiac conduction: Fast block of sodium channels during the action potential with slow recovery from block during diastole. Anesthesiology 1985;62:396-405.

Covino BG, Marx GF, Finster M, Zsigmond EK. Prolonged sensory/motor deficits following inadvertent spinal anesthesia (editorial). Anesth Analg 1980;59:399-400.

Covino BG, Vassallo HL. Local anesthetics: Mechanisms of Action and Clinical Use. New York, Grune and Stratton, 1976.

Datta S, Lambert DH, Gergus J, Gissen AJ, Covino BJ. Differential sensitivities of mammalian nerve fibers during pregnancy. Anesth Analg 1983;62:1070-2.

Denson DD, Coyle DE, Santos D, Turner PA, Myers JA, Knapp R. Bupivacaine protein binding in the term parturient: Effects of lactic acidosis. Clin Parmacol Ther 1984a;35:409-15.

Denson DD, Santos DJ, Coyle DE. The effect of elevated progesterone on the serum protein binding of bupivacaine. Anesthesiology 1984b;61:A235.

deOliveira LF, Heavner JE, deJong RH. 5-Hydroxytryptophan intensifies local anesthetic-induced convulsions. Arch Inter Pharmacodyn Ther 1974;207:333-9.

DiFazio CA, Niederlehner JR, Burney RG. The anesthetic potency of lidocaine in the rat. Anesth Analg 1976;55:818-21.

Finster M. Toxicity of local anesthetics in the fetus and the newborn. Bull NY Acad Med 1976;52:222-5.

Foldes FF, Davidson GM, Duncalf D, Kuwabara S. The intravenous toxicity of local anesthetic agents in man. Clin Pharmcol Ther 1965;6:328-35.

Franz DN, Perry RS. Mechanisms for differential block among single myelinated and non-myelinated axons by procaine. J Physiol 1974;236:193-210.

Geddes DM, Nesbitt K, Traill T, Blackburn JP. First pass uptake of ^{14}C-propranolol by the lung. Thorax 1979;34:810-3.

Gross JB, Caldwell CB, Shaw LM, Apfelbaum JL. The effect of lidocaine infusion on the ventilatory response to hypoxia. Anesthesiology 1984;61:662-5.

Harris WH. Choice of anesthetic agents for intravenous regional anesthesia. Acta Anaesthesiol Scand 1969;36:47-52.

Hille B. Local anesthetics: Hydrophilic and hydrophobic pathways for the drug receptor interaction. J Gen Physiol 1977;69:497-515.

Incaudo G, Schatz M, Patterson R, Rosenberg M, Yamamoto F, Hamburger RN. Administration of local anesthetics to patients with a prior adverse reaction. J. Allergy Clin Immunol 1978;61:339-45.

Inoue R, Suganuma T, Echizen H, Ishizaki T, Kushida K, Tomona Y. Plasma concentrations of lidocaine and its principal metabolites during intermittent epidural anesthesia. Anesthesiology 1985;63:304-10.

Jorfeldt L. Lewis DH, Lofstrom JB, Post C. Lung uptake of lidocaine in man. Regional Anesthesia 1980;5:6-7.

Kaniaris P, Fassoulaki A, Liarmakopoulou K, Dermitzakis E. Serum cholinesterase levels in patients with cancer. Anesth Analg 1979;58:82-4.

Kaplan JA, Miller ED, Gallagher EG. Postoperative analgesia for thoracotomy patients. Anesth Analg 1975;54:773-7.

Kasten GW, Martin ST: Bupivacaine cardiovascular toxicity: Comparison of treatment with bretylium and lidocaine. Anesth Analg 1985;64:911-6.

Kendig JJ. Barbiturates: Active form and site of action at node ofRanvier sodium channels. J. Pharmacol Exp Ther 1981;218:175-81.

Kendig JJ. Clinical implications of the modulated receptor hypothesis: Local anesthetics and the heart (editorial). Anesthesiology 1985;62:382-4.

Kerr JH. Intravenous regional analgesia. Anaesthesia 1967;22:562-7.

Kotelko DM, Shnider SM, Dailey PA, et al,. Bupivacaine-induced cardiac arrhythmias in sheep. Anesthesiology 1984;60:10-8.

Kuhnert BR, Kuhnert PM, Philipson EH, Syracuse CD, Kaine CJ, Chang-hyon Y. The half-life of 2-chloroprocaine. Anesth Analg 1986a;65-273-8.

Kuhnert BR, Kuhnert PM, Prochaska BS, Gross TL. Plasma levels of 2-chloroprocaine in obstetric patients and their neonates after epidural anesthesia. Anesthesiology 1980;53:21-5.

Kuhnert BR, Philipson EH, Pimental R, Kuhnert PM, Zuspan KJ, Syracuse CD. Lidocaine disposition in mother, fetus, and nenonate after spinal anesthesia. Anesth Analg 1986b;65:139-44.

Lalka D, Vicuna N, Burrow SR, et al,. Bupivacaine and

other amide local anesthetics inhibit the hydrolysis of chloroprocaine by human serum. Anesth Analg 1978;57:534-9.

Miska AL, Patel MN, Alluri VR, Mule SJ, Nyak PK. Disposition and metabolism of ($_3$H) cocaine in acutely and chronically treated dogs. Xenobiotica 1976;6:537-52.

Moore DC, Crawford RD, Scurlock JE. Severe hypoxia and acidosis following local anesthetic-induced convulsions. Anesthesiology 1980;53:259-60.

Morishima HO, Pederson H, Finster M, et al,. Bupivacaine toxicity in pregnant and nonpregnant ewes. Anesthesiology 1985;63:134-9.

Munson ES, Paul WL, Embro WJ: Central-nervous-system toxicity of local anesthetic mixtures in monkeys. Anesthesiology 1977;46:179-83.

Negre I, Labaille T, Samii K, Noviant Y. Ventilatory response to carbon dioxide following axillary blockade with bupivacaine. Anesthesiology 1985;63:401-3.

Prescott LF, Adejepon-Yamoah KK, Talbot RG: Impaired lignocaine metabolism in patients with myocardial infarction and cardiac failure. Br Med J 1976;1:939-41.

Ramanathan J, Bottorff M, Jeter JN, Khalil M, Sibai BM. The pharmacokinetics and maternal and neonatal effects of epidural lidocaine in preeclampsia. Anesth Analg 1986;65-120-6.

Ravindran RS, Bond VK, Tasch MD, Gupta CD, Luerssen TG. Prolonged neural blockade following regional analgesia with 2-chloroprocaine. Anesth Analg 1980;59:447-51.

Reidenberg MM, James M, Drign LG. The rate of procaine hydrolysis in serum of normal subjects and diseased patients. Clin Pharmacol Ther 1972;13:279-84.

Reisner LS, Hochman BN, Plumer MH: Persistent neurologic deficit and adhesive arachnoiditis following intrathecal 2-chloroprocaine injection. Anesth Analg 1980;59:452-4.

Reynolds F. A comparison of the potential toxicity of bupivacaine, lignocaine and mepivacaine during epidural blockade. Br J Anaesth 1971;43:567-72.

Ritchie JM, Greengard AG. On the mode of action of local anesthetics. Ann Rev Pharmacol 1966;6:405-30.

Rothstein P, Cole J, Pitt BR. Pulmonary extraction of bupivacaine is dose dependent. Anesthesiology 1984;61:A236.

Rothstein P, Pitt BR. Pulmonary extraction of bupivacaine and its modification by propranolol. Anesthesiology 1983;59:A189.

Sakabe T, Maekawa T, Ishikawa T, Takeshita H. The effects of lidocaine on canine cerebral metabolism and circulation related to the electroencephalogram. Anesthesiology 1974;40:433-41.

Scott DB, Jebson PJR, Braid B, Ortengren B, Frisch P. Factors affecting plasma levels of lignocaine and prilocaine. Br J Anaesth 1972;44:1040-9.

Stoelting RK. Circulatory changes during direct laryngoscopy and tracheal intubation: Influence of duration of laryngoscopy with or without prior lidocaine. Anesthesiology 1977;47:381-3.

Thomas J, Long G, Moore G, Morgan D. Plasma protein binding and placental transfer of bupivacaine. Clin Pharmacol Ther 1976;19:426-34.

Thomson PD, Melman KL, Richardson JA, et al. Lidocaine pharmacokinetics in advanced heart failure; liver disease, and renal failure in humans. Ann Intern Med 1973;78:499-508.

Tucker GT, Mather LE. Clinical pharmacokinetics of local anesthetics. Clin Pharmacokinet 1979;4:241-78.

Viegas O, Stoelting RK. Lidocaine in arterial blood after laryngotracheal administration. Anesthesiology 1975;43:491-3.

Winnie AP, LaValley DA, DeSosa B, Mazud KZ. Clinical pharmacokinetics of local anesthetics. Can Anaesth Soc J 1977a;24:252-62.

Winnie AP, Tay C-H, Patel KP, Ramamurthy S, Durrani Z. Pharmacokinetics of local anesthetics during plexus blocks. Anesth Analg 1977b;56:852-61.

Yukioka H, Yoshimoto N, Nishimura K, Fujimori M. Intravenous lidocaine as a suppressant of coughing during tracheal intubation. Anesth Analg 1985;64:1189-92.

C H A P T E R 8

Neuromuscular Blocking Drugs

INTRODUCTION

The major pharmacologic effect of neuromuscular blocking drugs is the interruption of transmission of nerve impulses at the neuromuscular junction. On the basis of distinct electrophysiologic differences in their mechanisms of action, these drugs can be classified as depolarizing neuromuscular blocking drugs, long-acting nondepolarizing neuromuscular blocking drugs, and intermediate-acting nondepolarizing neuromuscular blocking drugs (Table 8-1). These drugs produce phase I depolarizing neuromuscular blockade, phase II depolarizing neuromuscular blockade, or nondepolarizing neuromuscular blockade.

Clinically, the most reliable method for determining the type and degree of neuromuscular blockade present is to observe or record the skeletal muscle responses that are evoked by a supramaximal electrical stimulus delivered from a peripheral nerve stimulator. Most often contraction of the adductor pollicis muscle (e.g., twitch response) following electrical stimulation of the ulnar nerve is used to assess the effect of neuromuscular blocking drugs. It is important to recognize that the dose of neuromuscular blocking drug necessary to produce a given degree of neuromuscular blockade at the diaphragm is about twice the dose required to produce similar blockade of the adductor pollicis muscle (Donati et al, 1986). The electromyogram serves the same purpose as the peripheral nerve stimulator. A single twitch response evoked using a peripheral nerve stimulator reflects events at the postjunctional membrane (Lee et al, 1977). Conversely, the response to continuous stimulation or train-of-four stimulation reflects events at the presynaptic membrane. The differences in effects of nondepolarizing neuromuscular blocking drugs on responses to single stimulus versus multiple or continuous stimulation most likely reflect differences in the magnitude of presynaptic and postsynaptic effects of these drugs (Bowman, 1980).

HISTORY

Modern clinical use of neuromuscular blocking drugs dates from 1932 when purified fractions of d-tubocurarine were administered to control skeletal muscle spasms in patients with tetanus (West, 1932). In 1940, d-tubocurarine was administered as an adjuvant to drug-induced electroshock therapy (Bennett, 1940). The first use of d-tubocurarine to produce skeletal muscle relaxation during surgery and general anesthesia was in 1942 (Griffith and Johnson, 1942).

The use of curarized animals in experiments conducted on succinylcholine in 1906 masked the neuromuscular blocking properties of this drug (Hunt and Taveau, 1906). Indeed, the neuromuscular blocking effects of succinycholine were not recognized until 1949.

Table 8-1
Classification of Neuromuscular Blocking Drugs

Depolarizers
Succinylcholine
Decamethonium
Nondepolarizers
Long-acting
d-Tubocurarine
Metocurine
Gallamine
Pancuronium
Intermediate-acting
Atracurium
Vecuronium

CLINICAL USES

Today, the principal uses of neuromuscular blocking drugs are (1) to provide skeletal muscle relaxation to facilitate intubation of the trachea and (2) to provide optimal surgical working conditions (see the section entitled Drug Selection). It must be recognized that neuromuscular blocking drugs lack central nervous system depressant and analgesic effects. Therefore, these drugs cannot substitute for anesthetic drugs. Furthermore, ventilation of the lungs must be mechanically provided whenever substantial neuromuscular blockade is produced by these drugs. Clinically, evaluation of the degree of neuromuscular blockade is typically provided by monitoring the evoked skeletal muscle responses produced by an electrical stimulus delivered from a peripheral nerve stimulator. Other indicators of residual neuromuscular blockade include grip strength, ability to sustain head lift, vital capacity measurement, and generation of negative inspiratory pressure.

Drug Selection

The choice between depolarizing and nondepolarizing neuromuscular blocking drugs is influenced by the speed of onset, duration of action, and possibility of drug-induced side effects due to actions of these drugs at sites other than the neuromuscular junction. A rapid onset and brief duration of neuromuscular blockade, as provided by succinylcholine, is useful when intubation of the trachea is the reason for administering a neuromuscular blocking drug. When longer periods of neuromuscular blockade are needed, succinylcholine can be administered as a continuous intravenous infusion, or nondepolarizing neuromuscular blocking drugs are selected. Likewise, when a rapid onset of neuromuscular blockade is not considered necessary, skeletal muscle relaxation to facilitate intubation of the trachea can be provided by nondepolarizing neuromuscular blocking drugs.

Sequence of Onset of Neuromuscular Blockade

Small, rapidly moving muscles such as those of the eyes and digits are affected by neuromuscular blocking drugs before those of the trunk and abdomen. Ultimately, intercostal muscles and finally the diaphragm are paralyzed. Recovery of skeletal muscles usually occurs in the reverse order to that of paralysis such that the diaphragm is the first to regain function.

Intravenous injection of a nondepolarizing neuromuscular blocking drug to a person who is awake initially produces difficulty in focusing and weakness in the mandibular muscles followed by ptosis, diplopia, and dysphagia. Relaxation of the small muscles of the ears improves acuity of hearing. Consciousness and sensorium remain undisturbed even in the presence of complete neuromuscular blockade.

STRUCTURE ACTIVITY RELATIONSHIPS

Neuromuscular blocking drugs have structural similarities to the endogenous neurotransmitter, acetylcholine (Fig. 8-1). For example, succinylcholine is two molecules of acetylcholine linked through acetate methyl groups (Fig. 8-1). The long, slender, and flexible structure of succinylcholine allows it to bind to and activate cholinergic receptors. Bulky and rigid molecules characteristic of nondepolarizing neuromuscular blocking drugs, although containing portions similar to acetylcholine cannot activate the nicotinic cholinergic receptor (Fig. 8-1). Pancuronium is most closely related structurally to acetylcholine. The acetylcholine-like fragments of pancuronium

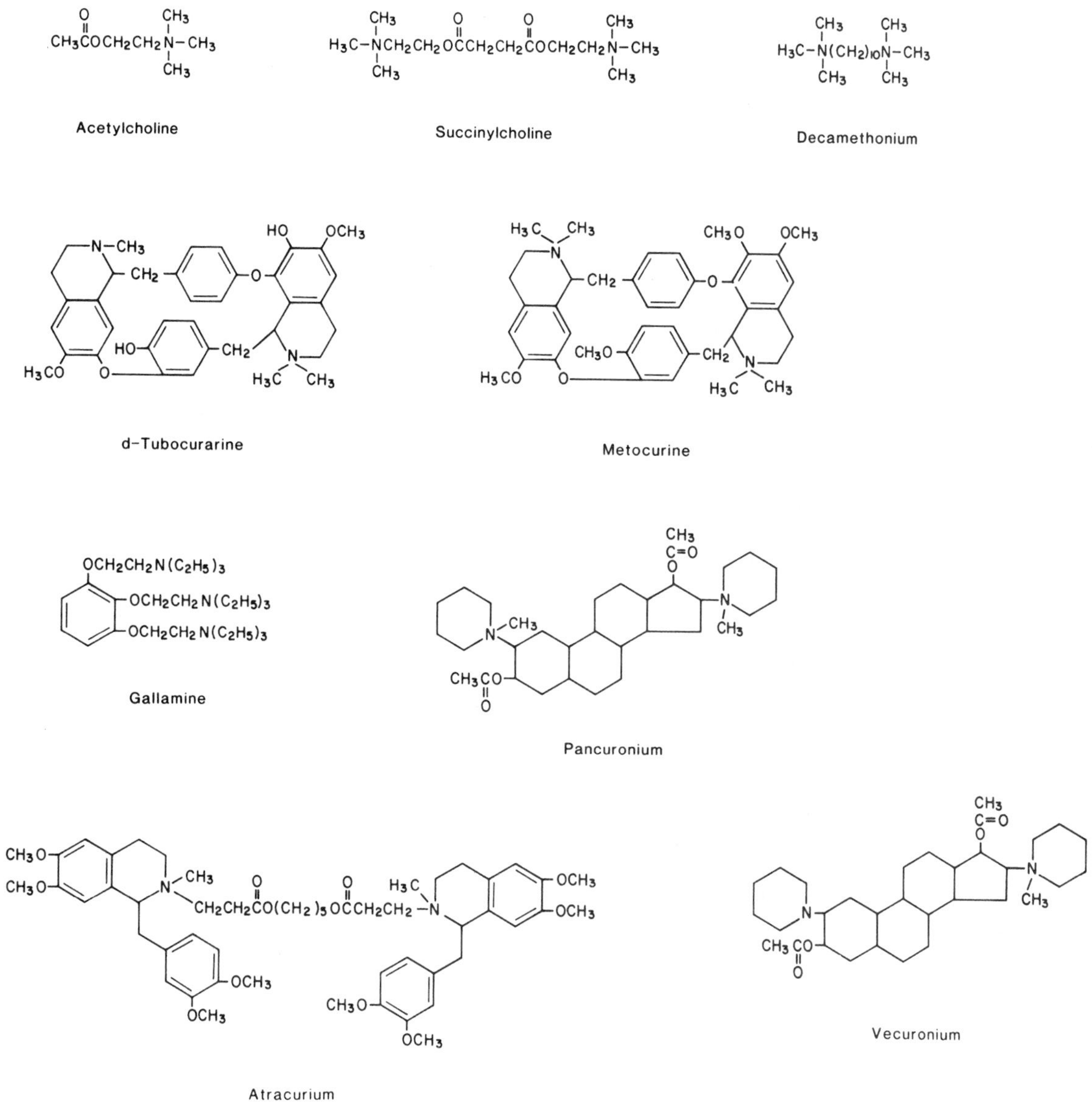

FIGURE 8-1. Acetylcholine and neuromuscular blocking drugs.

confer upon the steroidal molecule its high neuro-muscular blocking activity and its plasma cholin-esterase-inhibiting action.

Acetylcholine has a positively charged quater-nary ammonium group (i.e., four carbons attached to one nitrogen) which is attracted to the nega-tively charged cholinergic receptor (Fig. 8-1). This same feature is common to neuromuscular

blocking drugs which all contain one or more pos-itively charged quaternary ammonium groups. For example, d-tubocurarine and vecuronium are monoquaternary; metocurine, pancuronium, and atracurium are bisquaternary; and gallamine is tri-quaternary (Fig. 8-1). Pancuronium is an aminos-teroid with no hormonal activity. The bisquater-nary ammonium structure of most of these drugs suggests that an electrostatic association occurs between two ionized cationic centers of the drug and anionic groups on the cholinergic receptor.

It is no longer tenable to propose that optimal nondepolarizing neuromuscular blocking activity is dependent on an optimal distance between quaternary ammonium groups. Indeed, d-tubocurarine and vecuronium contain only one quaternary ammonium group. It is likely, however, that an interquaternary distance of 1.25 nm confers optimal depolarizing neuromuscular blocking activity.

The electrostatic attraction of the negatively charged cholinergic receptor for the positively charged quaternary ammonium group occurs at cholinergic sites other than the neuromuscular junction including cardiac muscarinic receptors and autonomic ganglia nicotinic receptors. This lack of specificity for the neuromuscular junction means neuromuscular blocking drugs could produce cardiovascular effects particularly as reflected by changes in blood pressure and heart rate (see the section entitled Cardiovascular Effects of Neuromuscular Blocking Drugs).

The specificity of a drug for the autonomic ganglia nicotinic receptor versus the neuromuscular junction is influenced by the length of the carbon chain separating the two positively charged ammonium groups. Maximal autonomic ganglion blockade occurs when the positive charges are separated by six carbon atoms (*e.g.,* hexamethonium) while neuromuscular blockade occurs when ten carbon atoms are present (*e.g.,* decamethonium). As a bulky monoquaternary molecule, d-tubocurarine is more likely to produce autonomic ganglion blockade than is a bisquaternary drug. Indeed, methylation of d-tubocurarine to the bisquaternary ammonium drug, metocurine, dramatically reduces the autonomic ganglion blocking properties associated with production of neuromuscular blockade. Likewise, bisquaternary ammonium neuromuscular blocking drugs such as metocurine and pancuronium are less likely than the monoquaternary d-tubocurarine to evoke the release of histamine. Presumably, the histamine-releasing properties of d-tubocurarine are due to the presence of the tertiary amine. The increased efficacy of d-tubocurarine in the presence of acidosis most likely reflects increased ionization of the tertiary amino group as the plasma *p*H declines. Gallamine possesses marked vagolytic effects presumably due to the presence of three quaternary ammonium nitrogens.

NEUROMUSCULAR JUNCTION

The neuromuscular junction consists of a prejunctional motor nerve ending separated from a highly folded postjunctional membrane of the skeletal muscle by a synaptic cleft that is 20 to 30 nm wide and filled with extracellular fluid (Fig. 8-2) (Drachman, 1978) (see Chapter 55). The nonmyelinated nerve ending contains mitochondria, endoplasmic reticulum, and synaptic vesicles necessary for the synthesis of the neurotransmitter, acetylcholine. The resting transmembrane potential of about −90 mv across nerve and skeletal muscle membranes is maintained by the unequal distribution of potassium and sodium ions across the membranes (see Chapter 39). Nicotinic cholinergic receptors are situated on both the presynaptic and postsynaptic membranes.

Acetylcholine

Acetylcholine, a quaternary ammonium ester, is the neurotransmitter at the neuromuscular junc-

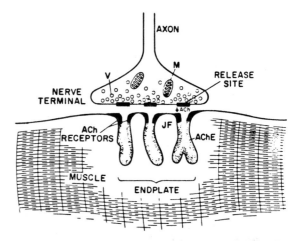

FIGURE 8-2. Schematic depiction of neuromuscular junction. Acetylcholine (ACh) is present in vesicles (V) of the axon for release in response to nerve impulses. The neurotransmitter diffuses across the synaptic cleft to attach to receptors that are concentrated on the junctional folds (JF) of the skeletal muscle endplate. Acetylcholinesterase (AChE) is present in the JF to facilitate rapid hydrolysis of ACh. (From Drachman DA. Myasthenia gravis. N Engl J Med 1978;298:136–42. Reprinted by permission of the New England Journal of Medicine 1978;298:136–42.)

tion. Synthesis of acetylcholine in motor nerve endings is by the acetylation of choline under the control of the enzyme, choline acetylase. This acetylcholine is stored in synaptic vesicles in motor nerve endings and released into the synaptic cleft as packets (quanta) each of which contains at least 1000 molecules of acetylcholine. Arrival of a nerve impulse causes the release of hundreds of quanta of acetylcholine which bind to nicotinic cholinergic receptors on postsynaptic membranes causing a change in membrane permeability to ions. This change in permeability causes a decline in the transmembrane potential from about -90 mv to -45 mv (threshold potential) at which point a propagated action potential spreads over the surfaces of skeletal muscle fibers leading to a muscular contraction. In the absence of action potentials, quanta of acetylcholine are randomly released producing miniature endplate potentials of less than 1 mv that are insufficient to trigger depolarization. Calcium ions must be present for the release of acetylcholine from synaptic vesicles into the synaptic cleft. It is speculated that a nerve action potential activates adenylate cyclase in membranes of nerve terminals leading to the formation of cyclic AMP which subsequently opens calcium channels causing synaptic vesicles to fuse with the nerve membrane and to release acetylcholine (Standaert and Dretchen, 1981). Indeed, drugs such as aminophylline, which stimulate formation of cyclic AMP, facilitate neuromuscular transmission while calcium channel blocking drugs, such as verapamil, interfere with neuromuscular transmission.

Situated in close proximity to cholinergic receptors is the enzyme, acetylcholinesterase. This enzyme is responsible for the rapid hydrolysis (within 15 msec) of acetylcholine to acetic acid and choline. Choline can reenter the motor nerve ending to again participate in the synthesis of new acetylcholine. The rapid hydrolysis of acetylcholine prevents sustained depolarization at the neuromuscular junction.

Postjunctional Nicotinic Receptors

The postjunctional membrane possesses two types of receptors that respond to neuromuscular blocking drugs (Standaert, 1984). Nicotinic cholinergic receptors are present in large numbers on postjunctional membranes. Extrajunctional cholinergic receptors appear throughout skeletal muscle whenever there is deficient stimulation of the skeletal muscle by the nerve.

Nicotinic Cholinergic Receptors

The postjunctional nicotinic cholinergic receptor is a glycoprotein with a molecular weight of 250,000 daltons (Raftery *et al*, 1980; Standaert, 1984). Each receptor consists of five subunits designated alpha, beta, gamma, and delta (Fig. 8-3) (Taylor, 1985). There are two alpha subunits weighing about 40,000 daltons each; the other subunits weigh 50,000 to 65,000 daltons. Electron micrographs of nicotinic cholinergic receptors show these receptors to be particularly concentrated on the shoulders of the postjunctional membrane folds, which places them precisely opposite prejunctional release sites for acetylcholine.

Nicotinic cholinergic receptors extend through the entire cell membrane but continue for only about 2 nm into the cytoplasm (Stroud, 1983). The subunits of the receptor are arranged such that a channel is formed that allows the flow of ions along a concentration gradient (Fig. 8-3) (Taylor, 1985). For example, sodium and calcium ions move into skeletal muscle while potassium ions exit via these channels. These channels are open (*i.e.,* in the active state) only when an acetylcholine molecule occupies each of the alpha subunits causing the subunits to rotate into an open conformation that allows the flow of ions (Fig. 8-3) (Taylor, 1985). This flow of ions is the basis of normal neuromuscular transmission.

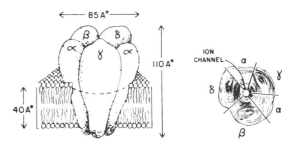

FIGURE 8-3. The postjunctional nicotinic cholinergic receptor consists of five subunits designated alpha, beta, gamma, and delta. (From Taylor P. Are neuromuscular blocking agents more efficacious in pairs? Anesthesiology 1985;63:1–3. Reproduced by permission of the author and publisher.)

The two alpha subunits, in addition to being the binding sites for acetylcholine, are the sites occupied by neuromuscular blocking drugs. For example, occupation of one or both alpha subunits by a neuromuscular blocking drug causes the channel to remain closed. As a result, ions do not flow in these channels, and depolarization cannot occur at these sites. If enough channels remain closed, there is blockade of neuromuscular transmission. A nondepolarizing neuromuscular blocking drug may show preference for one of the two alpha subunits. This might result in synergism if two neuromuscular blocking drugs with different selective preferences for each alpha subunit are administered simultaneously. Succinylcholine, by binding to each alpha subunit, causes the pore to remain open.

The extracellular end of the channel is larger than the portion that extends through the cell membrane. Large molecules can act to plug the channel and in this way prevent the normal flow of ions. Channel blockade may be the mechanism for a number of drug interactions that occur with neuromuscular blocking drugs. Similar channel blockade is produced by local anesthetics that plug sodium channels.

Extrajunctional Cholinergic Receptors

Extrajunctional cholinergic receptors are normally not present in large numbers because their synthesis is suppressed by neural activity. Whenever motor nerves are less active (*e.g.,* traumatized skeletal muscle, denervation) these extrajunctional cholinergic receptors proliferate rapidly (Pumplin and Fambrough, 1982). These extrajunctional cholinergic receptors appear over the entire postjunctional membrane rather than being confined to the area of the neuromuscular junction.

Extrajunctional cholinergic receptors are very responsive to agonists, such as acetylcholine or succinylcholine, and poorly responsive to antagonists, such as the nondepolarizing neuromuscular blocking drugs. Because extrajunctional cholinergic receptors are formed rapidly after slackening of neural influence on skeletal muscle and are degraded soon after the neural influence returns, mixtures of nicotinic cholinergic receptors and extrajunctional cholinergic receptors are present in many clinical situations and may account for some of the quantitative differences in response to neuromuscular blocking drugs among individuals and various disease states.

Prejunctional Nicotinic Receptors

Prejunctional nicotinic cholinergic receptors on motor nerve endings influence the release of neurotransmitters. These prejunctional receptors seem to be different from postjunctional nicotinic cholinergic receptors in (1) their chemical binding characteristics, (2) the nature of the ion channel they control, and (3) their preferential blockade during high-frequency stimulation. Prejunctional receptor or channel blockade as produced by d-tubocurarine diminishes the release of acetylcholine from nerves stimulated at high frequency and this contributes to diminished neuromuscular transmission (Standaert, 1982).

DEPOLARIZING NEUROMUSCULAR BLOCKING DRUGS

Depolarizing neuromuscular blocking drugs are represented by succinylcholine and decamethonium (Fig. 8-1). Succinylcholine in a dose of 0.5 to 1 mg kg^{-1} has a rapid onset (30–60 seconds) and short duration of action (3–5 minutes). These characteristics make succinylcholine ideal to provide skeletal muscle relaxation to facilitate intubation of the trachea. Based on measurements during halothane anesthesia, the estimated ED_{95} for succinylcholine is about 0.2 mg kg^{-1} (Miller *et al*, 1971). Succinylcholine has several associated adverse side effects that can limit or even contraindicate its use. Decamethonium is available but rarely used.

Mechanism of Action

Succinylcholine attaches to each of the alpha subunits of the nicotinic cholinergic receptor and mimics the action of acetylcholine thus producing depolarization of the postjunctional membrane. Compared with acetylcholine, the hydrolysis of succinylcholine is slow, resulting in sustained depolarization. Neuromuscular blockade develops because a depolarized postjunctional membrane cannot respond to subsequent release of acetylcholine (*i.e.,* depolarizing neuromuscular blockade). Depolarizing neuromuscular blockade is also referred to as phase I blockade. Succinylcholine has presynaptic effects, but these are considered to be minor when compared to postsynaptic actions (Standaert and Adams, 1965).

A single large dose (greater than 2 mg kg^{-1}), repeated doses, or a prolonged continuous infusion of succinylcholine may result in a postjunctional membrane that does not respond normally to acetylcholine even when the postjunctional membrane has become repolarized (*i.e.,* desensitization neuromuscular blockade). The mechanism for the development of desensitization neuromuscular blockade is unknown and, for this reason, phase II blockade, which does not infer a mechanism is preferred terminology (Hunter and Feldman, 1976). It is likely that combinations of receptor desensitization, channel blockade, and entrance of succinylcholine into the cytoplasm of skeletal muscle are responsible for the events that manifest as phase II blockade.

Depolarizing neuromuscular blocking drugs produce sustained opening of the receptor channels. This sustained opening of channels and resulting depolarization of the postjunctional membrane is associated with leakage of potassium ions from the interior of cells sufficient to produce an average 0.5 mEq L^{-1} increase in the serum potassium concentration. In addition to opening channels, a drug such as decamethonium can enter and block the channels or pass entirely through channels to enter the cytoplasm of skeletal muscle (Adams and Sakmann, 1978; Taylor *et al,* 1965).

Characteristics of Phase I Blockade

Electrically evoked mechanical responses, using a peripheral nerve stimulator, that are characteristic of phase I blockade include (1) decreased contraction in response to a single twitch stimulus, (2) decreased amplitude but sustained response to continuous stimulation, (3) train-of-four ratio greater than 70%, (4) absence of posttetanic facilitation, and (5) augmentation of neuromuscular blockade by anticholinesterase drugs. In addition, the onset of phase I blockade is accompanied by skeletal muscle fasciculations that reflect the generalized depolarization of postjunctional membranes produced by succinylcholine.

Characteristics of Phase II Blockade

Electrically evoked mechanical responses, using a peripheral nerve stimulator, that are characteristic

of phase II blockade resemble those considered typical of neuromuscular blockade produced by nondepolarizing neuromuscular blocking drugs (see the section entitled Characteristics of Nondepolarizing Neuromuscular Blockade). Furthermore, phase II blockade can be reversed with anticholinesterase drugs. Despite these similarities, it is likely that the mechanisms of nondepolarizing neuromuscular blockade and succinylcholine-induced phase II blockade differ.

The transition between phase I and phase II blockade is fairly abrupt occurring at a total dose of succinylcholine of 2 to 4 mg kg^{-1} (Fig. 8-4) (Lee, 1975). Clinically, the onset of phase II blockade is often initially manifested as tachyphylaxis and the need to increase the infusion rate of succinylcholine or to administer progressively larger incremental doses. At a single time, there may be varying degrees of phase I and phase II blockade that are present simultaneously (Ali and Savarese, 1976). When neuromuscular blockade is predominantly phase I, administration of an anticholinesterase drug will enhance neuromuscular

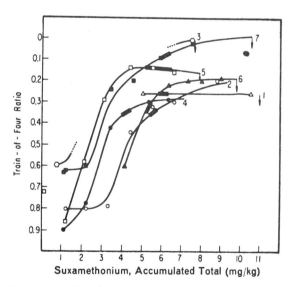

FIGURE 8-4. The transition between phase I and phase II blockade as depicted by the train-of-four ratio is fairly abrupt occurring at a total dose of succinylcholine (suxamethonium) of 2 to 4 mg kg^{-1}. (From Lee C. Dose relationship of phase II, tachyphylaxis and train-of-four fade on suxamethonium-induced dual neuromuscular block in man. Br J Anesth 1975;47:841–45. Reproduced by permission of the author and publisher.)

blockade. Conversely, an anticholinesterase drug will antagonize a predominant phase II blockade. A common practice is to observe the mechanical responses evoked by a peripheral nerve stimulator following administration of a small dose of anticholinesterase drug such as edrophonium (0.1–0.2 mg kg^{-1}). If this small dose of anticholinesterase drug improves neuromuscular transmission, it is likely that additional anticholinesterase drug will antagonize, rather than enhance, neuromuscular blockade produced by succinylcholine.

Duration of Action and Metabolism

The brief duration of action of succinylcholine (3–5 minutes) is principally due to its hydrolysis by plasma cholinesterase (pseudocholinesterase) enzyme (Fig. 8-5). The initial metabolite, succinylmonocholine, is a much weaker neuromuscular blocker (1/20 to 1/80 as potent) than the parent drug. Succinylmonocholine is subsequently hydrolyzed to succinic acid and choline. Plasma cholinesterase has an enormous capacity to hydrolyze succinylcholine at a rapid rate such that only a small fraction of the original intravenous dose of drug actually reaches the neuromuscular junction. Because plasma cholinesterase is not present at

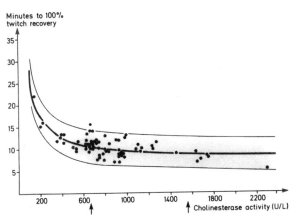

FIGURE 8-6. The duration of succinylcholine-induced neuromuscular blockade parallels activity of plasma cholinesterase enzyme. (From Viby-Mogensen J. Correlation of succinylcholine duration of action with plasma cholinesterase activity in subjects with the genotypically normal enzyme. Anesthesiology 1980;53:517–20. Reproduced by permission of the author and publisher.)

the neuromuscular junction, neuromuscular blockade produced by succinylcholine is terminated by its diffusion away from the neuromuscular junction into extracellular fluid. Therefore, plasma cholinesterase influences the duration of action of succinylcholine by controlling the amount of neuromuscular blocking drug that is hydrolyzed before reaching the neuromuscular junction.

Rapid hydrolysis makes it difficult to obtain pharmacokinetic data for succinylcholine. Nevertheless, based on isolated tourniquet techniques, it seems likely that significant succinylcholine is still circulating even 3 minutes after injection (Holst-Larsen, 1976).

Reductions in the hepatic production of plasma cholinesterase, drug-induced reductions in plasma cholinesterase activity, or the genetically determined presence of atypical plasma cholinesterase result in slow or absent hydrolysis of succinylcholine and corresponding prolongation of the neuromuscular blockade produced by this drug (Fig. 8-6) (Viby-Mogensen, 1980). Liver disease must be severe before reductions in plasma cholinesterase production sufficient to prolong succinylcholine-induced neuromuscular blockade occur (Foldes *et al*, 1956). Potent anticholin-

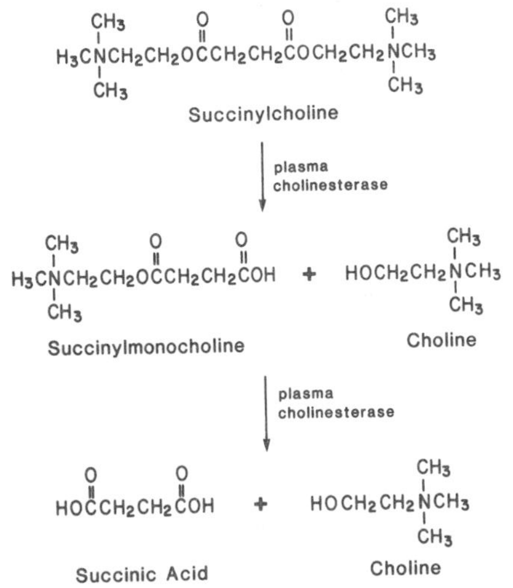

FIGURE 8-5. The brief duration of action of succinylcholine is principally due to its rapid hydrolysis in the plasma by cholinesterase enzyme to inactive metabolites.

esterase drugs, as used in insecticides, and occasionally in the treatment of glaucoma and myasthenia gravis as well as chemotherapeutic drugs such as nitrogen mustard and cyclophosphamide may so reduce plasma cholinesterase activity that prolonged neuromuscular blockade follows administration of succinylcholine. High estrogen levels, as observed in parturients at term, are associated with up to 40% decreases in plasma cholinesterase activity. Paradoxically, the duration of action of succinylcholine-induced skeletal muscle paralysis is not prolonged presumably reflecting an increased volume of distribution of the drug at term (Leighton *et al,* 1986).

The presence of atypical plasma cholinesterase is often recognized only after an otherwise healthy patient experiences prolonged neuromuscular blockade (1–3 hours) following a conventional dose of succinylcholine. Determination of the dibucaine number permits diagnosis of the presence of atypical plasma cholinesterase (Kalow and Genest, 1957). Dibucaine, a local anesthetic with an amide linkage, inhibits the activity of normal plasma cholinesterase about 80% compared with only about 20% inhibition of the activity of the atypical enzyme (Table 8-2). A dibucaine number of 80 (*i.e.,* percent inhibition) confirms the presence of normal plasma cholinesterase while about 1 in every 3200 patients is homozygous for the atypical plasma cholinesterase and has a dibucaine number of 20. About 1 in every 480 patients is heterozygous for atypical plasma enzyme and has a dibucaine number of 40 to 60 (Table 8-2). These heterozygous patients may manifest a modestly prolonged duration of neuromuscular blockade following administration of succinylcholine.

There are many other genetically determined variants of plasma cholinesterase although the dibucaine-related variants are the most important. It is important to recognize that the dibucaine number reflects the quality of plasma cholinesterase (*i.e.,* ability to metabolize succinylcholine) and not the quantity of enzyme that is circulating in the plasma. For example, reductions in plasma cholinesterase activity due to liver disease or anticholinesterase drugs are associated with a normal dibucaine number (about 80).

Four isoenzymes of plasma cholinesterase have been electrophoretically separated. In addition, some persons have a fifth isoenzyme and experience a shorter duration of action of succinylcholine than do those who lack this component (Sugimori, 1986).

Adverse Side Effects

Adverse side effects that may accompany the administration of succinylcholine include (1) cardiac dysrhythmias, (2) hyperkalemia, (3) myalgia, (4) myoglobinuria, (5) increased intragastric pressure, (6) increased intraocular pressure, (7) increased intracranial pressure, and (8) sustained skeletal muscle contraction. These side effects may limit or even contraindicate the administration of succinylcholine.

Administration of a nonparalyzing dose of nondepolarizing neuromuscular blocking drug (*e.g.,* pretreatment) may attenuate or prevent the occurrence of cardiac dysrhythmias, myalgia, and elevations of intragastric and intraocular pressure (Miller and Way, 1971; Miller *et al,* 1968; Stoelting, 1977; Stoelting and Peterson, 1975). Pretreat-

Table 8-2

Variants of Plasma Cholinesterase Enzyme and Response to Succinylcholine

	Duration of Succinylcholine-Induced Neuromuscular Blockade	Dibucaine Number (% inhibition of enzyme activity)	Incidence
Homozygous	5–10 minutes	80	Normal
Heterozygous	Modestly prolonged	40–60	1 in 480
Homozygous atypical	Greatly prolonged	20	1 in 3200

ment, however, does not influence the magnitude of potassium release evoked by succinylcholine (Stoelting and Peterson, 1975).

Cardiac Dysrhythmias

Sinus bradycardia, junctional rhythm, and even sinus arrest may follow the administration of succinylcholine. These cardiac effects reflect the action of succinylcholine at cardiac muscarinic cholinergic receptors where this drug mimics the normal effects of acetylcholine. Cardiac dysrhythmias are most likely to occur when a second intravenous dose of succinylcholine is administered about 5 minutes after the first dose. This relationship to the second dose suggests a possible role of the metabolites of succinylcholine (*e.g.,* succinylmonocholine and choline) in enhancing the slowing of heart rate (Schoenstadt and Whitcher, 1963). Administration of gallamine, 0.3 mg kg⁻¹, about 3 minutes before the first dose of succinylcholine greatly reduces the incidence of heart rate slowing following the first or second intravenous dose of succinylcholine (Table 8-3) (Stoelting, 1977). A similar protective effect is not provided by intravenous atropine, 6 μg kg⁻¹ (Table 8-3) (Stoelting, 1977).

In contrast to actions at cardiac muscarinic cholinergic receptors, effects of succinylcholine at autonomic nervous system ganglia may produce ganglionic stimulation and associated elevations in heart rate and blood pressure. This ganglionic stimulation reflects an effect of succinylcholine on autonomic ganglia that resembles that of the normal neurotransmitter, acetylcholine.

Hyperkalemia

Hyperkalemia may occur following administration of succinylcholine to patients with (1) unhealed third degree burns, (2) denervation leading to skeletal muscle atrophy, (3) upper motor neuron lesions, and (4) severe intra-abdominal infections (Cooperman *et al*, 1970; Gronert and Theye, 1975; Kohlschutter *et al*, 1976; Stone *et al*, 1970). This vulnerability to hyperkalemia most likely reflects a proliferation of extrajunctional cholinergic receptors providing more sites for potassium ions to leak outward from cells during depolarization. The potential for excessive potassium release develops within 2 days of injury and may persist for an indefinite period up to 2 years or more. Pretreatment with a nonparalyzing dose of a nondepolarizing neuromuscular blocking drug does not influence the magnitude of potassium release evoked by succinylcholine (Stoelting and Peterson, 1975).

Myalgia

Postoperative skeletal muscle myalgia in the muscles of the neck, back, and abdomen can occur

---

Table 8-3
Succinylcholine-Induced Cardiac Rhythm Changes with Prior Gallamine or Atropine

	Gallamine (0.3 mg kg⁻¹)	Atropine (0.006 mg kg⁻¹)
Heart rate 15% less than control 1 minute after succinylcholine		
First succinylcholine injection	1 of 40 patients	1 of 40 patients
Second succinylcholine injection *	1 of 39 patients	14 of 40 patients
Junctional rhythm present 1 minute after succinylcholine		
First succinylcholine injection	1 of 40 patients	1 of 40 patients
Second succinylcholine injection *	none of 39 patients	none of 40 patients

* Second injection 5 minutes after first injection
(Data from Stoelting RK. Comparison of gallamine and atropine as pretreatment before anesthetic induction and succinylcholine administration. Anesth Analg 1977;56:493–5.)

after administration of succinylcholine especially to young adults undergoing minor surgical procedures that permit early ambulation (Waters and Mapleson, 1971). It is speculated that unsynchronized contractions of skeletal muscle fibers associated with generalized depolarization produced by succinylcholine lead to myalgia. Indeed, prevention of succinylcholine-induced skeletal muscle fasciculations with the prior administration of a nonparalyzing dose of d-tubocurarine prevents or attenuates the incidence of myalgia following administration of succinylcholine (Table 8-4) (Stoelting and Peterson, 1975).

Myoglobinuria

Damage to skeletal muscle is suggested by the occurrence of myoglobinuria following administration of succinylcholine to pediatric patients (Ryan *et al*, 1971). Presumably, myoglobinuria reflects skeletal muscle damage associated with succinylcholine-induced fasciculations. For reasons that are not clear, myoglobinuria rarely occurs in adults receiving succinylcholine.

Increased Intragastric Pressure

Succinylcholine produces inconsistent elevations in intragastric pressure (Fig. 8-7) (Miller and Way,

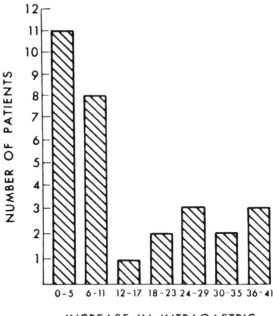

FIGURE 8-7. Succinylcholine produces inconsistent and unpredictable elevations of intragastric pressure. (From Miller RD, Way WL. Inhibition of succinylcholine-induced increased intragastric pressure by nondepolarizing muscle relaxants and lidocaine. Anesthesiology 1971;34:185–8. Reproduced by permission of the authors and publisher.)

1971). When intragastric pressure increases, it seems to be related to the intensity of skeletal muscle fasciculations induced by succinylcholine. Indeed, prevention of skeletal muscle fasciculations by prior administration of a nonparalyzing dose of nondepolarizing neuromuscular blocking drug prevents increases in intragastric pressure produced by the subsequent administration of succinylcholine (Miller and Way, 1971). The risk of increased intragastric pressure (gastroesophageal sphincter can open spontaneously at pressures above 28 cm H_2O) is passage of gastric fluid into the esophagus and pharynx and subsequent inhalation into the lungs. Minimal to absent skeletal muscle fasciculations in children are consistent with the absence of appreciable increases in intragastric pressure that accompany ad-

Table 8-4
Skeletal Muscle Myalgia Following Administration of Succinylcholine With or Without d-Tubocurarine Pretreatment

	Number of Patients Complaining of Myalgia 24 Hours After Administration of Succinylcholine
Control	None of 20 patients
Succinylcholine (1 mg kg^{-1})	8 of 20 patients
d-Tubocurarine (0.04 mg kg^{-1}) Succinylcholine (1 mg kg^{-1})	None of 20 patients
d-Tubocurarine (0.04 mg kg^{-1}) Succinylcholine (2 mg kg^{-1})	5 of 20 patients

(Data from Stoelting RK, Peterson C. Adverse effects of increased succinylcholine dose following d-tubocurarine pretreatment. Anesth Analg 1975;54:282–8.)

ministration of succinylcholine to this age group (Salem *et al*, 1972).

Increased Intraocular Pressure

Succinylcholine causes a maximum increase in intraocular pressure 2 to 4 minutes after its administration (Pandey *et al*, 1972). This increase in intraocular pressure is transient lasting only 5 to 10 minutes. The mechanism by which succinylcholine increases intraocular pressure has not been clearly defined but presumably involves contraction of tonic myofibrils or transient dilation of choroidal blood vessels. For these reasons, succinylcholine should not be administered to a patient with an open eye injury or a recent ocular incision. Intraocular pressure may decline following administration of nondepolarizing neuromuscular blocking drugs presumably reflecting the effect of paralysis of extraocular muscles.

Increased Intracranial Pressure

In halothane anesthetized animals, succinylcholine, 1 mg kg^{-1} administered intravenously, produces evidence of arousal on the electroencephalogram that is associated with substantial increases in cerebral blood flow and corresponding elevations in intracranial pressure (Lanier *et al*, 1986). In anesthetized patients with brain tumors, succinylcholine increases intracranial pressure an average 4.9 mmHg with some patients experiencing increases of 9 mmHg or greater (Minton *et al*, 1986).

Sustained Skeletal Muscle Contraction

Skeletal muscle contraction that is sustained accompanies the administration of succinylcholine to patients with myotonia congenita or myotonia dystrophica (Mitchell *et al*, 1978). This sustained skeletal muscle contraction may interfere with ventilation of the lungs and become life-threatening. Contraction, rather than relaxation of skeletal muscles is also an early manifestation of succinylcholine-induced malignant hyperthermia.

LONG-ACTING NONDEPOLARIZING NEUROMUSCULAR BLOCKING DRUGS

Long-acting nondepolarizing neuromuscular blocking drugs. such as d-tubocurarine, metocur-

ine, gallamine, and pancuronium, are characterized by an onset of maximum neuromuscular blockade in 3 to 5 minutes and a duration of action of 90 to 120 minutes (Fig. 8-1) (Table 8-5) (Savarese *et al*, 1977).

Dose response curves for d-tubocurarine, metocurine, and pancuronium in adult patients 19 to 67 years old anesthetized with nitrous oxide, thiopental, and morphine do not deviate from parallelism (Fig. 8-8) (Savarese *et al*, 1977). The dose of neuromuscular blocking drug necessary to depress twitch can be determined from such dose response curves. Indeed, the dose of nondepolarizing neuromuscular blocking drug necessary to depress twitch 50% (ED$_{50}$) and 95% (ED$_{95}$) is frequently used as an index of equal potency for comparisons between drugs (Table 8-5).

Mechanism of Action

Nondepolarizing neuromuscular blocking drugs are classically thought to act by combining with nicotinic cholinergic receptors but not causing any activation of the receptors. Specifically, these drugs can act competitively with acetylcholine at the alpha subunits of the postjunctional nicotinic

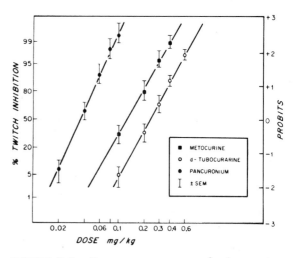

FIGURE 8-8. Dose response curves for long-acting neuromuscular blocking drugs do not deviate from parallelism. (From Savarese JJ, Ali HH, Antonio RP. The clinical pharmacology of metocurine: Dimethyltubocurarine revisited. Anesthesiology 1977;47:277–84. Reproduced by permission of the authors and publisher.)

Table 8-5
Comparative Pharmacology of Long-Acting Nondepolarizing Neuromuscular Blocking Drugs

	ED_{95} (mg kg^{-1})	Onset to Maximum Twitch Depression (minutes)	Volume of Distribution (L kg^{-1})	Clearance (ml kg^{-1} min^{-1})	Renal Excretion (% unchanged)	Biliary Excretion (% unchanged)	Hepatic Degradation	Elimination Half-Time (hours)
d-Tubocurarine	0.51	3–5	0.30	2.25	45	10–40	Insignificant	2.0
Metocurine	0.28	3–5	0.51	1.2	43	<2	Insignificant	5.8
Gallamine		3–5	0.21	1.2	>95	0	Insignificant	2.3
Pancuronium	0.07	3–5	0.26	1.90	80	5–10	10%–40%	2.4

cholinergic receptor without causing a conformational change in the receptor. In addition, these drugs can act by causing blockade of the channels (see the section entitled Postjunctional Nicotinic Receptors). Even though neuromuscular blocking drugs may act at both the alpha subunits and the channels, a given drug may preferentially act at one site or the other. For example, it requires a higher concentration of pancuronium to affect channels than receptor sites while gallamine acts at both sites at all concentrations. d-Tubocurarine, at low concentrations, is a relatively selective receptor blocker at the alpha subunits while high doses also act at channels. Nondepolarizing neuromuscular blocking drugs also act at prejunctional nicotinic receptors. Nevertheless, it is the actions at the postjunctional sites that are most important.

Occupation of as many as 70% of the nicotinic cholinergic receptors by a neuromuscular blocking drug does not produce evidence of neuromuscular blockade as reflected by the twitch response to a single stimulus (Fig. 8-9) (Waud and Waud, 1971). Neuromuscular transmission, however, fails when 80% to 90% of the receptors are blocked. This confirms the wide margin of safety of neuromuscular transmission and forms the basis for the techniques of clinical monitoring of neuromuscular blockade.

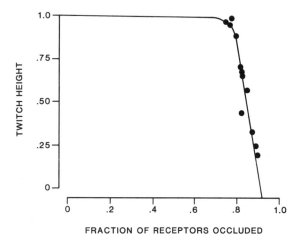

FIGURE 8-9. Schematic depiction of the number of receptors that must be occupied (receptor occupancy theory) before existence of neuromuscular blockade is evident as a decrease in twitch height.

Characteristics of Nondepolarizing Neuromuscular Blockade

Characteristic skeletal muscle responses in the presence of nondepolarizing neuromuscular blockade, as evoked by electrical stimulation from a peripheral nerve stimulator, include (1) decreased twitch response to a single stimulus, (2) nonsustained response (fade) during continuous stimulation, (3) train-of-four ratio less than 70%, (4) posttetanic potentiation, (5) potentiation by other nondepolarizing neuromuscular blocking drugs, and (6) antagonism by anticholinesterase drugs. In addition, skeletal muscle fasciculations do not accompany the onset of nondepolarizing neuromuscular blockade.

Skeletal muscle contraction is an all or none phenomenon. Each muscle fiber either contracts maximally or does not contract at all. Therefore, when twitch response is reduced, some fibers are contracting normally while others are completely blocked. Fade of skeletal muscle contraction in response to continuous electrical stimulation suggests that some fibers are more susceptible to being blocked by neuromuscular blocking drugs and need a greater sustained release of acetylcholine to trigger their responses.

Pharmacokinetics

Nondepolarizing neuromuscular blocking drugs, because of their quaternary ammonium groups, are highly ionized at physiologic pH and possess limited lipid solubility (Shanks, 1986). As a result of these two characteristics, the volume of distribution of neuromuscular blocking drugs is small ($80-140$ ml kg^{-1}), being limited principally to the extracellular fluid (Table 8-5). In addition, neuromuscular blocking drugs cannot easily cross lipid membrane barriers such as the blood–brain barrier, renal tubular epithelium, gastrointestinal epithelium, or placenta. Therefore, neuromuscular blocking drugs do not produce central nervous system effects, renal tubular reabsorption is minimal, oral administration is not effective, and maternal administration does not affect the fetus.

The rate of disappearance of long-acting nondepolarizing neuromuscular blocking drugs from the plasma is characterized by an initial rapid decline followed by a slower decline. Distribution of neuromuscular blocking drugs to tissues is the major cause of the initial rapid decrease in the plasma concentration while the slower decline is due to hepatic and renal clearance mechanisms. Many of the variable patient responses evoked by neuromuscular blocking drugs can be explained by differences in pharmacokinetics.

Pharmacokinetic factors that should be considered in predicting the response to nondepolarizing neuromuscular blocking drugs include (1) size of the initial dose, (2) renal disease, (3) biliary and hepatic disease, (4) protein binding, (5) anesthetic drugs, and (6) advanced age. The relative impact of these various factors varies among the neuromuscular blocking drugs (Table 8-5).

Pharmacokinetics of nondepolarizing neuromuscular blocking drugs are calculated following bolus intravenous injection of the drug. If the volume of distribution is reduced, as by decreased protein binding, dehydration, or acute hemorrhage, the same dose of drug produces a greater plasma concentration and the apparent potency of the drug is augmented.

Size of the Initial Dose

The size of the initial dose of d-tubocurarine, and presumably other nondepolarizing neuromuscular blocking drugs, does not influence the pharmacokinetics or pharmacodynamics of the drug. For example, there is no significant difference in the dose of d-tubocurarine required to maintain the same degree of neuromuscular blockade whether the drug is administered as a single bolus, intermittent injection, or continuous infusion (Ham *et al*, 1979). Clearly, the size of the initial dose or supplemental doses of nondepolarizing neuromuscular blocking drugs determines the resulting plasma concentration of drug. The magnitude of neuromuscular blockade, as characterized by twitch response, is proportional to the plasma concentration of the neuromuscular blocking drug (Matteo *et al*, 1974; Shanks *et al*, 1979). For example, twitch response begins to reappear at a plasma d-tubocurarine concentration of about 0.7 μg ml^{-1}, twitch response is 50% when the plasma concentration is 0.45 μg ml^{-1}, and recovery of twitch response is complete at a plasma concentration of 0.2 μg ml^{-1} (Fig. 8-10) (Matteo *et al*, 1974).

Renal Disease

Renal disease can greatly affect the pharmacokinetics of long-acting nondepolarizing neuromus-

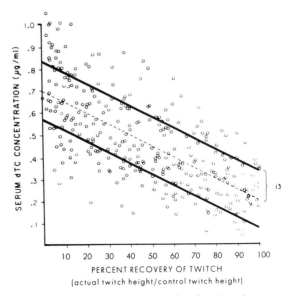

FIGURE 8-10. d-Tubocurarine (dTc)-induced neuromuscular blockade parallels the plasma (serum) concentration of the drug. (From Matteo RS, Spector S, Horowitz PE. Relation of serum d-tubocurarine concentration to neuromuscular blockade in man. Anesthesiology 1974;41:440–3. Reproduced by permission of the authors and publisher.)

cular blocking drugs. The rate at which the plasma concentration of pancuronium decreases is more influenced by renal failure than is the rate of decline in the plasma concentrations of d-tubocurarine or metocurine (Fig. 8-11) (Brotherton and Matteo, 1981; McLeod *et al*, 1976; Miller *et al*, 1977). Indeed, an estimated 80% of a single dose of pancuronium is eliminated unchanged in the urine. Conversely, about 45% of an administered dose of d-tubocurarine is recovered unchanged in the urine during the first 24 hours following its administration. Only an additional 7% more drug is recovered in the urine after 96 hours. Therefore, it is likely that d-tubocurarine is stored in inactive tissue sites, perhaps for prolonged periods of time. Similarly, about 43% of metocurine is recovered unchanged in the urine. Because biliary excretion and metabolism of metocurine are not significant, it is presumed this drug, like d-tubocurarine, is stored for prolonged periods of time in inactive tissue sites.

Renal failure does not alter the distribution half-time of nondepolarizing neuromuscular

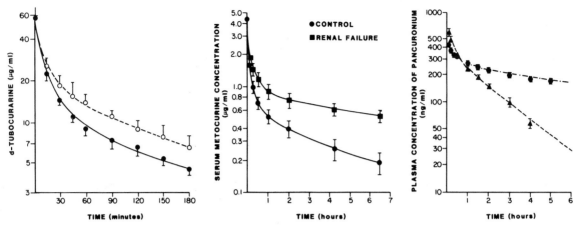

FIGURE 8-11. The rate at which the plasma concentration of pancuronium decreases is more influenced by renal failure than is the rate of decline in the plasma concentrations of d-tubocurarine or metocurine. Mean ± SE. (From Brotherton WP, Matteo RS. Pharmacokinetics and pharmacodynamics of metocurine in humans with and without renal failure. Anesthesiology 1981;55:273 – 6; McLeod K, Watson MJ, Rawlings MD. Pharmacokinetics of pancuronium in patients with normal and impaired renal function. Br J Anaesth 1976;48:341 – 5; Miller RD, Matteo R, Benet LZ, Sohn YJ. Influence of renal failure on the pharmacokinetics of d-tubocurarine in man. J Pharmacol Exp Ther 1977;202:1 – 7; © by American Society for Pharmacology and Experimental Therapeutics. Redrawn by permission of the authors and publishers.)

blocking drugs because this phase reflects passage of drug to tissues independent of clearance mechanisms. Likewise, plasma concentrations of neuromuscular blocking drugs necessary to produce a given degree of neuromuscular blockade are not altered by renal failure. Predictably, the elimination half-time of these drugs is prolonged in the presence of renal failure paralleling the magnitude of drug normally eliminated unchanged in the urine.

Biliary and Hepatic Disease

Patients with total biliary obstruction and hepatic cirrhosis have (1) increased volume of distribution, (2) reduced plasma clearance, and (3) prolonged elimination half-time for pancuronium (Table 8-6) (Duvaldestin *et al,* 1978). The large volume of distribution means a greater initial dose of pancuronium will be required to produce the same plasma concentration but the resulting neuromuscular blockade may be prolonged because of decreased clearance.

An estimated 10% to 40% of a dose of pancuronium undergoes hepatic deacetylation to 3-hydroxypancuronium, 17-hydroxypancuronium, and 3,17 hydroxypancuronium (Agoston *et al,* 1973). The 3-hydroxypancuronium metabolite is about 50% as potent as pancuronium at the neuromuscular junction while the other metabolites have only minimal activity (Miller *et al,* 1978a).

In normal patients, an estimated 10% of d-tubocurarine is eliminated unchanged in the bile. This percentage of biliary elimination may increase to about 40% in the presence of renal failure. Therefore, d-tubocurarine disappears from the neuromuscular junction and plasma even in the absence of renal function. Biliary excretion of metocurine is minimal (estimated less than 2% of an injected dose) regardless of the state of renal function. Unlike pancuronium, d-tubocurarine and metocurine do not undergo significant hepatic metabolism (Stanski *et al,* 1979).

Protein Binding

The extent and importance of protein binding of the various nondepolarizing neuromuscular blocking drugs are not clearly defined. Various studies demonstrate binding to both albumin and

Table 8-6
Pharmacokinetics of Pancuronium and Hepatic Dysfunction

	Normal Hepatic Function	Cirrhosis
Volume of distribution (ml kg^{-1})	279	416*
Clearance (ml kg^{-1} min^{-1})	1.9	1.5*
Elimination half-time (minutes)	114	208*

* P < 0.05 compared with normal hepatic function
(Data from Duvaldestin P, Agoston S, Henzel E, Kersten UW, Desmonts JM. Pancuronium pharmacokinetics in patients with liver cirrhosis. Br J Anaesth 1978;50:1131–6.)

gamma globulin (Skivington, 1972). Protein binding of d-tubocurarine is not altered by renal or hepatic disease despite the fact these diseases are well known to be associated with altered protein binding to other drugs (Ghoneim *et al,* 1973). Previously, it had been speculated that increased binding of d-tubocurarine to gamma globulin was responsible for resistance to the effects of this drug in patients with severe cirrhosis of the liver.

Anesthetic Drugs

Despite changes in the distribution of blood flow, inhaled anesthetics have little or no effect on the pharmacokinetics of neuromuscular blocking drugs. For example, the distribution and elimination half-time of d-tubocurarine, and presumably the other nondepolarizing neuromuscular blocking drugs, are not significantly different during nitrous oxide-opioid or nitrous oxide-halothane anesthesia (Ramzan *et al,* 1981). Enhancement of neuromuscular blockade by volatile anesthetics reflects a pharmacodynamic action as manifested by reduced plasma concentrations of neuromuscular blocking drugs required to produce a given degree of neuromuscular blockade in the presence of a volatile anesthetic (see the section entitled Causes of Altered Responses, Volatile Anesthetics).

Advanced Age

Aging is associated with a decreased rate of decline in the plasma concentrations of d-tubocurarine, metocurine, and pancuronium (Fig. 8-12)

(Duvaldestin *et al,* 1982; Matteo *et al,* 1985). These prolonged elimination half-times reflect declining renal function in the elderly and manifest as a prolonged duration of neuromuscular blockade. The absence of an age-related change in responsiveness of the neuromuscular junction (*e.g.,* changes in pharmacodynamics) is confirmed by similar dose-response curves in elderly and young adults for all three of the long-acting nondepolarizing neuromuscular blocking drugs (Fig. 8-13) (Duvaldestin *et al,* 1982; Matteo *et al,* 1985).

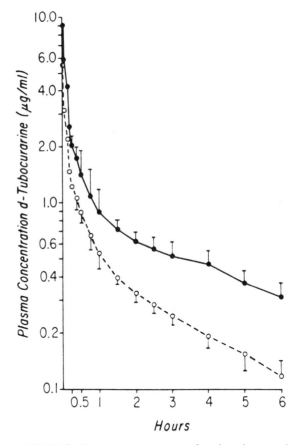

FIGURE 8-12. Aging is associated with a decreased rate of decline in the plasma concentrations of long-acting neuromuscular blocking drugs. Mean ± SD. (From Matteo RS, Backus WW, McDaniel DD, Brotherton WP, Abraham R, Diaz J. Pharmacokinetics and pharmacodynamics of d-tubocurarine and metocurine in the elderly. Anesth Analg 1985;64:23–9. Reproduced by permission of the authors and the International Anesthesia Research Society.)

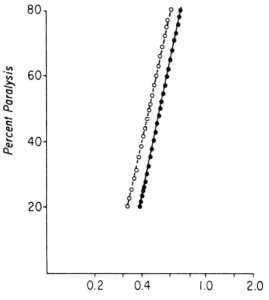

FIGURE 8-13. Absence of age-related changes in the responsiveness of the neuromuscular junction to long-acting neuromuscular blocking drugs is confirmed by the similarity of plasma concentrations necessary to produce comparable responses in young adults (clear symbols) and elderly individuals (solid symbols). (From Matteo RS, Backus WW, McDaniel DD, Brotherton WP, Abraham R, Diaz J. Pharmacokinetics and pharmacodynamics of d-tubocurarine and metocurine in the elderly. Anesth Analg 1985;64:23–9. Reproduced by permission of the authors and the International Anesthesia Research Society.)

Central Nervous System

Despite being highly ionized, detectable amounts of d-tubocurarine are present in the cerebrospinal fluid (Fig. 8-14) (Matteo *et al,* 1977). Gallamine and d-tubocurarine have been shown to increase the dose of lidocaine administered to animals that is necessary to evoke a seizure (Munson and Wagman, 1973). Finally, pancuronium administered to patients reduces the anesthetic requirement for halothane by 25% (Fig. 8-15) (Forbes *et al,* 1979).

Response of Pediatric Patients

The plasma concentration of d-tubocurarine necessary to depress twitch response 50% during ni-

trous oxide-halothane anesthesia is age-dependent, being lowest in the neonate and greatest in the adult (Table 8-7) (Fisher *et al,* 1982b). Conversely, the elimination half-time of d-tubocurarine is longer in neonates than adults. Since plasma clearance is not different between pediatric and adult patients, the prolonged elimination half-time of d-tubocurarine reflects the greater volume of distribution in younger patients. Based on these observations, it is clear that neonates and infants are more sensitive to d-tubocurarine, and presumably other nondepolarizing neuromuscular blocking drugs. This increased sensitivity to nondepolarizing neuromuscular blocking drugs demonstrated by neonates is an example of age-related differences in pharmacodynamics. Nevertheless, the initial dose administered to achieve the same plasma concentration of neuromuscular blocking drug is similar in both age groups because the greater volume of distribution in neonates offsets the impact of increased sensitivity of the neuromuscular junction (Fisher *et al,* 1982b).

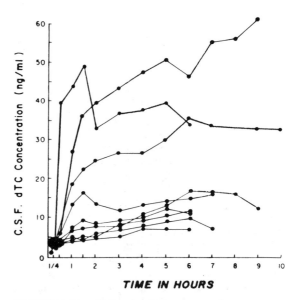

FIGURE 8-14. Following intravenous administration, d-tubocurarine (dTc) is detectable in the cerebrospinal fluid (CSF). (From Matteo RS, Pua EK, Khambatta HJ, Spector S. Cerebrospinal fluid levels of d-tubocurarine in man. Anesthesiology 1977;46:396–9. Reproduced by permission of the authors and publisher.)

Cardiovascular Effects

Neuromuscular blocking drugs may exert cardiovascular effects by virtue of (1) drug-induced release of histamine or other vasoactive substances from circulating mast cells, (2) effects at cardiac muscarinic receptors, or (3) effects at nicotinic receptors at autonomic ganglia (Table 8-8) (Scott and Savarese, 1985) (see the sections entitled Structure Activity Relationships and Adverse Ef-

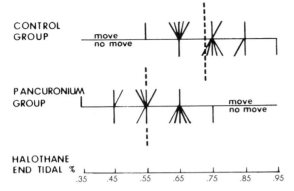

FIGURE 8-15. Pancuronium reduces anesthetic requirements for halothane *(broken vertical line)* by about 25%. (From Forbes AR, Cohen NH, Eger EI. Pancuronium reduces halothane requirement in man. Anesth Analg 1979;58:497–9. Reproduced by permission of the authors and the International Anesthesia Research Society.)

fects of Succinylcholine). There is considerable species difference with respect to mechanisms responsible for circulatory effects of neuromuscular blocking drugs. It is likely that relative importance varies from patient to patient according to factors such as underlying autonomic system activity, preoperative medication, drugs administered for maintenance of anesthesia, and concurrent drug therapy.

The difference between the dose of neuromuscular blocking drug that produces neuromuscular blocking and circulatory effects is the autonomic margin of safety (Hughes and Chapple, 1976). Doses of d-tubocurarine (*e.g.*, ED_{95}) that produce neuromuscular blockade also produce circulatory changes, and the autonomic margin of safety is narrow. Conversely, metocurine, atracurium, and vecuronium have wide autonomic margins of safety because the dose necessary to produce neuromuscular blockade is less than that which evokes circulatory changes.

d-Tubocurarine

Rapid intravenous injection of an ED_{95} dose of d-tubocurarine can evoke sufficient histamine release and, to a lesser extent, blockade of sympathetic and parasympathetic ganglia to cause significant (20% or greater) reductions in mean arterial pressure (Fig. 8-16) (Stoelting, 1972). Diminished venous return due to loss of skeletal muscle

Table 8-7
Pharmacokinetics and Pharmacodynamics of d-Tubocurarine

	Volume of Distribution	Clearance ($ml\ kg^{-1}\ min^{-1}$)	Elimination Half-Time (minutes)	Plasma Concentration Necessary to Maintain 50% Twitch Depression ($\mu g\ ml^{-1}$)
Neonates	0.74*	3.7	174†	0.18‡
Infants	0.52	3.3	130	0.27‡
Children	0.41	4.0	90	0.42
Adults	0.31	3.0	89	0.53

* P < 0.05 compared with infants, children and adults
† P < 0.05 compared with children and adults
‡ P < 0.05 compared with children and adults
(Data from Fisher DM, O'Keefe C, Stanski DR, Cronnelly R, Miller RD, Gregory GA. Pharmacokinetics and pharmacodynamics of d-tubocurarine in infants, children, and adults. Anesthesiology 1982b;57:203–8.)

Table 8-8
Mechanisms of Neuromuscular Blocking Drug-Induced Cardiovascular Effects

ED_{95} Dose	Histamine Release	Cardiac Muscarinic Receptors	Nicotinic Receptors at Autonomic Ganglia
Succinylcholine	Slight	Modest stimulation	Modest stimulation
d-Tubocurarine	Moderate	None	Moderate blockade
Metocurine	Modest	None	Modest blockade
Gallamine	None	Moderate blockade	None
Pancuronium	None	Modest blockade	None
Atracurium	Slight	None	None
Vecuronium	None	None	None

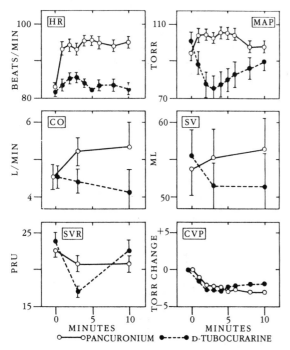

○—○ PANCURONIUM ●--● D-TUBOCURARINE

FIGURE 8-16. Rapid intravenous administration of d-tubocurarine (0.4 mg kg^{-1}) during halothane anesthesia results in a decline in mean arterial pressure (MAP) and a corresponding reduction in peripheral (systemic) vascular resistance (SVR). Under the same conditions, pancuronium causes an increase in mean arterial pressure, heart rate, and cardiac output. HR — heart rate; CO — cardiac output; SV — stroke volume; CVP — central venous pressure. Mean ± SE. (From Stoelting, RK. The hemodynamic effects of pancuronium and d-tubocurarine in anesthetized patients. Anesthesiology 1972; 136:612–5. Reproduced by permission of the author and publisher.)

tone and the effects of positive airway pressure also contribute to reductions in blood pressure. The maximum decline in mean arterial pressure following administration of d-tubocurarine occurs at a time when the cardiac output is unchanged confirming that blood pressure reductions parallel declines in peripheral vascular resistance (Fig. 8-16) (Stoelting, 1972). This peripheral vasodilation is most likely due to d-tubocurarine-induced release of histamine while blockade of autonomic ganglia occurs at higher doses. Indeed, d-tubocurarine produces a dose-dependent increase in the plasma concentration of histamine that parallels the reduction in blood pressure (Fig. 8-17) (Moss et al, 1981). Direct cardiac depressant effects of d-tubocurarine do not occur.

The magnitude of blood pressure reduction depends on the dose of d-tubocurarine administered as well as the depth of anesthesia (Fig. 8-18) (Munger et al, 1974; Stoelting and Longnecker, 1972a). Furthermore, the injection of d-tubocurarine over 90 seconds rather than as a bolus minimizes the subsequent decline in blood pressure (Fig. 8-19) (Stoelting et al, 1980). This rate-related phenomenon is consistent with histamine release evoked by a rapid, but not slow, injection of d-tubocurarine. In addition, pretreatment with an antihistamine drug, such as promethazine, attenuates blood pressure reductions evoked by d-tubocurarine in some patients (Stoelting and Longnecker, 1972b). The dependence of blood pressure changes on dose of d-tubocurarine and volatile anesthetic (specifically halothane) most likely reflects drug-related production of ganglionic blockade and/or cardiac depression.

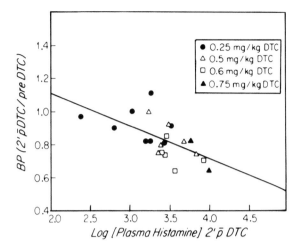

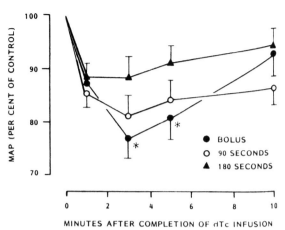

FIGURE 8-17. Blood pressure (BP) reductions following intravenous administration of d-tubocurarine (DTC) parallel the plasma concentration of histamine. (From Moss J, Rosow CE, Savarese JJ, Philbin DM, Kniffen KJ. Role of histamine in the hypotensive action of d-tubocurarine in humans. Anesthesiology 1981;55:19–25. Reproduced by permission of the authors and publisher.)

FIGURE 8-19. The rate of injection of d-tubocurarine (dTc) influences the magnitude of drug-induced reduction in mean arterial pressure (MAP). Mean ± SE. (From Stoelting RK, McCammon RL, Hilgenberg JC. Changes in blood pressure with varying rates of administration of d-tubocurarine. Anesth Analg 1980;59:697–9. Reproduced by permission of the authors and the International Anesthesia Research Society.)

Metocurine

In the presence of a volatile anesthetic, such as halothane, an ED_{95} dose of metocurine reduces mean arterial pressure about one half as much (10%) as an equivalent dose of d-tubocurarine (Fig. 8-20) (Stoelting, 1974). During nitrous oxide, thiopental, opioid anesthesia, the administration of metocurine produces minimal dose-related changes in mean arterial pressure and heart rate (Fig. 8-21) (Savarese et al, 1977). These lesser circulatory effects compared with d-tubocurarine are consistent with a reduced ability of the bisquaternary ammonium structure of metocurine to evoke the release of histamine or produce autonomic ganglion blockade (Fig. 8-1).

Pancuronium

Pancuronium, in contrast to d-tubocurarine, produces a modest 10% to 15% increase in heart rate, mean arterial pressure, and cardiac output (Fig. 8-16) (Stoelting, 1972). These cardiovascular effects are attributed to selective cardiac vagal blockade (i.e., atropine-like effect limited to cardiac muscarinic receptors) and activation of the sympathetic nervous system (Domenech et al, 1976). Both release of norepinephrine from ad-

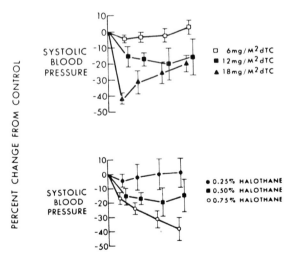

FIGURE 8-18. The magnitude of blood pressure reduction produced by d-tubocurarine (dTc) parallels the dose of drug administered and the depth of anesthesia. Mean ± SE. (From Munger WL, Miller RD, Stevens WC. The dependence of d-tubocurarine-induced hypotension on alveolar concentration of halothane, dose of d-tubocurarine, and nitrous oxide. Anesthesiology 1974;40:442–8. Reproduced by permission of the authors and publisher.)

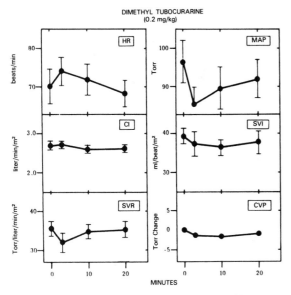

FIGURE 8-20. Rapid intravenous administration of metocurine (dimethyltubocurarine) during halothane anesthesia decreases mean arterial pressure (MAP) about one-half the magnitude produced by a comparable dose of d-tubocurarine. Mean ± SE. (See Fig. 8-16.) (From Stoelting RK. Hemodynamic effects of dimethyltubocurarine during nitrous oxide-halothane anesthesia. Anesth Analg 1974;53:513–5. Reproduced by permission of the author and the International Anesthesia Research Society.)

renergic nerve endings and blockade of uptake of norepinephrine back into postganglionic nerve endings have been proposed as mechanisms for the activation of the sympathetic nervous system by pancuronium (Ivankovich *et al*, 1975; Vercruyse *et al*, 1979). Pancuronium may also interfere with activity of muscarinic receptors that normally inhibit the release of norepinephrine. Likewise, pancuronium may produce blockade at muscarinic receptors that normally release dopamine thus facilitating transmission through ganglia by inactivating the inhibitory influence of the dopaminergic cell loop (Scott and Savarese, 1985). The increase in circulating plasma concentrations of catecholamines following intravenous administration of pancuronium supports a drug-induced activation of the sympathetic nervous system (Domenech *et al*, 1976).

Pancuronium increases heart rate principally by blocking vagal muscarinic receptors in the si-

noatrial node as evidenced by the ability of prior administration of atropine to block this response. A sympathomimetic effect of pancuronium apparently plays a minor role in heart rate responses. Indeed, heart rate responses evoked by pancuronium still occur in patients treated with beta-adrenergic antagonists (Morris *et al*, 1983). The magnitude of heart rate increase evoked by pancuronium seems more dependent on the preexisting heart rate (an inverse relationship) than the dose of drug administered. Marked increases in heart rate seem more likely to occur in patients with altered atrioventricular conduction of cardiac impulses as characteristic of atrial fibrillation.

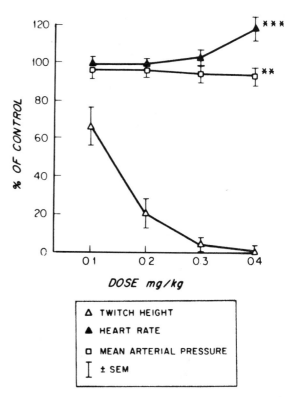

FIGURE 8-21. During nitrous oxide, thiopental, opioid anesthesia, the intravenous administration of metocurine produces minimal, although statistically significant, changes in heart rate and mean arterial pressure. **P<0.01 ***P<0.001. (From Savarese JJ, Ali HH, Antonio RP. The clinical pharmacology of metocurine: Dimethyltubocurarine revisited. Anesthesiology 1977; 47:277–84. Reproduced by permission of the authors and publisher.)

The modest increase in blood pressure following the administration of pancuronium reflects the effect of heart rate on cardiac output in the absence of changes in peripheral vascular resistance. Direct inotropic effects of pancuronium have not been demonstrated (Scott and Savarese, 1985).

An increased incidence of cardiac dysrhythmias has been observed following administration of pancuronium, but not succinylcholine, to patients being chronically treated with digitalis (see Chapter 13). Cardiac dysrhythmias may reflect sudden changes in the balance of autonomic nervous system activity in favor of the sympathetic nervous system. Cardiac stimulating effects of pancuronium may also increase the incidence of myocardial ischemia in patients with coronary artery disease (Thompson and Putnins, 1985). Histamine release and autonomic ganglion blockade are not produced by pancuronium.

Gallamine

Gallamine produces selective cardiac vagal blockade (atropine-like effect limited to cardiac muscarinic receptors). Heart rate increases are dose-dependent with the maximum effect being a 30% to 40% elevation following administration of paralyzing doses of gallamine (1 mg kg^{-1} or greater) (Fig. 8-22) (Stoelting, 1973). Paralyzing doses of gallamine do not, however, produce complete vagal blockade because atropine can still increase heart rate. Nevertheless, nonparalyzing doses of gallamine (0.3 mg kg^{-1}) as used for pretreatment prior to the administration of succinylcholine increase heart rate as much or more than intravenous atropine (Stoelting, 1977). Gallamine-induced heart rate increases persist even when effects at the neuromuscular junction are waning or absent. Heart rate increases evoked by gallamine result in modest elevations in cardiac output and mean arterial pressure (Fig. 8-22) (Stoelting, 1973).

Like pancuronium, gallamine may activate the sympathetic nervous system (Brown and Crout, 1970). Cardiac dysrhythmias following administration of gallamine may reflect a sudden change in the balance of autonomic nervous system activity in favor of the sympathetic nervous system. Gallamine does not alter activity of autonomic ganglia or evoke the release of histamine.

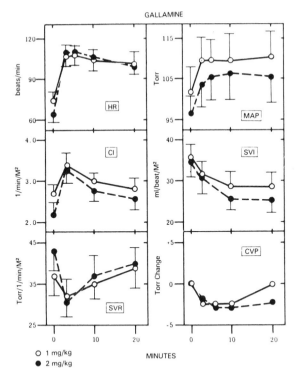

FIGURE 8-22. Circulatory effects following intravenous administration of gallamine 1 mg kg^{-1} *(clear circles)* or 2 mg kg^{-1} *(solid circles)* to patients anesthetized with nitrous oxide-halothane. (From Stoelting RK. Hemodynamic effects of gallamine during halothane-nitrous oxide anesthesia. Anesthesiology 1973;39:645–7. Reproduced by permission of the author and publisher.)

Causes of Altered Responses

Drugs administered in the perioperative period may enhance the effects of long-acting nondepolarizing neuromuscular blocking drugs at the neuromuscular junction. Examples of drugs that can enhance neuromuscular blockade include (1) volatile anesthetics, (2) aminoglycoside antibiotics, (3) local anesthetics, (4) cardiac antidysrhythmic drugs, (5) diuretics, (6) magnesium, (7) lithium, and (8) ganglionic blocking drugs. Changes unrelated to concurrent drug therapy such as (1) hypothermia, (2) acid–base alterations, (3) changes in the serum potassium concentration, (4) adrenocortical dysfunction, (5) burn injury, and (6) allergic reactions may also influence the characteristics of neuromuscular blockade produced by nondepolarizing neuromuscular blocking drugs. Finally, combinations of nondepolarizing neuromuscular blocking drugs may produce a degree of neuromuscular blockade that is different from that which would be produced by either drug alone.

Volatile Anesthetics

Volatile anesthetics produce dose-dependent enhancement of the magnitude and duration of neuromuscular blockade due to nondepolarizing neuromuscular blocking drugs (Fogdall and Miller, 1975; Miller *et al,* 1971). The enhancement of neuromuscular blockade is greatest with enflurane and isoflurane, intermediate with halothane, and least with nitrous oxide plus an opioid (Fig. 8-23) (Ali and Savarese, 1976). For example, 1.25 MAC halothane decreases d-tubocurarine dose requirements about 50% compared with the dose necessary to produce the same degree of neuro-

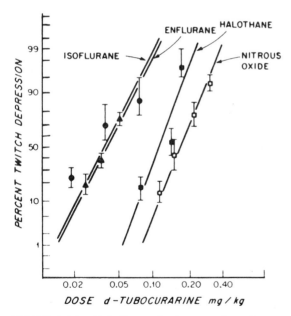

FIGURE 8-23. Volatile anesthetics cause dose-dependent and drug-specific enhancement of neuromuscular blockade produced by long-acting nondepolarizing neuromuscular blocking drugs. Mean ± SE. (From Ali HH, Savarese JJ. Monitoring of neuromuscular function. Anesthesiology 1976;45:216–49. Reproduced by permission of the authors and publisher.)

muscular blockade during nitrous oxide plus an opioid. A 1.25 MAC dose of enflurane and isoflurane reduces d-tubocurarine dose requirements about 70%. These same volatile anesthetics also reduce atracurium and vecuronium dose requirements, but the magnitude (10%–30%) is much less than observed with the long-acting neuromuscular blocking drugs (see the section entitled Intermediate-Acting Neuromuscular Blocking Drugs).

Enhancement of neuromuscular blockade produced by halothane is not dependent on the duration of administration of halothane as measured between 10 and 160 minutes of inhalation of the drug (Fig. 8-24) (Miller *et al,* 1976a; Stanski *et al,* 1980). In contrast, the ability of enflurane to enhance neuromuscular blockade is time-dependent as reflected by about a 10% increase per hour in the magnitude of neuromuscular blockade despite a constant plasma concentration of d-tubocurarine (Fig. 8-24) (Stanski *et al,* 1980). It is speculated that halothane acts on the highly perfused neuromuscular junction accounting for its early onset of maximal effect. In addition to this action at the neuromuscular junction, it is speculated that enflurane also acts directly on skeletal muscle where blood flow is less. As a result, a longer time is required for enflurane to achieve its maximal enhancement of nondepolarizing neuromuscular blockade.

MECHANISM. Volatile anesthetics most likely enhance the effects of nondepolarizing neuromuscular blocking drugs by virtue of anesthetic-induced depression of the central nervous system, which reduces the tone of skeletal muscles (Waud and Waud, 1975). In addition, volatile anesthetics may reduce the sensitivity of postjunctional membranes to depolarization (Waud, 1979). This decrease in end-plate sensitivity depends on the specific volatile anesthetic and the dose administered. Twitch response is decreased by volatile anesthetics alone when the concentration is sufficient to depress depolarization by 50% (1.25–1.57 MAC enflurane or 2.83–3.67 MAC halothane) (Waud and Waud, 1979). Increased skeletal muscle blood flow, as a means to deliver more drug to the neuromuscular junction, is probably important only for the enhanced neuromuscular blockade seen in the presence of isoflurane (Vitez *et al,* 1974). Inhaled anesthetics do not enhance neuromuscular blockade by decreasing the release of acetylcholine from the motor nerve ending or by

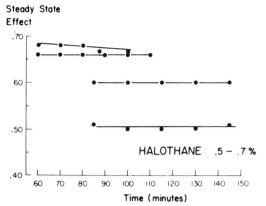

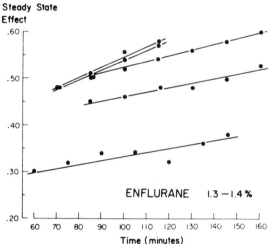

FIGURE 8-24. Enhancement of neuromuscular blockade produced by halothane does not change with time whereas the magnitude of neuromuscular blockade produced by enflurane increases with time. (From Stanski DR, Ham J, Miller RD, Sheiner LB. Time-dependent increase in sensitivity to d-tubocurarine during enflurane anesthesia in man. Anesthesiology 1980;52:483 – 7. Reproduced by permission of the authors and publisher.)

altering the configuration of the cholinergic receptor (Waud and Waud, 1973).

Antibiotics

Several types of antibiotics have been shown to enhance neuromuscular blockade produced by nondepolarizing neuromuscular blocking drugs (see Chapter 28). Prominent among the antibiotics that produce this enhancement are the aminoglycoside antibiotics. Antagonism of antibiotic-potentiated neuromuscular blockade by an anticholinesterase drug or calcium is unpredictable. Antibiotics devoid of neuromuscular blocking effects are the penicillins and cephalosporins.

MECHANISM. Antibiotics may exert effects on the prejunctional membranes similar to magnesium resulting in decreased release of acetylcholine (Sokoll and Gergis, 1981). Likewise, the same antibiotics may stabilize postjunctional membranes emphasizing that attempts to propose a common mechanism for antibiotic-induced enhancement of neuromuscular blockade are probably not possible.

Inhibition of the presynaptic release of acetylcholine by antibiotics may reflect competition of these drugs with calcium. Indeed, intravenous injection of calcium may at least transiently reverse the enhanced neuromuscular blockade associated with administration of antibiotics. Nevertheless, in addition to facilitating the prejunctional release of acetylcholine, calcium at the same time stabilizes postjunctional membranes to the effects of acetylcholine. These different effects of calcium at the neuromuscular junction are consistent with the unpredictable effects of calcium in antagonizing antibiotic-induced enhancement of neuromuscular blockade produced by nondepolarizing neuromuscular blocking drugs.

Local Anesthetics

Small doses of local anesthetics can enhance neuromuscular blockade produced by nondepolarizing neuromuscular blocking drugs, while in large doses local anesthetics can block neuromuscular transmission (see Chapter 7). Depending on the dose, local anesthetics (1) interfere with the prejunctional release of acetylcholine, (2) stabilize postjunctional membranes, and (3) directly depress skeletal muscle fibers. In addition, ester local anesthetics compete with other drugs for plasma cholinesterase thus introducing the possibility of a prolonged drug effect from succinylcholine.

Cardiac Antidysrbythmic Drugs

Lidocaine, as administered intravenously to treat cardiac dysrhythmias could augment preexisting neuromuscular blockade (Harrah *et al*, 1970) (see the section entitled Local Anesthetics). This potential drug interaction should be considered when administering lidocaine to patients recovering from general anesthesia that included use of a nondepolarizing neuromuscular blocking drug.

Quinidine potentiates neuromuscular blockade produced by nondepolarizing and depolarizing neuromuscular blocking drugs presumably by interfering with the prejunctional release of acetylcholine (Miller *et al*, 1967). As with lidocaine, this drug interaction may manifest when quinidine is administered to treat cardiac dysrhythmias in patients who have previously received neuromuscular blocking drugs during general anesthesia.

Diuretics

Furosemide, 1 mg kg^{-1} intravenously, enhances neuromuscular blockade produced by nondepolarizing neuromuscular blocking drugs (Miller *et al*, 1976b). This effect most likely reflects furosemide-induced inhibition of cyclic AMP production leading to reduced prejunctional output of acetylcholine. Conversely, large doses of furosemide may inhibit phosphodiesterase making more cyclic AMP available and leading to antagonism of nondepolarizing neuromuscular blocking drugs (Azar *et al*, 1980). Azathioprine also antagonizes nondepolarizing neuromuscular blockade presumably by inhibition of phosphodiesterase (Dretchen *et al*, 1976). This same drug augments neuromuscular blockade produced by succinylcholine.

Mannitol does not influence the degree of neuromuscular blockade produced by nondepolarizing neuromuscular blocking drugs even in the presence of diuresis (Matteo *et al*, 1980). This emphasizes that renal clearance of neuromuscular blocking drugs depends on glomerular filtration. Osmotic diuretics increase urine output independent of glomerular filtration rate.

Chronic hypokalemia due to treatment with diuretics reduces dose requirements for pancuronium and increases the dose of neostigmine necessary to reverse neuromuscular blockade (Miller and Roderick, 1978a) (see the section entitled Serum Potassium Concentration).

Magnesium

Magnesium enhances neuromuscular blockade produced by nondepolarizing neuromuscular blocking drugs and to a lesser extent that pro-

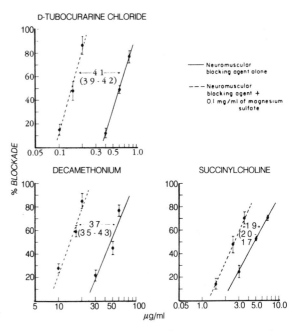

FIGURE 8-25. Magnesium enhances neuromuscular blockage produced by nondepolarizing neuromuscular blocking drugs and to a lesser extent that produced by succinylcholine. Mean ± SE. (From Ghoneim MM, Long JP. The interaction between magnesium and other neuromuscular blocking agents. Anesthesiology 1970;32:23 – 7. Reproduced by permission of the authors and publisher.)

duced by succinylcholine (Fig. 8-25) (Ghoneim and Long, 1970). There is a suggestion that the interaction between magnesium and vecuronium is more pronounced than that occurring with d-tubocurarine (Sinatra *et al*, 1985). Speculated mechanisms for this interaction include (1) decreased prejunctional release of acetylcholine and (2) decreased sensitivity (stabilization) of postjunctional membranes to acetylcholine. These effects of magnesium are consistent with enhancement of neuromuscular blockade produced by nondepolarizing neuromuscular blocking drugs as administered to patients with toxemia of pregnancy being treated with magnesium. The mechanism by which these effects of magnesium enhance neuromuscular blockade produced by succinylcholine, is not apparent. It is possible that phase II blockade occurs more readily when succinylcholine is administered in the presence of elevated plasma concentrations of magnesium.

Lithium

Lithium, as used to treat psychiatric depression, may enhance the neuromuscular blocking effects of depolarizing and nondepolarizing neuromuscular blocking drugs (Havdala *et al*, 1979).

Phenytoin

Patients treated chronically with phenytoin are resistant to the neuromuscular effects of metocurine, and presumably other nondepolarizing neuromuscular blocking drugs (Ornstein *et al*, 1985). This resistance seems to be related to a pharmacodynamic mechanism because the plasma concentration of metocurine required to produce a given level of neuromuscular blockade in phenytoin-treated patients is nearly double that necessary to produce the same response in untreated patients.

Ganglionic Blocking Drugs

Ganglionic blocking drugs, such as trimethaphan, can influence responses produced by neuromuscular blocking drugs by virtue of (1) decreases in skeletal muscle blood flow, (2) inhibition of plasma cholinesterase activity, and (3) decreased sensitivity of postjunctional membranes (Sklar and Lanks, 1977). Theoretically, a reduction in skeletal muscle blood flow would delay the onset and prolong the duration of neuromuscular blockade.

Hypothermia

Hypothermia prolongs neuromuscular blockade produced by d-tubocurarine and pancuronium reflecting delayed biliary and urinary excretion (Ham *et al*, 1978; Miller *et al*, 1978b). Pancuronium-induced neuromuscular blockade is also further enhanced by hypothermia-induced reductions in hepatic enzyme activity responsible for the metabolism of the drug. Finally, hypothermia also appears to increase sensitivity of the neuromuscular junction to pancuronium but not d-tubocurarine.

Acid – Base Changes

Respiratory acidosis enhances d-tubocurarine and pancuronium-induced neuromuscular blockade and opposes their reversal with neostigmine (Miller and Roderick, 1978b). Changes produced by metabolic acidosis and respiratory and metabolic alkalosis have not been consistent.

Serum Potassium Concentration

An acute decrease in the extracellular concentration of potassium will increase the transmembrane potential causing hyperpolarization of cell membranes. This change manifests as resistance to the effects of depolarizing neuromuscular blocking drugs and increased sensitivity to nondepolarizing neuromuscular blocking drugs. Conversely, hyperkalemia lowers the resting transmembrane potential and thus partially depolarizes cell membranes. This change increases the effects of depolarizing neuromuscular blocking drugs and opposes the action of nondepolarizing neuromuscular blocking drugs.

Adrenocortical Dysfunction

Cortisol or adrenocorticotropic hormone can improve neuromuscular function in patients with myasthenia gravis. In patients with inadequate adrenocortical function, nondepolarizing neuromuscular blocking drugs may produce prolonged neuromuscular blockade (Meyers, 1977).

Burn Injury

Burn injury is accompanied by a greater than threefold increase in the dose and nearly a fivefold increase in the plasma concentration of d-tubocurarine required to produce the same degree of neuromuscular blockade as in normal patients (Figs. 8-26 and 8-27) (Martyn *et al*, 1980). It is speculated that burn injury is accompanied by a proliferation of extrajunctional cholinergic receptors that are responsive to acetylcholine. As such, the apparent resistance to d-tubocurarine and other neuromuscular blocking drugs in the presence of burn injury is due to a change in pharmacodynamics and not pharmacokinetics. This resistance has been observed as long as 463 days following a 35% third degree burn (Fig. 8-28) (Martyn *et al*, 1982). The prolonged duration of resistance has implications for the use of succinylcholine in burn patients because it is presumed that hyperkalemia after administration of this drug reflects an increased number of receptor sites for potassium exchange to occur during succinylcholine-induced depolarization.

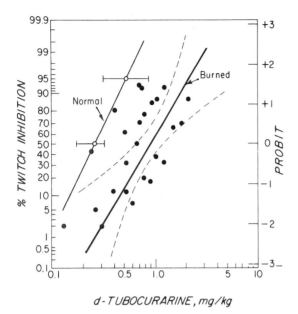

d - TUBOCURARINE , mg/kg

FIGURE 8-26. The dose-response curve for d-tubocurarine is displaced to the right (resistance) by burn injury. (From Martyn JAJ, Szyfelbein SK, Ali HH, Matteo RS, Savarese JJ. Increased d-tubocurarine requirement following major thermal injury. Anesthesiology 1980;52:352–5. Reproduced by permission of the authors and publisher.)

Paresis or Hemiplegia

Monitoring neuromuscular blockade with a peripheral nerve stimulator attached to the arm on the side affected by a cerebral vascular accident reveals resistance (decreased sensitivity) to the effects of the neuromuscular blocking drug compared with responses observed on the unaffected side (Iwasaki *et al,* 1985; Moorthy and Hilgenberg, 1980). Furthermore, even the unaffected arm shows resistance to the effects of neuromuscular blocking drugs compared with responses observed in normal patients (Fig. 8-29) (Shayevitz and Matteo, 1985). As a result, monitoring neuromuscular blockade with a peripheral nerve stimulator following a cerebral vascular accident may underestimate the degree of neuromuscular blockade present at muscles of respiration.

Resistance to neuromuscular blocking drugs in the affected arm may reflect proliferation of acetylcholine-responsive extrajunctional cholinergic receptor sites. This proliferation of receptor sites can occur within 48 to 72 hours following

denervation (Shayevitz and Matteo, 1985). In addition, collateral reinnervation of individual skeletal muscle fibers by surviving lower motor neurons occurs after about 6 months, further increasing the number of acetylcholine-responsive receptors.

Allergic Reactions

Anaphylactic and anaphylactoid reactions occur occasionally following the intravenous administration of nondepolarizing neuromuscular blocking drugs and succinylcholine (Stoelting, 1983). There may be cross-sensitivity between succinylcholine and nondepolarizing neuromuscular blocking drugs especially in patients with circulating IgE antibodies to quaternary ammonium groups of succinylcholine (Harle *et al,* 1984). Furthermore, there may be cross-sensitivity between long-acting and intermediate-acting nondepolarizing neuromuscular blocking drugs (Harle *et al,* 1985).

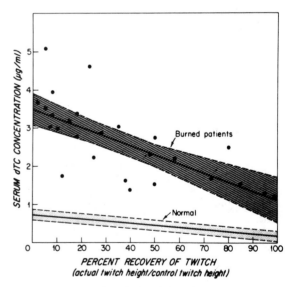

PERCENT RECOVERY OF TWITCH
(actual twitch height/control twitch height)

FIGURE 8-27. The plasma (serum) concentration of d-tubocurarine (dTc) associated with a given level of twitch recovery is greater in burned patients than in normal patients. (From Martyn JAJ, Szyfelbein SK, Ali HH, Matteo RS, Savarese JJ. Increased d-tubocurarine requirement following major thermal injury. Anesthesiology 1980;52:352–5. Reproduced by permission of the authors and publisher.)

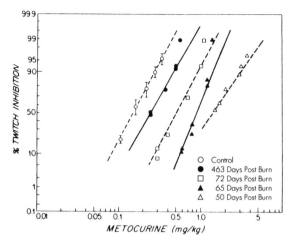

FIGURE 8-28. Resistance to the effects of drug-induced neuromuscular blockade in burn patients, as reflected by rightward displacement of the dose-response curve, may persist for several months. (From Martyn JAJ, Matteo RS, Szyfelbein SK, Kaplan RF. Unprecedented resistance to neuromuscular blocking effects of metocurine, with persistence and complete recovery in a burned patient. Anesth Analg 1982;61:614 – 7. Reproduced by permission of the authors and the International Anesthesia Research Society.)

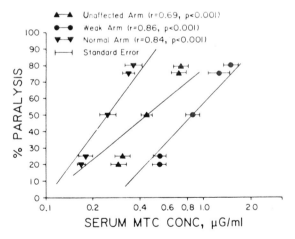

FIGURE 8-29. Resistance to the effects of nondepolarizing neuromuscular blocking drugs is detectable in both the paretic and unaffected arms of patients following a cerebral vascular accident compared with normal patients. Mean ± SE. (From Shayevitz JR, Matteo RS. Decreased sensitivity to metocurine in patients with upper motorneuron disease. Anesth Analg 1985; 64:767 – 72. Reproduced by permission of the authors and the International Anesthesia Research Society.)

Cross-sensitivity between neuromuscular blocking drugs emphasizes structural similarities of these drugs, especially the presence of one or more antigenic quaternary ammonium groups. A drug with a single quaternary ammonium group, such as vecuronium, may be less likely to cause cross-sensitivity. Anaphylactic reactions that occur following the first exposure to a neuromuscular blocking drug may reflect sensitization that occurs from prior contact with cosmetics and soaps that also contain antigenic quaternary ammonium groups.

Succinylcholine Followed by a Nondepolarizing Neuromuscular Blocking Drug

Administration of a nondepolarizing neuromuscular blocking drug following use of succinylcholine, as used to facilitate intubation of the trachea, results in a prolonged effect of the nondepolarizing drug (Katz, 1971). This is unexpected because succinylcholine and a nondepolarizing neuromuscular blocking drug should be antagonistic. Presumably, postjunctional membranes remain desensitized by succinylcholine resulting in a prolonged effect produced by nondepolarizing neuromuscular blocking drugs.

Combinations of Neuromuscular Blocking Drugs

The combination of pancuronium with metocurine or d-tubocurarine produces neuromuscular blockade that is greater than the additive effects of the individual drugs (Fig. 8-30) (Lebowitz et al, 1980). This greater than additive neuromuscular blocking effect does not occur when metocurine is combined with d-tubocurarine. Despite the enhancement of neuromuscular blockade produced by combinations of pancuronium with metocurine or d-tubocurarine, the duration of neuromuscular blockade is shorter than that produced by pancuronium alone. It is possible that this potentiation of neuromuscular blockade reflects simultaneous prejunctional and postjunctional receptor blockade (Taylor, 1985). Two neuromuscular blocking drugs, such as d-tubocurarine and metocurine, that act principally at the same prejunctional site would not be expected to produce more than additive effects when administered in combination (Bowman, 1980; Robbins et al, 1984). Pre-

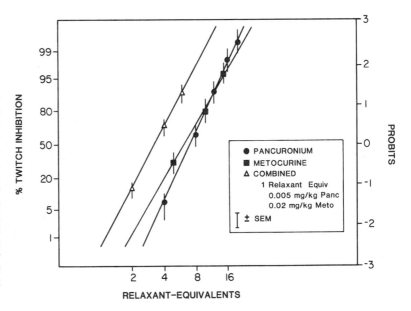

FIGURE 8-30. The combination of pancuronium with metocurine or d-tubocurarine produces neuromuscular blockade that is greater than the additive effects of the individual drugs. (From Lebowitz PW, Ramsey FM, Savarese JJ, Ali HH. Potentiation of neuromuscular blockade in man produced by combinations of pancuronium and metocurine or pancuronium and d-tubocurarine. Anesth Analg 1980;59:604–9. Reproduced by permission of the authors and the International Anesthesia Research Society.)

sumably, decreased release of acetylcholine from prejunctional sites due to these drugs would increase the potency of neuromuscular blocking drugs that act principally at postjunctional sites (Duncalf *et al*, 1983). Nevertheless, there is also evidence that this potentiation can be entirely due to postjunctional actions of the neuromuscular blocking drugs (Waud and Waud, 1985).

The combination of nondepolarizing neuromuscular blocking drugs permits achievement of the same degree of neuromuscular blockade with a smaller dose of each drug which results in fewer dose-related side-effects (Lebowitz *et al*, 1981). Indeed, blood pressure and heart rate effects of the combination of pancuronium and metocurine are less than with pancuronium alone (Fig. 8-31) (Lebowitz *et al*, 1981).

INTERMEDIATE-ACTING NONDEPOLARIZING NEUROMUSCULAR BLOCKING DRUGS

Atracurium and vecuronium are intermediate-acting nondepolarizing and noncumulative neuromuscular blocking drugs (Miller *et al*, 1984; Shanks, 1986; Stoelting, 1985). As such, these drugs are useful alternatives to succinylcholine and long-acting nondepolarizing neuromuscular

blocking drugs especially when intubation of the trachea and/or skeletal muscle relaxation are needed for short operations, such as outpatient procedures. Compared with long-acting nondepolarizing neuromuscular blocking drugs, these drugs have (1) a similar rate of onset of maximum neuromuscular blockade, (2) about one-third the duration of action (hence the designation intermediate-acting), (3) a 30% to 50% more rapid rate of recovery, (4) minimal to absent cumulative effects, and (5) minimal to absent cardiovascular effects (Basta *et al*, 1982a; Fahey *et al*, 1981b). The intermediate duration of action of both these drugs is due to their rapid clearance from the circulation. Because of their slow onset, atracurium or vecuronium are usually not acceptable substitutes for succinylcholine when intubation of the trachea must be accomplished within 60 seconds of rendering the patient unconscious.

Neuromuscular blockade produced by intermediate-acting neuromuscular blocking drugs is reliably antagonized by anticholinesterase drugs often within 20 minutes of administering a paralyzing dose of these drugs (Gencarelli and Miller, 1982). Spontaneous recovery from neuromuscular blockade may negate the need for pharmacologic antagonism assuming the peripheral nerve stimulator also documents a sustained response to continuous stimulation for 5 seconds or a normal train-of-four response.

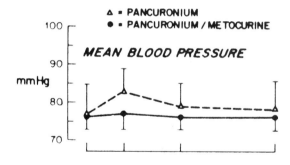

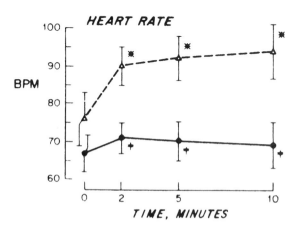

FIGURE 8-31. Blood pressure and heart rate effects of the combination of pancuronium and metocurine are less than with pancuronium alone. (From Lebowitz PW, Ramsey FM, Savarese JJ, Ali HH, deBros FM. Combination of pancuronium and metocurine: Neuromuscular and hemodynamic advantages over pancuronium alone. Anesth Analg 1981;60:12–7. Reproduced by permission of the authors and the International Anesthesia Research Society.)

Chemical Structure

Atracurium

Atracurium is a bisquaternary ammonium neuromuscular blocking drug with a bulky structure unlike that of any other neuromuscular blocking drug (Fig. 8-1). This drug was designed specifically to undergo spontaneous *in vivo* degradation (Hofmann elimination) at normal body temperature and pH (Stenlake *et al,* 1983). The iodide salt, besylate, provides water solubility, and commercial preparation in any aqueous solution adjusted to a pH of 3.25 to 3.65 minimizes *in vitro* Hofmann elimination. In view of its acid pH *in vitro*, atracu-

rium probably should not be mixed with alkaline drugs such as barbiturates or exposed to solutions with pH near 7.4 as present in delivery tubing used for infusion of intravenous fluids. Exposure of atracurium to an increased pH prior to vascular injection could theoretically result in premature breakdown of the drug. The potency of atracurium stored at room temperature declines about 5% every 30 days.

Vecuronium

Vecuronium is a monoquaternary analogue of pancuronium (Fig. 8-1). Clinically, vecuronium is pancuronium without the quaternary methyl group in the A ring of the steroid nucleus. The absence of this quaternary methyl group reduces the acetylcholine-like character of vecuronium as compared with pancuronium. Indeed, the vagolytic property of vecuronium is reduced about 20-fold. The monoquaternary structure of vecuronium increases its lipid solubility compared to pancuronium. Vecuronium is unstable in solution and for this reason is supplied as a lypophilized powder which must be dissolved in sterile water prior to its use.

Metabolism

Atracurium

Atracurium undergoes spontaneous metabolism at normal body temperature and pH by a base-catalyzed reaction termed Hofmann elimination (Fig. 8-32) (Stenlake *et al,* 1983). A second and simultaneously occurring route of metabolism is ester hydrolysis (Fig. 8-32) (Stenlake *et al,* 1983). These two routes of metabolism are independent of hepatic and renal function as well as plasma cholinesterase activity (Merrett *et al,* 1983). In addition to Hofmann elimination and ester hydrolysis, there is evidence that substantial atracurium clearance (up to 60%) occurs by hepatic or other nonrenal mechanisms (Fisher *et al,* 1986). Despite this potential importance of hepatic clearance, liver failure does not substantially prolong the response to atracurium (see the section entitled Hepatic Dysfunction). The duration of atracurium-induced neuromuscular blockade is intermediate and similar in normal patients or those with impaired or absent renal function or atypical plasma cholinesterase. Hofmann elimination and

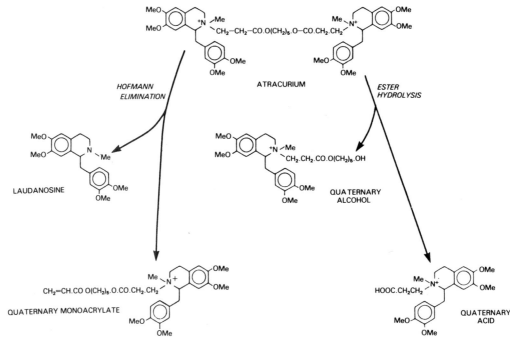

FIGURE 8-32. Atracurium undergoes spontaneous metabolism at normal body temperature and *p*H by Hofmann elimination and ester hydrolysis. (From Stenlake JB, Waigh RD, Urwin J, Dewar GH, Coker GG. Atracurium: Conception and inception. Br J Anaesth 1983;55:3S–10S. Reproduced by permission of the authors and publisher.)

ester hydrolysis also account for the lack of cumulative drug effect with repeated doses or continuous infusion of atracurium.

HOFMANN ELIMINATION. Hofmann elimination (*e.g.,* fission) begins to occur immediately after atracurium enters the circulation. In the presence of mild alkalosis (*i.e.,* *p*H 7.4) Hofmann elimination occurs at the quaternary nitrogen of the alphatic side chain of atracurium to yield laudanosine as the primary metabolite. The rate of Hofmann elimination is slowed by acidosis (*i.e.,* *p*H below 7.4) or reductions in body temperature below 37°C. The reverse changes will speed metabolism of atracurium by Hofmann elimination.

LAUDANOSINE. Peak plasma concentrations of laudanosine in humans occur 2 minutes after a rapid intravenous injection of atracurium and remain at about 75% of peak levels for nearly 15 minutes (Fahey *et al*, 1985). Laudanosine readily crosses the blood–brain barrier (peak cerebro-

spinal fluid concentrations in 3–10 minutes) and can produce seizures in laboratory animals. Administration of atracurium, 1 to 2.5 mg kg⁻¹, to dogs breathing subanesthetic concentrations of halothane is followed by evidence of arousal on the electroencephalogram in the absence of changes in cerebral blood flow, cerebral metabolic oxygen requirements, or intracranial pressure (Lanier *et al*, 1985). Cerebral stimulation is largely eliminated by 1 MAC halothane. It is presumed this arousal on the electroencephalogram reflects central nervous system stimulating effects of laudanosine derived from the metabolism of atracurium. Further evidence of central nervous system effects is up to a 30% increase in halothane MAC in rabbits receiving infusions of laudanosine to produce plasma concentrations of the metabolite similar to those observed in patients with renal failure receiving atracurium, 0.5 mg kg⁻¹ (Fahey *et al*, 1985; Shi *et al*, 1985) (see the section entitled Renal Dysfunction). Indeed, laudanosine is excreted unchanged by the kidneys, and its elimination half-time in animals is 113 minutes (Hennis *et al,* 1986).

Laudanosine resulting from metabolism of atracurium probably will not produce evidence of seizure activity in anesthetized patients because skeletal muscle paralysis from atracurium would preclude movement. Furthermore, inhaled anesthetics or injected drugs such as thiopental would tend to suppress any laudanosine-evoked central nervous system stimulation. In the absence of central nervous system depression produced by anesthetics, as in the postoperative period or in the critical care unit, it is theoretically possible that plasma concentrations of laudanosine associated with evidence of central nervous system stimulation could occur (Shi *et al,* 1985). In addition, the possibility of intraoperative awareness may be greater in lightly anesthetized patients if anesthetic requirements are simultaneously increased by laudanosine resulting from metabolism of atracurium (Shi *et al,* 1985). A transient and modest (14%) decrease in blood pressure follows the intravenous administration of laudanosine, 1 mg kg^{-1}, to halothane-anesthetized dogs (Hennis *et al,* 1986). Laudanosine is inactive at the neuromuscular junction.

ESTER HYDROLYSIS. Ester hydrolysis of atracurium occurs by nonspecific esterases that are unrelated to plasma cholinesterase. The activity of these enzymes is species-dependent with animals such as rats possessing greater enzyme activity than humans (Nigrovic *et al,* 1985). For this reason, it is likely that Hofmann elimination, or other reactions, are more important than ester hydrolysis in metabolism of atracurium in patients. As with Hofmann elimination, laudanosine is also a metabolite of ester hydrolysis.

Prolonged neuromuscular blockade does not follow administration of atracurium to patients with atypical plasma cholinesterase, emphasizing the dependence of ester hydrolysis of atracurium on nonspecific esterases that are unrelated to plasma cholinesterase. In contrast to Hofmann elimination, the rate of ester hydrolysis of atracurium is enhanced by reductions in blood pH below 7.4.

Vecuronium

Increased lipid solubility of vecuronium as compared with pancuronium facilitates entrance of vecuronium into hepatocytes where it undergoes deacetylation to 3-hydroxyvecuronium, 17-hydroxyvecuronium, and 3,17-dihydroxyvecuronium (Savage *et al,* 1980). The 3-hydroxyvecuronium derivative is about one-half as potent as the parent compound but is rapidly converted to the 3,17-dihydroxyvecuronium derivative. The 3,17-dihydroxyvecuronium and 17-hydroxyvecuronium derivatives have less than one-tenth the neuromuscular blocking potencies of vecuronium.

Increased lipid solubility also facilitates biliary excretion of vecuronium. For example, in patients an estimated 50% of the intravenous dose of vecuronium may be present in the liver 30 minutes after injection, and about 40% of the drug is excreted unchanged in the bile in the first 24 hours (Bencini *et al,* 1986a). About 30% of an administered dose of vecuronium appears in the urine as unchanged drug and metabolites in the first 24 hours (Bencini *et al,* 1986b). The extensive hepatic uptake of vecuronium may account for the rapid decline in vecuronium plasma concentration and its relatively short duration of action.

Onset and Duration of Action

Atracurium and vecuronium, like the long-acting neuromuscular blocking drugs, manifest a dose-dependent onset and duration of action with a rate of spontaneous recovery that is independent of the total dose of neuromuscular blocking drug (Table 8-9). The onset of action of atracurium and vecuronium is similar to the long-acting neuromuscular blocking drugs, but the duration of action is about one-third that of the long-acting drugs. A rapid onset of action similar to succinylcholine may be achieved by administering an initial subparalyzing dose of atracurium or vecuronium (about 10% of the total dose) followed in 3 to 6 minutes by the larger remaining portion of the dose (Gergis *et al,* 1983; Mehta *et al,* 1985; Schwarz *et al,* 1985). For example, administration of vecuronium, 0.01 mg kg^{-1}, intravenously 4 minutes prior to 0.1 mg kg^{-1} is the optimal dose and time interval for speeding the onset of neuromuscular blockade produced by this drug (Taboada *et al,* 1986). This divided dose technique is known as the priming principle and may serve as a useful alternative when administration of succinylcholine is best avoided. Conceptually, it is presumed, the initial subparalyzing dose decreases the margin of safety of neuromuscular transmission allow-

Table 8-9

Comparative Pharmacology of Intermediate-Acting Neuromuscular Blocking Drugs

	Atracurium	*Vecuronium*
ED_{95} (mg kg^{-1})	0.15–0.30	0.04–0.07
Onset of maximal twitch depression (minutes)	3–5	3–5
Time to 25% recovery of twitch height (minutes)	20–35	20–35
Recovery index* (minutes)	15–25	15–25
Dose for continuous infusion (μg kg^{-1} min^{-1})	6.2	1
Volume of distribution (L kg^{-1})	0.20	0.27
Clearance (ml kg^{-1} min^{-1})	5.5	5.2
Active metabolites	No	Slight
Degradation Dependent on:		
Body temperature	Yes	Yes
Blood pH	Yes	No
Renal function	No	Yes
Hepatic function	No?	Yes

* Recovery of twitch height from 25% to 75% of control

ing a more rapid onset of effect after the second larger dose. A similar more rapid onset occurs with divided doses of long-acting nondepolarizing neuromuscular drugs or the combination of long- and intermediate-acting neuromuscular blocking drugs (Mehta *et al*, 1985).

The rate of recovery from 10% to 25% of control twitch response is more rapid with intermediate-acting than with long-acting nondepolarizing neuromuscular blocking drugs. This rate of recovery is clinically important because abdominal musculature is adequately relaxed at 10% but not 25% of control twitch response. Typically, neuromuscular blockade can be antagonized 20 to 30 minutes after initial injection of two times the ED_{95} dose of atracurium or vecuronium. Supplemental doses of these drugs (usually about one-third the initial dose) can usually be antagonized 10 to 30 minutes later, providing spontaneous recovery of twitch response has begun.

Atracurium

The distribution half-time, elimination half-time, and clearance of atracurium in anesthetized patients are consistent with the drug's intermediate duration of action (Table 8-9) (Ward and Wright, 1983). The elimination half-time of about 22 minutes reflects rapid metabolism and is about one-third the elimination half-time for long-acting neuromuscular blocking drugs. An estimated 82% of atracurium is bound to plasma protein, presumably albumin (Foldes and Deery, 1983).

The site of action of atracurium, like other nondepolarizing neuromuscular blocking drugs is on both presynaptic and postsynaptic nicotinic cholinergic receptors (Hughes and Payne, 1983). Atracurium may also produce neuromuscular blockade by directly interfering with passage of ions through channels of nicotinic cholinergic receptors.

During nitrous oxide-thiopental-fentanyl anesthesia, the ED_{95} dose of atracurium is 0.2 mg kg^{-1} (Basta *et al*, 1982a). Spontaneous recovery to 95% twitch response after the ED_{95} dose is 44 minutes compared with 137 minutes for d-tubocurarine. The onset of maximum twitch depression after the ED_{95} dose of 4 minutes is similar to long-acting neuromuscular blocking drugs.

Vecuronium

The elimination half-time and rate of clearance of vecuronium are consistent with its intermediate duration of action compared with pancuronium (Table 8-9) (Cronnelly *et al*, 1983). This reflects rapid hepatic metabolism and biliary excretion of vecuronium. Even though the elimination half-time of vecuronium (71 minutes) is greater than atracurium (22 minutes), the two drugs have similar durations of action. The onset of maximum neuromuscular blockade following administration of vecuronium is similar to pancuronium, but the duration of neuromuscular blockade is shorter and rate of recovery more rapid after vecuronium (Fahey *et al*, 1981b). Despite its greater lipid solubility, the volume of distribution of vecuronium does not differ from pancuronium perhaps explaining the similar onset of action of both drugs (Table 8-5) (Cronnelly *et al*, 1983).

The plasma concentration of vecuronium necessary to depress twitch 50% is similar to the plasma concentration of pancuronium producing the same degree of twitch depression (Cronnelly *et al*, 1983). This observation suggests that pancuronium and vecuronium are equally potent and by extrapolation, the ED_{95} for vecuronium would be 0.07 mg kg^{-1} (*i.e.*, the same as the ED_{95} for pancuronium). Nevertheless, other studies have de-

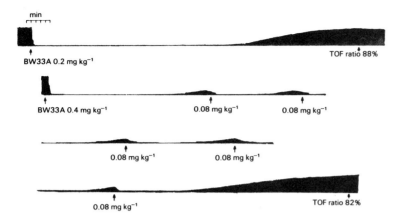

FIGURE 8-33. Repeated doses of atracurium (BW33A) do not produce a cumulative drug effect as evidenced by the unchanging time intervals between doses for the same degree of recovery from neuromuscular blockade to occur. (From Ali HH, Savarese JJ, Basta SJ, Sunder N, Gionfriddo M. Evaluation of cumulative properties of three new nondepolarizing neuromuscular blocking drugs. BW A444U, atracurium and vecuronium. Br J Anaesth 1983; 55:107S – 11S. Reproduced by permission of the authors and publisher.)

scribed vecuronium as being 15% to 50% more potent than pancuronium (Fahey *et al,* 1981b; Miller *et al,* 1984). The reasons for these discrepancies may reflect failure to control precisely the depth of anesthesia or the use of cumulative dose response curves to determine the ED_{95} (Gramstad and Lilleaasen, 1982). For example, the rapid clearance of intermediate-acting neuromuscular blocking drugs makes it difficult to derive valid ED_{95} values from dose-response techniques based on repeated dose techniques (Fisher *et al,* 1982a; Gibson *et al,* 1985).

Lack of Cumulative Effects

Consistency of onset to recovery intervals after repeated supplemental doses of atracurium is a unique characteristic of this drug that reflects the absence of cumulative drug effect (Fig. 8-33) (Ali *et al,* 1983). This absence of a cumulative drug effect is due to rapid metabolism of atracurium which is independent of redistribution or hepatic and renal clearance mechanisms. Lack of a cumulative drug effect minimizes the likelihood of persistent residual neuromuscular blockade when prolonged surgical procedures require repeated doses of atracurium.

Repeated supplemental doses of vecuronium produce slight but detectable increases in the duration of neuromuscular blockade (Fig. 8-34) (Fahey *et al,* 1981b). This cumulative effect is more than that observed with atracurium but much less than that produced by pancuronium. Following a single dose of vecuronium or pancuronium, plasma concentrations decrease rapidly because

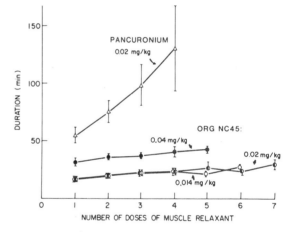

FIGURE 8-34. Repeated doses of vecuronium produce slight evidence of a cumulative drug effect which is greater than that observed after administration of atracurium (see Fig. 8-33) but less than that associated with pancuronium. (From Fahey MR, Morris RB, Miller RD, Sohn YJ, Cronnelly R, Gencarelli P. Clinical Pharmacology of ORG NC45 [Norcuron]: A new nondepolarizing muscle relaxant. Anesthesiology 1981;55:6 – 11. Reproduced by permission of the authors and publisher.)

of redistribution from the central to peripheral compartments. With subsequent doses, any drug in the peripheral compartment limits the distribution phase and thus also the rate of decline in the plasma concentrations of neuromuscular blocking drugs. Thus, both pancuronium and to a lesser extent, vecuronium can be demonstrated to have cumulative effects. The lack of a significant cumulative drug effect permits continuous infusion of atracurium or vecuronium with little likelihood of unexpected prolonged neuromuscular blockade. It is important to recognize that the noncumulative effects of atracurium, and to a lesser extent vecuronium, are dependent on the size of the supplemental doses. For example, supplemental doses of either drug that exceed the rate of plasma clearance would likely result in cumulative drug effects.

Pharmacologic and Physiologic Interactions

Drugs (volatile anesthetics, succinylcholine, antibiotics) and physiologic changes known to enhance neuromuscular blockade produced by long-acting neuromuscular blocking drugs also interact in a similar manner with intermediate-acting neuromuscular blocking drugs. The magnitude of these interactions, however, may differ between long-acting and intermediate-acting neuromuscular blocking drugs (Stoelting, 1985).

Volatile Anesthetics

Volatile anesthetics enhance neuromuscular blockade produced by atracurium and vecuronium, but the potentiation is less than that produced by the long-acting neuromuscular blocking drugs. For example, enflurane and isoflurane augment a d-tubocurarine and pancuronium neuromuscular blockade about twice as much as does an equally potent concentration of halothane. In contrast, the augmentation of atracurium or vecuronium-induced neuromuscular blockade by enflurane or isoflurane is only 20% to 30% compared with that present during halothane (Figs. 8-35 and 8-36) (Rupp et al, 1984; Rupp et al, 1985). Augmentation of neuromuscular blocking effects produced by vecuronium in the presence of halothane is evidenced by the decreased rate of drug infusion required to maintain an unchanging level of neuromuscular blockade compared with nitrous oxide-fentanyl (Fig. 8-37) (Swen et al, 1985).

The impact of volatile anesthetics on the onset and duration of action of intermediate-acting neuromuscular blocking drugs is inconsistent. Most often, the rate of onset is not influenced by the volatile anesthetic while the duration of action may be prolonged compared with a nitrous oxide-

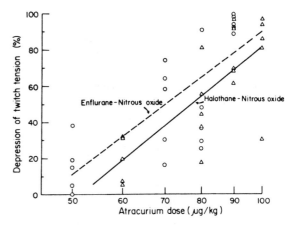

FIGURE 8-35. Atracurium-induced neuromuscular blockade is enhanced by volatile anesthetics, but the magnitude of this enhancement is less than observed with long-acting nondepolarizing neuromuscular blocking drugs (see Fig. 8-23). (From Rupp SM, McChristian JW, Miller RD. Neuromuscular effects of atracurium during halothane-nitrous oxide and enflurane-nitrous oxide anesthesia in humans. Anesthesiology 1985;63:16–9. Reproduced by permission of the authors and publisher.)

opioid anesthetic (Fahey et al, 1981b; Payne and Hughes, 1981).

Changes in the alveolar concentration of volatile anesthetic also have less impact on neuromuscular blockade produced by intermediate-acting compared with long-acting neuromuscular blocking drugs. For example, increasing the anesthetic concentration from 1.2 to 2.2 MAC decreases the ED_{50} of vecuronium 51%, 33%, and 18% during enflurane, isoflurane, and halothane anesthesia, respectively (Rupp et al, 1984). In contrast, the ED_{50} for pancuronium is decreased 57% for similar increases in the halothane concentration.

The advantage of lessened augmentation of intermediate-acting neuromuscular blocking drugs by volatile anesthetics is a more predictable degree of neuromuscular blockade in the absence of precise knowledge of the alveolar (e.g., brain) partial pressure of the anesthetic. Conversely, a disadvantage is that existing neuromuscular blockade is not easily enhanced by increasing the delivered concentration of volatile anesthetic. The reasons for atracurium and vecuronium being less influenced by the specific volatile anesthetic and its concentration are not known.

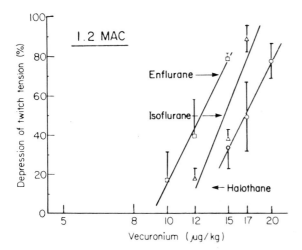

FIGURE 8-36. Vecuronium-induced neuromuscular blockade is enhanced by volatile anesthetics, but the magnitude of this enhancement is less than observed with long-acting nondepolarizing neuromuscular blocking drugs (see Fig. 8-23). (From Rupp SM, Miller RD, Gencarelli P. Vecuronium-induced neuromuscular blockade during enflurane, isoflurane, and halothane anesthesia in humans. Anesthesiology 1984;60:102–5. Reproduced by permission of the authors and publisher.)

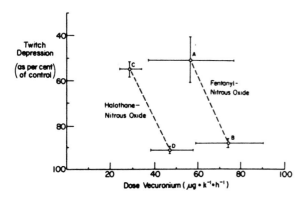

FIGURE 8-37. Augmentation of neuromuscular blocking effects produced by vecuronium in the presence of halothane-nitrous oxide is evidenced by the decreased rate of drug infusion required to maintain an unchanging level of neuromuscular blockade compared with fentanyl-nitrous oxide. Mean ± SD. (From Swen J, Gencarelli PJ, Koot HWJ. Vecuronium infusion dose requirements during fentanyl and halothane anesthesia in humans. Anesth Analg 1985;64:411–14. Reproduced by permission of the authors and the International Anesthesia Research Society.)

Succinylcholine

As with long-acting neuromuscular blocking drugs, the prior administration of succinylcholine, 1 mg kg^{-1}, enhances the magnitude of twitch response depression produced by the subsequent administration of atracurium or vecuronium even when evidence of neuromuscular blockade produced by succinylcholine has waned (Krieg *et al*, 1981; Stirt *et al*, 1983). Despite this initial enhancement, the subsequent duration of action of neuromuscular blockade is not prolonged by the prior administration of succinylcholine. A smaller dose of succinylcholine, 0.5 mg kg^{-1}, does not enhance subsequent neuromuscular blocking effects of vecuronium (Fisher and Miller, 1983a).

Combination with Long-Acting Neuromuscular Blocking Drugs

The combination of vecuronium with d-tubocurarine is significantly more potent than would be expected from a simple additive effect of the drugs administered individually (Mirakhur *et al*, 1985). This response is similar to the potentiation of neuromuscular blockade produced when combinations of long-acting nondepolarizing neuromuscular blocking drugs are administered (see the section entitled Combinations of Neuromuscular Blocking Drugs). Potentiation produced by combinations of neuromuscular blocking drugs is presumed to reflect different principal sites of action (prejunctional versus postjunctional).

Antibiotics

Aminoglycoside antibiotics prolong neuromuscular blockade produced by atracurium or vecuronium (Chapple *et al*, 1983).

Hypothermia

Hypothermia prolongs the duration of action of atracurium and decreases the rate of continuous infusion necessary to maintain a constant degree of neuromuscular blockade (Flynn *et al*, 1983). Presumably, this enhanced neuromuscular blocking effect reflects decreased metabolism of atracurium by Hofmann elimination and ester hydrolysis. Hypothermia also increases the duration of action of vecuronium presumably reflecting temperature-induced slowing of hepatic clearance mechanisms (Buzello *et al*, 1985a).

Acid – Base Changes

ATRACURIUM. Despite pH-dependent Hofmann elimination (accelerated by alkalosis and slowed by acidosis), it is unlikely that the range of pH changes encountered clinically is sufficiently great to alter the rate of Hofmann elimination and thus the duration of atracurium-induced neuromuscular blockade (Payne and Hughes, 1981). Furthermore, pH changes influence the rate of ester hydrolysis in a direction opposite to the change in the rate of Hofmann elimination such that slowed Hofmann elimination in the presence of acidosis is theoretically offset by an accelerated rate of ester hydrolysis.

VECURONIUM. The impact of acid–base changes on vecuronium-induced neuromuscular blockade depends on whether the changes in blood pH precede or follow the administration of vecuronium (Gencarelli et al, 1983). For example, changes in $PaCO_2$ that precede the administration of vecuronium do not alter the magnitude of neuromuscular blockade. Conversely, hypercarbia introduced after the establishment of vecuronium-induced neuromuscular blockade significantly enhances the effects of the neuromuscular blocking drug. For this reason, the onset of hypoventilation, as may occur in the early postoperative period could enhance residual neuromuscular blockade. A similar enhancement can occur when respiratory acidosis occurs in the presence of residual d-tubocurarine neuromuscular blockade.

Histamine

It is estimated that the plasma concentration of histamine must double before cardiovascular changes manifest. This degree of histamine release occurs with the ED_{95} dose of d-tubocurarine and two times the ED_{95} dose of metocurine (Basta et al, 1982b). Atracurium does not evoke sufficient histamine release to cause cardiovascular changes until three times the ED_{95} dose is administered (Basta et al, 1982b). In contrast, histamine release, and thus cardiovascular changes, do not occur with even three and one-half times the ED_{95} dose of vecuronium (Basta et al, 1983).

Renal Dysfunction

The duration of action of long-acting neuromuscular blocking drugs can be greatly enhanced by renal dysfunction. In contrast, the impact of renal dysfunction on neuromuscular blockade produced by even large doses of atracurium or vecuronium is negligible to absent (Fahey et al, 1981a; Hunter et al, 1984). About 30% of an administered dose of vecuronium appears in the urine as unchanged drug and metabolites in the first 24 hours (Bencini et al, 1986b). This modest dependence on renal clearance does slow the rate of disappearance of vecuronium from the plasma of patients with renal failure but is not sufficient to significantly increase the duration of action of vecuronium. An apparent tolerance to vecuronium in patients with renal failure is suggested by higher plasma concentrations of vecuronium at 25% and 75% recovery compared to patients with normal renal function (Bencini et al, 1986b). This tolerance is consistent with a slower onset of action of vecuronium in patients with renal failure. A similar but less prominent degree of tolerance may also occur following administration of atracurium to patients in renal failure (Hunter et al, 1984). Plasma concentrations of laudanosine following a single dose of atracurium, 0.5 mg kg^{-1}, are greater in patients in renal failure compared with normal patients (Fahey et al, 1985).

Hepatic Dysfunction

Hepatic failure does not alter the elimination half-time of atracurium compared with normal patients (Ward and Neill, 1983). The elimination half-time of vecuronium, 0.2 mg kg^{-1}, is increased from 58 minutes to 84 minutes and plasma clearance is decreased 50% when administered to patients with cirrhosis of the liver (Fig. 8-38) (Lebrault et al, 1985). This prolongation is consistent with the dependence of vecuronium on hepatic clearance mechanisms. When the dose of vecuronium is 0.1 mg kg^{-1}, the presence of cirrhosis of the liver does not influence elimination half-time (Bell et al, 1985). It is possible that other elimination mechanisms such as renal clearance or diffusion of drug onto nonspecific receptors (e.g., cartilage) offset the effect of impaired hepatic function when lower doses of vecuronium are administered. In patients with cholestasis undergoing bili-

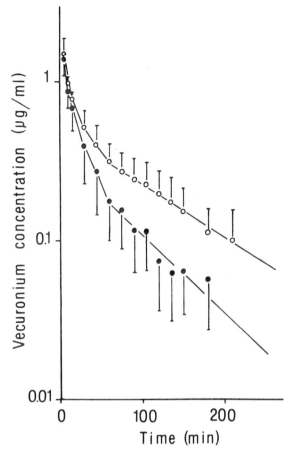

FIGURE 8-38. Disappearance of vecuronium from the plasma is slowed in patients with hepatic cirrhosis *(clear circles)* compared with normal patients *(solid circles)* Mean ± SD. (From Lebrault C, Berger JL, D'Hollander AA, Gomeni R, Henzel D, Duvaldestin P. Pharmacokinetics and pharmacodynamics of vecuronium [ORG NC45] in patients with cirrhosis. Anesthesiology 1985;62:601–5. Reproduced by permission of the authors and publisher.)

ary surgery, the administration of 0.2 mg kg^{-1} of vecuronium results in a prolonged elimination half-time and increased duration of action of the drug (Lebrault *et al*, 1986).

Circulatory Effects

Long-acting nondepolarizing neuromuscular blocking drugs produce predictable and often clinically significant reductions in blood pressure and peripheral vascular resistance (d-tubocurarine, metocurine) or increases in heart rate (gallamine, pancuronium). These circulatory effects may be undesirable in the presence of hypovolemia, valvular heart disease, or coronary artery disease. In this regard, a major advantage of vecuronium, and to a lesser extent atracurium, is the absence of circulatory effects after administration of these drugs. Conversely, bradycardia associated with opioid-based anesthetics, which is masked by heart rate-accelerating effects of pancuronium, will not be offset by intermediate-acting nondepolarizing neuromuscular blocking drugs (Salmenpera *et al*, 1983).

Atracurium

Blood pressure and heart rate changes do not accompany the rapid intravenous administration of atracurium in doses up to two times the ED$_{95}$ with background anesthetics including nitrous oxide, fentanyl, halothane, enflurane, and isoflurane (Fig. 8-39) (Basta *et al*, 1982a; Hilgenberg *et al*, 1983; Rupp *et al*, 1983a; Sokoll *et al*, 1983). During nitrous oxide-fentanyl anesthesia a two and one-half and three times the ED$_{95}$ dose of atracurium increases heart rate 5.5% and 8.3% and decreases mean arterial pressure 13.3% and 21.5% respectively (Fig. 8-39) (Basta *et al*, 1982a). These circulatory changes are transient occurring 60 to 90 seconds after administration of atracurium and disappearing within 5 minutes. Facial and truncal flushing in some patients suggests release of histamine as the mechanism for the circulatory changes accompanying these high doses of atracurium. Indeed, plasma histamine concentrations increase transiently and parallel blood pressure and heart rate changes when atracurium (0.6 mg kg^{-1}) is administered rapidly (Scott *et al*, 1984). Conversely, the same dose of atracurium administered over 75 seconds does not alter plasma histamine concentrations, and blood pressure and heart rate do not change (Scott *et al*, 1984). Animal evidence also suggests that laudanosine may contribute to transient blood pressure reductions associated with rapid administration of large doses of atracurium (Hennis *et al*, 1986).

Vecuronium

Vecuronium is devoid of circulatory effects even at doses (0.28 mg kg^{-1}) that exceed three times the

FIGURE 8-39. Heart rate and blood pressure changes do not occur following the rapid intravenous administration of atracurium (BW 33A) up to doses equivalent to two times the ED_{95} (*e.g.*, 0.4 mg kg^{-1}). Larger doses of atracurium produce transient increases in heart rate and decreases in blood pressure. (From Basta SJ, Ali HH, Savarese JJ, *et al*. Clinical pharmacology of atracurium besylate [BW 33A]: A new non-depolarizing muscle relaxant. Anesth Analg 1982;61:723–9. Reproduced by permission of the authors and the International Anesthesia Research Society.)

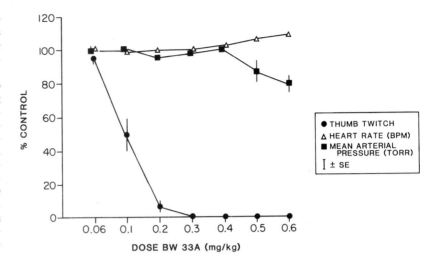

ED_{95}, emphasizing the lack of vagolytic effects or histamine release associated with administration of this drug (Morris *et al*, 1983). Bradycardia may accompany the concomitant injection of vecuronium and high doses of opioids, especially sufentanil (Salmenpera *et al*, 1983; Starr *et al*, 1986). It is not clear whether this represents a parasympathomimetic effect of vecuronium in certain patients or failure of vecuronium to offset inherent vagotonic effects of opioids.

Obstetric Patients

The short duration of action of atracurium and vecuronium makes these drugs attractive selections for production of skeletal muscle relaxation during general anesthesia for cesarean section. The slow onset of action, however, compared with succinylcholine detracts from their use when rapid intubation of the trachea is considered important. Like the long-acting neuromuscular blocking drugs, insufficient amounts of atracurium and vecuronium cross the placenta to produce significant effects in the fetus (Dailey *et al*, 1984; Frank *et al*, 1983). For example, the maternal to fetal ratio of vecuronium following administration of 0.04 to 0.08 mg kg^{-1} to the mother is 0.11. Concentrations of atracurium in umbilical venous blood are below the sensitivity limits of the assay. The clearance of vecuronium may be accelerated during late pregnancy, possibly re-

flecting stimulation of hepatic microsomal enzymes by progesterone as well as by cardiovascular changes and fluid shifts that occur during pregnancy (Eadie *et al*, 1977).

Pediatric Patients

Atracurium

Effective doses of atracurium are similar in adults and children (2–16 years of age) when differences in extracellular fluid volume are minimized by calculating the dose on a mg m^{-2} rather than mg kg^{-1} basis (Brandom *et al*, 1984). Conversely, infants 1 to 6 months of age require about one-half the dose of atracurium given to older children to achieve the same degree of neuromuscular blockade (Brandom *et al*, 1983). This implies that infants are more sensitive than children or adults to the neuromuscular blocking effects of atracurium. A similar sensitivity occurs in infants to d-tubocurarine (Fisher *et al*, 1982b). Recovery from atracurium-induced neuromuscular blockade, however, is more rapid in infants (23 minutes) than adolescents (29 minutes) (Brandom *et al*, 1983).

Vecuronium

The potency of vecuronium in infants (7–45 weeks), children (1–8 years), and adults (18–38 years) is similar during nitrous oxide-halothane

Table 8-10

Comparison of Vecuronium-Induced Neuromuscular Blockade in Pediatric and Adult Patients

	Vecuronium (mg kg^{-1})	Onset of Maximum Twitch Depression (minutes)	Duration (minutes to 90% twitch recovery)	Recovery Index (minutes for twitch response to recover from 25%–75% of control)
Infants	0.07	1.5*	73*	20†
Children	0.07	2.4	35	9
Adults	0.07	2.9	54	13

* P < 0.05 compared with adults
† P < 0.05 compared with children
(Data from Fisher DM, Miller RD. Neuromuscular effects of vecuronium [ORG NC 45] in infants and children during N_2O halothane anesthesia. Anesthesiology 1983;58:519–23.)

anesthesia (Table 8-10) (Fisher and Miller, 1983b). Onset of action is shorter in infants than in adults whereas duration is longest in infants and shortest in children (Table 8-10) (Fisher and Miller, 1983b). Presumably, a high cardiac output in infants speeds the onset of vecuronium-induced neuromuscular blockade while the longer duration of action reflects immaturity of the neonate's liver and/or increased volume of distribution. An increased volume of distribution means more drug is sequestered in peripheral compartments and inaccessible to hepatic and renal clearance mechanisms. Age-related changes in biliary clearance may also contribute to a longer duration of vecuronium-induced neuromuscular blockade in infants.

Elderly Patients

Atracurium

Increasing age has no effect on the continuous rate of intravenous infusion of atracurium necessary to maintain a constant degree of neuromuscular blockade (D'Hollander *et al*, 1983). Likewise, the rate of recovery and thus the duration of neuromuscular blockade is similar in young adults and the elderly. This lack of influence of aging on dose requirements of atracurium most likely reflects the independence of Hofmann elimination and ester hydrolysis from age-related effects on renal and hepatic function. Furthermore, changes in

volume of distribution that occur with aging will not influence the clearance of atracurium from the plasma.

Vecuronium

Increasing age is associated with decreases in the continuous rate of intravenous infusion of vecuronium necessary to maintain a constant degree of neuromuscular blockade (D-Hollander *et al*, 1982). Presumably this reflects decreased plasma clearance of vecuronium due to age-related reductions in hepatic and renal blood flow and possibly decreased hepatic microsomal enzyme activity. Furthermore, when the continuous infusion of vecuronium is discontinued, the rate of recovery of twitch response is prolonged in the elderly compared with young adults. This delayed rate of recovery could manifest as a prolonged duration of vecuronium-induced neuromuscular blockade in the elderly. In contrast to the detectable impact of aging during and following the continuous intravenous infusion of vecuronium, dose-response curves as determined from twitch responses produced by single intravenous doses of vecuronium are not influenced by increasing age (O'Hara *et al*, 1985).

In patients 70 to 80 years of age, the volume of distribution and plasma clearance of vecuronium are decreased compared with younger patients (Rupp *et al*, 1983b). The decrease in distribution volume is consistent with age-related reductions in skeletal muscle mass and total body water, whereas, reductions in plasma clearance most likely reflect decreased hepatic blood flow in the elderly. Evidence of unchanged responsiveness of the neuromuscular junction despite increasing age is the similarity of the plasma concentration of vecuronium necessary to depress twitch response 50% in elderly patients and young patients (Rupp *et al*, 1983b).

Intracranial Pressure

Intracranial pressure is not changed following the administration of atracurium or vecuronium to anesthetized patients undergoing surgery for expansive brain lesions (Rosa *et al*, 1986a; Rosa *et al*, 1986b). These data suggest atracurium may be utilized for skeletal muscle relaxation during neurosurgical operations despite its potential for histamine release and stimulation of the central nervous system.

Malignant Hyperthermia

Malignant hyperthermia does not follow the administration of atracurium or vecuronium to sensitive swine (Buzello *et al*, 1985b; Skarpa *et al*, 1983). Prolonged vecuronium-induced neuromuscular blockade has been reported in a malignant hyperthermia-susceptible patient pretreated with dantrolene (Driessen *et al*, 1985). This could reflect dantrolene-induced reductions in neurotransmitter mobilization at the neuromuscular junction due to impaired release of calcium ions from storage sites within cholinergic nerve terminals (Durant *et al*, 1980). It seems likely that similar prolongation of neuromuscular blockade could occur with other neuromuscular blocking drugs administered in the presence of dantrolene.

REFERENCES

Adams PR, Sakmann B. Decamethonium both opens and blocks endplate channels. Proc Natl Acad Sci 1978;75:2992–8.

Agoston S, Vermeer GA, Kersten UW, Meijer DKF. The fate of pancuronium bromide in man. Acta Anaesth Scand 1973;17:267–75.

Ali HH, Savarese JJ. Monitoring of neuromuscular function. Anesthesiology 1976;45:216–49.

Ali HH, Savarese JJ, Basta SJ, Sunder N, Gionfriddo M. Evaluation of cumulative properties of three new nondepolarizing neuromuscular blocking drugs BW A444U, atracurium and vecuronium. Br J Anaesth 1983;55:107S–11S.

Azar I, Cottrell J, Gupta B, Turndorf H. Furosemide facilitates recovery of evoked twitch response after pancuronium. Anesth Analg 1980;59:55–7.

Basta SJ, Ali HH, Savarese JJ, *et al*. Clinical pharmacology of atracurium besylate (BW 33A): A new nondepolarizing muscle relaxant. Anesth Analg 1982a;61:723–9

Basta SJ, Savarese JJ, Ali HH, *et al*. Vecuronium does not alter serum histamine within the clinical dose range. Anesthesiology 1983;59:A273.

Basta SJ, Savarese JJ, Ali HH, Moss J, Gionfriddo BA. Histamine-releasing potencies of atracurium besylate (BW 33A), Dimethyltubocurarine and d-tubocurarine. Anesthesiology 1982b;57:A261.

Bell CF, Hunter JM, Jones RS, Utting JE. Use of atracurium and vecuronium in patients with oesophageal varices. Br J Anaesth 1985;57:160–8.

Bencini AF, Scaf AHJ, Sohn YJ, Kersten-Kleff UW, Agoston S. Hepatobiliary disposition of vecuronium bromide in man. Br J Anaesth 1986a;58:988–95.

Bencini AF, Scaf AHJ, Sohn YJ *et al*. Disposition and urinary excretion of vecuronium bromide in anesthetized patients with normal renal function or renal failure. Anesth Analg 1986b;65:245–51.

Bennett AE. Preventing traumatic complications in convulsive shock therapy by curare. JAMA 1940;114:322–4.

Bowman WC. Prejunctional and post-junctional cholinoceptors at the neuromuscular junction. Anesth Analg 1980;59:935–43.

Brandom BW, Rudd GD, Cook DR. Clinical pharmacology of atracurium in paediatric patients. Br J Anaesth 1983;55:117S–21S.

Brandom BW, Woelfel SK, Cook DR, Fehr BL, Rudd GD. Clinical pharmacology of atracurium in infants. Anesth Analg 1984;63:309–12.

Brotherton WP, Matteo RS. Pharmacokinetics and pharmacodynamics of metocurine in humans with and without renal failure. Anesthesiology 1981;55:273–6.

Brown BB, Crout JR. The sympathomimetic effect of gallamine on the heart. J Pharmacol Exp Ther 1970;172:216–23.

Buzello W, Schluermann D, Schindler M, Spillner F. Hypothermic cardiopulmonary bypass and neuromuscular blockade by pancuronium and vecuronium. Anesthesiology 1985a;62:201–4.

Buzello W, Williams CH, Chandra P, Watkins ML, Dozier SE. Vecuronium and porcine malignant hyperthermia. Anesth Analg 1985b;64:515–9.

Chapple DJ, Clark JS, Hughes R. Interaction between

atracurium and drugs used in anaesthesia. Br J Anaesth 1983;55:17S – 22S.

Cooperman LH, Strobel GE, Kennell EM. Massive hyperkalemia after administration of succinylcholine. Anesthesiology 1970;32:161 – 4.

Cronnelly R, Fisher DM, Miller RD, Gencarelli P, Nguyen-Gruenka L, Castagnoli N. Pharmacokinetics and pharmacodynamics of vecuronium (ORG NC45) and pancuronium in anesthetized humans. Anesthesiology 1983;58:405 – 8.

Dailey PA, Fisher DM, Shnider SM, et al. Pharmacokinetics, placental transfer, and neonatal effects of vecuronium and pancuronium administered during cesarean section. Anesthesiology 1984;60: 569 – 74.

D'Hollander AA, Luyckx C, Barvais L, Deville A. Clinical evaluation of atracurium besylate requirement for a stable muscle relaxation during surgery: Lack of age-related effects. Anesthesiology 1983;59:237 – 40.

D'Hollander AA, Massaux F, Nevelsteen M, Agoston S. Age-dependent dose-response relationship of ORG NC45 in anaesthetized patients. Br J Anaesth 1982;54:653 – 7.

Domenech JS, Garcia RC, Sasiain JMR, Loyola AQ, Oroz JS. Pancuronium bromide: An indirect sympathomimetic agent. Br J Anaesth 1976;48:1143 – 8.

Donati F, Antzaka C, Bevan DR. Potency of pancuronium at the diaphragm and the adductor pollicis muscle in humans. Anesthesiology 1986;65:1 – 5.

Drachman DA. Myasthenia gravis. N Engl J Med 1978; 298:136 – 42.

Dretchen KL, Morgenroth VH, Standaert FG, Walts LF. Azathioprine: Effects on neuromuscular transmission. Anesthesiology 1976;45:604 – 9.

Driessen JJ, Wuis EW, Gielen JM. Prolonged vecuronium neuromuscular blockade in a patient receiving orally administered dantrolene. Anesthesiology 1985;62:523 – 4.

Duncalf D, Chaudry I, Aoki T, Nagashima H, Foldes FF. Potentiation of pancuronium, vecuronium and atracurium by d-tubocurarine or metocurine. Anesthesiology 1983;59:A292.

Durant NN, Lee C, Katz RL. The action of dantrolene on transmitter mobilization at the rat neuromuscular junction. Eur J Pharmacol 1980;68:403 – 8.

Duvaldestin P, Agoston S, Henzel E, Kersten UW, Desmonts JM. Pancuronium pharmacokinetics in patients with liver cirrhosis. Br J Anaesth 1978; 50:1131 – 6.

Duvaldestin P, Saada J, Berger JL, D'Hollander A, Desmonts JM. Pharmacokinetics, pharmacodynamics, and dose-response relationship of pancuronium in control and elderly subjects. Anesthesiology 1982;56:36 – 40.

Eadie MJ, Lander CM, Tyrer JH. Plasma drug level monitoring in pregnancy. Clin Pharmacokinet 1977; 2:427 – 36.

Fahey MR, Morris RB, Miller RD, Nguyen T-L, Upton RA. Pharmacokinetics of ORG NC45 (Norcuron) in patients with and without renal failure. Br J Anaesth 1981a;53:1049 – 52.

Fahey MR, Morris RB, Miller RD, Sohn YJ, Cronnelly R, Gencarelli P. Clinical pharmacology of ORG NC45 (Norcuron): A new nondepolarizing muscle relaxant. Anesthesiology 1981b;55:6 – 11.

Fahey MR, Rupp SM, Canfell C, et al. Effect of renal function on laudanosine excretion in man. Br J Anaesth 1985;57:1049 – 51.

Fisher DM, Canfell PC, Fahey MR, Rosen JI, Rupp SM, Sheiner LB, Miller RD. Elimination of atracurium in humans: Contribution of Hofmann elimination and ester hydrolysis versus organ-based elimination. Anesthesiology 1986;65:6 – 12.

Fisher DM, Fahey MR, Cronnelly R, Miller RD. Potency determination for vecuronium (ORG NC45). Comparison of cumulative and single dose techniques. Anesthesiology 1982a;57:309 – 10.

Fisher DM, O'Keeffe C, Stanski DR, Cronnelly R, Miller RD, Gregory GA. Pharmacokinetics and pharmacodynamics of d-tubocurarine in infants, children, and adults. Anesthesiology 1982b;57:203 – 8.

Fisher DM, Miller RD: Interaction of succinylcholine and vecuronium during N_2O-halothane anesthesia. Anesthesiology 1983a;59:A278.

Fisher DM, Miller RD: Neuromuscular effects of vecuronium (ORG NC45) in infants and children during N_2O, halothane anesthesia. Anesthesiology 1983b; 58:519 – 23.

Flynn PJ, Hughes P, Walton B. The use of atracurium in cardiopulmonary bypass with induced hypothermia. Anesthesiology 1983;59:A262.

Fogdall RP, Miller RD. Neuromuscular effects of enflurane, alone and combined with d-tubocurarine, pancuronium, and succinylcholine, in man. Anesthesiology 1975;42:173 – 7.

Foldes FF, Deery A. Protein binding of atracurium and other short acting neuromuscular blocking agents and their interaction with human cholinesterase. Br J Anaesth 1983;55:31S – 4S.

Foldes FF, Rendell-Baker L, Birch JH. Causes and prevention of prolonged apnea with succinylcholine. Anesth Analg 1956;35:609 – 13.

Forbes AR, Cohen NH, Eger EI. Pancuronium reduces halothane requirement in man. Anesth Analg 1979;58:497 – 9.

Frank M, Flynn PJ, Hughes R. Atracurium in obstetric anaesthesia. Br J Anaesth 1983;55:113S – 14S.

Gencarelli PJ, Miller RD. Antagonism of Org NC45 (vecuronium) and pancuronium neuromuscular blockade by neostigmine. Br J Anaesth 1982; 54:53 – 6.

Gencarelli PJ, Siven J, Koot HWJ, Miller RD. The effects of hypercarbia and hypocarbia on pancuronium and vecuronium neuromuscular blockades in anesthetized humans. Anesthesiology 1983;59:376 – 80.

Gergis SD, Sokoll MD, Mehta M, Kemmotsuo O, Rudd GD. Intubation conditions after atracurium and suxamethonium. Br J Anaesth 1983;55:83S.

Ghoneim MM, Kramer E, Bannow R, Pandya H, Routh JI. Binding of d-tubocurarine to plasma proteins in normal man and in patients with hepatic or renal disease. Anesthesiology 1973;39:410 – 5.

Ghoneim MM, Long JP. The interaction between magnesium and other neuromuscular blocking agents. Anesthesiology 1970;32:23 – 7.

Gibson FM, Mirakhur RK, Lavery GG, Clarke RSJ. Potency of atracurium: A comparison of single dose and cumulative dose techniques. Anesthesiology 1985;62:657 – 9.

Gramstad L, Lilleaasen P. Dose-response relation of atracurium, ORG NC45 and pancuronium. Br J Anaesth 1982;54:647 – 51.

Griffith HR, Johnson GE. The use of curare in general anesthesia. Anesthesiology 1942;3:418 – 20.

Gronert GA, Theye RA. Pathophysiology of hyperkalemia induced by succinylcholine. Anesthesiology 1975;43:89 – 99.

Ham J, Miller RD, Benet LZ, Matteo RS, Roderick LL. Pharmacokinetics and pharmacodynamics of d-tubocurarine during hypothermia in the cat. Anesthesiology 1978;49:324 – 9.

Ham J, Miller RD, Sheiner LB, Matteo RS. Dosage-schedule independence of d-tubocurarine pharmacokinetics and pharmacodynamics, and recovery of neuromuscular function. Anesthesiology 1979; 50:528 – 33.

Harle DG, Baldo BA, Fisher MM. Detection of IgE antibodies to suxamethonium after anaphylactoid reactions during anaesthesia. Lancet 1984;1:930 – 2.

Harle DG, Baldo BA, Fisher MM. Cross-reactivity of metocurine, atracurium, vecuronium and fazadinium with IgE antibodies from patients unexposed to these drugs but allergic to other myoneural blocking drugs. Br J Anaesth 1985;57:1073 – 6.

Harrah MD, Way WL, Katzung BG. The interaction of d-tubocurarine with antiarrhythmic drugs. Anesthesiology 1970;33:406 – 10.

Havdala HS, Borison RL, Diamond BI. Potential hazards and applications of lithium in anesthesiology. Anesthesiology 1979;50:534 – 7.

Hennis PJ, Fahe MR, Canfell PC, Shi W-Z, Miller RD. Pharmacology of laudanosine in dogs. Anesthesiology 1986;65:56 – 60.

Hilgenberg JC, Stoelting RK, Harris WA. Systemic vascular responses to atracurium during enflurane-nitrous oxide anesthesia in humans. Anesthesiology 1983;58:242 – 4.

Holst-Larsen H. The hydrolysis of suxamethonium in human blood. Br J Anaesth 1976;48:887 – 91.

Hughes R, Chapple DJ. Effects of nondepolarizing neuromuscular blocking agents on peripheral autonomic mechanisms in cats. Br J Anaesth 1976; 48:59 – 67.

Hughes R, Payne JP. Clinical assessment of atracurium using the single twitch and tetanic responses of the adductor pollicis muscles. Br J Anaesth 1983; 55:47S – 52S.

Hunt R, Taveau RM: On the physiological action of certain choline derivatives and new methods for detecting choline. Br Med J 1906;2:1788 – 91.

Hunter AR, Feldman SA. Muscle relaxants (editorial). Br J Anaesth 1976;48:277 – 8.

Hunter JM, Jones RS, Utting JE. Comparison of vecuronium, atracurium and tubocurarine in normal patients and in patients with no renal function. Br J Anaesth 1984;56:941 – 50.

Ivankovich AD, Miletich DJ, Albrecht RF, Zahed B. The effect of pancuronium on myocardial contraction and catecholamine metabolism. J Pharm Pharmacol 1975;27:837 – 41.

Iwasaki H, Namiki A, Omote K, Omote T, Takahashi T. Response differences of paretic and healthy extremities to pancuronium and neostigmine in hemiplegic patients. Anesth Analg 1985;64:864 – 6.

Kalow W, Genest K. A method for the detection of atypical forms of human serum cholinesterase. Determination of dibucaine numbers. Can J Biochem 1957;35:339 – 53.

Katz RL. Modification of the action of pancuronium by succinylcholine and halothane. Anesthesiology 1971;35:602 – 6.

Kohlschutter B, Bauer H, Roth F. Suxamethonium-induced hyperkalemia in patients with severe intraabdominal infections. Br J Anaesth 1976;48:557 – 62.

Krieg N, Hendrickx HH1, Crul JF. Influence of suxamethonium on the potency of ORG NC45 in anesthetized patients. Br J Anaesth 1981;53:259 – 62.

Lanier WL, Milde JH, Michenfelder JD: The cerebral effects of pancuronium and atracurium in halothane-anesthetized dogs. Anesthesiology 1985;63:589 – 97.

Lanier WL, Milde JH, Michenfelder JD. Cerebral stimulation following succinylcholine in dogs. Anesthesiology 1986;64:551 – 9.

Lebowitz PW, Ramsey FM, Savarese JJ, Ali HH. Potentiation of neuromuscular blockade in man produced by combinations of pancuronium and metocurine or pancuronium and d-tubocurarine. Anesth Analg 1980;59:604 – 9.

Lebowitz PW, Ramsey FM, Savarese JJ, Ali HH, deBros FM. Combination of pancuronium and metocurine: Neuromuscular and hemodynamic advantages over pancuronium alone. Anesth Analg 1981;60: 12 – 7.

Lebrault C, Berger JL, D'Hollander AA, Gomeni R, Henzel D, Duvaldestin P. Pharmacokinetics and pharmacodynamics of vecuronium (ORG NC45) in patients with cirrhosis. Anesthesiology 1985;62: 601 – 5.

Lebrault C. Duvaldestin P, Henzel D, Chauvin M, Guesnon P. Pharmacokinetics and pharmacodynamics of vecuronium in patients with cholestasis. Br J Anaesth 1986;58:983–7.

Lee C. Dose relationship of phase II, tachyphylaxis and train-of-four fade on suxamethonium-induced dual neuromuscular block in man. Br J Anaesth 1975;47:841–5.

Lee C, Chan D, Katz RL. Characteristics of nondepolarizing block. I. Post-junctional block by alpha-bungarotoxin. Can Anaesth Soc J 1977;24:212–9.

Leighton BL, Cheek TG, Gross JB *et al.* Succinylcholine pharmacodynamics in peripartum patients. Anesthesiology 1986;64:202–5.

Martyn JAJ, Matteo RS, Szyfelbein SK, Kaplan RF. Unprecedented resistance to neuromuscular blocking effects of metocurine, with persistence and complete recovery in a burned patient. Anesth Analg 1982;61:614–7.

Martyn JAJ, Szyfelbein SK, Ali HH, Matteo RS, Savarese JJ. Increased d-tubocurarine requirement following major thermal injury. Anesthesiology 1980;52:352–5.

Matteo RS, Backus WW, McDaniel DD, Brotherton WP, Abraham R, Diaz J. Pharmacokinetics and pharmacodynamics of d-tubocurarine and metocurine in the elderly. Anesth Analg 1985;64:23–9.

Matteo RS, Nishitateno K, Pua E, Spector S. Pharmacokinetics of d-tubocurarine in man: Effect of an osmotic diuretic on urinary excretion. Anesthesiology 1980;52:335–8.

Matteo RS, Pua EK, Khambatta HJ, Spector S. Cerebrospinal fluid levels of d-tubocurarine in man. Anesthesiology 1977;46:396–9.

Matteo RS, Spector S, Horowitz PE. Relation of serum d-tubocurarine concentration to neuromuscular blockade in man. Anesthesiology 1974;41:440–3.

McLeod K, Watson MJ, Rawlings MD. Pharmacokinetics of pancuronium in patients with normal and impaired renal function. Br J Anaesth 1976;48:341–5.

Mehta MP, Choi WW, Gergis SD, Sokoll MD, Adolphson AJ. Facilitation of rapid endotracheal intubations with divided doses of nondepolarizing neuromuscular blocking drugs. Anesthesiology 1985;62:392–5.

Merrett RA, Thompson CW, Webb FW. In vitro degradation of atracurium in human plasma. Br J Anaesth 1983;55:61–6.

Meyers EF. Partial recovery from pancuronium neuromuscular blockade following hydrocortisone administration. Anesthesiology 1977;46:148–50.

Miller RD, Agoston S, Booij LHDJ, Kersten U, Crul JF, Ham J. The comparative potency and pharmacokinetics of pancuronium and its metabolites in anesthetized man. J Pharmacol Exp Ther 1978a;207:539–43.

Miller RD, Agoston S, Van der Pol F, Booij LHDJ, Crul JF, Ham J. Hypothermia and pharmacokinetics and

pharmacodynamics of pancuronium in the cat. J Pharmacol Exp Ther 1978b;207:532–8.

Miller RD, Criqui M, Eger EI. The influence of duration of anesthesia on a d-tubocurarine neuromuscular blockade. Anesthesiology 1976a;44:207–10.

Miller, RD, Matteo R, Benet LZ, Sohn YJ. Influence of renal failure on the pharmacokinetics of d-tubocurarine in man. J Pharmacol Exp Ther 1977;202:1–7.

Miller RD, Roderick L. Diuretic-induced hypokalaemic pancuronium neuromuscular blockade and its antagonism by neostigmine. Br J Anaesth 1978a;50:541–4.

Miller RD, Roderick LL. Acid-base balance and neostigmine antagonism of pancuronium neuromuscular blockade. Br J Anaesth 1978b;50:317–24.

Miller RD, Rupp SM, Fisher DM, Cronnelly R, Fahey MR, Sohn YJ. Clinical pharmacology of vecuronium and atracurium. Anesthesiology 1984;61:444–53.

Miller RD, Sohn YJ, Matteo RS. Enhancement of d-tubocurarine neuromuscular blockade by diuretics in man. Anesthesiology 1976b;45:442–5.

Miller RD, Way WL. Inhibition of succinylcholine induced increased intragastric pressure by nondepolarizing muscle relaxants and lidocaine. Anesthesiology 1971;34:185–8.

Miller RD, Way WL, Dolan WM, Stevens WC, Eger EI. Comparative neuromuscular effects of pancuronium, gallamine, and succinylcholine during Forane and halothane anesthesia in man. Anesthesiology 1971;35:509–14.

Miller RD, Way WL, Hickey RL. Inhibition of succinylcholine induced increased intraocular pressure by nondepolarizing muscle relaxants. Anesthesiology 1968;29:123–6.

Miller RD, Way WL, Katzung BG. The potentiation of neuromuscular blocking agents by quinidine. Anesthesiology 1967;28:1036–41.

Minton MD, Grosslight K, Stirt JA, Bedford RF. Increases in intracranial pressure from succinylcholine: Prevention by prior nondepolarizing blockade. Anesthesiology 1986;65:165–9.

Mirakhur RK, Gibson FM, Ferres CJ. Vecuronium and d-tubocurarine combination: Potentiation of effect. Anesth Analg 1985;64:711–4.

Mitchell MM, Ali HH, Savarese JJ. Myotonia and neuromuscular blocking agents. Anesthesiology 1978;49:44–8.

Moorthy SS, Hilgenberg JC. Resistance to nondepolarizing muscle relaxants in paretic upper extremities of patients with residual hemiplegia. Anesth Analg 1980;59:624–7.

Morris RB, Cahalan MK, Miller RD, Wilkinson PL, Quasha AL, Robinson SL. The cardiovascular effects of vecuronium (ORG NC45) and pancuronium in patients undergoing coronary artery bypass grafting. Anesthesiology 1983;58:438–40.

Moss J, Rosow CE, Savarese JJ, Philbin DM, Kniffen KJ.

Role of histamine in the hypotensive action of d-tubocurarine in humans. Anesthesiology 1981; 55:19–25.

Munger WL, Miller RD, Stevens WC. The dependence of d-tubocurarine-induced hypotension on alveolar concentration of halothane, dose of d-tubocurarine, and nitrous oxide. Anesthesiology 1974;40: 442–8.

Munson ES, Wagman IH. Elevation of lidocaine seizure threshold by gallamine. Arch Neurol 1973;28:329–33.

Nigrovic V, Pandya JB, Auen M, Wajskol A. Inactivation of atracurium in human and rat plasma. Anesth Analg 1985;64:1047–52.

O'Hara DA, Fragen RJ, Shanks CA. The effects of age on the dose-response curves for vecuronium in adults. Anesthesiology 1985;63:542–4.

Ornstein E, Matteo RS, Young WL. Resistance to metocurine-induced neuromuscular blockade in patients receiving phenytoin. Anesthesiology 1985;63:294–8.

Pandey K, Badola RP, Kumar S. Time course of intraocular hypertension produced by suxamethonium. Br J Anaesth 1972;44:191–6.

Payne JP, Hughes R. Evaluation of atracurium in anesthetized man. Br J Anaesth 1981;53:45–56.

Pumplin DW, Fambrough DM. Turnover of acetylcholine receptors in skeletal muscle. Ann Rev Physiol 1982;44:319–35.

Raftery MA, Hunkapiller MW, Strader CD, Hood LE. Acetylcholine receptor: Complex of homologous subunits. Science 1980;208:1454–7.

Ramzan IM, Somogyi AA, Walker JS, Shanks CA, Triggs EJ. Clinical pharmacokinetics of the non-depolarizing muscle relaxants. Clin Pharmackin 1981;6:25–60.

Robbins R, Donati F, Bevan DR, Bevan JC. Differential effects of myoneural blocking drugs on neuromuscular transmission in infants. Br J Anaesth 1984;56:1095–9.

Rosa G, Orfei P, Sanfilippo M, Vilardi V. Gasparetto A. The effects of atracurium besylate (Tracrium) on intracranial pressure and cerebral perfusion pressure. Anesth Analg 1986a;65:381–4.

Rosa G, Sanfilippo M, Vilardi V, Orfei P, Gasparetto A. Effects of vecuronium bromide on intracranial pressure and cerebral perfusion pressure. Br J Anaesth 1986b;58:437–40.

Rupp SM, Fahey MR, Miller RD. Neuromuscular and cardiovascular effects of atracurium during nitrous oxide-isoflurane anaesthesia. Br J Anaesth 1983a;55:67S–70S.

Rupp SM, Fisher DM, Miller RD, Castagnoli K. Pharmacokinetics and pharmacodynamics of vecuronium in the elderly. Anesthesiology 1983b;59:A270.

Rupp SM, McChristian JW, Miller RD. Neuromuscular effects of atracurium during halothane-nitrous

oxide and enflurane-nitrous oxide anesthesia in humans. Anesthesiology 1985;63:16–9.

Rupp SM, Miller RD, Gencarelli P. Vecuronium-induced neuromuscular blockade during enflurane, isoflurane, and halothane anesthesia in humans. Anesthesiology 1984;60:102–5.

Ryan JF, Kagen LJ, Hyman AI. Myoglobinemia after a single dose of succinylcholine. N Engl J Med 1971;285:824–7.

Salem MR, Wong AY, Lin YH. The effect of suxamethonium on the intragastric pressure in infants and children. Br J Anaesth 1972;44:166–70.

Salmenpera M, Peltola K, Takkumen O, Heinonen J. Cardiovascular effects of pancuronium and vecuronium during high-dose fentanyl anesthesia. Anesth Analg 1983;62:1059–64.

Savage DS, Sleigh T, Carlyle I. The emergence of ORG NC45, 1 . . . (2 beta, 3 alpha, 5 alpha, 16 beta, 17 beta)-3,-17 bis (acetyloxy)-2-(1-piperidinyl)-androstan-16 y1) . . . -1-methyl piperidinium bromide from the pancuronium series. Br J Anaesth 1980;52:3S–10S.

Savarese JJ, Ali HH, Antonio RP. The clinical pharmacology of metocurine: Dimethyltubocurarine revisited. Anesthesiology 1977;47:277–84.

Schoenstadt DA, Whitcher CE. Observations on the mechanism of succinylcholine-induced cardiac arrhythmias. Anesthesiology 1963;24:358–62.

Schwarz S, Ilias W, Lackner F, Mayrhofer O, Foldes FF. Rapid tracheal intubation with vecuronium: The priming principle. Anesthesiology 1985;62:388–93.

Scott RPF, Savarese JJ. The cardiovascular and autonomic effects of neuromuscular blocking agents. Semi Anes 1985;3:319–34.

Scott RPF, Savarese JJ, Ali HH, *et al.* Atracurium: Clinical strategies for preventing histamine release and attenuating the hemodynamic response. Anesthesiology 1984;61:A287.

Shanks CA. Pharmacokinetics of the nondepolarizing neuromuscular relaxants applied to calculation of bolus and infusion dosage regimens. Anesthesiology 1986;64:72–86.

Shanks CA, Somogyi AA, Triggs EJ. Dose-response and plasma concentration - response relationships of pancuronium in man. Anesthesiology 1979;51: 111–8.

Shayevitz JR, Matteo RS. Decreased sensitivity to metocurine in patients with upper motorneuron disease. Anesth Analg 1985;64:767–72.

Shi W-Z, Fahey MR, Fisher DM, Miller RD, Canfell C, Eger EI. Laudanosine C (A metabolite of atracurium) increases the minimal alveolar concentration of halothane in rabbits. Anesthesiology 1985;63:584–8.

Sinatra RS, Philip BK, Naulty JS. Osthheimer GW. Prolonged neuromuscular blockade with vecuronium in a patient treated with magnesium sulfate. Anesth Analg 1985;64:1220–2.

Skarpa M, Dayan AD, Follenfant M, *et al.* Toxicity testing of atracurium. Br J Anaesth 1983;55:27S–9S.

Skivington MA. Protein binding of three tritiated muscle relaxants. Br J Anaesth 1972;44:1030–4.

Sklar GS, Lanks KW. Effects of trimethaphan and sodium nitroprusside on hydrolysis of succinylcholine in vitro. Anesthesiology 1977;47:31–3.

Sokoll MD, Gergis SD. Antibiotics and neuromuscular function. Anesthesiology 1981;55:148–59.

Sokoll MD, Gergis SD, Mehta M, Ali HH, Lineberry C. Safety and efficacy of atracurium (BW 33A) in surgical patients receiving balanced or isoflurane anesthesia. Anesthesiology 1983;58:450–5.

Standaert F. Release of transmitter at the neuromuscular junction. Br J Anaesth 1982;54:131–45.

Standaert FG. Donuts and holes: Molecules and muscle relaxants. Sem Anesth 1984;3:251–61.

Standaert FG, Adams JE. The actions of succinylcholine on the mammalian motor nerve terminal. J Pharmacol Exp Ther 1965;149:113–23.

Standaert FG, Dretchen KL. Cyclic nucleotides in neuromuscular transmission. Anesth Analg 1981;60:91–9.

Stanski DR, Ham J, Miller RD, Sheiner LB. Phramacokinetics and pharmacodynamics of d-tubocurarine during nitrous oxide-narcotic and halothane anesthesia in man. Anesthesiology 1979;51:235–41.

Stanski DR, Ham J, Miller RD, Sheiner LB. Time-dependent increase in sensitivity to d-tubocurarine during enflurane anesthesia in man. Anesthesiology 1980;52:483–7.

Starr NK, Sethna DH, Estafanous FG. Bradycardia and asystole following the rapid administration of sufentanil with vecuronium. Anesthesiology 1986;64:521–3.

Stenlake JB, Waigh RD, Urwin J, Dewar GH, Coker GG. Atracurium: Conception and inception. Br J Anaesth 1983;55:3S–10S.

Stirt JA, Katz RL, Murray AL, Guillot JP, Evreux JC. Modification of atracurium blockade by halothane and by suxamethonium. Br J Anaesth 1983;55:71S–7S.

Stoelting RK. The hemodynamic effects of pancuronium and d-tubocurarine in anesthetized patients. Anesthesiology 1972;36:612–5.

Stoelting RK. Hemodynamic effects of gallamine during halothane-nitrous oxide anesthesia. Anesthesiology 1973;39:645–7.

Stoelting RK. Hemodynamic effects of dimethyltubocurarine during nitrous oxide-halothane anesthesia. Anesth Analg 1974;53:513–5.

Stoelting RK. Comparison of gallamine and atropine as pretreatment before anesthetic induction and succinylcholine administration. Anesth Analg 1977;56:493–5.

Stoelting RK. Allergic reactions during anesthesia. Anesth Analg 1983;62:341–56.

Stoelting RK. Intermediate-acting neuromuscular blocking drugs. In: Stoelting RK, Barash PF, Gallagher TJ, eds. Advances in Anesthesia. Chicago, Year Book Medical Publishers, 1985:407.

Stoelting RK, Longnecker DE. Influence of end-tidal halothane concentration on d-tubocurarine hypotension. Anesth Analg 1972a;51:364–7.

Stoelting RK, Longnecker DE. Effects of promethazine on hypotension following d-tubocurarine use in anesthetized patients. Anesth Analg 1972b;51:509–13.

Stoelting RK, McCammon RL, Hilgenberg JC. Changes in blood pressure with varying rates of administration of d-tubocurarine. Anesth Analg 1980;59:697–9.

Stoelting RK, Peterson C. Adverse effects of increased succinylcholine dose following d-tubocurarine pretreatment. Anesth Analg 1975;54:282–8.

Stone WA, Beach TP, Hamelberg W. Succinylcholine — Danger in the spinal-cord-injured patient. Anesthesiology 1970;33:168–9.

Stroud RM. Acetylcholine receptor structure. Neurosci Comm 1983;1:124–38.

Sugimori T. Shortened action of succinylcholine in individuals with cholinesterase C₅ isozyme. Can Anaesth Soc J 1986;33:321–7.

Swen J, Gencarelli PJ, Koot HWJ. Vecuronium infusion dose requirements during fentanyl and halothane anesthesia in humans. Anesth Analg 1985;64:411–4.

Taboada JA, Rupp SM, Miller RD. Refining the priming principle for vecuronium during rapid-sequence induction of anesthesia. Anesthesiology 1986;64:243–7.

Taylor P. Are neuromuscular blocking agents more efficacious in pairs? Anesthesiology 1985;63:1–3.

Taylor DB, Creese R, Nedergaard PA, Case R. Labeling de-polarizing drugs in normal and denervated muscle. Nature 1965;208:901–2.

Thomson IR, Putnins CL. Adverse effects of pancuronium during high-dose fentanyl anesthesia for coronary artery bypass grafting. Anesthesiology 1985;62:708–13.

Vercruyse P, Bossuyt P, Hanegreffs G, Verbeuren TJ, Van Houtte PM. Gallamine and pancuronium inhibit pre- and post-junctional muscarinic receptors in canine saphenous veins. J Pharmacol Exp Ther 1979;209:225–30.

Viby-Mogensen J. Correlation of succinylcholine duration of action with plasma cholinesterase activity in subjects with the genotypically normal enzyme. Anesthesiology 1980;53:517–20.

Vitez TS, Miller RD, Eger EI, VanHyhuis LS, Way WL. Comparison in vitro of isoflurane and halothane potentiation of d-tubocurarine and succinylcholine neuromuscular blockades. Anesthesiology 1974; 41:53 – 6.

Ward S, Neill EAM. Pharmacokinetics of atracurium in acute hepatic failure (with acute renal failure). Br J Anaesth 1983;55:1169 – 72.

Ward S, Wright D. Combined pharmacokinetic and pharmacodynamic study of a single bolus dose of atracurium. Br J Anaesth 1983;55:35S – 8S.

Waters DJ, Mapleson WW. Suxamethonium pains: Hypothesis and observation. Anaesthesia 1971;26: 127 – 31.

Waud BE. Decrease in dose requirements of d-tubocurarine by volatile anesthetics. Anesthesiology 1979;51:298 – 302.

Waud BE, Waud DR. The relation between tetanic fade and receptor occlusion in the presence of competitive neuromuscular block. Anesthesiology 1971;35:456 – 64.

Waud BE, Waud DR. Comparison of drug-receptor dissociation constants at the mammalian neuromuscular junction in the presence and absence of halothane. J Pharmacol Exp Ther 1973;187:40 – 6.

Waud BE, Waud DR. The effects of diethyl ether, enflurane and isoflurane at the neuromuscular junction. Anesthesiology 1975;42:275 – 80.

Waud BE, Waud DR. Effects of volatile anesthesics on directly and indirectly stimulated muscle. Anesthesiology 1979;50:103 – 10.

Waud BE, Waud DR. Interaction among agents that block end-plate depolarization competitively. Anesthesiology 1985;63:4 – 15.

West R. Curare in man. Proc R Soc Med 1932;25:1107 – 16.

CHAPTER 9

Anticholinesterase Drugs and Cholinergic Agonists

Anticholinesterase drugs inhibit the enzyme, acetylcholinesterase (true cholinesterase) which is normally responsible for the hydrolysis of acetylcholine to choline and acetic acid. Acetylcholinesterase is one of the most efficient enzymes known with a single molecule having the capacity to hydrolyze an estimated 300,000 molecules of acetylcholine per minute (Taylor, 1985). Acetylcholinesterase is widely distributed in the body being present wherever acetylcholine is the neurotransmitter.

CLASSIFICATION

Anticholinesterase drugs are classified according to the mechanism by which they inhibit the activity of acetylcholinesterase (Fig. 9-1). Inhibition of acetylcholinesterase is by (1) reversible inhibition, (2) formation of carbamyl esters, and (3) irreversible inactivation by organophosphates.

Reversible Inhibition

Edrophonium is a quaternary ammonium anticholinesterase drug that lacks a carbamate group and thus produces reversible inhibition of acetylcholinesterase by virtue of its electrostatic attachment to the anionic site on the enzyme (Fig. 9-2). This binding is further stabilized by hydrogen bonding at the esteratic site on the enzyme (Fig. 9-2). The edrophonium-acetylcholinesterase enzyme com-

plex prevents the natural substrate, acetylcholine, from approximating correctly with enzyme. Because a true chemical bond is not formed, acetylcholine can easily compete with edrophonium for access to acetylcholinesterase, making the inhibition truly reversible. Indeed, the duration of action of edrophonium is considered to be brief, reflecting its reversible binding with acetylcholinesterase.

The predominant site of action of edrophonium appears to be presynaptic. This site of action may explain differences in dose-response relationships compared with longer-acting anticholinesterase drugs that presumably act principally at postsynaptic sites (Cronnelly et al, 1982).

Muscarinic effects of edrophonium are mild compared with longer-acting anticholinesterase drugs. Edrophonium is used to (1) antagonize the effects of nondepolarizing neuromuscular blocking drugs, (2) diagnose and assess therapy of myasthenia gravis and cholinergic crisis, and (3) evaluate the presence of dual blockade produced by succinylcholine.

Formation of Carbamyl Esters

Drugs such as physostigmine, neostigmine, and pyridostigmine produce reversible inhibition of acetylcholinesterase by formation of a carbamyl-ester complex at the esteratic site of the enzyme (Fig. 9-3). In contrast to edrophonium, these drugs act as competitive substrate substitutes for

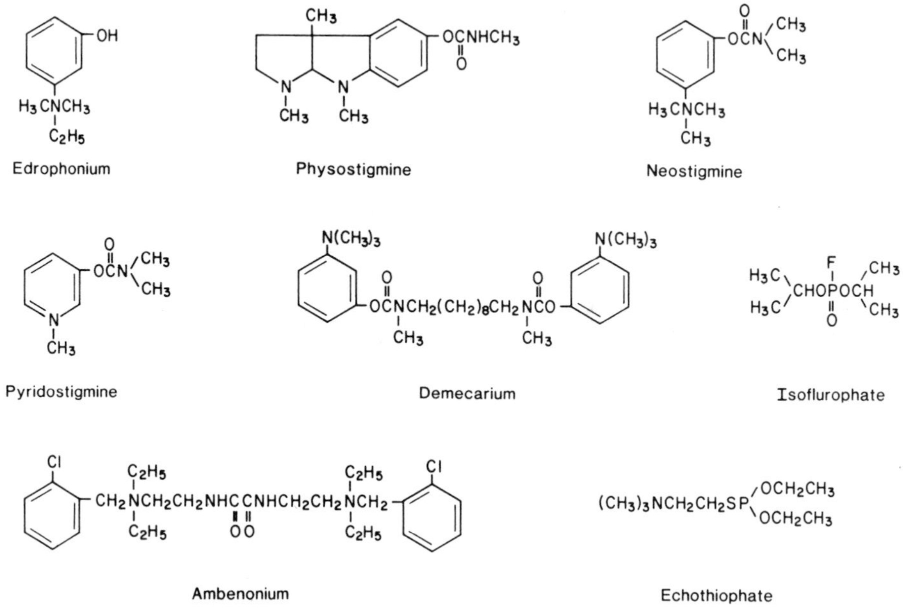

Edrophonium

Physostigmine

Neostigmine

Pyridostigmine

Demecarium

Isoflurophate

Ambenonium

Echothiophate

FIGURE 9-1. Anticholinesterase drugs.

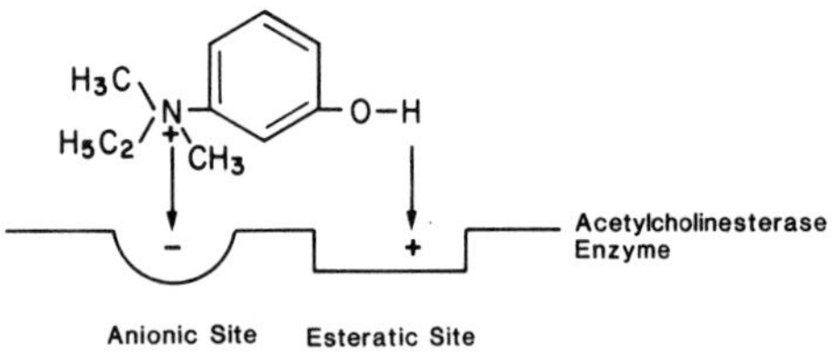

FIGURE 9-2. Edrophonium produces reversible inhibition of acetylcholinesterase by electrostatic attachment to the anionic site and hydrogen bonding at the esteratic site of the enzyme.

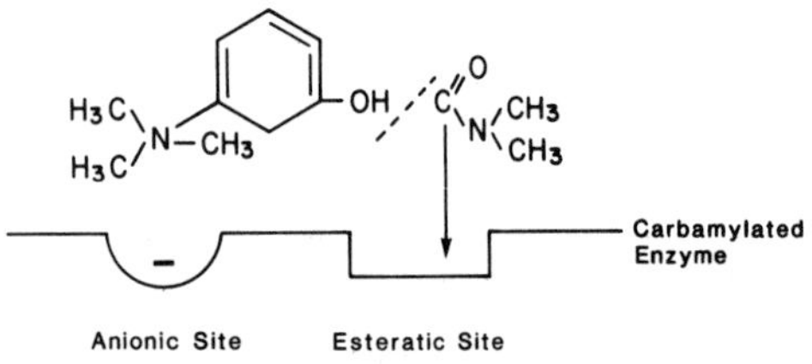

FIGURE 9-3. Drugs, such as physostigmine, neostigmine, and pyridostigmine, produce reversible inhibition of acetylcholinesterase by forming a carbamyl-ester complex at the esteratic site of the enzyme.

acetylcholine in the normal interaction with acetylcholinesterase. Indeed, the initial formation of drug-enzyme complex proceeds in the same way as the initial reaction between acetylcholine and anticholinesterase. Likewise, the next stage of formation of an intermediate acid-enzyme compound and first split product also proceeds normally. At this stage, there is transfer of a carbamate group to acetylcholinesterase at the esteratic site. This carbamylated acetylcholinesterase cannot hydrolyze acetylcholine until the carbamate-enzyme bond dissociates. Neostigmine also has presynaptic actions as manifested by an increased rate of repetitive firing following a single impulse. This repetitive firing also contributes to the buildup of acetylcholine at the neuromuscular junction.

Irreversible Inactivation

Organophosphate anticholinesterase drugs combine with acetylcholinesterase at the esteratic site to form a stable inactive complex that does not undergo hydrolysis (Fig. 9-4). Echothiophate interacts with both the esteratic and anionic subsites, thus accounting for its extreme potency.

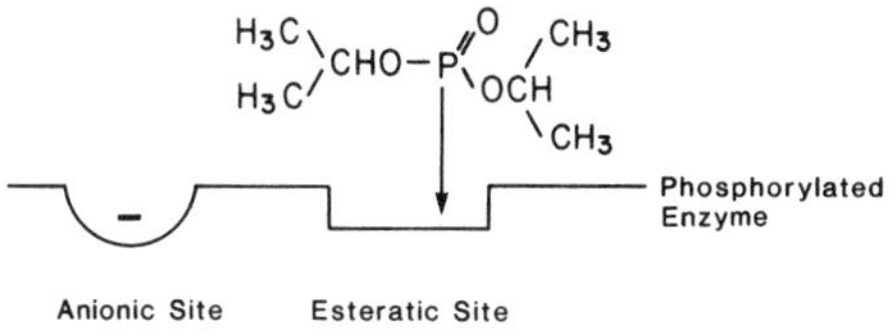

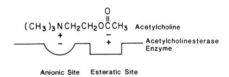

FIGURE 9-4. Organophosphate anticholinesterase drugs produce irreversible inhibition of acetylcholinesterase by forming a phosphorylate complex at the esteratic site of the enzyme.

Spontaneous regeneration of acetylcholinesterase either requires several hours or does not occur requiring synthesis of new enzyme.

Echothiophate is the only organophosphate anticholinesterase drug used clinically (Fig. 9-1) (see the section entitled Therapeutic Uses of Anticholinesterase Drugs). Other drugs such as parathion and malathion are used as insecticides. Malathion is a selective insecticide because enzymes necessary for its metabolism are absent in insects. In mammals and birds, malathion undergoes extensive hydrolysis by enzymes known as phosphorylphosphatases before excretion in the urine. Nerve gases such as tabum, saran, and soman are extremely lipid-soluble organophosphate inhibitors, and absorption can occur even through intact skin.

STRUCTURE ACTIVITY RELATIONSHIPS

Acetylcholinesterase consists of an anionic and esteratic site which are so arranged that they are complementary to the natural substrate, acetylcholine (Fig.9-5). The anionic site of the enzyme binds the quaternary nitrogen of acetylcholine. This binding serves to orient the ester linkage of acetylcholine to the esteratic site of acetylcholinesterase (Fig. 9-5). Thus, acetylcholinesterase has an optimum substrate concentration and is less effective against longer chain substrates.

Neostigmine is a quaternary ammonium derivative of physostigmine having a greater stability and equal or greater potency (Fig. 9-1). Pyridostigmine is a closely related congener of neostigmine (Fig. 9-1). An increase in anticholinesterase potency and duration of action occurs from linking two quaternary ammonium nuclei by a chain of appropriate structure and length. For ex-

ample, the potent anticholinesterase drug, demecarium, is two molecules of neostigmine connected at the carbamate nitrogen atoms by a series of 10 methylene groups (Fig. 9-1). Another bis-quaternary compound is ambenonium which binds strongly to acetylcholinesterase and exerts direct effects at both prejunctional and postjunctional membranes (Fig. 9-1).

PHARMACOKINETICS

Edrophonium, neostigmine, and pyridostigmine do not differ in terms of their pharmacokinetics (Table 9-1) (Cronnelly *et al,* 1979; Cronnelly *et al,* 1980; Cronnelly and Morris, 1982; Morris *et al,* 1981). The similarity in pharmacokinetics among these anticholinesterase drugs means that differences in potency are most likely explained on a pharmacodynamic basis. Affinity for acetylcholinesterase is probably of major importance in determining the relative potency of these drugs as anticholinesterase inhibitors. The fact that edrophonium dose response curves are not parallel to those for neostigmine and pyridostigmine suggests that different mechanisms of action may be involved for the different anticholinesterase drugs (Fig. 9-6) (Cronnelly *et al,* 1982).

Lipid Solubility

Anticholinesterase drugs containing a quaternary ammonium group (edrophonium, neostigmine, pyridostigmine) are poorly lipid soluble and thus do not easily penetrate lipid cell membrane barriers such as the gastrointestinal tract or blood–brain barrier. Lipid-soluble drugs, such as tertiary amines (*e.g.,* physostigmine) and organophosphates, are readily absorbed from the gastrointes-

$$(CH_3)_3 N CH_2 CH_2 O \overset{O}{\overset{\|}{C}} CH_3 \quad \text{Acetylcholine}$$

Acetylcholinesterase Enzyme

Anionic Site   Esteratic Site

FIGURE 9-5. The anionic and esteratic sites of acetylcholinesterase are so arranged that they are complimentary to the quaternary nitrogen and ester linkage of acetylcholine respectively.

Table 9-1

Comparative Characteristics of Anticholinesterase Drugs Administered to Antagonize Nondepolarizing Neuromuscular Blockade

	Elimination Half-Time (minutes)		Volume of Distribution ($L\ kg^{-1}$)		Clearance ($ml\ kg^{-1}\ min^{-1}$)		Renal Contribution to Total Clearance (%)	Speed of Onset	Duration (minutes)	Principal Site Of Action	Dose of Atropine ($\mu g\ kg^{-1}$)
	Normal	Anephric	Normal	Anephric	Normal	Anephric					
Edrophonium ($0.5\ mg\ kg^{-1}$)	110	206	1.1	0.7	9.6	2.7	66	Rapid	60	Presynaptic	7
Neostigmine ($0.043\ mg\ kg^{-1}$)	80	183	0.7	0.8	9.0	3.4	54	Intermediate	60	Presynaptic Postsynaptic	15
Pyridostigmine ($0.35\ mg\ kg^{-1}$)	112	379	1.1	1.0	8.6	2.1	76	Delayed	90	Postsynaptic	15

(Data from Cronnelly R, Stanski DR, Miller RD, Sheiner LB, Sohn YJ. Renal function and the pharmacokinetics of neostigmine in anesthetized patients. Anesthesiology 1979;51:222–6; Cronnelly R, Stanski DR, Miller RD, Sheiner LB. Pyridostigmine kinetics with and without renal function. Clin Pharmacol Ther 1980;28:78–81; Cronnelly R, Morris RB: Antagonism of neuromuscular blockade. Br J Anaesth 1982;54:183–93; Morris RB, Cronnelly R, Miller RD, Stanski DR, Fahey MR. Pharmacokinetics of edrophonium and neostigmine when antagonizing d-tubocurarine neuromuscular blockade in man. Anesthesiology 1981;54:399–402.)

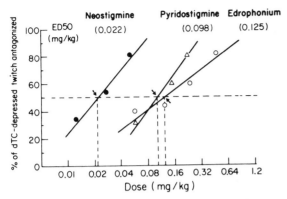

FIGURE 9-6. The dose response curve for edrophonium is not parallel to the curves for neostigmine and pyridostigmine suggesting different mechanisms of action for the various anticholinesterase drugs. (From Cronnelly R, Morris RB, Miller RD. Edrophonium: Duration of action and atropine requirement in humans during halothane anesthesia. Anesthesiology 1982;57:261–6. Reproduced by permission of the authors and publisher.)

(*i.e.,* acetylcholinesterase inhibition) action whereas the postsynaptic action is predominant for neostigmine and pyridostigmine (Fig. 9-7) (Blabler, 1972; Cronnelly *et al,* 1982; Miller *et al,* 1974). It is also possible that onset times could reflect differences in rate constants at presynaptic and postsynaptic sites of action. The slower onset of action of neostigmine and pyridostigmine compared with edrophonium is not related to the need to form active metabolites (Hennis *et al,* 1984).

Renal Clearance

Renal excretion accounts for about 50% of the elimination of neostigmine and about 75% of the elimination of edrophonium and pyridostigmine. This large proportion of renal clearance suggests a role for renal tubular secretory mechanisms as well as glomerular filtration. The elimination half-times of these anticholinesterase drugs are greatly prolonged by renal failure (Table 9-1) (Cronnelly

tinal tract or across mucous membranes and have predictable effects on the central nervous system.

Volume of Distribution

The large volume of distribution of quaternary ammonium anticholinesterase drugs compared with nondepolarizing neuromuscular blocking drugs is surprising because these drugs would not be expected to easily cross lipid membranes (Table 9-1). Presumably, this large volume of distribution reflects extensive tissue storage in organs such as the liver or kidneys. The liver, as a site of this tissue uptake, is suggested by the presence of unchanged volumes of distribution in anephric patients (Table 9-1).

Onset of Action

Because the pharmacokinetics of anticholinesterase drugs are similar, it is likely that differences in onset of action reflect a pharmacodynamic mechanism. For example, the more rapid onset of action of edrophonium may reflect a presynaptic (*i.e.,* acetylcholine release) rather than a postsynaptic

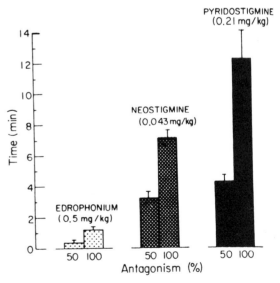

FIGURE 9-7. Comparison of the onset of action of anticholinesterase drugs as reflected by antagonism of drug-induced neuromuscular blockade. Mean ± SE. (From Cronnelly R, Morris RB, Miller RD. Edrophonium: Duration of action and atropine requirement in humans during halothane anesthesia. Anesthesiology 1982;57:261–6. Reproduced by permission of the authors and publisher.)

et al, 1979; Cronnelly et al, 1980). As a result, plasma clearance of anticholinesterase drugs will be delayed as long as, if not longer than, the nondepolarizing neuromuscular blocking drugs, making the occurrence of recurarization unlikely.

Metabolism

In the absence of renal function, hepatic metabolism accounts for 50% of a dose of neostigmine, 30% of edrophonium, and 25% of pyridostigmine. The principal metabolite of neostigmine is 3-hydroxyphenyltrimethylammonium which has about one-tenth the antagonist activity of the parent compound (Hennis et al, 1984). The principal metabolite of pyridostigmine is 3-hydroxy-N-methylpyridinium which lacks pharmacologic activity. Edrophonium undergoes conjugation to edrophonium glucuronide which is presumed to be pharmacologically inactive. Physostigmine is hydrolyzed at its ester linkage, and renal excretion is of minor importance.

Influence of Patient Age

The time course of onset and duration of antagonism produced by equipotent doses of neostigmine is similar in infants, children, and adults (Fisher et al, 1983). However, the dose of neostigmine required to produce 50% antagonism of d-tubocurarine-induced neuromuscular blockade is less in neonates and children (13.1–15.5 μg kg^{-1}) than adults (22.9 μg kg^{-1}) (Fisher et al, 1983). Conversely, dose requirements for edrophonium are not different for infants, children, and adults (Fisher et al, 1984). This difference between edrophonium and neostigmine further supports the concept that they antagonize neuromuscular blockade by different mechanisms (Cronnelly and Morris, 1982). It is likely that the age-related differences for dose requirements of neostigmine are related to pharmacodynamic mechanisms since the pharmacokinetics are similar in pediatric and young adult age groups (Fisher et al, 1983). Conversely, the duration of the maximum response produced by neostigmine is prolonged in elderly compared with younger patients reflecting a smaller extracellular fluid volume in elderly patients (Young et al, 1984). Pharmacodynamics are not altered as emphasized by similar responses evoked by neostigmine at the same plasma concentration in middle-aged and elderly adults.

PHARMACOLOGIC EFFECTS

Pharmacologic effects of anticholinesterase drugs are predictable and reflect the accumulation of acetylcholine at muscarinic and nicotinic cholinergic receptor sites. Depending on the reason for administration of anticholinesterase drugs, these effects may be considered therapeutic or undesirable.

Muscarinic cholinergic effects, such as bradycardia, salivation, miosis, and hyperperistalsis are evoked by lower concentrations of acetylcholine than are required for production of nicotinic effects at autonomic ganglia and the neuromuscular junction. For this reason, the use of an anticholinesterase drug to reverse nondepolarizing neuromuscular blocking drugs also includes administration of an anticholinergic drug to prevent adverse muscarinic cholinergic effects that would otherwise be associated with the high dose of anticholinesterase drug (see the section entitled Reversal of Neuromuscular Blockade). The anticholinergic drug selectively blocks the effects of acetylcholine at muscarinic cholinergic receptors while leaving intact responses to acetylcholine at the nicotinic cholinergic receptors. Neostigmine and pyridostigmine, but not edrophonium, produce marked and prolonged inhibition of plasma cholinesterase activity (Mirakhur, 1986). Indeed, prolonged effects of succinylcholine that is administered shortly following reversal of nondepolarizing neuromuscular blockade may reflect this enzyme inhibition.

Cardiovascular System

Cardiovascular effects of anticholinesterase drugs reflect effects of accumulated acetylcholine on the heart and blood vessels by actions at autonomic ganglia and postganglionic cholinergic nerve fibers. The predominant effect on the heart from the peripheral actions of accumulated acetylcholine is bradycardia due to slowed conduction velocity of the cardiac impulse through the atrioventricular node. Typically, blood vessels are dilated, although the coronary and pulmonary circulations may manifest an opposite response. Reductions in blood pressure that accompany accumulation of acetylcholine presumably reflect decreases in peripheral vascular resistance.

Gastrointestinal Tract

Anticholinesterase drugs enhance gastric fluid secretion by parietal cells and increase motility of the entire gastrointestinal tract, particularly the large intestine. For example, neostigmine counters inhibition of gastric motility induced by atropine and enhances the stimulatory effect of morphine. The lower portion of the esophagus is stimulated by neostigmine, resulting in a beneficial increase in tone and peristalsis in patients with achalasia. Neostigmine, 0.5 to 1 mg subcutaneously, is often effective in treatment of paralytic ileus or atony of the urinary bladder. This treatment, however, should not be used when there is mechanical obstruction of the gastrointestinal tract or urinary bladder. Actions of anticholinesterase drugs on gastrointestinal motility most likely reflect effects of accumulated acetylcholine at the ganglion cells of Auerbach's plexus and on smooth muscle fibers (see Chapter 54).

Anticholinesterase drugs applied topically to the cornea cause constriction of the sphincter of the iris (miosis) and ciliary muscle. Constriction of the ciliary muscle manifests as inability to focus for near vision. This spasm of accommodation is usually shorter in duration than is miosis. Intraocular pressure declines due to facilitation of outflow of aqueous humor (see the section entitled Treatment of Glaucoma).

Salivary Glands

Anticholinesterase drugs augment production of secretions of glands that are innervated by postganglionic cholinergic fibers. Such glands include bronchial, lacrimal, sweat, salivary, gastric, intestinal, and acinar pancreatic glands. Smooth muscle fibers of bronchioles and ureters are contracted by anticholinesterase drugs.

Beta-Adrenergic Blockade

Theoretically, beta-adrenergic blockade would result in a predominance of parasympathetic nervous system activity at the heart which might be exaggerated by the subsequent administration of an anticholinesterase drug to reverse nondepolarizing neuromuscular blockade (Sprague, 1975; Prys-Roberts, 1979). Nevertheless, bradycardia does not accompany mixtures of atropine and neostigmine or pyridostigmine administered to animals with acutely produced beta-adrenergic blockade using propranolol (Wagner *et al*, 1982).

CLINICAL USES

The principal clinical uses of anticholinesterase drugs are for (1) reversal of neuromuscular blockade as produced by nondepolarizing neuromuscular blockings drugs, (2) treatment of central nervous system effects produced by certain drugs, (3) treatment of myasthenia gravis, and (4) treatment of glaucoma.

Reversal of Neuromuscular Blockade

Antagonism of drug-induced neuromuscular blockade by neostigmine, pyridostigmine, or edrophonium reflects increased availability of acetylcholine at the neuromuscular junction by virtue of inhibition of acetylcholinesterase which is necessary for the hydrolysis of acetylcholine. Physostigmine is not used for reversal of neuromuscular blockade as the dose required is excessive. Increased amounts of acetylcholine in the region of the neuromuscular junction improve the chances that two acetylcholine molecules will bind to the alpha subunits of the nicotinic cholinergic receptor (Standaert, 1984). This tips the balance of the competition between acetylcholine and a nondepolarizing neuromuscular blocking drug in favor of the neurotransmitter and restores neuromuscular transmission. In addition, anticholinesterase drugs may generate antidromic action potentials and repetitive firing of motor nerve endings (*e.g.,* presynaptic effects) (Donati *et al,* 1983). These postsynaptic and presynaptic mechanisms are dose-related and operate simultaneously to restore neuromuscular transmission in the presence of nondepolarizing neuromuscular blocking drugs.

In comparison with neostigmine, edrophonium is more and pyridostigmine is less effective at presynaptic receptors (Donati *et al,* 1983). Conceivably, matching the principal site of action of the anticholinesterase drug with that of the neuromuscular blocking drug (*i.e.,* presynaptic versus postsynaptic) would result in more selective antagonism with a minimum dose of anticholinesterase drug.

Onset and Duration of Action

Edrophonium, 0.5 mg kg^{-1}, produces antagonism of neuromuscular blockade that is equal in magnitude to that produced by neostigmine, 0.043 mg kg^{-1}, or pyridostigmine, 0.21 mg kg^{-1} (Fig. 9-8) (Cronnelly *et al*, 1982; Miller *et al*, 1974). Edrophonium has the most rapid onset of action, followed by neostigmine and pyridostigmine (Fig. 9-7) (Cronnelly *et al*, 1982; Miller *et al*, 1974). When twitch height is depressed 90% or greater, the dose of edrophonium may need to be increased to 1 mg kg^{-1} to produce as rapid an onset as neostigmine (Rupp *et al*, 1986). Although edrophonium in the past has been considered a short-acting drug, controlled studies in anesthetized patients have documented that the duration of action of edrophonium does not differ from neostigmine (Cronnelly *et al*, 1982). Because neostigmine, pyridostigmine, and edrophonium have similar elimination half-times but pyridostigmine has a longer duration of action, the time course of reversal of neuromuscular blockade may

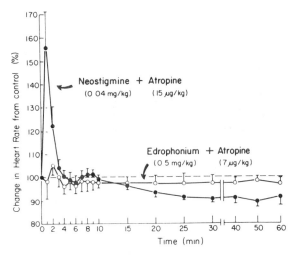

FIGURE 9-9. Heart rate changes are less following the administration of edrophonium-atropine than following administration of neostigmine-atropine. Mean ± SE. (From Cronnelly R, Morris RB, Miller RD. Edrophonium: Duration of action and atropine requirement in humans during halothane anesthesia. Anesthesiology 1982;57:261–6. Reproduced by permission of the authors and publisher.)

be unrelated to the clearance of anticholinesterase drugs from the plasma.

Mixture with Anticholinergic Drugs

Reversal of neuromuscular blockade requires only the nicotinic cholinergic effects of the anticholinesterase drug. Therefore, muscarinic cholinergic effects of the anticholinesterase drug are prevented by the concurrent administration of an anticholinergic drug such as atropine or glycopyrrolate (Table 9-1). For example, neostigmine and pyridostigmine both require atropine, 15 μg kg^{-1}, to prevent bradycardia and excessive salivation (Fogdall and Miller, 1973). Initial tachycardia observed when atropine is administered simultaneously with neostigmine or pyridostigmine reflects the slower onset of these anticholinesterase drugs relative to atropine. The lesser muscarinic stimulant effects of edrophonium and its more rapid onset of action result in less variation in heart rate when administered with atropine (Fig. 9-9) (Cronnelly *et al*, 1982). Indeed, edrophonium requires less atropine (7 μg kg^{-1}) to prevent associated heart rate changes.

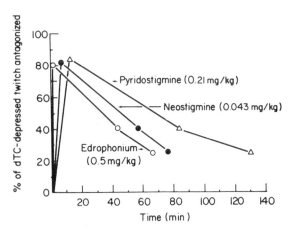

FIGURE 9-8. Edrophonium produces antagonism of drug-induced neuromuscular blockade that is similar in magnitude to that produced by neostigmine or pyridostigmine. (From Cronnelly R, Morris RB, Miller RD. Edrophonium: Duration of action and atropine requirement in humans during halothane anesthesia. Anesthesiology 1982;57:261–6. Reproduced by permission of the authors and publisher.)

The more delayed onset of cardiac vagal effects of glycopyrrolate is appropriately matched for the slower onset of action of neostigmine and pyridostigmine, while the more rapid onset of vagolytic activity provided by atropine more closely parallels the onset of activity produced by edrophonium (Azar *et al,* 1983; Ramamurthy *et al,* 1972). Indeed, a mixture of neostigmine and glycopyrrolate (7 μg kg⁻¹) results in less tachycardia than a mixture of neostigmine and atropine. Conversely, bradycardia is likely following administration of an edrophonium–glycopyrrolate mixture but not an edrophonium–atropine mixture (Fig. 9-10) (Azar *et al,* 1983). A mixture of edrophonium and atropine is also superior to a mixture of edrophonium and glycopyrrolate because edrophonium and atropine have similar durations of action. Furthermore, late bradycardia is more likely when short-acting atropine rather than long-acting glycopyrrolate is combined with neostigmine. This emphasizes the value of matching both the onset and duration of action of the anticholinergic drug to the anticholinesterase drug.

Excessive Neuromuscular Blockade

Once acetylcholinesterase is maximally inhibited, administration of additional anticholinesterase

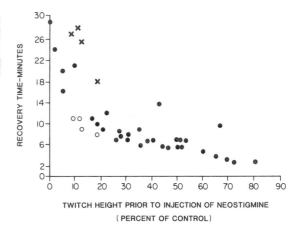

FIGURE 9-11.   The rate of antagonism of drug-induced neuromuscular blockade parallels the magnitude of blockade present just before administration of the anticholinesterase drug. (From Katz RL. Clinical neuromuscular pharmacology of pancuronium. Anesthesiology 1971;34:550–6. Reproduced by permission of the author and publisher.)

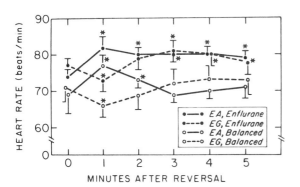

FIGURE 9-10.   Bradycardia is more likely to occur following the administration of edrophonium-glycopyrrolate (EG) than following administration of edrophonium-atropine (EA). Mean ±SE. *P<0.05 compared with heart rate at zero time just before administration of the drug combination. (From Azar I, Pham AN, Karambelkar DJ, Lear E. The heart rate following edrophonium-atropine and edrophonium-glycopyrrolate mixtures. Anesthesiology 1983;59:139–41. Reproduced by permission of the authors and publisher.)

drug does not further antagonize nondepolarizing neuromuscular blockade. For this reason, persistence of neuromuscular blockade despite large doses of anticholinesterase drugs (neostigmine, 70 μg kg⁻¹, or equivalent doses of the other anticholinesterase drugs) is often an indication to mechanically ventilate the lungs until neuromuscular blockade dissipates with time.

Events that Influence Reversal of Neuromuscular Blockade

The speed and extent of reversal of neuromuscular blockade by anticholinesterase drugs are influenced by a number of factors including the (1) intensity of the preexisting neuromuscular blockade and (2) nondepolarizing neuromuscular blocking drug being antagonized. For example, the rate of antagonism directly parallels the magnitude of neuromuscular blockade present just before administration of the anticholinesterase drug (Fig. 9-11) (Katz, 1971). Comparable degrees of neuromuscular blockade due to gallamine are reversed less rapidly by neostigmine than is neuromuscular blockade produced by d-tubocurarine or pancuronium (Miller *et al,* 1972).

Antagonism of neuromuscular blockade by anticholinesterase drugs may be inhibited or even prevented by (1) certain antibiotics, (2) hypothermia, (3) respiratory acidosis associated with a $PaCO_2$ above 50 mmHg, (4) hypokalemia and metabolic alkalosis (Fig. 9-12) (Miller *et al,* 1975).

4-Aminopyridine

4-Aminopyridine has advantages over neostigmine and pyridostigmine for reversing neuromuscular blockade. These advantages include (1) longer duration of action, (2) absence of muscarinic effects, and (3) effectiveness in antagonizing antibiotic-potentiated neuromuscular blockade. This drug is presumed to enhance the presynaptic release of acetylcholine by facilitating the entry of calcium ions into nerve endings (Molgo *et al,* 1977). The dose of 4-aminopyridine necessary to antagonize neuromuscular blockade (1 mg kg^{-1}), however, produces central nervous system stimulation. For this reason, 4-aminopyridine has been combined with anticholinesterase drugs in an attempt to reduce the dose of both drugs and thus minimize side effects. Indeed, 0.35 mg kg^{-1} of 4-aminopyridine reduces by 68% to 75% the amount of anticholinesterase drug required to reliably antagonize nondepolarizing neuromuscular blockade (Fig. 9-13) (Miller *et al,* 1979). 4-Aminopyridine has also been used to treat Eaton-Lambert syndrome, botulism, and myasthenia gravis (Lundh *et al* 1979).

Treatment of Central Nervous System Effects of Certain Drugs

Physostigmine, a tertiary amine, crosses the blood–brain barrier and is thus effective in antagonizing adverse central nervous system effects of certain drugs.

Anticholinergic Drugs

Physostigmine, 10 to 30 μg kg^{-1}, administered intravenously is effective in antagonizing restlessness and confusion (*e.g.,* central anticholinergic syndrome) due to atropine or scopolamine (see Chapter 10). Presumably, physostigmine increases concentrations of acetylcholine in the brain making more neurotransmitter available for interaction with cholinergic receptors. The duration of action of physostigmine is shorter than that of anticholinergic drugs. For this reason, it may be necessary to repeat the dose of physostigmine used in the treatment of central anticholinergic syndrome.

Opioids

Physostigmine may reverse the depression of the ventilatory response to carbon dioxide but not analgesia produced by prior administration of morphine (Snir-Mor *et al,* 1983; Weinstock *et al,* 1982). It is speculated that opioids diminish the ventilatory response to carbon dioxide by reducing the amounts of acetylcholine in the area of the respiratory center that would normally be released in response to hypercarbia. Other data, however, do not support an antagonist effect of physostigmine on opioid-induced depression of ventilation (Bourke *et al,* 1984).

Benzodiazepines

Physostigmine may increase the state of consciousness in patients sedated by diazepam (Bidwai *et al,* 1979). Considering the selective anticholinesterase effect of physostigmine, it is surprising that the effects of benzodiazepines, which facilitate the gamma-aminobutyric acid neurotransmitter system, would be altered. Despite partial reversal of sedation, the administra-

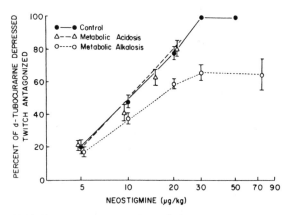

FIGURE 9-12. Antagonism of drug-induced neuromuscular blockade by anticholinesterase drugs is impaired by metabolic alkalosis. Mean $\pm$ SE. (From Miller RD *et al.*: Anesthesiology 1975;42:377–83. Reproduced by permission of the authors and publisher.)

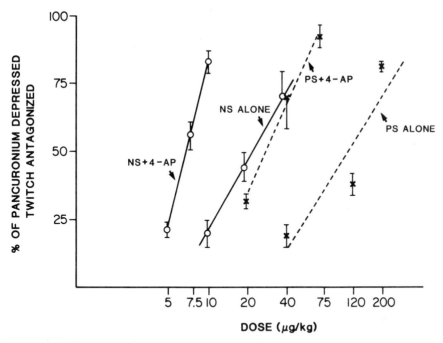

FIGURE 9-13. Dose response curves for reversal of pancuronium-induced neuromuscular blockade with neostigmine (NS) or pyridostigmine (PS) alone or combined with 4-aminopyridine (4-AP). Mean ±SE. (From Miller RD, Booij LDHJ, Agoston S, Crul JF. Aminopyridine potentiates neostigmine and pyridostigmine in man. Anesthesiology 1979;50:416–20. Redrawn by permission of the authors and publisher).

tion of physostigmine may, at the same time, further decrease the ventilatory response to carbon dioxide associated with diazepam (Spaulding *et al,* 1984).

Anesthetics

Physostigmine reduces postoperative somnolence following anesthesia with a volatile anesthetic (Hill *et al,* 1977). Furthermore, physostigmine produces electroencephalographic evidence of arousal during administration of halothane (Roy and Stullken, 1981). Perhaps physostigmine is acting by permitting accumulation of acetylcholine at muscarinic cholinergic receptors in the ascending reticular activating system. Reversal of the adverse central nervous system effects of ketamine by physostigmine while analgesia remains intact have been described (Balmer and Wyte, 1977). Sedative effects of other drugs, including phenothiazines and tricyclic antidepressants, may also be reversed by physostigmine.

Treatment of Myasthenia Gravis

Neostigmine, pyridostigmine, and ambenonium are the standard anticholinesterase drugs used in the symptomatic treatment of myasthenia gravis. These drugs increase the response of skeletal muscles to repetitive impulses presumably by increasing the availability of endogenous acetylcholine.

The quaternary ammonium structure of neostigmine and pyridostigmine limits the oral absorption of these drugs. For example, the oral dose of neostigmine is about 30 times greater than the intravenous dose. The interval between oral doses is usually 2 to 4 hours for neostigmine and 3 to 6 hours for pyridostigmine or ambenonium.

Muscarinic cardiovascular and gastrointestinal side effects are controlled as necessary with anticholinergic drugs.

In the assessment of anticholinesterase drug therapy of myasthenia gravis, intravenous edrophonium is used in 1 mg increments administered every 1 to 2 minutes until a change in symptoms is observed. Inadequate anticholinesterase drug therapy is diagnosed if there is a decrease in myasthenic symptoms. Conversely, patients with excess anticholinesterase drug therapy experiencing a cholinergic crisis develop increased skeletal muscle weakness with administration of edrophonium.

Treatment of Glaucoma

Anticholinesterase drugs reduce intraocular pressure in patients with narrrow-angle and wide-angle glaucoma reflecting a decrease in the resistance to outflow of aqueous humor. Treatment of glaucoma with long-acting anticholinesterase drugs (echothiophate, demecarium, isoflurophate) for 6 months or longer carries the risk of cataract formation. For this reason, short-acting miotic anticholinesterase drugs are used initially with introduction of long-acting miotic anticholinesterase drugs only when the therapeutic response to the short-acting drugs is not effective. Beta-adrenergic antagonists, such as timilol, do not produce miosis, but do reduce intraocular pressure by decreasing the secretion of aqueous humor (see Chapter 14).

OVERDOSE OF ANTICHOLINESTERASE DRUGS

Effects of acute intoxication by anticholinesterase drugs manifest as muscarinic and nicotinic symptoms on peripheral and central nervous system sites. Muscarinic symptoms include miosis, difficulty focusing, salivation, bronchoconstriction, bradycardia, abdominal cramps, and loss of bladder and rectal control. Nicotinic actions at the neuromuscular junction range from skeletal muscle weakness to overt paralysis with resulting apnea. Central nervous system actions include confusion, ataxia, seizures, coma, and depression of ventilation.

The diagnosis of anticholinesterase drug overdose is made by the history of exposure and characteristic signs and symptoms. Organophosphate anticholinesterases, as present in insecticides, are rapidly absorbed by the lungs, skin, and gastrointestinal tract and may be the cause of toxic symptoms. Accidental posioning from these drugs most often occurs by inhalation or dermal absorption. The high lipid solubility of organophosphate anticholinesterases ensures that these drugs will cross the blood–brain barrier easily and produce intense effects on the central nervous system.

Treatment

Treatment of anticholinesterase drug overdose is with atropine occasionally supplemented by an acetylcholinesterase reactivator, pralidoxime (Fig. 9-14). Atropine (35–70 μg kg^{-1} administered intravenously every 3–10 minutes until muscarinic symptoms disappear) is specific for reversing the muscarinic effects of excess acetylcholine but has no impact on nicotinic actions at the neuromuscular junction. Effects of excess acetylcholine at the neuromuscular junction and, to a lesser extent, effects at autonomic ganglia can be reversed by intravenous administration over 2 minutes of pralidoxime, 15 mg kg^{-1}. This dose is repeated after 20 minutes if skeletal muscle weakness is not reversed. Central nervous system effects are not antagonized by pralidoxime.

Pralidoxime is more effective in countering the effects of drugs that phosphorylate acetylcholinesterase than against drugs that carbamylate the enzyme. Furthermore, pralidoxime may not be effective unless it is administered within minutes after exposure to the potent anticholinesterase drug.

In addition to specific pharmacologic antagonism, treatment of anticholinesterase drug overdose includes supportive measures such as intubation of the trachea and mechanical ventilation of the lungs. Seizures may require suppression with drugs such as thiopental.

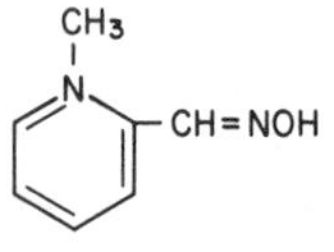

FIGURE 9-14. Pralidoxime.

SYNTHETIC CHOLINERGIC AGONISTS

Synthetic cholinergic agonist drugs have as their primary action the activation of cholinergic receptors that are innervated by postganglionic parasympathetic nerves. Additional actions are exerted on ganglia and on cells that do not receive extensive parasympathetic innervation but, nevertheless, possess cholinergic receptors.

Acetylcholine has no therapeutic application because of its diffuse sites of action and rapid hydrolysis by acetylcholinesterase and to a lesser extent by plasma cholinesterase. Derivatives of acetylcholine have been synthesized that have more selective effects and prolonged durations of action. Of the synthetic acetylcholine derivatives, only methacholine, carbachol, and bethanechol have clinical usefulness (Fig. 9-15). The muscarinic actions of all these drugs are blocked selectively by atropine.

These drugs are administered orally, subcutaneously, or topically to the eye. Asthma, coronary artery disease, and peptic ulcer disease are examples of diseases which could be exacerbated by cholinergic agonists. For example, bronchoconstriction produced by these drugs could produce an asthmatic attack. Vasodilation and resulting reductions in diastolic blood pressure may reduce coronary blood flow sufficiently to evoke myocardial ischemia in vulnerable patients. Finally, enhanced secretion of acidic gastric fluid may aggravate the symptoms of peptic ulcer.

Methacholine

Methacholine has a longer duration of action than acetylcholine because its rate of hydrolysis by acetylcholinesterase is slower than for acetylcholine. Furthermore, methacholine is almost totally resistant to hydrolysis by plasma cholinesterase. Its greater selectivity than acetylcholine is manifested by a lack of significant nicotinic and predominance of muscarinic actions. This drug is rarely used clinically because of the unpredictable nature of its muscarinic effects especially on the cardiovascular system.

Carbachol and Bethanechol

Carbachol and bethanechol are totally resistant to hydrolysis by acetylcholinesterase or plasma cho-

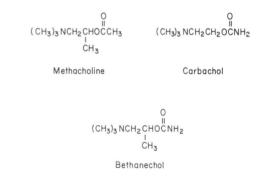

FIGURE 9-15. Synthetic acetylcholine derivatives.

linesterase. Bethanechol has mainly muscarinic actions but both drugs act with some selectivity on the smooth muscle of the gastrointestinal tract and urinary bladder. Carbachol retains a high level of nicotinic activity particularly on autonomic ganglia which may reflect drug-induced release of endogenous acetylcholine from the terminals of cholinergic fibers. In contrast to methacholine, the cardiovascular effects of carbachol and bethanechol are less prominent than effects on the gastrointestinal and urinary tracts.

Effects on the gastrointestinal tract include increased peristalsis and enhanced secretory activity. Nausea, vomiting, and defecation are manifestations of increased gastrointestinal motility. Selective effects of carbachol and bethanechol include stimulation of ureteral peristalsis and contraction of the detrusor muscle of the urinary bladder. In addition, the trigone and external sphincter are relaxed. These effects evoke evacuation of a neurogenic bladder.

Secretions are increased from all glands that receive parasympathetic nervous system innervation including the lacrimal, tracheobronchial, salivary, digestive, and exocrine sweat glands. Effects on the respiratory system, in addition to increased tracheobronchial secretion, include bronchoconstriction and stimulation of the chemoreceptors of the carotid and aortic bodies. Instilled into the eye, these drugs produce miosis.

Bethanechol is used as a stimulant of the smooth muscle of the gastrointestinal tract and the urinary bladder. For example, oral bethanechol may relieve adynamic ileus or gastric atony following bilateral vagotomy. Bethanechol may be useful in combating urinary retention when mechanical obstruction is absent as in the postoperative

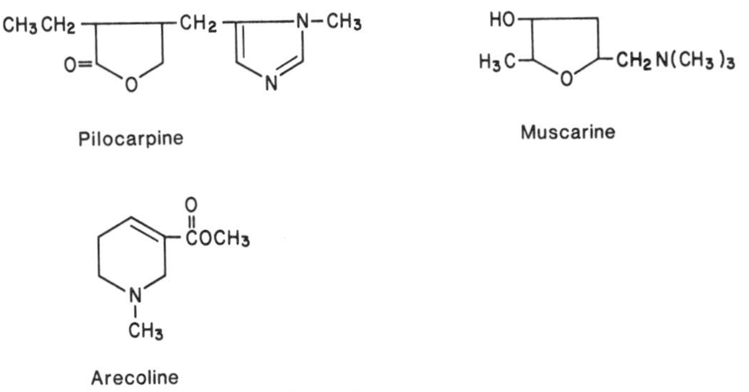

FIGURE 9-16. Cholinomimetic alkaloids.

and postpartum period and in certain cases of neurogenic bladder thus avoiding the risk of infection attendant with catheterization. For acute urinary retention, the usual adult dose of bethanechol is 5 mg injected subcutaneously which can be repeated after 15 to 30 minutes if necessary.

Carbachol is not used for its actions on the gastrointestinal tract and urinary bladder because of its relatively greater nicotinic action at autonomic ganglia. Instead, carbachol is useful as a topical solution in the chronic therapy of narrow-angle glaucoma and to produce miosis during intraocular surgery.

Pilocarpine, Muscarine, and Arecoline

Pilocarpine, muscarine, and arecoline are examples of cholinomimetic alkaloids (Fig. 9-16). The sties of actions of these drugs and pharmacologic actions are the same as for choline agonists. Pilocarpine has a dominant muscarinic action, and sweat glands are particularly sensitive to this drug. Muscarine acts almost exclusively at muscarinic cholinergic receptors. Arecoline acts in addition at nicotinic cholinergic receptors. The clinical use of these drugs is largely limited to the topical administration of pilocarpine as a miotic. Pilocarpine when applied topically to the eye causes miosis, paralysis of accommodation, and a sustained reduction in intraocular pressure. Miosis may persist for several hours, but cycloplegia usually wanes within 2 hours. Pilocarpine is useful for overcoming mydriasis produced by atropine.

REFERENCES

Azar I, Pham AN, Karambelkar DJ, Lear E. The heart rate following edrophonium-atropine and edrophonium-glycopyrrolate mixtures. Anesthesiology 1983;59:139 – 41.

Balmer HGR, Wyte SR. Antagonism of ketamine by physostigmine (letter). Br J Anaesth 1977;49:510.

Bentz EW, Stoelting RK. Prolonged response to succinylcholine following pancuronium reversal with pyridostigmine. Anesthesiology 1976;44:258 – 60.

Bidwai AV, Stanley TH, Rogers C, Riet EK. Reversal of diazepam-induced postanesthetic somnolence with physostigmine. Anesthesiology 1979;51: 256 – 9.

Blabler LC: The mechanism of the facilitory action of edrophonium on cat skeletal muscle. Br J Pharmacol 1972;46:498 – 507.

Bourke DL, Rosenberg M. Allen PD. Physostigmine: Effectiveness as an antagonist of respiratory depression and psychomotor effects caused by morphine or diazepam. Anesthesiology 1984;61:523 – 8.

Cronnelly R, Morris RB: Antagonism of neuromuscular blockade. Br J Anaesth 1982;54:183 – 93.

Cronnelly R, Morris RB, Miller RD. Edrophonium: Duration of action and atropine requirement in humans during halothane anesthesia. Anesthesiology 1982;57:261 – 6.

Cronnelly R, Stanski DR, Miller RD, Sheiner LB, Sohn YJ, Renal function and the pharmacokinetics of neostigmine in anesthetized patients. Anesthesiology 1979;51:222 – 6.

Cronnelly R, Stanski DR, Miller RD, Sheiner LB. Pyridostigmine kinetics with and without renal function. Clin Pharmacol Ther 1980;28:78 – 81.

Donati F, Ferguson A, Bevan DR. Twitch depression and train-of-four ratio after antagonism of pancuronium with edrophonium, neostigmine, or pyridistigmine. Anesth Analg 1983;62:314 – 6.

Fisher DM, Cronnelly R, Miller RD, Sharma M. The neuromuscular pharmacology of neostigmine in infants and children. Anesthesiology 1983;59:220 – 5.

Fisher DM, Cronnelly R. Sharma M. Miller RD. Clinical pharmacology of edrophonium in infants and children. Anesthesiology 1984;61:428 – 33.

Fogdall RP, Miller RD. Antagonism of d-tubocurarine

and pancuronium-induced neuromuscular blockades by pyridostigmine in man. Anesthesiology 1973;39:504–9.

Hennis PJ, Cronnelly R, Sharma M, Fisher DM, Miller RD. Metabolites of neostigmine and pyridostigmine do not contribute to antagonism of neuromuscular blockade in the dog. Anesthesiology 1984;61:534–9.

Hill GE, Stanley TH, Sentker CR. Physostigmine reversal of postoperative somnolence. Can Anaesth Soc J 1977;24:707–11.

Katz RL. Clinical neuromuscular pharmacology of pancuronium. Anesthesiology 1971:34:550–6.

Lundh H, Milsson O, Rosen I. Effects of 4-aminopyridine in myasthenia gravis. J Neuro, Neurosurg, Psychiatry 1979;42:171–5.

Miller RD, Booij LDHJ, Agoston S, Crul JF. Aminopyridine potentiates neostigmine and pyridostigmine in man. Anesthesiology 1979;50:416–20.

Miller RD, Larson CP, Way WL. Comparative antagonism of d-tubocurarine, gallamine-, and pancuronium-induced neuromuscular blockade by neostigmine. Anesthesiology 1972;37:503–9.

Miller RD, Van Nyhius LS, Eger EI, Vitez TS, Way WL. Comparative times to peak effect and duration of action of neostigmine and pyridostigmine. Anesthesiology 1974;41:27–33.

Miller RD, Van Nyhuis LS, Eger EI, Way WL. The effect of acid–base balance on neostigmine antagonism of d-Tubocurarine-induced neuromuscular blockade. Anesthesiology 1975;42:377–83.

Mirakhur RK. Edrophonium and plasma cholinesterase activity. Can Anaesth Soc J 1986;33:588–90.

Molgo L, Lemeignan M, Lechat P. Effects of 4-aminopyridine at the frog neuromuscular junction. J Pharmacol Exp Ther 1977;203:653–63.

Morris RB, Cronnelly R, Miller RD, Stanski DR, Fahey MR. Pharmacokinetics of edrophonium and neostigmine when antagonizing d-tubocurarine neuromuscular blockade in man. Anesthesiology 1981;54:399–402.

Prys-Roberts C. Hemodynamic effects of anesthesia and surgery in renal hypertensive patients receiving large doses of β-receptor antagonists. Anesthesiology 1979;51:S122.

Ramamurthy S, Shaker MH, Winnie AP. Glycopyrrolate as a substitute for atropine in neostigmine reversal of muscle relaxants. Can Anaesth Soc J 1972;19:399–411.

Roy RC, Stullken EH. Electroencephalographic evidence of arousal in dogs from halothane after doxapram, physostigmine, or naloxone. Anesthesiology 1981;55:392–7.

Rupp SM, McChristian JW, Miller RD, Taboada JA, Cronnelly R. Neostigmine and edrophonium antagonism of varying neuromuscular blockade induced by atracurium, pancuronium, or vecuronium. Anesthesiology 1986;64:711–7.

Snir-Mor I, Weinstock M, Davidson JT, Bahar M. Physostigmine antagonizes morphine-induced respiratory depression in human subjects. Anesthesiology 1983;59:6–9.

Spaulding BC, Choi SD, Gross JB, Apfelbaum JL, Broderson H. The effect of physostigmine on diazepam-induced ventilatory depression: a double-blind study. Anesthesiology 1984;61:551–4.

Sprague DH. Severe bradycardia after neostigmine in a patient taking propranolol to control paroxysmal atrial tachycardia. Anesthesiology 1975;42:208–10.

Standaert FG. Donuts and holes: Molecules and muscle relaxants. Semin Anes 1984;3:251–61.

Taylor P. Anticholinesterase agents. In: Gilman AG, Goodman LS, Rall TW, Murad F, eds. The Pharmacological Basis of Therapeutics. New York, Macmillan Publishing Co 1985:110.

Wagner DL, Moorthy SS, Stoelting RK. Administration of anticholinesterase drugs in the presence of beta-adrenergic blockade. Anesth Analg 1982;61:153–4.

Weinstock M, Davidson JT, Rosin AJ, Schnieden H. Effect of physostigmine on morphine-induced postoperative pain and somnolence. Br J Anaesth 1982;54:429–34.

Young WL, Backus W, Matteo RS, Ornstein E, Diaz T. Pharmacokinetics and pharmacodynamics of neostigmine in the elderly. Anesthesiology 1984;61:A300.

Anticholinergic Drugs

INTRODUCTION

Anticholinergic drugs competitively antagonize the effects of the neurotransmitter, acetylcholine, at cholinergic postganglionic sites designated as muscarinic receptors. Muscarinic cholinergic receptors are present in the heart, salivary glands, and smooth muscle of the gastrointestinal tract and genitourinary tract. Acetylcholine is also the neurotransmitter at postganglionic nicotinic receptors located at the neuromuscular junction and autonomic ganglia. In contrast to muscarinic receptors, usual doses of anticholinergic drugs exert little to no effect at nicotinic cholinergic receptors. As such, anticholinergic drugs may be considered to be selectively antimuscarinic.

Naturally occurring tertiary amine anticholinergic drugs represented by atropine and scopolamine are alkaloids of belladonna plants. Semisynthetic congeners of the belladonna alkaloids represented by glycopyrrolate are usually quaternary ammonium derivatives. These quaternary ammonium derivatives are often more potent than their parent compounds with respect to peripheral anticholinergic effects but lack central nervous system activity because of poor penetrance into the brain.

STRUCTURE ACTIVITY RELATIONSHIPS

Naturally occurring anticholinergic drugs (atropine and scopolamine) are esters formed by the combination of tropic acid and a complex organic base, either tropine or scopine (Fig. 10-1). Structurally, these drugs resemble cocaine, and, in fact, atropine has weak analgesic actions. Atropine and scopolamine consist of mixtures of equal parts of dextrorotatory and levorotatory isomers but the anticholinergic effect is almost entirely due to the levorotatory form. Synthetic anticholinergic drugs such as glycopyrrolate contain mandelic acid rather than tropic acid (Fig. 10-1). Like acetylcholine, anticholinergic drugs contain a cationic portion that can fit into the muscarinic cholinergic receptor.

MECHANISM OF ACTION

Anticholinergic drugs reversibly combine with muscarinic cholinergic receptors and thus prevent access of the neurotransmitter, acetylcholine, to these sites. In contrast to acetylcholine, the combination of an anticholinergic drug to the muscarinic receptor does not result in cell membrane changes that lead to a cholinergic response. Anticholinergic drugs do not prevent the liberation of acetylcholine nor do they react with acetylcholine.

There are variations in the sensitivity of different muscarinic cholinergic receptors as well as differences in potency among the anticholinergic drugs (Eger, 1962). For example, muscarinic cholinergic receptors controlling salivary and bronchial secretions are inhibited by lower doses of

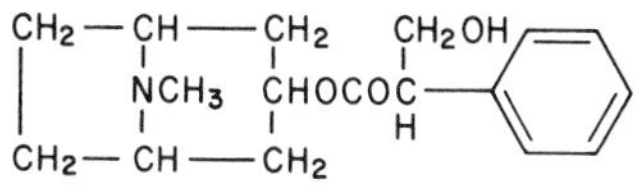

FIGURE 10-1. Naturally occurring and synthetic anticholinergic drugs.

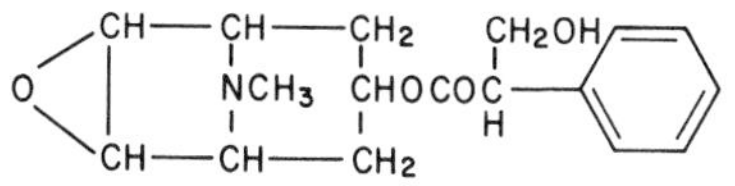

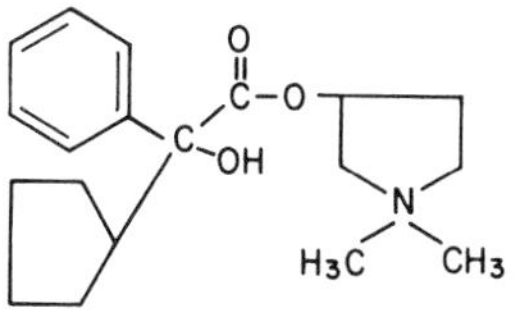

anticholinergic drugs than necessary to inhibit receptors that regulate acetylcholine effects on the heart and eye. Even larger doses of anticholinergic drugs inhibit cholinergic control of the gastrointestinal tract and genitourinary tract thus decreasing the tone and motility of the intestine and inhibiting micturition. Still larger doses of anticholinergic drugs are required to inhibit gastric secretion of hydrogen ions. As a result, a dose of anticholinergic drug that inhibits gastric secretion of hydrogen ions invariably affects salivary secretion, heart rate, ocular accommodation, and micturition.

Examples of differences in anticholinergic potency between drugs is the greater antisialagogue and ocular effects of scopolamine compared with atropine (Table 10-1) (Eger, 1962). Conversely, atropine has greater anticholinergic effects at the heart, bronchial smooth muscle, and gastrointestinal tract than scopolamine does (Table 10-1) (Herxheimer, 1958).

Evidence that anticholinergic drugs are not pure muscarinic cholinergic receptor antagonists is the observation that small doses of atropine, scopolamine, and glycopyrrolate can produce heart rate slowing even when the drug is administered in the presence of bilateral vagotomy (Flacke and Flacke, 1986). This heart rate slowing reflects a weak peripheral muscarinic cholinergic receptor agonist effect of the anticholinergic drug. Previous speculation that heart rate slowing following administration of atropine reflected central vagal action before the peripheral blocking effects could occur is not supported by similar heart rate changes following administration of glycopyrrolate which cannot easily cross the blood–brain barrier (see the section entitled Pharmacokinetics).

An additional indirect effect of anticholinergic drugs can result from interference by these drugs with the normal inhibition of the release of endogenous norepinephrine (Levy and Blattberg, 1976). This indirect effect may manifest as a sympathomimetic effect of atropine.

PHARMACOKINETICS

Oral absorption of even the tertiary amine anticholinergic drugs is not sufficiently predictable to recommend their administration by this route in the perioperative period. Intramuscular or intravenous administration is most often utilized for administration of anticholinergic drugs. Despite attempts to develop anticholinergic drugs with greater specificity for certain functions, the sequence of muscarinic cholinergic blockade is similar for all drugs (see the section entitled Mechanism of Action).

Atropine and scopolamine are lipid-soluble tertiary amines that easily penetrate the blood–brain barrier. In contrast, glycopyrrolate is a poorly lipid-soluble quaternary ammonium compound with minimal ability to cross the blood–brain barrier and produce central nervous system effects. Quaternary ammonium compounds usually have a somewhat more prolonged duration of action, and these anticholinergic drugs have a greater potency at nicotinic cholinergic receptors as emphasized by the occasional occurrence of impotence or orthostatic hypotension in patients taking these drugs.

About 50% of an injected dose of atropine appears unchanged in the urine, and another 30% can be recovered as tropine and tropic acid reflecting hydrolysis of atropine to inactive metabolites. Minimal amounts of atropine are destroyed in human plasma compared with certain animals, such as the rabbit, which possess a specific plasma

Table 10-1
Comparative Effects of Anticholinergic Drugs

	Sedation	Antisialagogue	Increase Heart Rate	Relax Smooth Muscle	Mydriasis Cycloplegia	Prevent Motion Sickness	Decrease Gastric Hydrogen Ion Secretion	Alter Fetal Heart Rate
Atropine	+	+	+++	++	+	+	∓	0
Scopolamine	+++	+++	+	+	+++	+++	±	?
Glycopyrrolate	0	++	++	++	0	0	±	0

0 none
 + mild
 ++ moderate
+++ marked

enzyme, atropine esterase, capable of hydrolyzing atropine. Conversely, scopolamine is nearly entirely broken down in the body with only about 1% appearing unchanged in the urine.

CLINICAL USES

Anticholinergic drugs are utilized in a wide variety of clinical conditions and situations. The lack of selectivity, however, of these drugs makes it difficult to obtain desired therapeutic responses without concomitant side effects (Table 10-1). The most important uses of anticholinergic drugs in the perioperative period are (1) preoperative medication, (2) treatment of reflex-mediated bradycardia, and (3) protection against the muscarinic effects of anticholinesterase drugs as used to antagonize nondepolarizing neuromuscular blocking drugs (see Chapter 9). Other less frequent uses of anticholinergic drugs are for (1) bronchodilation, (2) biliary and ureteral smooth muscle relaxants, (3) production of mydriasis and cycloplegia, (4) antagonists of gastric hydrogen ion secretion, (5) prevention of motion-induced nausea, and (6) constituents in nonprescription cold remedies.

Preoperative Medication

Historically, intramuscular atropine was administered prior to the induction of anesthesia to protect the heart from vagal reflexes and to prevent excessive secretions. Currently used inhaled or injected anesthetic drugs are not predictably associated with these effects, and it is not mandatory to include an anticholinergic drug in the preoperative medication. When an anticholinergic drug is included in the preoperative medication, the therapeutic goals are to produce sedation and/or an antisialagogue effect. Anticholinergic drugs in traditional doses used for preoperative medication in adults do not alter gastric fluid pH or volume (Table 10-2) (Stoelting, 1978) (see Chapter 26).

The patient with glaucoma and the parturient present special considerations in using anticholinergic drugs for preoperative medication. For example, the mydriatic effects of scopolamine are greater than atropine suggesting caution in the use of scopolamine in patients with glaucoma (Garde et al, 1978). Intramuscular atropine, 0.4 mg, or intravenous atropine, 1 mg, as administered with an anticholinesterase drug seem safe as little or no change in pupil size occurs (Balamoutsos, 1980). Glycopyrrolate has the least effect on pupil size of all the anticholinergic drugs used for preoperative medication. Both atropine and scopolamine can cross the placenta, but fetal heart rate is not significantly changed following intravenous administration of either atropine or glycopyrrolate (Fig. 10-2) (Abboud et al, 1983; Murad et al, 1981).

Sedation

Scopolamine is selected when sedation is the reason for including an anticholinergic drug in the preoperative medication. Indeed, scopolamine is about 100 times more potent than atropine in depressing the reticular activating system. Scopola-

Table 10-2

Gastric Fluid pH *and Volume Without or With Inclusion of an Anticholinergic Drug in the Preoperative Medication*

	Gastric Fluid pH Below 2.5 (% of patients)	Gastric Fluid Volume Above 20 ml (% of patients)
Morphine (n − 75)	63	27
Morphine–atropine (n − 75)	57	27
Morphine–glycopyrrolate (n − 75)	49	23

n = number of patients

(Data from Stoelting RK. Responses to atropine, glycopyrrolate, and Riopan of gastric fluid pH and volume in adult patients. Anesthesiology 1978;48:367–9.)

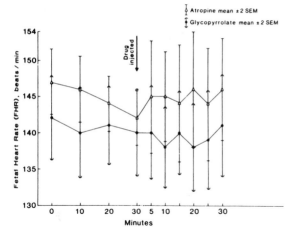

FIGURE 10-2. Atropine or glycopyrrolate do not alter fetal heart rate following intravenous administration to the mother. Mean ±2 SEM. (From Abboud T, Raya J, Sadri S, Grobler N, Stine L, Miller F. Fetal and maternal cardiovascular effects of atropine and glycopyrrolate. Anesth Analg 1983;62:426–30. Reproduced by permission of the authors and the International Anesthesia Research Society.)

mine, in addition to depressing the cerebral cortex, also affects other areas of the brain causing amnesia. Small intramuscular doses of scopolamine (0.3–0.5 mg) usually cause sedation while similar doses of atropine produce minimal central nervous system effects. Glycopyrrolate, which does not easily cross the blood–brain barrier, is devoid of sedative effects. Scopolamine also greatly enhances sedative effects of concomitantly administered drugs especially opioids and benzodiazepines (Frumin *et al,* 1976). Indeed, the combination of morphine and scopolamine is favored by many anesthesiologists when a reliable sedative effect from the preoperative medication is desired.

Occasionally central nervous system effects of anticholinergic drugs, especially scopolamine, cause symptoms ranging from restlessness to somnolence (see the section entitled Central Anticholinergic Syndrome). These symptoms may be more likely to occur in elderly patients and should be considered as a possible explanation for delayed awakening from anesthesia or agitation in the early postoperative period. Inhaled anesthetics can potentiate the central nervous system effects of anticholinergic drugs leading to an increased incidence of postoperative restlessness or somnolence (Holzgrafe *et al,* 1973). Physostigmine is effective in reversing restlessness or somnolence due to central nervous system effects of tertiary amine anticholinergic drugs.

Antisialagogue Effect

Scopolamine is about three times more potent as an antisialagogue than atropine. For this reason, scopolamine is often selected when both an antisialagogue effect and sedation are desired results of preoperative medication. In equivalent antisialagogue doses, scopolamine, 0.3 to 0.5 mg, is less likely than atropine, 0.4 to 0.6 mg, to produce heart rate changes. Glycopyrrolate is selected when an antisialagogue effect, in the absence of sedation, is desired. As an antisialogogue, glycopyrrolate is about twice as potent as atropine and its duration of action is longer (Murad *et al*, 1981).

Treatment of Reflex-Mediated Bradycardia

Administered intravenously, atropine, 15 to 70 $\mu g\ kg^{-1}$, and, to a lesser extent, scopolamine and glycopyrrolate, increase the heart rate by blocking the effects of acetylcholine on the sinoatrial node (Gravenstein *et al*, 1964; Meyers and Tomeldan, 1979). Indeed, the maximum increase in heart rate produced by atropine is an indication of the degree of control normally exerted by the vagus nerve on the sinoatrial node. On the electrocardiogram, the effect of anticholinergic drugs is to shorten the P–R interval.

In young adults, in whom vagal tone is greatest, the influence of atropine on heart rate is most marked, while in infants or elderly patients even large doses may fail to increase heart rate. During anesthesia that includes a volatile drug, the dose of atropine required to increase heart rate may be reduced compared with an awake patient. Intramuscular administration, in contrast to intravenous injection, is occasionally associated with heart rate slowing reflecting a peripheral agonist effect of the anticholinergic drug (see the section entitled Mechanisms of Action).

Bronchodilation

Anticholinergic drugs can relax bronchial smooth muscles by blocking the constrictor effects of the vagus nerves. The resulting relaxation of bronchial smooth muscle lowers airway resistance and increases dead space particularly in patients with bronchial asthma or chronic bronchitis (Butler *et al*, 1960; Severinghaus and Stupfel, 1955). For example, clinical doses of scoplamine decrease airway resistance and increase dead space by about one third, but this effect depends largely on the degree of preexisting bronchomotor tone. Glycopyrrolate is equally effective as a bronchodilator and is devoid of central nervous system effects and evokes minimum heart rate effects (Fig. 10-3) (Gal and Suratt, 1981).

Bronchodilation is more likely to occur when anticholinergic drugs are administered by inhala-

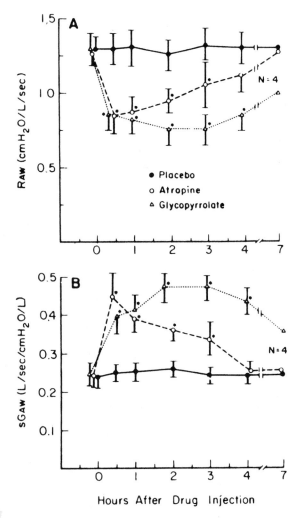

FIGURE 10-3. Atropine and glycopyrrolate are equally effective in lowering airway resistance (Raw) and increasing airway conductance (sGAW). (From Gal TJ, Suratt PM. Atropine and glycopyrrolate effects on lung mechanics in normal man. Anesth Analg 1981;60:85–90. Reproduced by permission of the authors and the International Anesthesia Research Society.)

tion as aerosols. For example, ipratropium, a derivative of methylatropine, is as effective as isoproterenol as a bronchodilator when administered by inhalation. An advantage of aerosol administration is the absence of adverse cardiovascular side effects that are more likely to accompany systemic administration.

Administration of anticholinergic drugs for

preanesthetic medication could result in inspissation of secretions leading to the possibility of airway obstruction rather than decreases in airway resistance. Nevertheless, it seems unlikely that a single dose of anticholinergic drug would predictably produce these adverse effects.

Biliary and Ureteral Smooth Muscle Relaxation

Atropine decreases the tone of the smooth muscle of the biliary tract and ureter. This modest antispasmodic action, however, is unlikely to overcome opioid-induced spasm of the sphincter of Oddi. Conversely, atropine may prevent spasm of the ureter produced by morphine supporting the custom of administering atropine with an opioid for the management of pain due to a renal stone (e.g., renal colic). Therapeutic doses of atropine are thought to diminish the tone of the fundus of the bladder and to increase the tone of the vesical sphincter possibly contributing to urinary retention.

Mydriasis and Cycloplegia

Circular muscles of the iris which constrict the pupil are innervated by cholinergic fibers from the third cranial nerve while fibers from the same nerve cause contraction of the ciliary muscles allowing the lens to become more convex (see Chapter 41). Anticholinergic drugs placed topically on the cornea block the action of acetylcholine at both these sites resulting in mydriasis and cycloplegia. Complete recovery from mydriasis and cycloplegia produced by topical atropine requires 7 to 14 days. In patients with glaucoma, relaxation of the ciliary muscle produced by an anticholinergic drug occludes the angular space while mydriasis obstructs passage of fluid into the venous circulation resulting in potentially hazardous elevations of intraocular pressure.

Doses of atropine used for preoperative medication are probably inadequate to elevate intraocular pressure even in susceptible patients assuming medications being used to treat glaucoma are continued. Indeed, mydriasis produced by any anticholinergic drug is completely offset by topical corneal placement of an anticholinesterase drug such as pilocarpine. Nevertheless, intramuscular scopolamine is a more potent mydriatic than either atropine or glycopyrrolate suggesting the need for caution in using this anticholinergic drug for preoperative medication of a patient with glaucoma (Garde et al, 1978) (see the section entitled Preoperative Medication).

Antagonists of Gastric Hydrogen Ion Secretion

Anticholinergic drugs have been utilized in the management of peptic ulcer disease. Indeed, glycopyrrolate was originally introduced as an anticholinergic drug to control gastric acidity (Sun, 1962). Nevertheless, none of the anticholinergic drugs are selective for this effect, and the high doses required to inhibit gastric hydrogen ion secretion are often associated with unacceptable secretory, ocular, and cardiac side effects. Furthermore, the efficacy of H_2 receptor antagonists for reducing gastric hydrogen ion secretion has largely negated the use of anticholinergic drugs for this purpose (see Chapter 21).

Anticholinergic drugs have predictable effects on the tone and motility of the gastrointestinal tract because the parasympathetic nervous system provides almost exclusive motor innervation to this organ. As with suppression of gastric hydrogen ion secretion, however, large doses of anticholinergic drugs are necessary to alter gastrointestinal motility often introducing unacceptable side effects. Nevertheless, high doses of anticholinergic drugs do prevent excess peristalsis of the gastrointestinal tract that would otherwise be associated with reversal of nondepolarizing neuromuscular blocking drugs using anticholinesterase drugs.

Prevention of Motion-Induced Sickness

Transdermal absorption of scopolamine provides sustained therapeutic plasma concentrations that protect against motion-induced nausea without introducing prohibitive side effects such as sedation, cycloplegia, or drying of secretions (Price et al, 1981; Schmitt et al, 1981). For example, a postauricular application of scopolamine delivers the drug at 5 μg hr^{-1} for 72 hours (i.e., total absorbed dose <0.5 mg). Protection against motion-induced nausea is greatest if the transdermal application of scopolamine is initiated at least 4 hours before the noxious stimulus. Administration of transdermal scopolamine after the onset of symptoms is less effective than prophylactic administration. Similar protection against motion-induced nausea utilizing oral or intravenous administration of scopolamine would require large doses resulting in undesirable side effects and subsequent poor patient acceptance. It is presumed that scopolamine blocks transmission to the medulla of impulses arising from overstimulation of the vestibular apparatus of the inner ear.

Constituents of Nonprescription Cold Remedies

Anticholinergic drugs are common constituents of nonprescription cold remedies. The apparent efficacy of these drugs is most likely due to inhibition of production of upper airway secretions. With the exception of allergic mechanisms, it is also likely that contributions of antihistamines in cold remedies are also primarily due to their anticholinergic effects (see Chapter 21).

CENTRAL ANTICHOLINERGIC SYNDROME

Scopolamine, and to a lesser extent atropine, can enter the central nervous system and produce symptoms characterized as the central anticholinergic syndrome. Symptoms range from restlessness and hallucinations to somnolence and unconsciousness (Duvoisin and Katz, 1968) (see the section entitled Preoperative Medication). Presumably, these responses reflect blockade of muscarinic cholinergic receptors in the central nervous system. Glycopyrrolate does not easily cross the blood–brain barrier and, thus, is not likely to cause a central anticholinergic syndrome. Indeed, arousal in the first 30 minutes following cessation of anesthesia is delayed following administration of atropine–neostigmine but not glycopyrrolate–neostigmine mixtures as used to reverse the effects of nondepolarizing neuromuscular blocking drugs (Baraka et al, 1980).

Physostigmine, a tertiary amine anticholinesterase drug, administered in intravenous doses of 15 to 60 μg kg^{-1} is a specific treatment for the central anticholinergic syndrome (see Chapter 9). Neostigmine and pyridostigmine are not effective antidotes because the quaternary ammonium structure prevents these drugs from easily entering the central nervous system.

OVERDOSE

Deliberate or accidental overdose with an anticholinergic drug produces a rapid onset of symptoms characteristic of muscuranic cholinergic receptor blockade. The mouth becomes dry, swallowing and talking are difficult, vision is blurred, photophobia is present, and tachycardia is prominent. The skin is dry and flushed and a rash may appear especially over the face, neck, and upper chest (i.e., blush area). Even therapeutic doses of anticholinergic drugs may occasionally selectively dilate cutaneous vessels in the blush area. Body temperature is likely to be elevated by anticholinergic drugs especially when the environmental temperature is also increased. This rise in body temperature largely reflects inhibition of sweating by anticholinergic drugs emphasizing that innervation of sweat glands is by sympathetic nervous system nerves that release acetylcholine as the neurotransmitter. Small children are particularly vulnerable to drug-induced elevations in body temperature with "atropine fever" occasionally occurring in this age group following administration of even a therapeutic dose of anticholinergic drug. Minute ventilation may be slightly increased due to central nervous system stimulation and the impact of an enlarged physiologic dead space due to bronchodilation. Blood gases are usually unchanged (Nunn and Bergman, 1964). Skeletal muscle weakness and orthostatic hypotension, when present, reflect nicotinic cholinergic receptor blockade. Fatal events due to an overdose of anticholinergic drug include seizures, coma, and medullary ventilatory center paralysis.

Small children and infants seem particularly vulnerable to developing life-threatening symptoms following an overdose of anticholinergic drug. Physostigmine administered intravenously in doses of 15 to 60 μg kg^{-1} is the specific treatment for reversal of symptoms. Because physostigmine is rapidly metabolized, repeated doses of this anticholinesterase drug may be necessary to prevent a recurrence of symptoms.

REFERENCES

Abboud T, Raya J, Sadri S, Grobler N, Stine L, Miller F. Fetal and maternal cardiovascular effects of atropine and glycopyrrolate. Anesth Analg 1983; 62:426-30.

Balamoutsos NG, Drossou Fr, Alevizou Fr, Tjvairi E, Pa-

pastephanou C, Marios A. Pupil size during reversal of muscle relaxants. Anesth Analg 1980;59:615-6.

Baraka A, Yared J-P, Karam A-M, Winnie A. Glycopyrrolate-neostigmine and atropine-neostigmine mixtures affect postanesthetic arousal times differently. Anesth Analg 1980;59:431-4.

Butler J, Caro CG, Alcala R, Dubois AB. Physiologic factors affecting airway resistance in normal subjects and in patients with obstructive respiratory disease. J. Clin Invest 1960;39:584-91.

Duvoisin RC, Katz RL. Reversal of central anticholinergic syndrome in man by physostigmine. JAMA 1968;206:1963-5.

Eger EI. Atropine, scopamine and related compounds. Anesthesiology 1962;23:365-83.

Flacke WE, Flacke JW. Cholinergic and anticholinergic agents. In: Smith NT, Corbascio AN, eds. Drug Interactions in Anesthesia. Philadelphia, Lea and Febiger 1986:160.

Frumin MJ, Herekar VR, Jarvik ME. Amnesic actions of diazepam and scopolamine in man. Anesthesiology 1976;45:406-12.

Gal TJ, Suratt PM. Atropine and glycopyrrolate effects on lung mechanics in normal man. Anesth Analg 1981;60:85-90.

Garde JF, Aston R, Endler GC, Sison OS. Racial mydriatic response to belladonna premedication. Anesth Analg 1978;57:572-6.

Gravenstein JS, Andersen TW, DePadua CB. Effects of atropine and scopolamine on the cardiovascular system in man. Anesthesiology 1964;25:123-30.

Herxheimer A. A comparison of some atropine-like drugs in man, with particular reference to their end-organ specificity. Br J Pharmacol 1958;13:184-9.

Holzgrafe RE, Vondrell JJ, Mintz SM. Reversal of postoperative reactions to scopolamine with physostigmine. Anesth Analg 1973;52:921-5.

Levy MN, Blattberg B. Effect of vagal stimulation on the overflow of norepinephrine into the coronary sinus during cardiac sympathetic nerve stimulation in the dog. Circ Res 1976;38:81-5.

Meyers EF, Tomeldan SA. Glycopyrrolate compared with atropine in prevention of the oculocardiac reflex during eye muscle surgery. Anesthesiology 1979;51:350-2.

Murad SHN, Conklin KA, Tabsh KMA, Brinkman CR, Erkkola R, Nuwayhid B. Atropine and glycopyrrolate: Hemodynamic effects and placental transfer in the pregnant ewe. Anesth Analg 1981;60:710-4.

Nunn JF, Bergman NA. The effect of atropine on pulmonary gas exchange. Brit J Anaesth 1964;36:68-73.

Price NM, Schmitt LG, McGuire J, Shaw JE, Trobough G. Transdermal scopolamine in the prevention of motion sickness at sea. Clin Pharmacol Ther 1981;29:414-9.

Schmitt LG, Shaw JE, Carpenter PF, Chandrasekaran SK. Comparison of transdermal and intravenous administration of scopolamine. Clin Pharmacol Ther 1981;29:282.

Severinghaus JW, Stupfel M. Respiratory dead space increase following atropine in man, and atropine, vagal, or ganglionic blockade and hypothermia in dogs. J Appl Physiol 1955;8:81-7.

Stoelting RK. Responses to atropine, glycopyrrolate, and Riopan of gastric fluid pH and volume in adult patients. Anesthesiology 1978;48:367-9.

Sun DCH. Comparative study of the effect of glycopyrrolate and propantheline on basal gastric secretion. Ann NY Acad Sci 1962;99:153-7.

C H A P T E R   11

Nonopioid and Nonsteroidal Analgesic, Antipyretic, and Anti-Inflammatory Drugs

INTRODUCTION

Aspirin (acetylsalicylic acid) is the prototype of the nonopioid analgesic, antipyretic, and anti-inflammatory drugs (Fig. 11-1). Despite great variations in chemical structure, these drugs often share therapeutic activities, side effects, and mechanisms of action. Aspirin and related drugs do not bind to opioid receptors.

Aspirin and aspirin-like drugs are most often administered as (1) analgesics for the symptomatic relief of low intensity pain associated with headache and with musculoskeletal disorders such as osteoarthritis, and rheumatoid arthritis, (2) antipyretics, and (3) inhibitors of platelet aggregation in patients vulnerable to vascular obstruction from emboli. Prostaglandins may play a role in the maintenance of a patent ductus arteriosus, and drugs that inhibit synthesis of prostaglandins, such as indomethacin, have been used with limited success in neonates to evoke closure of the ductus arteriosus (Heymann *et al,* 1976) (see the section entitled Mechanism of Action). Excessive production of prostaglandins is present in Bartter's syndrome and aspirin-like drugs have been used successfully in treatment (Norby, 1976).

Unlike opioids, aspirin-like drugs do not produce cardiovascular effects or lead to tolerance or physical dependence. The analgesic action of aspirin-like drugs is confined to a small dose range below which there is little effect and above which

an increase in dose produces toxic effects with little increase in analgesia.

MECHANISM OF ACTION

Aspirin-like drugs produce analgesia by virtue of their ability to inhibit the activity of cyclooxygenase (prostaglandin synthetase) enzyme leading to a decrease in the synthesis and release of prostaglandins from cells (Metz, 1981; Moncada and Vane, 1979) (see Chapter 20). Individual drugs have differing modes of inhibitory activity on the cyclooxygenase enzyme. For example, aspirin acetylates an active site of the enzyme (Roth and Siok, 1978). Platelets are especially vulnerable to this enzyme inhibition, because unlike most other cells, they are not capable of regenerating cyclooxygenase. Presumably, this reflects the inability of platelets to independently synthesize proteins. This means that a single dose of aspirin will inhibit cyclooxygenase enzyme in platelets for the life span of the platelet which is 8 to 11 days. In contrast to aspirin, salicylic acid (orthohydroxybenzoic acid) lacks acetylating capacity and produces its inhibition of prostaglandin synthesis in a different manner (Fig. 11-1) (Metz, 1981; Moncada and Vane, 1979). Aspirin is rapidly hydrolyzed to salicylic acid suggesting that this drug may inhibit prostaglandin synthesis by a nonacetylation as well as acetylation mechanism. Indomethacin inhibition of cyclooxygenase is com-

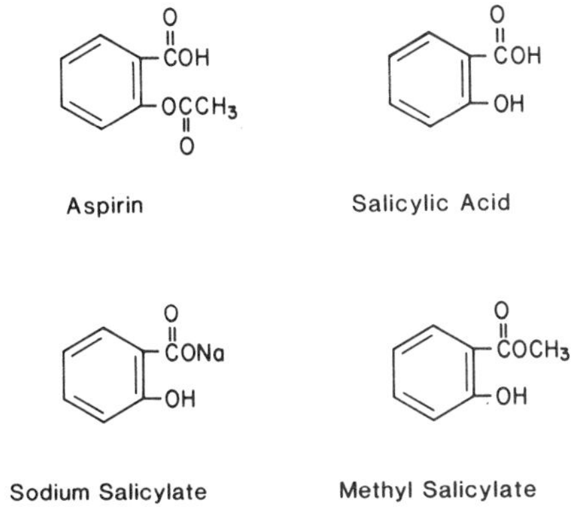

FIGURE 11-1.   Salicylates.

plex and likely involves a site on the enzyme different from that which is acetylated by aspirin. Aspirin-like drugs have little effect on the release of histamine or 5-hydroxytryptamine.

In contrast to opioids which act centrally, analgesia produced by aspirin-like drugs is principally a peripheral phenomenon. For example, aspirin seems to be effective as an analgesic only when prostaglandins are produced locally around sensitive nerve endings. Indeed, local production of prostaglandins is characteristic of inflammation that typically accompanies pain that is relieved by aspirin-like drugs. Aspirin-like drugs are not effective as analgesics when inflammation (*e.g.,* prostaglandins) is not present or against sharp stabbing pain (*e.g.,* visceral pain) caused by direct stimulation of sensory nerves.

Aspirin is effective as an antipyretic presumably by virtue of its ability to prevent pyrogen-induced release of prostaglandins in the central nervous system, including the hypothalamus. This is consistent with the known temperature-regulating role of the hypothalamus and the pyrogenic effect of most prostaglandins.

SALICYLATES

The two most frequently used preparations of salicylates are aspirin and salicylic acid (Fig. 11-1). Aspirin is about 50% more effective and toxic than salicylic acid. Among the nonopioid analgesics, aspirin serves as the standard of comparison for analgesic, antipyretic, and anti-inflammatory effects. There is often a great deal of individual varia-

tion in the response to different aspirin-like drugs, and the choice of drug may be largely empirical especially in the treatment of patients with arthritis.

Pharmacokinetics

Orally administered salicylates are rapidly absorbed from the small intestine and to a lesser extent from the stomach. Rate of absorption is influenced by (1) dissolution rates of the administered tablets and (2) gastric emptying time. If gastric *p*H is increased, salicylate is more ionized and the rate of absorption is decreased. The presence of food also delays gastric absorption of salicylates. There is no conclusive evidence that sodium bicarbonate given with aspirin (*e.g.,* buffered aspirin) has a faster onset of action, greater peak intensity, or longer analgesic effect. In fact, alkalinization of the urine may increase urinary excretion of the salicylate requiring administration of a larger dose of aspirin to achieve the same plasma concentration. Aspirin available in buffered effervescent preparations, however, undergoes more rapid systemic absorption and achieves higher plasma concentrations than the corresponding tablet formulations. These effervescent preparations also cause less gastrointestinal irritation.

Salicylates cross the blood–brain barrier slowly, reflecting the highly ionized nature of these drugs at physiologic *p*H. Conversely, salicylates seem to readily cross the placenta (Turner and Collins, 1975).

Protein Binding

Salicylic acid is highly bound to albumin (80%–90%). Conversely, aspirin is less avidly bound by albumin. There is competition between salicylic acid and protein binding sites for thyroxine, triiodothyronine, penicillin, phenytoin, and thiopental. Aspirin-like drugs may displace other drugs such as warfarin, oral hypoglycemics, and methotrexate from protein binding sites. The interaction with warfarin is accentuated because most of the aspirin-like drugs also disturb normal platelet function.

Clearance

Aspirin absorbed into the systemic circulation is rapidly hydrolyzed in the liver to salicylic acid. As a result of this rapid hydrolysis, plasma concentrations of aspirin rarely exceed 20 μg ml^{-1}. Nevertheless, aspirin is pharmacologically active and does not require hydrolysis to salicylic acid for its effects. Metabolism of salicylic acid also occurs in the liver where the acid is conjugated with glycine to form salicyluric acid. Salicyluric acid is excreted in the urine along with free salicylic acid. Renal excretion of free salicylic acid is highly variable from up to 85% of the ingested drug when the urine is alkaline to as low as 5% in acidic urine. The plasma concentration of salicylic acid is increased in the presence of renal dysfunction that is characterized by decreased glomerular filtration rate or decreased secretory activity of proximal renal tubules. The elimination half-time for aspirin is about 15 minutes and for salicylic acid 2 to 3 hours.

Side Effects

Side effects associated with administration of salicylates are numerous and include (1) gastric irritation and ulceration, (2) prolongation of bleeding time, (3) central nervous system stimulation, (4) hepatic dysfunction, (5) renal dysfunction, (6) metabolic alterations, (7) uterine effects, and (8) allergic reactions (Settipane, 1981). Epidemiologic evidence has suggested the possibility of an association between the use of aspirin in the treatment of fever in children and the development of Reye's syndrome.

Gastric Irritation and Ulceration

Salicylates may cause gastric irritation and ulceration. Reduction in prostaglandin synthesis, which normally inhibits gastric acid secretion, contributes to gastric mucosa ulceration. Resulting hemorrhage manifests as hematest positive stools and iron deficiency anemia. For example, plasma salicylate concentrations in the usual range for anti-inflammatory therapy (i.e., 12–35 mg dl^{-1} produced by 4–5 g of aspirin daily) result in an average daily fecal blood loss of 3 to 8 ml (Leonards and Levy, 1973).

Prolongation of Bleeding Time

Aspirin-induced platelet dysfunction reflects prevention of formation of thromboxane A2 which is a potent platelet aggregating prostaglandin

(Smith and Willis, 1971) (see Chapter 20). Bleeding time nearly doubles in response to 650 mg of aspirin presumably reflecting acetylation of platelet cyclooxygenase. This inhibition lasts for the normal life span of platelets which is 8 to 11 days. Furthermore, large doses of aspirin chronically decrease production of prothrombin leading to prolonged prothrombin time. Aspirin should be avoided in patients with severe hepatic dysfunction, vitamin K deficiency, hypoprothrombinemia, or hemophilia because inhibition of platelet aggregation in these patients can result in hemorrhage.

Central Nervous System Stimulation

Excessive doses of salicylates (plasma concentration greater than 50 mg dl^{-1}) produce stimulation of the central nervous system manifesting as seizures and hyperventilation. Hyperventilation is due to direct stimulation of the medullary ventilatory center. Initially, these changes result in respiratory alkalosis which is promptly compensated for by renal excretion of bicarbonate, sodium, and potassium ions with return of the pH towards normal. Ultimately, however, salicylate overdose is likely to progress to metabolic and respiratory acidosis. Metabolic acidosis reflects depression of renal function with accumulation of strong metabolic acids plus derangement of carbohydrate metabolism leading to an increased formation of pyruvic, lactic, and acetoacetic acids. Adults, in contrast to children, however, rarely develop metabolic acidosis regardless of the severity of the overdose. Hyperthermia and dehydration may be life-threatening results of salicylate overdose.

Tinnitus associated with elevated plasma concentrations of salicylates reflects drug-induced increases in labyrinthine pressure or an effect on hair cells of the cochlea. This side effect is the earliest sign of salicylate overdose. Nausea and vomiting are due to irritation of gastric mucosa at low doses and stimulation of the medullary chemoreceptor trigger zone by large doses.

Correction of metabolic acidosis is crucial in the treatment of salicylate overdose because a decrease in pH causes a shift of salicylic acid from plasma into the central nervous system. Metabolic alkalosis produced by the intravenous administration of sodium bicarbonate reverses the direction of transfer of salicylic acid and increases renal excretion (Hill, 1973). Diuretic-induced diuresis combined with intravenous sodium bicarbonate is effective in speeding renal excretion of salicylic acid.

Hepatic Dysfunction

Salicylates can be associated with elevated plasma concentrations of transaminase enzymes indicative of hepatic damage (Halla, 1976). This drug-induced hepatic dysfunction is reversible and is most likely to occur when the plasma concentration of salicylates exceeds 25 mg dl^{-1}. Patients with preexisting liver disease are more likely to develop changes in hepatic function in response to salicylates. In severe salicylate intoxication, fatty infiltration of the liver and kidneys may occur.

Renal Dysfunction

Chronic use of large doses of salicylates may lead to renal papillary necrosis and chronic interstitial nephritis often initially manifesting as reduced urine concentrating ability (Arger *et al*, 1976). This renal effect may reflect loss of the normal function of prostaglandins in the control of renal circulation. Salicylates produce a dose-dependent (greater than 5 g) uricosuric action. Even small doses of salicylates negate the effects of probenecid and other uricosuric drugs.

Metabolic Alterations

Large doses of salicylates may cause hyperglycemia, glycosuria, and may deplete liver and skeletal muscle glycogen. Salicylates reduce lipogenesis by partially blocking incorporation of free fatty acids.

Uterine Effects

Prolongation of labor by salicylates may reflect loss of the normal uterotropic effects of prostaglandins. Certainly, aspirin should be discontinued prior to the anticipated time of parturition to avoid prolonging labor or increasing postpartum hemorrhage.

Allergic Reactions

Allergic reactions to aspirin, although rare, can be life-threatening. Clinical manifestations may appear within minutes of ingestion and can include vasomotor rhinitis, laryngeal edema, bronchoconstriction, and cardiovascular collapse. Aspirin is more likely than salicylic acid to be associated with an allergic reaction. Despite the resemblance of the response to anaphylaxis, there is no evidence of an immunologic mechanism (Abrishami and Thomas, 1977). Nasal polyps develop in about 10% of patients who exhibit asthmatic-like allergic reactions to aspirin. Patients who are allergic to aspirin cross-react to all inhibitors of prostaglandin synthesis.

PHENYLBUTAZONE

Phenylbutazone is an effective anti-inflammatory drug that is useful in the therapy of acute gout and treatment of rheumatoid arthritis (Fig. 11-2). Acute exacerbations of these conditions respond well to this drug, and its use should be reserved for such episodes. Phenylbutazone is an effective alternative to colchicine in acute gout providing control in 85% of patients within 24 to 36 hours. Because of its toxicity, this drug should be given for short periods not exceeding 7 days (see the section entitled Side Effects). Certainly, phenylbutazone should not be used routinely as an analgesic or antipyretic.

Pharmacokinetics

Phenylbutazone is rapidly and completely absorbed from the gastrointestinal tract. Plasma protein binding approaches 98%. Metabolism of phenylbutazone is extensive involving glucuronidation and hydroxylation of the phenyl rings or the butyl side chain (Faigle and Dieterle, 1977). Oxyphenbutazone is a metabolite of phenylbutazone with anti-inflammatory activity similar to the parent drug. Phenylbutazone and oxyphenbutazone are slowly excreted in the urine because extensive plasma protein binding limits glomerular

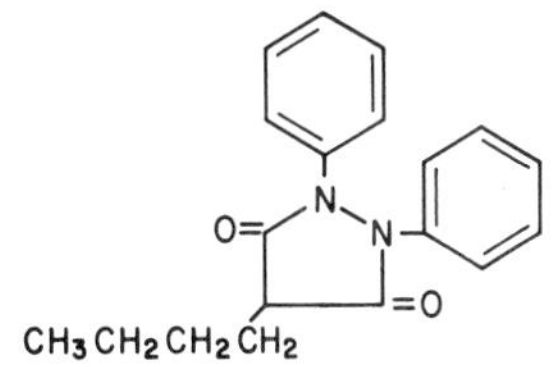

FIGURE 11-2. Phenylbutazone.

filtration. The elimination half-time of phenylbutazone is 50 to 100 hours, and significant plasma concentrations may persist in synovial spaces of joints for up to 3 weeks after treatment is discontinued.

Side Effects

Serious side effects of phenylbutazone therapy are frequent and include anemia and granulocytosis which limit the usefulness of this drug. Nausea, vomiting, epigastric discomfort, and skin rashes are frequent. Phenylbutazone causes significant sodium retention due to a reversible direct effect on renal tubules. This renal tubular effect is accompanied by decreased urine output. Plasma volume increases as much as 50%, and pulmonary edema may occur in patients with poor cardiac function. Weight gain and the appearance of dilutional anemia reflect drug-induced fluid retention.

Phenylbutazone displaces drugs including warfarin, oral hypoglycemics, and sulfonamides from protein binding sites. Displacement of thyroid hormone from protein binding sites complicates interpretation of thyroid function tests. Phenylbutazone reduces uptake of iodine by the thyroid gland presumably by inhibition of synthesis of organic iodine compounds.

PARA-AMINOPHENOL DERIVATIVES

Phenacetin and its active metabolite, acetaminophen, are useful alternatives to aspirin as analgesics and antipyretics especially in patients in whom salicylates are contraindicated (e.g., those with peptic ulcer disease) or when prolongation of bleeding time would be a disadvantage (Fig. 11-3). Indeed, para-aminophenol derivatives, unlike salicylates, do not produce gastric irritation or alter aggregation characteristics of platelets. Furthermore, unlike salicylates, these drugs do not antagonize the effects of uricosuric drugs permitting their administration to patients with gouty arthritis who are taking a uricosuric. Acetaminophen (325–650 mg every 4 hours in adults) has somewhat less overall toxicity and is usually preferred over phenacetin.

The anti-inflammatory effects of phenacetin and acetaminophen are weak (e.g., no significant antirheumatic effects) presumably reflecting the

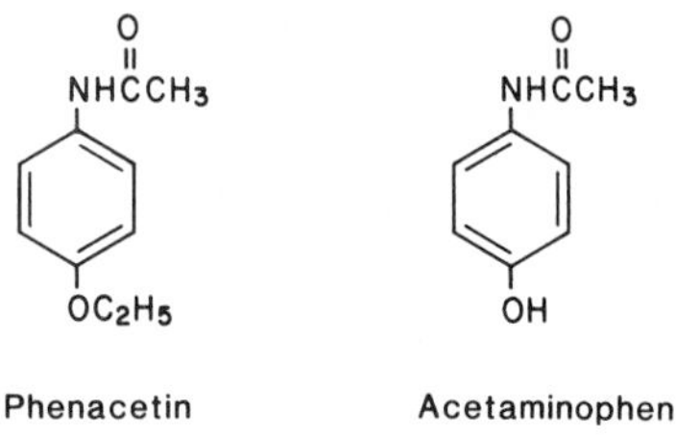

FIGURE 11-3. Para-aminophenol derivatives.

modest peripheral inhibiting effects on prostaglandin synthesis produced by these drugs. Conversely, strong central inhibition of prostaglandin synthesis confers analgesic and antipyretic effects.

Pharmacokinetics

The systemic absorption of phenacetin and acetaminophen after oral absorption is nearly complete. Significant binding to serum proteins does not occur.

Metabolism

About 75% of phenacetin is dealkylated to acetaminophen in the liver. Acetaminophen is converted by conjugation and hydroxylation in the liver to inactive metabolites with only small amounts of drug being excreted unchanged. High doses of acetaminophen result in formation of N-acetyl-p-benzoquinone which is believed to be responsible for hepatotoxicity (Levy, 1981) (see the section entitled Side Effects). Genetically determined limitations to metabolize phenacetin to acetaminophen result in formation of other metabolites with the potential to produce methemoglobinemia and hemolysis (see the section entitled Side Effects).

Side Effects

Methemoglobinemia following administration of phenacetin to susceptible persons and hepatic necrosis after an overdose of acetaminophen are the most serious side effects of para-aminophenol derivatives. Patients who are allergic to salicylates may also exhibit sensitivity to these drugs. Phenacetin may produce a sedative effect. Acid–base changes do not accompany administration of phenacetin or acetaminophen.

Methemoglobinemia

Phenacetin may cause methemoglobinemia and hemolytic anemia in patients with a genetic deficiency of glucose-6-phosphate enzyme in erythrocytes. Hemolysis and subsequent jaundice associated with administration of phenacetin are presumed to be due to metabolites that oxidize glutathione and components of erythrocyte membranes leading to shortened erythrocyte survival. Anuria may accompany severe intravascular hemolysis.

Hepatic Necrosis

Hepatic necrosis and death may accompany a single dose of acetaminophen that exceeds 15 g. Renal failure and hypoglycemia may also occur (Prescott, 1982). Clinical manifestations of hepatic damage, including jaundice and coagulation defects, occur 2 to 6 days after the overdose. Liver biopsy reveals centrilobular necrosis. Acetylcysteine administered early after an acetaminophen overdose may be effective in restoring hepatic stores of glutathione and preventing drug-induced hepatic necrosis (Prescott *et al,* 1976; Rumack *et al,* 1981).

INDOMETHACIN

Indomethacin is a methylated indole derivative with analgesic, antipyretic, and anti-inflammatory effects comparable to salicylates (Fig. 11-4). This drug is one of the most potent inhibitors of cyclooxygenase enzyme known. Its anti-inflammatory effects are useful in the management of patients with arthritis. Indomethacin provides anti-inflammatory effects comparable to cholchicine in the treatment of acute attacks of gouty arthritis. Conversely, indomethacin does not correct hyperuricemia and is, therefore, not useful in management of patients with chronic gout. Cardiac failure in neonates caused by patent ductus arteriosus may be controlled with single doses of indomethacin emphasizing the ability of this drug to inhibit synthesis of prostaglandins. Indomethacin also appears to be more effective than aspirin in relieving the pain of dysmenorrhea. Finally, patients with Bartter's syndrome have been successfully treated with indomethacin as well as with other inhibitors of prostaglandin synthesis (Norby *et al,* 1976).

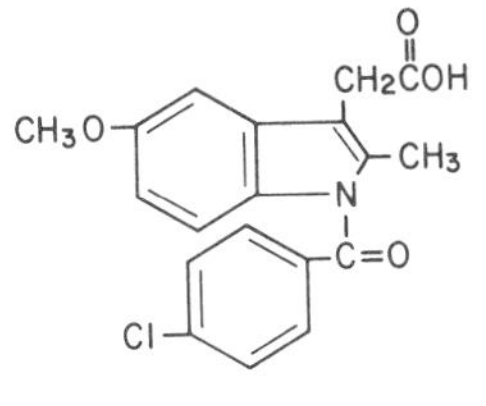

Pharmacokinetics

Indomethacin is rapidly and almost completely absorbed from the gastrointestinal tract following oral administration (Alvan *et al,* 1975). Protein binding is extensive, approaching 90%. Hepatic metabolism converts indomethacin to inactive substances.

Side Effects

Side effects associated with chronic administration of indomethacin limit its usefulness as an analgesic (Boardman and Hart, 1967). Up to 50% of patients receiving usual therapeutic doses of indomethacin experience unpleasant symptoms with severe frontal headaches being most frequent. Allergic reactions may occur, and cross-sensitivity with salicylates is likely. Neutropenia, thrombocytopenia, and aplastic anemia are rare.

PROPIONIC ACID DERIVATIVES

Ibuprofen, naproxen, and fenoprofen are nonsteroidal proprionic acid derivatives with prominent analgesic, antipyretic, and anti-inflammatory effects as a reflection of inhibition of prostaglandin synthesis (Fig. 11-5) (Miller, 1981; Sturge *et al,* 1977; Willkens, 1975). Proprionic acid derivatives are as useful as salicylates in treatment of various forms of arthritis including osteoarthritis, rheumatoid arthritis, and acute gouty arthritis. Naproxen is unique in that its longer elimination half-time makes twice daily administration effective.

Gastrointestinal irritation and mucosal ulceration are usually less severe than that which may accompany administration of salicylates. Platelet function is altered similarly to that produced by

FIGURE 11-4.   Indomethacin.

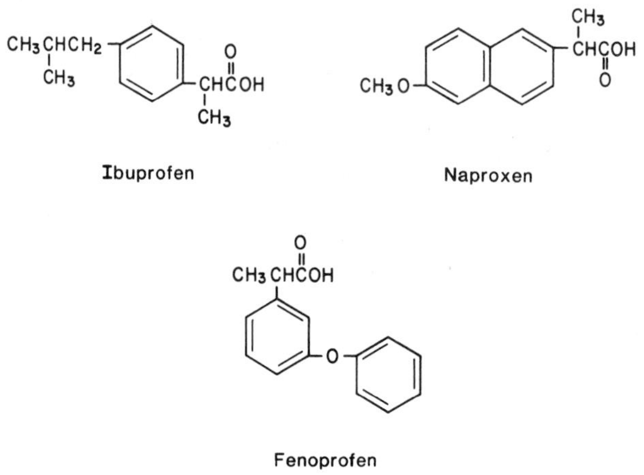

FIGURE 11-5.
Propionic acid derivatives.

Ibuprofen

Naproxen

Fenoprofen

salicylates. It should be assumed that any patient who is hypersensitive to salicylates may also be allergic to propionic acid derivatives.

Adverse drug interactions often reflect the extensive plasma protein binding to albumin of proprionic acid derivatives. For example, the dose of warfarin must be reduced because of its displacement from protein binding sites as well as alterations in platelet aggregation. Ibuprofen, however, is an exception, presumably because it occupies only a small number of binding sites on albumin. Hematopoietic suppression characterized by agranulocytosis and bone marrow granulocytic aplasia has been associated with chronic administration of ibuprofen (Mamus *et al*, 1986).

TOLMETIN

Tolmetin is an analgesic, antipyretic, and anti-inflammatory drug, that, like salicylates, causes gastric irritation and prolongs bleeding time (Fig. 11-6). It is more potent than salicylates and less potent than indomethacin or phenylbutazone (Aylward *et al*, 1976). After oral administration absorption is rapid and binding to plasma proteins is extensive (99%). Most of tolmetin is inactivated by decarboxylation.

ZOMEPIRAC

Zomepirac is a close analogue of tolmetin and possesses similar analgesic, antipyretic, and anti-inflammatory properties (Fig. 11-7) (Lewis,

1981). It relieves moderate postoperative pain presumably by inhibiting prostaglandin synthesis (Dunn *et al*, 1983). After oral administration of 100 mg, the onset of analgesia is in about 30 minutes with a duration of action of 4 to 6 hours. The analgesic effectiveness of zomepirac, 100 mg, is greater than codeine, 60 mg. Zomepirac reduces the need to use opioids in patients with chronic pain.

The incidence of gastrointestinal bleeding with zomepirac is less than with salicylates. Platelet adhesiveness and aggregation are decreased but, in contrast to the irreversible effects of aspirin on platelets, those of zomepirac are transient and normal function returns 24 to 48 hours after the drug is discontinued.

Zomepirac is eliminated primarily by the kidneys, and renal function should be evaluated peri-

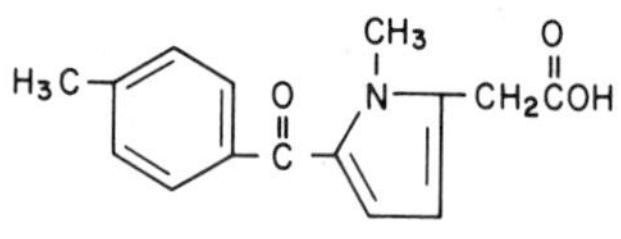

FIGURE 11-6. Tolmetin.

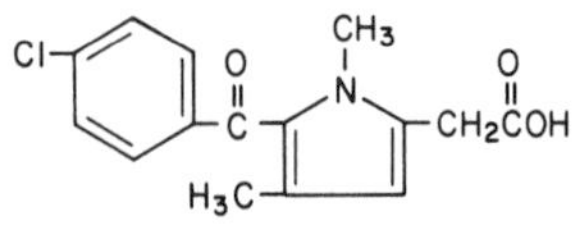

FIGURE 11-7. Zomepirac.

odically during long-term use. Allergy to salicylates is likely to manifest as cross-sensitivity with zomepirac. Although zomepirac is highly bound (98.5%) to plasma proteins, it does not interfere with the protein binding of warfarin and does not alter the prothrombin time of patients being treated with warfarin.

DIFLUNISAL

Diflunisal is a salicylic acid derivative that differs chemically from salicylates but possesses analgesic, antipyretic, and anti-inflammatory effects (Fig. 11-8) (Borgden *et al*, 1980). Like salicylates, this drug inhibits the synthesis of prostaglandins. Diflunisal, 500 to 1000 mg, is useful as an analgesic for the treatment of mild to moderate pain. Antiarthritic effects are prominent while antipyretic actions, although present, are not clinically useful. Diflunisal also has a uricosuric effect (Dresse *et al*, 1979).

Pharmacokinetics

Oral absorption of diflunisal is rapid. Like salicylic acid, diflunisal exhibits nonlinear pharmacokinetics characterized by more than a doubling of the plasma concentration when the dose is doubled. Metabolism of diflunisal is to glucuronide conjugates which are excreted in the urine.

Side Effects

The most frequent side effects of diflunisal are nausea, vomiting, and gastrointestinal irritation. The effect of diflunisal on platelet function and bleeding time is dose-related but reversible. Acute interstitial nephritis, perhaps due to inhibition of prostaglandin synthesis, may occur. Elevations in plasma concentrations of transaminase

enzymes occur in about 15% of patients, but severe hepatic dysfunction associated with jaundice is rare. Drowsiness is the most common symptom observed with an overdose of diflunisal.

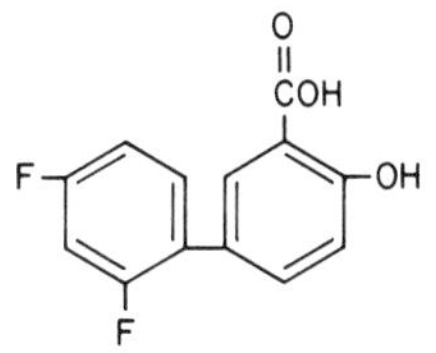

GOLD

Gold may be preferred to glucocorticoids in the treatment of rheumatoid arthritis producing symptomatic relief most likely by its uptake into macrophages and subsequent inhibition of phagocytosis and the activities of lysosomal enzymes (Jessop *et al*, 1973). Gold also reduces immunologic responses (Gottlieb *et al*, 1975). Water-soluble gold salts are rapidly absorbed after intramuscular injection. With chronic use, gold is concentrated in the synovium of affected joints. Renal excretion accounts for 60% to 90% of the administered gold and the remainder is lost via the bile.

Side Effects

Side effects of gold involve the skin and mucous membranes, usually of the mouth. Cutaneous reactions may vary in severity from simple erythema to severe exfoliative dermatitis. Glossitis is common and may extend to the pharynx, trachea, and gastrointestinal tract. A gray to blue pigmentation (chrysiasis) may occur in the skin and mucous membranes especially in areas exposed to light.

Thrombocytopenia is the most frequent cause of mortality and reflects accelerated degradation of platelets (Levin *et al,* 1975). Leukopenia, agranulocytosis, and aplastic anemia may also occur. Eosinophilia is common during therapy with gold. Proteinuria is frequent, reflecting damage to proximal renal tubules. Nephrosis characterized by membranous glomerulonephritis may develop. Rare but other serious complications include encephalitis, peripheral neuritis, hepatitis, and pulmonary infiltrates. Regular examination of the skin and buccal mucosa and performance of platelet counts and renal function tests are indicated to detect early gold-induced toxicity.

COLCHICINE

Colchicine reduces inflammation and thus relieves pain in acute gouty arthritis (Fig. 11-9). This drug is unique in that its beneficial anti-inflammatory effects are limited to the treatment of acute

FIGURE 11-8.   Diflunisal.

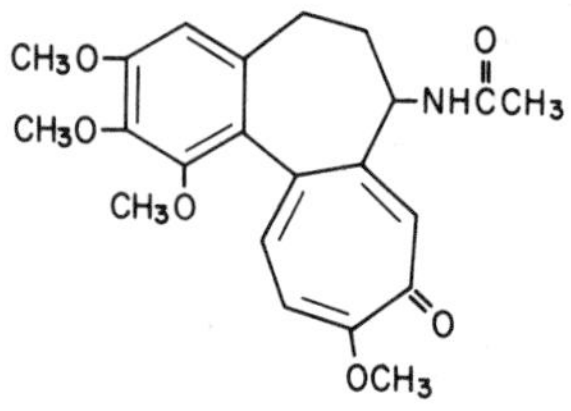

FIGURE 11-9. Colchicine.

attacks of gout as well as prophylaxis against such attacks (Malawista, 1975). Relief of pain and inflammation usually occurs within 24 to 48 hours after oral administration. Colchicine is not an analgesic and does not provide relief of other types of pain or inflammation.

Mechanism of Action

Colchicine does not influence the renal excretion of uric acid but instead alters fibrillar microtubules in granulocytes resulting in inhibition of the migration of these cells into inflamed areas (Spilberg *et al*, 1979). This effect reduces the release of lactic acid and other inflammation-producing enzymes. As a result, the cycle that leads to the inflammatory response evoked by crystals of sodium urate that are deposited in joint tissue is inhibited. Large amounts of colchicine and its metabolites are excreted in the bile with lesser amounts appearing in the urine (Halkin *et al*, 1980).

Side Effects

Nausea, vomiting, diarrhea, and abdominal pain are the most common side effects of colchicine occurring in about 80% of patients. Gastrointestinal intolerance tends to protect the patient from toxic doses of colchicine. Indeed, oral administration of colchicine must be discontinued as soon as gastrointestinal symptoms appear because hemorrhagic gastroenteritis can result in severe fluid and electrolyte losses. Gastrointestinal side effects may be minimized by administering colchicine intravenously. Colchicine enhances effects produced by central nervous system depressants and sympathomimetics. The medullary ventilatory center is depressed. Severe colchicine toxicity may manifest as bone marrow depression with leukopenia and thrombocytopenia.

ALLOPURINOL

Allopurinol is the preferred drug for the therapy of primary hyperuricemia of gout and that which occurs during therapy with chemotherapeutic drugs (Fig. 11-10). In contrast to uricosuric drugs that facilitate renal excretion of urate, allopurinol interferes with the terminal steps of uric acid synthesis by virtue of inhibition of xanthine oxidase, the enzyme that converts xanthine to uric acid.

Allopurinol is readily absorbed after oral administration and is rapidly converted to oxipurinol with less than 10% to 30% of the drug appearing unchanged in the urine. Most of the oxipurinol is excreted unchanged by the kidney. Oxipurinol is also an inhibitor of xanthine oxidase activity and has an elimination half-time of about 21 hours compared with 1.3 hours for allopurinol.

The most common side effect of allopurinol is a maculopapular rash, frequently preceded by pruritus. Fever and myalgia may occur. These hypersensitivity-like syndromes may be due to allopurinol acting as a hapten to produce immune complex dermatitis. Pruritus is an indication to discontinue therapy with allopurinol. Allopurinol, acting as a hapten, could also result in nephritis and vasculitis. Hepatic dysfunction, ranging from increases in plasma concentrations of transaminase enzymes to hepatitis are common in patients treated will allopurinol.

Allopurinol inhibits the enzymatic inactivation of 6-mercaptopurine and azathioprine such that doses of these drugs must be reduced. Hepatic drug metabolizing enzymes are inhibited by allopurinol which may result in unexpected prolonged effects produced by drugs that are extensively metabolized including the oral anticoagulants.

URICOSURIC DRUGS

Uricosuric drugs, such as probenecid and sulfinpyrazone, act directly on renal tubules to increase the rate of excretion of uric acid and other organic

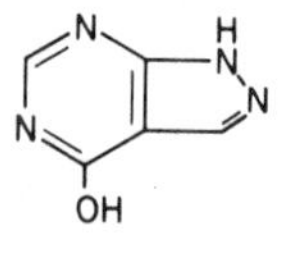

FIGURE 11-10. Allopurinol.

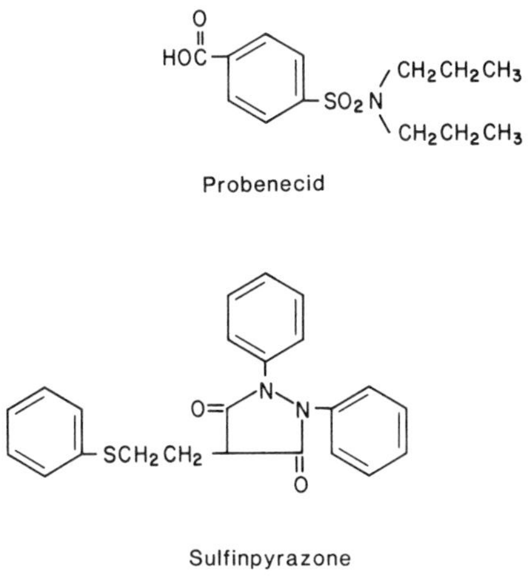

Probenecid

Sulfinpyrazone

FIGURE 11-11. Uricosuric drugs.

acids including penicillin (Fig. 11-11). These drugs are also useful for the control of hyperuricemia resulting from the use of chemotherapeutic drugs or from diseases that are associated with the accelerated destruction of erythrocytes. Salicylates antagonize the uricosuric action of probenecid but not its capacity to inhibit the renal tubular excretion of penicillin. Biliary excretion of rifampin is reduced by probenecid making it possible to achieve higher plasma concentrations of this antituberculosis drug.

Probenecid

Probenecid is completely absorbed after oral administration with peak plasma concentrations occurring in 2 to 4 hours. The elimination half-time is about 8 hours. About 90% of probenecid is bound to plasma albumin. A total adult daily dose of 1 g of probenecid in four divided doses is necessary to block effectively the renal excretion of penicillin. The plasma concentration of penicillin achieved in the presence of probenecid is at least twice the level achieved with the antibiotic alone.

Mild allergic reactions characterized as cutaneous rashes occur in 2% to 4% of patients treated with probenecid. This rash is a diagnostic dilemma when probenecid is administered in conjunction with penicillin. Hepatic dysfunction can occur but is rare.

Sulfinpyrazone

Sulfinpyrazone is an organic congener of phenylbutazone that lacks anti-inflammatory effects but instead is a potent inhibitor of the renal tubular reabsorption of uric acid (Margulies *et al,* 1980). This uricosuric action of sulfinpyrazone is antagonized by salicylates. Renal tubular secretion of many drugs is also reduced. For example, sulfinpyrazone may induce hypoglycemia by decreasing the excretion of oral hypoglycemics.

Sulfinpyrazone is well-absorbed after oral administration. Protein binding approaches 98%. The drug undergoes secretion by proximal renal tubules as protein binding limits its glomerular filtration. About 90% of sulfinpyrazone appears unchanged in the urine. The remainder of the drug is metabolized to the parahydroxyl analogue which also has uricosuric activity.

Gastrointestinal irritation occurs in 10% to 15% of patients treated with sulfinpyrazone suggesting caution in the administration of this drug to patients with peptic ulcer disease. Allergic reactions, characterized by rash and fever, occur infrequently. Sulfinpyrazone inhibits platelet function.

REFERENCES

Abrishami MA, Thomas J. Aspirin intolerance—a review. Ann Allergy 1977;39:28–37.

Alvan G, Orme M, Bertilsson L, Ekstrand R, Palmer L. Pharmacokinetics of indomethacin. Clin Pharmacol Ther 1975;18:364–73.

Arger PH, Bluth EI, Murray T, Goldberg M. Analgesic abuse nephrotoxicity. Urology 1976;7:123–8.

Aylward M, Maddock J, Parker RJ, Thomas SR, Holly F. Evaluation of tolmetin in the treatment of active chronic rheumatoid arthritis: open and controlled double blind studies. Curr Med Res Opin 1976;4:158–69.

Boardman RL, Hart ED. Clinical measurement of the anti-inflammatory effects of salicylates in rheumatoid arthritis. Br Med J 1967;4:264–8.

Brogden RN, Heel RC, Pakes GE, Speight TM, Avery GS. Diflunisal: Review of its pharmacological properties and therapeutic use in pain and musculoskeletal strain and sprains and pain in osteoarthritis. Drugs 1980;19:84–106.

Dresse A, Fisher P, Gerard MA, et al. Uricosuric properties of diflunisal in man. Br J Clin Pharmac 1979;7:267–72.

Dunn GL, Morison DH, Fargas-Babjak AM, Goldsmith CH. A comparison of zomepirac and codeine as analgesic premedicants in short-stay surgery. Anesthesiology 1983;58:265–9.

Faigle JW, Dieterle W. The biotransformation of phenylbutazone (butazolidin). J Int Med Res 1977;5:2–14.

Gottlieb NL, Kiem IM, Penneys NS, Schultz DR. The influence of chrysotherapy on serum protein and immunoglobulin levels, rheumatoid factor, and antiepithelial antibody titers. J Lab Clin Med 1975;86:962–72.

Halkin H, Dany S, Greenwald M, Shnaps Y, Tirosh M. Colchicine kinetics in patients with familial mediterranean fever. Clin Pharmacol Ther 1980;28:82–7.

Halla JT. Aspirin, liver, and rheumatic diseases. J Med Assoc State Ala 1976;46:23–5.

Heymann MA, Rudolph AM, Silverman NH. Closure of the ductus arteriosus in premature infants by inhibition of prostaglandin synthesis. N Engl J Med 1976;295:530–3.

Hill JB. Salicylate intoxication. N Engl J Med 1973;288:1110–3.

Jessop JD, Vernon-Roberts B, Harris J. Effects of gold salts and prednisolone on inflammatory cells. Phagocytic activity of macrophages and polymorphs in inflammatory exudates studied by a skin-window technique in rheumatoid and control patients. Ann Rheum Dis 1973;32:294–300.

Leonards JR, Levy G. Gastrointestinal blood loss during prolonged aspirin administration. N Engl J. Med 1973;289:1020–2.

Levin HA, McMillan R, Tavassoli M, Longmire RL, Yelenosky R, Sacks PV. Thrombocytopenia associated with gold therapy: observations on the mechanism of platelet destruction. Am J Med 1975;59:274–80.

Levy G. Comparative pharmacokinetics of aspirin and acetaminophen. Arch Intern Med 1981;141:279–81.

Lewis JR. Zomepirac sodium: New nonaddicting analgesic. JAMA 1981;246:377–9.

Malawista SE. The action of colchicine in acute gouty arthritis. Arthritis Rheum 1975;6:835–46.

Mamus SW, Burton JW, Groat JD, Schulte DA, Lobell M, Zanjani ED. Ibuprofen-associated pure white-cell aplasia. N Engl J Med 1986;314:624–5.

Margulies EH, White AM, Sherry S. Sulfinpyrazone: Review of its pharmacological properties and therapeutic use. Drugs 1980;20:179–97.

Metz SA. Anti-inflammatory agents as inhibitors of prostaglandin synthesis in man. Med Clin North Am 1981;65:713–57.

Miller RR. Evaluation of analgesic efficacy of ibuprofen. Pharmacotherapy 1981;1:21–7.

Moncada S, Vane JR. Mode of action of aspirin-like drugs. Adv Intern Med 1979;24:1–22.

Norby L, Flamenbaum W, Lentz R, Ramwell P. Prostaglandins and aspirin therapy in Bartter's syndrome. Lancet 1976;2:604–6.

Prescott LF. Analgesic nephropathy. Reassessment of role of phenacetin and other analgesics. Drugs 1982;23:75–149.

Prescott LF, Park J, Sutherland GR, Smith IJ, Proudfood AT. Cysteamine, methionine, and penicillamine in the treatment of paracetamol poisoning. Lancet 1976;2:109–13.

Roth GR, Siok CJ. Acetylation of the NH_2-terminal serine of prostaglandin synthetase by aspirin. J Biol Chem 1978;253:3782–4.

Rumack BH, Peterson RC, Koch GG, Amara IA. Acetaminophen overdose: 662 cases with evaluation of oral acetylcysteine treatment. Arch Intern Med 1981;141:380–5.

Settipane GA. Adverse reactions to aspirin and related drugs. Arch Intern Med 1981;141:328–32.

Smith JB, Willis AL. Aspirin selectively inhibits prostaglandin production in human platelets. Nature 1971;231:235–7.

Spilberg I, Mandell B, Mehta J, Simchowitz L, Rosenberg D. Mechanism of action of colchicine in acute urate crystal-induced arthritis. J Clin Invest 1979;64:775–80.

Sturge RA, Scott JT, Hamilton EBD, et al. Multicentre trial of naproxen and phenylbutazone in acute gout. Ann Rheum Dis 1977;36:80–2.

Turner G, Collins E. Fetal effects of regular salicylate ingestion in pregnancy. Lancet 1975;2:338–9.

Willkens RF. Treatment of acute gout with naproxen. J Clin Pharmacol 1975;15:363–6.

CHAPTER 12

Sympathomimetics

INTRODUCTION

Sympathomimetics include naturally occurring (endogenous) catecholamines, synthetic catecholamines, and synthetic noncatecholamines that are further subdivided as indirect-acting and direct-acting (Table 12-1). These drugs evoke physiologic responses similar to that produced by endogenous activity of the sympathetic nervous system. For example, pharmacologic effects of sympathomimetics, although quantitatively different, may include (1) vasoconstriction, especially in the cutaneous and renal circulations, (2) vasodilation in skeletal muscle, (3) bronchodilation, (4) cardiac stimulation characterized by increased heart rate, myocardial contractility, and vulnerability to cardiac dysrhythmias, (5) hepatic glycogenolysis, (6) liberation of free fatty acids from adipose tissue, (7) modulation of secretion of insulin, renin, and pituitary hormones, and (8) central nervous system stimulation (Lawson and Wallfisch, 1986; Smith and Corbascio, 1970; Smith and Oldershaw, 1984). The net effect of sympathomimetics on cardiac function is influenced by baroreceptor-mediated reflex responses.

CLINICAL USES

Clinically, sympathomimetics are used most often as (1) positive inotropes to improve myocardial contractility or (2) vasopressors to elevate blood pressure from unacceptably low levels as may accompany sympathetic nervous system blockade produced by regional anesthesia. A pulmonary artery catheter permitting measurement of atrial filling pressures and cardiac output as well as calculation of peripheral and pulmonary vascular resistances is useful when sympathomimetics are administered to improve myocardial contractility. Sympathomimetics may also be used as vasopressors to maintain blood pressure during the time needed to eliminate excess inhaled anesthetic or restore intravascular fluid volume. The prolonged administration of sympathomimetics to support blood pressure in the presence of hypovolemia is not recommended. Indeed, the only time a vasopressor should be administered is when blood pressure must be increased immediately to prevent pressure-dependent reductions in blood flow and resulting organ ischemia. Disadvantages of using sympathomimetics that lack significant beta-1 adrenergic effects to maintain blood pressure include intense vasoconstriction and associated blood pressure elevations that evoke reflex-mediated bradycardia that lowers cardiac output. Other uses of selected sympathomimetics include (1) treatment of bronchospasm in patients with asthma, (2) management of life-threatening allergic reactions, and (3) addition to local anesthetic solutions to retard systemic absorption of the local anesthetic (see Chapter 7).

Table 12-1
Classification and Comparative Pharmacology of Sympathomimetics

| | Receptors Stimulated | | | Mechanism of Action | Cardiac Effects | | | Peripheral Vascular Resistance | Renal Blood Flow | Mean Arterial Pressure | Airway Resistance | Central Nervous System Stimulation | Single Intravenous Dose (70-kg adult) | Continuous Infusion Dose (70-kg adult) |
	Alpha	Beta-1	Beta-2		Cardiac Output	Heart Rate	Dys-rhythmias							
Natural Catecholamines														
Epinephrine	+	++	++	Direct	++	++	+++	±	––	+	––	Yes	200–350 µg	1–20 µg min⁻¹
Norepinephrine	+++	++	0	Direct	–	–	+	+++	–––	+++	NC	No	Not used	4–16 µg min⁻¹
Dopamine	++	++	+	Direct	+++	+	+	+	+++	+	NC	No	Not used	2–20 µg kg⁻¹ min⁻¹
Synthetic Catecholamines														
Isoproterenol	0	+++	+++		+++	+++	+++	––	–	±	–––	Yes	1–4 µg	1–5 µg min⁻¹
Dobutamine	0	+++	0		+++	+	±	NC	++	+	NC	No	Not used	2–10 µg kg⁻¹ min⁻¹
Synthetic Noncatecholamines														
Indirect-Acting														
Ephedrine	++	+	+	Indirect, some direct	++	++	++	+	––	++	––	Yes	10–25 mg	Not used
Mephentermine	++	+	+	Indirect	++	++	++	+	––	++	–	Yes	10–25 mg	Not used
Amphetamines	++	+	+	Indirect	+	+	+	++	––	+	NC	Yes	Not used	Not used
Metaraminol	++	+	+	Indirect, direct	–	–	+	+++	–––	+++	NC	No	1.5–5 mg	40–500 µg min⁻¹
Direct Acting														
Phenylephrine	+++	0	0	Direct	–	–	NC	+++	––––	+++	NC	No	50–100 µg	20–50 µg min⁻¹
Methoxamine	+++	0	0	Direct	–	–	NC	+++	–––	+++	NC	No	5–10 mg	Not used

0 none; + minimal increase; ++ moderate increase; +++ marked increase; – minimal decrease; –– moderate decrease; ––– marked decrease; NC No Change

STRUCTURE ACTIVITY RELATIONSHIPS

All sympathomimetics are derived from beta-phenylethylamine (Fig. 12-1). The presence of hydroxyl groups on the 3 and 4 positions of the benzene ring (*e.g.,* dihydroxybenzene) of beta-phenylethylamine is designated a catechol and drugs with this composition are designated catecholamines. For example, 3,4-dihydroxylphenyl-ethylamine is the endogenous catecholamine, dopamine. Hydroxylation of the beta carbon of dopamine results in the endogenous catecholamine and neurotransmitter, norepinephrine. The third endogenous catecholamine, epinephrine, results from methylation of the terminal amine of norepinephrine. Addition of an isopropyl group rather than a methyl group to the terminal amine results in the synthetic catecholamine, isoproterenol. The other synthetic catecholamine, dobutamine, possesses a bulky aromatic substituent on the terminal amine. Synthetic noncatecholamines include the beta-phenylethylamine structure but lack hydroxyl groups on the 3 and/or 4 positions of the benzene ring (Fig. 12-2).

The dextrorotatory forms of norepinephrine and epinephrine are about one-half as active as the levorotatory isomer. The levorotatory isomer of isoproterenol is more than 1000 times as active as the dextrorotatory isomer.

Receptor Selectivity

The relative selectivity of sympathomimetics for various adrenergic receptors depends on the chemical structure of the drug. Maximal alpha- and beta-adrenergic receptor activity depends on the presence of hydroxyl groups on the 3 and 4 positions of the benzene ring of beta-phenylethyl-amine (*e.g.,* catecholamine). Epinephrine has the optimal structure for producing alpha- and beta-adrenergic effects (Fig. 12-1). Any change in chemical structure compared with epinephrine results in a compound that is less active at alpha-

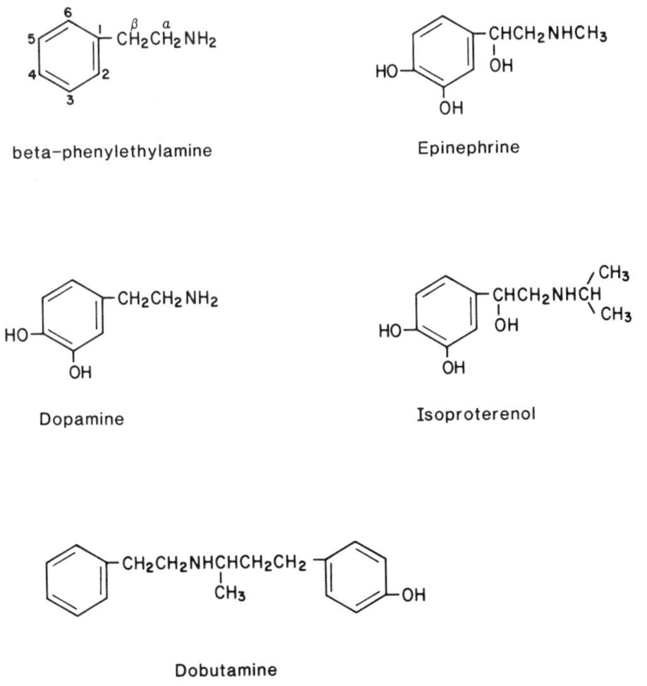

FIGURE 12-1. Sympathomimetics are derived from beta-phenylethylamine with a catecholamine being any compound that has hydroxyl groups on the 3 and 4 positions of the benzene ring.

and beta-adrenergic receptors. Indeed, phenylephrine, which lacks the 4-hydroxyl group, is less potent than epinephrine on both alpha- and beta-adrenergic receptors (Fig. 12-2). Despite decreased potency, the removal of this 4-hydroxyl group increases the alpha-1 selectivity of phenylephrine. Substitution on the terminal amine of beta-phenylethylamine increases activity of the drug at beta receptors. For example, norepinephrine possesses minimal beta-2 agonist activity while this activity is greatly accentuated in epinephrine with the addition of a methyl group to the terminal amine. Beta-1 and beta-2 receptor activity are maximal in isoproterenol which contains an isopropyl group on the terminal amine.

Hydroxyl groups in the 3 and 5 positions of the benzene ring confer selective beta-2 agonist activity on compounds with long chain substituents (Fig. 12-3). Thus, metaproterenol, terbutaline, and albuterol relax bronchial smooth muscle without evoking significant beta-1 cardiac effects.

Central Nervous System Stimulation

Central nervous system stimulation is prominent with synthetic noncatecholamines that lack substitutents on the benzene ring (e.g., methamphetamine) (Fig. 12-2). Substitution of a hydroxyl group on the beta carbon of the ethylamine side chain (e.g., ephedrine) reduces central nervous system stimulant effects presumably by decreasing lipid solubility. Such a substitution, however, enhances alpha- and beta-adrenergic receptor agonist activity. Thus, ephedrine is less potent than methamphetamine as a central nervous system

stimulant but is more potent as a bronchodilator and cardiac stimulant. Catecholamines have limited lipid solubility and thus are not likely to cross the blood–brain barrier in sufficient amounts to cause central nervous system stimulation.

MECHANISM OF ACTION

Sympathomimetics exert their pharmacologic effects by activating either directly or indirectly alpha-adrenergic, beta-adrenergic, or dopaminergic receptors (see Chapter 42). Production of cyclic AMP by stimulation of the enzyme adenylate cyclase is the speculated mechanism by which sympathomimetics produce pharmacologic effects considered to reflect beta-adrenergic receptor stimulation (Maze, 1981). For example, increased cyclic AMP stimulates protein kinases which phosphorylate substrates and enhance inward calcium flux which may manifest as myocardial stimulation (e.g., beta-1 effects). Conversely, beta-2 receptor activation, characterized by relaxation of bronchial and vascular smooth muscle, reflects hyperpolarization of cell membranes and reduced inward calcium flux. Alpha-1 receptor stimulation increases inward flux of calcium ions and also probably facilitates the release of bound intracellular calcium. These actions may be mediated by increased membrane turnover of phosphatidylinositol (Fain and Garcia-Sainz, 1980). Alpha-2 receptor stimulation inhibits adenylate cyclase activity. Dopamine-mediated activation of adenylate cyclase and subsequent increased intracellular concentrations of cyclic AMP is responsible for renal artery dilatation that follows activa-

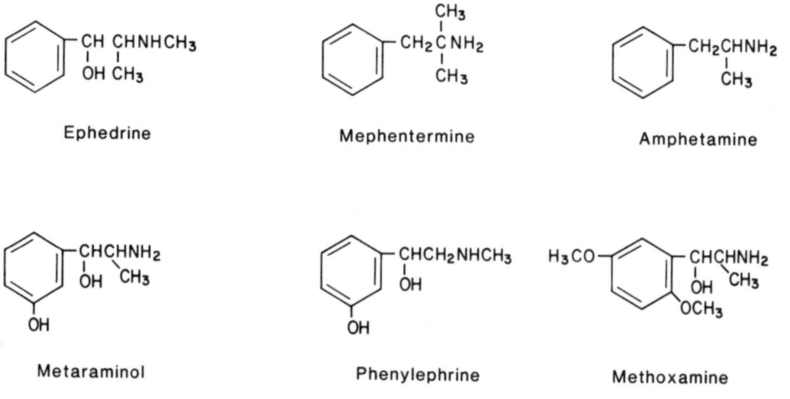

FIGURE 12-2. Indirect-acting and direct-acting synthetic non-catecholamines.

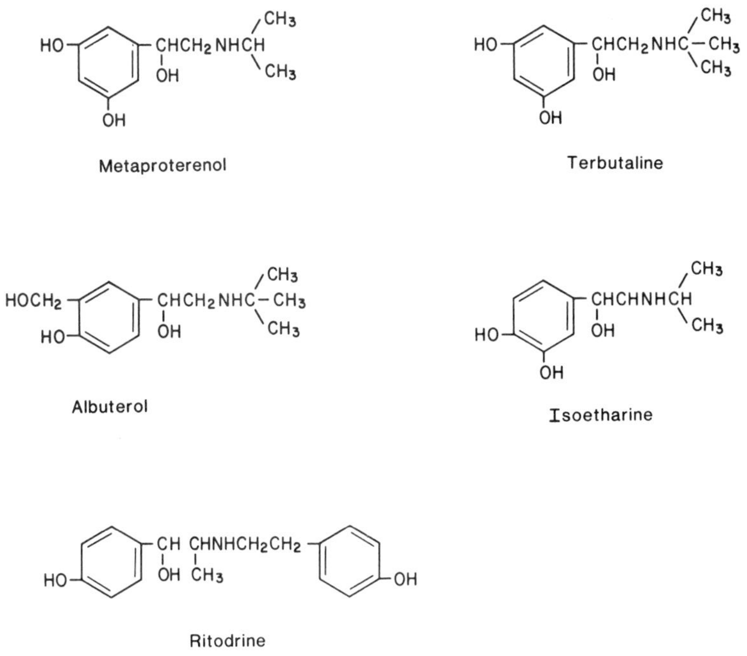

Metaproterenol

Terbutaline

Albuterol

Isoetharine

Ritodrine

FIGURE 12-3. Selective beta-2 agonists.

tion of dopamine-1 receptors (Gilbert *et al,* 1975).

Cyclic AMP is often referred to as the second messenger while the water-soluable sympathomimetic which activates adenylate cyclase to catalyze the conversion of adenosine triphosphate to cyclic AMP is referred to as the first messenger. The intracellular level of cyclic AMP is also controlled by phosphodiesterase which hydrolyzes cyclic AMP to an inactive molecule.

An important factor in the pharmacologic response elicited by a sympathomimetic is the density of alpha- and beta-adrenergic receptors in tissues. There is an inverse relationship between the concentration of available sympathomimetic and the number of receptors (Roth *et al,* 1979). For example, increased plasma concentrations of norepinephrine result in a decrease in the density of beta-adrenergic receptors in cell membranes (i.e., down regulation). Likewise, chronic treatment of patients with bronchial asthma, utilizing a beta-2 agonist, results in tachyphylaxis presumably reflecting decreased receptor density.

The anatomical distribution of alpha- and beta-adrenergic receptors influences the pharmacologic response evoked by sympathomimetics (Table 12-1). For example, norepinephrine has minimal effects on airway resistance because adrenergic receptors in bronchial smooth muscle are principally beta-2 receptors and are not stimulated by this catecholamine. Conversely, epinephrine and isoproterenol are potent bronchodilators as a result of their ability to activate beta-2 receptors. Cutaneous blood vessels possess alpha-adrenergic receptors almost exclusively resulting in vasoconstriction when activated by norepinephrine or epinephrine. Smooth muscle of blood vessels supplying skeletal muscle contains both beta-2 and alpha-1 receptors such that low doses of epinephrine produce beta-mediated vasodilation and high doses evoke alpha-mediated vasoconstriction which overrides evidence of beta stimulation. Beta-1 receptors are equally responsive to epinephrine and norepinephrine while beta-2 receptors are more sensitive to epinephrine than norepinephrine (Maze, 1981).

Indirect-Acting Sympathomimetics

Indirect-acting sympathomimetics are synthetic noncatecholamines that activate adrenergic receptors by evoking the release of the endogenous neurotransmitter, norepinephrine, from postganglionic sympathetic nerve endings (Table 12-1) (Fig. 12-2). Presumably, these drugs enter postganglionic sympathetic nerve endings from which they displace norepinephrine outward into the synaptic cleft (Burn and Rand, 1958). Denervation or depletion of neurotransmitter, as with repeated doses of sympathomimetics, blunts the pharmacologic responses normally evoked by these drugs. For some synthetic noncatecholamines, such as ephedrine, pharmacologic effects may reflect combinations of direct and indirect actions.

Indirect-acting sympathomimetics are characterized mostly by alpha- and beta-1 agonist effects because norepinephrine is a weak beta-2 agonist (Table 12-1). The blood pressure response to indirect-acting sympathomimetics is reduced by drugs that decrease central nervous system sympathetic

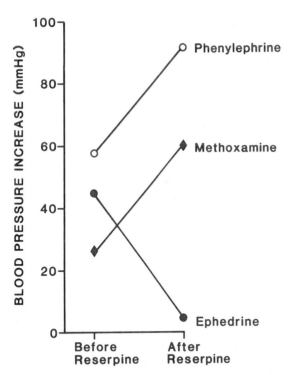

FIGURE 12-4. Reserpine blunts blood pressure-elevating effects of an indirect-acting sympathomimetic (ephedrine) while blood pressure responses to direct-acting sympathomimetics (phenylephrine and methoxamine) are enhanced. (Data from Eger EI, Hamilton WK. The effect of reserpine on the action of various vasopressors. Anesthesiology 1959;20:641–5; with permission of the authors and publisher.)

nervous system activity (Figs. 12-4 and 12-5) (Eger and Hamilton, 1959; Miller *et al,* 1968).

Direct-Acting Sympathomimetics

Direct-acting sympathomimetics include catecholamines and synthetic noncatecholamines, phenylephrine, and methoxamine (Table 12-1) (Fig. 12-2). These sympathomimetics activate adrenergic receptors directly although the potency of direct-acting synthetic noncatecholamines is less than catecholamines. Denervation or depletion of neurotransmitter does not prevent the activity of these drugs. Most direct-acting sympathomimetics activate both alpha- and beta-adrenergic receptors, but the magnitude of alpha and beta activity varies greatly among drugs from almost pure alpha agonist activity for phenylephrine to almost pure beta agonist activity for isoproterenol (Table 12-1).

Sympathetic nervous system blockade which deprives alpha-adrenergic receptor sites of tonic impulses results in increased sensitivity of these sites to norepinephrine. As a result, exaggerated blood pressure increases can follow the administration of direct-acting sympathomimetics (Fig. 12-4) (Eger and Hamilton, 1959).

METABOLISM

Catecholamines

All drugs containing the 3,4-dihydroxybenzene structure (*e.g.,* catecholamines) are rapidly inactivated by the enzymes monoamine oxidase (MAO) and/or catechol-O-methyltransferase (COMT). MAO is an enzyme present in the liver, kidneys, and gastrointestinal tract that catalyzes oxidative deamination. COMT is capable of methylating a hydroxyl group of catecholamines. The resulting inactive methylated metabolites are conjugated with glucuronic acid and appear in the urine as 3-methoxy-4-hydroxymandelic acid, metanephrine (derived from epinephrine), and normetanephrine (derived from norepinephrine).

Despite the importance of enzymatic degradation of catecholamines, the biologic actions of these substances are terminated principally by uptake back into postganglionic sympathetic nerve endings. Inhibition of this uptake mechanism produces a greater potentiation of the effects of epi-

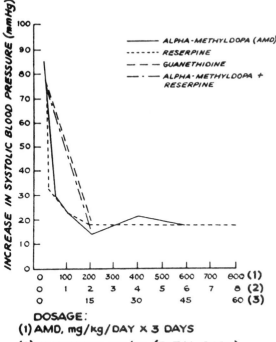

FIGURE 12-5. Pretreatment with methyldopa (AMD), reserpine, or guanethidine prevents the increase in blood pressure normally evoked by intravenous administration of ephedrine. (From Miller RD, Way WL, Eger EI. The effects of alpha-methyldopa, reserpine, guanethidine, and iproniazid on minimum alveolar anesthetic requirement [MAC]. Anesthesiology 1968; 29:1153–8. Reproduced by permission of the authors and publisher.)

nephrine than does inhibition of either enzyme. The completeness of this uptake mechanism and metabolism is emphasized by the appearance of only minimal amounts of unchanged catecholamines in the urine.

Circulating concentrations of dopamine and epinephrine are not altered in passage across the lungs while norepinephrine is removed to a large extent (Junod, 1977). Because epinephrine traverses the lungs without change, the same concentration exists in arterial and venous blood. In animals, halothane and nitrous oxide decrease removal of norepinephrine from the blood by the lungs (Naito and Gillis, 1973). It is possible that

inhaled anesthetics interfere with the amine transport system necessary to deliver norepinephrine into pulmonary cells.

Synthetic Noncatecholamines

Synthetic noncatecholamines lacking a 3-hydroxyl group are not affected by COMT and thus depend on MAO for their metabolism. Metabolism of these sympathomimetics, however, is often slower than that of catecholamines, and inhibition of MAO may even further prolong their duration of action. For this reason, patients treated with monoamine oxidase inhibitors may manifest exaggerated responses when treated with synthetic noncatecholamines (see Chapter 19).

The presence of an alpha methyl group, as with ephedrine or amphetamine, inhibits deamination by MAO. Ephedrine may be excreted unchanged in the urine. Urinary excretion of unchanged drug is even greater if the urine is acidified, emphasizing the fact that many synthetic noncatecholamines have pK values above 9.

ROUTE OF ADMINISTRATION

Oral administration of catecholamines is not effective, presumably reflecting the metabolism of these compounds by enzymes in the gastrointestinal mucosa and liver before reaching the systemic circulation. For this reason, epinephrine is administered subcutaneously or intravenously. Dopamine and norepinephrine are administered only intravenously. Absence of one or both of the 3,4-hydroxyl groups or the presence of an alpha methyl group, as characteristic of synthetic noncatecholamines, increases their oral absorption.

NATURALLY OCCURRING CATECHOLAMINES

Naturally occurring catecholamines are epinephrine, norepinephrine and dopamine (Table 12-1) (Fig. 12-1).

Epinephrine

Epinephrine is the prototype drug among the sympathomimetics. Its natural functions upon release from the adrenal medulla include regulation of (1) myocardial contractility, (2) heart rate, (3) vascular and bronchial smooth muscle tone, (4) glandular secretions, and (5) metabolic processes such as glycogenolysis and lipolysis. It is the most potent activator of alpha-adrenergic receptors being two to ten times more active than norepinephrine and more than 100 times more potent that isoproterenol. Epinephrine also activates beta-1 and beta-2 receptors. Oral administration is not effective because epinephrine is rapidly metabolized in the gastrointestinal mucosa and liver. Therefore, the route of administration of epinephrine is subcutaneous or intravenous. Absorption after subcutaneous injection is slow because of local vasoconstriction. Epinephrine is poorly lipid soluble preventing its ready entrance into the central nervous system and accounting for the lack of cortical effects.

Clinical Uses

Clinical uses of epinephrine include (1) addition to local anesthetic solutions so as to reduce systemic absorption and prolong the duration of action of the anesthetic, (2) treatment of life-threatening allergic reactions, (3) production of course ventricular fibrillation during cardiopulmonary resuscitation, and (4) continuous intravenous infusion to increase myocardial contractility.

Cardiovascular Effects

Cardiovascular effects of epinephrine result from epinephrine-induced stimulation of alpha- and beta-adrenergic receptors (Table 12-1). Small intravenous doses of epinephrine ($1-2$ μg min^{-1}) administered to adults stimulate principally beta-2 receptors in peripheral vasculature. Stimulation of beta-1 receptors occurs at somewhat greater doses (4 μg min^{-1}) while large doses of epinephrine ($10-20$ μg min^{-1}) stimulate both alpha- and beta-adrenergic receptors with the effects of alpha stimulation predominating in most vascular beds including the cutaneous and renal circulations. A single rapid intravenous injection of epinephrine, 2 to 8 μg, produces transient cardiac stimulation lasting 1 to 5 minutes usually without an overshoot of blood pressure or heart rate. During continuous infusion the concomitant administration of a vasodilator can offset epinephrine-induced vasocon-

striction especially in the splanchnic and renal circulations.

Epinephrine stimulates beta-1 receptors to cause an increase in systolic blood pressure, heart rate, and cardiac output. There is a modest reduction in diastolic blood pressure reflecting vasodilation in skeletal muscles due to activation of beta-2 receptors. The net effect of the blood pressure changes is an increase in pulse pressure and minimal change in mean arterial pressure. Because mean arterial pressure does not change greatly, there is little likelihood that baroreceptor activation will occur to produce reflex bradycardia. Epinephrine speeds heart rate by accelerating the rate of spontaneous phase 4 depolarization which also increases the likelihood of cardiac dysrhythmias. Increased cardiac output reflects epinephrine-induced increases in heart rate, myocardial contractility, and venous return. Repeated doses of epinephrine produce similar cardiovascular effects in contrast to tachyphylaxis that accompanies administration of synthetic noncatecholamines that evoke the release of norepinephrine.

Epinephrine predominantly stimulates alpha-1 receptors in the skin, mucosa, and hepatorenal vasculature producing intense vasoconstriction. In skeletal muscles, epinephrine principally stimulates beta-2 receptors producing vasodilation. The net effect of these peripheral vascular changes is preferential distribution of cardiac output to skeletal muscles and decreased peripheral vascular resistance. Renal blood flow is substantially reduced by epinephrine even in the absence of changes in blood pressure. Indeed, epinephrine is estimated to be two to ten times more potent than norepinephrine for increasing renal vascular resistance. The secretion of renin is increased due to epinephrine-induced stimulation of beta receptors in the kidneys. In usual therapeutic doses, epinephrine has no significant vasoconstrictive effect on cerebral arterioles. Coronary blood flow is enhanced by epinephrine even at doses that do not alter blood pressure.

Chronic elevations in the plasma concentration of epinephrine, as in patients with pheochromocytoma, result in a reduction of plasma volume due to loss of protein-free fluid to the extracellular space. Arterial wall damage and local areas of myocardial necrosis may also accompany chronic circulating excesses of epinephrine. Conventional doses of epinephrine, however, do not produce these effects.

Airway Smooth Muscle

Smooth muscles of the bronchi are relaxed by virtue of epinephrine-induced activation of beta-2 receptors. This bronchodilator effect of epinephrine is converted to bronchoconstriction in the presence of beta-adrenergic blockade reflecting activity of alpha receptors. Beta-2 stimulation, by increasing intracellular concentrations of cyclic AMP, reduces release of vasoactive mediators associated with symptoms of bronchial asthma.

Metabolic Effects

Epinephrine has the most significant effects of all the catecholamines on metabolism. Beta-1 receptor stimulation by epinephrine increases liver glycogenolysis and adipose tissue lipolysis while alpha-1 receptor stimulation inhibits release of insulin. Liver glycogenolysis results from epinephrine-induced activation of hepatic phosphorylase enzyme. Lipolysis is due to epinephrine-induced activation of triglyceride lipase which accelerates the breakdown of triglycerides to form free fatty acids and glycerol. Infusions of epinephrine usually increase plasma concentrations of cholesterol, phospholipids, and low-density lipoproteins.

Release of epinephrine and resulting glycogenolysis and inhibition of insulin secretion is the most likely explanation for the hyperglycemia that commonly occurs during the perioperative period. In addition, epinephrine can produce inhibition of glucose uptake by peripheral tissues which is also due, in part, to inhibition of insulin secretion. Increased plasma concentrations of lactate presumably reflect glycogenolysis in skeletal muscle due to epinephrine.

Selective beta-2 agonist effects of low-dose infusion of epinephrine (0.05 μg kg^{-1} min^{-1}) are speculated to reflect activation of the sodium–potassium pump in skeletal muscles leading to transfer of potassium ions into cells (Fig. 12-6) (Brown *et al*, 1983). This epinephrine-induced hypokalemia could contribute to cardiac dysrhythmias that occasionally accompany stimulation of the sympathetic nervous system. Conversely, epinephrine may stimulate the release of potassium from the liver tending to offset the decrease in extracellular concentrations of this ion produced by entrance into skeletal muscles.

Among the exocrine glands, only the salivary glands respond significantly to epinephrine producing thick sparse secretions.

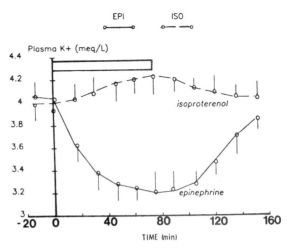

FIGURE 12-6. Selective beta-2 agonist effects of epinephrine are responsible for stimulating the movement of potassium into cells with a resulting decrease in the serum concentration of potassium. (From Brown MJ, Brown DC, Murphy MB. Hypokalemia from beta$_2$-receptor stimulation by circulating epinephrine. N Engl J Med 1983;309:1414–9. Reprinted by permission of the New England Journal of Medicine 1983;309:1414–9.)

Ocular Effects

Epinephrine causes contraction of the radial muscle of the iris producing mydriasis. Contraction of orbital muscles produces an appearance of exophthalmus considered characteristic of hyperthyroidism. Adrenergic receptors responsible for these ocular effects are probably alpha receptors because norepinephrine is less potent than epinephrine and isoproterenol has practically no ocular effects.

Gastrointestinal and Genitourinary Effects

Epinephrine, norepinephrine, and isoproterenol produce relaxation of gastrointestinal smooth muscle. Activation of beta-adrenergic receptors relaxes the detrusor muscle of the bladder while activation of alpha-adrenergic receptors contracts the trigone and sphincter muscles.

Coagulation

Epinephrine increases the total leukocyte count but at the same time causes eosinopenia. Blood coagulation is accelerated by epinephrine presumably due to increased activity of factor V, (Forwell and Ingram, 1957).

Norepinephrine

Norepinephrine is the endogenous neurotransmitter released from postganglionic sympathetic nerve endings. It is approximately equal in potency to epinephrine for stimulation of beta-1 receptors but unlike epinephrine, norepinephrine has little agonist effect at beta-2 receptors (Table 12-1). Norepinephrine is a potent alpha agonist producing intense arterial and venous vasoconstriction in all vascular beds and lacks bronchodilating effects on airway smooth muscle. Hyperglycemia is unlikely to occur as a result of norepinephrine infusion.

Cardiovascular Effects

A continuous intravenous infusion of norepinephrine, 4 to 16 μg min^{-1} may be used to treat refractory hypotension as may occur in the early period following ligation of the vascular supply to a pheochromocytoma. Placement of norepinephrine in a 5% dextrose solution provides sufficient acidity to prevent oxidation of the catecholamine. Extravasation during intravenous infusion can produce severe local vasoconstriction and possible necrosis.

Intravenous administration of norepinephrine results in intense vasoconstriction in skeletal muscles, liver, kidneys, and skin. The resulting increase in peripheral vascular resistance reduces venous return to the heart and elevates systolic, diastolic, and mean arterial pressure (Table 12-1). Reduced venous return to the heart combined with baroreceptor-mediated reflex decreases in heart rate due to the marked increase in mean arterial pressure tend to reduce cardiac output despite beta-1 effects of norepinephrine. Peripheral vasoconstriction may so reduce tissue blood flow that metabolic acidosis occurs. Chronic infusion of norepinephrine or elevated circulating concentrations of this catecholamine, as may be associated with a pheochromocytoma, cause precapillary vasoconstriction and loss of protein-free fluid to the extracellular space.

Dopamine

Dopamine is an important neurotransmitter in the central nervous system and peripheral nervous system. In the central nervous system, especially in basal ganglia, this neurotransmitter acts via presynaptic dopamine-1 receptors. In the peripheral nervous system, dopamine acts on vasodilating postsynaptic dopamine-2 receptors in the renal and mesenteric vasculature (Kebabian and Calne, 1979). Rapid metabolism of dopamine mandates its use as a continuous intravenous infusion of 1 to 20 μg kg^{-1} min^{-1} to maintain therapeutic plasma concentrations. Dopamine should be dissolved in 5% dextrose in water for intravenous administration so as to avoid inactivation of the catecholamine that may occur in an alkaline solution.

Depending on the dose, dopamine stimulates principally dopaminergic receptors (1–2 μg kg^{-1} min^{-1}) in the renal vasculature to produce renal vasodilation, beta-1 receptors (2–10 μg kg^{-1} min^{-1}) in the heart, and alpha receptors (above 10 μg kg^{-1} min^{-1}) in the peripheral vasculature. Extravasation of dopamine, like norepinephrine, produces intense local vasoconstriction which should be treated by the local infiltration of phentolamine. Dopamine is not effective orally nor does it cross the blood–brain barrier in sufficient amounts to cause central nervous system effects. The immediate precursor of dopamine, L-dopa, is absorbed from the gastrointestinal tract and readily crosses the blood–brain barrier (see Chapter 31).

Clinical Uses

Dopamine is used clinically to increase cardiac output in the patient with low blood pressure, increased atrial filling pressures, and low urine output. It is unique among the catecholamines in being able to simultaneously increase (1) myocardial contractility, (2) renal blood flow, (3) glomerular filtration rate, (4) excretion of sodium, and (5) urine output. There is evidence that dopamine inhibits renal tubular solute reabsorption suggesting that diuresis and natriuresis that frequently accompany dopamine administration may occur independently of the effect on renal blood flow (Hilberman *et al*, 1984). Nevertheless, the renal effects of dopamine are abolished by a dopamine receptor antagonist, such as droperidol, but not by a beta-adrenergic receptor antagonist. Inhibition of aldosterone secretion may contribute to increased sodium excretion produced by dopamine. Hyperglycemia that is commonly present in patients receiving a continuous intravenous infusion of dopamine is likely to reflect drug-induced inhibition of insulin secretion.

Cardiovascular Effects

Dopamine increases cardiac output by stimulation of beta-1 receptors. This increase in cardiac output is usually accompanied by only modest elevations in heart rate, blood pressure, and peripheral vascular resistance. A portion of the positive inotropic effect of dopamine is due to stimulation of release of endogenous norepinephrine which may predispose to the development of cardiac dysrhythmias. Nevertheless, dopamine is less arrhythmogenic than epinephrine. The release of norepinephrine caused by dopamine may be an unreliable mechanism for increasing cardiac output when cardiac catecholamine stores are depleted as in the patient in chronic cardiac failure.

Infusion rates of dopamine above 8 μg kg^{-1} min^{-1} may increase the pulmonary artery occlusion pressure despite concomitant increases in myocardial contractility (Fig. 12-7) (Hess *et al*, 1979). This paradoxical effect may be a reflection of reduced left ventricular compliance or increased venous return due to venous constriction. Indeed, concomitant infusion of nitroglycerin prevents the effect of high doses of dopamine on atrial filling pressure.

SYNTHETIC CATECHOLAMINES

The two clinically useful synthetic catecholamines are isoproterenol and dobutamine (Table 12-1) (Fig. 12-1).

Isoproterenol

Isoproterenol is the most potent activator of all the sympathomimetics at beta-1 and beta-2 receptors, being two to ten times more potent than epinephrine and at least 100 times more active than norepinephrine. In clinical doses, isoproterenol is devoid of alpha agonist effects. Metabolism of isoproterenol in the liver by COMT is rapid necessi-

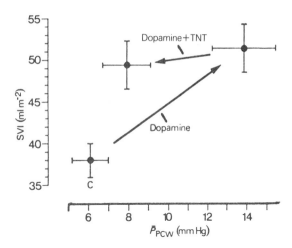

FIGURE 12-7. Plots of left ventricular function (mean ± SE) during the control period (C), during infusion of dopamine, 8 μg kg^{-1} min^{-1}, and during the infusion of the combination of dopamine with nitroglycerin (TNT) (mean dose 0.5 μg kg^{-1} min^{-1}). (From Hess W, Klein W, Mueller-Busch C, Tarnow J. Haemodynamic effects of dopamine and dopamine combined with nitroglycerin in patients subjected to coronary bypass surgery. Br J Anaesth 1979;51:1063–9. Reproduced by permission of the authors and publisher.)

tating a continuous intravenous infusion to maintain a therapeutic plasma concentration. Uptake of isoproterenol into postganglionic sympathetic nerve endings is minimal.

Clinical Uses

Clinical uses of isoproterenol include (1) administration as an intravenous infusion or as an aerosol to produce bronchodilation, (2) continuous intravenous infusion of 1 to 5 μg min^{-1} to increase heart rate in the presence of complete heart block, and (3) continuous intravenous infusion to decrease pulmonary vascular resistance in patients with pulmonary hypertension (Elliott and Gorlin, 1966). More specific beta-2 agonists, however, have largely replaced isoproterenol as a bronchodilator.

Cardiovascular Effects

Cardiovascular effects of isoproterenol reflect activation of beta-1 receptors in the heart and beta-2 receptors in the vasculature of skeletal muscle.

For example, continuous intravenous infusion of isoproterenol, 1 to 5 μg min^{-1}, greatly increases heart rate, myocardial contractility, and cardiac automaticity while vasodilation in skeletal muscles reduces peripheral vascular resistance. The net effect of these changes is an increase in cardiac output which is usually sufficient to increase systolic blood pressure. The mean arterial pressure, however, may decline due to the decrease in peripheral vascular resistance and associated reduction in diastolic blood pressure. Decreased diastolic blood pressure and cardiac dysrhythmias induced by isoproterenol may decrease coronary blood flow at the same time myocardial oxygen requirements are elevated by tachycardia and increased myocardial contractility. This combination of events is undesirable in patients with coronary artery disease. Compensatory baroreceptor-mediated reflex slowing of the heart rate does not occur during infusion of isoproterenol because mean arterial pressure is not elevated.

Dobutamine

Dobutamine is a synthetic catecholamine that acts as a selective beta-1 agonist. Rapid metabolism of dobutamine dictates its administration as a continuous intravenous infusion at 2 to 10 μg kg^{-1} min^{-1} to maintain therapeutic plasma concentrations. Like dopamine, dobutamine should be dissolved in 5% dextrose in water for intravenous infusion so as to avoid inactivation of the catecholamine that may occur in an alkaline solution.

Clinical Uses

Dobutamine is used to improve cardiac output in patients in cardiac failure, particularly if heart rate and peripheral vascular resistance are elevated. Combinations of drugs may be useful to increase the spectrum of activity and improve the distribution of cardiac output. For example, dobutamine may be used to increase cardiac output and a low dose of dopamine may be added to favor renal perfusion. Vasodilators may be combined with dobutamine or dopamine to reduce afterload to optimize cardiac output in the presence of increased peripheral vascular resistance.

Cardiovascular Effects

Dobutamine produces dose-dependent increases in cardiac output and reductions in atrial filling pressures without marked increases in heart rate or blood pressure. The usual small increase in heart rate compared with dopamine reflects a lesser effect of dobutamine on the sinoatrial node. Peripheral and pulmonary vascular resistance may be decreased but usually are not greatly altered. Indeed, dobutamine may be ineffective in patients who require increased peripheral vascular resistance rather than augmentation of cardiac output to improve blood pressure. Minimal effects on heart rate and blood pressure reduce the likelihood of adverse increases in myocardial oxygen requirements during infusion of dobutamine. Unlike dopamine, dobutamine does not act indirectly by stimulating the release of endogenous norepinephrine from the heart nor does this catecholamine activate dopaminergic receptors to increase renal blood flow. Renal blood flow, however, improves as a result of increased cardiac output.

High doses of dobutamine (greater than 10 μg kg^{-1} min^{-1}) may predispose to tachycardia and cardiac dysrhythmias. Nevertheless, cardiac dysrhythmias are unlikely presumably because of the absence of endogenous catecholamine release. Conduction velocity through the atrioventricular node, however, is increased by dobutamine raising the possibility that excessive increases in heart rate could occur in patients in atrial fibrillation.

SYNTHETIC NONCATECHOLAMINES

Synthetic noncatecholamines that possess potential clinical usefulness include, but are not limited to, ephedrine, mephentermine, amphetamine, metaraminol, phenylephrine, and methoxamine (Table 12-1) (Fig. 12-2) (Smith and Corbascio, 1970).

Ephedrine

Ephedrine is a nonselective synthetic noncatecholamine acting on alpha- and beta-adrenergic receptors. The drug owes part of its pharmacologic effects to endogenous release of norepinephrine (*i.e.* indirect-acting), but it also has direct stimulant effects on adrenergic receptors (*i.e.,* direct-acting). Ephedrine is resistant to metabolism by MAO in the gastrointestinal tract thus permitting unchanged drug to be absorbed into the circulation following oral administration. Intramuscular injection of ephedrine is also acceptable as local vasoconstriction is insufficient to greatly delay systemic absorption. Up to 40% of a single dose of ephedrine is excreted unchanged in the urine. Some ephedrine is deaminated by MAO in the liver, and conjugation also occurs. The slow inactivation and excretion of ephedrine are responsible for the prolonged duration of action of this sympathomimetic.

Ephedrine, unlike epinephrine, does not produce marked hyperglycemia. Mydriasis accompanies the administration of ephedrine, and central nervous system stimulation, although less than produced by amphetamine, does occur.

Clinical Uses

Ephedrine, 10 to 25 mg administered intravenously to adults, is a commonly selected sympathomimetic when drug therapy is utilized to increase blood pressure in the presence of sympathetic nervous system blockade produced by a regional anesthetic or hypotension due to inhaled or injected anesthetics. Indeed, in an animal model, ephedrine more specifically corrects the noncardiac circulatory changes produced by spinal anesthesia than does either a selective alpha- or beta-agonist drug (Butterworth *et al*, 1986). Uterine blood flow is not greatly altered when ephedrine is administered to restore normal maternal blood pressure following production of sympathetic nervous system blockade (Fig. 12-8) (Ralston *et al*, 1974). This contrasts with selective alpha-agonists which restore blood pressure but, at the same time, decrease uterine flow because of vasoconstriction (Fig. 12-8) (Ralston *et al*, 1974). Ephedrine can be used as chronic oral medication in the treatment of bronchial asthma reflecting its bronchodilating effects by virtue of activation of beta-2 receptors. Compared to epinephrine, the onset of action of ephedrine is slow becoming complete only an hour or more after administration. A decongestant effect accompanying oral administration of ephedrine produces symptomatic relief from acute coryza.

Cardiovascular Effects

The cardiovascular effects of ephedrine resemble epinephrine, but the blood pressure-elevating response is less intense and lasts about ten times longer. It requires about 250 times more ephedrine than epinephrine to produce equivalent

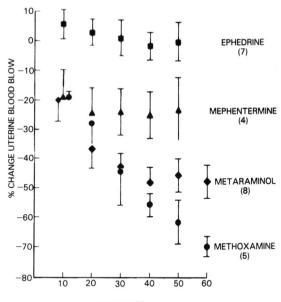

FIGURE 12-8. Ephedrine-induced increases in mean arterial pressure produce the least changes in uterine blood flow. Mephentermine has an intermediate effect, and increases in blood pressure produced by metaraminol and methoxamine result in substantial reductions in uterine blood flow. (From Ralston DH, Shnider SM, deLorimer AA. Effects of equipotent ephedrine, metaraminol, mephentermine and methoxamine on uterine blood flow in the pregnant ewe. Anesthesiology 1970;40:354–70. Reproduced by permission of the authors and publisher.)

blood pressure responses. Intravenous administration of ephedrine results in elevations in systolic and diastolic blood pressure, heart rate, and cardiac output. Renal and splanchnic blood flows are decreased whereas coronary and skeletal muscle blood flows are increased. Peripheral vascular resistance may be minimally altered as vasoconstriction in some vascular beds is offset by vasodilation (*e.g.,* beta-2 stimulation) in other areas. These cardiovascular effects are due, in part, to alpha receptor-mediated peripheral vasoconstriction. The principal mechanism, however, for cardiovascular effects produced by ephedrine, is increased myocardial contractility due to activation of beta-1 receptors.

A second dose of ephedrine produces a less intense blood pressure response than the first dose. This phenomenon, known as tachyphylaxis, occurs with many sympathomimetics and is related to the duration of action of these drugs. Tachyphylaxis probably represents a persistent blockade of adrenergic receptors. For example, ephedrine-induced activation of adrenergic receptors persists even after blood pressure has returned to near predrug levels by virtue of compensatory cardiovascular changes. When ephedrine is administered at this time, the receptors still occupied by ephedrine limit available sites and the blood pressure response is less. Alternatively, tachyphylaxis may be due to depletion of norepinephrine stores.

Mephentermine

Mephentermine is an indirect-acting synthetic noncatecholamine that stimulates alpha- and beta-adrenergic receptors. It is closely related structurally to methylamphetamine but has only modest central nervous system-stimulating qualities. Administered intravenously, mephentermine produces cardiovascular effects that resemble ephedrine (Udhoji and Weil, 1965) (see the section entitled Ephedrine). Despite its positive inotropic effect, however, mephentermine exerts an antidysrhythmic effect (Wilson *et al,* 1958).

Amphetamines

Amphetamine and related sympathomimetics (dextroamphetamine and methamphetamine) resemble ephedrine in evoking alpha- and beta-adrenergic receptor stimulation but differ from ephedrine in producing significant central nervous system stimulation. The central nervous system stimulant effects as well as appetite suppressant actions reflect release of norepinephrine from storage sites in the central nervous system. Tachyphylaxis is prominent, and drug dependence is predictable considering the ability of these drugs to stimulate the central nervous system.

Acute intravenous administration of dextroamphetamine to dogs increases anesthetic requirements presumably reflecting the release of norepinephrine into the central nervous system (Johnston *et al,* 1974). Conversely, chronic administration of dextroamphetamine decreases central nervous system stores of catecholamines

and anesthetic requirements may be reduced (Johnston *et al,* 1974). Excretion of amphetamine is negligible in alkaline urine (2%–3%) because the drug exists predominantly in the nonionized fraction that is readily reabsorbed by renal tubules. For this reason, treatment of amphetamine overdose includes acidification of the urine.

Metaraminol

Metaraminol is a synthetic noncatecholamine that, like ephedrine, acts on alpha- and beta-adrenergic receptors by indirect and direct effects. This sympathomimetic undergoes uptake into postganglionic sympathetic nerve endings where it substitutes for norepinephrine and acts as a weak false neurotransmitter. Indeed, chronically administered metaraminol (2–3 hours by continuous intravenous infusion) lowers blood pressure in hypertensive patients reflecting the lesser vasoconstrictor potency (estimated to be one tenth) of this sympathomimetic compared with norepinephrine. Sudden withdrawal of a metaraminol infusion can lead to profound hypotension until the nerve ending stores of norepinephrine are replenished. Metaraminol is not a substrate for MAO or COMT.

Cardiovascular Effects

Metaraminol produces more intense peripheral vasoconstriction and less increase in myocardial contractility than ephedrine. Intravenous administration of metaraminol, 1.5 to 5 mg to adults, produces a sustained increase in systolic and diastolic blood pressure that is due almost entirely to peripheral vasoconstriction emphasizing the predominant alpha agonist effect of this sympathomimetic. Vasoconstriction decreases renal and cerebral blood flow. Reflex bradycardia often accompanies drug-induced increases in blood pressure resulting in a decline in cardiac output. If heart rate slowing is prevented by atropine, metaraminol can increase cardiac output similar to ephedrine.

Phenylephrine

Phenylephrine is a synthetic noncatecholamine that activates principally alpha-adrenergic receptors by a direct effect with only a small part of the pharmacologic response being due to its ability to release norepinephrine (*e.g.,* indirect action). There is a minimal effect on beta-adrenergic receptors. The dose of phenylephrine necessary to stimulate alpha-1 receptors is far less than that which stimulates alpha-2 receptors. Resulting venoconstriction is greater than arterial constriction. Structurally, phenylephrine is 3-hydroxyphenylethylamine differing from epinephrine only in lacking a 4-hydroxyl group on the benzene ring (see the section entitled Structure Activity Relationships). Clinically, phenylephrine mimics the effects of norepinephrine but is less potent and longer lasting. Central nervous system stimulation is minimal.

Clinical Uses

Phenylephrine, 50 to 100 μg, is often administered intravenously to adults to treat blood pressure reductions that accompany sympathetic nervous system blockade produced by a regional anesthetic or peripheral vasodilatation that accompanies administration of injected or inhaled anesthetics. This drug has been used as a continuous infusion (20–50 μg min^{-1}) in adults to sustain blood pressure at normal levels as during cardiopulmonary bypass or at artificially elevated levels during carotid endarterectomy. The reflex vagal effects produced by phenylephrine can be used to slow heart rate in the presence of hemodynamically significant supraventricular tachydysrhythmias. Topically applied, phenylephrine is a nasal decongestant and produces mydriasis without cycloplegia.

Cardiovascular Effects

Intravenous phenylephrine produces intense peripheral vasoconstriction, increased systolic and diastolic blood pressure, and reflex bradycardia. Reflex heart rate slowing can result in a decrease in cardiac output. Renal, splanchnic, and cutaneous blood flows are reduced, but coronary blood flow is increased. Pulmonary arterial pressure is elevated.

Methoxamine

Methoxamine is a synthetic noncatecholamine that acts directly and selectively on alpha-adrenergic receptors. Beta-adrenergic receptor stimulation is absent. Administered intravenously to adults methoxamine, 5 to 10 mg, causes intense arterial vasoconstriction that manifests as increased systolic and diastolic blood pressure and baroreceptor-mediated reflex bradycardia that contributes to a reduction in cardiac output. Venoconstriction is minimal following administration of methoxamine. Renal blood flow is reduced to a greater extent than after equally potent doses of norepinephrine. Conversely, coronary blood flow may increase as a result of increased perfusion pressure and increased time for blood flow due to reflex bradycardia. Atropine prevents reflex bradycardia and the associated decrease in cardiac output. Methoxamine exerts a modest antidysrhythmic effect by an unknown mechanism.

SELECTIVE BETA-2 AGONISTS

Selective beta-2 agonists specifically relax bronchiole and uterine smooth muscle, but in contrast to isoproterenol generally lack stimulating (beta-1) effects on the heart (Table 12-2) (Fig. 12-3). In addition to the treatment of reversible bronchospasm, these drugs have been administered as continuous intravenous infusions to stop uterine contractions in premature labor. Associated sustained beta-2 agonist stimulation may produce hyokalemia by driving potassium intracellularly (Hurlbert *et al,* 1981; Moravec and Hurlbert, 1980).

Metaproterenol

Metaproterenol is a selective beta-2 agonist that resembles isoproterenol chemically, except that the two hydroxyl groups are attached at the meta positions on the benzene ring rather than at the meta and para positions (Fig. 12-3). This structure makes metaproterenol resistant to methylation by COMT. The drug is excreted in the urine principally as conjugates with glucuronic acid.

Administered by inhalation, metaproterenol, 0.65 mg, produces a prompt and sustained reduction in previously elevated airways resistance in adults. Tolerance, however, may occur with repeated administration. Oral administration of metaproterenol, 200 mg, produces improvement in breathing for up to 4 hours.

Table 12-2
Comparative Pharmacology of Selective Beta-2 Agonists

	Peak Effect (min)	*Duration of Action (hr)*	*Method of Administration*
Metaproterenol	30–60	3–4	Spray
Terbutaline	60	4–6	Solution
Albuterol (Salbutamol)	30–60	4–6	Spray
Isoetharine	15–60	2–4	Spray
Ritodrine	30–60	4–6	Intravenous Oral

Terbutaline

Terbutaline is a selective beta-2 agonist that is administered orally or subcutaneously for the treatment of reversible airways obstruction. Administered orally, 5 mg produces bronchodilatation in adults after about 1 hour and lasts for about 7 hours. Onset of bronchodilation is sooner following subcutaneous administration (0.25 mg), but beta-2 selectivity is less with beta-1 cardiac effects also manifesting. Continuous intravenous infusion of terbutaline, as used to stop uterine contractions of premature labor, has been associated with tachycardia, pulmonary edema, and hypokalemia (Hurlbert *et al,* 1981; Moravec and Hurlbert, 1980; Ravindran *et al,* 1980; Wheeler *et al,* 1981). Hypokalemia presumably reflects beta-2 agonist effects which drive potassium into the cells. Ventricular cardiac dysrhythmias may occur when terbutaline is administered subcutaneously to treat bronchospasm in patients anesthetized with halothane (Thiagarajah *et al,* 1986).

Albuterol (Salbutamol)

Albuterol is a selective beta-2 agonist that promptly reduces airways resistance for prolonged periods (4 to 6 hours) when administered to adults as an aerosol (100 μg per inhalation). Cardiac effects are unlikely when the aerosol dose of albuterol is kept below 400 μg. For example, albuterol and isoproterenol are approximately equally potent as bronchodilators when given by aerosol whereas ten times the dose of albuterol is necessary to cause equal cardiac stimulant effects. Administered intravenously, beta-1 cardiac

effects begin to manifest and hypokalemia may develop. As with other beta-agoinsts, chronic administration leads to tachyphylaxis.

Isoetharine

Isoetharine structurally resembles isoproterenol but has less beta-1 activity. It is as effective as isoproterenol as a bronchodilator and has a low incidence of side effects. Administration is by inhalation with one to four inhalations usually producing a therapeutic response that lasts up to 4 hours. When used for nebulization, the usual dose in adults is 5 mg inhaled over 15 to 20 minutes.

Ritodrine

Ritodrine is the beta-2 agonist most often used to stop uterine contractions of premature labor. This action on uterine activity reflects stimulation of beta-2 receptors through activation of adenylate cyclase. Although ritodrine predominantly stimulates beta-2 receptors, it also has some beta-1 effects manifesting as tachycardia. Ritodrine is administered intravenously at doses up to 350 μg min^{-1} until uterine contractions are inhibited for at least 12 hours. This is followed by oral ritodrine until delivery of a mature infant is assured. Teratogenic effects have not been shown to accompany the prenatal use of ritodrine after 20 weeks of gestation.

Ritodrine readily crosses the placenta such that cardiovascular and metabolic effects occur in both the mother and fetus. Tachycardia and hypertension are common in mother and fetus when the drug is administered intravenously. Pulmonary edema due to excessive tachycardia seems to be more likely when ritodrine and corticosteroids are administered concurrently. The concentration of insulin in the cord blood may be increased resulting in neonatal hypoglycemia. Maternal hypokalemia is associated with intravenous infusion of ritodrine. The possibility of an additive effect with potassium-depleting diuretics should be considered. Exaggerated blood pressure reductions are possible when ritodrine is given with other drugs that can cause hypotension, such as volatile anesthetics.

Ritodrine as administered intravenously for inhibition of premature labor in insulin-dependent diabetics, has been followed by ketoacidosis despite prior subcutaneous doses of insulin (Mordes *et al,* 1982). Concomitant administration of glucocorticoids to promote fetal lung maturity is also likely to aggravate the diabetic state in these patients and contribute to the beta agonist actions of ritodrine in promoting glycogenolysis and lipolysis. Nevertheless, abrupt metabolic deterioration is not common in diabetics who receive glucocorticoids without ritodrine. Continuous infusion of insulin may be indicated in the diabetic parturient receiving intravenous ritodrine. Maximum rates of ritodrine infusion may result in at least doubling of previous insulin requirements. Oral ritodrine is not associated with an apparent increase in insulin requirements. Certainly, plasma glucose and potassium concentrations should be monitored during intravenous administration of ritodrine.

Theophylline

Theophylline is a methylxanthine derivative that inhibits phosphodiesterase, the enzyme responsible for the inactivation of cyclic AMP (Fig. 12-9). As a result, cyclic AMP accumulates and beta-adrenergic effects occur including bronchodilation and cardiac stimulation. Aminophylline, a water-

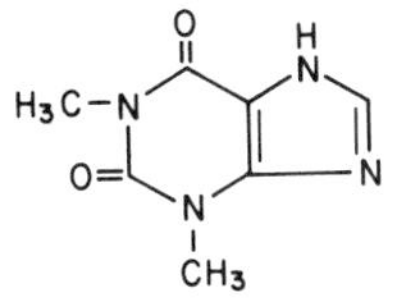

FIGURE 12-9. Theophylline.

soluble salt of theophylline, is administered orally ($3 - 6$ mg kg^{-1}) or intravenously (loading dose, 5 mg kg^{-1}, followed by $0.5 - 1$ mg kg^{-1} hr^{-1}) for initial treatment of moderate to severe reversible bronchospasm. Because aminophylline increases cardiac output and decreases peripheral vascular resistance, it is beneficial in the management of pulmonary edema due to left ventricular failure.

Therapeutic plasma concentrations of theophylline are between 10 and 20 μg ml^{-1} with toxic responses becoming more prevalent above 20 μg ml^{-1}. Toxic responses include cardiac dysrhythmias and seizures. In the presence of toxic plasma concentrations of aminophylline, the subsequent administration of halothane is more likely than enflurane or isoflurane to be associated with the development of cardiac dysrhythmias. Aminophylline readily crosses the placenta and may produce toxicity in infants of mothers receiving this drug during labor.

Frequent monitoring of plasma concentrations is indicated because there is great individual variation in rates of metabolism of theophylline. For example, metabolism is slowed in the presence of liver dysfunction due to cardiac failure or alcoholism, and treatment with cimetidine or beta-adrenergic receptor antagonists. Conversely, cigarette smoking speeds metabolism of theophylline. In the presence of normal rates of metabolism, the elimination half-time is about 6 hours.

Pentoxifylline

Pentoxifylline is a methylxanthine derivative that increases flexibility of erythrocytes and reduces viscosity of blood thereby improving capillary blood flow and associated tissue oxygenation. Patients with intermittent claudication due to chronic occlusive arterial disease of the limbs begin to experience improvement within 2 to 4 weeks after initiation of oral administration of pentoxifylline, 400 mg every 8 hours. This drug is not a vasodilator or anticoagulant and is unrelated to aspirin or dipyridamole.

Side effects are rare but may include hypotension, angina pectoris, and cardiac dysrhythmias. Bleeding and/or prolonged prothrombin time may occur in the presence of anticoagulants or platelet aggregation inhibitors. Pentoxifylline is compatible with digitalis and beta-adrenergic antagonists.

REFERENCES

Brown MJ, Brown DC, Murphy MB. Hypokalemia from Beta$_2$-receptor stimulation by circulating epinephrine. N Engl J Med 1983; 309:1414–9.

Burn JH, Rand MJ. The action of sympathomimetic amines in animals treated with reserpine. J Physiol 1958; 144:314–36.

Butterworth JF, Piccione W, Berrizbeitia LD, Dance G, Shemin RJ, Cohn LH. Augmentation of venous return by adrenergic agonists during spinal anesthesia. Anesth Analg 1986;65:612–6.

Eger EI, Hamilton WK. The effect of reserpine on the action of various vasopressors. Anesthesiology 1959;20:641–5.

Elliott WC, Gorlin R. Isoproterenol in treatment of heart disease: Hemodynamic effects of circulatory failure. JAMA 1966;197:93–8.

Fain JN, Garcia-Sainz JA. Role of phosphatidyl inositol turnover in alpha$_1$ and of adenylate cyclase inhibition in alpha$_2$ effects of catecholamines. Life Sci 1980;26:1183–94.

Forwell GD, Ingram GIC. The effect of adrenaline infusion on human blood coagulation. J Physiol 1957;135:371–83.

Gilbert JC, Murthy VV, Goldberg LI, Kuo JF. Dopamine-sensitive adenylate cyclase in dog renal artery. Adv Cyclic Nucleotide Res 1975;5:840.

Hess W, Klein W, Mueller-Busch C, Tarnow J. Haemodynamic effects of dopamine and dopamine combined with nitroglycerin in patients subjected to coronary bypass surgery. Br J Anaesth 1979;51:1063–9.

Hilberman M, Maseda J, Stinson EB, et al. The diuretic properties of dopamine in patients following open heart operations. Anesthesiology 1984;61:489–94.

Hurlbert BJ, Edelman JD, David K. Serum potassium levels during and after terbutaline. Anesth Analg 1981;60:723–5.

Johnston PR, Way WL, Miller RD. The effect of CNS catecholamine-depleting drugs on dextroamphetamine-induced elevation of halothane MAC. Anesthesiology 1974;41:57–61.

Junod AF. Metabolism of vasoactive agents in lung. Am Rev Resp Dis 1977;115:51–7.

Kebabian JW, Calne DB. Multiple receptors for dopamine. Nature 1979;277:93–6.

Lawson NW, Wallfisch HK. Cardiovascular pharmacology: A new look at the pressors. In: Stoelting RK, Barash PG, Gallagher TJ, eds. Advances in Anesthesia. Chicago. Year Book Medical Publishers, 1986:195–270.

Maze M. Clinical implications of membrane receptor function in anesthesia. Anesthesiology 1981; 55:160–71.

Miller RD, Way WL, Eger EI. The effects of alpha-methyldopa, reserpine, guanethidine, and iproniazid on minimum alveolar anesthetic requirement (MAC). Anesthesiology 1968;29:1153–8.

Moravec MA, Hurlbert BJ. Hypokalemia associated with terbutaline administration in obstetrical patients. Anesth Analg 1980;59:917–20.

Mordes D, Kreutner K, Metzger W, Colwell JA. Dangers of intravenous ritodrine in diabetic patients. JAMA 1982;248:973–5.

Naito H, Gillis CN. Effects of halothane and nitrous oxide on removal of norepinephrine from the pulmonary circulation. Anesthesiology 1973;39:575–80.

Ralston DH, Shnider SM, deLorimer AA. Effects of equipotent ephedrine, metaraminol, mephentermine and methoamine on uterine blood flow in the pregnant ewe. Anesthesiology 1974;40:354–70.

Ravindran R, Viegas OJ, Padilla LM, LaBlonde P. Anesthetic considerations in pregnant patients receiving terbutaline therapy. Anesth Analg 1980;59:391–2.

Roth J, Lesniak MA, Bar RS, et al. An introduction to receptors and receptor disorders. Proc Soc Exp Biol Med 1979;162:3–12.

Smith NT, Corbascio AN. The use and misuse of pressor agents. Anesthesiology 1970;33:58–101.

Smith LDR, Oldershaw PJ. Inotropic and vasopressor agents. Br J Anaesth 1984;56:767–80.

Thiagarajah S, Grynsztejn M, Lear E, Azar I. Ventricular arrhythmias after terbutaline administration to patients anesthetized with halothane. Anesth Analg 1986;65:417–8.

Udhoji VN, Weil MH. Vasodilator action of a "pressor amine," mephentermine (Wyamine), in circulatory shock. Am J Cardiol 1965;16:841–6.

Wheeler AS, Patel KF, Spain J. Pulmonary edema during beta-2-tocolytic therapy. Anesth Analg 1981; 60:695–6.

Wilson M, Perez-Arzola M, Oppenheimer MJ. Mephentermine and the arrhythmias. Am J Med Sci 1958;236:300–6.

C H A P T E R   13

Digitalis and Related Drugs

INTRODUCTION

Digitalis is the term used for cardiac glycosides that occur naturally in many plants including the foxglove plant. Digoxin, digitoxin, and ouabain are examples of clinically useful cardiac glycosides (Fig. 13-1). Nonglycoside and noncatecholamine drugs that may be administered for similar clinical purposes as cardiac glycosides are calcium, glucagon, and amrinone (Fig. 13-2).

CLINICAL USES

Cardiac glycosides are used almost exclusively to treat cardiac failure or to slow the ventricular response rate in patients with supraventricular tachydysrhythmias such as paraoxysmal atrial tachycardia, atrial fibrillation, or atrial flutter (Doherty and Kaul, 1975; Smith and Oldershaw, 1984). These drugs are particularly useful in patients with cardiac failure that results from essential hypertension, valvular heart disease, or atherosclerotic heart disease. Digitalis preparations may not be of benefit, however, in high output cardiac failure as caused by hyperthyroidism or thiamine deficiency. Before administering a cardiac glycoside to treat a supraventricular dysrhythmia, it is important to confirm that the cardiac dysrhythmia is not due to digitalis toxicity (see the section entitled Digitalis Toxicity).

Intravenous propranolol combined with digoxin may provide more rapid control of supraventricular tachydysrhythmias and minimize the likelihood of toxicity by permitting decreases in the dose of both drugs. Direct current cardioversion in the presence of digitalis may be hazardous because of an alleged increased risk for developing cardiac dysrhythmias including ventricular fibrillation. In about 30% of patients with Wolff-Parkinson-White syndrome, digitalis reduces refractoriness in the accessory conduction pathway to the point that rapid atrial impulses can cause ventricular fibrillation. Finally, digitalis may be harmful in patients with hypertrophic subaortic stenosis because increased myocardial contractility intensifies the resistance to ventricular ejection.

STRUCTURE ACTIVITY RELATIONSHIPS

The basic structure of cardiac glycosides is that of a steroid cyclopentenophenanthrene nucleus that consists of a glycone and an aglycone portion (Fig. 13-1). As such, cardiac glycosides are related chemically to bile acids and sex hormones. The glycone portion is a sugar, often glucose, but closely related sugars, such as digitoxose, may also be present. Glycones are pharmacologically inactive but are necessary to assure fixation of cardiac glycosides to cardiac muscle. It is the aglycone portion of cardiac glycosides that produces the pharmacologic activity on the heart characterized as digitalis-like.

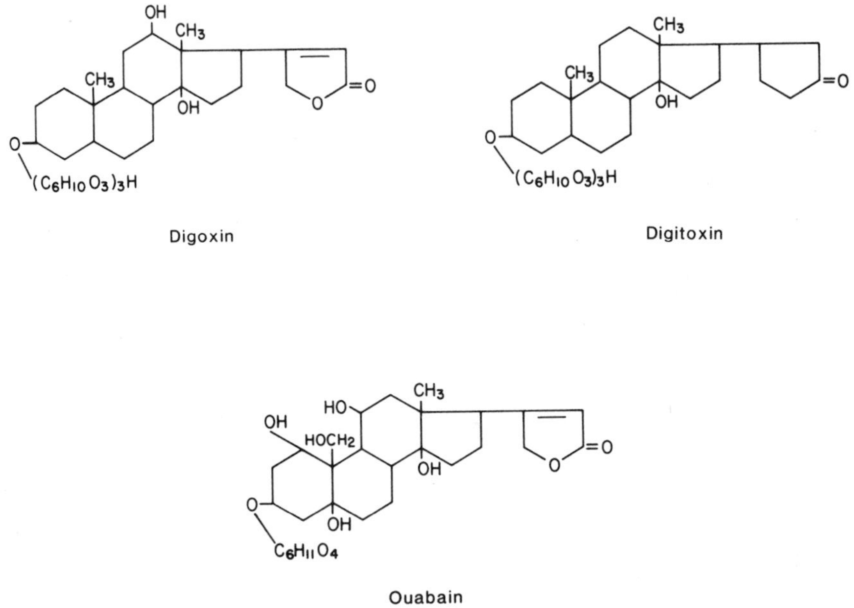

Digoxin

Digitoxin

Ouabain

FIGURE 13-1. Cardiac glycosides.

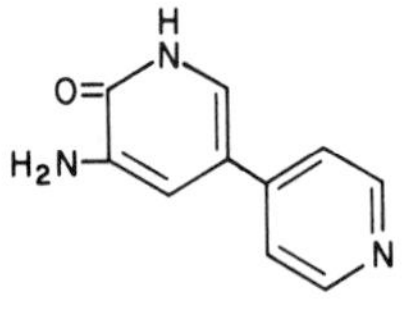

FIGURE 13-2. Amrinone.

MECHANISM OF ACTION

The mechanism of the positive inotropic effect evoked by cardiac glycosides is complex including (1) direct effects on the heart which modify its electrical and mechanical activity and (2) indirect effects evoked by reflex alterations in autonomic nervous system activity.

Direct Effects on the Heart

The most likely explanation for the direct positive inotropic effect of cardiac glycosides is drug-induced inhibition of the sodium:potassium ATPase ion transport system (*i.e.*, sodium pump) located in cardiac cell membranes (Akera *et al*, 1970).

Cardiac glycosides bind to ATPase enzyme inducing a conformational change that interferes with outward transport of sodium ions across cardiac cell membranes. The resulting increase in sodium ion concentration in cardiac cells leads to decreased extrusion of calcium ions by the sodium pump mechanism. It is presumed that this increased intracellular concentration of calcium ions is responsible for the positive inotropic effects of cardiac glycosides (Van Winkle and Schwartz, 1976).

Many of the known effects of cardiac glycosides on the cardiac action potential can be explained on the basis of drug-induced inhibition of the sodium:potassium ATPase ion transport system. Indeed, this ion transport system is essential for maintaining normal gradients for sodium and potassium ions that determine depolarization and excitability characteristics of cardiac cell membranes. For example, cardiac glycosides reduce resting transmembrane potentials and thus increase automaticity (*e.g.*, excitability) of cardiac cells by virtue of alterations in potassium ion gradients (Fig. 13-3) (Hoffman and Bigger, 1985). Automaticity is also accentuated by drug-induced increases in the slope of phase 4 depolarization.

Inhibition of outward transport of sodium ions decreases the slope of phase 0 of the cardiac action potential. The decrease in the duration of the cardiac action potential results largely from shortening of the duration of phase 2. Excessive digitalis-induced increases in intracellular calcium ion concentrations reduce the spread of excitatory current from one myocardial cell to another manifesting as impaired conduction of the cardiac impulse.

Alterations in Autonomic Nervous System Activity

Autonomic nervous system effects of cardiac glycosides include increased parasympathetic ner-

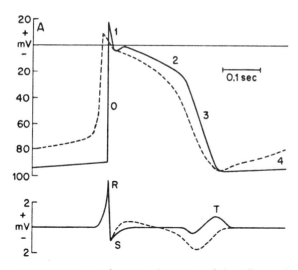

FIGURE 13-3. Schematic depiction of the effects of digitalis (broken line) on the transmembrane potential and electrocardiogram compared with recordings in the absence of digitalis. In the presence of digitalis, the resting transmembrane potential becomes less negative and the slope of spontaneous phase 4 depolarization is increased (*i.e.,* automaticity is enhanced). The change in the slope and duration of phases 2 and 3 results in changes in the S-T segment and T wave on the electrocardiogram, and the R-T interval is shortened. (Reproduced by permission of Hoffman BF, Bigger JT. Digitalis and allied cardiac glycosides. In: Gilman AG, Goodman LS, Rall TW, Murad F, eds. The Pharmacological Basis of Therapeutics, 7th ed. New York. Macmillan Publishing Co. 1985, 716.)

vous system activity due to sensitization of arterial baroreceptors (*e.g.,* carotid sinus) and activation of vagal nuclei and the nodose ganglion in the central nervous system (Gillis *et al,* 1975). Enhanced parasympathetic nervous system activity produced by therapeutic concentrations of digitalis results in (1) decreased activity of the sinoatrial node and (2) prolongation of the effective refractive period and thus the time for conduction of cardiac impulses through the atrioventricular node. The manifestation of these effects is a slowed heart rate especially in the presence of atrial fibrillation. Furthermore, the relative predominance of parasympathetic to sympathetic nervous system activity produced by digitalis is consistent with suppression of ectopic cardiac pacemakers. Indirect neurally mediated effects of therapeutic concentrations of digitalis on the specialized ventricular conduction system are less important than effects on the sinoatrial and atrioventricular node.

PHARMACOKINETICS

The assay of plasma concentrations of cardiac glycosides has greatly improved the understanding of the pharmacokinetics of these drugs (Butler, 1972; Doherty, 1973). At equilibrium, the concentration of cardiac glycosides in the heart is 15 to 30 times greater than those in the plasma. The concentration of cardiac glycosides in skeletal muscle is about one-half that in the heart.

Digoxin

Absorption of digoxin after oral administration is about 75% in the first hour with peak plasma concentrations occurring in 1 to 2 hours (Table 13-1) (Hoffman and Bigger, 1985). Intramuscular administration of digoxin is painful and absorption is often unpredictable. Therapeutic plasma concentrations of diogoxin can be achieved rapidly with intravenous administration of the drug (up to 10 μg kg^{-1} over about 30 min) producing an appreciable effect in 5 to 30 minutes. Following achievement of therapeutic plasma concentrations of digoxin by either the oral or intravenous route, the maintenance oral dose is adjusted according to the individual patient's response and the plasma concentration of digoxin.

Elimination of digoxin is primarily by the kid-

Table 13-1

Comparison of Digoxin and Digitoxin

	Digoxin	Digitoxin
Average digitalizing dose		
Oral	0.75–1.5 mg	0.8–1.2 mg
IV	0.5–1 mg	0.8–1.2 mg
Average daily maintenance dose		
Oral	0.125–0.5 mg	0.05–0.2 mg
IV	0.25 mg	0.1 mg
Onset of effect		
Oral	1.5–6 hours	3–6 hours
IV	5–30 minutes	30–120 minutes
Absorption from gastrointestinal tract	75%	90%–100%
Plasma protein binding	25%	95%
Route of elimination	Renal	Hepatic
Enterohepatic circulation	Minimal	Marked
Elimination half-time	31–33 hours	5–7 days
Therapeutic plasma concentration	0.5–2 ng ml^{-1}	10–35 ng ml^{-1}

(Adapted by permission of Hoffman BF, Bigger JT. Digitalis and allied cardiac glycosides. In Gilman AG, Goodman LS, Rall TW, Murad F, eds. The Pharmacological Basis of Therapeutics, 7th ed. New York, Macmillan Publishing Co. 1985, 716.)

neys with about one third of the drug excreted daily (Marcus, 1975). In the presence of renal dysfunction, the elimination of digoxin is depressed in proportion to the reduction in creatinine clearance. For example, elimination half-time of digoxin is 31 to 33 hours in the presence of normal renal function and up to 4.4 days in the absence of renal function. Metabolism of digoxin is minimal with a few patients forming an inactive metabolite, dihydrodigoxin.

In elderly patients with reduced renal function and skeletal muscle mass, the administration of usual doses of digoxin may result in unexpectedly high plasma concentrations of drug (Ewy *et al*, 1969). A rule of thumb is that the dose of digoxin should be reduced by 50% when the serum creatinine is 3 to 5 mg dl^{-1} and by 75% in the absence of renal function (Marcus, 1975).

The principal inactive tissue reservoir site for digoxin is skeletal muscle. A decrease in the size of this reservoir results in increased plasma and myocardial levels of the drug. Minimal amounts of digoxin accumulate in fat (Ewy *et al*, 1971). About 25% of digoxin is bound to protein. Occasionally, a patient forms antibodies to digoxin which prevents a therapeutic effect.

Digitoxin

Absorption of digitoxin after oral administration is 90% to 100% reflecting the greater lipid solubility of this cardiac glycoside compared with digoxin (Table 13-1) (Hoffman and Bigger, 1985). Digitoxin is actively metabolized by hepatic microsomal enzymes and one of these metabolites is digoxin. Only 8% of digitoxin appears unchanged in the urine (Marcus, 1975). The elimination half-time of digitoxin and its metabolites is 5 to 7 days. Elimination half-time is not appreciably altered by hepatic disease, emphasizing the large reserve capacity of the liver for metabolic degradation of digitoxin (Doherty and Kaul, 1975). Likewise, impaired renal function does not alter plasma concentrations of digitoxin (Rasmussen *et al*, 1971). The long elimination half-time of digitoxin is an advantage for maintaining therapeutic concentrations should a patient miss several doses.

Ouabain

Ouabain is administered intravenously in doses of 1.5 to 3 μg kg^{-1} to provide rapid increases in myocardial contractility or to reduce the heart rate in uncontrolled atrial fibrillation. It is unlikely, however, that ouabain offers any advantages over intravenous digoxin administered for the same reasons. The total adult intravenous dose of ouabain should not exceed 1 mg in 24 hours. Ouabain is rapidly excreted in the urine with about 50% of the unchanged drug being recovered in 8 hours. A longer acting digitalis preparation should be substituted for ouabain when maintenance therapy is indicated. Ouabain is not effective when administered orally reflecting destruction of its glycoside portion in the gastrointestinal tract.

CARDIOVASCULAR EFFECTS

The principal cardiovascular effect of digitalis glycosides administered to patients with cardiac failure is a dose-related increase in myocardial contractility that becomes significant with less than full digitalizing doses (Kim *et al,* 1975). This positive inotropic effect manifests as increased stroke volume, decreased heart size, and reduced left ventricular end-diastolic pressure. Indeed, cardiac glycosides can double stroke volume from a failing and dilated left ventricle. The ventricular function curve (Frank-Starling curve) is shifted to the left (Fig. 13-4). Improved renal perfusion due to the overall increase in cardiac output favors mobilization and excretion of edema fluid accounting for the diuresis that often accompanies the administration of cardiac glycosides to patients in cardiac failure. Excessive sympathetic nervous system activity that occurs as a compensatory response to cardiac failure is reduced with the improved circulation that accompanies administration of cardiac glycosides. The resulting decrease in peripheral vascular resistance further enhances forward left ventricular stroke volume.

In addition to positive inotropic effects, cardiac glycosides enhance parasympathetic nervous system activity leading to delayed conduction of cardiac impulses through the atrioventricular node and reductions in heart rate (see the section entitled Alterations in Autonomic Nervous System Activity). The magnitude of this negative dromotropic effect depends on the preexisting activity of the autonomic nervous system (Kim *et al,* 1975). Increased parasympathetic nervous system activity decreases contractility in the atria but direct positive inotropic effects of cardiac glycosides more than offset these negative inotropic effects on the ventricles.

Cardiac glycosides also increase myocardial contractility in the absence of cardiac failure. Nevertheless, the resulting tendency for cardiac output to increase may be offset by reductions in heart rate and direct vasoconstricting effects of cardiac glycosides on arterial, and to a lesser extent, on venous smooth muscle (Mason, 1966). Indeed, cardiac output is often unchanged or even decreased when cardiac glycosides are administered to patients with normal hearts.

ELECTROCARDIOGRAPHIC EFFECTS

The electrophysiologic effects of therapeutic plasma concentrations of cardiac glycosides manifest on the electrocardiogram as (1) a prolonged P–R interval due to delayed conduction of cardiac impulses through the atrioventricular node, (2) a shortened Q–T interval because of more rapid ventricular repolarization, (3) ST–T segment depression (scaphoid or scopped-out) due to a decreased slope of phase 3 repolarization of cardiac action potentials, and (4) diminished amplitude or inversion of the T wave. The P–R interval is rarely prolonged beyond 0.25 second, and the effect on the Q–T interval is independent of parasympathetic nervous system activity. Changes in the S-T segment and T wave do not correlate with therapeutic plasma concentrations of cardiac gly-

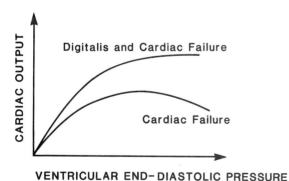

FIGURE 13-4. Cardiac glycosides shift the ventricular function curve of the failing myocardium to the left.

cosides. Furthermore, S – T segment and T wave changes may suggest myocardial ischemia. When digitalis is discontinued, the changes on the electrocardiogram disappear in about 20 days.

DIGITALIS TOXICITY

Cardiac glycosides have a narrow therapeutic range. Indeed, it is estimated that about 20% of patients who are being treated with cardiac glycosides experience some form of digitalis toxicity (Rodensky and Wasserman, 1961). Therapeutic effects of cardiac glycosides develop at about 35% of the fatal dose, and cardiac dysrhythmias typically manifest at about 60% of the fatal dose. The only difference between various cardiac glycosides when toxicity occurs is the duration of adverse effects.

There is general agreement that the toxic effects of cardiac glycosides result from inhibition of the sodium:potassium ATPase ion transport system leading to an accumulation of intracellular sodium ions and a corresponding reduction in intracellular potassium ions. The slope of phase 4 depolarization is enhanced by digitalis especially in the ventricles. A second mechanism for digitalis-induced increases in automaticity is oscillatory afterpotentials (Cranefield, 1977).

Causes

The most frequent cause of digitalis toxicity in the absence of renal dysfunction is the concurrent administration of diuretics that cause potassium depletion. During anesthesia, hyperventilation of the lungs can reduce the serum potassium concentration an average of 0.5 mEq L^{-1} for every 10 mmHg reduction in $PaCO_2$ (Edwards and Winnie, 1977). Hypokalemia probably increases myocardial binding of cardiac glycosides resulting in an excess drug effect (Smith and Haber, 1973a). Other electrolyte abnormalities that contribute to digitalis toxicity include hypercalcemia and hypomagnesemia (Neff et al, 1972). An increase in sympathetic nervous system activity as produced by arterial hypoxemia increases the likelihood of digitalis toxicity. Elderly patients with decreased skeletal muscle mass and reduced renal function are vulnerable to digitalis toxicity if the usual doses of digoxin are administered. Renal function may be altered during cardiopulmonary bypass re-

sulting in changes in electrolyte concentrations (e.g., hypokalemia, hypomagnesemia) that could predispose the patient to the development of digitalis toxicity (Coltart et al, 1971).

Diagnosis

Digitalis is often administered in situations in which the toxic effects of the drug are difficult to distinguish from the effects of the cardiac disease. For this reason, determination of the plasma concentration of the cardiac glycoside is used to indicate the likely presence of digitalis toxicity (Beller et al, 1971; Doherty, 1978). For example, a plasma digoxin concentration of less than 0.5 ng ml^{-1} eliminates the possibility of digitalis toxicity. Plasma concentrations between 0.5 and 2.5 ng ml^{-1} are usually considered therapeutic while levels above 3 ng ml^{-1} are definitely in a toxic range. Infants and children have an increased tolerance to cardiac glycosides, and the range of therapeutic concentrations for digoxin is 2.5 to 3.5 ng ml^{-1}.

It must be appreciated that the relationship between plasma concentrations and observed pharmacologic effects is not always consistent. For example, therapeutic plasma concentrations of digoxin, despite clinical symptoms of digitalis toxicity, are frequently observed in the presence of electrolyte disturbances and recent myocardial infarction. Conversely, high therapeutic plasma concentrations of digoxin, without symptoms of digitalis toxicity, are frequently observed in treatment of patients with supraventricular tachydysrhythmias which require large doses to reduce the ventricular response (Doherty, 1978).

Anorexia, nausea, and vomiting are early manifestations of digitalis toxicity. These symptoms, when present preoperatively in patients receiving cardiac glycosides, should arouse suspicion of digitalis toxicity. Excitation of the chemoreceptor trigger zone is the principal mechanism in the production of vomiting. Transitory amblyopia and scotomata have been observed. Pain simulating trigeminal neuralgia may be an early sign of digitalis toxicity. The extremities may also be a site of discomfort.

Electrocardiogram

There are no unequivocal features on the electrocardiogram that confirm the presence of digitalis toxicity (Smith and Haber, 1973b). Nevertheless, toxic plasma concentrations of digitalis typically cause atrial or ventricular cardiac dysrhythmias (*e.g.,* increased automaticity) and delayed conduction of cardiac impulses through the atrioventricular node (*e.g.,* prolonged P–R interval) culminating in heart block. Activity of the sinoatrial node may also be directly inhibited by high doses of cardiac glycosides. Conduction of cardiac impulses through specialized conducting tissues of the ventricles is not altered as evidenced by the lack of effects of even toxic plasma concentrations of digoxin on the duration of the QRS complex. Ventricular fibrillation is the most frequent cause of death from digitalis toxicity.

Treatment

Treatment of digitalis toxicity includes (1) correction of predisposing causes (*e.g.,* hypokalemia, arterial hypoxemia), (2) administration of drugs (phenytoin, lidocaine, atropine) to treat cardiac dysrhythmias, and (3) insertion of a temporary artificial transvenous cardiac pacemaker if complete heart block is present (Mason *et al,* 1971). Supplemental potassium decreases the binding of digitalis to cardiac tissue and thus directly antagonizes cardiotoxic effects of cardiac glycosides. Serum potassium concentrations should be determined before treatment because supplemental potassium, in the presence of a high preexisting level of potassium will intensify atrioventricular block and depress the automaticity of ectopic pacemakers in the ventricle leading to complete heart block. If renal function is normal and atrioventricular conduction block is not present, it is acceptable to administer 0.025 to 0.05 mEq kg^{-1} of potassium rapidly intravenously to treat life-threatening cardiac dysrhythmias associated with digitalis toxicity. Phenytoin (0.5–1.5 mg kg^{-1} over 5 minutes) or lidocaine (1–2 mg kg^{-1}) administered intravenously is effective in suppressing ventricular cardiac dysrhythmias caused by digitalis while phenytoin is also effective in suppressing atrial dysrhythmias (Bigger, 1972) (see Chapter 17). Atropine, 35 to 70 μg kg^{-1}, can be used to increase heart rate by offsetting excessive parasympathetic nervous system activity produced by toxic plasma concentrations of digitalis. Propranolol is effective in suppressing increased automaticity produced by digitalis toxicity, but its tendency to increase atrioventricular node refrac-

toriness limits its usefulness when conduction blockade is present (Bigger, 1972).

Life-threatening digitalis toxicity can be treated by administering antibodies (Fab fragments) to the drug thus decreasing the plasma concentration of cardiac glycoside available to attach to cardiac cell membranes (Ochs and Smith, 1977). The Fab-digitalis complex is eliminated by the kidneys.

PREOPERATIVE PROPHYLACTIC DIGITALIS

Preoperative prophylactic administration of digitalis to patients without signs of cardiac failure is controversial (Deutsch and Dalen, 1969; Selzer and Cohn, 1970). The obvious disadvantage of prophylactic digitalis is the administration of a drug with a narrow therapeutic-to-toxic dose difference to patients with no obvious need for the drug. Furthermore, there may be difficulty in differentiating anesthetic-induced cardiac dysrhythmias from those due to digitalis toxicity (Chung, 1981). Indeed, events such as alterations in renal function, decreases in serum potassium concentration due to hyperventilation of the lungs, and increases in sympathetic nervous system activity are likely to occur intraoperatively and thus increase the likelihood of an increased pharmacologic effect from circulating digitalis. Despite these theoretical disadvantages, there is evidence that patients with limited cardiac reserve may benefit from prophylactic digitalis. For example, the preoperative administration of oral digoxin (0.75 mg in divided doses the day before surgery and 0.25 mg before the induction of anesthesia) reduces the occurrence of postoperative supraventricular cardiac dysrhythmias in elderly patients undergoing thoracic or abdominal surgery (Chee *et al,* 1982). Prophylactic digoxin also reduces evidence of impaired cardiac function in patients with coronary artery disease recovering from anesthesia (Fig. 13-5) (Pinaud *et al,* 1983). Based on these observations, it may be reasonable to conclude that beneficial effects of prophylactic digitalis administered to appropriate selected patients in the preoperative period outweigh the potential hazards of digitalis toxicity. Certainly, there are no data to support discontinuing digitalis in any patient preoperatively including those undergoing cardiopulmonary bypass. It is particularly important to continue digitalis therapy through-

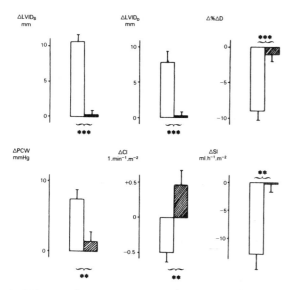

FIGURE 13-5. Preoperative and postoperative measurements (mean ± SE) of cardiac function in patients with coronary artery disease receiving (hashed bars) or not receiving (clear bars) digitalis. $LVID_s$ = end-systolic left ventricular internal dimension; $LVID_D$ = end-diastolic left ventricular internal dimension; $\%\Delta D$ = shortening fraction; PCW = pulmonary capillary occlusion pressure; Δ CI = change in cardiac index; Δ SI change in stroke index. **P<0.01,***P< 0.001. (From Pinaud, MLJ, Blanloeil YAG, Souron RJ. Preoperative prophylactic digitalization of patients with coronary artery disease—a randomized echocardiographic and hemodynamic study. Anesth Analg 1983;62:865–9. Reproduced by permission of the authors and the International Anesthesia Research Society.)

out the perioperative period in patients who are receiving the drug for heart rate control.

DRUG INTERACTIONS

Quinidine produces a dose-related increase in the plasma concentration of digoxin that becomes apparent within 24 hours after the first dose of the antidysrhythmic drug (Doering, 1979). This effect of quinidine may be due to displacement of digoxin from binding sites in tissues.

Succinylcholine, or any other drug that can abruptly increase parasympathetic nervous system activity, could theoretically have an additive effect with cardiac glycosides (Dowdy and Fabian, 1963). Cardiac dysrhythmias could also reflect succinylcholine-induced catecholamine release and resulting cardiac irritability. Despite these theoretical concerns, clinical experience does not support the occurrence of an increased incidence of cardiac dysrhythmias in patients treated with cardiac glycosides and receiving succinylcholine (Bartolone and Rao, 1983).

Sympathomimetics with beta-adrenergic agonist effects as well as pancuronium may increase the likelihood of cardiac dysrhythmias in the presence of cardiac glycosides (Bartolone and Rao, 1983; Solomon and Abrams, 1972). Calcium may precipitate cardiac dysrhythmias in patients receiving cardiac glycosides (Nola *et al,* 1970). Any drug that facilitates renal loss of potassium ions increases the likelihood of hypokalemia and associated digitalis toxicity. The simultaneous administration of an oral antacid and digitalis decreases the gastrointestinal absorption of the cardiac glycoside (Brown and Juhl, 1976).

Halothane can antagonize digitalis-induced cardiac dysrhythmias (Morrow and Townley, 1964). Fentanyl, enflurane, and, to a lesser extent, isoflurane protect against digitalis-enhanced cardiac automaticity (Ivankovich *et al,* 1976). The effect of anesthetics on automaticity due to oscillatory afterpotentials is not known.

NONCATECHOLAMINE NONGLYCOSIDE CARDIAC INOTROPES

Calcium

Calcium, when injected intravenously, produces an intense positive inotropic effect lasting 10 to 20 minutes and manifesting as increases in stroke volume and decreases in left ventricular end-diastolic pressure (Denlinger *et al,* 1975). Heart rate and peripheral vascular resistance decrease. The inotropic effects of calcium are enhanced in the presence of preexisting hypocalcemia. The risk of cardiac dysrhythmias when calcium is administered to patients receiving digitalis should be considered especially if hypokalemia is also present (Nola *et al,* 1970).

Calcium chloride, 5 to 10 mg kg^{-1} injected intravenously to adults, is often used to improve myocardial contractility and stroke volume at the conclusion of cardiopulmonary bypass. Indeed, myocardial contractility at the conclusion of cardiopulmonary bypass may be depressed by hypocalcemia due to (1) use of potassium-containing cardioplegia solutions, (2) administration of citrated stored whole blood, and (3) treatment of metabolic acidosis with sodium bicarbonate. A 10% solution of calcium chloride contains more calcium than a 10% calcium gluconate solution does although the availability of ionized calcium is prompt regardless of the preparation administered (see Chapter 35).

Glucagon

Glucagon is a polypeptide hormone produced by alpha cells of the pancreas (see Chapter 52). Like catecholamines, glucagon enhances the formation of cyclic AMP, but, unlike catecholamines, does not act via beta-adrenergic receptors. Glucagon also evokes the release of catecholamines, but this is not the predominant mechanism of its cardiovascular effects. The principal therapeutic cardiac indication for glucagon is to increase myocardial contractility and heart rate in the presence of intense drug-induced beta-adrenergic blockade (Kones and Phillips, 1971). Because glucagon is a peptide, it must be administered intravenously or intramuscularly.

Cardiovascular Effects

In adults, intravenous glucagon, as a rapid injection (1–5 mg) or as a continuous infusion (20 mg hr^{-1}) reliably increases stroke volume and heart rate independent of adrenergic receptor activation (Parmley *et al*, 1968). Tachycardia, however, may be sufficiently great to interfere with the augmented cardiac output. Abrupt increases in heart rate can occur when glucagon is administered to patients in atrial fibrillation. Mean arterial pressure may increase modestly, while peripheral vascular resistance is unchanged or reduced. In contrast to other sympathomimetics, glucagon enhances automaticity in the sinoatrial and atrioventricular nodes without increasing automaticity in the ventricle. The renal effect is similar to dopamine, but glucagon is less potent. In contrast to these acute cardiovascular effects, the chronic administration of glucagon is not effective in evoking sustained positive inotropic and chronotropic effects.

Side Effects

In awake patients, intravenous administration of glucagon often evokes nausea and vomiting. Hy-perglycemia is a predictable effect following intravenous administration of glucagon. Paradoxical hypoglycemia may occur in patients lacking sufficient hepatic glycogen stores to offset the increased insulin release caused by glucagon. Hypokalemia reflects increased secretion of insulin and subsequent intracellular transfer of glucose and potassium ions. Glucagon stimulates release of catecholamines and could evoke hypertension in a patient with an unrecognized pheochromocytoma. In this regard, glucagon, 1 to 2 mg administered intravenously, may be used as a provocative test in the differential diagnosis of pheochromocytoma. This dose of glucagon will evoke a three-fold or greater increase in the plasma concentration of catecholamines 1 to 3 minutes following administration to a patient with pheochromocytoma. A simultaneous increase in blood pressure of at least 20/15 mmHg is also likely.

Amrinone

Amrinone is a noncatecholamine nonglycoside bipyridine derivative that produces dose-dependent positive inotropic effects manifesting as increased cardiac output and decreased left ventricular end-diastolic pressure (Fig. 13-2) (LeJemtel *et al*, 1980; Wynne *et al*, 1980). Mild peripheral vasodilation is present, but blood pressure and heart rate are not significantly changed. Amrinone possesses neither antidysrhythmic nor arrhythmogenic properties.

Amrinone-induced inhibition of phosphodiesterase enzyme leads to increased intracellular concentrations of cAMP, which potentiates delivery of calcium ions to the myocardial contractile system (Kariya *et al*, 1982). Amrinone can be used in conjunction with digitalis without provoking digitalis toxicity suggesting the mechanism of action of these two drugs is different. Additive hemodynamic improvements are also noted when amrinone is administered in conjunction with hydralazine. The elimination half-time of amrinone is about 6 hours with the main route of excretion being that of unchanged drug in the urine.

Amrinone is effective when administered orally as well as intravenously. Administration of a single intravenous dose of 0.5 to 1.5 mg kg^{-1} increases cardiac output within 5 minutes with detectable positive inotropic effects persisting for about 2 hours (Wilmshurst *et al*, 1983). Following the initial injection, continuous intravenous infusion of 2 to 10 μg kg^{-1} min^{-1} produces positive inotropic effects that are maintained during the infusion (*e.g.,* tachyphylaxis does not occur) and for several hours following discontinuation of the infusion. The daily dose of amrinone should not exceed 10 mg kg^{-1} including the loading dose which may be repeated 30 minutes following the first injection.

Adverse side effects of amrinone include occasional hypotension due to vasodilation and thrombocytopenia with chronic therapy. In animals, chronic administration of amrinone has been associated with hepatic dysfunction. Overall the therapeutic index of amrinone is about 100 : 1 compared to 1.2 : 1 for cardiac glycosides.

REFERENCES

Akera T, Larsen FS, Brody TM. Correlation of cardiac sodium- and potassium-activated adenosine triphosphate activity with ouabain-induced inotropic stimulation. J Pharmacol Exp Ther 1970;173 : 145 – 51.

Bartolone RS, Rao TLK. Dysrhythmias following muscle relaxant administration in patients receiving digitalis. Anesthesiology 1983;58 : 567 – 9.

Beller GA, Smith TW, Abelmann WH, Haber E, Hood W. Digitalis intoxication: A prospective clinical study with serum level correlations. N Engl J Med 1971;284 : 989 – 97.

Bigger JT. Arrhythmias and antiarrhythmic drugs. Adv Intern Med 1972;18 : 251 – 81.

Brown DD, Juhl RP. Decreased bioavailability of digoxin due to antacids and kaolin-pectin. N Engl J Med 1976;295 : 1034 – 7.

Butler VP. Assays of digitalis in the blood. Prog Cardiovas Dis 1972;14 : 571 – 600.

Chee TP, Prakash NS, Desser KB, Benchimol A. Postoperative supraventricular arrhythmias and the role of prophylactic digoxin in cardiac surgery. Am Heart J 1982;104 : 974 – 7.

Chung DC: Anesthetic problems associated with the treatment ofcardiovascular disease: I. Digitalis toxicity. Can Anaesth Soc J 1981;28 : 6 – 16.

Coltart DJ, Chamberlain DA, Howard MR, Kettlewell MG, Mercer JL, Smith TW. Effect of cardiopulmonary bypass on plasma digoxin concentrations. Br Heart J 1971;33 : 334 – 8.

Cranefield PF. Action potentials, afterpotentials, and arrhythmias. Circ Res 1977;41 : 415 – 23.

Denlinger JP, Kaplan JA, Lecky JH, Wollman H. Cardiovascular responses to calcium administered intravenously to man during halothane anesthesia. Anesthesiology 1975;42 : 390 – 7.

Deutsch S, Dalen JE. Indications for prophylactic digitalization. Anesthesiology 1969;30 : 648 – 56.

Doering W. Quinidine-digoxin interaction: pharmacokinetics, underlying mechanism and clinical implications. N Engl J Med 1979;301 : 400 – 4.

Doherty JE. Digitalis glycosides. Pharmacokinetics and their clinical implications. Ann Intern Med 1973;79 : 229 – 38.

Doherty JE. How and when to use digitalis serum levels. JAMA 1978;239 : 2594 – 6.

Doherty JE, Kaul JJ. Clinical pharmacology of digitalis glycosides. Annu Rev Med 1975;26 : 159 – 66.

Dowdy EG, Fabian LW. Ventricular arrhythmias induced by succinylcholine in digitalized patients. Anesth Analg 1963;42 : 501 – 13.

Edwards R, Winnie AP, Ramamurphy S. Acute hypocapneic hypokalemia: An iatrogenic complication. Anesth Analg 1977;56 : 786 – 92.

Ewy GA, Groves BM, Ball MF, Nimmo L, Jackson B, Marcus F. Digoxin metabolism in obesity. Circulation 1971;44 : 810 – 4.

Ewy GA, Kapadia GG, Yao L, Lullin M, Marcus FI. Digoxin metabolism in the elderly. Circulation 1969;39 : 449 – 53.

Gillis RA, Pearle DL, Levitt B. Digitalis: A neuroexcitatory drug (editorial). Circulation 1975;52 : 739 – 42.

Hoffman BF, Bigger JT. Digitalis and allied cardiac glycosides. In: Gilman AG, Goodman LS, Rall TW, Murad F, eds. The Pharmacological Basis of Therapeutics, 7th ed. New York. Macmillan Publishing Co. 1985, 716.

Ivankovich AD, Miletich DJ, Grossman RK, Albrecht RF, El-Etr AA, Cairoli VJ. The effect of enflurane, isoflurane, fluroxene, methoxyflurane and diethyl ether anesthesia on ouabain tolerance in the dog. Anesth Analg 1976;55 : 360 – 5.

Kariya T, Wille LJ, Dage CD. Biochemical studies on the mechanism of cardiotonic activity of MDL 17,043. J Cardiovasc Pharmacol 1982;4:509 – 14.

Kim YI, Noble RJ, Zipes DP. Dissociation of the inotropic effect of digitalis from its effect on atrioventricular conduction. Am J Cardiol 1975;36:459 – 67.

Kones RJ, Phillips JH. Glucagon: Present status in cardiovascular disease. Clin Pharmacol Ther 1971;12 : 427 – 44.

LeJemtel TH, Keung E, Ribner HS, et al. Sustained beneficial effects of oral amrinone on cardiac and renal function in patients with severe congestive heart failure. Am J Cardiol 1980;45 : 123 – 9.

Marcus FI. Digitalis pharmacokinetics and metabolism. Am J Med 1975;58 : 452 – 9.

Mason DT. The cardiovascular effects of digitalis in normal man. Clin Pharmacol Ther 1966;7 : 1 – 16.

Mason Dt, Zelis R, Lee G, Hughes L, Spann JF, Amsterdam EA. Current concepts and treatment of digitalis toxicity. Am J Cardiol 1971;27 : 546 – 59.

Morrow DH, Townley NT. Anesthesia and digitalis toxicity: An experimental study. Anesth Analg 1964;43:510–19.

Neff MS, Mendelssohn S, Kim KE, Banach S, Swartz C, Seller RH. Magnesium sulfate in digitalis toxicity. Am J Cardiol 1972;29:377–82.

Nola GT, Pope S, Harrison DC. Assessment of the synergistic relationship between serum calcium and digitalis. Am Heart J 1970;79:499–507.

Ochs HR, Smith TW. Reversal of advanced digitoxin toxicity and modification of pharmacokinetics by specific antibodies and Fab fragments. J Clin Invest 1977;60:1303–13.

Parmley WW, Glick G, Sonnelblick EH. Cardiovascular effects of glucagon in man. N Engl J Med 1968;279:12–7.

Pinaud MLJ, Blanloeil YAG, Souron RJ. Preoperative prophylactic digitalization of patients with coronary artery disease — a randomized echocardiographic and hemodynamic study. Anesth Analg 1983;62:865–9.

Rasmussen K, Jewell J. Storstein L, Gjerdum K. Digitoxin kinetics in patients with impaired renal function. Clin Pharmacol Ther 1971;13:6–14.

Rodensky PL, Wasserman F. Observations on digitalis intoxication. Arch Intern Med 1961;108:171–88.

Selzer A, Cohn KE. Some thoughts concerning the prophylactic use of digitalis. Am J Cardiol 1970;26:214–6.

Smith LDR, Oldershaw PF. Inotropic and vasopressor agents. Br J Anaesth 1984;56:767–80.

Smith TW, Haber E. Digitalis. N Engl J Med 1973a;289:1063–72.

Smith TW, Haber E. Digitalis. N Engl J Med 1973b;289:1125–9.

Solomon HM, Abrams WB. Interactions between digitoxin and other drugs in man. Am Heart J 1972;83:277–80.

Van Winkle WG, Schwartz A. Ions and inotropy. Annu Rev Physiol 1976;38:247–72.

Wilmshurst PT, Thompson DS, Jenkins BS, Coltart DJ, Webb-Peploe M. Haemodynamic effects of intravenous amrinone in patients with impaired left ventricular function. Br Heart J 1983;49:77–82.

Wynn J, Malacoff RF, Benotti JR, et al. Oral amrinone in refractory congestive heart failure. Am J Cardiol 1980;45:1245–9.

CHAPTER 14

Alpha- and Beta-Adrenergic Receptor Antagonists

INTRODUCTION

Alpha- and beta-adrenergic receptor antagonists prevent the interaction of the endogenous neurotransmitter, norepinephrine, or sympathomimetics with the corresponding adrenergic receptor (Foex, 1984). Interference with normal adrenergic receptor function attenuates sympathetic nervous system homeostatic mechanisms and evokes predictable pharmacologic responses.

ALPHA-ADRENERGIC RECEPTOR ANTAGONISTS

Alpha-adrenergic receptor antagonists bind selectively to alpha-adrenergic receptors and interfere with the ability of catecholamines or other sympathomimetics to provoke alpha responses. Drug-induced alpha-adrenergic blockade prevents effects of catecholamines and sympathomimetics on the heart and peripheral vasculature and the inhibitory action of epinephrine on insulin secretion is blocked. Orthostatic hypotension, baroreceptor-mediated reflex tachycardia and impotence are invariable side effects of alpha-adrenergic blockade. Furthermore, absence of beta-adrenergic blockade permits maximum expression of cardiac stimulation from norepinephrine. These side effects prevent the use of nonselective alpha-adrenergic antagonists in the management of ambulatory essential hypertension.

Mechanism of Action

Phentolamine, prazosin (see Chapter 15), and yohimbine are competitive (*i.e.,* reversible binding with the receptor) alpha-adrenergic antagonists. In contrast, phenoxybenzamine binds covalently to the alpha-adrenergic receptor to produce an irreversible and insurmountable type of blockade. Once alpha blockade has been established with phenoxybenzamine even massive doses of sympathomimetics are ineffective until the effect of phenoxybenzamine is terminated by metabolism.

Phentolamine and phenoxybenzamine are nonselective alpha antagonists acting at postsynaptic alpha-1 receptors as well as presynaptic alpha-receptors. Prazosin is selective for alpha-1 receptors while yohimbine is selective for alpha-2 receptors.

Phentolamine

Phentolamine is a 2-substituted imidazoline derivative that produces transient nonselective alpha-adrenergic blockade (Fig. 14-1). Administered intravenously, phentolamine produces peripheral vasodilation and a decrease in blood pressure that manifests within 2 minutes and lasts 10 to 15 minutes. This vasodilation reflects alpha-1 receptor blockade and a direct action of phentolamine on vascular smooth muscle. Declines in blood pressure cause baroreceptor-mediated increases in sympathetic nervous system activity

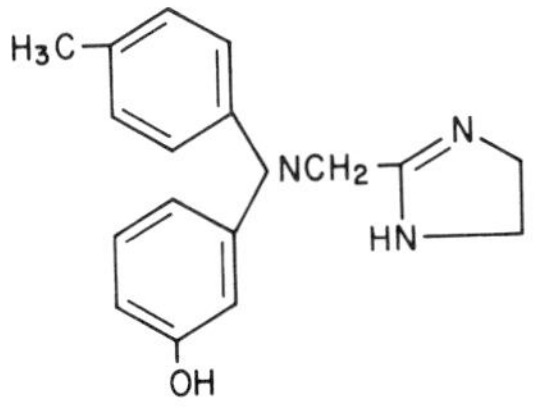

FIGURE 14-1. Phentolamine.

manifesting as cardiac stimulation. In addition to reflex stimulation, phentolamine-induced alpha-2 receptor blockade permits enhanced neural release of norepinephrine manifesting as increased heart rate and cardiac output. Indeed, cardiac dysrhythmias and angina pectoris may accompany the administration of phentolamine. Hyperperistalsis, abdominal pain, and diarrhea may be caused by a predominance of parasympathetic nervous system activity.

Clinical Uses

The principal use of phentolamine is treatment of acute hypertensive emergencies as may accompany intraoperative manipulation of a pheochromocytoma or autonomic hyperreflexia. Administration of phentolamine intravenously, 30 to 70 μg kg^{-1}, produces a prompt, but transient, reduction in blood pressure. A continuous intravenous infusion of phentolamine may be utilized to maintain normal blood pressure during intraoperative resection of a pheochromocytoma.

Local infiltration with a phentolamine-containing solution (2.5–5 mg in 10 ml) is appropriate when a sympathomimetic accidently is administered extravascularly.

Phenoxybenzamine

Phenoxybenzamine is a haloalkylamine derivative that acts as a nonselective alpha-adrenergic antagonist by combining covalently with alpha-adrenergic receptors (Fig. 14-2). Blockade at postsynaptic alpha-1 receptors is more intense than at alpha-2 receptors.

Pharmacokinetics

Absorption of phenoxybenzamine from the gastrointestinal tract is incomplete. Onset of alpha-

adrenergic blockade is slow taking up to 60 minutes to reach peak effect even following intravenous administration. This delay in onset is due to the time required for structural modification of the phenoxybenzamine molecule which is necessary to render the drug active. The elimination half-time of phenoxybenzamine is about 24 hours emphasizing the likelihood of cumulative effects with repeated doses.

Cardiovascular Effects

Phenoxybenzamine administered to a supine normovolemic patient in the absence of elevated sympathetic nervous system activity produces little change in blood pressure. Orthostatic hypotension, however, is prominent especially in the presence of preexisting hypertension or hypovolemia. In addition, impairment of compensatory vasoconstriction results in exaggerated blood pressure reductions in response to blood loss or vasodilating drugs such as volatile anesthetics. Despite reductions in blood pressure, cardiac output is often increased and renal blood flow is not greatly altered unless preexisting renal vasoconstriction was present. Cerebral and coronary vascular resistances are not changed.

Noncardiac Effects

Phenoxybenzamine blocks the inhibitory action of epinephrine on the secretion of insulin. Catecholamine-induced glycogenolysis in skeletal muscle or lipolysis is not altered.

Stimulation of the radial fibers of the iris are blocked and miosis is a prominent component of the response to phenoxybenzamine. Sedation may accompany chronic phenoxybenzamine therapy. Nasal stuffiness is due to unopposed vasodilation in mucous membranes in the presence of alpha-adrenergic blockade.

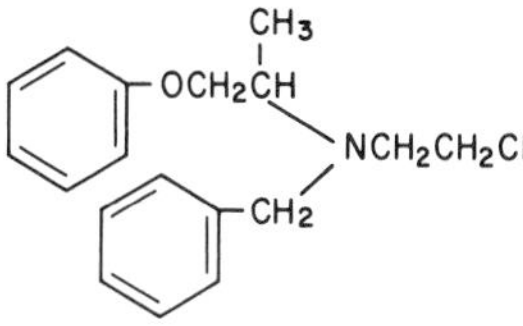

FIGURE 14-2. Phenoxybenzamine.

Clinical Uses

Oral phenoxybenzamine, 0.5 to 1 mg kg^{-1}, (or prazosin, see Chapter 15) is administered preoperatively to control blood pressure in patients with pheochromocytoma. Chronic alpha-adrenergic blockade, by relieving intense peripheral vasoconstriction, permits expansion of intravascular fluid volume as reflected by a decrease in the hematocrit. Excessive vasoconstriction with associated tissue ischemia as accompanies hemorrhagic shock may be reversed by phenoxybenzamine but only after intravascular fluid volume has been replenished.

Treatment of peripheral vascular disease characterized by intermittent claudication is not favorably influenced by alpha-adrenergic blockade since cutaneous, rather than skeletal muscle blood flow, is increased. The most beneficial clinical responses to alpha-adrenergic blockade are in diseases with a large component of vasoconstriction, such as Raynaud's syndrome.

Yohimbine

Yohimbine is a selective antagonist at presynaptic alpha-2 receptors leading to enhanced release of norepinephrine from the nerve ending. As a result, this drug may be useful in treatment of the rare patient suffering from idiopathic orthostatic hypotension.

Prazosin

Prazosin is a selective postsynaptic alpha-1 receptor antagonist leaving intact the inhibiting effect of alpha-2 receptor activity on norepinephrine release from the nerve ending (see Chapter 15). As a result, prazosin is less likely than nonselective alpha-adrenergic antagonists to evoke reflex tachycardia.

BETA-ADRENERGIC RECEPTOR ANTAGONISTS

Beta-adrenergic receptor antagonists bind selectively to beta-adrenergic receptors and interfere with the ability of catecholamines or other sympathomimetics to provoke beta responses. Drug-induced beta-adrenergic blockade prevents effects of catecholamines and sympathomimetics on the heart and smooth muscle of the airways and blood vessels. Beta antagonist drug therapy should be continued throughout the perioperative period to maintain desirable effects and to avoid the risk of sympathetic nervous system hyperactivity associated with abrupt discontinuation of these drugs (Boudoulas *et al*, 1977; Boudoulas *et al*, 1979) (see the section entitled Side Effects). Propranolol is the standard beta antagonist with which all other drugs are compared.

Mechanism of Action

Beta-adrenergic receptor antagonists exhibit selective affinity for beta-adrenergic receptors where they act by competitive inhibition. Binding of antagonist drug to the beta-adrenergic receptor is reversible such that the drug can be displaced from the receptor if sufficiently large amounts of agonist become available. Competitive antagonism causes a rightward displacement of the dose-response curve for the agonist, but the slope of the curve remains unchanged emphasizing that sufficiently large doses of the agonist may still exert a full pharmacologic effect.

Chronic administration of beta-adrenergic antagonists is associated with an increase in the number of beta-adrenergic receptors (Roth *et al*, 1979).

Structure Activity Relationships

Beta-adrenergic antagonists are derivatives of the beta-agonist drug, isoproterenol (Fig. 14-3). Substituents on the benzene ring determine whether the drug acts on the beta-adrenergic receptor as an antagonist or agonist. The levorotatory forms of beta-antagonists and agonists are more potent than the dextrorotatory forms. For example, the dextrorotatory isomer of propranolol has less than 1% of the potency of the levorotatory isomer for blocking beta-adrenergic receptors.

Classification

Beta-adrenergic receptor antagonists are classified as nonselective and selective for beta-1 and beta-2 receptors (Table 14-1). Beta-antagonists are further classified as partial or pure antagonists on the basis of the presence or absence of intrinsic sympathomimetic activity (Table 14-1). Antagonists with intrinsic sympathomimetic activity cause less direct myocardial depression and heart rate slowing than drugs that lack this intrinsic sympathomimetic activity. As a result, partial antagonists may be better tolerated than pure antagonists by patients with poor left ventricular function.

Selective beta-1 antagonists include metoprolol and atenolol. It is important to recognize that beta-1 selectivity is dose-dependent and is lost when large doses of the antagonist are administered. This emphasizes that selectivity should not be interpreted as specificity for a specific type of beta-adrenergic receptor.

Beta-adrenergic antagonists may produce some degree of membrane stabilization in the heart, and thus resemble quinidine (Table 14-1). This membrane stabilization effect, however, is detectable only at plasma concentrations that are far greater than needed to produce clinically adequate beta-adrenergic blockade. Indeed, bradycardia and direct myocardial depression produced by beta-adrenergic antagonists are due to removal of sympathetic nervous system innervation to the heart and not membrane stabilization (Foex, 1984).

Propranolol

Propranolol is a nonselective beta-adrenergic receptor antagonist that lacks intrinsic sympathomimetic activity (*i.e.,* a pure antagonist) (Table 14-1). Antagonism of beta-1 and beta-2 receptors produced by propranolol is about equal. As the first beta antagonist introduced clinically, propranolol remains the standard drug with which all other beta-antagonists are compared (see the sections entitled Clinical Uses and Side Effects).

Cardiac Effects

The most important pharmacologic effects of propranolol are on the heart. Propranolol, by virtue of beta-1 receptor blockade, decreases heart rate and cardiac output especially during exercise or in the presence of increased sympathetic nervous system activity. Heart rate slowing induced by propranolol lasts longer than the negative inotropic effects suggesting a possible subdivision of beta-1 receptors (Boudoulas, 1977). Concomitant blockade of beta-2 receptors by propranolol increases peripheral vascular resistance including coronary vascular resistance. While prolongation of systolic

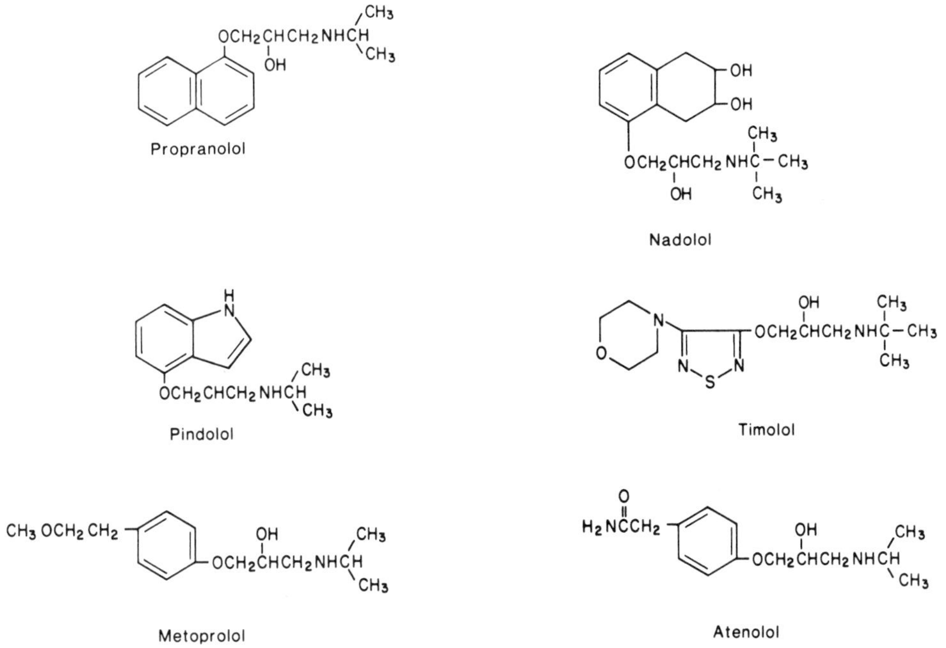

FIGURE 14-3. Beta-adrenergic antagonists.

Table 14-1
Comparative Characteristics of Beta-Adrenergic Receptor Antagonists

	Specificity	Potency (propranolol = 1)	Intrinsic Sympathomimetic Activity	Membrane Stabilizing Activity	Gastrointestinal Absorption (%)	Protein Binding (%)	Principal Method of Clearance	Elimination Half-Time (hours)	Adult Oral Dose (mg)
Propranolol	Nonselective	1	0	++	>90	90–95	Hepatic	2–6	40–1000
Nadolol	Nonselective	0.5–1	0	0	25		Renal	20–24	40–640
Pindolol	Nonselective	5–10	+	±	>90	40–60	Hepatic Renal	3–4	5–30
Timolol	Nonselective	5–10	±	0	>90	<50	Hepatic	3–4	5–45
Metoprolol	Selective, beta-1	0.5–2	0	±	>95	10	Hepatic	3–4	50–400
Atenolol	Selective, beta-1	1	0	0	40–50		Renal	6–9	50–300
Esmolol	Selective, beta-1						Plasma Hydrolysis	0.15	*100–300 μg kg^{-1} min^{-1}

* Intravenous dose

ejection and dilatation of the cardiac ventricles caused by propranolol increase myocardial oxygen requirements, the oxygen-sparing effects of decreased heart rate and myocardial contractility predominate. As a result, propranolol may relieve myocardial ischemia even though drug-induced increases in coronary vascular resistance oppose coronary blood flow.

Sodium retention associated with propranolol therapy most likely results from intrarenal hemodynamic changes that accompany drug-induced reductions in cardiac output (Nies *et al,* 1971).

Pharmacokinetics

Propranolol is rapidly and almost completely absorbed from the gastrointestinal tract, but systemic availability of the drug is limited by extensive hepatic first-pass metabolism which may account for up to 70% of the absorbed dose. Considerable individual variation in the magnitude of the hepatic first-pass effect exists accounting for the up to 20-fold differences in plasma concentrations of propranolol in patients after oral administration of comparable doses (Shand, 1975). First-pass hepatic metabolism is the reason the oral dose of propranolol must be substantially greater than the intavenous dose.

PROTEIN BINDING. Propranolol is extensively bound (90%–95%) to plasma proteins. Heparin-induced increases in plasma concentrations of free fatty acids due to elevated lipoprotein lipase activity results in decreased plasma protein binding of propranolol (Fig. 14-4) (Wood *et al,* 1979). In addition, hemodilution that occurs when cardiopulmonary bypass is initiated may alter protein binding of drugs because of the nonphysiologic protein concentration in the pump prime.

METABOLISM. Clearance of propranolol from the plasma is by hepatic metabolism. An active metabolite, 4-hydroxypropranolol, is detectable in the plasma after oral, but not intravenous, administration of propranolol (Nies and Shand, 1975). Indeed, cardiac beta-blocking activity following equivalent doses of propranolol is greater after oral than intravenous administration presumably reflecting the effects of this metabolite which is equivalent in activity to the parent compound. The elimination half-time of propranolol is 2 to 3 hours, whereas that of 4-hydroxypropranolol is even shorter. The plasma concentration of pro-

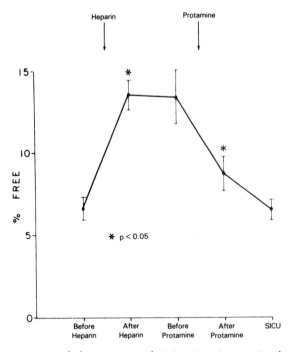

FIGURE 14-4. Heparin administration is associated with decreased plasma protein binding of propranolol manifesting as an increased plasma concentration of free (unbound) drug. Mean ± SE. (From Wood M, Shand DG, Wood AJJ. Propranolol binding in plasma during cardiopulmonary bypass. Anesthesiology 1979;51:512–6. Reproduced by permission of the authors and publisher.)

pranolol or the total dose administered does not correlate with its therapeutic effects.

Elimination of propranolol is greatly reduced when hepatic blood flow decreases. In this regard, propranolol may decrease its own elimination rate by decreasing cardiac output and hepatic blood flow. Alterations in hepatic enzyme activity may also influence the rate of hepatic metabolism. Renal failure does not alter the elimination half-time of propranolol, but accumulation of metabolites may occur.

Nadolol

Nadolol is a nonselective beta-adrenergic receptor antagonist that is unique in that its long duration of action permits once daily administration.

Pharmacokinetics

Nadolol is slowly and incompletely absorbed (an estimated 30%) from the gastrointestinal tract. Metabolism does not occur with about 75% of the drug being excreted unchanged in the urine and the remainder in the bile. Therefore, wide individual variations in plasma concentrations that occur with nadolol cannot be attributed to differences in metabolism as occurs with propranolol. The elimination half-time is 20 to 40 hours accounting for the need to administer this drug only once a day. The dosing interval should be extended beyond 14 hours in patients with renal dysfunction. The plasma concentration of nadolol, like propranolol, does not correlate with therapeutic effects of the drug.

Pindolol

Pindolol is a nonselective beta-adrenergic receptor antagonist with intrinsic sympathomimetic activity. Because it possesses intrinsic sympathomimetic activity, this drug causes minimal resting bradycardia. Also, because of this characteristic, large doses of the drug may cause an unexpected increase in blood pressure.

Pharmacokinetics

Pindolol is well absorbed from the gastrointestinal tract, but plasma concentrations of the drug vary greatly. Protein binding of pindolol is 40% to 60%. Approximately 40% to 50% of a single dose of pindolol can be recovered unchanged in the urine. No active metabolites have been identified. The elimination half-time of pindolol is 3 to 4 hours, and this is increased to greater than 11 hours in patients with renal failure.

Timolol

Timolol is a nonselective beta-adrenergic receptor antagonist that is as effective as propranolol for various therapeutic indications (see the section entitled Clinical Uses). In addition, timolol is effective in the treatment of glaucoma by virtue of its ability to decrease intraocular pressure presumably by reducing the production of aqueous humor. Timolol is administered as eye drops in the treatment of glaucoma, but systemic absorp-

tion may be sufficient to cause resting bradycardia and increased airway resistance. Indeed, bradycardia and hypotension that is refractory to treatment with atropine have been observed during anesthesia in pediatric and adult patients receiving topical timolol with or without pilocarpine (Mishra *et al*, 1983; Zimmerman *et al*, 1983). Pupil size is not altered by topical placement of timolol on the cornea.

Pharmacokinetics

Timolol is rapidly and almost completely absorbed after oral administration. Nevertheless, extensive hepatic first-pass metabolism limits the amount of drug reaching the systemic circulation to about 50% of that absorbed from the gastrointestinal tract. Protein binding of timolol is not extensive. The elimination half-time is about 4 hours.

Metoprolol

Metoprolol is a selective beta-1 antagonist that prevents inotropic and chronotropic responses to beta-adrenergic stimulation. Conversely, bronchodilator, vasodilator, and metabolic effects of beta-2 receptors remain intact such that metoprolol is less likely to cause adverse effects in patients with chronic obstructive airways disease or peripheral vascular disease and patients vulnerable to hypoglycemia. It is important to recognize, however, that selectivity is dose-related and large doses of metoprolol are likely to become nonselective, exerting antagonist effects at beta-2 receptors as well as beta-1 receptors. Indeed, airways resistance may increase in asthmatic patients treated with metoprolol although the magnitude of increase will be less than that evoked by propranolol. Furthermore, metoprolol-induced elevations in airway resistance are more readily reversed with beta-2 agonists such as terbutaline.

Pharmacokinetics

Metoprolol is readily absorbed from the gastrointestinal tract, but this is offset by substantial hepatic first-pass metabolism such that only about 40% of the drug reaches the systemic circulation. Protein binding is low being estimated to account for about 10% of the drug. None of the hepatic metabolites have been identified as active. Less than 10% of the drug appears unchanged in the urine. The elimination half-time of metoprolol is 3 to 4 hours. Plasma concentrations of metoprolol do not correlate with therapeutic effects of the drug.

Atenolol

Atenolol is a selective beta-1 receptor antagonist that may have specific usefulness in patients in whom the continued presence of beta-2 receptor activity is desirable (see the section entitled Metoprolol).

Pharmacokinetics

About 50% of an orally administered dose of atenolol is absorbed from the gastrointestinal tract. Atenolol undergoes little or no hepatic metabolism and is eliminated by renal excretion. The elimination half-time is 6 to 7 hours, and this may increase to more than 24 hours in patients with renal failure. Plasma concentrations of atenolol do not correlate with therapeutic effects of the drug.

Esmolol

Esmolol is a rapid onset and short-acting selective beta-1 receptor antagonist. These characteristics may make esmolol a useful drug for preventing or treating adverse blood pressure and heart rate responses that occur intraoperatively in response to noxious stimulation as during intubation of the trachea (Fig. 14-5) (Menkhaus et al, 1985). Administered as a continuous intravenous infusion (200 μg kg^{-1} min^{-1}) beginning 5 minutes before induction of anesthesia, esmolol prevents increases in heart rate associated with noxious stimulation in patients undergoing coronary artery bypass graft operations (Girard et al, 1986). In these anesthetized patients, esmolol does not change mean arterial pressure, atrial filling pressures, or cardiac output. Because beta-2 receptor function remains intact during administration of esmolol, there is minimal alteration in peripheral vascular resistance at the time blood pressure and heart rate responses are attenuated. This contrasts with nonselective beta receptor antagonists such as propranolol which not only attenuate circulatory responses but may also increase peripheral vascular resistance.

Pharmacokinetics

The short duration of effect of esmolol is due to hydrolysis by plasma esterases (Sum et al, 1983). Indeed, 5 minutes after discontinuing the drug, heart rate is unchanged from predrug values. The elimination half-time of esmolol is 9 to 10.5 minutes. Plasma concentrations of esmolol are usually not detectable 15 minutes after discontinuing the drug. Plasma esterases responsible for hydrolysis are distinct from plasma cholinesterase, and the duration of action of succinylcholine is not pro-

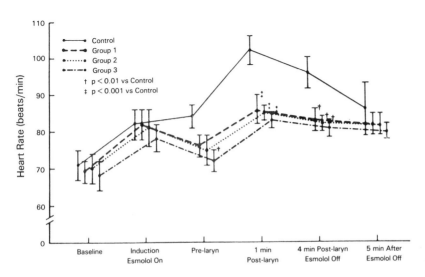

FIGURE 14-5. Esmolol administered as a continuous intravenous infusion attenuates heart rate responses to direct laryngoscopy. Groups 1, 2, and 3 received cumulative esmolol doses of 1100, 2000, and 1700 μg kg^{-1} respectively. Mean ± SE. (From Menkhaus PG, Reves JG, Kisson I, et al. Cardiovascular effects of esmolol in anesthetized humans. Anesth Analg 1985;64:327–34. Reproduced by permission of the authors and the International Anesthesia Research Society.)

longed in patients treated with esmolol (McCammon *et al,* 1985).

Side Effects

Side effects of beta antagonists are similar for all available drugs although the magnitude may differ depending on their selectivity and presence or absence of intrinsic sympathomimetic activity. Beta antagonists exert their most prominent pharmacologic effects as well as side effects on the cardiovascular system. These drugs may also alter airway resistance, carbohydrate and fat metabolism, and the distribution of extracellular potassium. Additive effects between drugs used for anesthesia and beta antagonists may occur. Beta antagonists penetrate the blood–brain barrier and cross the placenta. Gastrointestinal side effects of beta antagonists include nausea, vomiting, and diarrhea. Fever, rash, myopathy, alopecia, and thrombocytopenia have been associated with chronic beta antagonist administration. Beta antagonists have been reported to reduce plasma concentrations of high density lipoproteins and to increase triglyceride and uric acid levels.

The principal contraindication to administration of beta antagonists is preexisting atrioventricular heart block or cardiac failure not caused by tachycardia. Nonselective beta antagonists or high doses of selective beta antagonists should not be administered to patients with chronic obstructive airways disease. In patients with diabetes mellitus, there is the risk that beta-adrenergic blockade may mask the signs of hypoglycemia and thus delay its recognition.

Cardiovascular System

Beta antagonists produce negative inotropic and negative chronotropic effects. In addition, the speed of conduction of the cardiac impulse through the atrioventricular node is slowed and the rate of spontaneous phase 4 depolarization is decreased. Preexisting atrioventricular heart block due to any cause may be accentuated by beta antagonists.

The cardiovascular effects of beta-adrenergic blockade reflect removal of sympathetic nervous system innervation to the heart (*e.g.,* beta-1 blockade) and not membrane stabilization which occurs only at high plasma concentrations of the antagonist drug. In addition, nonselective beta-adrenergic blockade resulting in beta-2 receptor antagonism may impede left ventricular ejection due to unopposed alpha-adrenergic receptor-mediated peripheral vasoconstriction. The magnitude of cardiovascular effects produced by beta antagonists is greatest when preexisting sympathetic nervous system activity is increased as during exercise or in patients in cardiac failure. Indeed, the tachycardia of exercise is consistently prevented by beta antagonists. Furthermore, administration of a beta antagonist may precipitate cardiac failure in a patient who was previously compensated. Resting bradycardia is minimized and cardiac failure is less likely to occur when a partial beta antagonist with intrinsic sympathomimetic activity is administered. Acute cardiac failure is rare with oral administration of beta antagonists.

Classically, beta antagonists prevent the inotropic and chronotropic effects of isoproterenol as well as baroreceptor-mediated increases in heart rate evoked by decreases in blood pressure in response to vasodilator drugs. Conversely, the cardiac-stimulating effects of calcium, glucagon, and digitalis preparations are not detectably influenced by beta antagonists. Likewise, beta antagonists do not alter the response to alpha-adrenergic agonists such as epinephrine or phenylephrine. Indeed, the pressor effect of epinephrine is enhanced because nonselective beta antagonists prevent the beta-2 vasodilating effect of epinephrine and leave unopposed the alpha-adrenergic effect of this catecholamine. The presence of unopposed alpha-adrenergic-induced vasoconstriction may provoke paradoxical hypertension and even precipitate cardiac failure in a diseased myocardium that cannot respond to sympathetic nervous system stimulation because of beta-adrenergic blockade. Unexpected hypertension has occurred in patients receiving clonidine or alpha-methyldopa who subsequently receive a nonselective beta antagonist (Nies and Shand, 1973). Presumably, blockade of the vasodilating effect normally produced by activity of beta-2 receptors leaves unopposed alpha-adrenergic effects to provoke peripheral vasoconstriction with resulting hypertension.

Patients with peripheral vascular disease do not tolerate well peripheral vasoconstriction associated with beta-2 receptor blockade produced by nonselective beta antagonists. Indeed, the development of cold hands and feet is a common side effect of beta blockade. Vasospasm associated with Raynaud's disease is accentuated by propranolol.

The principal antidysrhythmic effect of beta-adrenergic blockade is to prevent the arrhythmogenic effect of endogenous or exogenous catecholamines or sympathomimetics. This reflects a reduction in sympathetic nervous system activity. Membrane stabilization is probably of little importance in the antidysrhythmic effects produced by usual doses of beta antagonists (Shand, 1975).

TREATMENT OF EXCESS MYOCARDIAL DEPRESSION. Excessive bradycardia and/or reductions in cardiac output due to drug-induced beta blockade should be treated initially with intravenous atropine in incremental doses of 70 μg kg^{-1}. Atropine is likely to be effective by blocking vagal effects on the heart and thus unmasking any residual sympathetic nervous system innervation. If atropine is ineffective, the use of drugs to produce direct positive chronotropic and inotropic effects is indicated. For example, continuous intravenous infusion of the nonselective beta agonist, isoproterenol, in doses sufficient to overcome competitive beta blockade, is appropriate. The necessary dose of isoproterenol may be 2 to 25 μg min^{-1} which is five to twenty times the necessary dose in the absence of beta blockade. When a pure beta antagonist is responsible for excessive cardiovascular depression, a pure beta-1 agonist such as dobutamine is recommended because isoproterenol, with beta-1 and beta-2 agonist effects, could produce vasodilation before the inotropic effect develops (Waagstein et al, 1978). Dopamine is not recommended because alpha-adrenergic-induced vasoconstriction is likely to occur with the high doses required to overcome beta blockade. Calcium chloride (250–1000 mg) or glucagon (1–5 mg) administered intravenously to adults effectively reverses myocardial depression produced by beta antagonists at normal doses because these drugs do not exert their effect by means of beta-adrenergic receptors (see Chapter 13). In the presence of life-threatening bradycardia the placement of a transvenous artificial cardiac pacemaker may be necessary.

Airway Resistance

Nonselective beta antagonists such as propranolol consistently increase airway resistance as a manifestation of bronchoconstriction due to blockade of beta-2 receptors. These airway resistance effects are exaggerated in patients with preexisting obstructive airways disease. Because bronchodilatation is a beta-2 agonist response, selective beta-1 antagonists, such as metoprolol, are less likely than propranolol to increase airway resistance.

Metabolism

Beta antagonists alter carbohydrate and fat metabolism. For example, nonselective beta antagonists, such as propranolol, interfere with glycogenolysis that ordinarily occurs in response to release of epinephrine during hypoglycemia. This emphasizes the need for beta-2 receptor activity in the occurrence of glycogenolysis. Furthermore, tachycardia that is an important warning sign of hypoglycemia in insulin-treated diabetics is blunted by beta antagonists. For this reason, nonselective beta antagonists are not recommended for administration to patients with diabetes mellitus who may be at risk for developing hypoglycemia because of treatment with insulin or oral hypoglycemics. Altered fat metabolism is evidenced by failure of sympathomimetics or sympathetic nervous system stimulation to increase plasma concentrations of free fatty acids in the presence of beta-adrenergic blockade.

Distribution of Extracellular Potassium

Distribution of potassium across cell membranes is influenced by sympathetic nervous system activity as well as insulin. Specifically, stimulation of beta-2 adrenergic receptors seems to facilitate movement of potassium ions intracellularly. As a result, beta-adrenergic blockade inhibits uptake of potassium ions into skeletal muscle and the plasma concentration of potassium is increased. Indeed, increases in the plasma concentration of potassium associated with intravenous infusion of this ion are greater in the presence of beta-adrenergic blockade produced by propranolol (Fig. 14-6) (Rosa et al, 1980). In animals, elevations in the plasma concentration of potassium following administration of succinylcholine last longer when beta-adrenergic blockade is present (McCammon and Stoelting, 1984). In view of the speculated role of beta-2 receptors in regulation of plasma concentrations of potassium, it is likely that selective beta-1 antagonists would impair skeletal muscle uptake of potassium ions less than nonselective beta antagonists.

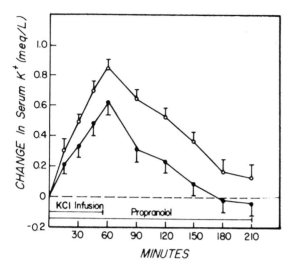

FIGURE 14-6. Increases in plasma (serum) potassium (K^+) concentration in response to infusion of potassium chloride (KCl) are greater in the presence of propranolol (clear circles) than in its absence (solid circles). Mean ± SE. (From Rosa RM, Silva P, Young JB, et al. Adrenergic modulation of extrarenal potassium disposal. N Engl J Med 1980;302:431–4. Reprinted by permission of the New England Journal of Medicine. 1980;302:431–4.)

Interactions with Anesthetics

Myocardial depression produced by inhaled or injected anesthetics could be additive with depression produced by beta antagonists. Nevertheless, clinical experience, as well as controlled studies in patients and animals, has confirmed that additive myocardial depression between anesthetics and beta antagonists is not excessive and treatment with beta antagonists may therefore be safely maintained up to the time of induction of anesthesia (Foex, 1984). An exception may be patients treated with topical timolol in whom profound bradycardia has been observed in the presence of inhaled anesthetics (see the section entitled Timolol).

Additive cardiovascular effects between inhaled anesthetics and beta antagonists seem to be greatest with enflurane, intermediate with halothane, and least with isoflurane (Foex, 1984; Kopriva et al, 1978; Philbin and Lowenstein, 1976; Roberts et al, 1976a). For example, cardiac output and blood pressure are similar with or without beta-adrenergic blockade in the presence of 1 or 2 MAC isoflurane (Philbin and Lowenstein, 1976). Even acute hemorrhage does not alter the interaction between isoflurane or halothane and beta antagonists (Horan et al, 1977a; Roberts et al, 1976b). In contrast, cardiac depression is more likely to occur in the presence of beta blockade when acute hemorrhage occurs in animals anesthetized with enflurane (Horan et al, 1977b). Cardiovascular responses to even high doses of opioids such as fentanyl, are not altered by preexisting beta-adrenergic blockade. In the presence of anesthetic drugs that increase sympathetic nervous system activity (e.g., ketamine) or when excessive sympathetic nervous system activity is present because of hypercarbia, the acute administration of a beta antagonist may unmask direct negative inotropic effects of concomitantly administered anesthetics with resulting reductions in blood pressure and cardiac output (Foex and Ryder, 1981).

Nervous System

Beta antagonists may cross the blood–brain barrier to produce side effects. For example, fatigue and lethargy are commonly associated with chronic propranolol therapy. Vivid dreams are frequent, but psychotic reactions are rare. Memory loss and mental depression are not infrequent. Peripheral paresthesias have been described. Atenolol and nadolol are less lipid soluble than other beta antagonists and thus may be associated with a lower incidence of central nervous system side effects.

Fetus

Beta antagonists can cross the placenta and cause bradycardia, hypotension, and hypoglycemia in newborn infants of mothers who are receiving the drug. Breast milk is also likely to contain beta antagonists administered to the mother.

Withdrawal Hypersensitivity

Acute discontinuation of beta antagonist therapy can result in excess sympathetic nervous system activity that manifests in 24 to 48 hours (Boudoulas et al, 1977). Presumably, this enhanced activity reflects an increase in the number of beta-adrenergic receptors (*e.g.,* up-regulation) during chronic therapy with beta antagonists (Roth *et al,* 1979). Continuous intravenous infusion of propranolol 3 mg hr^{-1} is effective in maintaining therapeutic plasma concentrations in adult patients who cannot take drugs orally during the perioperative period (Smulyan *et al,* 1982).

Clinical Uses

Clinical uses of beta-adrenergic antagonists are multiple but most often include (1) treatment of essential hypertension, (2) management of angina pectoris, (3) suppression of cardiac dysrhythmias, and (4) prevention of excess sympathetic nervous system activity. In appropriate doses, all beta antagonists seem to be equally effective in producing desired therapeutic effects.

Treatment of Essential Hypertension

Chronic therapy with beta antagonists results in gradual reductions in blood pressure. The antihypertensive effect of beta-adrenergic blockade is largely dependent on a reduction in cardiac output due to decreased heart rate. Large doses of beta antagonists may depress myocardial contractility as well. In many patients, peripheral vascular resistance remains unchanged. An important advantage in use of beta antagonists for the treatment of essential hypertension is the absence of orthostatic hypotension. Often a beta antagonist is used in combination with a vasodilator to minimize reflex baroreceptor-mediated increases in heart rate and cardiac output produced by the vasodilator. All beta antagonists appear to be equally effective antihypertensive drugs (Davidson *et al,* 1976).

Release of renin from the juxtaglomerular apparatus that occurs in response to stimulation of beta-2 receptors is blocked by nonselective beta antagonists such as propranolol. This may account for a portion of the antihypertensive effect of propranolol, especially in patients with high circulating plasma concentrations of renin (Buhler *et al,* 1972). Because drug-induced reductions in secretion of renin will lead to decreased release of aldosterone, beta antagonists will also prevent the compensatory sodium and water retention that accompanies treatment with a vasodilator.

Management of Angina Pectoris

Beta antagonists are equally effective in reducing the likelihood of myocardial ischemia manifesting as angina pectoris. This desirable response reflects drug-induced reductions in myocardial oxygen requirements secondary to decreased heart rate and cardiac output. Mortality after acute myocardial infarction is reduced by beta-adrenergic blockade (Hjalmarson *et al,* 1981; Julian *et al,* 1982).

Suppression of Cardiac Dysrhythmias

Beta antagonists reduce sympathetic nervous system activity to the heart with a resulting decrease in the rate of spontaneous phase 4 depolarization of ectopic cardiac pacemakers (see Chapter 17). In addition, decreased sympathetic nervous system activity due to beta blockade decreases activity of the sinoatrial node and slows conduction of the cardiac impulse through the atrioventricular node. Resting transmembrane potential and repolarization are not altered by beta antagonists.

The cardiac effects of beta blockade are responsible for the efficacy of beta antagonists in suppressing intraoperative supraventricular tachydysrhythmias as well as ventricular cardiac dysrhythmias (Foex, 1984; Manners and Walters, 1979) (see Chapter 17). For example, supraventricular and ventricular cardiac dysrhythmias are suppressed by the intravenous administration of propranolol, 5 to 15 μg kg^{-1}, especially if digitalis overdose is responsible for the abnormal rhythm. Seldom is a total dose of propranolol greater than 70 μg kg^{-1} required.

Prevention of Excess Sympathetic Nervous System Activity

Beta-adrenergic blockade is associated with decreased heart rate and blood pressure elevations in response to direct laryngoscopy and intubation of the trachea (Foex, 1984; Prys-Roberts *et al,* 1973) (see the section entitled Esmolol). Hypertrophic obstructive cardiomyopathies are often treated with beta antagonists. Tachycardia and cardiac dysrhythmias associated with pheochromocytoma and hyperthyroidism are effectively suppressed by propranolol. Cyanotic episodes in patients with tetralogy of Fallot are minimized by beta blockade. Propranolol has been used intraoperatively to prevent reflex baroreceptor-mediated increases in heart rate evoked by vasodilators administered to produce controlled hypotension (see Chapter 16). Even anxiety states associated with public speaking have been treated with propranolol.

REFERENCES

Boudoulas H. Differential time course of inotropic and chronotropic blockade after oral propranolol. Cardiovasc Med 1977;2:511 – 8.

Boudoulas H, Lewis RP, Kates RE, Dalamangas G, Dalamangas G. Hypersensitivity to adrenergic stimulation after propranolol withdrawal in normal subjects. Ann Intern Med 1977;87:433 – 6.

Boudoulas H, Lewis RP, Snyder GL, Karayannacos P, Vasko JS. Beneficial effect of continuation of propranolol through coronary bypass surgery. Clin Cardiol 1979;87:2 – 12.

Buhler FR, Laragh JH, Baer L, Vaughn DE, Brunner HR. Propranolol inhibition of renin secretion. N Engl J Med 1972;287:1209 – 14.

Davidson C, Thadani U, Singleton W, Taylor SH. Comparison of antihypertensive activity of beta-blocking drugs during chronic treatment. Br Med J 1976;2:7 – 9.

Foex P. Alpha- and beta-adrenoceptor antagonists. Br J Anaesth 1984;56:751 – 65.

Foex P, Ryder WA. Interactions of adrenergic beta-receptor blockade (oxprenolol) and PCO_2 in the anaesthetized dog: influence of intrinsic sympathomimetic activity. Br J Anaesth 1981;53:19 – 26.

Girard D, Shulman BJ, Thys DM, Mindich BP, Mikula SK, Kaplan JA. The safety and efficacy of esmolol during myocardial revascularization. Anesthesiology 1968;65:157 – 64.

Hjalmarson A, Elmfeldt D, Herlitz J, et al. Effect on mortality of metoprolol in acute myocardial infarction. Lancet 1981;2:823 – 6.

Horan BF, Prys-Roberts C, Roberts JG, Bennett MJ, Foex P. Haemodynamic responses to isoflurane anaesthesia and hypovolaemia in the dog, and their modification by propranolol. Br J Anaesth 1977a; 49:1179 – 87.

Horan BF, Prys-Roberts C, Hamilton WK, Roberts JG. Haemodynamic responses to enflurane anaesthesia and hypovolaemia in the dog, and their modification by propranolol. Br J Anaesth 1977b;49:1189 – 97.

Julian DG, Prescott RJ, Jackson FS, Szekely P. Controlled trial of sotalol for one year after myocardial infarction. Lancet 1982;1:1142 – 7.

Kopriva CJ, Brown ACD, Pappas G. Hemodynamics during general anesthesia in patients receiving propranolol. Anesthesiology 1978;48:28 – 33.

Manners JM, Walters FJM. Beta-adrenoceptor blockade and anaesthesia. Anaesthesia 1979;34:3 – 9.

McCammon RL, Hilgenberg JC, Sandage BW, Stoelting RK. The effect of esmolol on the onset and duration of succinylcholine-induced neuromuscular blockade. Anesthesiology 1985;63:A317.

McCammon RL, Stoelting RK. Exaggerated increase in serum potassium following succinylcholine in dogs with beta blockade. Anesthesiology 1984;61:723 – 5.

Menkhaus PG, Reves JG, Kisson I, et al. Cardiovascular effects of esmolol in anesthetized humans. Anesth Anal 1985;64:327 – 34.

Mishra P, Calvey TN, Williams NE, Murray GR. Intraoperative bradycardia and hypotension associated with timolol and pilocarpine eye drops. Br J Anaesth 1983;55:897 – 9.

Nies AS, McNeil JS, Schrier RW. Mechanism of increased sodium reabsorption during propranolol administration. Circulation 1971;44:596 – 604.

Nies AS, Shand DG. Hypertensive response to propranolol in a patient treated with methyldopa—a proposed mechanism. Clin Pharmacol Ther 1973;14:823 – 6.

Nies AS, Shand DG. Clinical pharmacology of propranolol. Circulation 1975;52:6 – 15.

Philbin DM, Lowenstein E. Lack of beta-adrenergic activity of isoflurane in the dog: A comparison of circulatory effects of halothane and isoflurane after propranolol administration. Br J Anaesth 1976;48:1165 – 70.

Prys-Roberts C, Foex P, Biro GP, Roberts JG. Studies of anaesthesia in relation to hypertension. V. Adrenergic beta-receptor blockade. Br J Anaesth 1973;45:671 – 81.

Roberts JG, Foex P, Clarke TNS, Bennett MJ. Haemodynamic interactions of high-dose propranolol pretreatment and anaesthesia in the dog. I. Halothane dose-response studies. Br J Anaesth 1976a; 48:315 – 25.

Roberts JG, Foex P, Clarke TNS, Bennett MJ, Saner CA. Haemodynamic interactions of high-dose propranolol pretreatment and anaesthesia in the dog. III. The effects of haemorrhage during halothane and trichlorethylene anaesthesia. Br J Anaesth 1976b;48:411 – 8.

Rosa RM, Silva P, Young JB, et al. Adrenergic modulation of extrarenal potassium disposal. N Engl J Med 1980;302:431 – 4.

Roth J, Lesniak MA, Bar RS, et al. An introduction to receptors and receptor disorders. Proc Soc Exp Biol Med 1979;162:3 – 12.

Shand DG. Drug therapy—propranolol. N Engl J Med 1975;293:280 – 5.

Smulyan H, Weinberg SE, Howanitz PJ. Continuous propranolol infusion following abdominal surgery. JAMA 1982;247:2539 – 42.

Sum CY, Yacobi A, Kartizinel R, Stampfli H, Davis CS, Lai CM. Kinetics of esmolol, an ultra-short-acting beta blocker, and of its major metabolite. Clin Pharmacol Ther 1983;34:427 – 34.

Waagstein F, Malek I, Hjalmarson A. The use of dobutamine in myocardial infarction for reversal of the cardiodepressive effect of metoprolol. Br J Clin Pharmacol 1978;5:515 – 9.

Wood M, Shand DG, Wood AJJ. Propranolol binding in plasma during cardiopulmonary bypass. Anesthesiology 1979;51:512 – 6.

Zimmerman TJ, Kooner JS, Morgan KS. Safety and efficacy of timolol in pediatric glaucoma. Surv Opthalmol 1983;28:262 – 4.

C H A P T E R 15

Antihypertensive Drugs

INTRODUCTION

All available antihypertensive drugs act to some extent by interfering with normal homeostatic mechanisms. Efficacy, toxicity, and suitable combinations of antihypertensive drugs can often be predicted by consideration of both the sites and mechanisms of action of the drugs. The effectiveness of a given drug, however, cannot necessarily be taken as evidence that its mechanism of action relates to the pathogenesis of the elevated blood pressure.

The potential adverse interaction between antihypertensive drugs and anesthetics has been exaggerated. When interactions are likely, they are usually predictable and can thus be avoided or their significance minimized. Specific concerns during administration of anesthesia to patients being treated with antihypertensive drugs include (1) attenuation of sympathetic nervous system activity, (2) modification of the response to sympathomimetic drugs, and (3) sedation. Attenuation of sympathetic nervous system activity is reflected preoperatively by orthostatic hypotension and exaggerated blood pressure reductions during anesthesia in response to (1) blood loss, (2) body position change, or (3) decreased venous return due to positive pressure ventilation of the lungs. Antihypertensive drugs that deplete norepinephrine or that act on peripheral vascular smooth muscle decrease the sensitivity to predominantly indirect-acting sympathomimetic drugs (Eger and Hamilton, 1959) (see Chapter 12). Conversely, sympathetic nervous system blockade, which deprives the alpha-adrenergic receptors of tonic impulses, results in exaggerated responses to catecholamines and direct-acting sympathomimetic drugs.

Patients remaining on antihypertensive therapy show less extreme swings in blood pressure and heart rate during anesthesia and are less likely to exhibit cardiac dysrhythmias (Prys-Roberts *et al,* 1971). It is an inescapable conclusion that antihypertensive drugs should be continued throughout the perioperative period. In this regard, the usual dose and unique pharmacology of each antihypertensive drug as well as the physiological reflexes that occur in response to drug-induced blood pressure changes must be considered when planning the management of anesthesia (Table 15-1) (Gottlieb and Chidsey, 1976).

METHYLDOPA

Methyldopa is an effective antihypertensive drug that acts in the central nervous system (Fig. 15-1). The average daily adult dose of methyldopa is 1 g with little additional effect with doses over 2 g. Methyldopa is given in divided doses, usually three times daily. Intravenous doses of methyldopa are 0.5 to 1 g.

Mechanism of Action

Methyldopa enters the central nervous system where it serves as an alternative substrate to dopa

Table 15-1
Principal Site of Action of Antihypertensive Drugs

Central Nervous System
Methyldopa
Clonidine
Reserpine
Guanabenz
Peripheral Vascular Smooth Muscle
Hydralazine
Prazosin
Minoxidil
Peripheral Sympathetic Nervous System
Guanethidine
Guanadrel
Peripheral Alpha- and Beta-Adrenergic Receptors
Labetalol
Angiotensin Converting Enzyme
Captopril
Angiotensin II Receptors
Saralasin
Tyrosine Hydroxylase Enzyme
Metyrosine

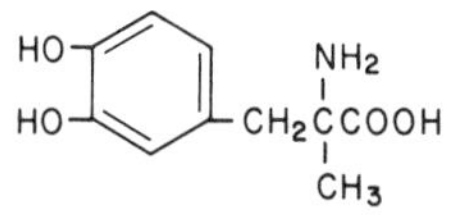

FIGURE 15-1. Methyldopa.

being decarboxylated to methyldopamine and beta-hydroxylated to alpha-methylnorepinephrine in central adrenergic neurons. When released, alpha-methylnorepinephrine intensely stimulates inhibitory alpha-2 adrenergic receptors in the hypothalamus which inhibits sympathetic nervous system outflow from the vasomotor center to the periphery (Frohlich, 1980). As a result, decreases in peripheral vascular resistance and blood pressure occur. Evidence that the centrally active substance is alpha-methylnorepinephrine is inhibition of antihypertensive effects by prevention of central nervous system decarboxylation or beta-hydroxylation of methyldopa.

Although the major mechanism of antihypertensive effect of methyldopa seems to be via the central nervous system, some impact of peripheral mechanisms cannot be ruled out. For example, a reduction in renal vascular resistance may be related to the fact that alpha-methylnorepinephrine

is a much weaker vasoconstrictor in this vascular bed than is norepinephrine (Finch and Haeusler, 1973).

Pharmacokinetics

The extent of absorption of methyldopa after oral administration is only about 25% (Myhre *et al*, 1982). Renal excretion of methyldopa or its conjugates accounts for about two thirds of the clearance of drug from the circulation. Nevertheless, there is no evidence that the dose should be substantially altered in the presence of hepatic or renal disease.

Cardiovascular Effects

Methyldopa produces significant reductions in blood pressure and peripheral vascular resistance while cardiac output and renal, cerebral, and myocardial blood flow are maintained (Safar *et al*, 1979). Predominance of parasympathetic nervous system activity may be manifested as bradycardia. The change in blood pressure is maximal within 4 to 6 hours after an oral dose and persists for as long as 24 hours. Secretion of renin is modestly decreased but is not necessary for the antihypertensive effect of the drug. Because methyldopa does not work solely by its effects on the sympathetic nervous system, a moderate decrease in supine blood pressure is usually not accompanied by orthostatic hypotension emphasizing the fact that compensatory sympathetic nervous system reflexes remain intact.

Decreased sympathomimetic responses following the administration of ephedrine have been documented in animals pretreated with methyldopa (Miller *et al*, 1969). Nevertheless, the clinical observation is that patients receiving methyldopa respond appropriately to ephedrine. Methyldopa is a logical choice in patients with renal disease, because this drug maintains or increases blood flow.

Side Effects

Side effects of methyldopa treatment include (1) sedation, (2) hepatic dysfunction, (3) development of a positive Coombs' test, (4) interactions with concomitantly administered drugs, and (5) rebound hypertension (Husserl and Messerli, 1981). In addition, methyldopa and its metabolites can interfere with some of the chemical tests for catecholamines producing false positive tests for pheochromocytoma. Depending on the chemical method used for analysis, methyldopa may also interfere with the measurement of serum creatinine, uric acid, and transaminase enzymes. Retention of sodium and water with weight gain and edema may occur during treatment with methyldopa. Methyldopa does not cause bradycardia or decreased salivary flow to the same extent as clonidine. Sexual dysfunction, primarily impotence, can occur. Orthostatic hypotension is possible but not frequent.

Sedation

Methyldopa predictably causes sedation, but this effect tends to decrease with chronic therapy. In animals, anesthetic requirements for volatile drugs are decreased 20% to 40% by methyldopa (Fig. 15-2) (Miller *et al,* 1969).

Hepatic Dysfunction

Methyldopa may be associated with elevations of plasma concentrations of transaminase enzymes and alkaline phosphatase especially during the first 6 to 12 weeks of treatment (Husserl and Messerli, 1981). Fever, malaise, and rarely jaundice may accompany this drug-induced hepatic dysfunction. Fatal hepatic necrosis has occurred with reexposure to the drug. Liver function tests should probably be performed at monthly intervals during the early periods of treatment with methyldopa.

Positive Coombs' Test

A positive Coombs' test develops in 10% to 20% of patients taking 1 g of methyldopa daily for 6 months or more (Hunter *et al,* 1971). Hemolytic anemia occurs in less than 5% of these patients and is generally reversible when the drug is discontinued. Nevertheless, the Coombs' test may remain positive for several months. Because most patients developing a positive Coombs' test do not also develop hemolytic anemia, a positive Coombs' test is not a contraindication to continued use of the drug. The principal problem presented by a positive Coombs' test is the difficulty in cross-

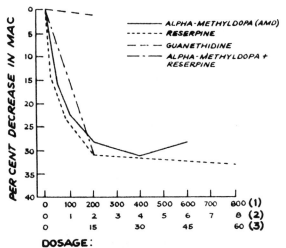

FIGURE 15-2. Methyldopa (AMD) and reserpine, but not guanethidine, produce dose-related reductions in anesthetic requirements (MAC). (From Miller RD, Way WL, Eger EI. The effects of alpha-methyldopa, reserpine, guanethidine, and iproniazid on minimum alveolar anesthetic requirement [MAC]. Anesthesiology 1969;29:1153–8. Reproduced by permission of the authors and publisher.)

matching blood. The antibody responsible for the positive Coombs' test is an immunoglobulin G directed at the erythrocyte membrane.

Drug Interactions

Dementia has been observed in patients treated with methyldopa who subsequently receive a butyrophenone drug such as haloperidol (Thornton, 1976). This dementia may be caused by the ability of both drugs to prevent dopamine from acting at a specific receptor in the central nervous system.

Propranolol elicits a pradoxical hypertensive response when administered to animals pretreated with methyldopa (Nies and Shand, 1973). This hypertensive response presumably reflects the ability of propranolol to block the beta-2 vasodilating component of alpha-methylnorepinephrine. As a result, only the alpha vasoconstricting effect of this metabolite is apparent.

Rebound Hypertension

Sudden withdrawal of methyldopa therapy can cause rebound hypertension. The incidence, however, of this complication seems to be less than that observed after discontinuation of other centrally acting antihypertensive drugs (see the section entitled Clonidine).

CLONIDINE

Clonidine is a centrally acting alpha-2 agonist that acts as an antihypertensive drug (Fig. 15-3) (Houston, 1982). The usual adult dose is 0.2 to 0.3 mg daily. A parenteral form of clonidine is not available. Transdermal clonidine administered once every 7 days lowers blood pressure in patients with mild to moderate hypertension (Weber et al, 1984).

In addition to treatment of patients with essential hypertension, clonidine has been used to aid in the diagnosis of pheochromocytoma (Bravo et al, 1981). For example, clonidine, 0.3 mg, will decrease the plasma concentration of catecholamines in normal patients but not in the presence of a pheochromocytoma. This reflects the ability of clonidine to suppress the release of neurogenically mediated catecholamines but not the diffusion of excess catecholamines into the circulation from a pheochromocytoma. Clonidine is also effective in suppressing the signs and symptoms of withdrawal from opioids (see Chapter 3). It is speculated that clonidine replaces opioid-mediated inhibition with alpha-2 mediated inhibition of central nervous system sympathetic activity (Gold et al, 1980). Finally, clonidine administered intrathecally is an analgesic and can be substituted for morphine when tolerance to the opioid develops (Milne et al, 1985).

Mechanism of Action

Clonidine stimulates alpha-2 inhibitory neurons in the medullary vasomotor center (VanZwieten,

FIGURE 15-3. Clonidine.

1973). As a result, there is a reduction of sympathetic nervous system outflow from the central nervous system to peripheral tissues. Reduced peripheral sympathetic nervous system activity is manifested as decreases in blood pressure, heart rate, and cardiac output.

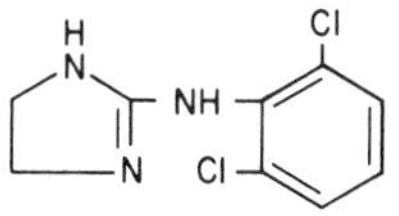

Pharmacokinetics

Clonidine is well absorbed after oral administration and about 60% of the drug appears unchanged in the urine. The duration of hypotensive effect after a single oral dose is about 8 hours. The elimination half-time averages 8.5 hours (Davies et al, 1977).

Cardiovascular Effects

The decline in systolic blood pressure produced by clonidine is more prominent than the decline in diastolic blood pressure. In patients treated chronically, peripheral vascular resistance is little affected and cardiac output, which is initially reduced, returns toward predrug levels. Homeostatic cardiovascular reflexes are maintained thus avoiding the problems of orthostatic hypotension or hypotension during exercise. The ability of clonidine to lower blood pressure without paralysis of compensatory homeostatic reflexes is highly desirable. Renal blood flow and glomerular filtration rate are maintained.

Side Effects

The most frequent side effects produced by treatment with clonidine are sedation and xerostomia which usually subside in intensity after 2 to 3 weeks of drug administration. Consistent with sedation is the observation in animals of a 42% to 48% decrease in halothane anesthetic requirements following intravenous administration of either 5 or 20 μg kg^{-1} of clonidine (Bloor and Flacke, 1983). In patients, 5 μg kg^{-1} administered orally 90 minutes before induction of anesthesia, substantially reduces the subsequent dose of fentanyl required to establish a known depth of anesthesia (Ghignone et al, 1986). This observation is consistent with a synergistic inhibitory action of clonidine and opioids on sympathetic outflow from the central nervous system. As with other antihypertensive drugs, retention of sodium and water often occurs such that combination of clonidine with a diuretic is often necessary. Skin rashes and constipation are frequent. Impotence occurs occasionally and orthostatic hypotension rarely.

Rebound Hypertension

Abrupt discontinuation of clonidine therapy can result in rebound hypertension as soon as 8 hours and as late as 36 hours after the last dose (Brodsky and Bravo, 1976; Bruce *et al*, 1979; Husserl and Messerli, 1981). Rebound hypertension is most likely to occur in patients who were receiving greater than 1.2 mg of clonidine daily. The increase in blood pressure is associated with more than a 100% increase in circulating concentrations of catecholamines and intense peripheral vasoconstriction (Hunyor *et al*, 1973). Symptoms of nervousness, diaphoresis, headache, abdominal pain, and tachycardia precede the actual rise in blood pressure. Beta-adrenergic blockade may exaggerate the magnitude of rebound hypertension by blocking the beta-2 vasodilating effects of catecholamines and leaving unopposed their alpha vasoconstricting actions (Briant *et al*, 1973). Likewise, tricyclic antidepressant therapy may exaggerate rebound hypertension associated with discontinuation of clonidine therapy (Briant *et al*, 1973; Stiff and Harris, 1983). Indeed, tricyclic antidepressants can potentiate the pressor effects of norepinephrine. Naloxone has also been observed to reverse the antihypertensive effects of clonidine in animals (Farsang and Kunos, 1979).

Rebound hypertension can usually be controlled by reinstituting clonidine therapy or by administering a vasodilating drug such as hydralazine, nitroprusside, or phentolamine. Beta-adrenergic blocking drugs are useful but should be administered only in the presence of alpha-adrenergic blockade. If clonidine therapy is interrupted because of surgery, the prior substitution of alternative drugs such as hydralazine or methyldopa alone or in conjunction with nitroprusside as necessary is effective (Bruce *et al*, 1979; Stiff and Harris, 1983). Alternatively, transdermal clonidine may provide continued drug effect for 7 days including the time oral administration is interrupted (White and Gilbert, 1985). For a planned withdrawal, clonidine dosage should be decreased gradually over 7 days or more.

Rebound hypertension following abrupt discontinuation of antihypertensive drugs is not unique to clonidine. Indeed, rebound hypertension similar to that observed after abrupt discontinuation of clonidine has also been observed following sudden cessation of treatment with methyldopa, reserpine, guanethidine, guanabenz, and beta-adrenergic receptor antagonists (Husserl and Messerli, 1981). Anihypertensive drugs that act independently of central nervous system and peripheral sympathetic nervous system mechanisms (*e.g.*, direct vasodilators, converting enzyme inhibitors) do not seem to be associated with rebound hypertension following sudden discontinuation of therapy.

RESERPINE

Reserpine depletes central nervous system stores of catecholamines and serotonin. Reduced concentrations of catecholamines can be measured within an hour after administration of reserpine, and depletion is maximal by 24 hours. The norepinephrine content of the heart is also reduced by reserpine. Despite rapid depletion of catecholamines, the antihypertensive effect of reserpine may not become maximal for up to 21 days. This antihypertensive effect is usually associated with a decreased cardiac output and bradycardia. Orthostatic hypotension is prominent.

Side Effects

Dose-related side effects of reserpine manifest principally on the central nervous system and gastrointestinal tract. For example, sedation and decreased requirements for volatile anesthetics presumably reflect central nervous system depletion of vital neurotransmitters (Miller *et al*, 1969). Mental depression also is most likely due to depletion of neurotransmitters. Signs of parasympathetic nervous system predominance include bradycardia, nasal stuffiness, xerostomia, increased gastric hydrogen ion secretion and exaggerated gastrointestinal motility manifesting as abdominal cramps and diarrhea. Nasal congestion is usually of minor importance but may occasionally cause signs of airway obstruction in neonates born of mothers treated with reserpine.

Increased sensitivity to catecholamines and direct-acting sympathomimetics may occur in patients treated chronically with reserpine. This response resembles denervation hypersensitivity. Conversely, the response to indirect-acting sympathomimetics is reduced in the presence of reserpine therapy (see Chaper 12).

GUANABENZ

Guanabenz is a guanidine derivative that lowers blood pressure by inhibiting sympathetic nervous sysem outflow from the central nervous system by activation of central alpha-adrenergic receptors (Fig. 15-4). Oral absorption is rapid with a single dose producing a peak plasma concentration in 4 hours. The duration of action of a single dose is 12 to 24 hours. Approximately 80% of an oral dose is excreted in the urine as metabolites.

Sedation and dryness to the mouth are the most common side effects of guanabenz therapy. Orthostatic hypotension is possible but less frequent than with guanethidine.

HYDRALAZINE

Hydralazine is a phthalazine derivative that lowers blood pressure by a direct relaxant effect on vascular smooth muscle, the dilatation effect on arterioles being greater than on veins (Fig. 15-5). Vasodilatation probably reflects hydralazine-related interference with calcium ion transport in vascular smooth muscle.

The usual adult oral dose of hydralazine is 20 to 40 mg administered four times daily. Concomitant administration with a beta-adrenergic antagonist to limit the reflex increase in sympathetic nervous system activity induced by hydralazine is common. Beta-adrenergic blockade effectively prevents cardiac stimulation and increased secretion of renin. Treatment of a hypertensive crisis can be accomplished with intravenous hydralazine 2.5 to 10 mg. This antihypertensive effect begins within 15 minutes after intravenous administration and lasts 3 to4 hours.

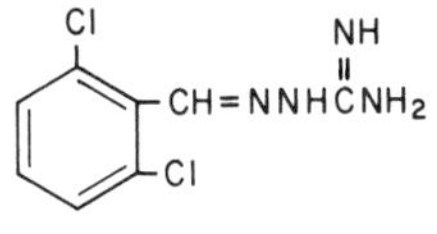

FIGURE 15-4. Guanabenz.

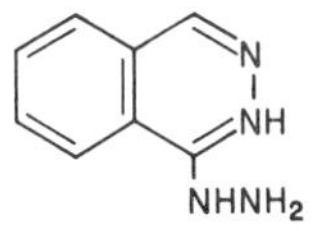

FIGURE 15-5. Hydralazine.

Pharmacokinetics

Extensive hepatic first pass metabolism limits availability of hydralazine following oral administration. Acetylation seems to be the major route of metabolism of hydralazine. Rapid acetylators have lower bioavailability (about 30%) than do slow acetylators (about 50%) following oral administration of hydralazine. During multiple oral dosing, slow acetylators attain higher concentrations of hydralazine in plasma than do those who acetylate the drug rapidly. The elimination half-time averages 3 hours. Following intravenous administration, less than 15% of the drug appears unchanged in the urine.

Cardiovascular Effects

Hydralazine often decreases diastolic blood pressure more than systolic blood pressure. Peripheral vascular resistance is reduced. Heart rate, stroke volume, and cardiac output increase reflecting reflex baroreceptor-mediated increases in sympathetic nervous system activity due to reductions in blood pressure. Nevertheless, tachycardia induced by hydralazine is greater than would be expected solely on a reflex basis and is poorly correlated with changes in blood pressure. This exaggerated heart rate response may reflect a direct effect of hydralazine on the heart and in the central nervous system in addition to baroreceptor-mediated responses.

The preferential dilatation of arterioles compared to veins minimizes orthostatic hypotension and promotes the increase in cardiac output. The effect of hydralazine develops gradually over about 15 minutes even after intravenous administration. Splanchnic, coronary, cerebral, and renal blood flow usually increase. Glomerular filtration rate, renal tubular function, and urine volume are not consistently affected. Renin activity is often increased presumably reflecting hydralazine-induced reflex increases in sympathetic nervous system activity leading to increased secretion of renin by the renal juxtaglomerular cells.

Side Effects

Like other vasodilators, hydralazine causes sodium and water retention if a diuretic is not given concomitantly. Other common side effects of hydralazine therapy include vertigo, diaphoresis, nausea, and tachycardia. Myocardial stimulation associated with hydralazine therapy can evoke angina pectoris and produces changes on the electrocardiogram that are characteristic of myocardial ischemia. Side effects are less frequent and less severe when the dose of hydralazine is increased slowly and tolerance may develop with continued administration. Drug fever, urticaria, polyneuritis, anemia, and pancytopenia are rare but require termination of hydralazine therapy. Peripheral neuropathies have been successfully treated with pyridoxine. Hydrazine-containing compounds, such as hydralazine, may lead to enhanced defluorination of enflurane (Mazze *et al*, 1982).

A lupus erythematosus-like syndrome occurs in 10% to 20% of patients treated chronically (greater than 6 months) with hydralazine especially if the dose exceeds 400 mg (Lee and Chase, 1975). The syndrome occurs predominantly in patients who are slow acetylators. Symptoms disappear when the drug is discontinued differentiating it from the true disease.

PRAZOSIN

Prazosin is a quinazoline derivative that produces peripheral vasodilation via selective and competitive postsynaptic alpha-1 receptor blockade (Fig. 15-6). Absence of a presynaptic alpha-2 effects leaves the normal inhibition of norepinephrine relese intact (Cambridge *et al*, 1977).

In addition to treating essential hypertension, prazosin may be of value for reducing afterload in patients with cardiac failure. Effectiveness of prazosin as a cardiac antidysrhythmic is evidenced by an increased dose of epinephrine necessary to evoke ventricular dysrhythmias during halothane anesthesia in animals (see Fig. 2-15) (Maze and Smith, 1983). This suggests a role for postsynaptic alpha-adrenergic receptors in the myocardium for halothane sensitization of the heart. Prazosin is often combined wih beta-adrenergic antagonist and/or a diuretic to maximize its antihypertensive effects at the lowest possible dose. In addition, prazosin is a useful alternative to phenoxybenz-

FIGURE 15-6. Prazosin.

amine in the preoperative preparation of patients with a pheochromocytoma.

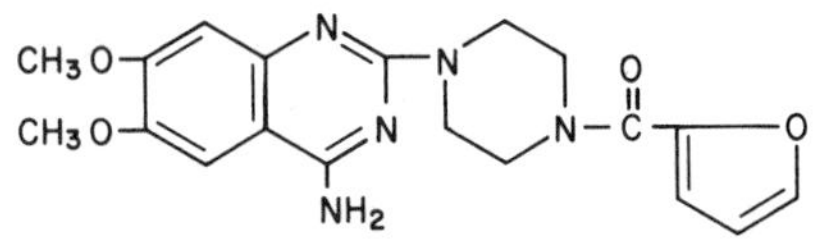

Pharmacokinetics

Prazosin is nearly completely metabolized and less than 60% bioavailability after oral administration suggests the occurrence of substantial hepatic first-pass metabolism. The elimination half-time is about 3 hours being prolonged by cardiac failure but not by renal dysfunction. The fact that this drug is metabolized in the liver permits its use in patients with renal failure without altering the dose.

Cardiovascular Effects

Prazosin reduces peripheral vascular resistance without causing reflex-induced tachycardia or increases in renin activity as occur with hydralazine or minoxidil. Failure to alter plasma renin activity reflects continued activity of alpha-2 receptors that normally inhibit release of renin. Vascular tone in both resistance and capacitance vessels is reduced resulting in decreased venous return and cardiac output. Because of its greater affinity for alpha receptors in veins than in arteries, prazosin produces hemodynamic changes (*e.g.,* orthostatic hypotension) that resemble nitroglycerin more than phentolamine or hydralazine.

Side Effects

Side effects of prazosin include vertigo, fluid retention, and orthostatic hypotension. Fluid retention requires the concomitant administration of a diuretic. Syncope may occur early in treatment with prazosin especially if the initial dose is greater than 1 mg every 8 hours and the patient is volume depleted. In most instances, this syncopal response is due to orthostatic hypotension presumably reflecting abrupt peripheral vasodilation.

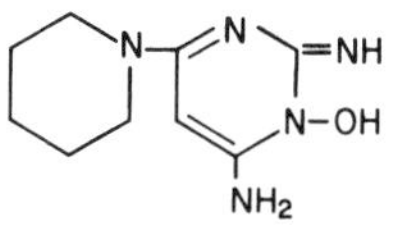

FIGURE 15-7. Minoxidil.

Eventually, patients may tolerate up to 20 mg daily of prazosin. The antihypertensive effect of prazosin can be abolished by the prostaglandin synthesis inhibitor, indomethacin. Dryness of the mouth, nasal congestion, nightmares, urinary frequency, lethargy, and sexual dysfunction may accompany treatment with this drug.

MINOXIDIL

Minoxidil is an orally active antihypertensive drug that reduces blood pressure by direct relaxation of arteriolar smooth muscle (Fig. 15-7) (Campese, 1981). There is little effect on venous capacitance vessels. Minoxidil is particularly effective in patients with renal disease complicated by accelerated hypertension.

Minoxidil should be used in combination with a beta-adrenergic antagonist and diuretic to minimize the dose (10 – 40 mg daily) and thus reduce the magnitude of cardiovascular stimulation and fluid retention that may accompany therapy with this drug.

Pharmacokinetics

About 90% of an oral dose of minoxidil is absorbed from the gastrointestinal tract, and peak plasma levels are attained within 1 hour. Metabolism to inactive minoxidil glucuronide is extensive and only 10% of the drug is recovered unchanged in the urine. The elimination half-time is about 4 hours.

Cardiovascular Effects

The hypotensive effect of minoxidil is accompanied by marked increases in heart rate and cardiac output. This same reflex stimulation of the sympathetic nervous system is also accompanied by increases in the plasma concentrations of norepinephrine and renin with associated sodium and

water retention. Orthostatic hypotension is not prominent in patients treated with minoxidil.

Side Effects

Fluid retention, manifesting as weight gain and edema, is a common side effect of minoxidil therapy. Furosemide or even dialysis may be necessary if fluid retention is unresponsive to less potent diuretics. Pulmonary hypertension associated with minoxidil is more likely due to fluid retention than a unique effect of this drug on pulmonary vasculature.

A potentially serious side effect of minoxidil therapy is the development of pericardial effusion and cardiac tamponade in about 3% of patients especially if severe renal dysfunction is present (Husserl and Messerli, 1981). Echocardiographic studies should be performed if pericardial effusion is suspected. Electrocardiographic abnormalities are characterized by flattening or inversion of the T wave and increased voltage of the QRS complex. During long-term therapy, T wave abnormalities generally disappear and the QRS voltage is reduced. Hypertrichosis, most notable around the face and arms is an unpleasant but harmless side effect which appears to some degree in nearly all patients treated for more than 1 month (Husserl and Messerli, 1981). This side effect cannot be attributed to any definite endocrine abnormality.

GUANETHIDINE

Guanethidine acts exclusively on the peripheral sympathetic nervous system and produces its antihypertensive effect by inhibiting the presynaptic release of the neurotransmitter, norepinephrine, in response to sympathetic nervous system stimulation (Fig. 15-8). With time, there is depletion of tissue concentrations of norepinephrine that persists for several days after the drug is discontinued. Uptake of guanethidine into adrenergic neurons by the same mechanism responsible for passage of

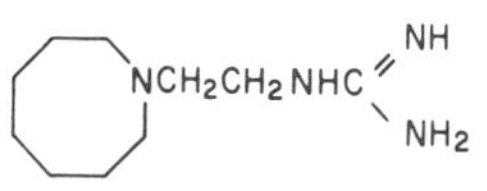

FIGURE 15-8. Guanethidine.

norepinephrine into the neurons is essential for the antihypertensive action of guanethidine.

Guanethidine is used in the treatment of essential hypertension that is resistant to less potent drugs. Another rare use of guanethidine is its intravenous injection into an extremity isolated from the circulation for the treatment of reflex sympathetic dystrophy (Hannington-Kiff, 1974).

Pharmacokinetics

Absorption of guanethidine after oral administration (25–50 mg daily) is variable ranging from 3% to 30% of the administered dose. Almost all of the guanethidine that enters the circulation in humans is eliminated in the urine as unchanged drug or inactive metabolites. Elimination half-time is prolonged averaging about 5 days allowing for a once daily dosing interval. Because of its long elimination half-time, the maximal hypotensive effect may not occur for 7 to14 days after initiating therapy. Furthermore, antihypertensive effects may persist for several days after guanethidine is discontinued.

Cardiovascular Effects

Guanethidine reduces blood pressure, heart rate, venous return, and cardiac output. Decreased venous return is most responsible for the decline in cardiac output. Orthostatic hypotension is prominent. Peripheral vascular resistance is usually decreased. Deterioration in renal function may occur. Cardiac output may return towards normal in association with sodium and water retention. Predominance of parasympathetic nervous system activity is often manifested as bradycardia.

Side Effects

Orthostatic hypotension is the most prominent side effect of treatment with guanethidine. Decreased sympathetic nervous system activity at the heart may precipitate cardiac failure particularly in the presence of fluid retention and preexisting cardiac disease. Fluid retention can lead to resistance to the antihypertensive effect if a diuretic is not administered concurrently. Diarrhea occurs in a high percentage of patients reflecting a predomi-

nance of parasympathetic nervous system activity in the presence of sympathetic nervous system blockade. The antihypertensive effect of guanethidine is prevented by drugs (tricyclic antidepressants, phenothiazines, amphetamines, cocaine) that prevent passage of norepinephrine as well as this drug into the postganglionic sympathetic nerve ending (Mitchell and Oates, 1970).

Chronic administration of guanethidine produces a denervation hypersensitivity phenomena. Indeed, hypertensive crisis can occur if direct-acting sympathomimetics are administered or if a patient with a pheochromocytoma receives guanethidine. Conversely, the response to indirect-acting sympathomimetics is attenuated.

Concentrations of catecholamines in the central nervous system are not altered by guanethidine reflecting the inability of this poorly lipid-soluble drug to cross the blood–brain barrier. Indeed, sedation and associated reductions in anesthetic requirements are not produced by guanethidine (Fig. 15-2) (Miller *et al*, 1969). Further evidence of lack of guanethidine entrance into the central nervous system is the absence of mental depression when this drug is administered.

GUANADREL

Guanadrel has a mechanism of action and hemodynamic effects similar to guanethidine, but it has a more rapid onset and shorter duration of action (Fig. 15-9). In contrast to guanethidine, guanadrel causes less orthostatic hypotension, diarrhea, and impotence.

Following oral administration, the maximal hypotensive effect occurs in 4 to 6 hours. Protein binding is estimated to be 20%. Unchanged drug and metabolites excreted in the urine account for 85% of an administered dose. The elimination half-time ranges from 5 to 45 hours.

LABETALOL

Labetalol is an antihypertensive drug that is unique in acting on alpha- and beta-adrenergic re-

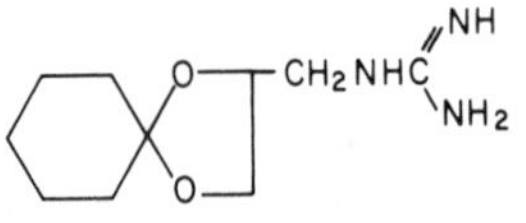

FIGURE 15-9. Guanadrel.

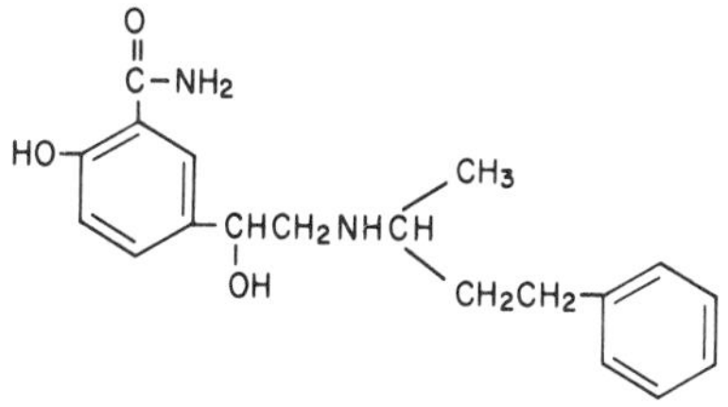

FIGURE 15-10. Labetalol.

ceptors (Fig. 15-10) (Wallin and O'Neill, 1983). Specifically, labetalol is a selective alpha-1 antagonist and nonselective antagonist at beta-1 and beta-2 receptors. Presynaptic alpha-2 receptors are spared by labetalol. This drug is about one-half as potent as phentolamine in its ability to block alpha receptors and about one-fourth as potent as propranolol as an antagonist at beta receptors. Antianginal effects of labetalol are less than those produced by propranolol. Like propranolol, labetalol lacks intrinsic sympathomimetic activity.

Pharmacokinetics

After oral administration, the bioavailability of labetalol is about 25% due to extensive hepatic first-pass metabolism. Cimetidine increases the bioavailability of labetalol. Metabolism is by conjugation to glucuronic acid with less than 5% of the drug recovered unchanged in the urine. The elimination half-time is 5 to 8 hours being prolonged in the presence of liver disease and unchanged by renal dysfunction.

Cardiovascular Effects

Chronic oral administration of labetalol maintains reductions in blood pressure principally due to decreases in peripheral vascular resistance as cardiac output is well-maintained. Heart rate does not increase in patients treated with labetalol.

Intravenous administration of labetalol (20 – 40 mg over 2 minutes) produces reductions in blood pressure because of simultaneous decreases in cardiac output and peripheral vascular resistance. The prompt reduction in blood pressure produced by intravenous labetalol makes this a useful drug in the treatment of hypertensive emergencies and production of controlled hypotension (Morel *et al,* 1982).

Side Effects

The most common side effect produced by labetalol is orthostatic hypotension. Fatigue, nausea, diarrhea, and dryness of the mouth may also occur. Fluid retention is the reason for often administering this drug with a diuretic. Bronchospasm is less likely to occur with labetalol than with other nonselective beta-adrenergic antagonists. Bradycardia can develop in patients receiving an overdose of labetalol.

CAPTOPRIL

Captopril is an orally effective antihypertensive drug that acts by competitive inhibition of angiotensin I-converting enzyme (*e.g.,* peptidyl dipeptidase) (Fig. 15-11) (Vidt *et al,* 1982). This is the enzyme that converts inactive angiotensin I to active angiotensin II (see Chapter 22). Angiotensin II is also responsible for stimulating secretion of aldosterone by the adrenal cortex. As a result of inhibition of this enzyme by captopril, there is a predictable decrease in circulating plasma concentrations of angiotensin II and aldosterone accompanied by a compensatory increase in angiotensin I and renin levels. The increase in plasma concentrations of renin reflects the loss of negative feedback control normally provided by angiotensin II. The decrease in aldosterone secretion results in a slight increase in serum potassium levels (Johnston *et al,* 1979). Patients with renovascular hypertension are particularly likely to respond to captopril. Nevertheless, this drug is often efficacious in treating hypertension even in patients who exhibit normal plasma renin activity. Part of this broad efficacy may reflect vasodilating effects of plasma kinins because the same converting enzyme inhibited by captopril is also responsible for the metabolism of bradykinin. Measures of general well-being (cognitive function, work performance, physical symptoms, sexual function)

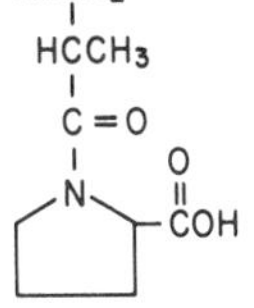

FIGURE 15-11. Captopril.

are better maintained in patients treated with captopril than in those treated with drugs acting on the central nervous system leading to improved patient compliance with drug therapy (Croog *et al*, 1986).

Pharmacokinetics

Captopril is well absorbed after oral administration with 25% to 30% of the drug reversibly bound to protein in the circulation. Inhibition of converting enzyme occurs within 15 minutes following oral administration. Excretion of unchanged drug in the urine accounts for about 50% of captopril. Indeed, renal dysfunction leads to drug retention.

Cardiovascular Effects

The antihypertensive effect of captopril is due to a decrease in peripheral vascular resistance as a result of decreased sodium and water retention. Typically, there are no concomitant changes in cardiac output or heart rate. Orthostatic hypotension does not occur. Simultaneous administration of captopril with a diuretic or beta-adrenergic antagonist is often utilized to increase antihypertensive effects.

Captopril may improve the efficacy of vasodilators in treating cardiac failure presumably by blocking vasodilator-induced increases in renin output (Gavras *et al*, 1978). Dramatic reversal of vascular and renal effects of scleroderma may follow the administration of captopril (Lopez-Overjero *et al*, 1979).

Side Effects

The most common side effect of captopril therapy occurring in about 10% of patients is a skin rash sometimes accompanied by fever and joint discomfort (Husserl and Messerli, 1981). Pruritus may accompany the rash. Loss of taste sensation occurs in about 7% of treated patients. Proteinuria has been observed in patients with preexisting renal disease treated for prolonged periods with high doses of captopril. Captopril may cause a marked elevation in the serum concentration of creatinine when administered to volume-depleted patients or those with renal disease. Elevated transaminase enzymes have been noted, but

a cause and effect relationship has not been established. Neutropenia has occurred in about 0.3% of patients being most frequent in patients with severe renal disease or those receiving immunosuppressive therapy. For this reason, white blood cell counts should be performed frequently during the first few months of captopril treatment.

Captopril increases serum potassium levels and may cause hyperkalemia, especially in patients with impaired renal function. The risk of hyperkalemia is increased if a potassium-sparing diuretic is given with captopril (Vidt *et al*, 1982).

Appearance of cough, and in patients with chronic obstructive airways disease an exacerbation of dyspnea and wheezing, may accompany the administration of captopril (Semple and Herd, 1986). It is speculated that these responses reflect potentiation of the effects of kinins due to captopril-induced inhibition of peptidyl dipeptidase activity (see Chapter 22).

The initial dose of captopril may cause an abrupt fall in blood pressure, particularly in patients who are volume depleted. Neurologic disturbances have been observed in patients receiving captopril and cimetidine concurrently. Indomethacin may antagonize the antihypertensive effect of captopril.

SARALASIN

Saralasin competitively and selectively blocks vascular smooth muscle receptors that mediate angiotensin II-induced vasoconstriction. As a result, there is a reduction in peripheral vascular resistance and a decline in blood pressure in patients with renin-dependent hypertension. Conversely, administration of this drug to hypertensive patients with subnormal plasma renin activity may evoke a pressor response reflecting intrinsic agonist activity of saralasin (Laragh *et al*, 1977). Another important agonist action of saralasin in the absence of elevated plasma renin activity is stimulation of the secretion of aldosterone. The elimination half-time of saralasin is brief (about 4 minutes) necessitating a continuous infusion to achieve a sustained effect.

METYROSINE

Metyrosine, 2 to 4 grams daily, administered to adults blocks catecholamine synthesis by inhibit-

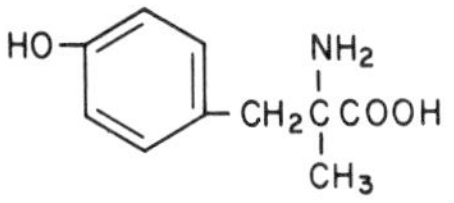

FIGURE 15-12. Metyrosine.

ing tyrosine hydroxylase, the enzyme that catalyzes the conversion of tyrosine to dopa (Fig. 15-12 and see Fig. 42-5). When administered to patients with pheochromocytoma, metyrosine reduces catecholamine production and usually decreases the frequency and severity of hypertensive attacks (Engelman *et al*, 1968). This drug is useful for the preoperative treatment of pheochromocytoma and for long-term therapy when surgery is not feasible. Metyrosine has not been compared to the traditional treatment regimen of alpha-adrenergic blockade with or without concomitant beta-adrenergic blockade in the preoperative preparation of patients with a pheochromocytoma. This drug is not consistently effective in the treatment of essential hypertension.

Pharmacokinetics

Metyrosine is well absorbed from the gastrointestinal tract with maximal biochemical effects occurring within 1 to 3 days after the initiation of therapy. The urinary concentration of catecholamines usually returns to pretreatment levels within 3 to 4 days after discontinuing the drug. Excretion of metyrosine is principally in the urine as unchanged drug.

Side Effects

Sedation is the most common side effect of metyrosine. Insomnia and psychic stimulation may occur when the drug is discontinued. Extrapyramidal reactions occur in about 10% of treated patients, and these effects may be potentiated by butyrophenones. Diarrhea may be severe in about 10% of patients. The risk of nephrolithiasis is reduced by increased water intake to achieve a daily urine output of at least 2 liters. Metyrosine should be discontinued if crystalluria persists despite an increase in water intake. Increased transaminase

levels and eosinophilia have been observed rarely.

REFERENCES

Bloor BC, Flacke WE. Reduction in halothane anesthetic requirements by clonidine, an alpha-adrenergic agonist. Anesth Analg 1982;61:741 – 5.

Bravo EL, Taraji RC, Fouad FM, Vidt DG, Gifford RW. Clonidine-suppression: A useful aid in the diagnosis of pheochromocytoma. N Engl J Med 1981;305:623 – 6.

Briant RH, Reid JL, Dollery CT. Interaction between clonidine and desipramine in man. Br Med J 1973;1:522 – 33.

Brodsky JB, Bravo JJ. Acute postoperative clonidine withdrawal syndrome. Anesthesiology 1976;44: 519 – 20.

Bruce DL, Croley TF, Lee JS. Preoperative clonidine withdrawal syndrome. Anesthesiology 1979;51: 90 – 2.

Cambridge D, Davey MJ, Messingham R. Prazosin a selective antagonist of post synaptic alpha adreno receptors. Br J Pharmacol 1977;59:514P – 5P.

Campese VM. Minoxidil: A review of its pharmacological properties and therapeutic use. Drugs 1981; 22:257 – 78.

Croog SH, Levine S, Testa MA et al. The effects of antihypertensive therapy on the quality of life. N Engl J Med 1986;314:1657 – 64.

Davies DS, Wing LMH, Reid JL, Neil E, Tippett P, Dollery CT. Pharmacokinetics and concentration-effect relationships of intravenous and oral clonidine. Clin Pharmacol Ther 1977;21:593 – 601.

Eger EI, Hamilton WK. The effect of reserpine on the action of various vasopressors. Anesthesiology 1959;20:641 – 5.

Engleman K, Horwitz D, Jequier E, Sjordsma A. Biochemical and pharmacologic effects of alpha methyltyrosine in man. J Clin Invest 1968;47:577 – 94.

Farsang C, Kunos G. Naloxone reverses the antihypertensive effect of clonidine. Br J Pharmacol 1979;67:161 – 4.

Finch L, Haeusler G. Further evidence for a central hypotensive action of alpha-methyldopa in both the rat and cat. Br J Pharmacol 1973; 47:217 – 28.

Frohlich ED. Methyldopa: Mechanisms and treatment 25 years later. Arch Intern Med 1980;140:954 – 9.

Gavras H, Brunner HR, Turini GA, et al. Antihypertensive effect of oral angiotensin converting-enzyme inhibitor SQ 14225 in man. N Engl J Med 1978;298: 991 – 5.

Ghignone M, Quintin L, Duke PC, Kehler CH, Calvillo O. Effects of clonidine on narcotic requirements and hemodynamic response during induction of fentanyl anesthesia and endotracheal intubation. Anesthesiology 1986;64:36 – 42.

Gold MS, Pottash AC, Sweeney DR, Kleber HD. Opiate

withdrawal using clonidine. A safe, effective and rapid nonopiate treatment. JAMA 1980;242:343 – 6.

Gottlieb TR, Chidsey CA. The clinician's guide to pharmacology of antihypertensive agents. Geriatrics 1976;31:99 – 110.

Hannington-Kiff G. Intravenous regional sympathetic block wih guanethidine. Lancet 1974;1:1019 – 20.

Houston MC. Clonidine hydrochloride. South Med J 1982;75:713 – 21.

Hunter E, Raik E, Gordon S, Taylor KB. Incidence of positive Coombs' test, LE cells and antinuclear factor in patients on alpha-methyldopa therapy. Med J Aust 1971;2:810 – 2.

Hunyor SN, Hansson L, Harrison TS, Hoobler SW. Effects of clonidine withdrawal: Possible mechanisms and suggestions for management. Br Med J 1973;2:209 – 21.

Husserl FE, Messerli FH. Adverse effects of antihypertensive drugs. Drugs 1981;22:188 – 210.

Johnston CI, Millar JA, McGrath BP, Matthews PG. Long-term effects of captopril (SQ14225) on blood-pressure and hormone levels in essential hypertension. Lancet 1979;2:493 – 6.

Laragh JH, Case DB, Wallace JM, Keim H. Blockade of renin or angiotensin for understanding human hypertension: A comparison of propranolol, saralasin and converting enzyme blockade. Fed Proc 1977;36:1781 – 7.

Lee SL, Chase PH. Drug-induced systemic lupus erythematosus: A critical review. Semin Arthritis Rheum 1975;5:83 – 103.

Lopez-Ovejero JA, Saal SD, D'Angelo WA, Cheigh JS, Stenzel KH, Laragh JH. Reversal of vascular and renal crises of scleroderma by oral angiotensin-converting-enzyme blockade. N Engl J Med 1979;300:1417 – 9.

Maze M, Smith CM. Identification of receptor mechanism mediating epinephrine-induced arrhythmias during halothane anesthesia in the dog. Anesthesiology 1983;59:322 – 6.

Mazze RI, Woodruff RE, Heerdt ME. Isoniazid-induced enflurane defluorination in humans. Anesthesiology 1982;57:5 – 8.

Miller RD, Way WL, Eger EI. The effects of alpha-methyldopa, reserpine, guanethidine and iproniazid on minimum alveolar anesthetic requirement (MAC). Anesthesiology 1969;29:1153 – 8.

Milne B, Cervenko FW, Jhamandas K, Sutak M. Local clonidine: Analgesia and effect on opiate withdrawal in the rat. Anesthesiology 1985;62:34 – 8.

Mitchell JR, Oates JA. Guanethidine and related agents. I. Mechanism of the selective blockade of adrenergic neurons and its antagonism by drugs. J Pharmacol Exp Ther 1970;172:100 – 7.

Morel DR, Forster A, Suter PM. I.V. labetalol in the treatment of hypertension following coronary-artery surgery. Br J Anaesth 1982;54:1191 – 6.

Myhre E, Rugsted HE, Hansen T. Clinical pharmacokinetics of methyldopa. Clin Pharmacokinet 1982;7:221 – 33.

Nies AS, Shand DG. Hypertensive response to propranolol in a patient treated with methyldopa—a proposed mechanism. Clin Pharmacol Ther 1973;14:823 – 6.

Prys-Roberts C, Meloche R, Foex P. Studies of anaesthesia in relation to hypertension. I: Cardiovascular responses to treated and untreated patients. Br J Anaesth 1971;43:122 – 37.

Safar ME, London GM, Levenson JA, Kheder MA, Abroas NE, Simon AC. Effect of alpha-methyldopa on cardiac output in hypertension. Clin Pharmacol Ther 1979;25:266 – 72.

Semple PF, Herd GW. Cough and wheeze caused by inhibitors of angiotensin-converting enzyme. N Engl J Med 1986;314:61.

Stiff JL, Harris DB. Clonidine withdrawal complicated by amitriptyline therapy. Anesthesiology 1983;59:73 – 4.

Thornton WE. Dementia induced by methyldopa with haloperidol. N Engl J Med 1976;194:1222.

VanZwieten PA. The central action of antihypertensive drugs mediated via central alpha receptors. J Pharm Pharmacol 1973;25:89 – 95.

Vidt DG, Bravo EL, Fouad FM. Captopril. N Engl J Med 1982;214 – 9.

Wallin JD, O'Neill WM. Labetalol. Current research and therapeutic status. Arch Intern Med 1983;143:485 – 90.

Weber MA, Drayer JIM, McMahon FG, Hamburger R, Shah AR, Kirk LN. Transdermal administration of clonidine for treatment of high BP. Arch Intern Med 1984;144:1211 – 3.

White WB, Gilbert JC. Transdermal clonidine in a patient with resistant hypertension and malabsorption. N Engl J Med 1985;313:1418.

CHAPTER 16

Peripheral Vasodilators

INTRODUCTION

Peripheral vasodilators are most frequently used clinically to (1) treat hypertensive crises, (2) produce controlled hypotension, and (3) facilitate left ventricular forward stroke volume, for example, in patients with regurgitant valvular heart lesions or acute cardiac failure (Chatterjee *et al,* 1973; Guiha *et al,* 1974; Kaplan *et al,* 1980). Peripheral vasodilators that are administered intravenously, often as a continuous infusion, include nitroprusside, nitroglycerin, trimethaphan, and diazoxide (Fig. 16-1). Conceptually, vasodilators lower blood pressure by decreasing peripheral vascular resistance (*i.e.,* arterial vasodilators) or by decreasing venous return and cardiac output (*i.e.,* venous vasodilators). Decreased peripheral vascular resistance also reduces the impedance to left ventricular ejection and allows for an increased forward left ventricular stroke volume, decreased left ventricular chamber size, and reduced myocardial oxygen requirements.

NITROPRUSSIDE

Nitroprusside is a direct-acting nonselective peripheral vasodilator causing relaxation of arterial and venous vascular smooth muscle (Fig. 16-1) (Kaplan *et al,* 1980; Tinker and Michenfelder, 1976). This drug lacks significant effects on other smooth muscle and on cardiac muscle. Its onset of action is almost immediate, and its duration of action is transient requiring continuous intravenous infusion to maintain a therapeutic effect. The extreme potency of nitroprusside necessitates careful titration of dosage as provided by continuous infusion devices and frequent monitoring of blood pressure, often by an intra-arterial catheter attached to a transducer.

Clinical Uses

Nitroprusside is used when prompt and reliable reduction in blood pressure is mandatory, as in treatment of hypertensive crises or production of controlled hypotension (Thompson *et al,* 1978). In addition, nitroprusside-induced decreases in left ventricular impedance, even in the absence of changes in blood pressure, can improve cardiac output in patients with acute cardiac failure due to myocardial ischemia or regurgitant valvular heart lesions.

Intravenous nitroprusside, 1 to 2 ug kg^{-1} as a rapid injection, is useful to offset blood pressure elevations produced by direct laryngoscopy for intubation at the trachea (Fig. 16-2) (Stoelting, 1979). Administration of nitroprusside, and presumably other vasodilators such as nitroglycerin, during the rewarming phase of cardiopulmonary bypass results in vasodilation that permits increased flow rates and thus improved heat delivery to peripheral tissues. As a result, the decline in nasopharyngeal temperature following cessation of cardiopulmonary bypass is minimized (Fig. 16-3) (Noback and Tinker, 1980).

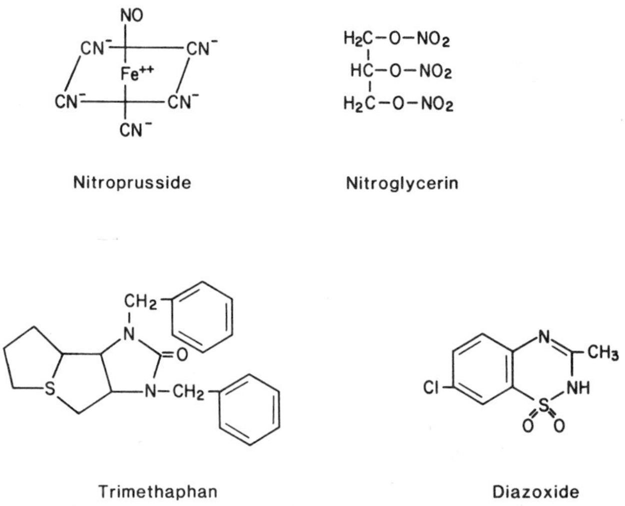

FIGURE 16-1. Peripheral vasodilators.

Mechanism of Action

Organic nitrates, such as nitroprusside, nitroglycerin, and hydralazine, can produce nitric oxide which activates the enzyme, guanylate cyclase (Rapoport and Murad, 1983). Guanylate cyclase results in increased concentrations of cyclic guanosine 3'5'-monophosphate (cyclic GMP) and subsequent relaxation of smooth muscle as present in veins and arteries. Support for the role of guanylate cyclase activation in the vasodilating effects of nitroso-containing drugs is the potentiation of the hypotensive effects of nitroprusside in dogs receiving aminophylline (Pearl *et al*, 1984). Presumably, aminophylline acting as a phosphodiesterase inhibitor, allows additional intracellular accumulation of cyclic GMP. This potential potentiation of the effects of peripheral vasodilators should be considered when administering these drugs to patients who are also receiving aminophylline.

Metabolism

Metabolism of nitroprusside begins with the transfer of an electron from the iron of oxyhemoglobin to nitroprusside yielding methemoglobin and an unstable nitroprusside radical (Fig. 16-4) (Smith and Kruszyna, 1974; Tinker and Michenfelder, 1976; Vesey *et al*, 1974). This electron transfer is independent of enzyme activity. The unstable nitroprusside radical promptly breaks down releasing all five cyanide ions, one of which reacts with methemoglobin to form cyanmethemoglobin. The remaining free cyanide ions are available to rhodanase enzyme in the liver and kidney for conversion to thiocyanate. Any free cyanide that is not rapidly converted to thiocyanate can bind to and inactivate tissue cytochrome oxidase and manifest as tissue hypoxia (see the section entitled Cyanide Toxicity). The breakdown of nitroprusside to cyanide by plasma glutathione or tissue sulfhydryl groups is too slow to be of any significance. The nonenzymatic release of cyanide from nitroprusside is not inhibited by hypothermia as may be present during cardiopulmonary bypass while enzymatic conversion of cyanide to thiocyanate may be delayed (Moore *et al*, 1985).

Because the conversion of nitroprusside to cyanide is independent of enzyme activity, the amount of cyanide release from nitroprusside depends entirely on the total dose of drug that is administered. The subsequent rate at which cyanide is converted to thiocyanate by rhodanase enzyme is dependent upon the availability of a sulfur donor for the enzyme (Smith, 1973). Usually, endogenous thiosulfate is the sulfur donor being derived from the amino acid cysteine.

Thiocyanate is cleared slowly by the kidney with an elimination half-time of 4 to 7 days (Bastron and Kaloyanides, 1972). Thus, thiocyanate accumulates with prolonged therapy or in the presence of renal failure. If the plasma concentration of thiocyanate exceeds 10 mg dl^{-1}, there may

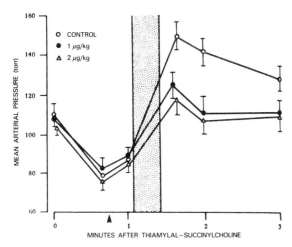

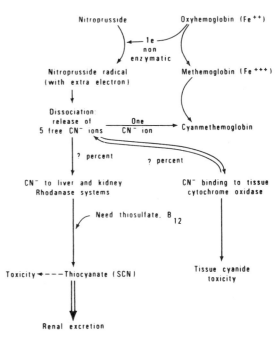

FIGURE 16-2. Intravenous nitroprusside attenuates the blood pressure response evoked by direct laryngoscopy (shaded area) and intubation of the trachea. Arrow denotes the injection of nitroprusside. (From Stoelting RK. Attenuation of blood pressure response to laryngoscopy and tracheal intubation with sodium nitroprusside. Anesth Analg 1979;58:116–9. Reproduced by permission of the author and the International Anesthesia Research Society.)

FIGURE 16-4. Metabolism of nitroprusside begins with the transfer of an electron from the iron of oxyhemoglobin to nitroprusside yielding methemoglobin and an unstable nitroprusside radical. (From Tinker JH, Michenfelder JD. Sodium nitroprusside: Pharmacology, toxicology and therapeutics. Anesthesiology 1976;45:340–54. Reproduced by permission of the authors and publisher.)

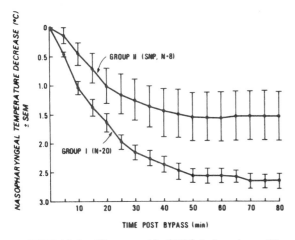

FIGURE 16-3. Nitroprusside (SNP)-induced vasodilation during the rewarming phase of cardiopulmonary bypass minimizes the subsequent decline in nasopharyngeal temperature (Group II) compared with untreated patients. (From Noback CR, Tinker JR. Hypothermia after cardiopulmonary bypass in man: amelioration by nitroprusside-induced vasodilation during rewarming. Anesthesiology 1980;53:277–80. Reproduced by permission of the authors and publisher.)

be skeletal muscle weakness, nausea, and mental confusion. Prolonged elevations of plasma thiocyanate concentrations can result in hypothyroidism since thiocyanate interferes with transport of iodine by the thyroid gland. Oxyhemoglobin can slowly oxidize thiocyanate back to sulfate and cyanide, but this is insufficient to cause cyanide toxicity (Smith, 1973).

Nitroprusside has been associated with methemoglobinemia in a patient receiving 321 mg of nitroprusside over 4 days (Bower and Peterson, 1975). Methylene blue, 1 to 2 mg kg^{-1} administered intravenously over 5 minutes, facilitates the conversion of methemoglobin to hemoglobin.

Cyanide Toxicity

There is a linear relationship between the plasma concentration of cyanide and the total dose of nitroprusside administered (Vesey *et al,* 1976). Cyanide toxicity from spontaneous breakdown of nitroprusside should be suspected in any patient who is resistant to the hypotensive effects of the drug despite adequate infusion rates (up to 8 μg kg^{-1} min^{-1}) or in a previously responsive patient who becomes unresponsive to the blood pressure-lowering effects of the drug despite increasing doses (*i.e.,* tachyphylaxis). Mixed venous PO$_2$ is elevated in the presence of cyanide toxicity indicating paralysis of cytochrome oxidase and inability of the tissues to utilize oxygen. At the same time, metabolic acidosis develops as a reflection of anaerobic metabolism in the tissues. Decreased cerebral oxygen utilization is evidenced by the increased cerebral venous oxygen content.

Blood cyanide levels are increased while thiocyanate levels are unchanged in patients who develop cyanide toxicity following short-term administration of nitroprusside (Vesey *et al,* 1976). Indeed, measurement of blood thiocyanate levels is of no value in the recognition of cyanide toxicity (Michenfelder and Tinker, 1977). Even measurement of plasma cyanide concentrations may be of limited value because circulating cyanide rapidly binds to tissue cytochrome oxidase.

The phenomenon of resistance to the therapeutic effects of nitroprusside may be related to an abnormality in the cyanide-thiocyanate pathway that allows cyanide to accumulate (Davies *et al,* 1975). For example, patients who have Leber's optic atrophy or tobacco ambylopia, manifest elevated blood concentrations of cyanide (Wilson, 1965). The mechanism by which cyanide results in resistance or tachyphylaxis to the blood pressure-lowering effects of nitroprusside is not confirmed but could reflect cyanide-induced stimulation of cardiac output which would tend to offset the hypotensive effects of the vasodilator. Furthermore, most patients who are resistant or develop tachyphylaxis to the hypotensive effects of nitroprusside are children or young adults. It is speculated that active baroreceptor reflexes in this age group evoke increases in sympathetic nervous system activity in response to drug-induced reductions in blood pressure. As a result, a larger initial dose or the subsequent need to increase the dose of nitroprusside is required to produce a reduction in blood pressure leading to the likelihood of dose-dependent cyanide toxicity. Propranolol can be administered to blunt these baroreceptor-mediated responses and thus minimize the total dose

of nitroprusside required to produce the desired blood pressure effect. Likewise, volatile anesthetics blunt baroreceptor reflex activity thus contributing to decreased dose requirements for nitroprusside (see the section entitled Dose).

There is no evidence that preexisting hepatic or renal disease increases the likelihood of cyanide toxicity. In fact, renal failure may prevent sulfate excretion which allows production of more thiosulfate to act as a sulfur donor and convert cyanide to thiocyanate (Fig. 16-5) (Tinker and Michenfelder, 1980).

Treatment of Cyanide Toxicity

Appearance of tachyphylaxis in a previously sensitive patient in association with metabolic acidosis and elevated mixed venous PO$_2$ mandates immediate discontinuation of nitroprusside administration. Sodium thiosulfate, 150 mg kg^{-1} administered intravenously over 15 minutes, is a recommended therapy for cyanide toxicity (Michenfelder and Tinker, 1977). Thiosulfate acts as a sulfur donor to convert cyanide to thiocyanate. If cyanide toxicity is severe, with deteriorating hemodynamics and metabolic acidosis, the treatment is the slow intravenous administration of sodium nitrate, 5 mg kg^{-1}, to convert hemoglobin to methemoglobin (Tinker and Michenfelder,

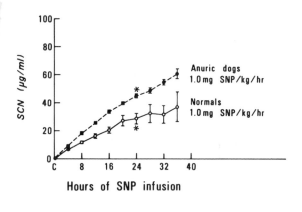

$* P < .05$

FIGURE 16-5. Plasma thiocyanate (SCN) concentrations are greater in anuric than normal dogs. (From Tinker JH, Michenfelder JD. Increased resistance to nitroprusside-induced cyanide toxicity in anuric dogs. Anesthesiology 1980;52:40–7. Reproduced by permission of the authors and publisher.)

1976). Methemoglobin acts as an antidote to cyanide toxicity, by converting cyanide to cyanmethemoglobin. Alternatively, administration of hydroxocobalamin, which reacts with cyanide to form cyanocobalamin, has been recommended (Cottrell *et al*, 1979).

Dose

Nitroprusside should be administered on the basis of total dose and not the blood pressure effect that is achieved. The maximum acceptable continuous intravenous infusion rate of nitroprusside is $8 \mu g \, kg^{-1} \, min^{-1}$ for a 1 to 3 hour administration or $0.5 \, mg \, kg^{-1} \, hr^{-1}$ for chronic infusion (Michenfelder and Tinker, 1977). Nevertheless, the vast majority of anesthetized patients do not require a dose near this maximum amount with the usual continuous perioperative intravenous infusion rate being 0.5 to $2 \mu g \, kg^{-1} \, min^{-1}$. Volatile anesthetics, which decrease baroreceptor sensitivity are associated with greatly reduced dose requirements for nitroprusside (Chen *et al*, 1982). Like volatile anesthetics, propanolol can also be utilized to blunt baroreceptor reflex responses and renin release thus minimizing the dose of nitroprusside required to produce desirable degrees of blood pressure reduction (Marshall *et al*, 1981). Conversely, hypotension produced by nitroprusside is followed by increased baroreceptor sensitivity (*e.g.,* baroreceptors are reset) which could contribute to subsequent increased dose requirements for nitroprusside to maintain blood pressure at a reduced level (Fig. 16-6) (Chen *et al*, 1982). Whenever the dose of nitroprusside approaches the maximum infusion rate, it is important to monitor arterial *p*H for evidence of metabolic acidosis as a manifestation of cyanide toxicity.

Effects on Organ Systems

The principal pharmacologic effects of nitroprusside are manifest on the (1) cardiovascular system, (2) blood flow to the central nervous system, and (3) hypoxic pulmonary vasoconstriction. Nitroprusside lacks direct effects on the central nervous system or autonomic nervous system. In animals, nitroprusside-induced reductions in blood pressure do not result in hepatic hypoxia or changes in hepatic blood flow (Gelman and Ernst, 1978; Si-

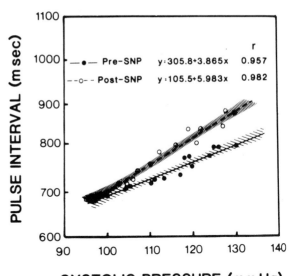

FIGURE 16-6. Baroreceptor sensitivity increases following nitroprusside-induced hypotension (post-SNP) compared with pre-SNP. (From Chen RYZ, Matteo RS, Fan F-C, *et al*. Resetting of baroreceptor sensitivity after induced hypotension. Anesthesiology 1982;56:29–35. Reproduced by permission of the authors and publisher.)

varajan *et al*, 1985). Furthermore, hepatic blood flow does not change when cardiac output is maintained in anesthetized patients despite 20% to 60% reductions in blood pressure produced by nitroprusside (Chauvin *et al*, 1985).

Cardiovascular System

Nitroprusside produces prompt reductions in blood pressure by virtue of arterial and venous vasodilation (Tinker and Michenfelder, 1976). Peripheral vascular resistance is decreased as evidence of arterial vasodilation while venous return is decreased because of vasodilation of venous capacitance vessels. It is likely that reductions in right atrial pressure reflect pooling of blood in veins. Baroreceptor-mediated reflex responses to nitroprusside-induced reductions in blood pressure manifest as tachycardia and increased myocardial contractility. Indeed, these reflex-mediated responses may offset the blood pressure-lowering effects of nitroprusside (see the sections entitled Cyanide Toxicity and Dose).

Although decreased venous return would tend to reduce cardiac output, the net effect is often an increase in cardiac output due to reflex-mediated increases in peripheral sympathetic nervous system activity combined with decreased impedance to left ventricular ejection. There is no evidence that nitroprusside exerts direct inotropic or chronotropic effects on the heart.

Nitroprusside-induced reductions in blood pressure often result in decreases in renal function (Tinker and Michenfelder, 1976). Release of renin may accompany blood pressure reductions produced by nitroprusside and contribute to blood pressure overshoots when the drug is discontinued (Khambatta et al, 1979; Miller et al, 1977). Indeed, infusion of saralasin, a competitive inhibitor of angiotensin II, prevents blood pressure overshoot following discontinuation of nitroprusside thus confirming the participation of the renin-angiotensin system in this response (Delaney and Miller, 1980). Increased plasma concentrations of catecholamines also accompany hypotension produced by nitroprusside but not trimethaphan (Fig. 16-7) (Knight et al, 1983) (see the section entitled Trimethaphan).

Nitroprusside has been reported to increase the area of damage associated with a myocardial infarction (Chiariello et al, 1976). It is speculated that nitroprusside causes an intracoronary steal of blood flow away from ischemic areas by arteriolar vasodilation (Becker, 1978). Clinical evidence of an intracoronary steal phenomena is the appearance of ischemic changes on the electrocardiogram. Reductions in diastolic blood pressure produced by nitroprusside may also contribute to myocardial ischemia by decreasing coronary blood flow (Sivarajan et al, 1985).

Cerebral Blood Flow

Nitroprusside is a direct cerebral vasodilator leading to increased cerebral blood flow and cerebral blood volume. These changes, when they occur in patients with reduced intracranial compliance, cause undesirable elevations of intracranial pressure (Turner et al, 1977). It is speculated that the rapidity of blood pressure reduction produced by nitroprusside exceeds the capacity of the cerebral circulation to autoregulate its blood flow such that intracranial pressure and blood pressure change simultaneously but in opposite directions (Rogers et al, 1979). Nevertheless, increases in intracranial pressure produced by nitroprusside are maxi-

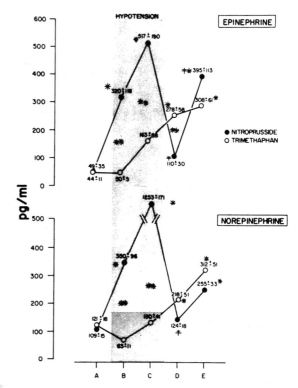

FIGURE 16-7. Increased plasma concentrations of epinephrine and norepinephrine accompany nitroprusside, but not trimethaphan-induced hypotension. (From Knight PR, Lane GA, Hensinger RN, et al. Catecholamine and renin-angiotensin response during hypotensive anesthesia induced by sodium nitroprusside or trimethaphan camsylate. Anesthesiology 1983;59:248–53. Reproduced by permission of the authors and publisher.)

mum during modest reductions (less than 30%) in mean arterial pressure. When nitroprusside-induced reductions in mean arterial pressure exceed 30% of the awake level, the intracranial pressure decreases below the awake value (Turner et al, 1977). Furthermore, lowering blood pressure over 5 minutes with nitroprusside in the presence of hypocarbia and hyperoxia negates the increase in intracranial pressure that accompanies the rapid infusion of nitroprusside (Fig. 16-8) (Marsh et al, 1979). Clearly, the potential adverse effects of nitroprusside on intracranial pressure are not present if this drug is administered after the dura is opened.

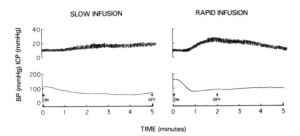

SLOW INFUSION   RAPID INFUSION

TIME (minutes)

FIGURE 16-8. Compared with rapid infusion, the slow intravenous administration of nitroprusside does not increase the intracranial pressure. (From Marsh ML, Aidinis SJ, Naughton KVH, Marshall LF, Shapiro HM. The technique of nitroprusside administration modifies the intracranial pressure response. Anesthesiology 1979;51:538–41. Reproduced by permission of the authors and publisher.)

Hypoxic Pulmonary Vasoconstriction

Reductions in the PaO_2 may accompany the infusion of nitroprusside and other peripheral vasodilators as used to produce controlled hypotension. Attenuation of hypoxic pulmonary vasoconstriction by peripheral vasodilators is the presumed mechanism for this effect on arterial oxygenation (Colley *et al*, 1979). Addition of propranolol to the vasodilator regimen does not alter the magnitude of reduction in PaO_2 (Miller *et al*, 1982). Furthermore, peripheral vasodilator-induced reductions in blood pressure may be more likely to increase the shunt fraction in patients with normal lungs than in those with chronic obstructive airways disease (Casthely *et al*, 1982). It is speculated that hypotension in the normal patients leads to decreased pulmonary artery pressure such that preferential perfusion of dependent but poorly ventilated alveoli occurs. In contrast, patients with chronic obstructive airways disease may develop destructive vascular changes that prevent alterations in distribution of pulmonary blood flow in response to vasodilation. The addition of positive end-expiratory pressure may reverse vasodilator-induced reductions in the PaO_2 (Berthelsen *et al*, 1986).

NITROGLYCERIN

Nitroglycerin is an organic nitrate that acts principally on venous capacitance vessels to produce peripheral pooling of blood, reduction of heart size, and decreased cardiac ventricular wall tension (Fig. 16-1) (Kaplan *et al*, 1980). As the dose of nitroglycerin is increased, there is also relaxation of arterial vascular smooth muscle. The most common clinical use of nitroglycerin is sublingual or intravenous administration for the treatment of angina pectoris due either to atherosclerosis of the coronary arteries or intermittent vasospasm of these vessels. Production of controlled hypotension has also been achieved with the continuous intravenous infusion of nitroglycerin.

Route of Administration

Sublingual administration of nitroglycerin results in peak plasma concentrations within 4 minutes. The elimination half-time is brief being 1 to 4 minutes. Only about 15% of the blood flow from the sublingual area passes through the liver which limits the initial first-pass metabolism of nitroglycerin.

Transdermal absorption of nitroglycerin (5–10 mg over 24 hours) provides sustained protection against myocardial ischemia. The plasma concentration resulting from transdermal absorption of nitroglycerin is low, and tolerance to the drug effect does not seem to occur.

Continuous intravenous infusion of nitroglycerin, via special delivery tubing to reduce absorption of the drug into plastic, is an ideal approach to maintain a constant plasma concentration of nitroglycerin.

Mechanism of Action

The ability of nitroglycerin to reduce myocardial oxygen requirements is the most likely mechanism by which this drug relieves angina pectoris in patients with atherosclerotic disease of the coronary arteries. For example, nitroglycerin-induced venodilatation and increased venous capacitance decreases venous return to the heart (*e.g.,* preload) resulting in reduced ventricular end-diastolic pressure and volume and, therefore, decreased myocardial oxygen requirements (Greenberg *et al*, 1975). In addition, any drug-induced reduction in peripheral vascular resistance decreases afterload and myocardial oxygen requirements. Nitroglycerin does not increase total coronary blood flow in patients with angina pectoris due to atherosclerosis (Garlin *et al*, 1959).

The ability of nitroglycerin to dilate selectively large coronary arteries may be an important mechanism in the relief of angina pectoris due to vasospasm. Specifically, nitroglycerin appears to cause redistribution of coronary blood flow to ischemic areas of subendocardium by selective dilatation of large epicardial vessels (Cowan *et al*, 1969). Indeed, nitroglycerin increases the rate of washout of radioactive xenon from ischemic areas of the ventricle indicating that blood flow to this region has increased (Horwitz *et al*, 1971). Nitroglycerin, in contrast to nitroprusside, has been reported to decrease the area of damage associated with a myocardial infarction, presumably by preferentially diverting blood flow to the ischemic area (Chiariello *et al*, 1976).

Metabolism

Nitroglycerin is metabolized in the liver by nitrate reductase (glutathione dependent) to glycerol dinitrate and nitrite which are excreted in the urine (Kaplan *et al*, 1980). Resulting denitrated metabolites of nitroglycerin are about ten times less potent as vasodilators. The nitrite metabolite of nitroglycerin is capable of converting hemoglobin to methemoglobin. Although significant methemoglobin formation is unlikely with total nitroglycerin doses less than 5 mg kg^{-1}, there are reports of methemoglobinemia in patients receiving lesser doses of nitroglycerin (Fibuch *et al*, 1979; Zurick *et al*, 1984). Treatment is with intravenous methylene blue, 1 to 2 mg kg^{-1} administered over 5 minutes, to facilitate the conversion of methemoglobin to hemoglobin.

Clinical Uses

Angina Pectoris

Sublingual nitroglycerin, 0.3 mg, is the most useful of the organic nitrates for the acute and chronic treatment and prevention of angina pectoris due to atherosclerotic coronary artery disease or coronary artery vasospasm. Failure of three sublingual tablets in a 15-minute period to relieve angina pectoris may reflect myocardial infarction. Other more expensive sublingual nitrates do not appear to be more effective than nitroglycerin. For example, isosorbide dinitrate, 5 to 10 mg orally, is no more effective than placebo in decreasing the frequency of angina pectoris or increasing the patient's exercise tolerance. Higher doses of isosorbide dinitrate, 20 to 40 mg orally every 4 hours, are effective but are also associated with an increased incidence of side effects. Application of 2% nitroglycerin ointment over an area of skin of 2.5 to 5 cm produces sustained protection from angina pectoris for up to 4 hours.

Continuous intravenous infusion of nitroglycerin, 0.25 to 1 μg kg^{-1} min^{-1} has been utilized intraoperatively as prophylaxis against myocardial ischemia in anesthetized patients with known coronary artery disease (Kaplan *et al*, 1976). Nevertheless, intravenous nitroglycerin, 0.5 to 1.0 μg kg^{-1} min^{-1} cannot be demonstrated to prevent changes of myocardial ischemia on the electrocardiogram of patients anesthetized with nitrous oxide-fentanyl and paralyzed with pancuronium (Gallagher *et al*, 1986; Thomson *et al*, 1984). Nitroglycerin does, however, reduce the incidence of hypertension as may occur during direct laryngoscopy and intubation of the trachea.

Headache is common and may be severe following administration of sublingual nitroglycerin. Presumably, headache reflects dilatation of meningeal vessels. Arterial dilatation in the face and neck manifests as facial flushing. Tolerance, which occurs with frequent exposure to high doses of organic nitrates, does not develop with the intermittent sublingual administration of nitroglycerin as used to treat angina pectoris (Danahy *et al*, 1977).

Cardiac Failure

Nitroglycerin primarily reduces preload and relieves pulmonary edema (Guiha *et al*, 1974). Intravenous infusion of nitroglycerin to patients with acute myocardial infarction can improve cardiac output, relieve pulmonary congestion, and decrease myocardial oxygen requirements thus limiting the size of the myocardial infarction (Chiariello *et al*, 1976).

Controlled Hypotension

Nitroglycerin can be used to produce controlled hypotension, but it is less potent than nitroprusside. For example, equivalent reductions in blood pressure are achieved by the continuous intravenous infusion of nitroglycerin, 4.7 μg kg^{-1} min^{-1}, and nitroprusside, 2.5 μg kg^{-1} min^{-1} (Fahmy,

1978). At comparable systolic blood pressures, the mean and diastolic blood pressures are higher with nitroglycerin than with nitroprusside. Evidence of myocardial ischemia may appear on the electrocardiogram during infusion of nitroprusside presumably reflecting the impact of decreased diastolic blood pressure on coronary blood flow (Fahmy, 1978). Because nitroglycerin acts predominantly on venous capacitance vessels, the production of controlled hypotension using this drug may be more dependent on intravascular fluid volume as compared with nitroprusside.

Acute Hypertension

Nitroglycerin may be effective in control of acute increases in blood pressure that may accompany noxious stimulation in the parturient as during cesarean section (Snyder *et al*, 1979). This drug crosses the placenta because of its low molecular weight (227) and nonionized state, but should not produce adverse metabolic or central nervous system effects in the fetus. Conversely, a theoretical concern exists as to the possible adverse effects of cyanide which is detectable in fetal blood following administration of nitroprusside to the mother (Lewis *et al*, 1977). Trimethaphan effectively controls maternal blood pressure but may produce undesirable autonomic nervous system effects in the newborn, including paralytic ileus.

Effects on Organ Systems

The principal pharmacologic actions of nitroglycerin manifest as cardiovascular effects. Nitroglycerin also acts on smooth muscle in the airways and gastrointestinal tract. For example, bronchial smooth muscle is relaxed regardless of the preexisting tone (Byrick *et al*, 1983). Smooth muscle of the biliary tract, including the sphincter of Oddi, is relaxed. Indeed, pain that mimics angina pectoris, but is due to opioid-induced biliary tract spasm, will often be relieved by nitroglycerin. Relief of this pain by nitroglycerin may lead to the incorrect conclusion that myocardial ischemia had been present. Esophageal muscle tone is reduced as is ureteral and uterine smooth muscle tone although these latter effects are somewhat unpredictable. Like nitroprusside, nitroglycerin is a cerebral vasodilator and may increase intracranial pressure in patients with decreased intracranial compliance (Gagnon *et al*, 1979).

Cardiovascular Effects

Nitroglycerin doses up to 2 μg kg^{-1} min^{-1} produce dilatation of veins that predominates over that produced in arterioles (Gerson *et al*, 1982). Venodilatation results in decreased left and right ventricular end-diastolic pressures. In normal individuals and patients with coronary artery disease, but in the absence of cardiac failure, nitroglycerin decreases cardiac output. This decreased cardiac output reflects reduced venous return as nitroglycerin is devoid of any direct inotropic effect on the heart. Heart rate is often not changed or only slightly increased during administration of nitroglycerin.

Nitroglycerin-induced reductions in blood pressure are more dependent on blood volume than are blood pressure changes produced by nitroprusside. Indeed, marked hypotension may occasionally follow sublingual administration of nitroglycerin especially if the patient is standing as this position augments venous pooling and further decreases cardiac output. Excessive reductions in diastolic blood pressure may decrease coronary blood flow. These reductions in diastolic blood pressure may also evoke baroreceptor-mediated reflex increases in sympathetic nervous system activity manifesting as tachycardia and increased myocardial contractility. The combination of decreased coronary blood flow and changes that increase myocardial oxygen requirements may provoke angina pectoris in susceptible patients.

Calculated peripheral vascular resistance is usually relatively unaffected by nitroglycerin. Pulmonary vascular resistance is, however, consistently decreased presumably reflecting a direct relaxant effect of nitroglycerin on pulmonary vasculature (Tinker and Michenfelder, 1976). Indeed, in an animal model for pulmonary hypertension, nitroglycerin, but not nitroprusside, was effective in decreasing pulmonary artery pressures and pulmonary vascular resistance (Pearl *et al*, 1983).

Nitroglycerin primarily dilates larger conductance vessels of the coronary circulation often leading to an increase in coronary blood flow to ischemic subendocardial areas. In contrast, nitroprusside may produce a coronary steal phenomena (see the section entitled Nitroprusside). Indeed, the frequency of S–T segment elevation during acute coronary artery occlusion in dogs is reduced by nitroglycerin but increased by nitroprusside (Chiariello *et al*, 1976). For these reasons, nitroglycerin has been recommended in favor of nitroprusside for the treatment of hypertension in patients with coronary artery disease (Kaplan *et al*, 1976).

Nitroglycerin produces a dose-related prolongation of bleeding time that parallels the decrease in blood pressure (Fig. 16-9) (Lichtenthal *et al*, 1985). Platelet aggregation is not altered suggesting that prolonged bleeding time is due to vasodilation and increased venous capacitance.

TRIMETHAPHAN

Trimethaphan is a peripheral vasodilator and ganglionic blocker that acts rapidly but so briefly that it must be given by continuous intravenous infusion (Fig. 16-1) (Vickers *et al*, 1984). Because trimethaphan directly relaxes capacitance vessels and blocks autonomic nervous system reflexes, it lowers blood pressure both by decreasing cardiac output and reducing peripheral vascular resistance (Harioka *et al*, 1984; Wang *et al*, 1977). Histamine release does not contribute to the reduction in blood pressure produced by trimethaphan (Fahmy and Soter, 1985). In contrast to nitroprusside, trimethaphan-induced reductions in blood pressure are not associated with increases in plasma concentrations of catecholamines and renin reflecting the effect of ganglionic blockade (Fig. 16-7) (Knight *et al*, 1983). Increases in heart rate secondary to administration of trimethaphan most likely reflect parasympathetic ganglionic blockade.

Ganglionic blockade produced by trimethaphan reflects occupation of receptors normally responsive to acetylcholine as well as stabilization of the postsynaptic membranes against the actions of acetylcholine liberated from presynaptic nerve endings. The route of metabolism of trimethaphan is unclear although hydrolysis by plasma cholinesterase has been implicated. As a quaternary ammonium drug, passage of trimethaphan across the blood–brain barrier is limited and central nervous system effects do not occur.

Clinical Uses

Trimethaphan is most often used as a continuous intravenous infusion ($10–200 \ \mu g \ kg^{-1} \ min^{-1}$) to produce controlled hypotension. Tachycardia may accompany drug-induced reductions in blood pressure, and cardiac output is likely to be reduced as a manifestation of decreased venous return (Harioka *et al*, 1984). Furthermore, tachycardia may offset the blood pressure-lowering effects of trimethaphan requiring the administration of propranolol. Indeed, patients who do not respond even initially to trimethaphan may be encountered (Stoelting *et al*, 1977).

Side Effects

A number of side effects may accompany the use of trimethaphan for production of controlled hypotension. Mydriasis, reduced gastrointestinal activity culminating in ileus, and urinary retention accompany ganglionic blockade produced by this drug. Mydriasis produced by trimethaphan may interfere with neurological evaluation of the patient following intracranial surgery. Deleterious cerebral metabolic disturbances in dogs characterized by decreased brain oxygen availability have occurred following production of controlled hypotension with trimethaphan but not nitroprusside (Michenfelder and Theye, 1977). In monkeys anesthetized with halothane-nitrous oxide, production of controlled hypotension by the administration of trimethaphan, but not nitroprusside, reduces cerebral blood flow while cerebral metabolic rate for oxygen remains unchanged (Fig. 16-10) (Sivarajan *et al*, 1985). These data are also consistent with decreased brain oxygen avail-

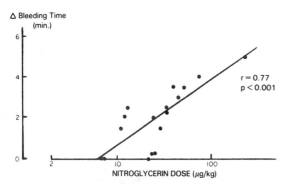

FIGURE 16-9. Nitroglycerin produces dose-related increases in bleeding time. (From Lichtenthal PR, Rossi EC, Louis G, *et al*. Dose-related prolongation of the bleeding time by intravenous nitroglycerin. Anesth Analg 1985;64:30–3. Reproduced by permission of the authors and the International Anesthesia Research Society.)

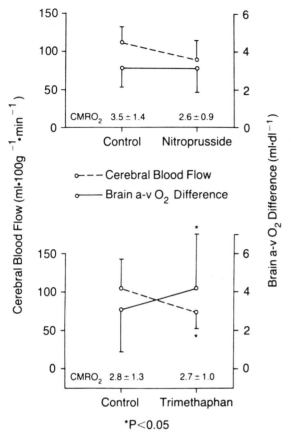

CMRO$_2$ 3.5 ± 1.4   2.6 ± 0.9

Control   Nitroprusside

◦– – – Cerebral Blood Flow

◦—— Brain a-v O$_2$ Difference

CMRO$_2$ 2.8 ± 1.3   2.7 ± 1.0

Control   Trimethaphan

*P<0.05

FIGURE 16-10. Hypotension produced by trimethaphan, but not nitroprusside, reduces cerebral blood flow while cerebral metabolic oxygen requirements, as reflected by an increased brain a-V oxygen difference, remain unchanged. (From Sivarajan M, Amory DW, McKenzie SM. Regional blood flows during induced hypotension produced by nitroprusside or trimethaphan in the rhesus monkey. Anesth Analg 1985;64:759–66. Reproduced by permission of the authors and the International Anesthesia Research Society.)

ability due to decreased oxygen delivery by reduced cerebral blood flow in the presence of unchanged oxygen utilization. Conversely, there is evidence that blood pressure reductions produced by trimethaphan evoke smaller increases in intracranial pressure than associated with comparable degrees of hypotension produced by nitroprusside or nitroglycerin (Turner *et al,* 1977). This may reflect a slower onset of action of tri-

methaphan allowing autoregulation of cerebral blood flow to occur.

Trimethaphan-induced controlled hypotension in animals is associated with decreased coronary blood flow but unchanged renal blood flow and hepatic blood flow (Sivarajan *et al,* 1985). Trimethaphan is a potent inhibitor of plasma cholinesterase such that the duration of action of succinylcholine is likely to be prolonged (Sklar and Lanks, 1977). Histamine release that may accompany the administration of trimethaphan makes administration of this drug to patients with pheochromocytoma questionable.

DIAZOXIDE

Diazoxide, a benzothiadiazene derivative, is closely related chemically to the thiazide diuretics (Fig. 16-1). This drug is used to treat acute blood pressure elevations as in patients with accelerated hypertension and severe hypertension associated with glomerulonephritis. For example, diazoxide, 1 to 3 mg kg^{-1} administered intravenously as a rapid injection to a hypertensive patient produces a decline in systolic and diastolic blood pressure within 1 to 2 minutes that lasts 6 or 7 hours. The drug can be repeated at intervals of 5 to 15 minutes. Previous recommendations that the drug had to be administered as a rapid intravenous injection to obtain a therapeutic effect are not true as an adequate response can be obtained with a less rapid injection (Garrett and Kaplan, 1982). Diazoxide is eliminated principally as unchanged drug by the kidneys. Although excessive blood pressure reductions are unlikely, a disadvantage of diazoxide, compared with nitroprusside, is the inability to adjust the dose of this drug in accordance with the patient's response.

Cardiovascular Effects

Diazoxide-induced reductions in blood pressure are associated with significant increases in cardiac output and often an elevation in heart rate. Peripheral vascular resistance is decreased. Because diazoxide increases cardiac output and left ventricular ejection velocity, this drug is unsuitable for the treatment of hypertension associated with a dissecting aortic aneurysm. Indeed, excessive hypotension and reflex sympathetic nervous system stimulation leading to myocardial ischemia may occur unpredictably. Conversely, the hypotensive effect of diazoxide may be accentuated in patients receiving a beta-adrenergic antagonist because baroreceptor-mediated reflex increases in sympathetic nervous system activity (*e.g.,* increased heart rate and cardiac output) are blocked. The principal site of action of diazoxide is on arteriolar resistance rather than venous capacitance vessels (Ogilvie and Mikulic, 1972).

Side Effects

Unlike thiazide diuretics, diazoxide causes sodium and water retention which may result in cardiac failure in susceptible patients. This effect may necessitate concomitant administration of a thiazide diuretic. Retention of sodium occurs independently of reductions in glomerular filtration rate and renal blood flow that predictably accompany diazoxide-induced reductions in blood pressure. Diazoxide is a powerful uterine relaxant being capable of stopping labor (Huddleston, 1982). Hyperglycemia can occur 4 to 5 hours after a single intravenous injection reflecting drug-induced alpha-adrenergic agonist-like inhibition of insulin release from the pancreas. Thiazide diuretics may enhance the hyperglycemic effects of diazoxide. Blood glucose concentrations should be monitored daily during chronic use of diazoxide as hyperglycemic, hyperosmolar, nonketoacidotic coma have occurred. Stimulation of catecholamine release prohibits the use of this drug in patients with pheochromocytoma.

DIPYRIDAMOLE

Dipyridamole is administered orally as prophylaxis against angina pectoris although convincing evidence of efficacy is not available (Fig. 16-11). In combination with warfarin, dipyridamole is administered to patients with prosthetic heart valves as prophylaxis against thromboemboli (Moncada and Korbut, 1978). This clinical use reflects the ability of dipyridamole, like aspirin, to inhibit platelet aggregation. Dipyridamole may interfere with platelet function by potentiating the effect of prostacyclin or by inhibiting phosphodiesterase enzyme activity thus increasing intracellular concentrations of cyclic AMP.

    Coronary vascular resistance is decreased while coronary blood flow and oxygen tension in

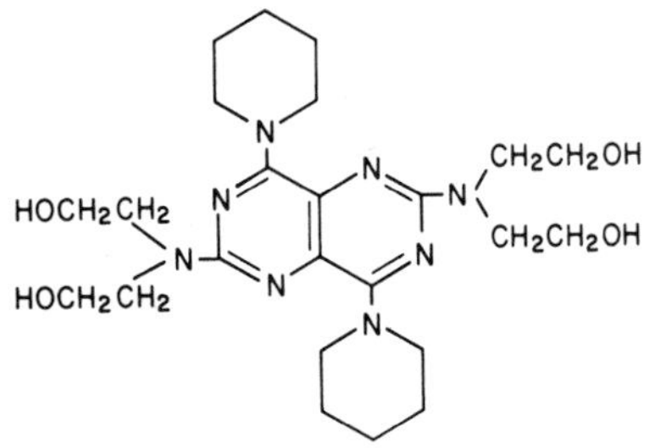

FIGURE 16-11. Dipyridamole.

coronary sinus blood are increased by dipyridamole. The drug appears to act principally on small resistance vessels in the coronary circulation with little effect on resistance to flow in ischemic areas of the myocardium where vessels are already maximally dilated. These actions of dipyridamole are linked to the metabolism and transport of adenosine and adenine nucleotides. Adenosine is released from ischemic myocardium acting as a vasodilator and an important signal for the autoregulation of coronary blood flow (see Chapter 47). Indeed, dipyridamole inhibits cellular uptake of adenosine.

PAPAVERINE

Papaverine is a nonspecific smooth muscle relaxant present in opium but unrelated chemically or pharmacologically to the opioid alkaloids (Fig. 16-12). It is possible that papaverine-induced vasodilatation is related to its ability to inhibit phosphodiesterase leading to an increased intracellular concentration of cyclic AMP. Papaverine has not been demonstrated to be efficacious in any condition.

PURINES

Purines represented by adenosine triphosphate (ATP) and adenine nucleotides are potent vasodilators. For example, ATP is an important endogenous vasodilator involved in the regulation of local blood flow in several vascular beds including the heart and brain (Olsson, 1981). ATP-induced controlled hypotension is characterized by rapid onset and stable level of blood pressure which is promptly reversed when the infusion is discontinued (Sollevi *et al,* 1984). Rapid recovery of blood pressure reflects the 10 to 20 minute elimination

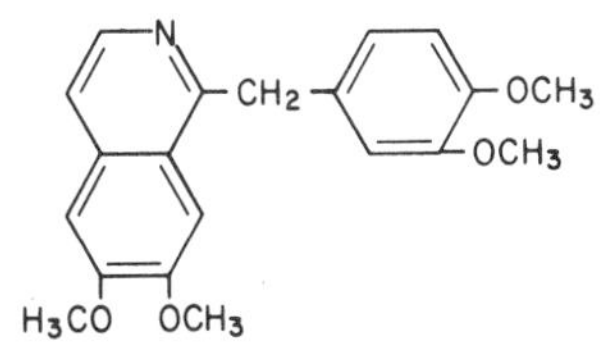

FIGURE 16-12. Papaverine.

half-time of ATP. The necessary dose of ATP can be minimized by pretreatment with an adenosine uptake inhibitor, such as dipyridamole. During controlled hypotension produced by ATP there is a marked reduction in peripheral vascular resistance and a modest increase in heart rate. Cardiac output is enhanced, coronary sinus blood flow is increased, and cardiac filling pressures are maintained suggesting minimal alteration in venous capacitance and venous return to the heart (Bloor *et al,* 1985). Glomerular filtration rate may be reduced by ATP as used to produce controlled hypotension (Osswald *et al,* 1982). The unchanging infusion requirements to maintain constant reductions in blood pressure for as long as 120 minutes confirm the absence of tachyphylaxis. Likewise, plasma concentrations of renin and catecholamines do not increase which is again consistent with unchanging dose requirements (Bloor *et al,* 1985).

REFERENCES

Bastron RD, Kaloyanides GJ. Effect of sodium nitroprusside on function in the isolated and intact dog kidney. J Pharmacol Exp Ther 1972;181:244–9.

Becker LC. Conditions for vasodilator-induced coronary steal in experimental myocardial ischemia. Circulation 1978;57:1103–10.

Berthelsen P, St Haxholdt O, Husum R, Rasmussen JP. PEEP reverses nitroglycerin-induced hypoxemia following coronary artery bypass surgery. Acta Anaesthesiol Scand 1986;30:243–6.

Bloor BC, Fukunaga AF, Ma C, et al. Myocardial hemodyamics during induced hypotension: A comparison between sodium nitroprusside and adenosine triphosphate. Anesthesiology 1985;63:517–25.

Bower PJ, Peterson JN. Methemoglobinemia after sodium nitroprusside therapy. N Engl J Med 1975; 292:865.

Byrick RJ, Hobbs EG, Martineau R, Noble WH. Nitroglycerin relaxes large airways. Anesth Analg 1983;62:421–5.

Casthely PA, Lear S, Cottrell JE, Lear E. Intrapulmonary shunting during induced hypotension. Anesth Analg 1982;61:231–5.

Chatterjee K, Parmley WW, Swan HJC, Berman G, Forrester J, Marcus HS. Beneficial effects of vasodilator agents in severe mitral regurgitation due to dysfunction of subvalvular apparatus. Circulation. 1973;48:684–90.

Chauvin M, Bonnet F, Montembault C, Lafay M, Curet P, Viars P. Hepatic plasma flow during sodium nitroprusside-induced hypotension in humans. Anesthesiology 1985;63:287–93.

Chen RYZ, Matteo RS, Fan F-C, Schuessler GB, Chien S. Resetting of baroreceptor sensitivity after induced hypotension. Anesthesiology 1982;56:29–35.

Chiariello M, Gold HK, Leinbach RC, Davis MA, Maroko PR. Comparison between the effects of nitroprusside and nitroglycerin on ischemic injury during acute myocardial infarction. Circulation 1976;54:766–73.

Colley PS, Cheney FW, Hlastala MP. Ventilation-perfusion and gas exchange effects of sodium nitroprusside in dogs with normal and edematous lungs. Anesthesiology 1979;50:489–95.

Cottrell JE, Casthely P, Brodie JD, Patel K, Klein A, Turndorf H. Prevention of nitroprusside-induced cyanide toxicity with hydroxocobalamin. N Engl J Med 1979;298:809–11.

Cowan C, Duran PVM, Corsini G, et al. The effects of nitroglycerin on myocardial blood flow in man. Am J Cardiol 1969;24:154–60.

Danahy DT, Burwell DT, Aronow WS, Prakash R. Sustained hemodynamic and antianginal effect of high dose oral isosorbide dinitrate. Circulation 1977;55:382–7.

Davies DW, Greiss L, Steward DJ. Sodium nitroprusside in children: Observations on metabolism during normal and abnormal responses. Can Anaesth Soc J 1975;22:553–60.

Delaney TJ, Miller ED. Rebound hypertension after sodium nitroprusside prevented by saralism in rats. Anesthesiology 1980;52:154–6.

Fahmy NR. Nitroglycerin as a hypotensive drug during general anesthesia. Anesthesioloy 1978;49:17–20.

Fahmy NR, Soter NA. Effects of trimethaphan on arterial blood histamine and systemic hemodynamics in humans. Anesthesiology 1985;62:562–6.

Fibuch EE, Cecil WT, Reed WA. Methemoglobinemia associated with organic nitrate therapy. Anesth Analg 1979;58:521–3.

Gagnon RL, Marsh ML, Smith RW, Shapiro HM. Intracranial hypertension caused by nitroglycerin. Anesthesiology 1979;51:86–7.

Gallagher JD, Moore RA, Jose AB, Botros SB, Clark DL. Prophylactic nitroglycerin infusions during coronary artery bypass surgery. Anesthesiology 1986;64:785–9.

Garlin R, Brachfield N, MacLeod C, Bopp P. Effect of nitroglycerin on the coronary circulation in patients with coronary artery disease or increased left ventricular work. Circulation 1959;19:705–18.

Garrett BN, Kaplan NM, Efficacy of slow infusion of diazoxide in treatment of severe hypertension without organ hypoperfusion. Am Heart J 1982; 103:390–4.

Gelman S, Ernst EA. Hepatic circulation during sodium nitroprusside infusion in the dog. Anesthesiology 1978;49:182–7.

Gerson JI, Allen FB, Seltzer JL, Parker FB, Markowitz AH. Arterial and venous dilation by nitroprusside and nitroglycerin—is there a difference? Anesth Analg 1982;61:256–60.

Greenberg H, Dwyer EM, Jameson AG, Dwyer EM, Jameson DG, Pinkernell BH. Effects of nitroglycerin on the major determinants of myocardial oxygen consumption. Am J Cardiol 1975;36:426–32.

Guiha NH, Cohn JN, Franciosa JA, Limas CJ. Treatment of refractory heart failure with infusion of nitroprusside. N Engl J Med 1974;291:587–92.

Harioka T, Hatano Y, Mori K, Toda N. Trimethaphan is a direct arterial vasodilator and an alpha-adrenoceptor antagonist. Anesth Analg 1984;63:290–6.

Horwitz LD, Garlin R, Taylor WJ, Kemp HG. Effects of nitroglycerin on regional myocardial blood flow in coronary artery disease. J Clin Invest 1971; 50:1578–84.

Huddleston JF. Preterm labor. Clin Obstet Gynecol 1982;25:123–36.

Kaplan JA, Dunbar RW, Jones EL. Nitroglycerin infusion during coronary artery surgery. Anesthesiology 1976;45:14–21.

Kaplan JA, Finlayson DC, Woodward S. Vasodilator therapy after cardiac surgery: a review of the efficacy and toxicity of nitroglycerin and nitroprusside. Can Anaesth Soc J 1980;27:154–8.

Khambatta HJ, Stone JG, Khan E. Hypertension during anesthesia on discontinuation of sodium nitroprusside-induced hypotension. Anesthesiology 1979;51:127–30.

Knight PR, Lane GA, Hensinger RN, Bolles RS, Bjoraker DJ. Catecholamine and renin-angiotensin response during hypotensive anesthesia induced by sodium nitroprusside or trimethaphan camsylate. Anesthesiology 1983;59:248–53.

Lewis PE, Cefalo RC, Naulty JS, Rodkey FL. Placental transfer and fetal toxicity of sodium nitroprusside. Gynecol Invest 1977;8:46.

Lichtenthal PR, Rossi EC, Louis G, et al. Dose-related prolongation of the bleeding time by intravenous nitroglycerin. Anesth Analg 1985;64:30–3.

Marsh ML, Aidinis SJ, Naughton KVH, Marshall LF, Shapiro HM. The technique of nitroprusside administration modifies the intracranial pressure response. Anesthesiology 1979;51:538–41.

Marshall WK, Bedford RF, Arnold WP, et al. Effects of propranolol on the cardiovascular and renin-angiotensin systems during hypotension produced by sodium nitroprusside in humans. Anesthesiology 1981;55:277–80.

Michenfelder JD, Theye RA. Canine systemic and cerebral effects of hypotension induced by hemorrhage, trimethaphan, halothane, or nitroprusside. Anesthesiology 1977;46:188–95.

Michenfelder JD, Tinker JH. Cyanide toxicity and thiosulfate protection during chronic administration of sodium nitroprusside in the dog: Correlation with a human case. Anesthesiology 1977;47:441–8.

Miller ED, Ackerly JA, Vaughn ED, Peach MJ, Epstein RM. The renin-angiotensin system during controlled hypotension with sodium nitroprusside. Anesthesiology 1977;47:257–62.

Miller JR, Benumof JL, Trousdale FR. Combined effects of sodium nitroprusside and propranolol on hypoxic pulmonary vasoconstriction. Anesthesiology 1982;57:267–71.

Moncada S, Korbut R. Dipyridamole and other phosphodiesterase inhibitors act as antithrombotic agents by potentiating endogenous prostacyclin. Lancet 1978;1:1286–9.

Moore RA, Geller EA, Gallagher JD, Clark DL. Effect of hypothermic cardiopulmonary bypass on nitroprusside metabolism. Clin Pharmacol Ther 1985;37:680–3.

Noback CR, Tinker JR. Hypothermia after cardiopulmonary bypass in man: amelioration by nitroprusside-induced vasodilation during rewarming. Anesthesiology 1980;53:277–80.

Ogilvie RI, Mikulic E. Effects of diazoxide and ethacrynic acid on sequential vascular segments in the canine gracilis muscle. J Pharmacol Exp Ther 1972;180:368–76.

Olsson RA, Local factors regulating cardiac and skeletal muscle blood flow. Ann Rev Physiol 1981;43:385–95.

Osswald H, Hermes HH, Nabakowski G. Role of adenosine in signal transmission of tubuloglomerular feedback. Kidney Int 1982;22:136–42.

Pearl RG, Rosenthal MH, Ashton JPA. Pulmonary vasodilator effects of nitroglycerin and sodium nitroprusside in canine oleic acid-induced pulmonary hypertension. Anesthesiology 1983;58:514–8.

Pearl RG, Rosenthal MH, Murad F, Ashton JPA. Aminophylline potentiates sodium nitroprusside-induced hypotension in the dog. Anesthesiology 1984;61: 712–3.

Rapoport RM, Murad F. Agonist-induced endothelium-dependent relaxation in rat thoracic aorta may be mediated through cGMP. Circ Res 1983;52:352–7.

Rogers MC, Hamburger C, Owen K, Epstein MH. Intracranial pressure in the cat during nitroglycerin-induced hypotension. Anesthesiology 1979;51: 227–9.

Sivarajan M, Amory DW, McKenzie SM. Regional blood

flows during induced hypotension produced by nitroprusside or trimethaphan in the rhesus monkey. Anesth Analg 1985;64:759 – 66.

Sklar GS, Lanks KW. Effects of trimethaphan and sodium nitroprusside on hydrolysis of succinylcholine in vitro. Anesthesiology 1977;47:31 – 3.

Smith RP. Cyanate and thiocyanate: Acute toxicity. Proc Soc Exp Biol Med 1973;142:1041 – 4.

Smith RP, Kruszyna H. Nitroprusside produces cyanide poisoning via a reaction with hemoglobin. J Pharmacol Exp Ther 1974;191:557 – 63.

Snyder SW, Wheeler AS, James FM. The use of nitroglycerin to control severe hypertension of pregnancy during cesarean section. Anesthesiology 1979;51:563 – 4

Sollevi A, Lagerkranser M, Irestedt L, Gordon E, Lindquist C. Controlled hypotension with adenosine in cerebral aneurysm surgery. Anesthesiology 1984; 61:400 – 5.

Stoelting RK. Attenuation of blood pressure response to laryngoscopy and tracheal intubation with sodium nitroprusside. Anesth Analg 1979;58:116 – 9.

Stoelting RK, Viegas O, Campbell RL. Sodium nitroprusside-produced hypotension during anesthesia and operation in the head-up position. Anesth Analg 1977;56:391 – 4.

Thompson GE, Miller RD, Stevens WC, Murray WR. Hypotensive anesthesia for total hip arthroplasty: A study of blood loss and organ function (brain, heart, liver, and kidney). Anesthesiology 1978;48:91 – 6.

Thomson IR, Mutch WAC, Culligan JD. Failure of intravenous nitroglycerin to prevent intraoperative myocardial ischemia during fentanyl-pancuronium anesthesia. Anesthesiology 1984;61:385 – 93.

Tinker JH, Michenfelder JD. Sodium nitroprusside: Pharmacology, toxicology and therapeutics. Anesthesiology 1976;45:340 – 54.

Tinker JH, Michenfelder JD. Increased resistance to nitroprusside-induced cyanide toxicity in anuric dogs. Anesthesiology 1980;52:40 – 7.

Turner JM, Powell D, Gibson RM, McDowell DG. Intracranial pressure changes in neurosurgical patients during hypotension induced with sodium nitroprusside or trimethaphan. Br J Anaesth 1977;49:419 – 24.

Vesey CJ, Cole PV, Linnell JC, Wilson J. Some metabolic effects of sodium nitroprusside in man. Br Med J 1974;2:140 – 2.

Vesey CJ, Cole PV, Simpson PJ. Cyanide and thiocyanate concentrations following sodium nitroprusside infusion in man. Br J Anaesth 1976;48:651 – 60.

Vickers MD, Schneiden H, Wood-Smith FG. Cardiovascular drugs (trimethaphan camsylate). Drugs in Anaesthesia Practice, 6th edition. London, Butterworths, 1984:344.

Wang HH, Liu LMP, Katz RL. A comparison of the cardiovascular effects of sodium nitroprusside and trimethaphan. Anesthesiology 1977;46:40 – 8.

Wilson L. Leber's hereditary optic atrophy: A possible defect in cyanide metabolism. Clin Sci 1965; 29:505 – 15.

Zurick AM, Wagner RH, Starr NJ, Lytle B, Estafanous FG. Intravenous nitroglycerin, methemoglobinemia, and respiratory distress in a postoperative cardiac surgical patient. Anesthesiology 1984;61:464 – 6.

C H A P T E R   17

Cardiac Antidysrhythmic Drugs

INTRODUCTION

Treatment of cardiac dysrhythmias and disturbances in conduction of the cardiac impulse with antidysrhythmic drugs is based on an understanding of the electrophysiologic basis of the abnormality and the mechanism of action of the therapeutic drug to be employed (see Chapter 48). Even when information is incomplete and the diagnosis uncertain, it is possible to treat most cardiac dysrhythmias and conduction disturbances by applying knowledge gained from prior clinical experience. Indeed, the selection of an antidysrhythmic drug may be empirical with the ultimate choice being determined by which drug proves to be effective with minimal side effects (Gettes, 1971; Kupersmith, 1976; Mason *et al,* 1970).

Patients may be taking antidysrhythmic drugs for chronic suppression of cardiac rhythm disturbances. These drugs pose little threat to the uneventful course of anesthesia and should be continued up to the time of induction of anesthesia.

The majority of cardiac dysrhythmias that occur during anesthesia do not require therapy. Cardiac dysrhythmias, however, do require treatment when (1) they cannot be corrected by removing the precipitating cause, (2) hemodynamic function is compromised, and (3) the disturbance predisposes to more serious cardiac rhythm changes. During the perioperative period, antidysrhythmic drugs are most often administered by the intravenous route.

The mechanism of cardiac dysrhythmias may

be different with or without anesthesia. For example, anesthetic-related cardiac dysrhythmias have been ascribed to abnormal pacemaker activity characterized by suppression of the sinoatrial node with the emergence of latent pacemakers within or below the atrioventricular tissues (Reynolds *et al,* 1970; Reynolds *et al,* 1971). Furthermore, development of reentry circuits is likely to be important in the mechanism of cardiac dysrhythmias that occur during anesthesia. Certainly anesthetics, particularly inhaled drugs, have effects on the specialized conduction system for the cardiac impulse (Atlee and Alexander, 1977; Atlee *et al,* 1978).

CLASSIFICATION

Antidysrhythmic drugs are classified into four groups based on their electrophysiologic effects (Table 17-1). Available drugs differ in their pharmacokinetics, effects on specialized areas of the heart, and efficacy in treating specific types of cardiac dysrhythmias (Tables 17-1 and 17-2) (Singh and Hauswirth, 1974).

Membrane Stabilizers

Membrane stabilizers are divided into two subgroups. The dominant electrophysiologic properties of group Ia drugs (quinidine and procainamide) are related to their ability to block the rapid

Table 17-1

Comparative Electrophysiological Effects and Pharmacokinetics of Cardiac Antidysrhythmic Drugs

	Automaticity (phase 4)	Excitability (phase 0)	Duration of Action Potential	Effective Refractory Period	P-R Interval	QRS Duration	Principal Clearance Mechanism	Protein Binding (%)	Elimination Half-Time (hours)	Therapeutic Plasma Concentration
Membrane Stabilizers										
Group 1a										
Quinidine	D	D	I	I	I	I	Hepatic	70–80	6	2–8 μg ml^{-1}
Procainamide	D	D	I	I	NC,I	I	Renal and hepatic	20	2.5–5	4–12 μg ml^{-1}
Group 1b										
Lidocaine	D	NC,D	D	D	NC	NC	Hepatic	55	1.5	1–5 μg ml^{-1}
Tocainide	D	NC,D	D	D	NC	NC				1–5 μg ml^{-1}
Phenytoin	D	NC,D	D	D	NC,D	NC	Hepatic	>90	24	8–16 μg ml^{-1}
Beta-adrenergic Antagonists										
Propranolol	D	D	I	I	NC,I	NC	Hepatic	90–95	2–4	10–30 ng ml^{-1}
Antiadrenergic Drugs										
Bretylium	NC	NC	I	I	NC,I	NC	Renal	?	13.5	75–100 ng ml^{-1}
Disopyramide	D	D	I	I	NC	NC	Renal	?	7–8	2–4 μg ml
Amiodarone	NC	NC	I	I	I	I	Hepatic	>90	29 days	
Calcium Entry Blockers										
Verapamil	D	NC	D	D	NC,I	NC	Renal	90	3–7 days	100–300 ng ml^{-1}

I—increase; D—decrease; NC—no change

Table 17-2
Efficacy of Antidysrhythmic Drugs for Treatment of Specific Cardiac Dysrhythmias

	Conversion of Atrial Fibrillation	Paroxysmal Supraventricular Tachycardia	Premature Ventricular Contractions	Ventricular Tachycardia
Quinidine	+	++	++	+
Procainamide	+	++	++	++
Lidocaine	0	0	++	++
Phenytoin	0	0	++	++
Propranolol	+	++	+	+
Bretylium	0	0	+	++
Disopyramide	+	++	++	++
Amiodarone	+	++	++	++
Verapamil	+	++	0	0

0—none; +—modest; ++—marked

inward flux of sodium ions during phase 0 depolarization. This effect causes a reduced level of membrane responsiveness and slowed conduction of the cardiac impulse. In addition to slowed conduction of the cardiac impulse, these drugs decrease the rate of spontaneous phase 4 depolarization resulting in reduced automaticity. Group Ia drugs induce a bidirectional block and thus interrupt reentry.

Group Ib drugs (lidocaine, tocainide, phenytoin) decrease automaticity by reducing the rate of spontaneous phase 4 depolarization. Unlike group Ia drugs, however, there is little effect on membrane responsiveness produced by these drugs. As a result, antegrade conduction can take place and thus interrupt reentry.

Quinidine

Quinidine is effective in the treatment of acute and chronic supraventricular dysrhythmias (Fig. 17-1). A frequent indication for quinidine is to prevent recurrence of supraventricular tachydysrhythmias or to suppress ventricular premature contractions. For example, quinidine is often administered to slow the atrial rate in the presence of atrial fibrillation. Indeed, about 25% of patients with atrial fibrillation will convert to normal sinus rhythm when treated with quinidine. Supraventricular tachydysrhythmias associated with Wolff-Parkinson-White syndrome are effectively suppressed by quinidine.

It is common to administer prior digitalis when treating atrial fibrillation with quinidine since an occasional patient will manifest a paradoxical increase in the rate of ventricular response when quinidine is administered. Of interest is an occasional patient in whom a previously stable plasma concentration of digoxin increases dramatically when quinidine is acutely added to the treatment regimen (Leahey *et al,* 1978). Apparently quinidine causes displacement of digoxin from myocardial and peripheral tissue stores. An associated reduction in renal excretion of digoxin is due to a decrease in the renal tubular secretion of digoxin.

Quinidine is most often administered orally in a dose of 300 to 500 mg four times daily. Oral absorption of quinidine is rapid with peak concentrations in the plasma attained in 60 to 90 minutes with an elimination half-time of about 6 hours. The therapeutic blood level of quinidine is 2 to 8 μg ml^{-1}. Intramuscular injection is not recommended because of associated pain at the injection site. The use of intravenous quinidine is limited because peripheral vasodilation and myocardial depression can occur (see the section entitled Side Effects).

MECHANISM OF ACTION. Quinidine is the dextrostereoisomer of quinine and, like quinine, has antimalarial and antipyretic effects. Unlike quinine, however, quinidine has intense effects on the heart. For example, quinidine decreases the

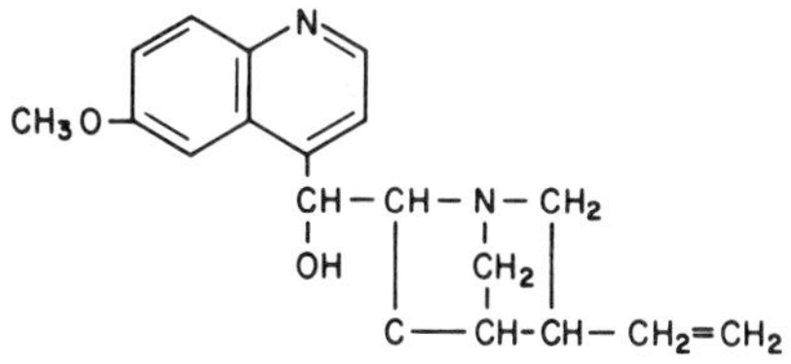

FIGURE 17-1. Quinidine.

slope of phase 4 depolarization explaining its effectiveness in suppressing cardiac dysrhythmias caused by enhanced automaticity. Quinidine increases the fibrillation threshold in atria and ventricles. Quinidine-induced slowing of the conduction of the cardiac impulse through normal and abnormal fibers may be responsible for the ability of quinidine to occasionally convert atrial flutter or fibrillation to normal sinus rhythm. This drug can abolish reentry dysrhythmias by prolonging conduction of the cardiac impulse in an area of injury thus converting one-way conduction blockade to two-way conduction blockade. Reduction of atrial rate during atrial flutter or fibrillation may reflect slowed conduction velocity and/or prolonged effective refractory period in the atria.

METABOLISM AND EXCRETION. Quinidine is hydroxylated in the liver to inactive metabolites which are excreted in the urine (Table 17-1). About 20% of quinidine is excreted unchanged in the urine. Enzyme induction significantly shortens the duration of action of quinidine (Data *et al,* 1976). As a result of its dependence on renal excretion and hepatic metabolism for clearance from the body, accumulation of quinidine or its metabolites may occur in the presence of impaired function of these organs.

About 70% to 80% of quinidine in plasma is bound to albumin. Quinidine accumulates rapidly in most tissues except the brain.

SIDE EFFECTS. Quinidine has a low therapeutic ratio and side effects are predictable if the plasma concentration of quinidine becomes excessive. As the plasma concentration increases above 2 μg ml^{-1}, the P–R interval, QRS complex, and Q–T interval on the electrocardiogram are prolonged emphasizing the importance of the electrocardiogram for monitoring patients being treated with quinidine (Table 17-1). A 50% increase in the duration of the QRS complex requires a reduction in dosage of quinidine or heart block may ensue. Occasionally, uniquely susceptible patients being treated with quinidine experience syncope or sudden death despite low plasma concentrations of drug. Quinidine syncope may reflect the occurrence of ventricular dysrhythmias due to delayed intraventricular conduction of the cardiac impulse (Selzer and Wray, 1964). Persons with a preexisting prolongation of the Q–T interval or evidence of atrioventricular heart block on the electrocardiogram should not be treated with quinidine (Koster and Wellens, 1976).

Quinidine can cause significant hypotension, particularly if administered intravenously. This response most likely reflects peripheral vasodilation from alpha-adrenergic blockade. High plasma concentrations depress myocardial contractility, and this is further accentuated by hyperkalemia.

Patients in normal sinus rhythm treated with quinidine may show an increase in heart rate which presumably is due either to an anticholinergic action and/or a reflex increase in sympathetic nervous system activity. This atropine-like action of quinidine opposes its direct depressant actions on the sinoatrial and atrioventricular node.

Fever may accompany administration of quinidine and disappears when the drug is withdrawn. Thrombocytopenia is a rare occurrence that is due to drug-platelet complexes that evoke production of antibodies. Discontinuation of quinidine results in return of the platelet count to normal in 2 to 7 days. Nausea, vomiting, and diarrhea occur in about one third of treated patients.

Like other cinchona alkaloids and salicylates, quinidine can cause cinchonism. Symptoms of cinchonism include tinnitus, decreased hearing acuity, blurring of vision, and gastrointestinal upset. In severe cases, there may be abdominal pain and mental confusion.

Since quinidine is an alpha-adrenergic blocking drug, it can interact in an additive manner with drugs that cause vasodilation. For example, nitroglycerin can cause orthostatic hypotension in patients being treated with quinidine.

Quinidine interferes with normal neuromuscular transmission and may accentuate the effect of neuromuscular blocking drugs (Harrah *et al,* 1970) (see Chapter 8). Recurrence of skeletal muscle paralysis in the immediate postoperative period has been observed in association with the administration of quinidine (Way *et al,* 1967).

Procainamide

Procainamide has similar therapeutic uses as quinidine (Table 17-2). Premature ventricular contractions and paroxysmal ventricular tachycardia are suppressed in most patients within a few minutes after intravenous administration. The effectiveness of procainamide against atrial dysrhythmias is comparable to that of quinidine.

Procainamide, 3 to 6 grams, is effectively absorbed following oral administration reaching peak concentrations in 45 to 75 minutes. The plasma concentration of procainamide associated with antidysrhythmic effects is 4 to 12 μg ml^{-1}. The probability of toxicity becomes greater when the plasma concentration of procainamide increases above 8 μg ml^{-1}. Intramuscular and intravenous routes of administration of procainamide are acceptable. For example, procainamide can be administered in doses of 1.5 mg kg^{-1} over 1 minute and repeated every 5 minutes until the cardiac dysrhythmia is controlled or the total dose reaches about 15 mg kg^{-1} (never more than 1000 mg). The total loading dose is never given as a single intravenous injection because it can cause hypotension. When the cardiac dysrhythmia is controlled, a constant rate of intravenous infusion is used to maintain a therapeutic plasma concentration of procainamide. Although procainamide and quinidine have a broader spectrum of antidysrhythmic effects than lidocaine (*e.g.*, useful in treatment of supraventricular and ventricular cardiac dysrhythmias), they are rarely used during anesthesia because of their propensity to produce hypotension.

MECHANISM OF ACTION. Procainamide differs from procaine only by replacement of the ester linkage by an amide (Fig. 17-2; see Fig. 7-2). This structural change provides a longer duration of action and increased cardiac effects relative to local anesthetic actions and actions on the central nervous system. In fact, procainamide is relatively ineffective in producing conduction blockade in nerve fibers.

Effects of procainamide on the electrical activity of the heart as manifested on the electrocardiogram are similar to quinidine (Table 17-1). The presence of preexisting abnormalities of conduction of the cardiac impulse increases the likelihood that procainamide will cause further conduction delay. Compared with quinidine, the anticholinergic action of procainamide is less, and this drug does not produce alpha-adrenergic blockade.

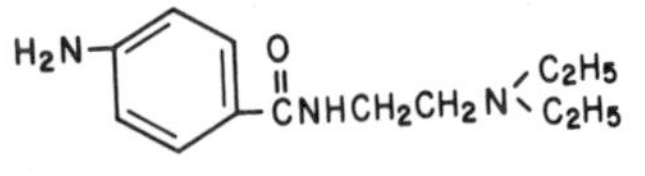

METABOLISM AND EXCRETION. Procainamide is eliminated by renal excretion and hepatic metabolism (Table 17-1) (Galiazzi *et al*, 1976). In humans, 40% to 60% of procainamide is excreted unchanged by the kidneys. In the liver, the remaining procainamide is acetylated to N-acetyl procainamide (NAPA), which is also eliminated by the kidneys. This metabolite is cardioactive and probably contributes to the antidysrhythmic effects of procainamide. In the presence of renal failure, plasma concentrations of NAPA may reach dangerous levels. Eventually, 90% of an administered dose of procainamide is recovered as unchanged drug or its metabolites.

The activity of the N-acetyltransferase enzyme responsible for the acetylation of procainamide is genetically determined (Reidenberg *et al*, 1975). In fast acetylators, the elimination half-time of procainamide is 2.5 hours compared with 5 hours in slow acetylators. The blood level of NAPA exceeds that of procainamide in rapid, but not slow acetylators.

Unlike its analogue procaine, procainamide is highly resistant to hydrolysis by plasma cholinesterase. Indeed, only 2% to 10% of an administered dose of procainamide is recovered unchanged in the urine as para-aminobenzoic acid.

Only about 20% of procainamide is bound to plasma proteins. Despite this limited binding in plasma, procainamide is avidly bound to tissue proteins with the exception of brain.

SIDE EFFECTS. The incidence of side effects is high when procainamide is used as an antidysrhythmic drug. Rapid intravenous injection of procainamide can cause hypotension while higher plasma concentrations slow conduction of the cardiac impulse through the atrioventricular node and intraventricular conduction system. Indeed, ventricular asystole or fibrillation may occur when procainamide is administered in the presence of heart block as associated with digitalis toxicity (Zapata-Diaz *et al*, 1952). Direct myocardial depression that occurs at high plasma concentrations

FIGURE 17-2. Procainamide.

of procainamide is exaggerated by hyperkalemia. As with quinidine, ventricular dysrhythmias may accompany excessive plasma concentrations of procainamide.

A syndrome resembling systemic lupus erythematosus most often manifesting as arthralgia and hepatomegaly may accompany chronic but not acute therapy with procainamide (Ladd, 1962). Antinuclear antibodies are present, and the LE cell preparation is often positive. Slow acetylators are more prone than rapid acetylators to develop these antinuclear antibodies. Symptoms disappear when procainamide is discontinued.

Fever may force the discontinuation of procainamide therapy. Agranulocytosis may occur in the early weeks of therapy emphasizing the need for monitoring periodically complete blood counts.

Gastrointestinal irritation is less frequent than observed during administration of quinidine. Central nervous system symptoms can occur but are less likely than when patients are treated with lidocaine.

Flecainide

Flecainide is a fluorinated local anesthetic analogue of procainamide that is effective in suppression of nonsustained ventricular dysrhythmias in patients with normal or nearly normal left ventricular function (Roden and Woosley, 1986a). Conversely, patients with recurrent sustained ventricular tachycardia or ventricular fibrillation may experience an exacerbation of their dysrhythmia when treated with this drug. In contrast to procainamide, flecainide prolongs the duration of the P-R and QRS intervals on the electrocardiogram. These changes suggest the possibility of atrioventricular or infranodal conduction block of the cardiac impulse. Furthermore, flecainide may depress sinus node function in a manner similar to that of calcium channel blocking drugs. Pacing threshold is increased emphasizing caution in the use of this drug in patients with artificial cardiac pacemakers.

Oral absorption of flecainide is excellent, and prolonged elimination half-time makes a twice daily dose of 100 to 200 mg acceptable. About 25% of flecainide is excreted unchanged by the kidney, and the remainder appears as weakly active metabolites. Vertigo and difficulty in visual accommodation are common dose-related side effects of flecainide therapy.

Lidocaine

Lidocaine is used principally for suppression of ventricular dysrhythmias having minimal effects on supraventricular dysrhythmias (Table 17-2; see Fig. 7-2). This drug is particularly effective in suppressing reentry dysrhythmias such as premature ventricular contractions and ventricular tachycardia (Table 17-2).

Rapid intravenous administration of lidocaine, 1.0 to 1.5 mg kg^{-1}, provides antidysrhythmic effects lasting 15 to 60 minutes. This short duration of action is related to rapid tissue redistribution and metabolism of lidocaine. Maintenance of a therapeutic plasma lidocaine concentration of 1 to 5 μg ml^{-1} following a single initial intravenous injection is most often achieved by the continuous intravenous infusion of 15 to 60 μg kg^{-1} min^{-1}. Decreased hepatic blood flow, as produced by anesthetics, shock, or congestive heart failure, may decrease by 50% the rate of intravenous infusion of lidocaine necessary to maintain therapeutic plasma levels (Nies *et al*, 1976).

Advantages of lidocaine compared with quinidine and procainamide include a more rapid onset and prompt disappearance of effects when the continuous intravenous infusion is terminated. This permits moment to moment titration of the infusion rate necessary to produce an antidysrhythmic effect. Lidocaine for intravenous injection differs from that used for local anesthesia by not containing a preservative.

Lidocaine is well absorbed after oral administration but is subject to extensive first-pass hepatic metabolism (Boyes *et al*, 1971). Indeed, only about one third of the drug reaches the circulation resulting in low and often unpredictable plasma concentrations.

Intramuscular absorption of lidocaine is nearly complete. In an emergency situation, an intramuscular dose of lidocaine, 4 to 5 mg kg^{-1}, will produce a therapeutic plasma concentration in about 15 minutes, and this level is maintained for about 90 minutes (Lie *et al*, 1978).

MECHANISM OF ACTION. Lidocaine delays the rate of spontaneous phase 4 depolarization by preventing or diminishing the gradual decrease in potassium permeability that normally occurs during this phase (Table 17-1). Higher doses of lidocaine result in slowing of phase 0 depolarization (the rapid spike phase). This effect is presumably due to inhibition of inward movement of sodium ions across membranes of cardiac cells. This is similar to the effect that produces conduction blockade (*e.g.,* local anesthesia) in peripheral nerves (see Chapter 7). Lidocaine reduces the disparity in the duration of action potentials in normal (shortens refractory period) and ischemic (prolongs refractory period) myocardial cells and thus improves the chances of a uniform spread of depolarization through the myocardium (Kupersmith, 1976). Retrograde conduction is inhibited, and reentry fails to occur.

Effectiveness of lidocaine in suppressing premature ventricular contractions reflects its ability to decrease the rate of spontaneous phase 4 depolarization. Ineffectiveness of lidocaine against supraventricular dysrhythmias presumably reflects its inability to alter the rate of spontaneous phase 4 depolarization in atrial cardiac cells.

METABOLISM AND EXCRETION. Metabolites of lidocaine may possess antidysrhythmic activity (see Chapter 7).

SIDE EFFECTS. Lidocaine is essentially devoid of effects on the electrocardiogram or cardiovascular system when the plasma concentration remains below 5 μg ml^{-1}. For example, in contrast to quinidine and procainamide, lidocaine does not alter the duration of the QRS complex on the electrocardiogram and activity of the sympathetic nervous system is not changed (Table 17-1). Toxic plasma concentrations of lidocaine (greater than 5 – 10 μg ml^{-1}) produce peripheral vasodilation and direct myocardial depression with resulting hypotension. In addition, slowing of conduction of the cardiac impulse manifests as bradycardia and a prolonged P – R interval and widened QRS complex on the electrocardiogram.

The principal side effects of lidocaine are on the central nervous system. Stimulation of the central nervous system occurs in a dose-related manner with symptoms appearing when the plasma concentrations of lidocaine exceed 5 μg ml^{-1}. Seizures are possible at plasma concentrations of lidocaine of 5 to 10 μg ml^{-1}. Central nervous system depression, apnea, and cardiac arrest are possible when plasma concentrations of lidocaine exceed 10 μg ml^{-1}. The convulsive threshold for lidocaine is reduced during arterial hypoxemia, hyperkalemia, or acidosis emphasizing the importance of monitoring these parameters during continuous intravenous infusion of li-

docaine to patients for suppression of cardiac dysrhythmias.

Tocainide

Tocainide is an orally effective amine analogue of lidocaine that is used for the suppression of symptomatic ventricular dysrhythmias (Fig. 17-3) (Roden and Woosley, 1986b). The addition of the amine side-group enables tocainide to avoid significant hepatic first-pass metabolism that limits the effectiveness of orally administered lidocaine. The usual daily adult maintenance dose is 800 to 2200 mg in three divided doses.

MECHANISM OF ACTION. Electrophysiologically, tocainide is similar to lidocaine, producing decreases in the effective refractory period and duration of the action potential with an unchanged QRS complex on the electrocardiogram (Table 17-1).

METABOLISM AND EXCRETION. Absorption of tocainide from the gastrointestinal tract is rapid and complete. About 40% of the drug is excreted unchanged in the urine, and the remainder undergoes hepatic metabolism to inactive metabolites. Therapeutic plasma concentrations are 3 to 10 μg ml^{-1}, and the elimination half-time is 6 to 8 hours.

SIDE EFFECTS. A modest negative inotropic effect accompanies use of this drug and there is a potential for aggravating cardiac failure. Headache, tremor, paresthesia, dizziness, and gastrointestinal irritation are not infrequent and may become intolerable to the patient. It is possible that lidocaine, as administered intravenously in the perioperative period to treat cardiac dysrhythmias or provide additional protection against noxious stimulation, would have an additive effect with circulating tocainide.

Phenytoin

Phenytoin is particularly effective 'n suppression of ventricular dysrhythmias associated with digitalis toxicity (Table 17-2) (see Fig. 30-1) (Atkinson and Davison, 1974). This drug is not effective in suppression of atrial tachycardia or fibrillation. Phenytoin should be administered orally or by intermittent intravenous injection. Intramuscular

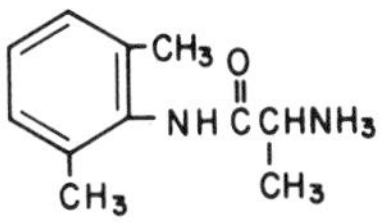

FIGURE 17-3. Tocainide.

absorption is too unreliable to treat cardiac dysrhythmias. The intravenous dose is 1.5 mg kg^{-1} every 5 minutes until the cardiac dysrhythmia is controlled or 10 to 15 mg kg^{-1} (maximum 1000 mg) have been administered (Bigger *et al,* 1968).

MECHANISM OF ACTION. The effects of phenytoin on automaticity and velocity of conduction of the cardiac impulse resemble lidocaine (Table 17-1) (Caracta *et al,* 1973). Like lidocaine, phenytoin has little effect on the electrocardiogram. Conduction through the atrioventricular node is improved, but activity of the sinus node may be depressed. The possible interaction with volatile anesthetics that also depress the sinoatrial node should be remembered if consideration is given to administering phenytoin during general anesthesia (see Chapter 2).

METABOLISM AND EXCRETION. Phenytoin is hydroxylated and then conjugated with glucuronic acid for excretion in the urine (see Chapter 30). The elimination half-time is about 24 hours.

SIDE EFFECTS. The most prominent effects of phenytoin during acute treatment of cardiac dysrhythmias are on the central nervous system. Symptoms of central nervous system toxicity include nystagmus, sedation, and ataxia. Neurological symptoms are usually indicative of plasma concentrations of phenytoin in excess of 20 μg ml^{-1}. Cardiac dysrhythmias that have not been suppressed at this concentration are unlikely to favorably respond to further increases in the dosage of phenytoin (Bigger *et al,* 1968).

Encainide

Encainide is a unique antidysrhythmic drug that combines the electrophysiologic effects of quinidine and lidocaine to suppress ventricular cardiac dysrhythmias. In contrast to quinidine, encainide has no consistent effect on the peripheral vasculature so alterations in blood pressure are uncommon after oral or intravenous administration. En-

cainide is rapidly absorbed following oral administration, and metabolism in the liver is rapid with an elimination half-time of about 2 hours. Despite this rapid elimination half-time the dosing interval is 6 hours reflecting the wide margin between therapeutic and toxic plasma concentrations and the likely presence of active metabolites. Side effects associated with chronic oral therapy include headache, dizziness, ataxia, and nausea.

Beta-Adrenergic Antagonists

Beta-adrenergic antagonists depress both automaticity and conduction of the cardiac impulse, with the latter effect being highly dependent on the degree of underlying sympathetic nervous system activity. At very high doses, certain beta-adrenergic antagonists, such as propranolol, also exhibit membrane depressant actions.

Propranolol

Propranolol is used principally to slow the ventricular response to atrial fibrillation or paroxysmal supraventricular tachycardia (Table 17-2) (see Fig. 14-3) (Nies and Shand, 1975). Premature ventricular contractions are also suppressed by propranolol. It is a useful drug for suppression in the prolonged Q – T interval syndrome. Propranolol abolishes ventricular dysrhythmias induced by digitalis, but it is associated with a greater incidence of side effects than are lidocaine or phenytoin.

Propranolol is given orally for long-term treatment of cardiac dysrhythmias. For emergency use, propranolol can be given intravenously during monitoring of the electrocardiogram and blood pressure. The usual intravenous dose of propranolol is 15 to 45 μg kg^{-1} to a total dose of 1 to 3 mg. The therapeutic plasma concentration of propranolol may vary from 10 to 30 ng ml^{-1}. The elimination half-time of propranolol is 2 to 4 hours, although the duration of antidysrhythmic activity usually persists for 6 to 8 hours.

MECHANISM OF ACTION. Antidysrhythmic effects of beta-adrenergic antagonists most likely reflect blockade of responses of beta receptors in the heart to sympathetic nervous system stimulation and circulating catecholamines. As a result, the rate of spontaneous phase 4 depolarization is decreased and the rate of sinoatrial discharge is reduced (Table 17-1). The electrical threshold of the atria and ventricles is minimally altered by propranolol. There is a substantial increase in the effective refractory period of the atrioventricular node due to beta-adrenergic receptor blockade. Reentry dysrhythmias are prevented by an increase in the refractoriness of the atrioventricular node.

In addition to beta-adrenergic blockade, propranolol causes alterations in the electrical activity of myocardial cells. This cell membrane effect is probably responsible for some of the antidysrhythmic effects of propranolol. Indeed, dextropropranolol, which lacks beta-adrenergic antagonist activity, is an effective antidysrhythmic.

METABOLISM AND EXCRETION. Orally administered propranolol is extensively metabolized in the liver, and a first-pass hepatic effect is responsible for the variation in plasma concentration of propranolol (see Chapter 14). The primary metabolite of propranolol is 4-hydroxypropranolol which possesses beta-adrenergic antagonist activity (Nies and Shand, 1975). This active metabolite most likely contributes to the antidysrhythmic activity following oral administration of propranolol.

SIDE EFFECTS. Propranolol often prolongs the P–R interval with a minimal effect on the QRS complex and Q–T interval recorded on the electrocardiogram (Table 17-1). In patients with chronic cardiac failure, a high level of sympathetic nervous system activity is essential for cardiac support. Treatment of cardiac dysrhythmias in these patients with propranolol reduces this vital compensatory mechanism and can result in accentuation of cardiac failure. The use of propranolol in the presence of preexisting atrioventricular blockade is not recommended.

Antiadrenergic Drugs

Antiadrenergic drugs (bretylium, disopyramide, amiodarone) that increase the duration of the action potential in ventricular and Purkinje fibers are effective in treating ventricular cardiac dysrhythmias. Absence of this effect on the duration of the action potential of atrial muscle is consistent with the ineffectiveness of these drugs in treating supraventricular cardiac dysrhythmias.

Bretylium

Bretylium is uniquely effective in the treatment of ventricular tachycardia and ventricular fibrillation (Table 17-2) (Fig. 17-4) (Hissenbuttel and Bigger, 1979). The usual intravenous dose is 5 to 10 mg kg^{-1}, and the duration of action is 8 to 24 hours. The most striking electrophysiologic effect of bretylium is prolongation of the ventricular action potential and refractory period explaining the effectiveness of this drug in suppressing ventricular dysrhythmias (Bigger and Jaffe, 1971). Bretylium initially causes the release of norepinephrine from postganglionic sympathetic nerve endings which can transiently lead to hypertension. Ultimately, the presence of bretylium in nerve endings prevents the release of norepinephrine and may lead to orthostatic hypotension and bradycardia.

The average elimination half-time of bretylium is 13.5 hours, which is directly related to renal clearance (Table 17-1). About 70% of the drug is excreted unchanged in the urine in the first 24 hours, and by 48 hours, 98% of the initially injected drug is recovered. Hepatic metabolism has not been demonstrated for bretylium. Prolonged and/or cumulative effects are predictable when bretylium is administered to patients with impaired renal function.

Disopyramide

Disopyramide is effective in the control of atrial and ventricular cardiac dysrhythmias (Table 17-2) (Fig. 17-5) (Luoma *et al*, 1978). The oral dose is 100 to 200 mg administered four times daily. About 90% of an oral dose is absorbed with peak plasma concentrations occurring in 1 to 2 hours. The elimination half-time is 7 to 8 hours.

Disopyramide resembles quinidine with respect to effects on the duration of the cardiac ac-

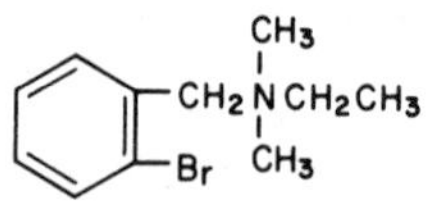

FIGURE 17-4. Bretylium.

FIGURE 17-5. Disopyramide.

tion potential and membrane responsiveness (Danilo and Rosen, 1976). There is little change in heart rate, and changes in the P–R interval, QRS complex, and Q–T interval on the electrocardiogram are less than observed with quinidine (Table 17-1).

About 50% of disopyramide is excreted unchanged by the kidney (Hinderling and Garrett, 1976). As a result, the elimination half-time is greatly prolonged in the presence of renal disease. A dealkylated metabolite with less antidysrhythmic and atropine-like activity than the parent compound accounts for about 20% of the drug.

The anticholinergic action of disopyramide produces a substantial incidence of dry mouth, blurred vision, and occasionally urinary retention. The potential for direct myocardial depression, especially in patients with preexisting left ventricular dysfunction, seems to be greater with this drug than with quinidine and procainamide (Jensen *et al*, 1975).

Amiodarone

Amiodarone is administered for the prevention of (1) recurrent paroxysmal supraventricular tachydysrhythmias such as atrial fibrillation that may accompany Wolff-Parkinson-White syndrome, and (2) recurrent ventricular tachycardia or ventricular fibrillation (Table 17-2) (Heger *et al*, 1981; Marcus *et al*, 1981). The usual daily adult oral dose is 3 to 5 mg kg^{-1}. The onset of action after an oral dose is slow, and full antidysrhythmic effects may not occur for several days. Administered intravenously over 2 to 5 minutes, a dose of 5 mg kg^{-1} produces a prompt antidysrhythmic effect that lasts up to 4 hours (Marcus *et al*, 1981).

Upon discontinuation, the therapeutic effects of amiodarone may persist for prolonged periods. Indeed, chronic oral administration of amiodarone results in an elimination half-time of 29 days (Fig. 17-6) (Kannan *et al*, 1982). This is the long-est elimination half-time of any antidysrhythmic drug. A pharmacologic effect of amiodarone lasts more than 45 days after its discontinuation.

MECHANISM OF ACTION. Amiodarone is a benzofurane derivative with a chemical structure that resembles thyroxine (Fig. 17-7). Like bretylium, amiodarone prolongs the duration of the action potential of atrial and ventricular muscle without altering the resting membrane potential, in effect delaying repolarization (Table 17-1). The effective refractory period is increased. Amiodarone depresses sinoatrial and atrioventricular nodal function and slows conduction of the cardiac impulse through the atrioventricular node. In most patients with the Wolff-Parkinson-White syndrome, amiodarone increases the refractory period of the accessory pathway accounting for the efficacy of this drug in the management of patients with this disorder (Rowland and Krikler, 1980).

FIGURE 17-6. Following discontinuation of amiodarone, the plasma concentration declines slowing resulting in an elimination half-time of 29 days. (From Kannan R, Nademanee K, Hendrickson JA, Rostami HJ, Singh BN. Amiodarone kinetics after oral doses. Clin Pharmacol Ther 1982;31:438–44. Reproduced by permission of the authors and publisher.)

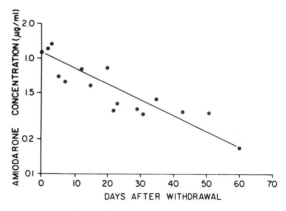

FIGURE 17-7. Amiodarone.

Amiodarone acts as an effective anti-anginal drug by dilating coronary arteries and increasing coronary blood flow. Anti-adrenergic effects of amiodarone most likely reflect noncompetitive blockade of alpha- and beta-adrenergic receptors.

METABOLISM AND EXCRETION. Amiodarone is minimally dependent on renal excretion as reflected by an unchanged elimination half-time in the absence of renal function (Kannan *et al*, 1982). It is not known if the metabolite, desmethylamiodarone, has any pharmacologic effects. Protein binding of the drug is extensive. There is an inconsistent relationship between the plasma concentration of amiodarone and its pharmacologic effects.

SIDE EFFECTS. Side effects of amiodarone are dose-dependent becoming most likely when the total daily dose exceeds 200 mg (Heger *et al*, 1981). Depressant effects on the heart are alleged to be minimal although an animal study suggests amiodarone is a direct myocardial depressant (MacKinnon *et al*, 1983). The heart rate often slows, and the Q – T interval on the electrocardiogram is prolonged. Heart rate slowing is resistant to the effects of atropine, and responsiveness to catecholamine and sympathetic nervous system stimulation is reduced by virtue of drug-induced inhibition of alpha- and beta-adrenergic receptors. Anti-adrenergic effects of amiodarone may be enhanced in the presence of general anesthesia manifesting as sinus arrest, atrioventricular heart block, low cardiac output, or hypotension. Drugs which inhibit automaticity of the sinoatrial node such as halothane and lidocaine could accentuate the effects of amiodarone and increase the likelihood of sinus arrest. The potential need for a temporary artificial cardiac (ventricular) pacemaker and administration of sympathomimetics such as isoproterenol should be considered in patients being treated with this drug and scheduled to undergo surgery (Liberman and Teasdale, 1985; Navalgund *et al*, 1986). Amiodarone may act as a coronary artery and peripheral vascular vasodilator. Indeed, intravenous administration of amiodarone may result in hypotension and atrioventricular heart block. Diffuse pulmonary fibrosis and neurologic abnormalities including proximal skeletal muscle weakness, gait abnormalities, tremor, and peripheral neuropathies have been reported (Heger *et al*, 1981).

Chronic amiodarone therapy is associated with an alteration in thyroid function causing either hypothyroidism or hyperthyroidism in 2% to 4% of patients (Jonckheer *et al*, 1973). Hyperthyroidism has occurred up to 5 months after discontinuation of amiodarone. Patients with preexisting thyroid dysfunction seem more likely to develop amiodarone related alterations in thyroid function.

Corneal microdeposits occur after several weeks in many patients, but visual impairment is unlikely. Photosensitivity and rash develop in up to 10% of patients. Rarely, there may be a cyanotic discoloration of the face that persists even after the drug is discontinued. Transient, mild elevations in plasma transaminase enzyme concentrations are common, and fatty liver infiltration has been observed (Heger *et al*, 1981). Amiodarone displaces digoxin from protein binding sites and may increase its plasma concentration as much as 70% (Moysey *et al*, 1981).

Calcium Entry Blockers

Group 4 drugs are the calcium entry blockers that specifically inhibit inward passage of calcium ions across the cardiac cell membranes (see Chapter 18).

Verapamil

Verapamil is uniquely effective in the suppression of reentrant supraventricular tachydysrhythmias (Table 17-2) (see Fig. 18-1). The usual intravenous dose of verapamil is 75 to 150 μg kg^{-1} infused over 1 to 3 minutes followed by a continuous infusion of about 5 μg kg^{-1} min^1 to maintain a sustained effect.

The oral dose of verapamil required for antidysrhythmic activity is about ten times the intravenous dose, emphasizing the extensive first-pass hepatic effect that occurs. The duration of action is 4 to 6 hours, which correlates with the elimination half-time of 3 to 7 hours (Table 17-1).

MECHANISM OF ACTION. Verapamil slows the rate of spontaneous phase 4 depolarization in sinoatrial and atrioventricular nodal tissue (Table 17-1). The action of verapamil on phase 4 depolarization is related to inhibition of the inward flux of calcium ions. In addition, the duration of the cardiac action potential and repolarization are shortened by verapamil. Calcium entry blockers are relatively ineffective in suppressing ectopic pace-maker activity of ventricular automatic cells.

METABOLISM AND EXCRETION. An estimated 70% of an injected dose of verapamil is eliminated by the kidneys while up to 15% may be present in the bile. A metabolite, norverapamil, may contribute to the parent drug's antidysrhythmic effects.

SIDE EFFECTS. Side effects of verapamil as used to treat cardiac dysrhythmias reflect extensions of the drug's pharmacologic effects (see Chapter 18). Atrioventricular heart block is more likely in patients with preexisting defects in the conduction of the cardiac impulse. Direct myocardial depression and reduced cardiac output are likely to be exaggerated in patients with poor left ventricular function. Peripheral vasodilation may contribute to hypotension. There may be potentiation of anesthetic-produced myocardial depression and effects of neuromuscular blocking drugs may be exaggerated (see Chapter 18).

REFERENCES

Atkinson AJ, Davison R. Diphenylhydantoin as an antiarrhythmic drug. Annu Rev Med 1974;25:99–113.

Atlee JL, Alexander SC. Halothane effects on conductivity of the AV node and His-Purkinje system in the dog. Anesth Analg 1977;56:378–86.

Atlee JL, Rusy BF, Kreul JF, Eby T. Supraventricular excitability in dogs during anesthesia with halothane and enflurane. Anesthesiology 1978;49:407–13.

Bigger JT, Jaffe CC. The effect of bretylium tosylate on the electrophysiological properties of ventricular muscle and Purkinje fibers. Am J Cardiol 1971;27:82–92.

Bigger JT, Schmidt DH, Kutt H. Relationship between the plasma level of diphenylhydantoin sodium and its cardiac antiarrhythmic effects. Circulation 1968;38:363–74.

Boyes RN, Scott DB, Jebson PJ, Goodman MJ, Julian DG. Pharmacokinetics of lidocaine in man. Clin Pharmacol Ther 1971;12:105–16.

Caracta AR, Damato AN, Josephson ME, Ricciutti MA, Gallagher JJ, Lau SH. Electrophysiologic properties of diphenylhydantoin. Circulation 1973;47:1234–41.

Danilo P, Rosen MR. Cardiac effects of disopyramide. Am Heart J 1976;92:532–6.

Data JL, Wilkinson GR, Nies AS. Interaction of quinidine with anticonvulsant drugs. N Engl J Med 1976;294:699–702.

Galiazzi RL, Sheiner LB, Lockwood T, Benet LZ. The renal elimination of procainamide. Clin Pharm Ther 1976;19:55–62.

Gettes LS. The electrophysiologic effects of antiarrhythmic drugs. Am J Cardiol 1971;28:526–35.

Harrah MD, Way WL, Katzung BG. The interaction of d-tubocurarine with antiarrhythmic drugs. Anesthesiology 1970;33:406–10.

Heger JJ, Prystowsky EN, Jackman WM, et al. Amiodarone. Clinical efficacy and electrophysiology during long-term therapy for recurrent ventricular tachycardia or ventricular fibrillation. N Engl J Med 1981;305:539–45.

Hinderling PH, Garrett ER. Pharmacokinetics of the antiarrhythmic disopyramide in healthy humans. J Pharmacokinet Biopharm 1976;4:199–230.

Hissenbuttel RH, Bigger JT. Bretylium tosylate: A newly available antiarrhythmic drug for ventricular arrhythmias. Ann Intern Med 1979;90:229–38.

Jensen G, Sigurd B, Uhrenholt A. Hemodynamic effects of intravenous disopyramide in heart failure. Eur J Clin Pharmacol 1975;8:167–73.

Jonckheer MH, Blockx P, Kawers R, Wyffels G. Hyperthyroidism as a possible complication of the treatment of ischemic heart disease with amiodarone. Acta Cardiol 1973;28:192–200.

Kannan R, Nademanee K, Hendrickson JA, Rostami HJ, Singh BN. Amiodarone kinetics after oral doses. Clin Pharmacol Ther 1982;31:438–44.

Koster RW, Wellens HJJ. Quinidine-induced ventricular flutter and fibrillation without digitalis therapy. Am J Cardiol 1976;38:519–23.

Kupersmith J. Antiarrhythmic drugs. Changing concepts. Am J Cardiol 1976;38:119–21.

Ladd AT. Procainamide-induced lupus erythematosus. N Engl J Med 1962;267:1357–8.

Leahey EB, Reiffel JA, Drusin RE, Hissenbuttel RH, Lovejoy WP, Bigger JT. Interaction between quinidine and digoxin. JAMA 1978;240:533–4.

Liberman BA, Teasdale SJ. Anaesthesia and amiodarone. Can Anaesth Soc J 1985;32:629–38.

Lie KI, Liem KL, Louridtz WJ, Janse MJ, Willebrands AF, Durrer D. Efficacy of lidocaine in preventing primary ventricular fibrillation within one hour after a 300 mg intramuscular injection. Am J Cardiol 1978;42:486–8.

Luoma PV, Kujala PA, Juustila HJ, Takkunen JT. Efficacy of intravenous disopyramide in the termination of supraventricular arrhythmias. J Clin Pharmacol 1978;18:293–301.

MacKinnon G, Landymore R, Marble A. Should oral amiodarone be used for sustained ventricular tachycardia in patients requiring open-heart surgery? Can J Surg 1983;26:355–7.

Marcus FI, Fontaine GH, Frank R, Grosgogeat Y. Clinical pharmacology and therapeutic applications of the antiarrhythmic agent, amiodarone. Am Heart J 1981;101:480–93.

Mason DT, Spann JF, Zelis R. The clinical pharmacology

and therapeutic applications of antiarrhythmic drugs. Clin Pharmacol Ther 1970;11:460–80.

Moysey JO, Jaggarao NSV, Grundy EW, Chamberlin DA. Amiodarone increases plasma digoxin concentrations. Br Med J 1981;282:272.

Navalgund AA, Alifimoff JK, Jakymec AJ, Bleyaert AL. Amiodarone-induced sinus arrest successfully treated with ephedrine and isoproterenol. Anesth Analg 1986;65:414–6.

Nies AS, Shand DG. Clinical pharmacology of propranolol. Circulation 1975;52:6–15.

Nies AS, Shand DG, Wilkinson GR. Altered hepatic blood flow and drug disposition. Clin Pharmokinet 1976;1:135–55.

Reidenberg MM, Drayer DE, Levy M, Warner H. Polymorphic acetylation of procainamide in man. Clin Pharmacol Ther 1975;17:722–30.

Reynolds AK, Chiz JF, Pasquet AF. Halothane and methoxyflurane: A comparison of their effects on cardiac pacemaker fibers. Anesthesiology 1970;33:602–10.

Reynolds AK, Chiz JF, Pasquet AF. Pacemaker migration and sinus node arrest with methoxyflurane and halothane. Can Anaesth Soc J 1971;18:137–44.

Roden DM, Woosley RL. Flecainide. N Engl J Med 1986a;315:36–41.

Roden DM, Woosley RL. Tocainide. N Engl J Med 1986b;315:41–5.

Rowland E, Krikler DM. Electrophysiological assessment of amiodarone in treatment of resistant supraventricular arrhythmias. Br Heart J 1980;44:82–90.

Selzer A, Wray HW. Quinidine syncope. Paroxysmal ventricular fibrillation occurring during treatment of chronic atrial arrhythmias. Circulation 1964;30:17–26.

Singh BN, Hauswirth O. Comparative mechanisms of action of antiarrhythmic drugs. Am Heart J 1974;87:367–82.

Way WL, Katzung BG, Larson CP. Recurarization with quinidine. JAMA 1967;200:163–4.

Zapata-Diaz J, Cabrera CE, Mendez R. An experimental and clinical study on the effects of procaineamide (Pronestyl) on the heart. Am Heart J 1952:43:854–70.

CHAPTER 18

Calcium Entry Blockers

INTRODUCTION

Calcium entry blockers (also known as calcium antagonists and calcium channel blockers) are a diverse group of structurally unrelated compounds which selectively interfere with inward calcium movement across cell membranes (Reves et al, 1982). Commonly used calcium entry-blockers are verapamil, nifedipine, and diltiazem (Fig. 18-1). Nifedipine is available only for oral administration.

MECHANISM OF ACTION

Channels with a system of gates exist in membranes of excitable cells for the inward transfer of calcium, sodium, and potassium ions (see Chapter 39). Conceptually, a slow calcium channel and fast sodium channel are present. Slow channels are 100 times more selective for calcium than for sodium or potassium ions. Two different gates are postulated to be present on slow calcium channels (Fig. 18-2) (Antman et al, 1980). The gate on the extracellular membrane is voltage dependent opening with depolarization and closing with repolarization. A second gate on the intracellular surface modulates calcium ion flux. Cyclic AMP allows widening of this gate which facilitates inward movement of calcium ions. Cyclic GMP causes narrowing of this gate.

Calcium entry blockers selectively interfere with inward transfer of calcium ions through slow calcium channels (Fleckenstein, 1977). Verapamil may act principally at the inner gate while nifedipine probably blocks the outer gate. Verapamil and diltiazem also have some blocking activity at fast sodium channels.

PHARMACOLOGIC EFFECTS

The pharmacologic effects of calcium blockers can be predicted from a consideration of the normal role of calcium ions in production of the cardiac action potential. For example, the slow plateau portion of the cardiac action potential (i.e., phase 2) is thought to be due to inward calcium ion flux (see Chapter 47). This phase of the action potential is particularly important in the excitation-contraction of cardiac muscle and vascular smooth muscle and to a lesser extent skeletal muscle (Adams and Schwartz, 1980; Fleckenstein, 1977). In addition, calcium ion movement during phase 2 of the cardiac action potential is responsible for depolarization in sinoatrial and atrioventricular nodal tissue. Based on these known effects of calcium ion transport on the action potential, it is predictable that calcium entry blockers will produce (1) decreased myocardial contractility, (2) decreased heart rate, (3) decreased rate of conduction of the cardiac impulse through the atrioventricular node, and (4) vascular smooth muscle relaxation with associated vasodilation and reductions in blood pressure (Reves et al, 1982). The relative abilities, however, of calcium entry

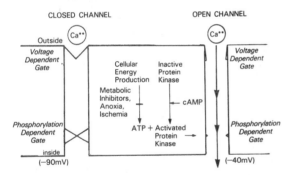

FIGURE 18-1. Calcium entry blockers.

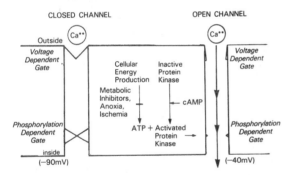

FIGURE 18-2. Schematic depiction of the slow calcium channel demonstrating a voltage-dependent gate on the extracellular membrane and a phosphorylation-dependent gate on the intracellular surface. (From Antman EM, Stone PH, Muller JE, Braunwald E. Calcium channel blocking agents in the treatment of cardiovascular disorders. Part 1 — Basic and clinical electrophysiologic effects. Ann Intern Med 1980;93:875 – 85. Reproduced by permission of the authors and publisher.)

blockers to evoke these pharmacologic effects differs among the drugs (Table 18-1) (Reves, 1984). In addition, verapamil and diltiazem also have some blocking activity at the fast sodium channels responsible for rapid phase 0 and phase 1 portions of the cardiac action potential. This ef-

fect on the fast sodium channels is consistent with the local anesthetic activity of these two drugs.

CLINICAL USES

Differences in cardiovascular effects produced by the various calcium entry blockers may influence the specific drug selected for individual patients (Table 18-1) (Reves, 1984). With this in mind, calcium entry blockers are particularly useful in the treatment of supraventricular tachydysrhythmias and management of angina pectoris due to coronary artery vasospasm or atherosclerosis. Other uses of calcium entry blockers may include (1) treatment of essential hypertension, (2) management of cerebral vasospasm, (3) cerebral protection after global ischemia, (4) myocardial protection during cardiopulmonary bypass, (5) production of controlled hypotension, (6) prevention of bronchospasm associated with exercise-induced asthma, and (7) treatment of esophageal spasms (Reves *et al*, 1982).

Supraventricular Tachydysrhythmias

Verapamil, but not nifedipine, is effective in terminating paroxysmal supraventricular tachycardia by delaying conduction of the cardiac impulse

Table 18-1
Comparative Effects of Calcium Channel Blockers

Decreased mean arterial pressure	nifedipine = verapamil = diltiazem
Increased heart rate	nifedipine > verapamil > diltiazem
Prolonged P–R interval	diltiazem ≥ verapamil > nifedipine
Decreased cardiac output	verapamil = diltiazem > nifedipine
Increased pulmonary artery occlusion pressure	nifedipine = verapamil = diltiazem
Decreased peripheral vascular resistance	nifedipine > verapamil = diltiazem

(Adapted from Reves JG. The relative hemodynamic effects of CA^{++} entry blockers. Anesthesiology 1984;61:3–5; by permission of the author and publisher.)

through the atrioventricular node (Smith *et al*, 1981; Waxman *et al*, 1981). The recommended intravenous dose of verapamil for treatment of supraventricular tachydysrhythmias is 75 to 150 μg kg^{-1} (5–10 mg for an adult) infused over 3 to 5 minutes. Diltiazem, 0.1 mg kg^{-1} administered intravenously, slows heart rate in patients with atrial fibrillation who develop supraventricular tachydysrhythmias intraoperatively (Iwatsuki *et al*, 1985).

Verapamil may be useful in the treatment of maternal and fetal tachydysrhythmias as well as premature labor (Murad *et al*, 1985a). Indeed, verapamil administered intravenously to the mother prolongs atrioventricular conduction in the fetus despite limited placental transport of the drug (ratio of umbilical vein to uterine artery verapamil concentrations 0.35 to 0.45). Fetal hepatic extraction of verapamil is substantial as evidenced by a plasma concentration in the fetal carotid artery less than in the umbilical vein. Verapamil may decrease uterine blood flow suggesting caution in the administration of this drug to parturients with impaired uteroplacental perfusion (Murad *et al*, 1985b).

Verapamil is as effective and more rapid in onset than digitalis in slowing the ventricular response in the presence of atrial flutter or fibrillation (Heng *et al*, 1975; Waxman *et al*, 1981). Reversion to sinus rhythm, however, is uncommon. In patients with mitral valve disease and rapid atrial fibrillation, verapamil may abruptly slow heart rate and relieve pulmonary congestion. The administration of oral verapamil to prevent recurrences of tachydysrhythmias appears to be safer than digitalis for use before electrical cardiover-

sion (Heng *et al*, 1975). Depending on conduction through the accessory pathway, verapamil may or may not be beneficial in the management of patients with preexcitation syndromes such as Wolff-Parkinson-White. In some of these patients, verapamil may actually increase the ventricular response during atrial fibrillation (Rinkenberger *et al*, 1980). Indeed, the rate of retrograde conduction of the cardiac impulse through accessory pathways is not altered by verapamil. Verapamil should probably be avoided in patients with sick sinus syndrome and in the presence of any degree of preexisting atrioventricular heart block.

Ventricular cardiac dysrhythmias are not predictably responsive to treatment with calcium entry blockers. A possible exception is ventricular tachycardia and fibrillation in patients with coronary artery vasospasm (Kapur *et al*, 1984b; Kinura *et al*, 1977). In addition, diltiazem administered to dogs increases the dose of epinephrine necessary to produce ventricular cardiac dysrhythmias during halothane anesthesia and abolishes premature ventricular contractions that appear spontaneously in patients anesthetized with halothane (Iwatsuki *et al*, 1985).

Coronary Artery Vasospasm

Coronary artery vasospasm is characterized by angina pectoris that occurs at rest in association with S–T changes on the electrocardiogram. Verapamil administered intravenously or nifedipine administered orally or sublingually are equally effective treatment for coronary artery vasospasm (Johnson *et al*, 1981). These drugs do not produce detectable coronary artery vasodilatation in patients who do not experience coronary artery vasospasm.

Exercise-Induced Angina Pectoris

Improvement in the balance of oxygen supply and demand is the presumed mechanism for the effectiveness of calcium entry blockers in the treatment of angina pectoris due to coronary atherosclerosis. For example, the beneficial effect of nifedepine in the treatment of exercise-induced angina pectoris appears to be due principally to its peripheral vasodilator action rather than to an effect on the coronary arteries.

Essential Hypertension

Calcium entry blockers are effective in treatment of essential hypertension, but it is unlikely these drugs offer significant advantages over other antihypertensive drugs (see Chapter 15). Oral nifedipine lowers blood pressure, but a reflex increase in heart rate and cardiac output may offset the antihypertensive effect unless blunted by the concomitant administration of a beta-adrenergic antagonist. Increased heart rate is not associated with verapamil administration as used to treat essential hypertension.

Cerebral Artery Vasospasm

Calcium entry blockers are potent cerebral as well as coronary artery vasodilators. In animals, cerebral artery vasodilation manifests as reductions in cerebral artery vasospasm as occurs with head trauma and subarachnoid hemorrhage. Increased intracranial pressure can accompany this drug-induced cerebral vasodilatation, especially if preexisting reductions in intracranial compliance are present (Giffin *et al*, 1983).

Cerebral Protection

Calcium entry blockers may be effective in ameliorating ischemic brain injury (White *et al*, 1984). This protection may be similar to protection from ischemia in the heart. The theoretical basis for considering calcium entry blockers is the observation that lack of oxygen interferes with maintenance of the normal calcium ion gradient across cell membranes leading to massive increases (at least 200-fold) in the intraneuronal concentrations of this ion.

Myocardial Protection

Calcium blockers may exert a protective effect during global myocardial ischemia associated with cardiopulmonary bypass by suppressing energy-dependent calcium ion-mediated myocardial activity. The combination of blockade of slow channels with a calcium entry blocker and fast channels with potassium may result in even a greater reduction in myocardial oxygen consumption than either intervention alone (Pinsky *et al*, 1981). High doses of calcium entry blockers, as used for this myocardial protection, however, could depress myocardial contractility in the period following cessation of cardiopulmonary bypass.

DRUG INTERACTIONS

The known pharmacologic effects of calcium entry blockers on cardiac, skeletal, and vascular smooth muscle as well as on the velocity of conduction of the cardiac impulse make drug interactions possible. For example, myocardial depression and peripheral vasodilation produced by volatile anesthetics could be exaggerated by similar actions of calcium entry blockers. Indeed, volatile anesthetics may interfere with calcium ion movement across cell membranes. Furthermore, delayed conduction of the cardiac impulse through the atrioventricular node produced by halothane may be, in part, due to calcium channel blockade (Lynch *et al*, 1980). The likelihood of adverse circulatory changes due to interactions between calcium entry blockers and anesthetic drugs would seem to be greater in patients with preexisting atrioventricular heart block or left ventricular dysfunction. In addition to the possibility of drug interactions on the cardiovascular system, calcium entry blockers may potentiate neuromuscular blocking drugs (van Poorten *et al*, 1984). Nevertheless, therapy with calcium entry blockers can be continued until the time of surgery without risk of significant drug interactions especially with respect to conduction of the cardiac impulse (Henling *et al*, 1984).

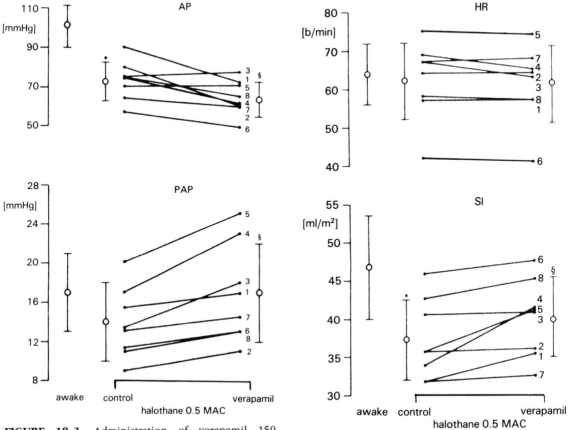

FIGURE 18-3. Administration of verapamil 150 μg kg^{-1} over 10 minutes to patients receiving chronic beta-adrenergic antagonist drug therapy and anesthetized with halothane produces modest decreases in arterial pressure (AP) while pulmonary arterial pressure (PAP) increases. Mean $\pm$ SD. (From Schulte-Sasse V, Hess W, Markschies-Harnung A, Tarnow J. Combined effects of halothane anesthesia and verapamil on systemic hemodynamics and left ventricular myocardial contractility in patients with ischemic heart disease. Anesth Analg 1984;63:791 – 8. Reproduced by permission of the authors and the International Anesthesia Research Society.)

FIGURE 18-4. Administration of verapamil 150 μg kg^{-1} over 10 minutes to patients receiving chronic beta-adrenergic antagonist drug therapy and anesthetized with halothane does not alter heart rate (HR) or stroke index (SI). Mean $\pm$ SD. (From Schulte-Sasse V, Hess W, Markschies-Harnung A, Tarnow J. Combined effects of halothane anesthesia and verapamil on systemic hemodynamics and left ventricular myocardial contractility in patients with ischemic heart disease. Anesth Analg 1984;63:791 – 8. Reproduced by permission of the authors and the International Anesthesia Research Society.)

Anesthetic Drugs

Calcium entry blockers are vasodilators and myocardial depressants. For these reasons, calcium entry blockers must be administered with caution during anesthesia especially to patients with impaired left ventricular function or hypovolemia. Nevertheless, intravenous administration of ver-

apamil, 150 μg kg^{-1} over 10 minutes, to patients with normal left ventricular function anesthetized with halothane does not produce adverse circulatory changes other than modest further reductions in blood pressure even in the presence of chronic low dose beta-adrenergic antagonist therapy (Figs. 18-3 and 18-4) (Schulte-Sasse *et al,* 1984). Conversely, in anesthetized patients with preexisting left ventricular dysfunction, administration of verapamil is associated with myocardial depression and decreased cardiac output (Chew *et al*, 1981). Treatment of cardiac dysrhythmias with calcium entry blockers in patients anesthetized with halothane produces only transient reductions in blood pressure and infrequent prolongation of the P–R interval on the electrocardiogram. Because of the tendency to produce atrioventricular heart block, verapamil should be used cautiously in patients taking digitalis or beta-adrenergic antagonists. Nevertheless, in patients without preoperative evidence of cardiac conduction abnormalities, the chronic combined administration of calcium entry blockers and beta-adrenergic antagonists is not associated with cardiac conduction abnormalities in the perioperative period (Table 18-2) (Henling *et al*, 1984).

In animals, continuous intravenous infusion of verapamil in the presence of anesthetic doses of halothane, enflurane, or isoflurane produces dose-dependent reductions in mean arterial pressure, heart rate, and cardiac index while the P–R interval on the electrocardiogram is increased (Fig. 18-5) (Kapur *et al*, 1984a). Reductions in blood pressure and the occurrence of conduction abnormalities are more prominent in animals anesthetized with enflurane than in those anesthetized with halothane or isoflurane (Kapur *et al*, 1984a). Dogs given nifedipine during halothane anesthesia develop exaggerated reductions in blood pressure, and increasing concentrations of halothane attenuate the usual reflex increases in heart rate produced by this drug.

Cardiovascular depression is accentuated in halothane anesthetized dogs rendered acutely hyperkalemic (Nugent *et al*, 1984). Administration of intravenous calcium is only partially effective in reversing this cardiovascular depression and of no value in antagonizing prolongation of the P–R interval on the electrocardiogram. Acute intravenous administration of verapamil to dogs in doses sufficient to prolong the P–R interval on the electrocardiogram lowers anesthetic requirements for halothane from 0.97% to 0.72% (Maze and Mason, 1983).

Table 18-2

Effect of Chronic Antianginal Therapy on Perioperative Heart Rate (beats min⁻¹) and P–R Interval (msec)

	Before Induction	After Induction	Ten Minutes After Cardiopulmonary Bypass
Control			
Heart rate	72	71	87
P–R interval	160	156	164
Calcium Entry Blockers			
Heart rate	69	70	86
P–R interval	168	169	175
Beta-Adrenergic Antagonists			
Heart rate	59	65	78
P–R interval	168	171	183
Nifedipine and Beta-Adrenergic Antagonists			
Heart rate	67	69	86
P–R interval	175	177	186

(Adapted from Henling CE, Slogoff S, Kodali SV, Arlund C. Heart block after coronary artery bypass—effect of chronic administration of calcium-entry blockers and beta blockers. Anesth Analg 1984;63:515–20; with permission of the authors and the International Anesthesia Research Society.)

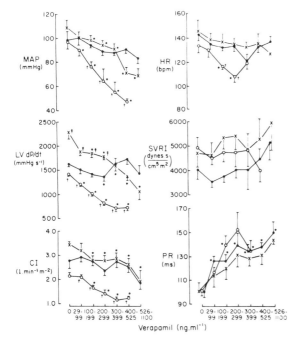

FIGURE 18-5. In animals, the continuous intravenous infusion of verapamil during halothane (solid circles), enflurane (clear circles) or isoflurane (x–x) produces dose-dependent medications in mean arterial pressure (MAP), heart rate (HR), left ventricular (LV) dp/dt, and cardiac index (CI). Peripheral vascular resistance is unchanged, and the P–R interval on the electrocardiogram is prolonged. *P < 0.05 compared with control. tP < 0.05 compared with both halothane and isoflurane. #P < 0.05 compared with halothane. Mean ± SE. (From Kapur PA, Bloor BC, Flacke WE, Olewine SK. Comparison of cardiovascular responses to verapamil during enflurane, isoflurane, or halothane anesthesia in the dog. Anesthesiology, 1984;61:156–60. Reproduced by permission of the authors and publisher.)

Neuromuscular Blocking Drugs

Calcium entry blockers alone do not produce a skeletal muscle relaxant effect as evidenced by failure to alter twitch height (Fig. 18-6) (Durant *et al*, 1984). Conversely, these drugs potentiate the effects of depolarizing and nondepolarizing neuromuscular blocking drugs (Fig. 18-6) (Durant *et al*, 1984). This potentiation resembles that produced by mycin antibiotics in the presence of neuromuscular blocking drugs (see Chapter 28). The

local anesthetic effect of verapamil, reflecting inhibition of sodium flux via fast sodium channels, may also contribute to the potentiation of neuromuscular blocking drugs. Observations of skeletal muscle weakness following administration of verapamil to a patient with muscular dystrophy is consistent with diminished release of neurotransmitter (Zalman *et al*, 1983). Therefore, the neuromuscular effects of verapamil may be more likely to manifest in patients with a compromised margin of safety of neuromuscular transmission.

Antagonism of neuromuscular blockade may be impaired because of diminished presynaptic release of acetylcholine in the presence of a calcium entry blocker (Lawson *et al*, 1983). Indeed, calcium is essential for the release of acetylcholine at the neuromuscular junction. In one report, edrophonium, but not neostigmine, was effective in antagonizing nondepolarizing neuromuscular blockade that was potentiated by verapamil (Jones *et al*, 1985).

Local Anesthetics

Verapamil has potent local anesthetic activity which may increase the risk of local anesthetic

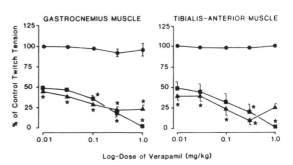

FIGURE 18-6. Infusion of verapamil in the absence of neuromuscular blocking drugs (circles) does not alter twitch height response (twitch tension) of indirectly stimulated rabbit skeletal muscle. When twitch tension is reduced to about 50% of control by the continuous infusion of pancuronium (squares) or succinylcholine (triangles), the addition of verapamil further reduces twitch tension. *P < 0.05 compared with the twitch tension before verapamil. Mean ± SE. (From Durant NN, Nguyen N, Katz R. Potentiation of neuromuscular blockade by verapamil. Anesthesiology, 1984;60:298–303. Reproduced by permission of the authors and publisher.)

toxicity when a regional block is administered to a patient being treated with this drug (Rosenblatt *et al*, 1984).

Potassium-Containing Solutions

Calcium entry blockers slow the inward movement of potassium ions. For this reason, hyperkalemia in patients treated with verapamil may occur after much smaller amounts of exogenous potassium infusion as associated with use of potassium chloride to treat hypokalemia or administration of stored whole blood (Nugent *et al*, 1984). In animals, however, pretreatment with verapamil does not alter the increase in serum potassium concentration following the administration of succinylcholine (Roth *et al*, 1985).

Dantrolene

The ability of both verapamil and dantrolene to inhibit intracellular calcium flux and excitation-contraction coupling would suggest this combination might be useful in the treatment of malignant hyperpyrexia. In swine, however, the administration of dantrolene in the presence of verapamil results in hyperkalemia and cardiovascular collapse (Fig. 18-7) (Saltzman *et al*, 1984). It is speculated that verapamil alters normal homeostatic mechanisms for regulation of serum potassium concentrations and results in hyperkalemia from a dantrolene-induced potassium release. Furthermore, there is evidence that verapamil does not influence the ability of known triggering agents to evoke malignant hyperthermia in susceptible animals (Gallant *et al*, 1985).

Platelet Function

Calcium entry blockers interfere with calcium-mediated platelet functions (Kiyomoto *et al*, 1983).

Digoxin

Calcium entry blockers may increase the plasma concentration of digoxin.

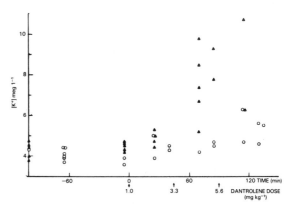

FIGURE 18-7. Administration of dantrolene to swine pretreated with verapamil *(triangles)* results in hyperkalemia (K) compared with animals receiving only dantrolene *(circles)*. (From Saltzman LS, Kates RA, Corke BC, Norfleet EA, Heath KR. Hyperkalemia and cardiovascular collapse after verapamil and dantrolene administration in swine. Anesth Analg 1984;63:473–8. Reproduced by permission of the authors and the International Anesthesia Research Society.)

VERAPAMIL

Verapamil is a synthetic derivative of papaverine that is supplied as a racemic mixture (Fig. 18-1). The dextro isomer is devoid of activity at slow calcium channels but instead acts on fast sodium channels accounting for the local anesthetic effects of verapamil (1.6 times as potent as procaine) (Kraynack *et al*, 1982). The levo isomer, however, is specific for slow calcium channels and the predominance of this action accounts for the classification of verapamil as a calcium entry blocker. Furthermore, it has been demonstrated that the parent drug of verapamil, papaverine, also possesses slow calcium channel blocking effects (Schneider *et al*, 1975).

Verapamil produces direct depressant effects on the sinoatrial node and delays antegrade transmission of the cardiac impulse through the atrioventricular node (Table 18-1) (Reves, 1984). Retrograde transmission of the cardiac impulse through the atrioventricular node or in accessory pathways is not significantly altered by verapamil (see the section entitled Clinical Uses). Negative inotropic effects of verapamil are not prominent except in patients with preexisting left ventricular dysfunction and possibly in those being treated with beta-adrenergic antagonists (see the section entitled Drug Interactions).

Verapamil, administered intravenously, is effective in the treatment of acute supraventricular tachydysrhythmias (see the section entitled Clinical Uses). Although the principal pharmacologic effect of verapamil is on the sinoatrial node and atrioventricular node, it also possesses mild vasodilating properties making this drug useful in the treatment of angina pectoris and essential hypertension. Verapamil is not as active as nifedipine in its effects on vascular smooth muscle and therefore, causes a less pronounced decrease in blood pressure and less reflex peripheral sympathetic nervous system activity (Table 18-1) (Reves, 1984). The concurrent administration of verapamil with a beta-adrenergic antagonist can produce atrioventricular heart block (Benaim, 1972; Singh and Roche, 1977) (see the section entitled Drug Interactions). Isoproterenol may be useful to acutely increase heart rate in the presence drug-induced heart block while life-threatening situations require temporary artificial cardiac pacing.

Intravenous administration of verapamil can produce hypotension especially when administered to patients with preexisting left ventricular dysfunction. Although verapamil is highly effective in some patients with hypertrophic cardiomyopathy, there have also been instances of drug-induced cardiovascular depression. Elevated plasma transaminase and alkaline phosphatase concentrations accompanied by hepatitis develop rarely.

Pharmacokinetics

Oral verapamil is almost completely absorbed, but extensive hepatic first-pass metabolism limits bioavailability to 10% to 20% (Table 18-3) (Reves *et al*, 1982). As a result, the oral dose (80 – 160 mg three times daily) is about ten times the intravenous dose. The therapeutic plasma concentration of verapamil is 100 to 300 ng ml^{-1}.

Table 18-3
Characteristics of Calcium Entry Blockers

	Verapamil	*Nifedipine*	*Diltiazem*
Dosage			
Oral	80 – 160 mg every 8 hours	10 – 20 mg every 8 hours	60 – 90 mg every 8 hours
Intravenous	75 – 150 μg kg^{-1}	5 – 15 μg kg^{-1}	75 – 150 μg kg^{-1}
Absorption (%)			
Oral	>90	>90	>90
Bioavailability	10 – 20	65 – 70	
Onset of Effect (minutes)			
Oral	<30	<20	<30
Sublingual		3	
Intravenous	1 – 3	1 – 3	1 – 3
Protein Binding (%)	90	90	80
Clearance Mechanisms			
Renal (%)	70	80	35
Fecal (%)	15	<15	60
Active Metabolites	Yes	No	No
Elimination Half-Time (hours)	2 – 7	4 – 6	4 – 6

(Adapted from Reves JG, Kissin I, Lell WA, Tosone S. Calcium entry blockers: Uses and implications for anesthesiologists. Anesthesiology 1982;57:504 – 18 with permission of the authors and publisher.)

Demethylated metabolites of verapamil predominate with norverapamil possessing sufficient activity to contribute to the antidysrhythmic properties of the parent drug (Henry, 1980). In view of the nearly complete hepatic metabolism of verapamil, almost none of the drug appears unchanged in the urine. Conversely, an estimated 70% of an injected dose of verapamil is recovered in the urine as metabolites and about 15% is excreted via the bile. Chronic oral administration of verapamil or renal dysfunction leads to the accumulation of norverapamil (Kates *et al*, 1981).

The elimination half-time of verapamil is 2 to 7 hours but may be prolonged to over 13 hours in patients with liver disease (Woodcock *et al*, 1981). Like nifedipine, verapamil is highly protein bound (90%), and the presence of other drugs (lidocaine, diazepam, propranolol) can increase the pharmacologically active unbound portion of the drug (Yong *et al*, 1980).

NIFEDIPINE

Nifedipine is a dihydropyridine derivative with greater coronary and peripheral arterial vasodilator properties than verapamil (Table 18-1) (Fig. 18-1) (Reves, 1984). There is minimal effect on venous capacitance vessels (Robinson *et al*, 1980). Unlike verapamil, nifedipine has little or no direct depressant effect on sinoatrial or atrioventricular nodal activity (Rowland *et al*, 1979). Peripheral vasodilation and the resulting decline in blood pressure produced by nifedipine activates baroreceptors leading to increased peripheral sympathetic nervous system activity most often manifesting as an elevated heart rate. This increased sympathetic nervous system activity counters the direct negative inotropic, chronotropic, and dromotropic effects of nifedipine. Nevertheless, nifedipine may produce excessive myocardial depression especially in patients with (1) aortic stenosis, (2) preexisting left ventricular dysfunction, or (3) beta-adrenergic antagonist therapy (see the section entitled Drug Interactions).

Nifedipine, 10 to 20 mg administered orally three times daily, is used to treat patients with angina pectoris especially that due to coronary artery vasospasm (see the section entitled Clinical Uses). The drug is oxidized by light and must, therefore, be protected during storage.

Pharmacokinetics

Absorption of an oral or sublingual dose of nifedipine is about 90% with onset of an effect being detectable within about 20 minutes after administration (Table 18-3) (Reves *et al*, 1982). Protein binding approaches 90%. Hepatic metabolism is nearly complete with elimination of inactive metabolites principally in the urine (about 80%) and to a lesser extent in the bile (Henry, 1980). The elimination half-time of nifedipine is 4 to 6 hours. Glucose intolerance and hepatic dysfunction occur rarely. Abrupt discontinuation of nifedipine has been associated with coronary artery vasospasm.

DILTIAZEM

Diltiazem is a calcium entry blocker derived from benzothiazapine (Fig. 18-1). Its cardiovascular effects are similar to those of verapamil (Table 18-1) (Reves, 1984). Resting heart rate is often decreased by diltiazem. Coronary arteries and peripheral arteries are dilated. Like other calcium entry blockers, diltiazem has a direct negative inotropic effect which could become prominent in patients with preexisting left ventricular dysfunction or those receiving beta-adrenergic antagonists. Intravenous infusion of diltiazem produces dose-related prolongation of the P–R interval on the electrocardiogram and decreases in blood pressure in dogs anesthetized with enflurane (Kapur et al, 1986).

Diltiazem is administered orally or intravenously for the management of patients with angina pectoris (Table 18-3). Oral absorption is excellent. Diltiazem is 80% bound to protein and is excreted as inactive metabolites principally in the bile (about 60%) and to a lesser extent in the urine (about 35%). The elimination half-time is 4 to 6 hours. The clinical uses and drug interactions for diltiazem are similar to verapamil.

REFERENCES

Adams RJ, Schwartz A. Comparative mechanisms for contraction of cardiac and skeletal muscle. Chest 1980;78:123–39.

Antman EM, Stone PH, Muller JE, Braunwald E. Calcium channel blocking agents in the treatment of cardiovascular disorders. Part 1—Basic and clinical electrophysiologic effects. Ann Intern Med 1980; 93:875–85.

Benaim ME. Asystole after verapamil. Br Med J 1972;2:169–70.

Chew CYC, Hecht HS, Collett JT, McAllister RG, Singh BN. Influence of severity of ventricular dysfunction on hemodynamic responses to intravenously administered verapamil in ischemic heart disease. Am J Cardiol 1981;47:917–22.

Durant NN, Nguyen N, Katz R. Potentiation of neuromuscular blockade by verapamil. Anesthesiology 1984;60:298–303.

Fleckenstein A. Specific pharmacology of calcium in myocardium, cardiac pacemakers, and vascular smooth muscle. Annu Rev Pharmacol Toxicol 1977;17:149–66.

Gallant EM, Foldes FF, Rempel WE, Gronert GA. Verapamil is not a therapeutic adjunct to dantrolene in porcine malignant hyperthermia. Anesth Analg 1985;64:601–6.

Giffin JP, Cottrell JE, Hartung J, Shiviry B. Intracranial pressure during nifedipine-induced hypotension. Anesth Analg 1983;62:1078–80.

Heng MK, Singh BN, Roche AHG, Norris RM, Mercer CJ. Effects of intravenous verapamil on cardiac arrhythmias and on the electrocardiogram. Am Heart J 1975;90:487–98.

Henling CE, Slogoff S, Kodali SV, Arlund C. Heart block after coronary artery bypass – effect of chronic administration of calcium-entry blockers and beta-blockers. Anesth Analg 1984;63:515–20.

Henry PD. Comparative pharmacology of calcium antagonists: Nifedipine, verapamil and diltiazem. Am J Cardiol 1980;46:1047–58.

Iwatsuki N, Katoh M, Ono K, Amaha K. Antiarrhythmic effect of diltiazem during halothane anesthesia in dogs and in humans. Anesth Analg 1985;64:964–70.

Johnson SM, Mauritson DR, Willerson JT, Hillis LD. Controlled trial of verapamil for Prinzmetal's variant angina. N Engl J Med 1981;304:862–6.

Jones RM, Cashman JN, Casson WR, Broadbent MP. Verapamil potentiation of neuromuscular blockade: Failure of reversal with neostigmine but prompt reversal with edrophonium. Anesth Analg 1985;64:1021–5.

Kapur PA, Bloor BC, Flacke WE, Olewine SK. Comparison of cardiovascular response to verapamil during enflurane, isoflurane, or halothane anesthesia in the dog. Anesthesiology 1984a;61:156–60.

Kapur PA, Campos JH, Buchea OC. Plasma diltiazem levels, cardiovascular function, and coronary hemodynamics during enflurane anesthesia in the dog. Anesth Analg 1986; 65:918–24.

Kapur PA, Norel E, Dajee H, Cimochowski G. Verapamil treatment of intractable ventricular arrhythmias

after cardiopulmonary bypass. Anesthesiology 1984b;1984;63:460–3.

Kates RE, Keefe DLD, Schwartz J, Harapat S, Kirsten EB, Harrison DC. Verapamil disposition kinetics in chronic atrial fibrillation. Clin Pharmacol Ther 1981;30:44–51.

Kinura E, Tanaka K, Mizuno K, Honda Y, Hashimoto H. Suppression of repeatedly occurring ventricular fibrillation with nifedipine in variant form of angina pectoris. Jpn Heart J 1977;18:736–42.

Kiyomoto A, Sasaki Y, Odawara A, Morita T. Inhibition of platelet aggregation by diltiazem: Comparison with verapamil and nifedipine and inhibitory potencies of diltiazem metabolites. Circ Res 1983;52:1115–9.

Kraynack BJ, Lawson NW, Gintautas J. Local anesthetic effect of verapamil in vitro. Reg Anesth 1982;7:114–7.

Lawson NW, Kraynack BJ, Gintautas J. Neuromuscular and electrocardiographic responses to verapamil in dogs. Anesth Analg 1983;62:50–4.

Lynch C, Vogel S, Sperelakis N. Halothane depresses cardiac slow action potentials. Anesthesiology 1980;53:S420.

Maze M, Mason DM. Verapamil decreases the MAC for halothane in dogs. Anesth Analg 1983;62:274.

Murad SHN, Tabsh KMA, Conklin KA, et al. Verapamil: Placental transfer and effects on maternal and fetal hemodynamics and atrioventricular conduction in the pregnant ewe. Anesthesiology 1985a;62:49–53.

Murad SHN, Tabsh KMA, Shilyanski G, et al. Effects of verapamil on uterine blood flow and maternal cardiovascular function in the awake pregnant ewe. Anesth Analg 1985b;64:7–10.

Nugent M, Tinker JH, Moyer TP. Verapamil worsens rate of development and hemodynamic effects of acute hyperkalemia in halothane-anesthetized dogs: Effects of calcium therapy. Anesthesiology 1984;60:435–9.

Pinsky WW, Lewis RM, McMillin-Wood JB, et al. Myocardial protection from ischemic arrest: Potassium and verapamil cardioplegia. Am J Physiol 1981;240: H326–35.

Reves JG. The relative hemodynamic effects of CA^{++} entry blockers. Anesthesiology 1984;61:3–5.

Reves JG, Kissin I, Lell WA, Tosone S. Calcium entry blockers: Uses and implications for anesthesiologists. Anesthesiology 1982;57:504–18.

Rinkenberger RL, Prystowsky EN, Heger JJ, Troup PJ, Jackman WM, Zipes DP. Effects of intravenous and chronic oral verapamil administration in patients with supraventricular tachyarrhythmias. Circulation 1980;62:996–1010.

Robinson BF, Dobbs RJ, Kelsey CR. Effects of nifedipine on resistance vessels, arteries and veins in man. Br J Clin Pharmacol 1980;10:433–8.

Rosenblatt RM, Weaver JM, Wang Y, Tallman RD. Verapamil potentiates the toxicity of local anesthetics. Anesth Analg 1984;63:269.

Roth JL, Nugent M, Gronert GA. Verapamil does not alter succinylcholine-induced increases in serum potassium during halothane anesthesia in normal dogs. Anesth Analg 1985;64:1202–4.

Rowland E, Evans T, Krikler D. Effect of nifedipine on atrioventricular conduction as compared with verapamil. Br Heart J 1979;42:124–7.

Saltzman LS, Kates RA, Corke BC, Norfleet EA, Heath KR. Hyperkalemia and cardiovascular collapse after verapamil and dantrolene administration in swine. Anesth Analg 1984;63:473–8.

Schneider JA, Brooker G, Sperelakis N. Papaverine blockade of an inward slow Ca^{2+} current in guinea pig heart. J Mol Cell Cardiol 1975;7:867–76.

Schulte-Sasse U, Hess W, Markschies-Harnung A, Tarnow J. Combined effects of halothane anesthesia and verapamil on systemic hemodynamics and left ventricular myocardial contractility in patients with ischemic heart disease. Anesth Analg 1984;63:791–8.

Singh BN, Roche AHG. Effects of intravenous verapamil on hemodynamics in patients with heart disease. Am Heart J 1977;94:593–99.

Smith WJ, Wenger TL, Grant AO, Strauss HC. The antiarrhythmic spectrum of verapamil. Drug Therapy 1981;11:44–61.

van Poorten JF, Dhasmana KM, Kuypers SM, Erdmann W. Verapamil and reversal of vecuronium neuromuscular blockade. Anesth Analg 1984;63:155–7.

Waxman HL, Myerberg RJ, Appel R, Sung RJ. Verapamil for control of ventricular rate in paroxysmal supraventricular tachycardia and atrial fibrillation or flutter. Ann Intern Med 1981;94:1–6.

White BC, Wiegenstein JG, Winegar CD. Brain ischemic anoxia. Mechanisms of injury. JAMA 1984;251:1586–90.

Woodcock BG, Rietbrock I, Vohringer HF, Rietbrock N. Verapamil disposition in liver disease and intensive care patients: Kinetics, clearance, and apparent blood flow relationships. Clin Pharmacol Ther 1981;29:27–34.

Yong CL, Kunka RL, Bates TR. Factors affecting the plasma protein binding of verapamil and norverapamil in man. Res Commun Chem Pathol Pharmacol 1980;30:329–479.

Zalman F, Perloff JK, Durant NN, Campion DS. Acute respiratory failure following intravenous verapamil in Duchenne's muscular dystrophy. Am Heart J 1983;105:510–1.

Drugs Used in Treatment of Psychiatric Disease

INTRODUCTION

Classes of drugs effective in the symptomatic treatment of psychiatric disease include (1) phenothiazines and structurally similar thioxanthenes, (2) butyphenones, (3) lithium, (4) tricyclic antidepressants, and (5) monoamine oxidase inhibitors (MAOI) (Table 19-1). Phenothiazines, thioxanthenes, and butyrophenones are most often administered for the treatment of schizophrenia, which accounts for their frequent designation as antipsychotics. Treatment of mania is with antipsychotics or lithium. Tricyclic antidepressants and MAOI are most often used in the treatment of depression.

PHENOTHIAZINES AND THIOXANTHENES

Phenothiazines and thioxanthenes have a high therapeutic index and a relatively flat dose-response curve, accounting for the remarkable safety of these drugs over a wide dose range. Even large overdoses are unlikely to cause life-threatening depression of ventilation. These drugs do not produce physical dependence, although abrupt discontinuation may be accompanied by skeletal muscle discomfort. In addition to their use in the treatment of psychiatric disease, phenothiazines and thioxanthenes possess other clinically useful properties, including antiemetic and antihistaminic effects and potentiation of analgesics.

Structure Activity Relationships

Phenothiazines have a three-ring structure in which two benezene rings are linked by a sulfur and nitrogen atom (Fig. 19-1). If the nitrogen atom at position 10 is replaced by a carbon atom with a double bond to the side chain, the compound becomes a thioxanthene (Fig. 19-1). Phenothiazines and thioxanthenes used to treat psychiatric disease have three carbon atoms interposed between position 10 of the central ring and the first amino nitrogen atom of the side chain at this position. In addition, the amine is always tertiary. This structure contrasts with that of antihistamine phenothiazines (*e.g.,* promethazine) or strongly anticholinergic phenothiazines (*e.g.,* ethopropazine, diethazine), which have only two carbon atoms separating the amino group from position 10 of the central ring. Loss of a methyl group or other substituents on the tertiary amino group, as can occur during metabolism, results in a loss of pharmacologic activity.

Mechanism of Action

Phenothiazines and thioxanthenes most likely produce their neuroleptic actions by virtue of antagonism of dopamine as a synaptic neurotransmitter in the basal ganglia and limbic portions of the forebrain (Baldessarini and Tarsy, 1978). Indeed, most phenothiazines and thioxanthenes are potentially associated with extrapyramidal side effects as evidence of interference with the normal actions of dopamine.

Pharmacokinetics

Phenothiazines and thioxanthenes often display erratic and unpredictable patterns of absorption following oral administration. These drugs are highly lipid soluble and accumulate in well-perfused tissues such as the brain. Passage across the placenta and accumulation of drug in the fetus is possible. Avid binding to protein in plasma and tissues limits effectiveness of hemodialysis in removing these drugs.

Metabolism

Metabolism of phenothiazines and thioxanthenes is principally by oxidation in the liver followed by conjugation. Most oxidative metabolites are pharmacologically inactive, with a notable exception being 7-hydroxychlorpromazine. Metabolites appear primarily in the urine and to a lesser extent in the bile. Typical elimination half-times of these drugs are 10 to 20 hours, permitting once daily dosing intervals. Elimination half-times may be prolonged in the fetus and in the elderly, who have decreased capacity to metabolize these drugs.

Side Effects

Side effects produced by treatment with phenothiazine or thioxanthenes are common and include (1) cardiovascular effects, (2) extrapyramidal symptoms, (3) endocrine changes, (4) neuroleptic malignant syndrome, (5) obstructive jaundice, (6) antiemetic effects, (7) anticholinergic effects, (8) sedation, (9) hypothermia, (10) altered seizure threshold, (11) skeletal muscle relaxation, (12) cutaneous reactions, and (13) drug interactions. Many of these side effects also accompany administration of butyrophenones.

Cardiovascular Effects

Intravenous administration of chlorpromazine causes a reduction in blood pressure resulting from (1) depression of vasomotor reflexes mediated by the hypothalamus or brain stem, (2) pe-

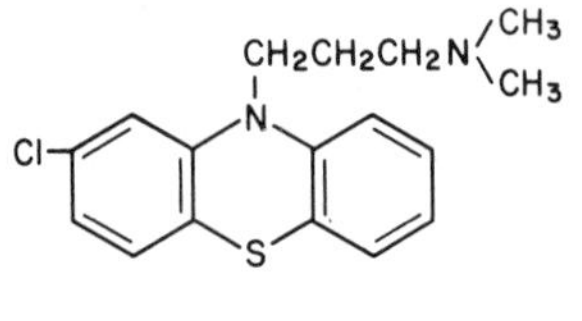

Table 19-1
Classification of Drugs Useful in the Treatment of Psychiatric Disease

> **Phenothiazines**
> Chlorpromazine
> Thioridazine
> Fluphenazine
> Perphenazine
> Trifluoperazine
> **Thioxanthenes**
> Chlorprothixene
> Thiothixene
> **Butyrophenones**
> Droperidol
> Haloperidol
> **Lithium**
> **Tricyclic Antidepressants**
> Imipramine
> Desipramine
> Amitriptyline
> Nortriptyline
> Doxepin
> Protriptyline
> **Monoamine Oxidase Inhibitors**
> Phenelzine
> Isocarboxazid
> Tranylcypromine
> Deprenyl

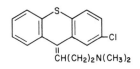

Chlorpromazine (A)

Chlorprothixene (B)

FIGURE 19-1. Phenothiazines (A) and thioxanthenes (B).

ripheral alpha-adrenergic blockade, (3) direct relaxant effects on vascular smooth muscle, and (4) direct cardiac depression. Alpha-adrenergic blockade produced by chlorpromazine is sufficient to prevent the pressor effects of epinephrine. Miosis that occurs predictably may also be due to alpha-adrenergic blockade. A cardiac antidysrhythmic effect of chlorpromazine may reflect the potent local anesthetic activity of this drug. Changes on the electrocardiogram include prolongation of the P-R and Q-T intervals and depression of the S-T segment.

Oral administration of these drugs is associated with less pronounced blood pressure – lowering effects. Indeed, tolerance develops to the hypotensive effect so that after several weeks of therapy, the blood pressure returns toward normal. Nevertheless, some element of orthostatic hypotension may persist for the duration of therapy.

Extrapyramidal Effects

Acute dystonic reactions characterized as facial grimacing and torticollis may be seen with the initiation of therapy with phenothiazines or thioxanthenes. Tardive dyskinesia is a late developing neurologic syndrome that has been associated with these drugs (Baldessarini and Tracy, 1978). This syndrome is characterized by involuntary movements such as smacking of the lips, lateral jaw movements, and sudden forward thrusts of the tongue. There may be choreiform and purposeless movements of all extremities that disappear during sleep. Compensatory increases in the function of dopamine activity in the basal ganglia may be responsible for the development of tardive dyskinesia.

Endocrine Changes

Prolactin secretion is stimulated by phenothiazines, presumably reflecting inhibition of the actions of dopamine at the hypothalamus and pituitary. Galactorrhea and gynecomastia may accompany excess prolactin secretion. Amenorrhea is a possible, but rare, complication of therapy. Decreased secretion of corticosteroids may be due to diminished corticotropin release from the pituitary. Chlorpromazine may impair glucose tolerance and the release of insulin in some patients (Erle *et al,* 1977).

Neuroleptic Malignant Syndrome

Neuroleptic malignant syndrome occurs in 0.5% to 1% of all patients treated with antipsychotic drugs (Diamond and Santos, 1982). Abrupt withdrawal of levodopa therapy in patients with Parkinson's disease has also been associated with this syndrome. The syndrome typically develops over 24 to 72 hours in young males and is characterized by (1) hyperthermia, (2) generalized hypertonicity of skeletal muscles, (3) instability of the autonomic nervous system manifesting as alterations in blood pressure, tachycardia, and cardiac dysrhythmias, and (4) fluctuating levels of consciousness (Guze and Baxter, 1985). Autonomic nervous system dysfunction may precede the onset of other symptoms. Increased skeletal muscle tone may so reduce chest-wall compliance that it becomes necessary to provide mechanical support of ventilation. Creatine phosphokinase is often elevated, and liver transaminase enzymes are increased. Mortality is 20% to 30% with common causes of death being ventilatory failure, cardiac failure and/or dysrhythmias, renal failure, and thromboembolism.

Malignant hyperthermia associated with anesthesia and the central anticholinergic syndrome may mimic the neuroleptic malignant syndrome (Guze and Baxter, 1985). A distinguishing feature is the ability of nondepolarizing neuromuscular blocking drugs, such as pancuronium, to produce flaccid paralysis in patients with neuroleptic malignant syndrome but not in those persons experiencing malignant hyperthermia (Sangal and Dimitrijevic, 1985). The cause of neuroleptic malignant syndrome is not known and, as a result, its treatment is empirical and includes symptomatic measures and the administration of dantrolene. The reported efficacy of dopamine agonists, such as bromocriptine and amantadine, in treatment of the associated skeletal muscle rigidity as well as the onset of the syndrome with abrupt withdrawal of levodopa therapy suggests a role of dopamine receptor blockade in the development of this syndrome Granato *et al,* 1983).

Obstructive Jaundice

Obstructive jaundice that is considered to be an allergic reaction occurs rarely 2 to 4 weeks after the administration of phenothiazines or thioxanthenes. Indeed, there is prompt recurrence of jaundice if the offending drug, usually chlorpromazine, is again administered. If jaundice is not observed in the first month of therapy, it is unlikely to occur at a later date.

Antiemetic Effects

Antiemetic effects of antipsychotic drugs reflect their interaction with dopaminergic receptors in the chemoreceptor trigger zone of the medulla. Motion sickness is not controlled. A high incidence of extrapyramidal side effects limits the usefulness of these drugs as antiemetics.

Anticholinergic Effects

Chlorpromazine has moderate anticholinergic effects manifesting as blurring of vision, decreased gastric hydrogen ion secretion, and reduced gastrointestinal motility. Decreased sweating and salivation are additional manifestations of anticholinergic effects.

Sedation

Phenothiazines and thioxanthenes, particularly chlorpromazine, produce sedative effects that are often most intense early in the treatment phase. With chronic therapy, tolerance develops to the sedative effects produced by these drugs.

Hypothermia

An effect of chlorpromazine on the hypothalamus is most likely responsible for the poikilothermic effect of this drug. In the past, this effect was used to facilitate the production of surgical hypothermia.

Seizure Threshold

Many antipsychotic drugs lower the seizure threshold and produce a pattern on the electroencephalogram similar to that associated with seizure disorders. Chlorpromazine causes a slowing of the electroencephalogram pattern, with some increase in burst activity and spiking (Fink, 1969). Sensory evoked potentials are often decreased in amplitude, and there is an increase in latency.

Skeletal Muscle Relaxation

Chlorpromazine causes skeletal muscle relaxation in some types of spastic conditions, presumably by actions on the central nervous system, as the drug is devoid of actions at the neuromuscular junction.

Cutaneous Reactions

Cutaneous reactions manifesting as urticaria or photosensitivity occur in about 5% of patients treated with chlorpromazine. Contact dermatitis may occur in personnel who handle chlorpromazine.

Drug Interactions

Ventilatory depressant effects of opioids are likely to be exaggerated by antipsychotic drugs. Likewise, the miotic and sedative effects of opioids are increased, and the analgesic actions are likely to be potentiated. These drugs may interfere with the actions of exogenously administered dopamine, and the effects of alcohol are enhanced.

BUTYROPHENONES

Butyrophenones, such as droperidol and haloperidol, structurally resemble and evoke pharmacologic effects similar to phenothiazines and thioxanthenes (Fig. 19-2). Like these drugs, butyrophenones can reduce the anxiety accompanying psychoses. Conversely, butyrophenones are less effective against acute situational anxiety such as that present in the preoperative period (see the section entitled Side Effects).

Droperidol is the butyrophenone most often administered in the perioperative period. Haloperidol has a longer duration of action than droperidol and lacks significant alpha-adrenergic antagonist effects such that reductions in blood pressure are unlikely. The principal use of haloperidol is as a long-acting antipsychotic drug.

Mechanism of Action

Butyrophenones act at postsynaptic receptor sites to decrease the neurotransmitter function of dopa-

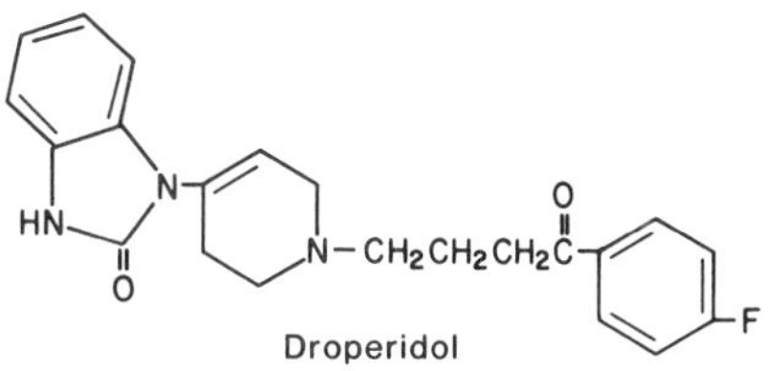

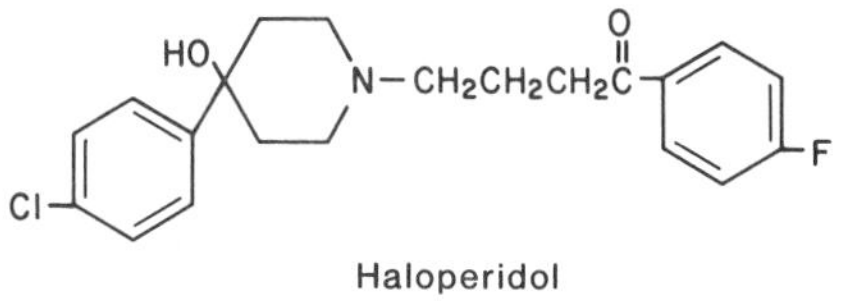

Droperidol

Haloperidol

FIGURE 19-2. Butyrophenones.

mine. Conceptually, there are two distinct binding sites on a single postsynaptic receptor (Richter, 1981). Dopamine binds to one site, and dopamine antagonists, such as droperidol, bind to the other site. Presumably, antipsychotic effects of butyrophenones reflect antagonism of dopaminergic receptors in various areas of the central nervous system. Droperidol is metabolized in the liver, with maximal excretion of metabolites during the first 24 hours.

Pharmacokinetics

In patients anesthetized with nitrous oxide – fentanyl, the elimination half-time of droperidol, 150 μg kg^{-1}, is 104 minutes, clearance 14.1 ml kg^{-1} min^{-1} and the volume of distribution 2.04 L kg^{-1} (Fischler *et al*, 1986). The total body clearance of droperidol is similar to hepatic blood flow, emphasizing the importance of hepatic metabolism. In this regard, potential accumulation of droperidol would occur when the hepatic blood flow is decreased rather than with an alteration in hepatic enzyme activity. The short elimination half-time is not consistent with the prolonged central nervous system effects of droperidol, which may reflect slow dissociation of the drug from receptors or retention of droperidol in the brain.

Clinical Uses

Clinical uses of droperidol are principally limited to production of neuroleptanalgesia and use as an antiemetic.

Neuroleptanalgesia

Droperidol combined with fentanyl is administered for the production of neuroleptanalgesia. A commercially available 50:1 combination of droperidol with fentanyl is known as Innovar. This fixed combination of drugs is not associated with enhanced depression of ventilation as compared with either drug alone (Harper *et al*, 1976). Droperidol does not enhance analgesia produced by fentanyl but rather prolongs its duration of action. Orthostatic hypotension and dysphoria are more likely to occur following the administration of Innovar compared with fentanyl alone.

Neuroleptanalgesia is characterized by trance-like (cateleptic) immobility in an outwardly tranquil patient dissociated and indifferent to the surroundings. Analgesia is intense allowing performance of a variety of diagnostic and minor surgical procedures (*e.g.,* bronchoscopy, cystoscopy). Disadvantages of neuroleptanalgesia are prolonged central nervous system depression and failure to predictably depress sympathetic nervous system responses to painful stimulation.

Antiemetic

Droperidol is a powerful antiemetic by virtue of inhibition of dopaminergic receptors in the chemoreceptor trigger zone of the medulla. For example, droperidol, 1.2 to 2.5 mg administered intravenously before the conclusion of surgery, decreases the incidence of postoperative nausea and vomiting (Fig. 19-3) (Santos and Datta, 1984). Use of droperidol in this manner, however, delays recovery from anesthesia and increases the incidence of postoperative vertigo (Cohen *et al,* 1984). Labyrinthine-induced vomiting (*e.g.,* motion sickness) is not influenced by droperidol.

Side Effects (also see section entitled Phenothiazines and Thioxanthenes)

As a dopamine antagonist, droperidol evokes extrapyramidal reactions in about 1% of patients

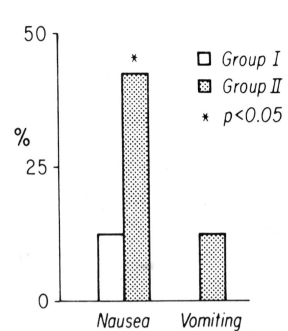

FIGURE 19-3. Droperidol 1.2 to 2.5 mg administered intravenously to group I patients before the conclusion of surgery decreases the incidence of nausea and vomiting. Group II patients did not receive droperidol but underwent similar surgery. (From Santos A, Datta S. Prophylactic use of droperidol for control of nausea and vomiting during spinal anesthesia for cesarean section. Anesth Analg 1984;63:85 – 7. Reproduced by permission of the authors and the International Anesthesia Research Society.)

(Rivera *et al,* 1975; Wicklund and Ngai, 1971). For this reason, droperidol should not be administered to patients being treated for Parkinson's disease. Intravenous diphenhydramine is an effective treatment for droperidol-induced extrapyramidal reactions.

The outwardly calming effect of droperidol may mask an overwhelming fear of surgery. This possible dysphoric reaction detracts from the use of droperidol in preoperative medication (Lee and Yeakel, 1975). Droperidol may be of value in reducing shivering associated with deliberate hypothermia.

Central Nervous System Effects

Droperidol is a cerebral vasoconstrictor leading to a reduction in cerebral blood flow while cerebral metabolic rate is not greatly altered. Failure to lower metabolic rate despite reduced cerebral blood flow could be undesirable in patients with cerebral vascular disease. The reticular activating system is not depressed and alpha rhythm persists on the electroencephalogram. Droperidol does not produce amnesia, nor does it have an anticonvulsant action.

Cardiovascular Effects

Droperidol can decrease blood pressure as a result of actions in the central nervous system and by peripheral alpha-adrenergic blockade (Whitwam and Russell, 1971). The decline in blood pressure is usually minimal, although occasionally, a patient may experience marked hypotension. Peripheral and pulmonary vascular resistances are only modestly and transiently reduced. Myocardial contractility is not altered by droperidol.

Extreme hypertension has been reported following administration of droperidol to patients with pheochromocytoma (Bittar, 1979; Sumikawa and Amakata, 1977). This blood pressure response reflects droperidol-induced release of catecholamines from the adrenal medulla as well as inhibition of catecholamine uptake into the chromaffin granules (Fig. 19-4) (Sumikawa *et al,* 1985).

Droperidol is a cardiac antidysrhythmic and protects against epinephrine-induced dysrhythmias (Bertolo *et al,* 1972). The mechanism for this cardiac antidysrhythmic effect has not been established but may reflect blockade of alpha-adrenergic receptors in the myocardium, stabilization of excitable membranes of myocardial cells by local anesthetic effects, and decreases in blood pressure that reduce the likelihood of pressure-dependent cardiac dysrhythmias. Large doses of droperidol ($0.2 - 0.6$ mg $\cdot$ kg^{-1}) depress conduction of the cardiac impulse along accessory pathways responsible for tachydysrhythmias that occur in patients with Wolff – Parkinson – White syndrome (Fig. 19-5) (Gomez – Arnau *et al,* 1983).

Ventilation

Resting ventilation and the ventilatory response to carbon dioxide are not altered by droperidol (Soroker *et al,* 1978). Furthermore, intravenous droperidol augments the ventilatory response evoked by arterial hypoxemia, presumably by blocking

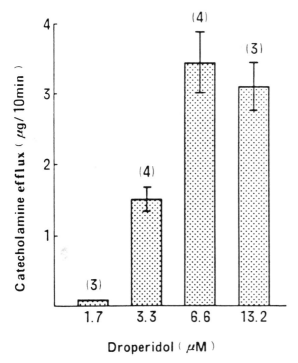

FIGURE 19-4. Catecholamine efflux (mean ±SE) from the perfused dog adrenal medulla is increased by droperidol. The number of experiments is indicated by the figure in parenthesis. (From Sumikawa K, Hirano H, Amakata Y, Kashimoto T, Wada A, Izumi F. Mechanism of the effect of droperidol to induce catecholamine efflux from the adrenal medulla. Anesthesiology 1985;62:17–22. Reproduced by permission of the authors and publisher.)

the action of the inhibitory neurotransmitter, dopamine, at the carotid body (Fig. 19-6) (Ward, 1984). In addition, the depression of the ventilatory response to arterial hypoxemia produced by dopamine is reversed by droperidol (Ward, 1984). For these reasons, droperidol may be an acceptable preoperative medication in patients with chronic obstructive airways disease who are dependent on carotid body drive to prevent hypoventilation.

LITHIUM

Lithium is used for the treatment of mania and for the prevention of recurrent attacks of manic-de-

pressive illness (Havdala *et al,* 1979). When given to manic patients who characteristically sleep very little, lithium corrects the sleep disorder as the mania abates. These changes are associated with diffuse slowing on the electroencephalogram.

The optimal plasma concentration of lithium is 0.8 to 1.5 mEq L^{-1}. This plasma concentration is usually achieved following daily oral lithium doses of 900 to 1500 mg. Monitoring of the plasma concentration of lithium is indicated, as the therapeutic and toxic concentrations do not differ greatly (see the section entitled Toxicity).

Mechanism of Action

At the cellular level, lithium ions act as imperfect substitutes for sodium ions. For example, lithium ions can replace sodium ions in supporting a single action potential, but they are not an adequate substrate for the sodium–potassium pump and cannot, therefore, maintain transmembrane potentials (see Chapter 39). Furthermore, once in the cell, lithium ions can be extruded at a rate only

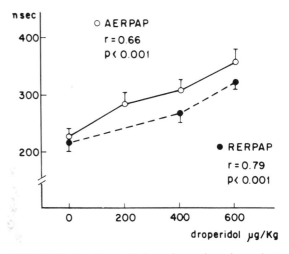

FIGURE 19-5. Droperidol produces dose-dependent prolongation of the antegrade and retrograde effective refractory period of accessory pathways. (From Gomez-Arnau J, Marquez-Montes J, Avello F. Fentanyl and droperidol effects on the refractoriness of the accessory pathway in the Wolff-Parkinson-White syndrome. Anesthesiology 1983;58:307–13. Reproduced by permission of the authors and publisher.)

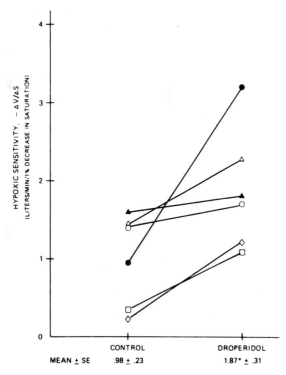

FIGURE 19-6. The ventilatory response to arterial hypoxemia (*i.e.,* hypoxic sensitivity) is enhanced by droperidol. Solid symbols represent repeated experiments on the same subjects as those represented by the open symbols. (From Ward DS. Stimulation of hypoxic ventilatory drive by droperidol. Anesth Analg 1984;63:106–10. Reproduced by permission of the author and the International Anesthesia Research Society.)

10% that of sodium ions. The resulting intracellular accumulation of lithium ions appears to interfere with the ability of several hormones to activate adenylate cyclase and produce cyclic AMP. Reduced availability of cyclic AMP would be associated with decreased responses of receptors to neurotransmitters and reduced cellular activity.

Pharmacokinetics

Lithium is almost completely absorbed from the gastrointestinal tract, with peak concentrations in plasma occurring 2 to 4 hours after an oral dose. Initial distribution is in the extracellular fluid, with subsequent accumulation in various tissues.

Passage across the blood–brain barrier is slow, but ultimately, the concentration of lithium in the cerebrospinal fluid is about 40% of the concentration in plasma. There is no evidence of lithium binding to plasma proteins.

Approximately 95% of a single dose of lithium is eliminated in the urine. About one third to two thirds of an acute dose is excreted during a 6- to 12-hour initial phase of excretion followed by a slow excretion over the next 10 to 14 days. Since 80% of the filtered lithium ions are reabsorbed by renal tubules, lithium clearance by the kidney is about 20% of that for creatinine. Most of the renal tubular reabsorption of the lithium seems to occur in proximal convoluted tubules. Sodium loading produces a small enhancement of lithium excretion, but sodium depletion promotes a clinically important degree of retention of the ion. Indeed, reabsorption of lithium back into the circulation can be produced by any diuretic (*e.g.,* thiazides, furosemide) that causes increased renal elimination of sodium ions (see the section entitled Toxicity). Triamterene may increase excretion of lithium, suggesting that some reabsorption of the ion may occur in distal renal tubules. Conversely, spironolactone does not increase the excretion of lithium.

Side Effects

Sodium is retained, and, in some cases, peripheral edema manifests in the initial phases of lithium therapy. An occasional lithium-treated patient develops benign diffuse thyroid enlargement. Rarely, lithium inhibits the release of thyroid hormones to the extent that hypothyroidism develops.

Polydipsia and polyuria may occur in patients treated with lithium. Indeed, nephrogenic diabetes insipidus has occurred in patients maintained chronically with therapeutic plasma concentrations of lithium (Burroughs *et al,* 1978). The mechanism of polyuria may involve inhibition of the action of antidiuretic hormone on renal adenylate cyclase resulting in reduced stimulation for reabsorption of water across the renal tubules.

Prolonged use of lithium causes a benign and reversible depression of the T wave on the electrocardiogram. This effect is not related to depletion of sodium or potassium ions (Demers and Heninger, 1971). An increase in the circulating concentration of leukocytes occurs during chronic treatment with lithium.

The association of sedation with lithium therapy suggests that anesthetic requirements for injected and inhaled drugs could be reduced. High plasma concentrations of lithium may delay recovery from central nervous system depressant effects of barbiturates (Mannisto and Saarnivaara, 1976). Responses to depolarizing and nondepolarizing neuromuscular blocking drugs may be prolonged in the presence of lithium (Hill *et al,* 1977).

Toxicity

The therapeutic range for lithium is narrow, with plasma concentrations below 0.8 mEq L^{-1} often being ineffective, whereas levels above 1.5 mEq L^{-1} may produce toxicity. Mild lithium toxicity is reflected by sedation, nausea, skeletal muscle weakness, and changes on the electrocardiogram characterized by widening of the QRS complex. Atrioventricular heart block, hypotension, cardiac dysrhythmias, and seizures may occur when the plasma concentration of lithium exceeds 2 mEq L^{-1}. It is not uncommon for elderly patients who excrete lithium slowly to become confused even in the presence of therapeutic plasma concentrations of this ion (Davis *et al,* 1973).

Diuretics that stimulate renal loss of sodium ions cause retention of lithium ions. Indeed, even short-term administration of thiazide diuretics or furosemide can quickly cause lithium toxicity (Macfie, 1975). In pregnancy, concomitant use of diuretics and low sodium diets contribute to maternal and neonatal lithium intoxication (Goldberg and Weinstein, 1973).

Treatment of lithium intoxication is supportive. If renal function is adequate, excretion of lithium ions can be modestly accelerated by osmotic diuresis and intravenous administration of sodium bicarbonate. Hemodialysis is also effective in removing excess lithium ions from the body.

TRICYCLIC ANTIDEPRESSANTS

The efficacy of tricyclic antidepressants in alleviating mental depression is well established. These drugs may also be used in the treatment of chronic pain, presumably reflecting a link between serotonin and nociception and the ability of tricyclic antidepressants to block the uptake of this neurotransmitter (Rosenblatt *et al,* 1984).

Structure Activity Relationships

The structure of tricyclic antidepressants resembles that of phenothiazines (Fig. 19-7). Imipramine is a dibenzazepine that differs from the phenothiazines only by replacement of the sulfur atom with an ethylene linkage to produce a seven-membered central ring. The other dibenzazepine is desipramine, which is also a major metabolite of imipramine. Dibenzocycloheptadienes are amitriptyline and its N-demethylated product nortriptyline. Doxepin is a dibenzoxepine, and protriptyline is a dibenzocycloheptatriene.

Mechanism of Action

Tricyclic antidepressants potentiate the action of norepinephrine in the central nervous system by prevention of its uptake (reuptake) back into postganglionic sympathetic nerve endings. The role of this effect, if any, in reversing mental depression is not convincingly documented, despite its frequent proposal as a likely explanation. Prevention of uptake of serotonin and/or potent anticholinergic effects may also be involved in the antidepressant effects of these drugs. Indeed, physostigmine may aggravate mental depression. Nevertheless, other potent anticholinergic drugs, such as atropine and scopolamine, are not effective antidepressants.

Pharmacokinetics

Tricyclic antidepressants are efficiently absorbed from the gastrointestinal tract after oral administration, reflecting their high lipid solubility. Peak plasma concentrations occur within 2 to 8 hours after oral administration. Therapeutic plasma concentrations (parent compound plus the pharmacologically active demethylated metabolites) are 100 to 300 ng ml^{-1}, whereas toxicity is likely at levels above 500 ng ml^{-1} (see the section entitled Metabolism). Tricyclic antidepressants are strongly bound to plasma and tissue proteins, which, in combination with high lipid solubility, results in a large volume of distribution (up to 50 L kg^{-1}) for these drugs. The long elimination half-

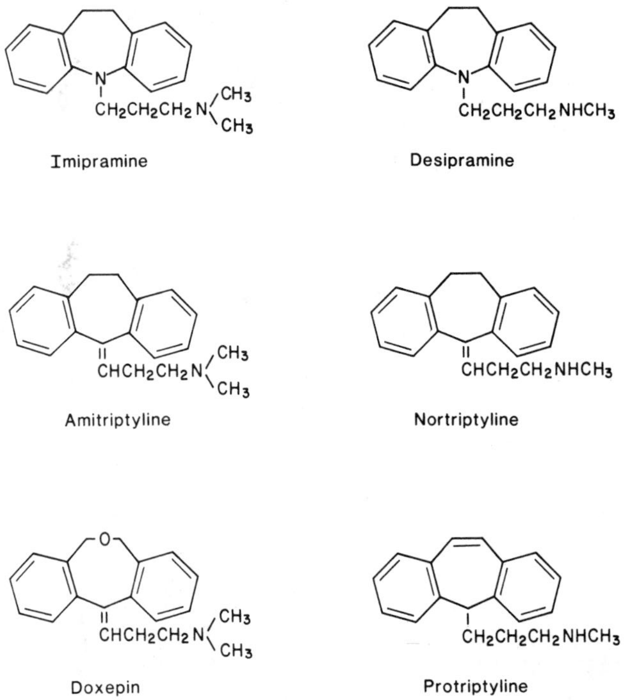

Imipramine

Desipramine

Amitriptyline

Nortriptyline

Doxepin

Protriptyline

FIGURE 19-7. Tricyclic antidepressants.

times (17 to 30 hours) and wide range of therapeutic plasma concentrations make once-daily–dosing intervals effective.

Metabolism

Tricyclic antidepressants are oxidized by microsomal enzymes in the liver, with subsequent conjugation with glucuronic acid. This inactivation and elimination of tricyclic antidepressants occurs over several days, with 1 week or longer required for excretion.

Imipramine is metabolized to the active compound, desipramine. Both these active compounds are inactivated by oxidation to hydroxy metabolites and by conjugation with glucuronic acid. Nortriptyline, which is a pharmacologically active demethylated metabolite of imipramine and amitriptyline, can accumulate to levels that exceed the precursors. Doxepin also appears to be converted to an active metabolite, nordoxepin, by demethylation (Ziegler *et al,* 1978).

Side Effects

Side effects of tricyclic antidepressants are frequent, most commonly manifesting as (1) anticholinergic effects, (2) cardiovascular effects, (3) central nervous system effects, and (4) drug interactions. Marked individual variation in the incidence and type of side effects may be related to the plasma concentrations of tricyclic antidepressant and its active metabolites. Weakness and fatigue are attributable to central nervous system effects and may resemble those seen with phenothiazines. Extrapyramidal reactions are rare, although a fine tremor develops in about 10% of patients, especially the elderly. These drugs produce insignificant effects on ventilation.

Anticholinergic Effects

Anticholinergic effects of tricyclic antidepressants, in contrast to the antipsychotic drugs, are prominent, especially at high doses. Amitriptyline causes the highest incidence of anticholinergic effects (*i.e.,* dry mouth, blurred vision, tachycardia, urinary retention, gastric emptying slowed) whereas desipramine produces the fewest such effects (Table 19-2). For this reason, desipramine is often selected when tachycardia would be undesirable.

Cardiovascular Effects

Previous suggestions that tricyclic antidepressants increase the risk of cardiac dysrhythmias and sudden death have not been substantiated in the absence of drug overdose (Moir *et al,* 1973; Thompson *et al,* 1983). Furthermore, in the absence of severe preexisting cardiac dysfunction, tricyclic antidepressants lack adverse effects on left ventricular function and may even possess cardiac antidysrhythmic properties (Veith *et al,* 1982). With the exception of doxepin, tricyclic antidepressants produce depression of conduction of cardiac impulses through the atria and ventricles, manifesting on the electrocardiogram as prolongation of the P-R interval, widening of the QRS complex, and flattening or inversion of the T wave (Hollister, 1978). Nevertheless, these electrocardiographic changes are probably benign and may gradually disappear with continued therapy (Thompson *et al,* 1983). Atropine is useful when tricyclic antidepressants slow atrioventricular or interventricular conduction of cardiac impulses. Orthostatic hypotension is a common side effect of tricyclic antidepressant therapy.

Direct cardiac depressant effects may reflect quinidine-like actions on the heart. For this reason, tricyclic antidepressants must be used with caution in patients with preexisting heart disease.

Conceivably, there could also be enhancement of depressant cardiac effects of anesthetics by tricyclic antidepressants.

Central Nervous System Effects

Sedation associated with tricyclic antidepressant therapy may be desirable for management of agitated patients. For this purpose, amitriptyline and doxepin produce the greatest degree of sedation (Table 19-2). Tricyclic antidepressants produce evidence of seizure activity on the electroencephalogram, introducing the question as to the safety of administering these drugs to patients with seizure disorders or to those receiving drugs that may produce seizures (see the section entitled Drug Interactions). Children seem to be especially vulnerable to the seizure-inducing effects of tricyclic antidepressants.

Drug Interactions

The anticholinergic and catecholamine uptake blocking properties of the tricyclic antidepressants are most likely to be responsible for drug interactions. Drug interactions may be prominent with (1) sympathomimetics, (2) inhaled anesthetics, (3) anticholinergics, (4) antihypertensives, and (5) opioids. Binding of tricyclic antidepressants to plasma albumin can be reduced by competition from other drugs, including phenytoin, aspirin, and scopolamine.

SYMPATHOMIMETICS. Tricyclic antidepressants, by virtue of inhibiting uptake of norepinephrine into postganglionic sympathetic nerve endings, make more neurotransmitter available to act at postsynaptic adrenergic receptors. As a result, the pressor response evoked by an indirect-acting sympathomimetic, such as ephedrine, is increased two- to tenfold in the presence of tricyclic antidepressants. Even epinephrine present in a local anesthetic solution could evoke hypertension if administered to a patient being treated with a tricyclic antidepressant (Boakes *et al,* 1973). If a sympathomimetic is required, a direct-acting drug, such as phenylephrine in reduced doses, would be an acceptable choice.

INHALED ANESTHETICS. An increased incidence of cardiac dysrhythmias, including sinus tachycardia, ventricular tachycardia, and ventricu-

Table 19-2
Comparative Pharmacology of Tricyclic Antidepressants

	Anticholinergic Effect	Sedative Effect
Imipramine	Moderate	Minimal
Desipramine	Minimal	Minimal
Amitriptyline	Marked	Marked
Nortriptyline	Moderate	Moderate
Doxepin	Moderate	Marked

lar fibrillation, has been observed in halothane-anesthetized dogs pretreated with imipramine and receiving pancuronium (Fig. 19-8) (Edwards *et al*, 1979). Presumably, there is an interaction between the tricyclic antidepressant and the anticholinergic and/or sympathetic nervous system stimulating effects of pancuronium (Fig. 19-9) (Edwards *et al*, 1979). Similar cardiac dysrhythmias do not occur in animals anesthetized with enflurane (Fig. 19-8) (Edwards *et al*, 1979). Theoretically, ketamine might produce a similar adverse response as pancuronium when administered in the presence of tricyclic antidepressants.

Induction of anesthesia may be associated with an increased incidence of cardiac dysrhythmias in patients being treated with tricyclic antidepressants. Likewise, the dose of exogenous epinephrine necessary to produce cardiac dysrhythmias during anesthesia with a volatile anesthetic, such as halothane, is reduced by tricyclic

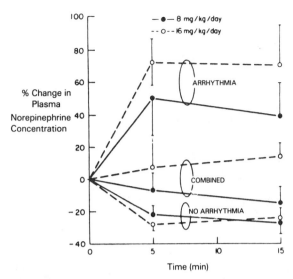

FIGURE 19-9. Dogs pretreated with imipramine that developed cardiac dysrhythmias following administration of pancuronium during halothane anesthesia also manifested increased plasma concentrations of norepinephrine. (From Edwards RP, Miller RD, Roizen MF, *et al.* Cardiac responses to imipramine and pancuronium during anesthesia with halothane or enflurane. Anesthesiology 1979;50:421–5. Reproduced by permission of the authors and publisher.)

antidepressants (Wong *et al*, 1980). Theoretically, increased availability of norepinephrine in the central nervous system could result in increased anesthetic requirements for inhaled drugs. Treatment with tricyclic antidepressants may enhance the central nervous system stimulating effects of enflurane (Sprague and Wolf, 1982).

ANTICHOLINERGICS. Because anticholinergic side effects of drugs may be additive, the use of centrally active anticholinergic drugs for preoperative medication of patients being treated with tricyclic antidepressants could increase the likelihood of postoperative delirium and confusion (*e.g.*, central anticholinergic syndrome) (see Chapter 10). Glycopyrrolate would be unlikely to evoke this drug interaction in patients being treated with tricyclic antidepressants.

ANTIHYPERTENSIVES. Tricyclic antidepressants prevent the antihypertensive effect of guanethidine, presumably by interfering with uptake of

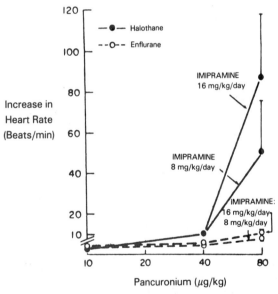

FIGURE 19-8. Correlation between dose of pancuronium and maximum increase in heart rate in dogs during halothane or enflurane anesthesia. Dogs were pretreated with 8 or 16 mg kg⁻¹ day⁻¹ of imipramine for 15 days. (From Edwards RP, Miller RD, Roizen MF, *et al.* Cardiac responses to imipramine and pancuronium during anesthesia with halothane or enflurane. Anesthesiology 1979;50:421–5. Reproduced by permission of the authors and publisher.)

guanethidine into postganglionic sympathetic nerve endings. These drugs can also block the centrally mediated antihypertensive action of alpha-methyldopa and clonidine (Briant *et al,* 1973; Kale and Satoskar, 1970). Rebound hypertension following abrupt discontinuation of clonidine may be accentuated and prolonged by concomitant tricyclic antidepressant therapy (Stiff and Harris, 1983). Conceivably, increased plasma concentrations of clonidine can persist for longer periods in the presence of tricyclic antidepressants that prevent uptake of norepinephrine back into the postganglionic sympathetic nerve endings. The combination of a tricyclic antidepressant and an MAOI has been associated with central nervous system toxicity manifesting as hyperpyrexia, seizures, and coma (Goldberg and Thornton, 1978).

OPIOIDS. In animals, tricyclic antidepressants augment the analgesic and ventilatory depressant effects of opioids. Likewise, the sedative and depressant effects of barbiturates are increased in animals (Dobkin, 1960). If these responses also occur in patients, it is predictable that doses of these drugs should be reduced so as to avoid exaggerated and/or prolonged depressant effects.

Tolerance

Tolerance to anticholinergic effects (*i.e.,* dry mouth, blurred vision, tachycardia) and orthostatic hypotension develops during chronic therapy with tricyclic antidepressants. Conversely, tolerance to desirable effects often fails to develop. Abrupt discontinuation of high doses of tricyclic antidepressants may be associated with a mild withdrawal syndrome characterized by malaise, chills, coryza, and skeletal muscle aching.

Overdose

In contrast to the antipyschotic drugs, overdose with tricyclic antidepressants is life threatening. Severe overdose is present with the acute ingestion of 1 g of imipramine or the equivalent of any other tricyclic antidepressant. Presenting features of an overdose include restlessness and seizures followed by coma, depression of ventilation, hy-potension, hypothermia, and striking signs of anticholinergic effects, including mydriasis, flushed dry skin, urinary retention, and tachycardia. The QRS complex on the electrocardiogram may be prolonged to greater than 100 msec. Indeed, the likelihood of seizures and ventricular dysrhythmias is increased when the duration of the QRS complex exceeds 100 msec (Boehnert and Lovejoy, 1985). Conversely, plasma concentrations of tricyclic antidepressants do not allow prediction of the likely occurrence of seizures or cardiac dysrhythmias (Boehnert and Lovejoy, 1985).

The comatose phase of tricyclic antidepressant overdose lasts 24 to 72 hours. Even after this phase passes, the risk of life-threatening cardiac dysrhythmias persists for up to 10 days, necessitating continued monitoring of the electrocardiogram in these patients (Vohra and Burrows, 1974).

Treatment

Treatment of a life-threatening overdose of tricyclic antidepressants is supportive, often including intubation of the trachea. Gastric lavage is sometimes used early in treatment, but this is most safely performed with a cuffed tracheal tube already in place. Nevertheless, rapid gastric emptying limits the value of gastric lavage, whereas avid protein binding of tricyclic antidepressants negates any therapeutic value of hemodialysis or drug-induced diuresis. Administration of activated charcoal, however, may absorb some drug in the gastrointestinal tract.

Physostigmine, 0.5 to 2 mg administered intravenously, may be effective in alleviating the toxic effects of tricyclic antidepressants (Baldessarini and Gelenberg, 1979). Repeat doses of physostigmine are likely to be necessary every 30 to 90 minutes. Diazepam has been used to control seizures produced by tricyclic antidepressants. Propranolol is recommended to control drug-induced tachycardia (Marshall and Green, 1968). In the presence of high plasma concentrations of tricyclic antidepressants, the effects of alpha-adrenergic agonists may be inhibited, resulting in difficulty in reversing hypotension with sympathomimetics.

MONOAMINE OXIDASE INHIBITORS

MAOI constitute a heterogeneous group of drugs that have in common the ability to prevent oxida-

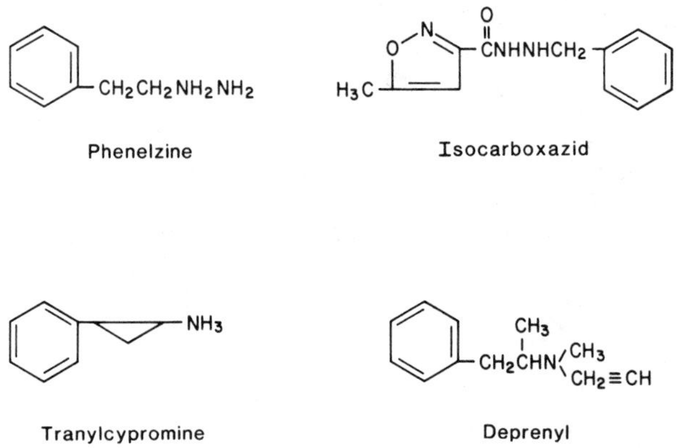

FIGURE 19-10. Monoamine oxidase inhibitors.

tive deamination of naturally occurring mono-amines (Fig. 19-10). As a result, these drugs lead to increased intraneuronal concentrations of amine neurotransmitters, including dopamine, norepinephrine, epinephrine, and serotonin.

Clinically used MAOI are classified as hydrazine or nonhydrazine derivatives, with a further subdivision based on the presence or absence of selectivity for the A or B form of the enzyme (Table 19-3) (Michaels *et al*, 1984; Roth, 1976) (see the section entitled Mechanism of Action). These durgs are administered only by the oral route, being readily absorbed from the gastrointestinal tract.

Clinical Uses

The use of MAOI is limited by serious drug interactions and hepatotoxicity. Furthermore, tricyclic antidepressants seem more effective than MAOI in the treatment of mental depression. Occasionally, the MAOI, pargyline, is administered to treat essential hypertension (see the section entitled Mechanism of Action). Effectiveness of MAOI in treatment of narcolepsy is consistent with the ability of these drugs to suppress the rapid eye movement phase of sleep (see Chapter 41).

Mechanism of Action

Monoamine oxidase is the principal intraneuronal enzyme responsible for the oxidative deamination of amine neurotransmitters, including dopamine, norepinephrine, epinephrine, and serotonin. As a result of inactivation of monoamine oxidase by MAOI, there is accumulation of these amines in the cytoplasm of nerve terminals. It is this intraneuronal accumulation of neurotransmitters in the central nervous system that is speculated to produce antidepressant effects.

Two forms of monoamine oxidase (MAO-A and MAO-B) have been defined on the basis of differences in substrate preferences (Table 19-3) (Michaels *et al*, 1984; Roth, 1976). Type A enzyme preferentially deaminates serotonin, dopamine, and norepinephrine (Fig. 19-11) (Michaels *et al*, 1984). Inhibition of MAO-A is clinically relevant, because serotonin and norepinephrine are important neurotransmitters in psychiatric disorders. Type B enzyme preferentially deaminates phenethylamine and tyramine (Fig. 19-11) (Michaels *et al*, 1984). Human brain contains approximately 80% MAO-B. Theoretically, use of selective MAOI could reduce the incidence of side effects that accompany the administration of nonselective MAOI (see the section entitled Side Effects).

Hypotensive effects of MAOI are attributed to accumulation of a false neurotransmitter, octopamine, in postganglionic sympathetic nerve endings. Release of this false neurotransmitter in response to a neural stimulus produces less vasoconstriction than does norepinephrine. As a result, blood pressure declines as a manifestation of a decrease in peripheral vascular resistance.

Side Effects

The ability of MAOI to inhibit activity of monoamine oxidase in the liver and gastrointestinal

Table 19-3
Drug Selectivity for MAO Enzymes

	MAO-A	MAO-B
Hydrazine Compound		
Phenelzine	+	+
Isocarboxazid	+	+
Iproniazid	+	+
Nonhydrazine Compound		
Tranylcypromine	+	+
Pargyline	?	+
Clorgyline	+	0
Deprenyl	?	+

(Data from Michaels I, Serrins M, Shier NQ, Barash PG. Anesthesia for cardiac surgery in patients receiving monoamine oxidase inhibitors. Anesth Analg 1984;63:1041–4; with permission.)

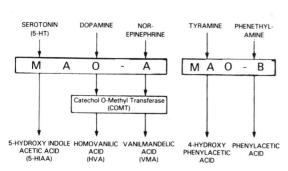

FIGURE 19-11. The two forms of monoamine oxidase enzyme (MAO-A and MAO-B) exhibit substrate selectivity. (From Michaels I, Serrins M, Shier NQ, Barash PG. Anesthesia for cardiac surgery in patients receiving monoamine oxidase inhibitors. Anesth Analg 1984;63:1041–4. Reproduced by permission of the authors and the International Anesthesia Research Society.)

tract is responsible for predictable side effects that accompany use of these drugs (Jenkins and Graves, 1976). Hepatotoxicity associated with hydrazine-containing compounds has led to discontinuation of the use of several MAOI. Peripheral neuropathy following use of MAOI may be related to pyridoxine deficiency. Effects of MAOI on the electroencephalogram are slight and not seizure-like, which contrasts with tricyclic antidepressants. Also, in contrast with tricyclic antidepressants, is the failure of MAOI to produce cardiac dysrhythmias (Wong *et al,* 1980).

Since enzyme inhibition of monoamine oxidase is often irreversible, it is commonly recommended that MAOI be discontinued at least 14 to 21 days prior to elective surgery so as to permit synthesis of new enzyme. Regeneration of new enzyme, however, may be more rapid following discontinuation of tranycypromine or pargyline, as these drugs do not irreversibly bind to monoamine oxidase. Indeed, a pharmacologic effect is no longer detectable 24 hours after discontinuing these drugs. Even patients receiving irreversible enzyme inhibitors may be safely anesthetized without waiting 14 to 21 days for regeneration of new enzyme to occur (El–Ganzouri *et al,* 1985; Michaels *et al,* 1984).

Sympathomimetics

The actions of indirect-acting and, to a lesser extent, direct-acting sympathomimetics are exaggerated by MAOI. This reflects the fact that MAOI act primarily intraneuronally such that more neurotransmitter becomes available for release by indirect-acting sympathomimetics. If hypotension occurs in a patient receiving a MAOI, direct-acting sympathomimetics such as phenylephrine, in reduced doses, are recommended. MAOI may have less potentiating effects on exogenously administered catecholamines since metabolism by catechol-O-methyltransferase and neuronal uptake partially offset the reduced activity of monoamine oxidase (Boakes *et al,* 1973).

Tyramine in Food

Monoamine oxidase is widely distributed in the body, with high concentrations of the enzyme being present in the liver and gastrointestinal tract. Ingestion of tyramine-containing foods (cheese, chicken liver, chocolate, beer, wine) may evoke hypertensive crisis, since tyramine is no longer inactivated in the gastrointestinal tract or liver. This allows tyramine to evoke the release of endogenous catecholamines that are present in excess amounts. Headache may be the first sign of life-threatening hypertension due to this food–drug interaction. The precipitous hypertension resembles that which occurs with release of catecholamines from a pheochromocytoma. Treatment of hypertension is with a peripheral vasodilator (nitroprusside) or an alpha-adrenergic antagonist (phentolamine). Cardiac dysrhythmias that persist after control of blood pressure are treated with lidocaine or propranolol.

Orthostatic Hypotension

Orthostatic hypotension occurs with all MAOI, possibly reflecting the accumulation of the false neurotransmitter, octopamine, in the cytoplasm of sympathetic nerve terminals. Release of this less potent neurotransmitter and vasoconstrictor in response to neural impulses is the most likely explanation for orthostatic hypotension as well as the antihypertensive effects associated with chronic administration of MAOI.

Hyperpyrexia

Hyperpyrexia may accompany the administration of meperidine to a patient receiving MAOI (Lewis, 1965). Evidence for a role of serotonin is the prevention of this hyperthermic response in animals pretreated with inhibitors of serotonin (Rogers, 1971). In addition to hyperpyrexia, there may be hypertension, hypotension, depression of ventilation, skeletal muscle rigidity, seizures, and coma. Meperidine is the most often incriminated opioid, but other opioids may cause similar responses (Brown and Cass, 1979). For this reason, postoperative pain management in the patient being treated with MAOI may be best provided by regional anesthetic techniques. Dantrolene has been reported to be useful in the treatment of skeletal muscle rigidity and associated symptoms of hypermetabolism following an overdose of a MAOI (Kaplan et al, 1986).

Inhibition of Hepatic Enzymes

Inhibition of hepatic enzymes other than monoamine oxidase by MAOI has been proposed as an explanation for exaggerated depressant effects produced by opioids and barbiturates (Eade and Renton, 1970). For this reason, the dose of opioid should be decreased to one fourth the usual amount (Janowsky et al, 1981). Exaggerated effects of antihistamines, anticholinergics, and tricyclic antidepressants may also reflect slow metabolism resulting from MAOI-induced decreases in enzyme activity. Prolonged responses to succinylcholine have been observed, suggesting inhibition of plasma cholinesterase by MAOI (Bodley et al, 1969).

Anesthetic Requirements

In animals, anesthetic requirements for volatile drugs are increased, presumably reflecting accumulation of norepinephrine in the central nervous system (Miller et al, 1968).

DISULFIRAM

Disulfiram is a thiuram derivative that inhibits acetaldehyde dehydrogenase activity necessary for the oxidation of acetaldehyde, which results from breakdown of alcohol by alcohol dehydrogenase. As a result, ingestion of alcohol in the presence of disulfiram leads to accumulation of acetaldehyde in the plasma, manifesting as flushing, vertigo, nausea, hyperventilation, tachycardia, and diaphoresis. Symptoms usually last 30 to 60 minutes but in some patients may persist for several hours. Sedation is predictable following waning of symptoms. Severe reactions occur less frequently and include hypoventilation, hypotension, cardiac dysrhythmias, cardiac failure, syncope, and seizures. Hypotension may reflect the ability of disulfiram to inhibit dopamine beta-hydroxylase activity necessary for the synthesis of norepinephrine from dopamine. The unpleasantness of symptoms that accompany ingestion of alcohol in the presence of inhibition of acetaldehyde dehydrogenase activity is the basis for the use of disulfiram as an adjunctive drug with psychiatric counseling to decrease consumption of alcohol. Compliance with long-term oral disulfiram therapy is often poor.

Management of anesthesia in patients being treated with disulfiram should consider the potential presence of disulfiram-induced sedation and hepatotoxicity. Preoperative determination of liver function tests seems prudent. Decreased drug requirements could reflect an additive effect with preexisting sedation or the ability of disulfiram to inhibit metabolism of drugs other than alcohol. For example, disulfiram may result in potentiation of the effects of benzodiazepines. Acute and otherwise unexplained hypotension during general anesthesia could reflect inadequate stores of norepinephrine due to disulfiram-induced inhibition of dopamine beta-hydroxylase (Diaz and Hill, 1979). This hypotension responds to ephedrine although a direct-acting sympathomimetic such as phenylephrine would seem more logical for treatment of hypotension due to depletion of norepinephrine. Use of regional anesthesia may be influenced by the occasional patient treated with disulfiram who develops polyneuropathy. Alcohol-containing solutions, as used for skin cleansing, should be avoided in these patients.

REFERENCES

Baldessarini RJ, Gelenberg AJ. Use of physostigmine in antidepressant-induced intoxication. Am J Psychiatry 1979;136:1608 – 9.

Baldessarini RJ, Tarsy D. Tardive dyskinesia. In: Lipton MA, DiMascio A, Killam KF, eds. Psychopharmacology: A Generation of Progress. New York, Raven Press, 1978;993.

Bertolo L, Novakovic L, Penna M. Antiarrhythmic effects of droperidol. Anesthesiology 1972;37:529 – 35.

Bittar DA. Innovar-induced hypertensive crisis in patients with pheochromocytoma. Anesthesiology 1979;50:366 – 9.

Boakes AJ, Laurence DR, Teoh PC, Barar FSK, Benedikter LT, Prichard BNC. Interactions between sympathomimetic amines and antidepressant agents in man. Br Med J 1973;1:311 – 5.

Bodley PO, Halwax K, Potts L. Low serum pseudocholinesterase levels complicating treatment with phenelzine. Br Med J 1969;3:510 – 2.

Boehnert MT, Lovejoy FH. Value of the QRS duration versus the serum drug level in predicting seizures and ventricular arrhythmias after an acute overdose of tricyclic antidepressants. N Engl J Med 1985;313:474 – 9.

Briant RH, Reed JL, Dollery CT. Interaction between clonidine and desipramine in man. Br Med J 1973;1:522 – 3.

Brown TCK, Cass NM. Beware – the use of MAO inhibitors is increasing again. Anaesth Intensive Care 1979;7:65 – 8.

Burroughs GD, Davies B, Kincaid – Smith P. Unique tubular lesion after lithium (letter). Lancet 1978;1:1310.

Cohen SE, Woods WA, Wyner J. Antiemetic efficacy of droperidol and metoclopramide. Anesthesiology 1984;60:67 – 9.

Davis JM, Janowsky DS, El – Yousef MK. The use of lithium in clinical psychiatry. Psychiatric Annals 1973;3:78 – 83.

Demers RG, Heninger GR. Electrocardiographic T-wave changes during lithium carbonate treatment. JAMA 1971;218:381 – 6.

Diamond JM, Santos AB. Unusual complications of antipsychotic drugs. Am Fam Physician 1982;26: 153 – 7.

Diaz JH, Hill GE. Hypotension with anesthesia in disulfiram-treated patients. Anesthesiology 1979;51: 366 – 8.

Dobkin AB. Potentiation of thiopental anaesthesia by derivatives and analogues of phenothiazine. Anesthesiology 1960;21:292 – 6.

Eade NR, Renton KW. The effect of phenelzine and tranylcypromine in the degradation of meperidine. J Pharmacol Exp Ther 1970;173:31 – 6.

Edwards RP, Miller RD, Roizen MF, et al. Cardiac responses to imipramine and pancuronium during anesthesia with halothane or enflurane. Anesthesiology 1979;50:421 – 5.

El – Ganzouri AR, Ivankovich AD, Braverman B, McCarthy R. Monoamine oxidase inhibitors: Should they be discontinued preoperatively? Anesth Analg 1985;64:592 – 6.

Erle G, Basso M, Federspil G, Sicolo N, Scandellari C. Effect of chlorpromazine on blood glucose and plasma insulin in man. Eur J Clin Pharmacol 1977;11:15 – 18.

Fink M. EEG and human psychopharmacology, Annu Rev Pharmacol 1969;9:241 – 58.

Fischler M, Bonnet F, Trang H et al. The pharmacokinetics of droperidol in anesthetized patients. Anesthesiology 1986;64:486 – 9.

Goldberg RB, Thornton WE. Combined tricyclic-MAOI therapy for refractory depression: A review with guidelines for appropriate usage. J Clin Pharmacol 1978;18:143 – 7.

Goldberg MD, Weinstein MR. Lithium carbonate in obstetrics — guidelines for clinical use. Am J Obstet Gynecol 1973;116:15 – 22.

Gomez – Arnau J, Marquez – Montes J, Avello F. Fentanyl and droperidol effects on the refractoriness of the accessory pathway in the Wolff – Parkinson – White syndrome. Anesthesiology 1983;58:307 – 13.

Granato JE, Stern BJ, Ringel A, et al. Neuroleptic malignant syndrome — successful treatment with dantrolene and bromocriptine. Ann Neurol 1983;14:89 – 90.

Guze BH, Baxter LR. Neuroleptic malignant syndrome. N Engl J Med 1985;313:163 – 6.

Harper MH, Hickey RF, Cromwell TH, Linwood S. The magnitude and duration of respiratory depression produced by fentanyl and fentanyl plus droperidol in man. J Pharmacol Exp Ther 1976;199:464 – 8.

Havdala HS, Borison RL, Diamond BI. Potential hazards and applications of lithium in anesthesiology. Anesthesiology 1979;50:534 – 7.

Hill GE, Wong KC, Hodges MR. Lithium carbonate and neuromuscular blocking agents. Anesthesiology 1977;46:122 – 6.

Hollister LE. Trycyclic antidepressants. N Engl J Med 1978;299:1106 – 9;1168 – 71.

Janowsky EC, Risch C, Janowsky DS. Effect of anesthesia on patients taking psychotropic drugs. J Clin Psychopharmacol 1981;1:14 – 20.

Jenkins LC, Graves HB. Potential hazards of psychoactive drugs in association with anaesthesia. Can Anaesth Soc J 1976;23:334.

Kale AK, Satoskar RS. Modification of the central hypotensive effect of methyldopa by reserpine, imipramine and tranylcypromine. Eur J Pharmacol 1970;9:120 – 3.

Kaplan RF, Feinglass NG, Webster W, Mudra S. Phenelzine overdose treated with dantrolene sodium. JAMA 1986;255:642 – 4.

Lee CM, Yeakel AE. Patients refusal of surgery following Innovar premedication. Anesth Analg 1975;54:224 – 6.

Lewis E. Hyperpyrexia with antidepressant drugs. Br Med J 1965;2:1671 – 2.

Macfie AC. Lithium poisoning precipitated by diuretics. Br Med J 1975;1:516.

Mannisto PT, Saarnivaara L. Effect of lithium and rubidium on the sleeping time caused by various anaesthetics in the mouse. Br J Anaesth 1976;48:185 – 9.

Marshall LJ, Green VA. Propranolol and diazepam for imipramine poisoning. Lancet 1968;2:1249.

Michaels I, Serrins M, Shier NQ, Barash PG. Anesthesia for cardiac surgery in patients receiving monoamine oxidase inhibitors. Anesth Analg 1984;63:1041 – 4.

Miller RD, Way WL, Eger EI. The effects of alpha-methyldopa, reserpine, guanethidine, and iproniazid on minimum alveolar anesthetic requirement (MAC). Anesthesiology 1968;29:1153 – 8.

Moir DC, Dingwall – Fordyce I, Weir RD. A follow-up study of cardiac patients receiving amitriptyline. Eur J Clin Pharmacol 1973;6:98 – 101.

Richter JJ. Current theories about the mechanisms of benzodiazepines and neuroleptic drugs. Anesthesiology 1981;54:66 – 72.

Rivera VM, Keichian AH, Oliver RE. Persistent parkinsonism following neuroleptanalgesia. Anesthesiology 1975;42:635 – 7.

Rogers KJ. Role of brain monoamines in the interaction between pethidine and tranylcypromine. Eur J Pharmacol 1971;14:86 – 8.

Rosenblatt RM, Reich J, Dehring D. Tricyclic antidepressants in treatment of depression and chronic pain. Anesth Analg 1984;63:1025 – 32.

Roth JA. Multiple forms of monoamine oxidase and their interaction with tricyclic psychomimetic drugs. Gen Pharmacol 1976;7:381 – 6.

Sangal R, Dimitrijevic R. Neuroleptic malignant syndrome. Successful treatment with pancuronium. JAMA 1985;254:2795 – 6.

Santos A, Datta S. Prophylactic use of droperidol for control of nausea and vomiting during spinal anesthesia for cesarean section. Anesth Analg 1984;63:85 – 7.

Soroker D, Barjilay E, Konichezky S, Bruderman. I. Respiratory function following premedication with droperidol or diazepam. Anesth Analg 1978;57:695 – 9.

Sprague DH, Wolf S. Enflurane seizures in patients taking amitriptyline. Anesth Analg 1982;61:67 – 8.

Stiff JL, Harris DB. Clonidine withdrawal complicated by amitriptyline therapy. Anesthesiology 1983;59:73 – 4.

Sumikawa K, Amakata Y. The pressor effect of droperidol on a patient with pheochromocytoma. Anesthesiology 1977;46:359 – 61.

Sumikawa K, Hirano H, Amakata Y, Kashimoto T, Wada A, Izumi F. Mechanism of the effect of droperidol to induce catecholamine efflux from the adrenal medulla. Anesthesiology 1985;62:17 – 22.

Thompson TL, Moran MG, Nies AS. Psychotropic drug use in the elderly. N Engl J Med 1983;308:194 – 8.

Veith RC, Raskind MA, Caldwell JH, Barnes RF, Gumbrecht G, Ritchie JL. Cardiovascular effects of tricyclic antidepressants in depressed patients with chronic heart disease. N Engl J Med 1982;306:954 – 9.

Vohra J, Burrows GD. Cardiovascular complications of tricyclic antidepressant overdosage. Drugs 1974;8:432 – 7.

Ward DS. Stimulation of hypoxic ventilatory drive by droperidol. Anesth Analg 1984;63:106 – 10.

Whitwam JG, Russell WJ. The acute cardiovascular changes and adrenergic blockade by droperidol in man. Br J Anaesth 1971;581 – 90.

Wiklund RA, Ngai SH. Rigidity and pulmonary edema after Innovar in a patient on levodopa therapy: Report of a case. Anesthesiology 1971;35:545 – 7.

Wong KC, Puerto AX, Puerto BA, Blatnick RA. Influence of imipramine and pargyline on the arrythmogenicity of epinephrine during halothane, enflurane or methoxyflurane anesthesia in dogs. Anesthesiology 1980;53:S25.

Ziegler VE, Biggs JT, Wylie LT. Doxepin kinetics. Clin Pharmacol Ther 1978;23:573 – 9.

CHAPTER 20

Prostaglandins

INTRODUCTION

Prostaglandins are among the most prevalent of the naturally occurring physiologically active endogenous substances (*i.e.*, autacoids) having been detected in almost every tissue and body fluid. No other autacoids (*e.g.*, histamine, serotonin, angiotensin II, plasma kinins) show more numerous and diverse effects than do prostaglandins (see Chapters 21 and 22). The production of prostaglandins increases in response to diverse stimuli, with minute amounts producing a broad array of effects. Inhibition of synthesis of prostaglandins is recognized as a mechanism of action of numerous drugs, including many of the nonsteroidal anti-inflammatory analgesics (see Chapter 11).

NOMENCLATURE AND STRUCTURE ACTIVITY RELATIONSHIPS

The designation of a substance as a prostaglandin reflects the initial observation that human semen contained a lipid-soluble acid that caused the uterus to relax (Euler, 1936; Kurzrok and Lieb, 1930). The generic term *eicosanoids* refers to the 20 carbon hairpin-shaped fatty acid chain that includes a cyclopentane ring, characteristic of prostaglandins (Fig. 20-1).

The letters PG denote the word *prostaglandin*. The third letter indicates the structure of the cyclopentane ring, such that PGE has a different ring structure than PGF. A subscript that follows the third letter denotes the number of double bonds in the structure as well as the fatty acid precursor of the prostaglandin. For example, PGE_1 has one double bond, whereas PGE_2 has two double bonds. The subscript 2 also designates arachidonic acid as the fatty acid precursor. Indeed, arachidonic acid is the most common fatty acid precursor of prostaglandins in man. Alpha or beta following the subscript indicates the direction of the hydroxyl group at the number 9 carbon in relation to the plane of the cyclopentane ring.

SYNTHESIS

Prostaglandins are derived principally from the polyunsaturated 20 carbon essential fatty acid, arachidonic acid. Arachidonic acid is a ubiquitous component of cell membranes and is released by the action of phospholipase enzyme. The enzyme is activated by various physical and chemical stimuli and inhibited by corticosteroids. Inhaled anesthetics, by virtue of their solubility in lipid cell membranes, may increase availability of arachidonic acid as a substrate (Shayevitz *et al*, 1985). Once released, arachidonic acid becomes available to serve as a substrate for production of prostaglandins via either the cyclooxygenase or lipoxygenase pathway (Fig. 20-2).

Cyclooxygenase

Cyclooxygenase is a widely distributed complex of microsomal enzymes necessary for the initial synthesis of prostaglandins (PGG_2 and PGH_2) known as endoperoxides (Fig. 20-2). Subsequent conversion of PGH_2 to thromboxane (TXA_2) and prostacyclin (PGI_2) requires the activity of tissue specific enzymes, thromboxane synthetase and prostacyclin synthetase (Fig. 20-2). In contrast to the wide tissue distribution of cyclooxygenase, thromboxane synthetase is principally present in platelets and the lungs, whereas prostacyclin synthetase is principally present in vascular endothelium.

Thromboxane and prostacyclin are highly active but unstable compounds, having brief elimination half-times (3–6 minutes) before nonenzymatic conversion to stable and inactive compounds (see the section entitled Metabolism). Indeed, estimates of plasma concentrations of thromboxane and prostacyclin are determined by measurement of the more stable inactive metabolites, thromboxane B_2 and 6-keto-prostaglandin $F_{1\alpha}$.

Lipoxygenase

Lipoxygenase enzymes are localized principally in platelets, vascular endothelium, lung, and leukocytes. Compounds formed by these enzymes

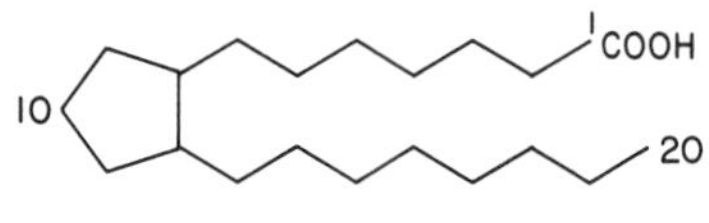

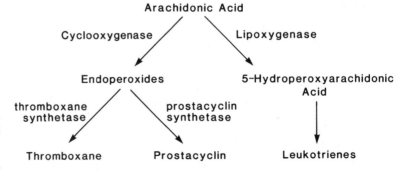

FIGURE 20-1. A 20 carbon hairpin-shaped fatty acid chain is characteristic of prostaglandins.

from arachidonic acid include 5-hydroperoxyarachidonic acid (HPETE) (Fig. 20-2) and its degradation product, 12-hydroxyarachidonic acid (HETE). Leukotrienes result from lipoxygenation of arachidonic acid and further addition of water-soluble substituents. Elevated concentrations of leukotrienes have been measured in several disease states, including bronchial asthma, neonatal hypoxemia with pulmonary hypertension, and the adult respiratory distress syndrome (Matthay *et al,* 1984). Leukotriene D (formerly designated slow reacting substance of anaphylaxis) has preferential effects on peripheral airways and is a more potent bronchoconstrictor than histamine. Furthermore, leukotriene-induced increases in vascular permeability occur at lower concentrations than histamine. Leukotriene B released from alveolar macrophages and other leukocytes stimulates neutrophil adhesion to endothelial cells, with subsequent degranulation, enzyme release, and superoxide generation (Samuelsson, 1983).

MECHANISM OF ACTION

In many tissues, prostaglandins act on specific receptors to stimulate snythesis of cyclic AMP by virtue of activation of adenylate cyclase. The acidic lipid nature of prostaglandins is unique among the autacoids and other substances that react with specific cell membrane receptors. Stimulation of smooth muscle by prostaglandins appears to be associated with the depolarization of cellular membranes and the release of calcium.

METABOLISM

Initial metabolism of prostaglandins to inactive substances is rapid, being catalyzed by specific

FIGURE 20-2. Synthesis of prostaglandins from arachidonic acid occurs via a cyclooxygenase pathway and lipoxygenase pathway.

enzymes that are widely distributed in the body, in such organs as the lungs, kidneys, liver, and the gastrointestinal tract (see the section entitled Cyclooxygenase). For example, 95% of infused PGE_2 is inactivated during one passage through the lungs (Ferreira and Vane, 1967). The unique position of the pulmonary circulation between the venous and arterial circulations allows the lungs to act as a filter for many of the prostaglandins, thus protecting the cardiovascular system and other organs from prolonged effects due to recirculation of these substances.

The initial rapid metabolism of prostaglandins is followed by a slower breakdown, during which the existing inactive metabolites are oxidized by enzymes responsible for oxidation of most fatty acids. The liver is the major site for this oxidation, and the resulting metabolites appear in the urine. For example, dicarboxylic acid is excreted in the urine as the major metabolite of both PGE_1 and PGE_2.

EFFECTS ON ORGAN SYSTEMS

The possible roles of prostaglandins as mediators of effects on organ systems depend on the system under consideration. For example, inhibitors of prostaglandin synthesis usually have little effect on the cardiovascular system or lungs, suggesting a negligible role of prostaglandins in the basal regulation of these systems. Conversely, normal platelet function and hemostasis are likely to be under strict regulation of prostaglandins as emphasized by the ability of nonsteroidal anti-inflammatory drugs to interfere with normal platelet aggregation (see Chapter 11).

Hematologic System

Prostaglandins exert powerful effects on platelets. For example, thromboxane acts as an intense stimulus for platelet aggregation, presumably reflecting inhibition of adenylate cyclase and subsequent reduced cyclic AMP snythesis in platelets (Gorman *et al,* 1978). Conversely, vascular endothelium opposes platelet aggregation by release of prostacyclin. Prostacyclin stimulates platelet production of cyclic AMP, leading to decreased platelet adhesiveness and prolonged platelet survival.

A normal thromboxane to prostacyclin ratio is important in maintaining platelet activity and co-agulation. An increase in this ratio, as may occur when atherosclerotic plaques release substances that inhibit synthesis of prostacyclin, results in a predominance of thromboxane activity manifesting as platelet aggregation and vasoconstriction (Brooks *et al,* 1971). This sequence of events could lead to reduced blood flow in the area of an atherosclerotic plaque manifesting as ischemia or infarction in organs such as the heart, brain, and kidneys. A similar imbalance in the ratio of thromboxane to prostacyclin in the venous circulation could lead to venous thromboembolism.

Bleeding disorders are likely in the presence of thromboxane depletion or excess prostacyclin. The speculated role for platelet aggregation in myocardial ischemia suggests a potentially useful role for prostacyclin in both dilating coronary arteries and preventing aggregation of platelets. These same effects of prostacyclin could be useful in the treatment of acute ischemic pain in extremities and to promote healing of ischemic ulcerations.

Prostacyclin present in low concentrations in the plasma may be responsible for preventing aggregation of normal platelets. A break in the vascular endothelium releases thromboxane, causing intense local vasoconstriction and platelet aggregation leading to formation of a hemostatic plug (Moncada *et al,* 1978). It seems likely that cyclooxygenase enzyme in the platelets that synthesizes thromboxane is more sensitive to inhibition by aspirin than is the same enzyme in vascular endothelium that synthesizes prostacyclin (McGiff and Stollermhan, 1980). As a result, thromboxane production in platelets is stopped by small doses of aspirin, whereas large doses of aspirin inhibit both thromboxane and prostacyclin production. If a patient is on low-dose aspirin, thromboxane is no longer present to oppose prostacyclin, and platelet aggregation does not occur.

Platelets are activated and consumed when blood passes over the surfaces of materials utilized for extracorporeal circulation. Continuous intravenous infusion of prostacyclin during extracorporeal circulation minimizes the degree of thrombocytopenia, and maintenance of platelet function is suggested by reduced postoperative bleeding (Fig. 20-3) (Longmore *et al,* 1981).

Iloprost

Iloprost is a prostacyclin analog that acts as a potent inhibitor of platelet aggregation but lacks sig-

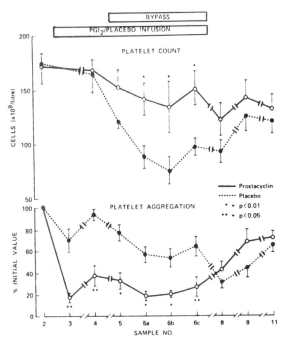

FIGURE 20-3. Variations in platelet count and platelet aggregation with prostacyclin (PGI₂) *(solid lines)* and without prostacyclin *(broken lines)*. (From Longmore DB, Bennett JG, Hoyle PM, *et al*. Prostacyclin administration during cardiopulmonary bypass in man. Lancet 1981;1:800 – 804. Reproduced by permission of the authors and publisher.)

nificant cardiovascular effects. Added to the cardiopulmonary bypass circuit, this prostaglandin preserves the circulating platelet count and prevents platelet granule release during simulated extracorporeal circulation (Addonizio *et al*, 1985).

Cardiovascular System

The effects of prostaglandins on cardiac function are complex, being dependent on direct inotropic effects, the activity of the sympathetic nervous system relative to the parasympathetic nervous system, and the metabolic status of the heart (Hintze *et al*, 1979; Kot *et al*, 1975). For example, PGE₂ produces an increase in heart rate and contractility by direct inotropic effects as well as by increasing reflex sympathetic nervous system activity. The in-

travenous administration of prostacyclin causes a reduction in blood pressure as a result of a decline in peripheral vascular resistance reflecting vasodilation in several vascular beds, including coronary, renal, mesenteric, and skeletal muscle circulations. Prostacyclin is not inactivated in the lungs and is thus an effective vasodilator when administered intravenously (Szczeklik *et al*, 1978). The effects of prostacyclin on heart rate are variable, apparently depending on the basal level of autonomic nervous system activity.

The activity of vascular smooth muscle in various vascular beds may be modulated by the relative magnitude of vasoconstriction and vasodilation produced by thromboxane and prostacyclin, respectively. For example, events leading to coronary artery spasm and thrombosis may arise from a deficiency of prostacyclin-induced vasodilation relative to thromboxane-induced vasoconstriction.

Local generation of PGE₂ and prostacyclin may participate in the transition of the fetal circulation to that of a normal newborn. Indeed, prostaglandin synthesis inhibitors may contribute to the closure of the ductus arteriosus (Olley and Coceani, 1981).

Alprostadil

Alprostadil (PGE₁) has a variety of pharmacologic effects, among which the most important are vasodilation, inhibition of platelet aggregation, and stimulation of gastrointestinal and uterine smooth muscle (Fig. 20-4). This drug is a potent relaxant of the smooth muscle of the ductus arteriosus and preserves ductal patency in neonates when infused intravenously before anatomic closure has occurred (Cole *et al*, 1981). For this reason, alprostadil is used in neonates with ductal-dependent congenital heart disease (pulmonary atresia, tretralogy of Fallot) so as to maintain patency of the ductus arteriosus until surgery can be performed.

Alprostadil is metabolized so rapidly that it

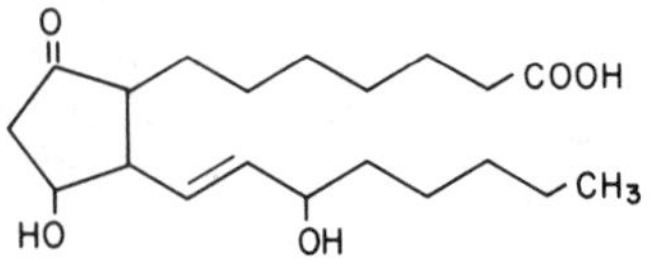

FIGURE 20-4. Aprostadil (prostaglandin E₂).

must be administered as a continuous intravenous infusion. Nearly 70% of circulating alprostadil is metabolized in one passage through the lungs, and the metabolites are excreted by the kidneys. Depression of ventilation, bronchoconstriction, flushing, bradycardia, and hyperpyrexia may be evoked by continuous intravenous infusion of this drug (Lewis *et al*, 1981). Alprostadil should not be administered to infants with respiratory distress syndrome.

Pulmonary Circulation

Pulmonary vasoconstriction may be related to increased circulating concentrations of thromboxane, PGE_2, and $PGE_{2\alpha}$ (Frolich *et al*, 1979). In an animal model, administration of PGE_1 and prostacyclin attenuated pulmonary hypertension and interstitial pulmonary edema induced by *Escherichia coli* endotoxin (Smith *et al*, 1982). In this regard, certain prostaglandins may become useful in the management of acute respiratory failure. Likewise, inhibitors of prostaglandin synthesis, such as indomethacin, may be useful in the treatment of pulmonary edema that does not respond to conventional therapy.

Release of prostacyclin from the lungs into the pulmonary circulation could prevent aggregation of platelets. This effect would provide a physiologic mechanism for dispersing clumps of platelets trapped in small pulmonary blood vessels (Moncada *et al*, 1978).

As a potent pulmonary vasoconstrictor, $PGF_{2\alpha}$ has been shown to enhance vasoconstriction in an atelectatic lung, diverting pulmonary blood flow to ventilated alveoli and increasing the PaO_2 (Scherer *et al*, 1985). In essence, $PGF_{2\alpha}$ is capable of potentiating hypoxic pulmonary vasoconstriction and thus improving arterial oxygenation. Since 70% to 98% of this prostaglandin is inactivated in one passage across the lung, it is possible, with the proper infusion rate, to selectively produce effects on the pulmonary vasculature to the exclusion of the systemic circulation.

Lungs

The lungs are a major site of prostaglandin synthesis. Prostaglandins may produce bronchoconstriction or bronchodilatation. Indeed, an imbalance between production of thromboxane and prosta-

cyclin in the lungs has been proposed as a mechanism of bronchial asthma (Boot *et al*, 1978). Asthmatic patients experience increased airway resistance with far lower inhaled amounts of $PGF_{2\beta}$ than do normal patients (Mathe and Hedqvist, 1975). Leukotriene D is several thousand times more potent as a constrictor of bronchial smooth muscle than is histamine (Drazen *et al*, 1980). Both PGE_1 and PGE_2 produce bronchodilatation when given by aerosol, but the associated irritant effect of this inhalation offsets their clinical usefulness.

Kidneys

The kidneys are a major site of synthesis of prostaglandins (Bolger *et al*, 1978). For example, the antihypertensive effect of normally functioning kidneys may be related to their capacity to synthesize and release into the circulation PGE_2 or prostacyclin, which causes diuresis, natriuresis, and a decrease in blood pressure. These effects of prostaglandins may be due to a direct action on renal tubular transport processes or a change in the distribution of renal blood flow (Grenier and Smith, 1978). Renal vasodilation produced by PGE_2 may offset renal vasoconstriction produced by events such as drug-induced increases in sympathetic nervous systemic activity. Prostacyclin and PGE_2 influence angiotensin-induced vasoconstriction by virtue of their ability to increase the release of renin from the kidney. Indeed, drugs such as aspirin and indomethacin that inhibit synthesis of prostaglandins by way of the cyclooxygenase enzyme pathway are effective in the treatment of primary hyperreninemia (Bartter's syndrome) (Gill *et al*, 1976). Certain prostaglandins may induce erythropoiesis by stimulating the release of erythropoietin from the renal cortex.

Gastrointestinal Tract

Certain prostaglandins, including prostacyclin, inhibit gastric acid secretion evoked by histamine or gastrin (Whittle *et al*, 1978). Methylated analogs of prostaglandins have been shown to decrease the volume of gastric fluid and its acidity after oral or intravenous administration (Karim, 1972). Nausea, vomiting, and diarrhea associated with the use of PGE_2 to induce abortion reflect stimulation of smooth muscle of the gastrointestinal tract as well as the uterus.

Uterus

The nongravid and gravid uterus are predictably contracted by PGE_2 and $PGF_{2\alpha}$, leading to the speculation that these prostaglandins are important in the initiation and maintenance of labor (Horton and Poyser, 1976). Intravenous infusion results in prompt and dose-dependent elevations in uterine muscle tone. In contrast to oxytocin, this effect of prostaglandins is observed at all stages of pregnancy, accounting for the usefulness of PGE_2 or $PGF_{2\alpha}$ for inducing abortion as well as labor. Prompt depression of progesterone output and resorption of the corpus luteum follow parenteral injection of $PGF_{2\alpha}$ to animals. This effect interrupts early pregnancy, which is dependent on luteal rather than placental progesterone.

Increased synthesis of prostaglandins in the endometrium is speculated to be a possible cause of dysmenorrhea. Indeed, inhibitors of prostaglandin synthesis such as aspirin or indomethacin reduce pain associated with dysmenorrhea. Chronic use of aspirin increases the average length of gestation and the duration of spontaneous labor. Likewise, these inhibitors of prostaglandin synthesis reduce contractions of the uterus in premature labor and could increase the likelihood of postpartum uterine atony.

Prostaglandins may be important in the control of uteroplacental circulation (Rankin, 1978). Changes in the production of prostaglandins have been implicated in the pathophysiology of preeclampsia.

Carboprost

Carboprost is a synthetic analog of naturally occurring $PGF_{2\alpha}$ (Fig. 20-5). The addition of a methyl group at carbon 15 results in a longer duration of action. Drug-induced uterine contractions are similar to those that accompany labor. Induction of elective abortion with carboprost is successful in more than 90% of patients between 12 and 20 weeks of gestation. Mean time to abortion is 16 hours following an average intramuscular dose of carboprost, which is 2.6 mg. Adverse effects are common but usually are not serious. Vomiting and diarrhea occur in more than 60% of patients. Body temperature elevation of 1°C to 2°C occurs in nearly 10% of patients and must be differentiated from that resulting from endometritis. Delivery of a live fetus with carboprost-induced abortion is possible.

Dinoprost

Dinoprost is $PGF_{2\alpha}$ and is administered intra-amniotically to induce uterine contractions (Fig. 20-6). The mean abortion time is about 20 hours. Nausea and vomiting occur in most patients and can often be ameliorated by antiemetics. Bronchospasm may occur in asthmatic patients. Grand mal seizures are possible in patients prone to epilepsy. Inadvertent intravenous administration produces immediate bronchospasm, tetanic uterine contraction, and hypotension or hypertension.

Dinoprostone

Dinoprostone is PGE_2 and produces physiologic-like uterine contractions (Fig. 20-7). Therapeutically, this prostaglandin is used to induce labor for elective abortion. Side-effects are similar to those produced by other prostaglandins used to induce abortion.

Immune System

Prostaglandins such as prostacyclin contribute to the signs and symptoms of inflammation, accentuating the pain and edema produced by bradykinin. Conversely, other prostaglandins suppress the release of chemical mediators from mast cells of patients experiencing allergic reactions.

Antibody responses may be decreased by PGE_1, possibly allowing greater acceptance of tissue transplants (Pelus and Strausser, 1977). Indeed, immunosuppressant effects of certain

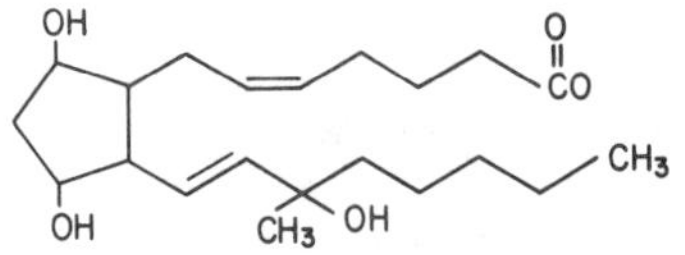

FIGURE 20-5. Carboprost.

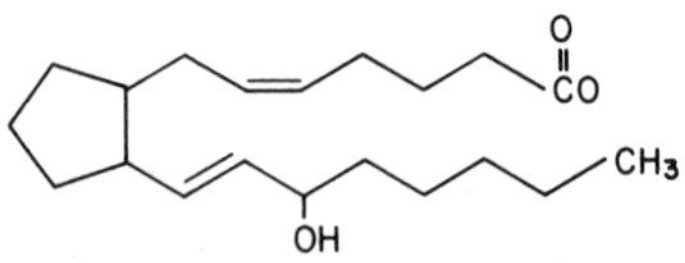

FIGURE 20-6. Dinoprost.

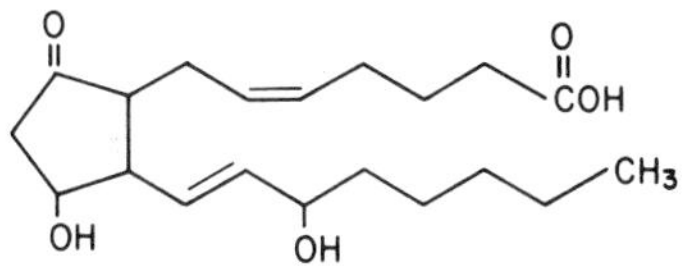

FIGURE 20-7. Dinoprostone.

tumors may reflect their ability to produce prostaglandins. Hypercalcemia associated with a tumor may reflect osteolytic activity of certain prostaglandins.

REFERENCES

Addonizio VP, Fisher CA, Jenkin BK, Strauss JF, Musial JF, Edmunds LH. Iloprost (ZK 36374), a stable analogue of prostacyclin, preserves platelets during simulated extracorporeal circulation. J Thorac Cardiovasc Surg 1985;89:926–33.

Bolger PM, Eisner GM, Ramwell PW, Slotkoff LM, Renal actions or prostacyclin. Nature 1978;271:457–69.

Boot JR, Cockerill AF, Dawson W, Mallen DNB, Osborne DJ. Modification of prostaglandin and thromboxane release by immunological sensitization and successive immunological challenge for guinea pig lung. Int Arch Allergy Appl Immunol 1978;57:159–64.

Brooks CJW, Steel G, Gilbert D, Harland WA. Lipids of human atheroma. Atherosclerosis 1971;13:223–7.

Cole RB, Abman S, Aziz KU, Bharati S, Lev M. Prolonged prostaglandin E infusion: Histologic effects on patent ductus arteriosus. Pediatrics 1981;67:816–9.

Drazen JM, Austen KF, Lewis RA, et al. Comparative airway and vascular activities of leukotrienes C-1 and D in vivo and in vitro. Proc Natl Acad Sci USA;1980;77:4354–8.

Euler US von. On the specific vasodilating and plain muscle stimulating substance from accessory genital glands in man and certain animals (prostaglandin and vesiglandin). J Physiol 1936;88:213–34.

Ferreira SH, Vane JR. Prostaglandins: their disappearance and release into the circulation. Nature 1967;216:868–73.

Frolich JC, Ogletree, Peskar BA, et al. Pulmonary hypertension correlated to pulmonary thromboxane synthesis. In: Samuelsson PW, Ramwell R, Paoletti, eds. Advances in Prostaglandin and Thromboxane Research. New York, Raven Press, 1979;7:745.

Gill JR, Frolich JC, Bowden RE, et al. Bartter's syndrome, a disorder characterized by high urinary prostaglandins and a dependence of hyperreninemia on prostaglandin synthesis. Am J Med 1976;61:43–51.

Gorman RR, Fitzpatrick FA, Miller OV. Reciprocal regulation of human platelet cAMP levels by thromboxane A and prostacyclin. In: Ignarro WJ, ed. Advances in Cyclic Nucleotide Research. New York, Raven Press, 1978;9:597.

Grenier FC, Smith WL. Formation of 6-keto PGF, by collecting tubule cells isolated from rabbit renal papillae. Prostaglandins 1978;16:759–72.

Hintze TH, Martin EG, Messina EJ, Kaley G. Prostacyclin (PGI₂) elicits reflex bradycardia in dogs: evidence for vagal mediation. Proc Soc Exp Biol Med 1979;162:96–100.

Horton EW, Poyser NC. Uterine luteolytic hormone. A physiological role for prostaglandin F₂alpha. Physiol Rev 1976;56:595–651.

Karim SMM. Prostaglandins and human reproduction: physiological roles and clinical uses of prostaglandins in relation to human reproduction. In: Karim SMM, ed. The Prostaglandins: Progress in Research. New York, John Wiley and Sons, Inc. 1972;71.

Kot PA, Johnson M, Ramwell PW, Ross JC. Effects of ganglionic and β-adrenergic blockade on cardiovascular responses to the bisenoic prostaglandins and their precursor arachidonic acid. Proc Soc Exp Biol Med 1975;149:953–7.

Kurzrok R, Lieb CC. Biochemical studies of human semen. II. The action of semen on the human uterus. Proc Soc Exp Biol Med 1930;28:268–72.

Lewis AB, Scheinman MM, Gonzalez R, Hess D. Side-effects of therapy with prostaglandin E, in infants with critical congenital heart disease. Circulation 1981;64:893–8.

Longmore DB, Bennett JG, Hoyle PM, et al. Prostacyclin administration during cardiopulmonary bypass in man. Lancet 1981;1:800–4.

Mathe AA, Hedqvist P. Effect of prostaglandins F₂alpha and E₂ on airway conductance in healthy subjects and asthmatic patients. Am Rev Respir Dis 1975;111:313–20.

Matthay M, Eschenbacher W, Goetzl E. Elevated concentrations of leukotriene D4 in pulmonary edema fluid of patients with adult respiratory distress syndrome. J Clin Immunol 1984;4:479–83.

McGiff J, Stollermhan, eds. Thromboxane and prostacyclin: Implications for function and disease of the vasculature. Ad Intern Med 1980;25.

Moncada S, Korbut R, Bunting S, Vane JR. Prostacyclin is a circulating hormone. Nature 1978;273:767–8.

Olley PM, Coceani F. Prostaglandins and ductus arteriosus. Annu Rev Med 1981;32:375–85.

Pelus LM, Strausser HR. Prostaglandins and the immune response. Life Sci 1977;20:903–14.

Rankin JHG. Role of prostaglandins in the maintenance of the placental circulation. Adv Prostaglandin Thromboxane Leukotriene Res 1978;4:261–9.

Samuelsson B. Leukotrienes: mediators of immediate hypersensitivity reactions and inflammation. Science 1983;220:568–75.

Scherer RW, Vigfusson G, Hultsch E, Van Aken H, Lawin

P. Prostaglandin F_2 alpha improves oxygen tension and reduces ventilation admixture during one-lung ventilation in anesthetized paralyzed dogs. Anesthesiology 1985;62:23 – 8.

Shayevitz JR, Traystman RJ, Adkinson NF, Sciuto AM, Gurtner GH. Inhalation anesthetics augment oxidant-induced pulmonary vasoconstriction: Evidence for a membrane effect. Anesthesiology 1985;63:624 – 32.

Smith ME, Gunther R, Zaiss C, Demling RH. Prostaglandin infusion and endotoxin-induced lung injury. Arch Surg 1982;117:175 – 80.

Szczeklik A, Gryglewski RJ, Nizankowski R, Musial J, Pieton R, Mruk J. Circulatory and anti-platelet effects of intravenous prostacyclin in healthy men. Pharmacol Res Commun 1978;10:545 – 56.

Whittle BJR, Boughton – Smith NK, Moncada S, Vane JR. Actions of prostacyclin (PGI_2) and its product 6-oxo-PGE_1 on the rat gastric mucosa in vivo and in vitro. Prostaglandins 1978;15:955 – 67.

Histamine and Histamine Receptor Antagonists

HISTAMINE

Histamine is one of several endogenous and naturally occurring substances (*i.e.,* autacoids) that produces intense physiologic effects when released locally or into the circulation (Fig. 21-1). Other autacoids include prostaglandins, serotonin, angiotensin II, and plasma kinins (see Chapters 20 and 22). Histamine is present in most tissues but is particularly prominent in mast cells located in the skin, lungs, and gastrointestinal tract. Circulating basophils also contain large amounts of histamine.

Synthesis

Synthesis of histamine in tissues is by decarboxylation of histidine. Histamine is stored in vesicles in a complex with heparin. Stored histamine is subsequently released in response to stimuli such as trauma or administration of certain drugs. Histamine ingested with food is largely destroyed in the liver or lungs or excreted in the urine (see the section entitled Metabolism).

Metabolism

There are two pathways of histamine metabolism in man. The most important pathway involves methylation catalyzed by histamine-N-methyltransferase, resulting in N-methylhistamine, which is further degraded by monoamine oxidase. In the other pathway, histamine undergoes oxidative deamination catalyzed by diamine oxidase (histaminase), which is a nonspecific enzyme widely distributed in body tissues. Resulting metabolites from both pathways are pharmacologically inactive and are excreted in the urine.

Receptors

Histamine receptors are classified as H_1 or H_2. These receptors are presumed to be components of cell membranes (Maze, 1981).

H_1 Receptors

H_1 receptors mediate histamine-induced contraction of smooth muscle in the gastrointestinal tract and bronchi (Ash and Schild, 1966; Maze, 1981). The only cardiac effect mediated by these receptors is a delay in the conduction of the cardiac impulse through the atrioventricular node. Increased capillary permeability and relaxation of vascular smooth muscle is a reflection of histamine activation of both H_1 and H_2 receptors. Elevated intracellular concentrations of cyclic guanosine 3', 5'-monophosphate (cyclic GMP) may accompany activation of H_1 receptors. In many respects, the responses evoked by stimulation of H_1 receptors are analogous to those associated with activation of alpha-adrenergic receptors (*i.e.,* mediates constrictor responses). Histamine-induced

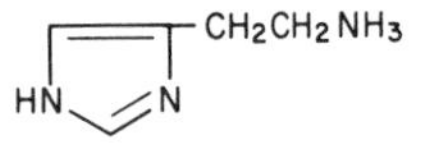

FIGURE 21-1. Histamine.

effects mediated by activation of H_1 receptors are suppressed by specific H_1 receptor antagonists such as diphenhydramine.

H_2 Receptors

H_2 receptors mediate histamine-induced secretion of gastric hydrogen ions (Hirschowitz, 1979; Maze, 1981). Increased myocardial contractility and heart rate is a reflection of histamine activation of these receptors in the heart. H_2 receptors are present in the central nervous system. Increased capillary permeability and relaxation of vascular smooth muscle is a reflection of histamine activation of both H_1 and H_2 receptors. Elevated intracellular concentrations of cyclic adenosine 3'5'-monophosphate (cyclic AMP) may accompany activation of H_2 receptors (Reinhardt et al, 1977). In many respects, the responses evoked by stimulation of H_2 receptors are analogous to those associated with activation of beta-adrenergic receptors (i.e., mediates dilator responses).

Histamine-induced effects mediated by activation of H_2 receptors are suppressed by specific H_2 receptor antagonists such as cimetidine and ranitidine. H_2 receptors in the central nervous system are blocked by lysergic acid diethylamide (Green et al, 1977). Similar actions of cimetidine would be consistent with confusional states noted in patients with renal dysfunction and in those receiving high doses of cimetidine (Schentag et al, 1979).

Effects on Organ Systems

Histamine exerts profound effects on the cardiovascular system, airways, and gastric hydrogen ion secretion. Histamine in large doses stimulates ganglion cells and chromaffin cells in the adrenal medulla, evoking the release of catecholamines. Central nervous system effects do not accompany peripheral release of histamine, because this compound cannot easily cross the blood–brain barrier.

Cardiovascular System

The predominant cardiovascular effects of histamine are due to dilatation of arterioles and capillaries, leading to (1) flushing, (2) decreased peripheral vascular resistance, (3) reductions in blood pressure, and (4) increased capillary permeability. Vascular dilatation results from a direct effect of histamine on the blood vessels mediated by both H_1 and H_2 receptors independent of autonomic nervous system innervation. Although peripheral vasodilatation is generalized, flushing is most obvious in the skin of the face and upper part of the body (i.e., the blush area). Increased capillary permeability is characterized as outward passage of plasma proteins and fluid into the extracellular space, manifesting as edema. This increased capillary permeability is due to histamine-induced contraction of capillary endothelial cells, thus exposing the freely permeable basement membranes of capillaries to protein containing intravascular fluid.

In addition to peripheral vasodilatation, histamine can produce inotropic, chronotropic, and antidromic effects (Bristow et al, 1982). Positive inotropic effects are due to histamine-mediated stimulation of H_2 receptors as well as the ability of histamine to evoke the release of catecholamines from the adrenal medulla. Positive chronotropic effects and the development of cardiac dysrhythmias reflect direct activation of H_2 receptors by histamine as well as an indirect effect due to histamine-induced catecholamine release (Powell and Brody, 1976). Slowed conduction of the cardiac impulse through the atrioventricular node is due to histamine activation of H_1 receptors. Changes in the threshold for ventricular fibrillation may be caused by the liberation of small amounts of histamine that are not detectable as changes in the plasma concentration (Trzeciakowski and Levi, 1982). It is conceivable that regional tissue release of histamine could contribute to cardiac dysrhythmias. Coronary artery vasoconstriction is mediated by H_1 receptors whereas coronary artery vasodilation is mediated by H_2 receptors (Bristow et al, 1982; Ginsberg et al, 1980).

The triple response elicited by histamine in the skin consists of (1) dilatation of capillaries in the injured area, (2) edema due to increased permeability of the capillaries, and (3) a flare consisting of dilated arteries surrounding the edema. The flare component of the triple response is an example of the ability of histamine to stimulate nerve endings. Histamine also causes pruritus when injected into superficial layers of the skin.

Reductions in blood pressure induced by histamine are prevented by the combination of H_1 and H_2 receptor antagonists (Philbin *et al*, 1981). Blockade of either receptor alone does not completely prevent the blood pressure – lowering effects of histamine.

Airways

Histamine activates H_1 receptors to constrict bronchial smooth muscle, whereas stimulation of H_2 receptors relaxes bronchial smooth muscle. In normal patients, the bronchoconstrictor action of histamine is negligible. Conversely, patients with obstructive airways disease, such as asthma or bronchitis, are more likely to develop increases in airway resistance in response to histamine.

Gastric Hydrogen Ion Secretion

Histamine evokes copious secretion of gastric fluid containing high concentrations of hydrogen ions. This response occurs in the presence of plasma concentrations of histamine that do not alter blood pressure. A doubling of the plasma histamine concentration is usually considered necessary to evoke changes in blood pressure (Rosow *et al,* 1980).

Increased gastric hydrogen ion secretion is believed to be a direct effect of histamine on gastric cells. Nevertheless, the presence of vagal activity results in even a higher rate of hydrogen ion secretion. For example, after vagotomy in man, the maximal secretory response to histamine decreases to about one third of its usual value. Cholinergic blockade, as produced by high doses of atropine, also decreases the gastric secretory response to histamine.

Allergic Reactions

During allergic reactions, histamine is only one of several chemical mediators released, and its relative importance in producing symptoms is greatly dependent on the species studied. Likewise, protection afforded by histamine receptor antagonists is highly variable and species-dependent. In humans, histamine receptor antagonists are effective in preventing edema formation and pruritus. Hypotension is attenuated but not totally blocked, whereas bronchoconstriction is not prevented, emphasizing the predominant role of leukotrienes in this response in humans.

Responses to histamine-releasing drugs are better controlled by histamine receptor antagonists than are allergic responses (Moss and Rosow, 1983; Philbin *et al*, 1981). Fewer chemical mediators are presumably involved in drug-induced responses, and histamine is relatively more important.

Clinical Uses

Histamine has been used to assess the ability of the stomach to secrete acid and to determine parietal cell mass. Antacidity or hyposecretion in response to histamine may reflect pernicious anemia, atropic gastritis, or gastric carcinoma. A hypersecretory response is present with Zollinger-Ellison syndrome and may be found in the presence of duodenal ulcer. Distressing side effects produced by histamine alone can be reduced by prior administration of an H_1 receptor antagonist that does not oppose histamine-induced gastric secretion. An alternative to histamine for gastric function tests is pentagastrin, a synthetic pentapeptide derivative of gastrin. Side effects from pentagastrin are minimal.

The fact that intradermal histamine causes a flare that is mediated by axon reflexes allows a test for the integrity of sensory nerves that may be of value in the diagnosis of certain neurologic conditions. The stimulant effect of histamine on chromaffin cells has been used in the past as a provocative test in patients with pheochromocytoma.

HISTAMINE RECEPTOR ANTAGONISTS

Depending on what responses to histamine are inhibited, drugs are classified as H_1 or H_2 receptor antagonists (Table 21-1). This classification is similar to terminology applied to drugs that act as antagonists at alpha or beta receptors. H_1 and H_2 receptor antagonists are presumed to act by occupying receptors on effector cell membranes, to the exclusion of agonist molecules, without themselves initiating a response. For histamine receptor antagonists, this is a competitive and reversible interaction (Maze, 1981). It is important to recognize that H_1 and H_2 receptor antagonists do not

Table 21-1
Effects Mediated by Activation of Histamine Receptors

	Receptor Subtype Activated
Increased intracellular cGMP	H_1
Slowed conduction of cardiac impulse through atrioventricular node	H_1
Coronary artery vasoconstriction	H_1
Bronchoconstriction	H_1
Increased intracellular cAMP	H_2
Central nervous system stimulation	H_2
Cardiac dysrhythmias	H_2
Increased myocardial contractility	H_2
Increased heart rate	H_2
Coronary artery vasodilatation	H_2
Bronchodilatation	H_2
Increased secretion of gastric fluid containing hydrogen ions	H_2
Increased capillary permeability	H_1, H_2
Vascular vasodilatation	H_1, H_2

inhibit release of histamine but rather attach to receptors and prevent responses mediated by histamine.

H_1 Receptor Antagonists

Several H_1 receptor antagonists (ethanolamines, ethylenediamines, alkylamines, piperazines, and phenothiazines) are available, but individual variability in responses makes it difficult to document unique effects or advantages of a single drug (Table 21-1). H_1 receptor antagonists resemble histamine in that they contain a substituted ethylamine (Fig. 21-2). Unlike histamine, the H_1 receptor antagonists contain a tertiary amino group linked to two aromatic substituents (Fig. 21-2). In addition to acting as antagonists at the H_1 receptor, those drugs that are classified as ethanolamines also possess some blocking activity at serotonin receptors (see Chapter 22).

Pharmacokinetics

H_1 receptor antagonists are readily absorbed from the gastrointestinal tract following oral adminis-

tration, reaching maximal plasma concentrations in 1 to 2 hours. Plasma concentrations parallel the pharmacologic effects of these drugs (Carruthers *et al*, 1978). The elimination half-time of most H_1 receptor antagonists is about 3.5 hours, with extensive metabolism occurring in the liver such that little if any drug is excreted unchanged in the urine.

Side Effects

The most common side effect is sedation, although the magnitude of this response varies among the H_1 receptor antagonists, being most prominent with ethanolamines represented by diphenhydramine (Table 21-2). Central nervous system sedation is less with ethylenediamines such as pyrilamine and the alkylamines represented by chlorpheniramine. Less commonly, small doses of H_1 receptor antagonists may evoke activation of the electroencephalogram and epileptiform seizures in patients with central nervous system disease.

Anticholinergic effects of H_1 receptor antagonists manifesting as dry mouth and increased heart rate may be prominent, with the exception of the ethylenediamine, pyrilamine (Table 21-2). Despite these anticholinergic effects, gastric secretion of hydrogen ions is not altered by H_1 receptor antagonists.

H_1 receptor antagonists possess local anesthetic activity but only at concentrations far greater than that necessary to antagonize the effects of histamine. Rapid intravenous injection of an H_1 receptor antagonist can transiently lower blood pressure, possibly reflecting this local anesthetic (*i.e.,* quinidine-like) effect. Oral administration of an H_1 receptor antagonist, however, does not usually alter blood pressure.

Smooth muscle responses in bronchi and peripheral vasculature are inhibited by H_1 receptor antagonists. In guinea pigs, protection is provided against bronchospasm that accompanies an allergic reaction, but this is not so in humans, in whom allergic bronchoconstriction is mediated less by histamine and more by leukotrienes (see the section entitled Allergic Reactions). On peripheral vascular smooth muscle, H_1 receptor antagonists inhibit both vasoconstrictor and vasodilator effects (Table 21-1). Residual vasodilation reflects the role of H_2 receptors, emphasizing the need to block both H_1 and H_2 receptors so as to prevent the decrease in blood pressure produced by hista-

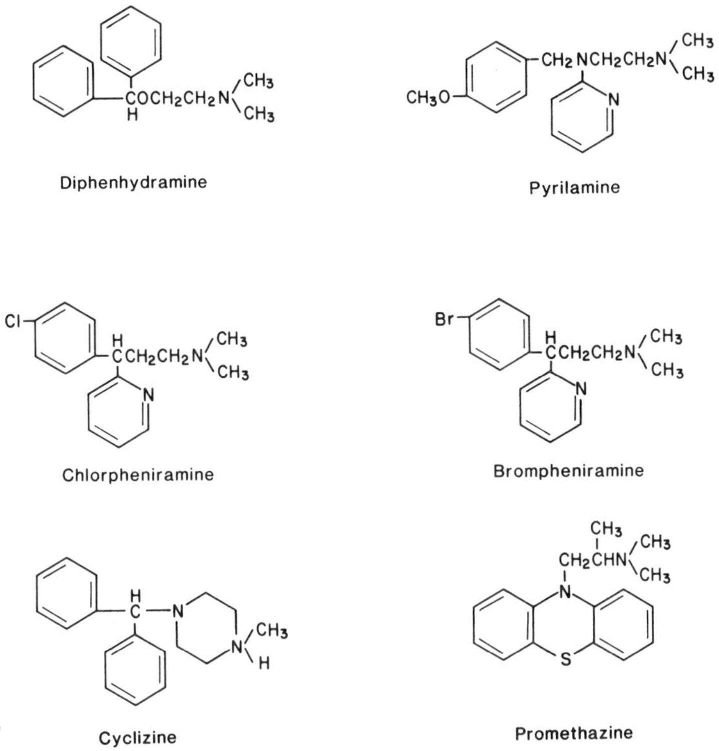

FIGURE 21-2. H_1 receptor antagonists.

mine. Allergic dermatitis is not uncommon with topical application of H_1 receptor antagonists such as those used to treat pruritus.

Acute overdose with an H_1 receptor antagonist, particularly if it occurs in small children, can produce central nervous system excitation culminating in seizures. Fixed dilated pupils with a flushed face and fever are common in children but not in adults. These latter symptoms are similar to atropine overdose. Ultimately, H_1 receptor antagonist overdose may progress to cardiopulmonary depression and coma. Treatment is symptomatic, with support of vital organ function.

Clinical Uses

H_1 receptor antagonists are effective in the symptomatic treatment of allergic disorders to pollens by virtue of their ability to antagonize the effects of subsequently released histamine. Sneezing, rhinorrhea, and conjunctivitis are predictably suppressed. These drugs are not effective in the treat-

ment of bronchial asthma, allergic reactions, or angioedema in which chemical mediators other than histamine are responsible for the symptoms.

H_1 receptor antagonists may be used for the prophylaxis and treatment of motion sickness. Diphenhydramine or promethazine are most effective in this regard, but scopolamine is even more efficacious (Table 21-2) (see Chapter 10). A possible explanation for the efficacy of these drugs in the management of motion sickness is central nervous system antagonism of acetylcholine similar to scopolamine.

Allergic dermatitis usually responds to H_1 receptor antagonists. These drugs prevent the action of histamine that results in increased capillary permeability and formation of edema as well as pruritus.

Sedative effects of H_1 receptor antagonists are used in nonprescription drugs used to treat insomnia. Even pyrilamine, which is considered to have mild central nervous system sedative effects, is a frequent component of these preparations.

Table 21-2
Classification of Histamine Receptor Antagonists

	Sedative Effects	Anticholinergic Activity	Antiemetic Effects	Duration of Action (hr)	Adult Dose (mg)
H_1 Antagonists					
Diphenhydramine	Marked	Marked	Moderate	3–6	50
Pyrilamine	Mild	None	None	3–6	25–50
Chlorpheniramine	Mild	Mild	None	4–12	2–4
Brompheniramine	Mild	Mild	None	4–12	4–8
Cyclizine	Moderate	Minimal	Mild	4–6	50
Promethazine	Moderate	Marked	Marked	4–24	25–50
H_2 Antagonists					
Cimetidine	Mild*	None	None	5–7	300
Ranitidine	None	None	None	8–12	150

* Manifests as confusion and agitation

H_2 Receptor Antagonists

The relationship between gastric hypersecretion of fluid containing high concentrations of hydrogen ions and peptic ulcer disease emphasizes the potential value of a drug that selectively blocks H_2 receptor–mediated secretion of acidic gastric fluid. Cimetidine and ranitidine are reversible and selective competitive antagonists of the actions of histamine on H_2 receptors. (Fig. 21-3). Despite the presence of H_2 receptors throughout the body, inhibition of histamine binding to the receptors of gastric parietal cells is the major beneficial clinical effect of H_2 receptor antagonists.

Cimetidine

Cimetidine is a selective and competitive H_2 receptor antagonist that blocks histamine-induced secretion of hydrogen ions by gastric parietal cells. The magnitude of this effect is dose-related and parallels the plasma concentration of cimetidine (Richardson, 1978). There is no significant effect of cimetidine on gastric emptying time, lower esophageal sphincter tone, or pancreatic secretions.

In addition to blockade of H_2 receptors, cimetidine also prevents the increase in gastric fluid secretion normally produced by gastrin and acetylcholine. The mechanism of this blockade is not clear but may reflect a final common mediator

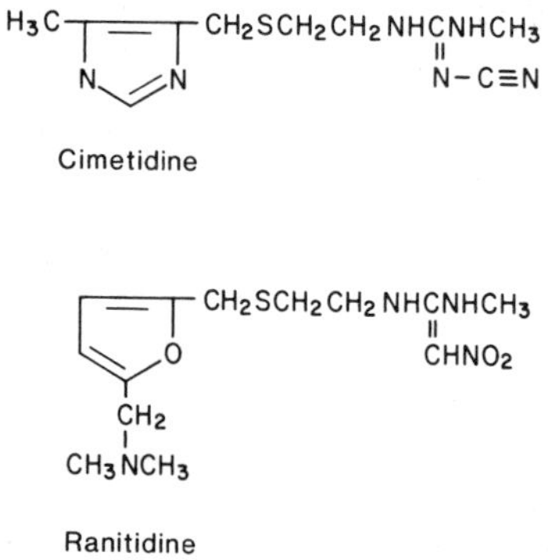

FIGURE 21-3. H_2 receptor antagonists.

phenomenon in which gastrin or acetylcholine render histamine more available to parietal cell H_2 receptors.

PHARMACOKINETICS. Cimetidine is readily absorbed from the small intestine following oral administration, with peak plasma concentrations occurring in 60 to 90 minutes. After an oral dose of 300 mg, therapeutic plasma concentrations of cimetidine are maintained for at least 4 hours, whereas 90% or greater suppression of gastric hydrogen ion secretion persists for 5 to 7 hours (Richardson, 1978). Cimetidine can also be administered intramuscularly or intravenously. This drug easily crosses lipid barriers such as the blood–brain barrier or placenta.

Cimetidine is rapidly filtered and excreted by the kidneys with 50% to 70% of the drug being excreted unchanged within 24 hours. Some reabsorption of cimetidine occurs in proximal renal tubules in addition to a small amount of tubular secretion. Hepatic inactivation occurs primarily by conversion of the side chain of cimetidine to a thioether or sulfoxide. These metabolites appear in the urine as a 5-hydroxymethyl and/or sulfoxide metabolites. Bacteria in the gastrointestinal tract, however, can convert some sulfoxide back to cimetidine. Only about 10% of cimetidine is excreted in the bile. The elimination half-time of cimetidine is 1.5 to 2 hours in the presence of normal renal function and is doubled in anephric patients (Ma *et al*, 1978).

CLINICAL USES. Cimetidine is of value in the treatment of duodenal ulcer disease associated with hypersecretion of gastric acid. The recommended dose is 300 mg orally four times a day. Zollinger-Ellison syndrome, characterized by hypersection of large amounts of acidic gastric fluid, is an indication for treatment with an H_2 receptor antagonist.

A number of investigators have confirmed the ability of cimetidine administered orally, intramuscularly, or intravenously to increase gastric fluid pH prior to the induction of anesthesia (Table 21-3) (Coombs *et al*, 1979; Stoelting, 1978; Weber and Hirschman, 1979). For this reason, cimetidine has been advocated as a useful drug in preoperative medication to reduce the risk of acid pneumonitis if inhalation of gastric fluid occurs in the perioperative period. A frequent approach is administration of cimetidine, 300 mg orally (*i.e.*, 3–4 mg kg⁻¹), 1.5 to 2 hours before the induction of anesthesia, with or without a similar dose the preceding evening. This dose may need to be increased to about 7.5 mg kg⁻¹ in pediatric patients and in obese adults (Goudsouzian *et al*, 1981). When a more rapid onset of effect is needed, the intramuscular or intravenous route is preferable to oral administration. The effects of cimetidine on gastric fluid volume are not consistent. Furthermore, cimetidine, in contrast to antacids, has no influence on the pH of the gastric fluid that is already in the stomach. Cimetidine crosses the placenta but does not adversely affect the fetus when administered prior to cesarean section (Hodgkinson *et al*, 1983; Johnston *et al*, 1983).

Preoperative preparation of the patient with an allergic history or the patient undergoing procedures associated with an increased likelihood of allergic reactions (*e.g.*, chymopapain injection, radiographic dye injection) may include prophylactic oral administration of an H_1 receptor antagonist (diphenhydramine, 0.5–1 mg kg⁻¹) and H_2 antagonist (cimetidine, 4 mg kg⁻¹) every 6 hours in the 24 hours preceding the possible triggering event (Stoelting, 1983). A corticosteroid, such as prednisone, 50 mg every 6 hours, may also be added to this regimen. The goal is to occupy receptors normally responsive to histamine such that subsequent release of this chemical mediator will be less likely to evoke life-threatening symptoms. Despite the logic of this approach, symptomatic allergic reactions to chymopapain and pre-

Table 21-3
Influence of Cimetidine on Gastric Fluid pH

	Gastric Fluid pH (percent of patients)		
	Below 2.5	*2.5–5*	*Above 5*
No cimetidine	60	34	6
Cimetidine (300 mg orally) evening before operation	22	38	40
Cimetidine (300 mg orally) with preanesthetic medication	16	24	60

(Data from Stoelting RK. Allergic reactions during anesthesia. Anesth Analg 1978;57:675)

sumably other triggering events may still occur (Bruno *et al,* 1984).

Drug-induced histamine release that may follow rapid intravenous administration of morphine, d-tubocurarine or atracurium is not altered by pretreatment with an H_1 receptor antagonist (diphenhydramine or chlorpheniramine) plus cimetidine (Moss *et al,* 1981; Philbin *et al,* 1981). The magnitude of the blood pressure reduction evoked by these drugs is, however, reduced, confirming that prior occupation of histamine receptors with an antagonist attenuates the cardiovascular effects of subsequently released histamine (Philbin *et al,* 1981). Treatment with diphenhydramine or cimetidine alone is not effective in preventing cardiovascular effects of released histamine, emphasizing the role of both H_1 and H_2 receptors in these responses.

SIDE EFFECTS. Side effects of cimetidine are frequent but predictable considering the widespread distribution of H_2 receptors (McGuigan, 1981).

Intravenous administration of cimetidine, 300 mg over 2 minutes to postoperative adult patients, often produces transient reductions in blood pressure that are maximal 2 minutes following the infusion (Iberti *et al,* 1986). The mechanism for this blood pressure decline appears to be a direct drug-induced peripheral vasodilation. Bradycardia, heart block, and even cardiac arrest have been observed following rapid intravenous administration of cimetidine to critically ill or elderly patients (Cohen *et al,* 1979; Shaw *et al,* 1980). Cardiovascular changes following intravenous administration of cimetidine are not surprising considering that cardiac effects of histamine are mediated principally by H_2 receptors (see Table 21-1). Cimetidine may increase airway resistance in patients with bronchial asthma, reflecting loss of H_2 receptor–mediated bronchodilatation, leaving unopposed H_1 receptor–mediated bronchoconstriction (see Table 21-1) (Nathan *et al,* 1981).

Since histamine is likely to be a neurotransmitter in the central nervous system, it is predictable that cimetidine, by virtue of its ability to cross the blood–brain barrier, could produce significant side-effects. Indeed, central nervous system dysfunction characterized by confusion, agitation, hallucinations, seizures, and coma have been observed, especially in elderly patients treated with cimetidine (Schentag *et al,* 1979). Central ner-

vous system dysfunction is more likely to occur in the presence of high plasma concentrations of cimetidine associated with renal dysfunction. Delayed awakening from anesthesia has been attributed to lingering central nervous system effects of cimetidine (Viegas *et al,* 1982). Physostigmine may reverse cimetidine-induced central nervous system dysfunction (Mogelnicki *et al,* 1979).

Prolonged H_2 receptor blockade and associated gastric achlorhydria may weaken the gastric barrier to bacteria and predispose to systemic infection (Cristiano and Paradisi, 1982). Likewise, pulmonary infections from inhaled secretions could be more likely if the acid-killing effect on bacteria in the stomach is altered. Sustained elevation of gastric fluid *p*H may lead to an overgrowth of other organisms such as *Candida albicans.* This may account for the occasional case of Candida peritonitis observed after peptic ulcer perforation in patients treated with cimetidine. Bacterial overgrowth in the colon leads to diarrhea. Prolonged elevation of gastric fluid *p*H also results in the production of nitroso compounds as a result of an increase in nitrate-reducing bacteria (Milton–Thompson *et al,* 1982). Nitroso derivatives are potent mutagens *in vitro,* but there is no evidence that this occurs *in vivo* in association with chronic cimetidine therapy.

Cimetidine has occasionally been associated with mild increases in serum transaminase and/or alkaline phosphatase enzymes (Lilly *et al,* 1978). Transient elevations in serum creatinine occur in about 3% of chronically treated patients, presumably reflecting a reversible interstitial nephritis. Cimetidine-induced neutropenia and thrombocytopenia are rare and usually reversible. Nevertheless, white blood cell counts should be monitored during chronic cimetidine therapy. A weak antiandrogen effect manifesting as gynecomastia in males has been observed during chronic therapy with high doses of cimetidine.

Cimetidine retards metabolism of drugs, such as lidocaine, propranolol, and diazepam, that normally undergo high hepatic extraction (Donovan *et al,* 1981; Klotz and Reimann, 1980). This reduced rate of metabolism may reflect cimetidine-induced reductions in hepatic blood flow as well as inhibition of the hepatic mixed function oxidase system by means of binding to microsomal cytochrome P_{450} enzymes (Feeley *et al,* 1981; Puurumen and Pelkonen, 1979). Indeed, benzodiazepines such as oxazepam and lorazepam that are eliminated almost entirely by glucuronidation are not altered by cimetidine-induced effects on P_{450} enzyme activity (Klotz and Reimann, 1980). Slowed metabolism and prolonged elimination half-times with associated exaggerated pharmacologic effects of propranolol and diazepam have been documented with only 24 hours of treatment with cimetidine (Figs. 21-4 and 21-5) (Feeley *et al,* 1981; Klotz and Reimann, 1980). Cimetidine modestly reduces defluorination of methoxyflurane and inhibits oxidative metabolism of halothane (Wood *et al,* 1986).

Ranitidine

Ranitidine is a selective and competitive H_2 receptor antagonist, which, unlike cimetidine, has a furan rather than imidazole structure (Fig. 21-3) (Zeldis *et al,* 1983). The imidazole ring present in histamine and cimetidine had previously been considered to be essential for antagonism of H_2 receptors. Ranitidine has the same clinical uses as cimetidine but is five to eight times more potent than cimetidine in antagonizing hydrogen ion se-

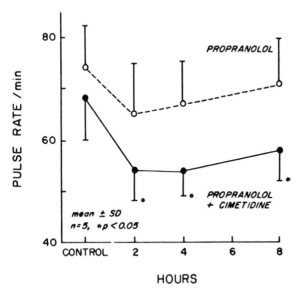

FIGURE 21-4. The effect of propranolol on resting heart rate is accentuated by the concomitant administration of cimetidine. (From Feely J, Wilkinson GR, Wood AJJ. Reduction of liver blood flow and propranolol metabolism by cimetidine. N Engl J Med 1981;304:692–5. Reprinted by permission of the New England Journal of Medicine 1981;304:692–5.)

cretion by gastric parietal cells (Fig. 21-6) (Francis and Kwik, 1982). Like cimetidine, ranitidine has no significant effect on gastric emptying time, lower esophageal sphincter tone, or pancreatic secretions.

PHARMACOKINETICS. Ranitidine is rapidly absorbed from the gastrointestinal tract, with an oral dose of 150 mg producing a peak plasma concentration in 30 to 60 minutes (Zeldis *et al,* 1983). Bioavailability of ranitidine is about 50% compared to 70% for cimetidine, reflecting a more significant hepatic first-pass effect for ranitidine. The duration of inhibition of gastric hydrogen ion secretion is prolonged, lasting 8 to 12 hours (Konturek *et al,* 1981).

About 50% of ranitidine is excreted by the kidney as unchanged drug. Up to 30% is metabolized in the liver to nitrogen oxide, sulfuric oxide, and desmethyl derivatives (Martin *et al,* 1982). The elimination half-time of ranitidine is 2 to 3 hours, and this is prolonged in the presence of renal dysfunction. For example, the elimination half-time of ranitidine is prolonged about 50% in elderly patients, presumably reflecting an age-related decline in glomerular filtration rate. Likewise, hepatic dysfunction increases the bioavailability and elimination half-time of ranitidine (Young *et al,* 1982). In patients with renal disease, therapeutic plasma concentrations of ranitidine can be achieved with one half the usual dose.

SIDE EFFECTS. Side effects may be less likely to follow administration of ranitidine than with cimetidine (Zeldis *et al,* 1983). For example, elderly patients and patients with renal or hepatic dysfunction may be less likely to develop central nervous system dysfunction during treatment with ranitidine. Presumably, this reflects minimal entrance of ranitidine into the central nervous system. In contrast to cimetidine, ranitidine does not bind to androgen receptors; thus, gynecomastia does not occur. Neutropenia and thrombocytopenia, which occur rarely during therapy with cimetidine, have not occurred with ranitidine treatment. Indeed, human lymphocytes have receptors for cimetidine but not ranitidine (Peden *et al,* 1981). Elevations in serum creatinine and interstitial nephritis seem to be less likely with ranitidine than with cimetidine therapy. As with cimetidine, transient increases in serum transaminase concentrations have been reported in patients treated with ranitidine (Barr and Piper, 1981). Adverse

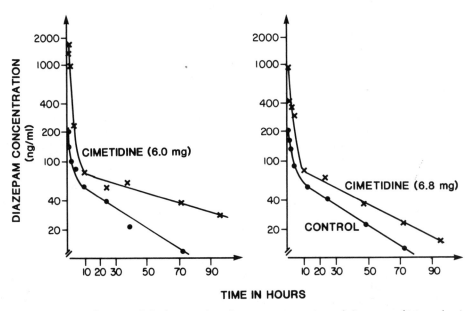

FIGURE 21-5. The rate of decline in the plasma concentration of diazepam (0.1 mg kg^{-1} intravenously) is slowed by the prior administration of cimetidine ($6-6.8$ mg kg^{-1}). (From Klotz U, Reimann I. Delayed clearance of diazepam due to cimetidine. N Engl J Med 1980;302:1012-4. Redrawn by permission of the New England Journal of Medicine 1980;302:1012-4.)

cardiac effects seem infrequent, but bradycardia has been observed after intravenous infusion of ranitidine (Cammari *et al,* 1982).

Ranitidine binds less avidly than cimetidine to hepatic microsomal P$_{450}$ enzymes. For this reason, ranitidine, in contrast to cimetidine, does not alter the rate of metabolism of drugs with a high hepatic extraction ratio. Both ranitidine and cimetidine, however, decrease hepatic blood flow.

CROMOLYN

Cromolyn inhibits antigen-induced release of histamine and other autacoids, including leukotrienes from pulmonary mast cells as well as from mast cells at other sites during antibody-mediated allergic responses (Fig. 21-7) (Cox, 1977). Cromolyn does not prevent the interaction between cell-bound immunoglobulin E and specific antigen, but, rather, it suppresses the secretory response elicited by the reaction. Release of histamine from basophils is not altered by cromolyn. Cromolyn does not relax bronchial or vascular smooth muscle.

The mechanism of action of cromolyn is not known but has been attributed to a membrane-stabilizing action that may reflect blockade of calcium channels. Oral absorption is poor, and the drug is therefore administered by inhalation. Drug absorbed into the circulation from the lung has an elimination half-time of about 80 minutes. Cromolyn is not metabolized, being excreted unchanged in the urine and bile in approximately equal amounts.

Side effects of cromolyn are rare and usually minor. Infrequent but more serious side effects, probably attributable to allergic reactions to the drug, include laryngeal edema, angioedema, urticaria, and anaphylaxis.

The principal use of cromolyn is in the prophylactic treatment of bronchial asthma. Given before an antigenic challenge, cromolyn will inhibit bronchoconstriction and prevent signs and

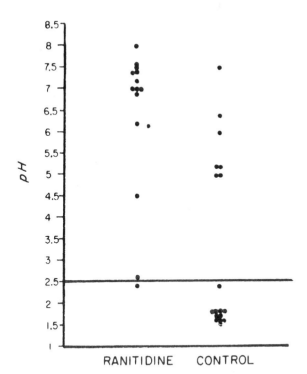

FIGURE 21-6. Distribution of *p*H values of gastric fluid in patients receiving ranitidine (150 mg orally the evening before and morning of surgery) compared with untreated patients. (From Francis RN, Kwik RSH. Oral ranitidine for prophylaxis against Mendelson's syndrome. Anesth Analg 1982;61:130–2. Reproduced by permission of the authors and the International Anesthesia Research Society.)

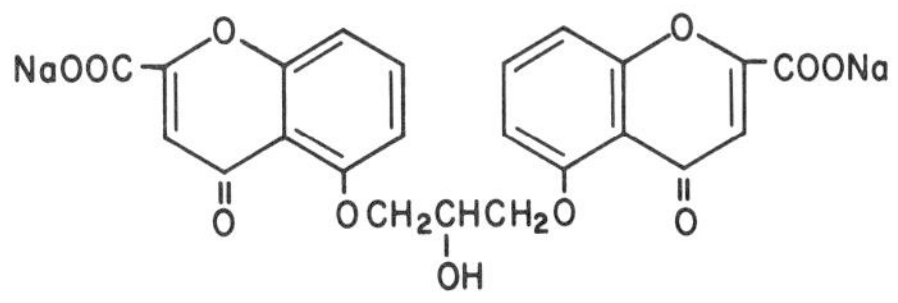

FIGURE 21-7. Cromolyn.

symptoms of an acute asthmatic attack. This protective effect can last for hours. Evidence that cromolyn has no role in the treatment of established bronchoconstriction is the observation that its administration as early as 1 minute after an antigen challenge is ineffective in altering the response.

REFERENCES

Ash ASF, Schild HO. Receptors mediating some actions of histamine. Br J Pharmacol 1966;27:427–39.

Barr GD, Piper DW. Possible ranitidine hepatitis. Med J Aust 1981;2:421.

Bristow MR, Ginsberg R, Harrison DC. Histamine and the human heart: The other receptor system. Am J Cardiol 1982;49:249–51.

Bruno LA, Smith DS, Bloom MJ, et al. Sudden hypotension with a test dose of chymopapain. Anesth Analg 1984;63:533–5.

Camarri E, Chirone E, Fanteria G, Zocchi M. Ranitidine induced bradycardia. Lancet 1982;2:160.

Carruthers SG, Shoeman DW, Hignite CE, Azarnoff DL. Correlation between plasma diphenhydramine level and sedative and antihistamine effects. Clin Pharmacol Ther 1978;23:375–82.

Cohen J, Weetman AP, Dargie HJ, Krikler DM. Life-threatening arrhythmias and intravenous injection of cimetidine. Br Med J 1979;2:768.

Coombs DW, Hooper D, Colton T. Acid aspiration prophylaxis by use of preoperative oral administration of cimetidine. Anesthesiology 1979;51:352–6.

Cox JSG, Cromolyn sodium. Pharmacol Biochem Prop Drug Subst 1977;1:277–310.

Cristiano P, Paradisi F. Can cimetidine facilitate infections by the oral route? Lancet 1982;2:45.

Donovan M, Hagerty A, Pael L, Castleden M, Pohl JEF. Cimetidine and bioavailability of propranolol. Lancet 1981;1:164.

Feely J, Wilkinson GR, Wood AJJ. Reduction of liver blood flow and propranolol metabolism by cimetidine. N Engl J Med 1981;304:692–5.

Francis RN, Kwik RSH. Oral ranitidine for prophylaxis against Mendelson's syndrome. Anesth Analg 1982;61:130–2

Ginsberg R, Bristow MR, Stinson EB, Harrison DC. Histamine receptors in the human heart. Life Sci 1980;26:2245–9.

Goudsouzian N, Cote CJ, Liu LMP, Dedrick DF. The dose–response effects of oral cimetidine on gastric *p*H and volume in children. Anesthesiology 1981;55:533–6.

Green JP, Johnson CL, Weinstein H, Maayani S. Antagonism of histamine-activated adenylate cyclase in brain D-lysergic acid diethylamide. Proc Natl Acad Sci 1977;74:5697–701.

Hirschowitz BI, H-2 histamine receptors. Ann Rev Pharmacol Toxicol 1979;19:203–44.

Hodgkinson R, Glassenberg R, Joyce TH, Coombs DW, Ostheimer GW, Gibbs CP. Comparison of cimetidine (Tagamet) with antacid for safety and effectiveness in reducing gastric acidity before elective cesarean section. Anesthesiology 1983;59:86–90.

Iberti TJ, Paluch TA, Helmer L, Murgolo VA, Benjamin E. The hemodynamic effects of intravenous cimetidine in intensive care patients: A double-blind, prospective study. Anesthesiology 1986;64:87–9.

Johnston JR, Moore J, McCaughey W, et al. Use of cimetidine as an oral antacid in obstetric anesthesia. Anesth Analg 1983;62:720–6.

Klotz U, Reimann I. Delayed clearance of diazepam due to cimetidine. N Engl J Med 1980;302:1012–4.

Konturek SJ, Obtulowicz W, Kwiecian N, Kopp B, Oleksy J. Kinetics and duration of action of ranitidine on gastric secretion and its effect on pancreatic secretion in duodenal ulcer patients. Scand J Gastroenterol 1981;69:91–9.

Lilly J, Hirch D, Javitt N. Cimetidine cholestatic jaundice in children. J Surg Res 1978;24:384–7.

Ma K, Brown D, Muscler D, Silvas S. Effects of renal failure on blood levels of cimetidine. Gastroenterology 1978;74:473–7.

Martin LE, Oxford J. Tanner RJN. Use of high-performance liquid chromatography–mass spectrometry for the study of the metabolism of ranitidine in man. J. Chromatogr 1982;251:215–24.

Maze M. Clinical implications of membrane receptor function in anesthesia. Anesthesiology 1981;55:160–71.

McGuigan JE. A consideration of the adverse effects of cimetidine. Gastroenterology 1981;80:181–92.

Milton–Thompson GJ, Lightfoot NF, Ahmet Z, et al. Intragastric acidity, bacteria, nitrite, and N-nitroso compounds before, during and after cimetidine treatment. Lancet 1982;1:1091–5.

Mogelnicki S, Waller J, Finalyson D. Physostigmine reversal of cimetidine-induced mental confusion. JAMA 1979;241:826–7.

Moss J, Rosow CE. Histamine release by narcotics and muscle relaxants in humans. Anesthesiology 1983;59:330–9.

Moss J, Rosow CE, Savarese JJ, Philbin DM, Kniffen KJ. Role of histamine in the hypotensive action of d-tubocurarine in man. Anesthesiology 1981;55:19–25.

Nathan R, Segall N, Schocket A. A comparison of the actions of H_1 and H-2 antihistamine on histamine-induced bronchoconstriction and cutaneous wheal response in asthmatic patients. J Allergy Clin Immunol 1981;67:171–7.

Peden NR, Robertson AJ, Boyd EJS, et al. Nitrogen stimulation of peripheral blood lymphocytes of duodenal ulcer patients during treatment with cimetidine or ranitidine. Gut 1981;23:398–403.

Philbin DM, Moss J, Akins CW, et al. The use of H_1 and H_2 histamine blockers with high dose morphine anes-

thesia: A double-blind study. Anesthesiology 1981;55:292–6.

Powell JR, Brody MJ. Identification and specific blockade of two receptors for histamine in the cardiovascular system. J Pharmacol Exp Ther 1976;196:1–14.

Puurumen J, Pelkonen O. Cimetidine inhibits microsomal drug metabolism in the rat. Eur J Pharmacol 1979;55:335–6.

Reinhardt D. Schmidt U, Bordle O-E, Schumann AJ. H-1 and H-2 receptor mediated responses to histamine on contractility and cyclic AMP of atrial and papillary muscles from guinea pig hearts. Agents Actions 1977;7:1–12.

Richardson CT. Effect of H-2 receptor antagonists on gastric acid secretion and serum gastrin concentration. Gastroenterology 1978;74:366–70.

Rosow CE, Basta SJ, Savarese JJ, Ali HH, Kniffen KJ, Moss J. Correlation of cardiovascular effects with increases in plasma histamine. Anesthesiology 1980;53:S270.

Schentag JJ, Cerra FB, Calleri G, DeGlopper E, Ross JQ, Bernhard H. Pharmacokinetic and clinical studies in patients with cimetidine associated mental confusion. Lancet 1979;1:177–81.

Shaw RG, Mashford ML, Desmond PV. Cardiac arrest after intravenous injection of cimetidine. Med J Aust 1980;2:629–30.

Stoelting RK. Gastric fluid pH in patients receiving cimetidine. Anesth Analg 1978;57:675–7.

Stoelting RK. Allergic reactions during anesthesia. Anesth Analg 1983;62:341–56.

Trzeciakowski J, Levi R. Analysis of receptors mediating histamine-induced decrease of ventricular fibrillation threshold in the guinea pig heart. Fed Proc 1982;40:692.

Viegas OJ, Stoops CA, Ravindran RS. Reversal of cimetidine-induced postoperative somnolence. Anesthesiol Rev 1982;9:30–1.

Weber L, Hirshman CA. Cimetidine for prophylaxis of aspiration pneumonitis: Comparison of intramuscular and oral dose schedules. Anesth Analg 1979;58:426–7.

Wood M, Vetrecht J, Pythyon JM et al. The effect of cimetidine on anesthetic metabolism and toxicity. Anesth Analg 1986;65:481–8.

Young CJ, Daneshmend TK, Roberts CJC. Effects of cirrhosis and aging on the elimination and bioavailability of ranitidine. Gut 1982;23:819–23.

Zeldis JB, Friedman LS, Isselbacher KJ. Ranitidine: A new H2 receptor antagonist. N Engl J Med 1983;309:1368–73.

CHAPTER 22

Renin, Plasma Kinins, and Serotonin

RENIN

Renin is a proteolytic enzyme that is synthesized and stored by juxtaglomerular cells that are present in the walls of renal afferent arterioles as they enter the glomeruli. The most important stimulus for the release of renin is a reduction in renal perfusion pressure associated with hemorrhage, dehydration, chronic sodium depletion, or renal artery stenosis. The secretion of renin is also increased by the sympathetic nervous system caused by activation of beta-adrenergic receptors.

Formation of Angiotensins

Release of renin initiates the formation of active hormones known as angiotensins. The first step is the reaction of renin with circulating angiotensinogen, a substrate formed in the liver, to form a decapeptide prohormone known as angiotensin I (Fig. 22-1). This prohormone is promptly hydrolyzed to the octapeptide, angiotensin II, by converting enzyme (peptidyl dipeptidase) that is present in highest concentrations in the lungs. Indeed, the lung converts 20% to 40% of angiotensin I to angiotensin II in a single circulation. This same converting enzyme is also responsible for the breakdown of plasma kinins, creating the situation in which the most potent endogenous vasoconstrictor (*i.e.,* angiotensin II) and vasodilator (*i.e.,* bradykinin) are cleared by the same enzyme (see the section entitled Plasma Kinins). Angio-

tensin II is metabolized to the heptapeptide angiotensin III by aminopeptidase enzyme (Fig. 22-1).

The renin–angiotensin–aldosterone system does not play an active role in the sodium-repleted patient but is of major importance in maintaining blood pressure and intravascular fluid volume during sodium deprivation or in the presence of hypovolemia. Furthermore, plasma renin activity is elevated in only about 15% of patients with essential hypertension. Nevertheless, the frequent efficacy of renin–angiotensin antagonists in treating essential hypertension suggests a much wider involvement than indicated solely by elevations in plasma renin activity (see Chapter 15).

Effects on Organ Systems

Vasoconstriction and stimulation of the synthesis and secretion of aldosterone by the adrenal cortex are the principal pharmacologic effects of angiotensin II. Aldosterone causes renal conservation of sodium ions with retention of water and loss of potassium and hydrogen ions. Other less intense effects include stimulation of the heart and sympathetic nervous system and increased release of antidiuretic hormone. Angiotensin III produces similar but less marked physiologic effects compared with angiotensin II. For example, its pressor effect is less than 50% of that of angiotensin II. Angiotensin III, however, is as potent or more so for evoking output of aldosterone when compared

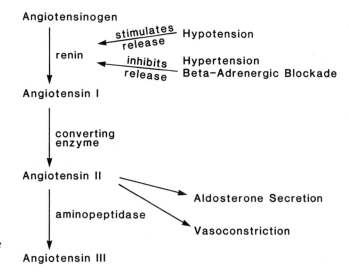

FIGURE 22-1. Schematic diagram of the renin–angiotensin–aldosterone system.

with angiotensin II (Peach, 1977). Angiotensin I has less than 1% of the activity of angiotensin II on vascular smooth muscle, heart, or adrenal cortex. Effects of angiotensin are most likely exerted through specific receptors on cell membranes (Devynck and Meyer, 1978).

Cardiovascular Effects

Angiotensin II produces vasoconstriction of pre-capillary arterioles and, to a lesser extent, postcapillary venules. Angiotensin II is the most powerful endogenous vasoconstrictor, being 40 times more potent than norepinephrine. This intense vasoconstriction reflects a direct action of angiotensin II on vascular smooth muscle and indirect activation of the sympathetic nervous system. The vasoconstrictive effect is greatest in skin, splanchnic vasculature, and kidneys, with blood flow being greatly reduced to these areas. Coronary artery vasoconstriction may jeopardize the adequacy of coronary blood flow (Gavras *et al,* 1977). Vasoconstriction is less in cerebral vessels and even weaker in skeletal muscle. In fact, total blood flow in these two regions may increase as the increased perfusion pressure more than offsets a modest increase in peripheral vascular resistance. Likewise, changes in pulmonary vascular pressures are usually modest.

Angiotensin II acts directly on cardiac cells to prolong the plateau phase of the cardiac action potential, which increases inward calcium movement that drives the contractile elements. Central and peripheral stimulant effects on the sympathetic nervous system may increase heart rate and myocardial contractility. Nevertheless, increased blood pressure may activate baroreceptors, which reflexively slow heart rate and decrease myocardial contractility. Changes in central venous pressure are modest, since angiotensin II has weak vasoconstrictor effects on large veins and thus reduces venous capacitance less than norepinephrine. The net result of all these changes is often a reduction in cardiac output.

Angiotensin II reduces intravascular fluid volume by virtue of loss of extracellular fluid in response to constriction of postcapillary venules, which increases capillary filtration pressure. In addition, angiotensin II increases vascular permeability in large arterioles by causing separation of the endothelial cells.

Central Nervous System

Central nervous system effects of angiotensin II occur despite the fact that peptides are generally regarded as being incapable of crossing the blood–brain barrier. Sustained hypertension reflects enhanced central outflow of sympathetic nervous system impulses by virtue of angiotensin

II effects on the medullary vasomotor center. Angiotensin II can also enhance release of adrenocorticotrophic hormone, presumably via a central nervous system action.

Peripheral Autonomic Nervous System

Peripheral autonomic nervous system effects of angiotensin II include stimulation of sympathetic nervous system ganglion cells and facilitation of ganglionic transmission. This may result in enhanced responsiveness of the innervated organ to norepinephrine as well as increased output of norepinephrine form the sympathetic nerve terminals (Zimmerman, 1978). Angiotensin-induced prolongation of the nerve action potential with influx of calcium ions may contribute to facilitation of norepinephrine release in response to each nerve impulse.

Angiotensin II stimulates release of catecholamines from the adrenal medulla by directly depolarizing the chromaffin cells. Resulting hypertension may be particularly marked in patients with pheochromocytoma.

Adrenal Cortex

Angiotensin II directly stimulates the synthesis and secretion of aldosterone from the adrenal cortex by facilitating the calcium-dependent mechanism necessary for the conversion of cholesterol to pregnenolone. This effect occurs with low concentrations of angiotensin II that lack effects on the blood pressure. Aldosterone subsequently acts on the kidneys to cause retention of sodium ions and excretion of potassium and hydrogen ions. The stimulant effects of angiotensin II on aldosterone secretion are enhanced when the plasma concentration of sodium ions is reduced or when plasma potassium concentration is elevated. These changes in responsiveness presumably reflect alterations in the number of receptors for angiotensin II on the zona glomerulosa cells (Davis and Freeman, 1976).

In addition to angiotensin II, hyponatremia, hyperkalemia, and adrenocorticotrophic hormone can stimulate the zona glomerulosa of the adrenal cortex to release aldosterone. Indeed, control of aldosterone secretion is not lost following bilateral nephrectomies, although responsiveness is blunted (Sealey *et al,* 1978).

Factors that Alter Plasma Renin Activity

Institution of positive end–expiratory pressure results in significant increases in plasma renin activity, plasma aldosterone concentration, and circulating levels of antidiuretic hormone (Annat *et al,* 1983). Nitroprusside-induced hypotension is associated with modest increases in plasma renin activity and marked elevations in the plasma concentration of antidiuretic hormone (Fig. 22-2) (Knight *et al,* 1983; Zubrow *et al,* 1983). Propranolol administered during nitroprusside-induced hypotension prevents the usual rise in plasma renin activity (Marshall *et al,* 1981). Plasma renin activity increases may contribute to tachyphylaxis during infusion of nitroprusside as well as overshoot of blood pressure above predrug levels when nitroprusside is discontinued (see Chapter 16). In contrast to nitroprusside, blood pressure

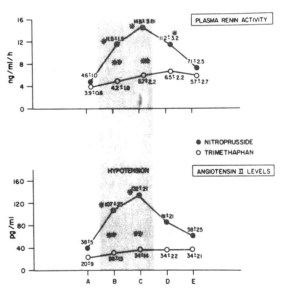

FIGURE 22-2. Plasma renin activity and angiotensin II concentrations are increased during sodium nitroprusside-induced hypotension *(clear circles)* but not during reductions in blood pressure produced by trimethaphan *(solid circles)*. (From Knight PR, Lane GA, Hensinger RN, Bolles RS, Bjoraker DG. Catecholamine and renin-angiotensin response during hypotensive anesthesia induced by sodium nitroprusside or trimethaphan camsylate. Anesthesiology 1983;59:248–53. Reproduced by permission of the authors and publisher.)

reductions produced by trimethaphan do not increase plasma renin activity, presumably because blockade of sympathetic nervous system ganglia by this vasodilator inhibits the release of renin (Fig. 22-2) (Knight *et al,* 1983) (see Chapter 16).

In sodium-repleted animals, plasma renin activity does not change during anesthesia with halothane, enflurane, or ketamine (Miller *et al,* 1978b). Conversely, in sodium-depleted animals, plasma renin activity increases during administration of these anesthetics (Miller *et al,* 1978a). Furthermore, subsequent infusion of saralasin to these animals accentuates blood pressure decreases, suggesting that the renin–angiotensin–aldosterone system is important in maintaining blood pressure in sodium-depleted and anesthetized animals. There is no evidence that anesthetics influence the rate of conversion of angiotensin I to angiotensin II (Miller *et al,* 1979).

Activation of the sympathetic nervous system may contribute to the release of renin via stimulation of beta-adrenergic receptors in the kidneys (Pettinger, 1978). Indeed, plasma renin activity and plasma concentrations of aldosterone increase dramatically during cardiopulmonary bypass (Fig. 22-3) (Bailey *et al,* 1975). Therefore, the renin–angiotensin–aldosterone system may play a role in blood pressure regulation during cardiopulmonary bypass, which could manifest as urinary excretion of potassium ions with associated hypokalemia.

Exogenous Infusion of Angiotensin II

Intravenous infusion of commercially available angiotensin II produces intense vasoconstriction and elevations in blood pressure. Too rapid infusion can elevate blood pressure to dangerous levels and produce myocardial ischemia. Compared with norepinephrine, angiotensin II has the following effects: (1) It is a more potent vasoconstrictor, (2) it produces a more sustained effect, (3) cardiac dysrhythmias are infrequent, and (4) hypotension is less likely to occur when a chronic infusion is abruptly discontinued. Spasm of the vein used for intravenous infusion does not occur, and tissue necrosis has not manifest, even with extravasation of angiotensin II. Like norepinephrine, angiotensin II diminishes intravascular fluid volume by promoting the loss of fluid from the circulation to tissues. As a constrictor of capacitance vessels, angiotensin II is less potent than

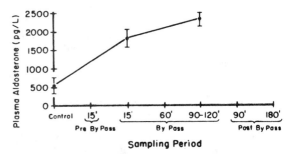

FIGURE 22-3. Plasma aldosterone concentrations increase dramatically during cardiopulmonary bypass. (From Bailey DR, Miller ED, Kaplan JA, Rogers PW. The renin–angiotensin–aldosterone system during cardiac surgery with morphine–nitrous oxide anesthesia. Anesthesiology 1975;42:538–44. Reproduced by permission of the authors and publisher.)

norepinephrine. The lack of a positive inotropic effect on the heart may be a disadvantage of angiotensin II compared with norepinephrine.

Antagonists of the Renin–Angiotensin–Aldosterone System

Antagonists of the renin–angiotensin–aldosterone system act by blocking receptors responsive to angiotensin II (*e.g.,* saralasin) and by inhibiting activity of the converting enzyme necessary for conversion of angiotensin I to angiotensin II (*e.g.,* captopril) (see Chapter 15). In addition, beta-adrenergic blockade prevents secretion of renin by sympathetic nervous system stimulation of juxtaglomerular cells. Furthermore, clonidine may decrease renin secretion by an action within the central nervous system (see Chapter 15).

PLASMA KININS

Plasma kinins are polypeptides that include kallidin and bradykinin (Schachter and Barton, 1979). These two kinins are the result of enzyme-induced cleavage of kinogens that exist in the plasma as α_2 globulins. These α_2 globulin enzymes are collectively referred to as kininogenases and include kallikreins, trypsin, and plasmin.

Plasma kinins are the most potent endogenous vasodilators known. Furthermore, in low plasma concentrations, kinins (1) increase capillary permeability, (2) produce edema, and (3) evoke intense burning pain by acting on nerve endings. Plasma kinins are about ten times more potent than histamine in causing vasodilation. Injected intravenously, plasma kinins cause flushing in the blush area and dilatation in renal, coronary, and cerebral arterioles. Vasodilation results in marked decreases in systolic and diastolic blood pressure. In contrast to effects on arterioles, plasma kinins tend to constrict large veins, leading to increased venous return. Increased venous return combined with reflexively increased baroreceptor reflex activity owing to diastolic hypotension results in increased heart rate and cardiac output. Increased capillary permeability produced by plasma kinins resembles that occurring in response to histamine and serotonin. Indeed, intradermal injections of plasma kinins produce a "wheal and flare response." Finally, plasma kinins may increase airway resistance in patients with reactive airways disease such as bronchial asthma.

Mechanism of Action

Specific plasma kinin receptors are postulated, whereas some responses to kinins may be mediated by production of prostaglandins (Barabe *et al,* 1977). Certain of the direct effects on blood vessels may reflect the ability of plasma kinins to evoke the release of histamine from mast cells.

Pharmacokinetics

The elimination half-time of plasma kinins is less than 15 seconds, with more than 90% being metabolized during a single passage through the lung. Other tissues are also capable of rapidly metabolizing the plasma kinins. The enzyme responsible for this rapid metabolism is known as *converting enzyme* (peptidyl dipeptidase) and is identical to the enzyme necessary for the conversion of angiotensin I to angiotensin II (see the section entitled Renin).

Bradykinin

Bradykinin (so-named because it produces slow contraction of the gastrointestinal tract) is formed from a high–molecular weight kinongen by the action of the enzyme, kallikrein. Typically, mini-mal amounts of bradykinin are formed because plasma kallikrein is present in an inactive form known as prekallikrein. Changes that activate prekallikrein and lead to the formation of bradykinin include alteration in pH or temperature and contact with negatively charged surfaces such as collagen when exposed by tissue damage. Indeed, many of the factors that activate prekallikrein are involved in factor XII–initiated coagulation and fibrinolysis (Chan *et al,* 1978; Coleman and Wong, 1977).

Hereditary angioedema is associated with the absence of the C_1 esterase inhibitor of the complement system, which is also an inhibitor of kallikrein. For this reason, it is speculated that episodes of edema that are characteristic of this disease may, in part, be due to excess formation of bradykinin (Donaldson *et al,* 1977). Other diseases that may be associated with excess formation of plasma kinins such as bradykinin include (1) septic shock, (2) allergic reactions, and (3) carcinoid syndrome. Conversely, inadequate amounts of bradykinin may be associated with essential hypertension. Indeed, accumulation of plasma kinins resulting from inhibition of the converting enzyme by captopril may contribute to the blood pressure–lowering effects of this drug (see Chapter 15).

Aprotinin

Aprotinin is a polypeptide inhibitor of kallikrein that may be useful in the treatment of acute pancreatitis and carcinoid syndrome (Haberland, 1978).

SEROTONIN

Serotonin (5-hydroxytryptamine) is a widely distributed vasoactive substance (*i.e.,* autacoid) that also serves as an inhibitory neurotransmitter in the central nervous system. About 90% of endogenous serotonin is present in enterochromaffin cells of the gastrointestinal tract. The remaining serotonin is present primarily in the central nervous system and in platelets. Mast cells of some species, but not humans, contain serotonin. The function of serotonin in platelets is unknown but may reflect an inactive storage site for serotonin that escapes from cells, particularly in the gastrointestinal tract. Indeed, the potentiating effect of serotonin on platelet aggregation is small, and platelets depleted of serotonin function normally.

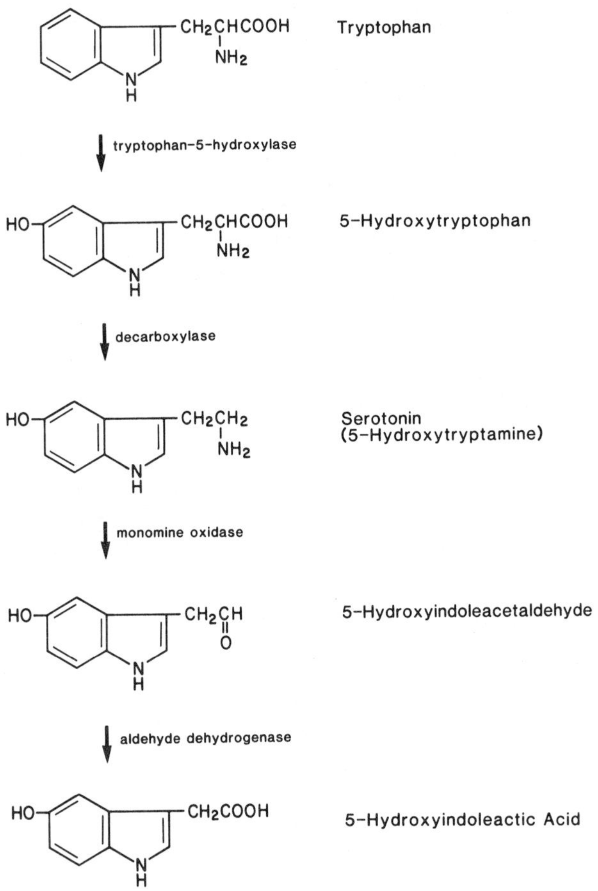

FIGURE 22-4. Synthesis and metabolism of serotonin.

Mechanism of Action

Receptors specific for serotonin are confirmed by the effectiveness of serotonin antagonist drugs. It is likely that subtypes of receptors that respond to serotonin exist, as emphasized by different responses exerted by various antagonist drugs. For example, methysergide and cyproheptadine antagonize effects of serotonin on peripheral tissues but do not act as antagonists in the central nervous system (see the section entitled Antagonists). Changes in cell membrane permeability to inorganic ions, including calcium ions, seem to be important in the function of serotonin receptors. Likewise, intracellular accumulation of cyclic AMP may be important in serotonin-induced responses.

Synthesis and Metabolism

Serotonin is synthesized in cells from tryptophan (Fig. 22-4). In cells, tryptophan is first hydroxylated to 5-hydroxytryptophan, which is then decarboxylated to serotonin (*i.e.,* 5-hydroxytryptamine) by the same nonspecific decarboxylase enzyme that is involved in the synthesis of catecholamines. Tryptophan ingested in food is not available for this endogenous synthesis of serotonin, because it is metabolized in the liver or lungs before it reaches tissue sites. An exception is platelets, which acquire tryptophan derived from exogenous sources during their passage through the gastrointestinal tract. In the cells, serotonin is stored in vesicles located in the cytoplasm for subsequent release.

Turnover rates of serotonin in the brain and gastrointestinal tract are about 1 and 17 hours, respectively. Carcinoid tumors that synthesize serotonin may divert so much tryptophan from protein synthesis to production of serotonin that hypoalbuminemia and pellegra results. Serotonin undergoes oxidative deamination by monoamine oxidase, ultimately resulting in the formation of 5-hydroxyindolacetic acid (Fig. 22-4). Patients with carcinoid tumors or those who have just ingested certain foods, such as bananas, manifest an elevated urinary excretion of this metabolite. Oral administration of serotonin followed by measurement of urinary excretion of 5-hydroxyindolacetic acid provides a method for testing the degree of inhibition of monoamine oxidase activity.

Effects on Organ Systems

Serotonin produces vasoconstriction of vascular smooth muscle, particularly in the splanchnic and renal circulations. Cerebral vasoconstriction may be marked. Pulmonary vasoconstriction induced by serotonin is less prominent in humans than in other species. Vasodilation occurs in skeletal muscles and skin, producing an intense flush response followed by cyanosis, presumably indicating stasis owing to venoconstriction. Indeed, serotonin acts as a potent constrictor of veins. Positive inotropic and chronotropic actions of serotonin are masked by reflex-mediated baroreceptor responses.

Bronchoconstriction is a prominent response to serotonin in animals but rarely in humans, except perhaps in patients with bronchial asthma (Rodbard and Kira, 1972). Motility of the gastrointestinal tract is greatly increased by circulating serotonin. Serotonin present in the peripheral circulation penetrates the blood–brain barrier poorly, producing minimal central nervous system effects.

Antagonists

Tricyclic antidepressants inhibit the uptake of serotonin back into tryptaminergic nerve endings similar to the effect exerted on catecholamines. A long-lasting depletion of serotonin is produced by the anorexiant drug fenfluramine. Lysergic acid derivatives are specific competitive antagonists at receptors normally responsive to serotonin. Other drugs that act as serotonin antagonists include H_1 receptor blockers of the ethylenediamine type; phenothiazines, especially chlorpromazine; and beta-haloalkylamines, such as phenoxybenzamine (Garattini and Samanin, 1978).

Methysergide

Methysergide is a congener of lysergic acid but lacks significant central nervous system effects (Fig. 22-5). It inhibits peripheral vasoconstriction evoked by serotonin. Clinical uses include prophylaxis against development of migraine and other vascular headaches. This drug is not effective after a headache has developed. Methysergide is useful in treating malabsorption and diarrhea in patients with carcinoid syndrome. It may also alleviate similar symptoms in patients with postgastrectomy dumping syndrome. Methysergide depresses prolactin secretion, perhaps by dopamine-like actions (Oppizzi *et al,* 1977).

An infrequent but serious side effect of treatment with methysergide is an inflammatory reaction that may manifest as retroperitoneal, pleuropulmonary, coronary, or endocardial fibrosis.

Cyproheptadine

Cyproheptadine resembles the structure of phenothiazine H_1 receptor antagonists and is able to block receptors for both histamine and serotonin (Fig. 22-6). In addition, this drug possesses weak

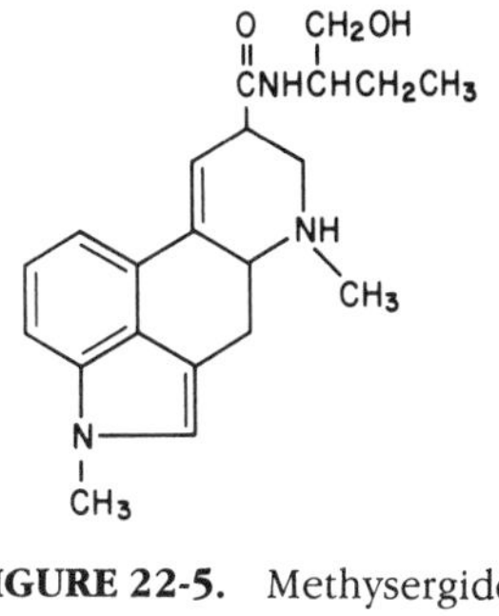

FIGURE 22-5. Methysergide.

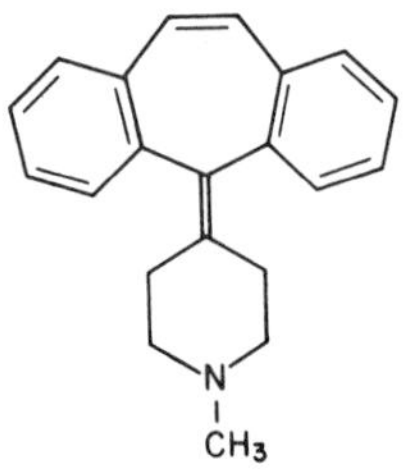

FIGURE 22-6. Cyproheptadine.

anticholinergic activity and mild central nervous system depressant properties (Stone *et al,* 1961).

The actions of cyproheptadine as an antagonist during allergic reactions are not relevant, because serotonin is not involved in human allergic responses. Uses of this drug are in the treatment of intestinal hypermotility associated with carcinoid syndrome and in the postgastrectomy dumping syndrome.

Side effects of cyproheptadine include sedation and dry mouth, as a reflection of H_1 receptor antagonism. Increased growth in children has been observed, perhaps as a result of altered secretion of insulin and growth hormone (Hintze *et al*, 1977).

REFERENCES

Annat G, Viale JP, Xuan BB, et al. Effect of PEEP ventilation on renal function, plasma renin, aldosterone, neurophysins and urinary ADH, and prostaglandins. Anesthesiology 1983;58:136–141.

Bailey DR, Miller ED, Kaplan JA, Rogers PW. The renin–angiotensin–aldosterone system during cardiac surgery with morphine–nitrous oxide anesthesia. Anesthesiology 1975;42:538–44.

Barabe J, Drouin J–N, Regoli D, Park WK. Receptors for bradykinin in intestinal and uterine smooth muscle. Can J Physiol Pharmacol 1977;55:2170–85.

Chan JYC, Burrowes CE, Movat HC. Surface activation of factor XII (Hageman factor) — critical role of high–molecular weight kininogen and another potentiator. Agents Actions 1978;8:65–72.

Coleman RW, Wong PY. Participation of Hageman factor–dependent pathways in human disease states. Thromb Haemost 1977;38:751–75.

Davis JO, Freeman RH. Mechanisms regulating renin release. Physiol Rev 1976;56:1–56.

Devynck MA, Meyer P. Angiotensin receptors. Biochem Pharmacol 1978;27:1–5.

Donaldson VH, Rosen FS, Bing DH. Role of the second component of complement (C_2) and plasmin in kinin release in hereditary angioneurotic edema (HANE) plasma. Trans Assoc Am Phys 1977;90:174–83.

Garattini S, Samanin R. Drugs affecting serotonin: a survey. In: Essman WB, ed. Physiologic Regulation and Pharmacological Action. Serotonin in Health and Disease. New York, Spectrum Publications, Inc, 1978;2:247–93.

Gavras H, Flessas A, Ryan TJ, Brunner HR, Faxon DP, Gavras I. Angiotensin II inhibition. Treatment of congestive cardiac failure in a high-renin hypertension. JAMA 1977;237:880–2.

Haberland GL. The role of kininogenases, kinin formation and kininogenase inhibition in post-traumatic shock and related conditions. Klin Wochenschr 1978;56:325–31.

Hintze KL, Grow AB, Fischer LJ. Cyproheptadine-induced alterations in rat insulin synthesis. Biochem Pharmacol 1977;26:2021–7.

Knight PR, Lane GA, Hensinger RN, Bolles RS, Bjoraker DG. Catecholamine and renin–angiotensin response during hypotensive anesthesia induced by sodium nitroprusside or trimethaphan camsylate. Anesthesiology 1983;59:248–53.

Marshall WK, Bedford RF, Arnold WP et al. Effects of propranolol on the cardiovascular and renin–angiotensin systems during hypotension produced by sodium nitroprusside in humans. Anesthesiology 1981;55:277–80.

Miller ED, Ackerly JA, Peach MJ. Blood pressure support during general anesthesia in a renin-dependent state in the rat. Anesthesiology 1978a;48:404–8.

Miller ED, Gianfagna W, Ackerly JA, Peach MJ. Converting-enzyme activity and pressure responses to angiotensin I and II in the rat awake and during anesthesia. Anesthesiology 1979;50:88–92.

Miller ED, Longnecker DE, Peach MJ. The regulatory function of the renin–angiotensin system during general anesthesia. Anesthesiology 1978b;48:399–403.

Oppizzi G, Verde G, Stefano L, et al. Evidence for a dopaminergic activity of methysergide in humans. Clin Endocrinol 1977;7:267–72.

Peach MJ. Renin–angiotensin system: biochemistry and mechanisms of action. Physiol Rev 1977;57:313–70.

Pettinger WA. Anesthetics and the renin–angiotensin–aldosterone axis (Editorial). Anesthesiology 1978;48:393–6.

Rodbard S, Kira S. Lobar, airway, and pulmonary vascular effects of serotonin. Angiology 1972;23:188–97.

Schachter M, Barton S. Kallikreins (Kininogenases) and

kinins. In: Cahill G, DeGroot LJ, eds. Endocrinology: Metabolic Basis of Clinical Practice. New York, Grune and Stratton, Inc., 1979.

Sealey JE, White RP, Laragh JH, Case DB, Rubin AL. Studies of plasma aldosterone in anephric people: evidence for the fundamental role of the renin system in maintaining aldosterone secretion. J Clin Endocrinol Metab 1978;47:52–60.

Stone CA, Wenger HC, Ludden CT, Stavorski IM, Ross CA. Antiserotonin–antihistaminic properties of cyproheptadine. J. Pharmacol Exp Ther 1961; 131:73–84.

Zimmerman BG. Actions of angiotensin on adrenergic nerve endings. Fed Proc 1978;37:199–202.

Zubrow AB, Daniel SS, Startk RI, Husain MK, James LS. Plasma renin, catecholamine, and vasopressin during nitroprusside-induced hypotension in ewes. Anesthesiology 1983;58:245–9.

C H A P T E R   23

Hormones as Drugs

INTRODUCTION

Preparations that contain active hormones secreted endogenously by endocrine glands may be administered as drugs. These synthetic hormones resemble the endogenous substances in structure and activity (see Chapter 52). Typically, the clinical application of these drugs is for hormone replacement (*i.e.,* a physiologic effect). In certain patients, however, large doses of the synthetic hormone are used to exert a pharmacologic effect. Recombinant deoxyribonucleic acid (DNA) technology permits the incorporation of synthetic genes that code for the synthesis of specific human hormones by bacteria, thus permitting production of pure hormones devoid of allerginic properties.

ANTERIOR PITUITARY HORMONES

Anterior pituitary hormones include growth hormone; prolactin; gonadotropins, including luteinizing hormone and follicle stimulating hormone; adrenocorticotrophic hormone (ACTH); and thyroid stimulating hormone (TSH) (see Chapter 52). Growth hormone, gonadotropins, and ACTH can be administered in the form of synthetic drugs.

Perioperative replacement of anterior pituitary hormones may be necessary for patients receiving exogenous hormone because of prior hypophysectomy. For example, cortisol must be

provided continuously. Conversely, thyroid hormone has such a long elimination half-time that it can be omitted for several days without adverse effects. Likewise, the loss of other anterior pituitary hormones has no immediate implications.

Growth Hormone

Growth hormone is used to treat hypopituitary dwarfism, based on documentation that the plasma concentration of the hormone is inadequate. In this regard, radioimmunoassays for growth hormone are used to measure plasma concentrations of the hormone. Treatment must be maintained for several months or years, corresponding to childhood. Injection of hormone at weekly intervals is usually adequate for treatment, despite an elimination half-time of about 20 minutes.

Gonadotropins

Gonadotropins are used most often for the treatment of infertility and cryptorchism. Induction of ovulation can be stimulated in females who are infertile because of pituitary insufficiency. Excessive ovarian enlargement and maturation of many follicles leading to multiple births is a possibility.

Gonadotropins are effective only by parenteral injection. Radioimmunoassays are useful in measuring the plasma and urine concentrations of gonadotropins.

Adrenocorticotrophic Hormone

The physiologic and pharmacologic effects of ACTH result from drug-induced secretion of corticosteroids from the adrenal cortex, principally cortisol. An important clinical use of ACTH is as a diagnostic aid in patients with suspected adrenal insufficiency. For example, a normal increase in the plasma concentration of cortisol in response to administration of ACTH rules out primary adrenocortical insufficiency. Furthermore, ACTH may be administered therapeutically to evoke the release of cortisol. Treatment of disease states with ACTH is not physiologically equivalent to administration of a specific hormone, because ACTH exposes the tissues to a mixture of glucocorticoids, mineralocorticoids, and androgens. Indeed, there may be associated retention of sodium, development of hypokalemic metabolic alkalosis, and appearance of acne, which are unlikely to accompany selective acting corticosteroids.

Absorption of ACTH after intramuscular injection is prompt. Following intravenous injection, ACTH disappears rapidly from the plasma with an elimination half-time of about 15 minutes. Maximal stimulation of the adrenal cortex is produced by ACTH, 25 units, absorbed over 8 hours. Allergic reactions ranging from mild fever to life-threatening anaphylaxis may be associated with administration of ACTH (Frossman and Mulder, 1973).

THYROID GLAND HORMONES

The thyroid gland is the source of triiodothyronine (T_3), thyroxine (T_4), and calcitonin (Fig. 23-1). Commercial preparations of T_3 and T_4 are available for treatment of hypothyroidism, as may be encountered in patients with a simple goiter.

The effectiveness of treatment is judged by the return of the plasma concentration of TSH to normal and a decrease in the size of the goiter. Certain carcinomas of the thyroid gland, particularly papillary tumors, may remain sensitive to TSH. Indeed, administration of thyroid hormones may suppress this responsiveness and cause regression of the malignant lesion.

Thyroid hormones enhance the effects of coumarin anticoagulants by increasing catabolism of vitamin K–dependent clotting factors. Cholestyramine binds orally administered thyroid hormone in the gastrointestinal tract.

Levothyroxine

Levothyroxine is the most frequently administered drug for treatment of diseases requiring thyroid hormone replacement. Oral administration is preferred, but intravenous injection is acceptable in emergency situations. Most patients can be maintained in a euthyroid state with 100 to 200 μg daily.

Liothyronine

Liothyronine is the levorotatory isomer of T_3, being 2.5 to 3 times as potent as levothyroxine. Its rapid onset and short duration of action preclude use of liothyronine for long-term thyroid replacement.

DRUGS THAT INHIBIT THYROID HORMONE SYNTHESIS

A large number of substances are capable of interfering with the synthesis of thyroid hormones. These compounds include (1) antithyroid drugs, (2) inhibitors of the iodide transport mechanism, (3) iodide, and (4) radioactive iodine.

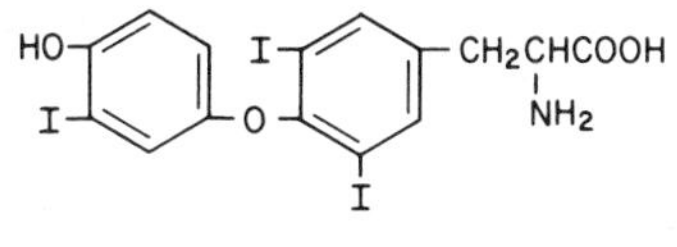

Triiodothyronine (T_3)

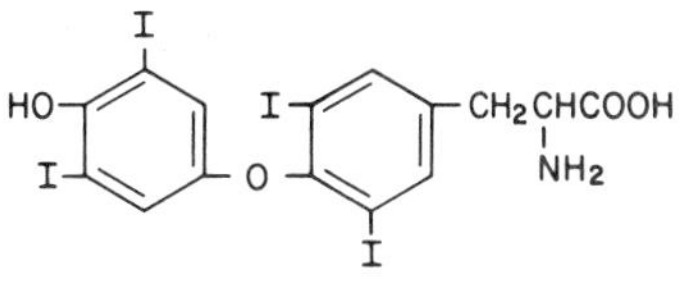

Thyroxine (tetraiodothyronine, T_4)

FIGURE 23-1. Thyroid gland hormones.

Antithyroid Drugs

Propylthiouracil and methimazole are antithyroid drugs that inhibit the formation of thyroid hormone by interfering with the incorporation of iodine into tyrosine residues of thyroglobulin (Fig. 23-2) (Cooper, 1984). In addition to blocking hormone synthesis, these drugs also inhibit the peripheral deiodination of T4 to T3 (Saberi *et al*, 1975). These drug-induced effects on thyroid hormone synthesis render antithyroid drugs useful in the treatment of hyperthyroidism prior to elective thyroidectomy.

Antithyroid drugs are not available as parenteral preparations, necessitating their administration by way of a gastric tube if drugs cannot be administered orally, such as during thyroid storm. Drug-induced reductions in excessive thyroid activity usually require several days, because preformed hormone must be depleted before symptoms begin to wane. In a few patients, especially those with severe hyperthyroidism, definite improvement is evident in 1 to 2 days.

Side Effects

The incidence of side effects produced by propylthiouracil and methiamazole are similar. The most common reaction is an urticarial or papular skin rash often associated with pruritus that occurs in about 3% of patients. This rash may disappear spontaneously without interrupting treatment. In others, this side effect necessitates changing to the other drug, since cross-sensitivity is not likely.

Granulocytopenia and agranulocytosis are serious but rare side effects that are most likely to occur in the first 2 months of therapy with an antithyroid drug. Periodic white blood cell counts, although helpful for detecting gradual reductions in the leukocyte count, should not be relied on to detect agranulocytosis because of the rapidity

with which this complication can develop. Fever or pharyngitis may be the earliest manifestation of the development of agranulocytosis. Recovery is likely if the antithyroid drug is discontinued at the first sign of this side effect.

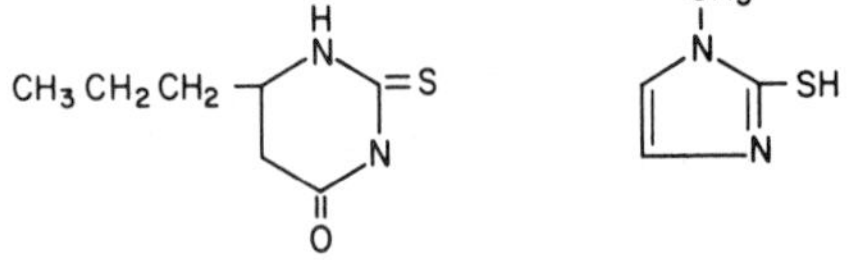

Antithyroid drugs cross the placenta and appear in breast milk. Placental passage, however, is limited for propylthiouracil, making it the preferred drug for use in the parturient.

Inhibitors of Iodine Transport Mechanisms

Inhibitors of iodide transport mechanisms are thiocyanate and perchlorate. These nonvalent ions are similar in size to iodide and, in some way, interfere with the uptake of iodide ions by the thyroid gland. Thiocyanate can result from the metabolism of nitroprusside or ingestion of cabbage, neither of which is likely to be clinically significant. Perchlorate is capable of producing aplastic anemia and is thus rarely used.

Iodide

Iodide is the oldest available therapy for hyperthyroidism, providing a paradoxical treatment that is effective for reasons that are not fully understood. The response of the patient with hyperthyroidism to iodide is often discernible within 24 hours, emphasizing that release of hormone into the circulation is quickly interrupted. Indeed, the most important clinical effect of high doses of iodide is inhibition of the release of thyroid hormone. This may reflect the ability of iodide to antagonize the ability of both TSH and cyclic AMP to stimulate hormone release (Pisarev *et al*, 1971).

Iodide is particularly useful in the treatment of hyperthyroidism prior to elective thyroidectomy. Indeed, the combination of oral potassium iodide and propranolol is a recommended approach for the preoperative preparation of the hyperthyroid patient (Feek *et al*, 1980). Vascularity of the thyroid gland is also reduced by iodide therapy. Chronic treatment with iodide, however, is often associated with a recurrence of previously suppressed excessive thyroid gland activity.

Allergic reactions may accompany treatment with iodide or administration of organic preparations that contain iodine. Angioedema and laryngeal edema may become life threatening.

FIGURE 23-2. Antithyroid drugs.

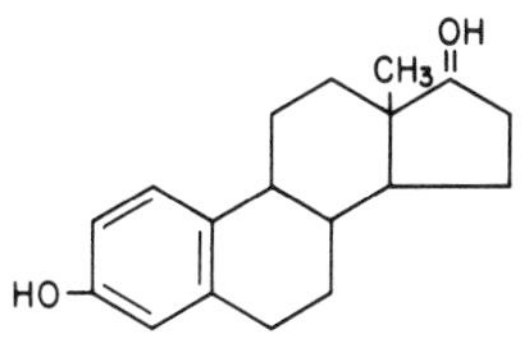

Estradiol

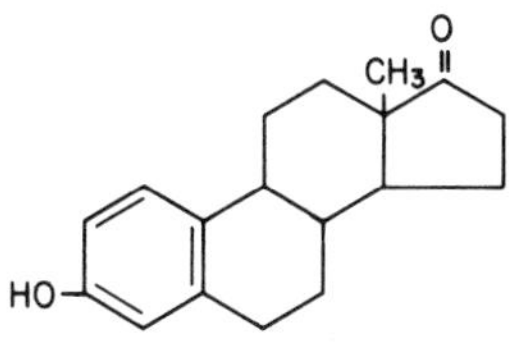

Estrone

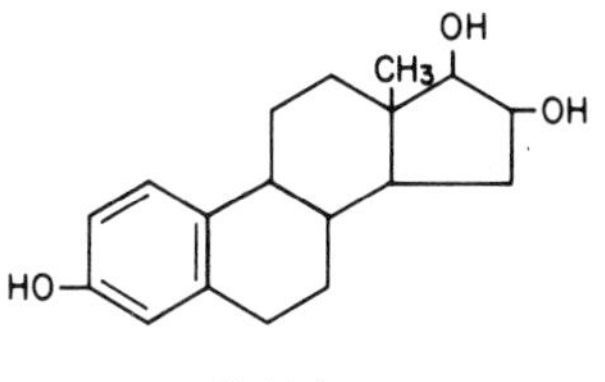

Estriol

FIGURE 23-3. Estrogens.

Radioactive Iodine

Among the radioactive isotopes of iodine, ^{131}I is the most frequently administered. This isotope is rapidly and efficiently trapped by thyroid gland cells, and the subsequent emission of destructive beta rays acts almost exclusively upon these cells with little or no damage to surrounding tissue. It is possible to completely destroy the thyroid gland with [131]I. Indeed, hypothyroidism occurs in about 10% of treated patients in the first year following ^{131}I administration and increases about 2% to 3% each year thereafter (Glennon *et al,* 1972). For this reason, iatrogenic hypothyroidism must be considered preoperatively in any patient who has previously been treated with [131]I.

Hyperthyroidism is treated with orally administered ^{131}I, with symptoms of excessive thyroid gland activity gradually abating over a period of 2 to 3 months. One half to two thirds of patients are cured by a single dose of isotope, and the remainder require an additional one to two doses. Despite the safety and effectiveness of ^{131}I, surgery is often selected for patients younger than 30 years of age because of the concern about potential carcinogenic effects of radiation. Nevertheless, there is no evidence that ^{131}I has ever caused cancer in adults.

The principal indication for ^{131}I treatment is hyperthyroidism in elderly patients and in those with heart disease. Indeed, hypothyroidism is not a common sequela following treatment with ^{131}I for toxic nodular goiter, the usual cause of hyper-

thyroidism in elderly patients. The use of ^{131}I is contraindicated during pregnancy, because the fetal thyroid gland would concentrate the isotope.

Most thyroid carcinomas except for follicular carcinoma accumulate little radioactive iodine. As a result, the therapeutic usefulness of ^{131}I for treatment of thyroid carcinoma is limited.

OVARIAN HORMONES

An understanding of the synthesis and action of ovarian hormones, including estrogens and progesterone, permits therapeutic interventions in certain disease states (see Chapter 52). Equally important is the therapeutic use of drugs that can mimic effects of these hormones and act as contraceptives.

Estrogens

Estrogens are effective in the treatment of unpleasant side-effects of menopause (Fig. 23-3). Senile or atrophic vaginitis responds to topical estrogen. There is no evidence that administration of estrogen delays the progression of atherosclerosis in postmenopausal women. Treatment of postmenopausal osteoporosis is as effective with calcium as with estrogens. Estrogens are administered to decrease milk production in the postpartum period. The presence of receptors for estrogen increases the likelihood of a palliative response to estrogen therapy in women with metastatic breast cancer. An important use of estrogens is in combination with progestins as oral contraceptives (see the section entitled Oral Contraceptives).

Route of Administration

The absorption of most estrogens and their derivatives from the gastrointestinal tract is prompt and nearly complete. Metabolism in the liver, however, limits the effectiveness of orally administered estrogens. Topical and intramuscular administration of estrogens is also effective. Radioimmunoassay methods are highly specific and sensitive for measuring the plasma concentrations of estrogens.

Side Effects (also see section entitled Oral Contraceptives)

The most frequent unpleasant symptom associated with the use of estrogens is nausea. Large doses of estrogens may cause retention of sodium and water, which is particularly undesirable in patients with cardiac or renal disease. There is an increased incidence of vaginal and cervical adenocarcinoma in female offspring of mothers treated with diethylstilbestrol or other synthetic estrogens during the first trimester of pregnancy. Most of the affected females have been 20 to 25 years of age when diagnosed. Use of estrogen by postmenopausal women increases the risk of developing endometrial carcinoma (Horwitz and Feinstein, 1978).

Antiestrogens

Clomiphene and tamoxifen act as antiestrogens by binding to estrogen receptors (Fig. 23-4). The subsequent loss of normal feedback inhibition of estrogen synthesis causes an increased secretion of gonadotropins. The most prominent effect of increased plasma concentrations of gonadotropins is enlargement of the ovaries and enhancement of fertility in otherwise infertile females.

Progesterone

Orally active derivatives of progesterone are designated progestins (Fig. 23-5). Progestins are often combined with estrogens as oral contraceptives (see the section entitled Oral Contraceptives). Dysfunctional uterine bleeding can be treated with small doses of a progestin for a few days, with the goal being induction of progesterone-withdrawal bleeding. Progestins, like estrogens, are effective in suppressing lactation in the immediate postpartum period. Palliative treatment of metastatic endometrial carcinoma is achieved with progestins. Absorption of progestins from the gastrointestinal tract is rapid, but metabolism is extensive during passage.

Oral Contraceptives

Oral contraceptives are most often a combination of an estrogen and a progestin. This combination inhibits ovulation, presumably by preventing release of follicle-stimulating hormone by estrogen and luteinizing hormone by progesterone.

Side Effects

Estrogens in combined preparations are believed to be responsible for most, if not all, the side effects of oral contraceptives. For example, estrogens seem to be responsible for the increased

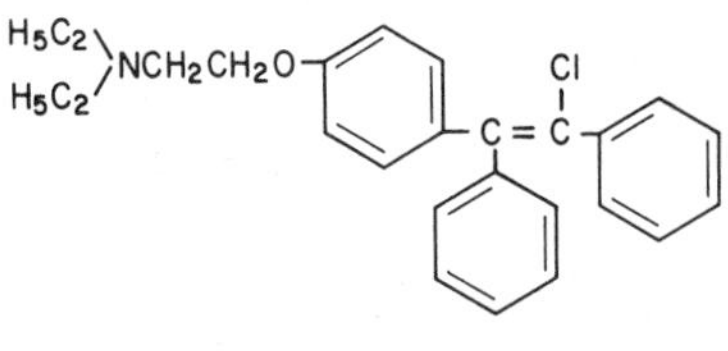

Clomiphene 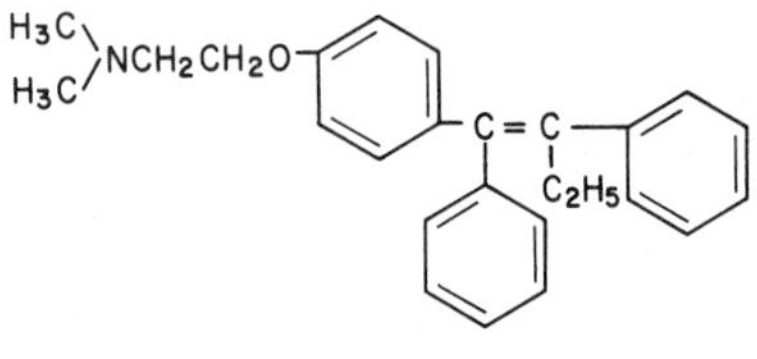   Tamoxifen

FIGURE 23-4. Antiestrogens.

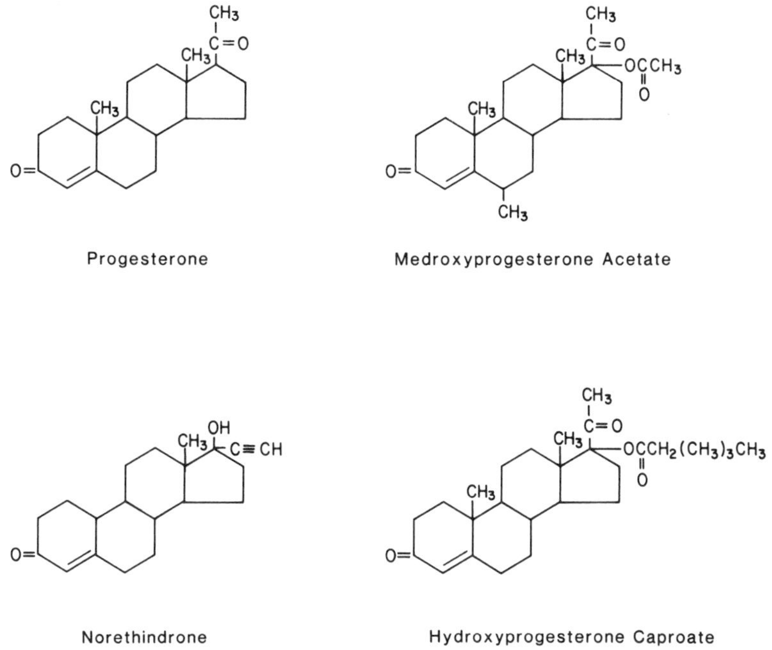

Progesterone

Medroxyprogesterone Acetate

Norethindrone

Hydroxyprogesterone Caproate

FIGURE 23-5. Progestins.

incidence of thrombophlebitis and thrombo-embolism (Kaplan, 1978). Indeed, patients taking estrogens manifest increased blood concentrations of some clotting factors as well as increased platelet aggregation. Nausea, vomiting, weight gain, and discomfort in the breasts resemble early pregnancy and are attributable to the estrogen component of oral contraceptives. The incidence of myocardial infarction and stroke is increased in patients who chronically take oral contraceptives (Kaplan, 1978; Mann et al, 1976). Hypertension occurs in about 5% of women taking oral contraceptives chronically (Laragh, 1976). This response probably reflects estrogen-induced increases in circulating plasma concentrations of renin and angiotensin, with associated retention of sodium and water.

Oral contraceptives containing high doses of estrogen may produce alterations in the glucose tolerance curve of patients with preclinical diabetes mellitus (Briggs, 1976). These drugs increase the concentration of cholesterol in bile, which is consistent with an increased incidence of cholelithiasis (Bennion et al, 1976). Benign hepatomas have been associated with the use of oral contraceptives (Baum et al, 1973). An increased incidence of breast tumors in patients tak-

ing estrogen-containing oral contraceptives has not been demonstrated (Kay, 1977). Depression of mood and fatigue have been attributed to the progestin component of oral contraceptives.

ANDROGENS

Androgens are most often administered to males to stimulate the development and/or maintenance of secondary sexual characteristics (Fig. 23-6). The most common indication for androgen therapy in females is palliative management of metastatic carcinoma of the breast. Androgens enhance erythropoiesis by stimulation of renal production of erythropoietin as well as by a direct dose-related stimulation of erythropoietin-sensitive elements in bone marrow. In addition, there is a drug-induced increase in 2, 3-diphosphoglycerate levels, which decreases hemoglobin affinity for oxygen, thus enhancing the availability of oxygen to tissues. For these reasons, androgen therapy is often instituted in the patient with aplastic anemia, hemolytic anemia, and anemia associated with chronic renal failure. Androgen-anabolic steroids have been used in the treatment of chronic debilitating diseases. These drugs promote a feel-

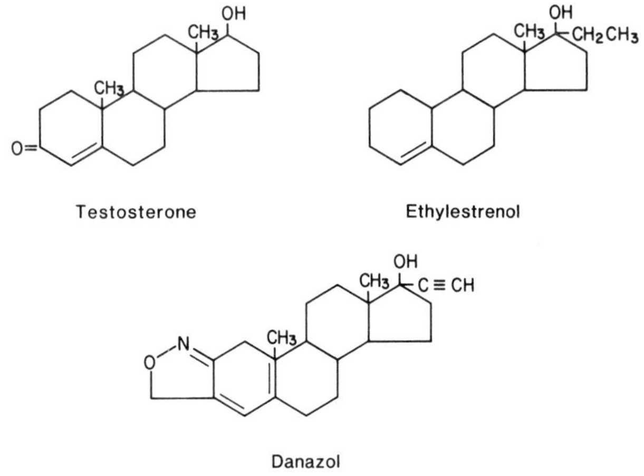

FIGURE 23-6. Androgens.

ing of well-being and may improve appetite when administered to patients with terminal illnesses. The efficacy of anabolic steroids to improve athletic performance is not documented and is condemned on ethical grounds. Finally, androgens are useful in the treatment of heredity angioedema (see the section entitled Danazol).

Route of Administration

Testosterone administered orally is readily absorbed but is metabolized so extensively by the liver that therapeutic effects do not occur. Alkylation of androgens at the 17 position retards their hepatic metabolism and permits such derivatives to be effective orally (Fig. 23-6). About 99% of testosterone circulating in the plasma is bound to sex hormone–binding globulin (Givens, 1978). As a result, this globulin determines the concentration of free testosterone in the plasma and thus its elimination half-time, which is 10 to 20 minutes.

Side Effects

Dose-related cholestatic hepatitis and jaundice are particularly likely to accompany androgen therapy for palliation in neoplastic disease. Elevations in plasma alkaline phosphatase and transaminase enzymes are also likely. Prolonged therapy (more than 1 year) with androgens, as for management of anemia, is associated with an increased incidence of hepatic adenocarcinoma (Henderson, et al, 1973). Retention of sodium and water is also likely to accompany palliative treatment of cancer with high doses of androgens.

Androgens increase the potency of coumarin anticoagulants and increase the likelihood of spontaneous hemorrhage. Androgens can decrease the concentration of thyroid binding globulin in plasma and thus influence thyroid function tests.

Danazol

The low androgenic activity of danazol makes it the preferred androgen for treatment of hereditary angioedema (Fig. 23-6). There is a remission of symptoms and increased production of previously deficient plasma protein factors. As with other androgens, danazol therapy has been associated with abnormal liver function tests and jaundice. Danazol also reduces breast pain and nodularity in many women with fibrocystic breast disease. Symptoms of endometriosis are reduced, and fertility is often restored by danazol. In patients with hemophilia A, danazol increases factor VIII activity and reduces the incidence of hemorrhage (Gralnick et al, 1985).

CORTICOSTEROIDS

The actions of corticosteroids are classified according to the potencies of these compounds to (1) evoke distal renal tubular reabsorption of so-

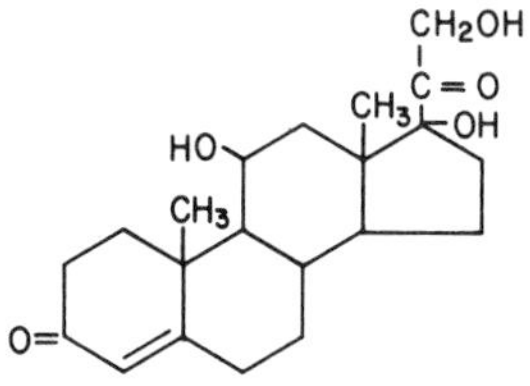

Cortisol

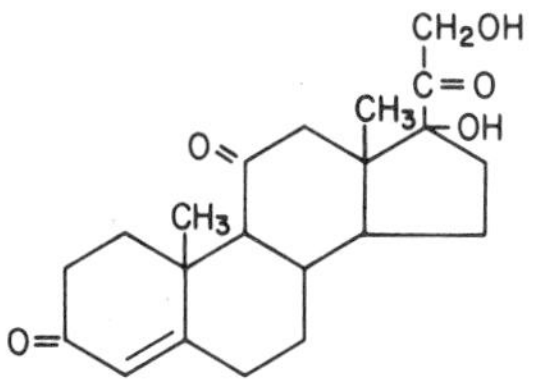

Cortisone

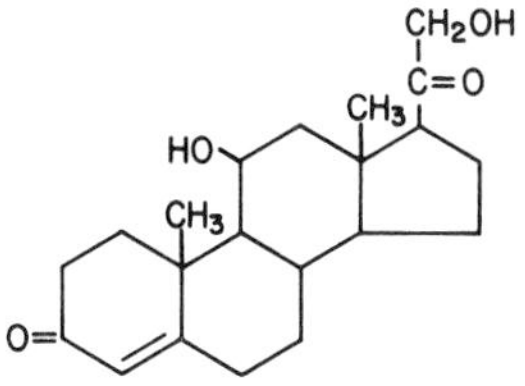

Corticosterone

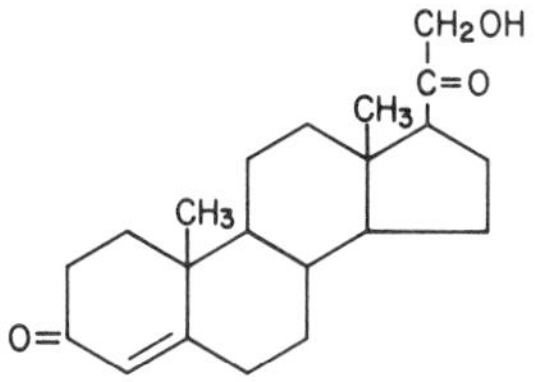

Desoxycorticosterone

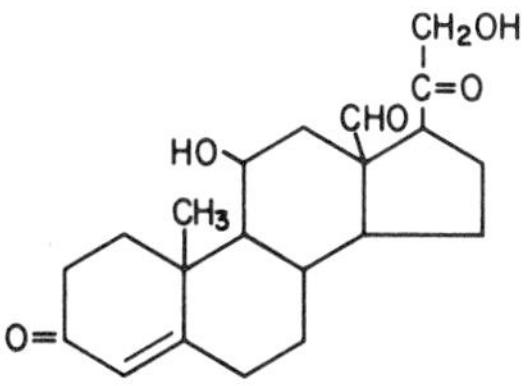

Aldosterone

FIGURE 23-7.   Endogenous corticosteroids.

dium in exchange for potassium ions (*i.e.,* mineralocorticoid effect), or (2) produce an anti-inflammatory response (*i.e.,* glucocorticoid effect) (see Chapter 52). Naturally occurring corticosteroids are cortisol (hydrocortisone), cortisone, corticosterone, desoxycorticosterone, and aldosterone (Fig. 23-7). Several synthetic corticosteroids are available, principally for use to produce anti-inflammatory effects (see the section entitled Synthetic Corticosteroids). Although it is possible to separate mineralocorticoid and glucocorticoid effects using synthetic drugs, it has not been possible to separate the various components of the glucocorticoid effects. Consequently, all synthetic corticosteroids when used in pharmacologic doses for their anti-inflammatory effects also produce less desirable effects, such as suppression of the hypothalamic–pituitary–adrenal axis, weight gain, and skeletal muscle wasting.

Structure Activity Relationships

All corticosteroids are constructed on the same primary molecular framework, designated as the steroid nucleus (Fig. 23-7). Changes in molecular structure may result in altered biologic responses owing to changes in absorption, protein binding, rate of metabolism, and intrinsic effectiveness of the drug at receptors. Modifications of structure, such as the introduction of a double bond in prednisolone and prednisone, have resulted in synthetic corticosteroids with more potent glucocorticoid effects than the two closely related natural hormones cortisol and cortisone, respectively (Table 23-1). At the same time, mineralocorticoid effects and the rate of hepatic metabolism of these synthetic drugs are less than those of the natural hormones. Despite increased anti-inflammatory effects, it has not been possible to separate this

Table 23-1
Comparative Pharmacology of Endogenous and Synthetic Corticosteroids

	Anti-Inflammatory Potency	Sodium Retaining Potency	Equivalent Dose (mg)	Elimination Half-Time (hr)	Duration of Action (hr)	Route of Administration
Cortisol	1	1	20	1.5–3	8–12	oral, IV, IM, IA
Cortisone	0.8	0.8	25	0.5	8–36	oral, IM
Prednisolone	4	0.8	5	2–4	12–36	oral, IV, IM, IA
Prednisone	4	0.8	5	3–4	18–36	oral
Methylprednisolone	5	0.5	4	2–4	12–36	oral, IV, IM, IA
Betamethasone	25	0	0.75	5	36–54	oral, IV, IM, IA
Dexamethasone	25	0	0.75	3.5–5	36–54	oral, IV, IM, IA
Triamcinolone	5	0	4	3.5	12–36	oral, IM, IA
Fludrocortisone	10	125	—	—	24	oral

* IV = intravenous; IM = intramuscular; IA = intra-articular.

response from alterations in carbohydrate and protein metabolism. This suggests that the multiple manifestations of drug-induced glucocorticoid effects are mediated by the same receptor.

Pharmacokinetics

Synthetic cortisol and its derivatives are effective orally (Table 23-1). Antacids, but not food, interfere with the oral absorption of corticosteroids. Water-soluble cortisol succinate can be administered intravenously to achieve prompt elevations in plasma concentrations. More prolonged effects are possible with intramuscular injection. Cortisone acetate may be given orally or intramuscularly but cannot be given intravenously. The acetate preparation is a slow-release preparation lasting 8 to 12 hours. After release, cortisone is converted into cortisol in the liver. Corticosteroids are also promptly absorbed after topical application or aerosol administration.

Cortisol is highly bound (90% or more) in the plasma to corticosteroid-binding globulin. Nevertheless, cortisol and related compounds readily cross the placenta. Small amounts of cortisol appear unchanged in the urine, but at least 70% is conjugated in the liver to inactive or poorly active metabolites. These water-soluble conjugated metabolites appear in the urine. The elimination half-time of cortisol is 1.5 to 3 hours (Table 23-1).

Synthetic Corticosteroids

Synthetic corticosteroids administered for their glucocorticoid effects include prednisolone, prednisone, methylprednisolone, betamethasone, dexamethasone, and triamcinolone (Table 23-1; Fig 23-8). Fludrocortisone is a synthetic halogenated derivative of cortisol, administered for its mineralocorticoid effect (Table 23-1; Fig. 23-8). Naturally occurring corticosteroids, such as cortisol and cortisone, are also available as synthetic drugs (Table 23-1; Fig. 23-7).

Prednisolone

Prednisolone is an analog of cortisol that is available as an oral or parenteral preparation. The anti-inflammatory effect of 5 mg of prednisolone is equivalent to that of 20 mg of cortisol. This drug and prednisone are suitable for sole replacement therapy in adrenocortical insufficiency because of the presence of glucocorticoid and mineralocorticoid effects (Table 23-1).

Prednisone

Prednisone is an analog of cortisone that is available as an oral or parenteral preparation. It is rapidly converted to prednisolone after its absorption from the gastrointestinal tract. Its anti-inflammatory effect and clinical uses are similar to those of prednisolone.

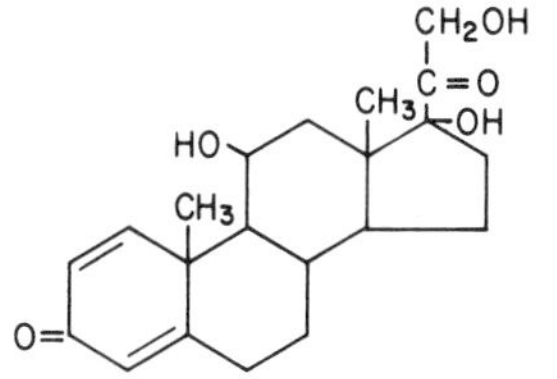

Prednisolone

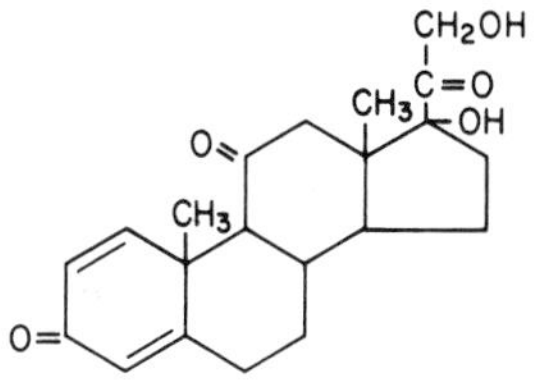

Prednisone

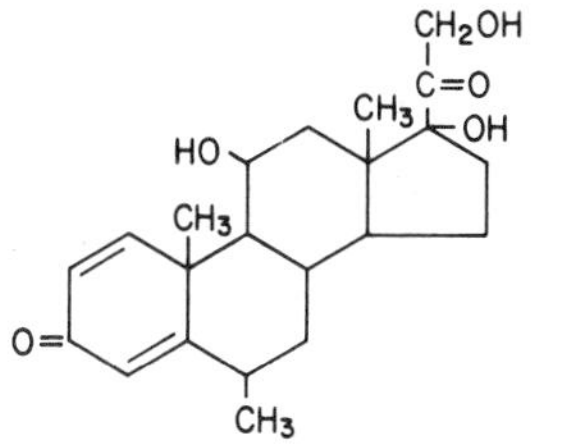

Methylprednisolone

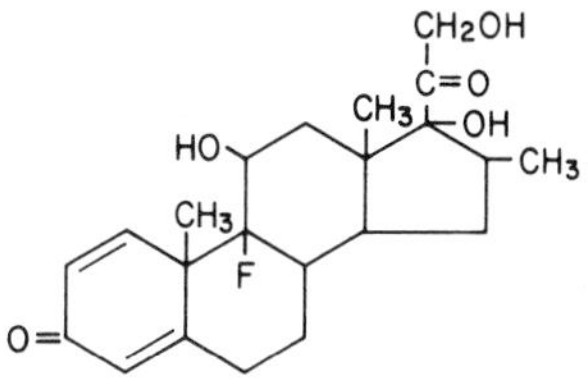

Betamethasone

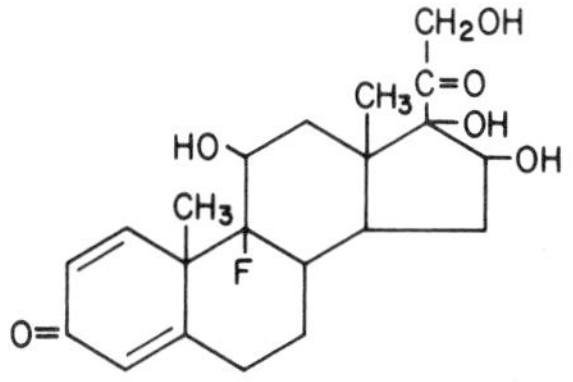

Triamcinolone

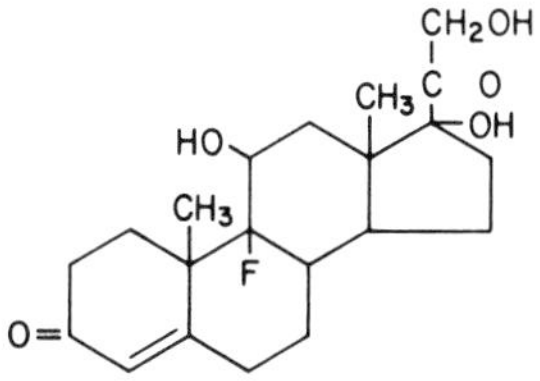

Fludrocortisone

FIGURE 23-8. Synthetic corticosteroids.

Methylprednisolone

Methylprednisolone is the methyl derivative of prednisolone. The anti-inflammatory effect of 4 mg of methylprednisolone is equivalent to that of 20 mg of cortisol. The acetate preparation administered intra-articularly has a prolonged effect. Methylprednisolone succinate is highly soluble in water and is used intravenously to produce an intense glucocorticoid effect.

Betamethasone

Betamethasone is a fluorinated derivative of prednisolone. The anti-inflammatory effect of 0.75 mg is equivalent to that of 20 mg of cortisol. Betamethasone lacks the mineralocorticoid properties of cortisol and, thus, is not acceptable for sole replacement therapy in adrenocortical insufficiency. Oral or parenteral administration is acceptable.

Dexamethasone

Dexamethasone is a fluorinated derivative of prednisolone and an isomer of betamethasone. The anti-inflammatory effect of 0.75 mg is equivalent to that of 20 mg of cortisol. Oral and parenteral preparations are available. The acetate preparation is used as a long-acting repository suspension. Dexamethasone sodium phosphate is water soluble, rendering it appropriate for parenteral use. This corticosteroid is commonly chosen to treat certain types of cerebral edema (see the section entitled Clinical Uses).

Triamcinolone

Triamcinolone is a fluorinated derivative of prednisolone. The anti-inflammatory effect of 4 mg is equivalent to that of 20 mg of cortisol. Triamcinolone has less mineralocorticoid effect than does prednisolone. Oral and parenteral preparations are available. The hexacetonide preparation injected intra-articularly may provide therapeutic effects for 3 months or longer. This drug is often used for epidural injections in the treatment of lumbar disc disease (see the section entitled Clinical Uses).

During the first days of treatment with triamcinolone, mild diuresis with sodium loss may occur. Conversely, edema may occur in patients with decreased glomerular filtration rate. Triamcinolone does not increase potassium ion loss except when administered in large doses.

Somewhat unique adverse side effects of triamcinolone include an increased incidence of skeletal muscle weakness. Likewise, anorexia rather than appetite stimulation and sedation rather than euphoria may accompany administration of triamcinolone.

Clinical Uses

The only universally accepted clinical use of corticosteroids and their synthetic derivatives is as replacement therapy for deficiency states (Plorn, 1966). With this exception, the use of corticosteroids in disease states is empirical and not curative, although anti-inflammatory responses exert an intense palliative effect. The safety of corticosteroids is such that it is acceptable to administer a single large dose in a life-threatening situation on the presumption that unrecognized adrenal or pituitary insufficiency may be present.

Prednisolone or prednisone are recommended when an anti-inflammatory effect is desired. The low mineralocorticoid potency of these drugs limits sodium and water retention when large doses are administered to produce the desired glucocorticoid effect (Table 23-1). It must be recognized, however, that the anti-inflammatory effect of corticosteroids is palliative, since the underlying cause of the response remains. Nevertheless, suppression of the inflammatory response may be lifesaving in some situations. Conversely, masking of the symptoms of inflammation may delay diagnosis of life-threatening illnesses such as peritonitis owing to perforation of a peptic ulcer.

Deficiency States

Acute adrenal insufficiency requires electrolyte and fluid replacement as well as supplemental corticosteroids. Cortisol is administered intravenously at a rate of 100 mg every 8 hours following an initial injection of 100 mg. Management of chronic adrenal insufficiency in adults is with the daily oral administration of cortisone, 25 to 37.5 mg. A typical regimen is 25 mg in the morning and 12.5 mg in the late afternoon. This schedule mimics the normal diurinal cycle of adrenal secretion. An orally effective mineralocorticoid such as fludrocortisone, 0.1 to 0.3 mg daily, is required by most patients.

Cerebral Edema

Corticosteroids in large doses are of value in the reduction or prevention of cerebral edema and the resulting increases in intracranial pressure that may accompany intracranial tumors and metastatic lesions. Cerebral edema owing to closed head injury is not predictably responsive to corticosteroids. There is doubt about the benefit of corticosteroids in the treatment of cerebral edema resulting from global ischemic injury. Dexamethasone, with minimal mineralocorticoid activity, is frequently selected to reduce cerebral edema and associated increases in intracranial pressure.

Aspiration Pneumonitis

The use of corticosteroids in the treatment of aspiration pneumonitis is controversial. There is evidence in animals that corticosteroids administered immediately after inhalation of acidic gastric fluid may be effective in reducing pulmonary damage (Dudley and Marshall, 1974). Conversely, other data show no beneficial effect or suggest that the use of corticosteroids may enhance the likelihood of gram-negative pneumonia (Downs et al, 1974; Wolfe et al, 1977; Wynne et al, 1981). Despite the absence of confirmatory evidence that corticosteroids are beneficial, it is not uncommon for the treatment of aspiration pneumonitis to include the empiric use of pharmacologic doses of these drugs.

Lumbar Disc Disease

An alternative to surgical treatment of lumbar disc disease is the epidural or subarachnoid placement of corticosteroids (Abram, 1978; Bullard and Houghton, 1977; Winnie *et al,* 1972). Corticosteroids may reduce inflammation and edema of the nerve root that has resulted from compression. A common regimen is epidural injection of 25 to 50 mg of triamcinolone or 40 to 80 mg of methylprednisolone, with 5 ml of lidocaine at the interspace corresponding to the distribution of pain. In animals, the epidural injection of triamcinolone, 2 mg kg^{-1}, interferes with the ability of the adrenal cortex to release cortisol in response to hypoglycemia for 4 weeks (Table 23-2) (Gorski *et al,* 1982). If this also occurs in patients receiving a single epidural injection of corticosteroid, it is conceivable that tolerance to stress would be reduced.

Organ Transplantation

In organ transplantation, high doses of corticosteroids are often administered at the time of surgery. Smaller maintenance doses of corticosteroids are continued indefinitely, and the dosage is increased if rejection of the transplanted organ is threatened.

CYCLOSPORIN A. Cyclosporin A is an immunosuppressant that inhibits the production of T-lymphocytes. The drug must be administered before T-lymphocyte cells undergo proliferation as a result of exposure to specific antigens as associated with organ transplants. The dose of other immunosuppressants, including prednisone and azathioprine, is reduced when cyclosporin A, 15 to 20 mg kg^{-1}, is administered concomitantly. Side-effects of cyclosporin A include gum hyperplasia, hirsutism, neurasthenias, hepatotoxicity, depressed renal function, and depressive psychoses.

Asthma

Corticosteroids are useful in the long-term treatment and suppression of asthma. The efficacy of corticosteroids in treatment of the acute phase of asthma is less well defined. Nevertheless, a controlled clinical study demonstrated that methylprednisolone, 125 mg administered intravenously to adults with acute bronchial asthma, reduces the need for subsequent hospitalization compared with placebo-treated patients (Littenberg and Gluck, 1986). Status asthmaticus can be treated with intravenous administration of a corticosteroid, such as cortisol, 50 to 100 mg every 8 hours, until the acute episode is suppressed. Subsequently, prednisone may be required for about 10 days, but the goal remains to gradually decrease the dose and ultimately discontinue the corticosteroid.

Severe chronic bronchial asthma that is uncontrolled by other measures may respond to aerosol administration of a corticosteroid. Aerosol therapy is predictably ineffective, however, in acute asthmatic attacks when airways may be

Table 23-2
Epidural Triamcinolone and Plasma Cortisol Response to Stress (Plasma Cortisol [µg · dl^{-1}] Before and After Hypoglycemia)

Control		Days After Administration of Epidural Triamcinolone (2 mg kg^{-1})									
		1		7		21		28		35	
Before	After	Before	After	Before	After	Before	After	Before	After	Before	After
5.1	7.4	2.3	2.2	2.7	2.3	2.5	2.1	2.5	2.9	4.8	8.3*

* P < 0.05 compared with Before
(Adapted from Gorski DW, Rao TLK, Glisson SN, Chinthagada M, El-Etr AA. Epidural triamcinolone and adrenal response to hypoglycemic stress in dogs. Anesthesiology 1982;57:364-6; with permission of the authors and publisher.)

plugged with mucus. Systemic effects are minimal with aerosol administration of corticosteroids, but pharyngeal candidiasis develops in a high percentage of patients (Webb–Johnson and Andrews, 1977).

Manifestations of allergic diseases that are of limited duration, such as hay fever, contact dermatitis, drug reactions, angioneurotic edema, and anaphylaxis can be suppressed by adequate doses of corticosteroids. Life-threatening allergic reactions, however, must be treated with epinephrine, since the onset of the anti-inflammatory effect produced by corticosteroids is delayed. Indeed, any beneficial effect of corticosteroids in the management of severe allergic reactions is probably related to suppression of the inflammatory response rather than to inhibition of production of immunoglobulins (Weston *et al,* 1973).

Arthritis

The criterion for initiating corticosteroid therapy in patients with rheumatoid arthritis is progressive disability despite maximal medical therapy. Corticosteroids are administered in the smallest dose possible that provides significant but not complete symptomatic relief. The usual initial dose is prednisone, 10 mg (or its equivalent), in divided doses.

Intra-articular injection of corticosteroids is recommended for treatment of episodic manifestations of acute joint inflammation associated with osteoarthritis. However, painless destruction of the joint is a risk of this treatment.

Collagen Diseases

Manifestations of collagen diseases, such as polymyositis, polyarteritis nodosa, and Wegener's granulomatosis, but not scleroderma, are reduced, and longevity is improved by chronic corticosteroid therapy. Fulminating systemic lupus erythematosus is a life-threatening illness that is aggressively treated initially with large doses of prednisone, 1 mg kg^{-1}, or its equivalent. Large doses of corticosteroids are effective for inducing a remission of sarcoidosis. In temporal arteritis, corticosteroid therapy is necessary to prevent blindness, which occurs in about 20% of untreated patients. Some forms of nephrotic syndrome respond favorably to corticosteroids. Rheumatic carditis may be suppressed by large doses of corticosteroids.

Ocular Inflammation

Corticosteroids are used to suppress ocular inflammation (*i.e.,* uveitis and iritis) and thus preserve sight. Instillation of corticosteroids into the conjunctival sac results in therapeutic concentrations in the aqueous humor. Topical corticosteroid therapy often increases intraocular pressure. For this reason, it is recommended that intraocular pressure be monitored when topical ocular corticosteroids are used for more than 2 weeks. Corticosteroids are contraindicated in herpes simplex (dendritic keratitis) of the eye. Topical corticosteroids should not be used for treatment of ocular abrasions, because delayed healing and infection may occur.

Cutaneous Disorders

Topical administration of corticosteroids is frequently effective in the treatment of skin diseases. Effectiveness is increased by application of the corticosteroid as an ointment under an occlusive dressing. Systemic absorption is also occasionally enhanced to the degree that suppression of the pituitary–adrenal axis occurs or manifestations of Cushing's syndrome appear. Corticosteroids may also be administered systemically for treatment of severe episodes of acute skin disorders and exacerbations of chronic disorders.

Postintubation Laryngeal Edema

Treatment of postintubation laryngeal edema may include intravenous administration of corticosteroids, such as dexamethasone, 0.1 to 0.2 mg kg^{-1}. Nevertheless, the efficacy of corticosteroids for treatment of this condition has not been proved.

Ulcerative Colitis

Corticosteroid therapy is indicated in selected patients with chronic ulcerative colitis. A disadvantage of this therapy is that signs and symptoms of intestinal perforation and peritonitis may be masked.

Myasthenia Gravis

Corticosteroids are usually reserved for patients with severe myasthenia gravis who are unresponsive to medical or surgical therapy. These drugs seem to be most effective after thymectomy. The mechanism of beneficial effects produced by corticosteroids is not known but may reflect drug-induced suppression of the production of an immunoglobulin that normally binds to the neuromuscular junction.

Respiratory Distress Syndrome

Administration of corticosteroids at least 24 hours before delivery reduces the incidence and severity of respiratory distress syndrome in neonates born after 26 to 34 weeks gestation.

Hypercalcemia

Pharmacologic doses of corticosteroids, by antagonizing the effects of vitamin D, are often effective in hypercalcemia caused by increased intestinal absorption of calcium ions. Corticosteroids also prevent hypercalcemia in patients with multiple myeloma by decreasing reabsorption of calcium ions from bone. These drugs are usually ineffective, however, when hypercalcemia is due to increased levels of parathyroid hormone, either from hyperparathyroidism or a neoplasm that secretes a parathyroid hormone – like substance.

Leukemia

The antilymphocytic effects of glucocorticoids are used to advantage in combination chemotherapy of acute lymphocytic leukemia and lymphomas, including Hodgkin's disease and mutliple myeloma. For example, prednisone and vincristine produce remissions in about 90% of children with lymphoblastic leukemia.

Septic Shock

Corticosteroids have been recommended as part of the therapeutic regimen, along with antibiotics and volume replacement in the treatment of septic shock (Schumer, 1976). Nevertheless, overall survival in patients with severe late septic shock treated with pharmacologic doses of corticosteroids is not improved (Sprung *et al,* 1984).

Side Effects

Side effects of chronic corticosteroid therapy include (1) suppression of the hypothalamic–pituitary–adrenal axis, (2) electrolyte and meta-bolic changes, (3) osteoporosis, (4) peptic ulcer disease, (5) skeletal muscle myopathy, (6) central nervous system dysfunction, (7) peripheral blood changes, and (8) inhibition of normal growth. Increased susceptibility to bacterial or fungal infection accompanies treatment with corticosteroids. Corticosteroid administration is associated with greater clearance of salicylates and reduced effectiveness of anticoagulants.

Suppression of the Hypothalamic – Pituitary – Adrenal Axis

Corticosteroid therapy may result in suppression of the hypothalamic–pituitary–adrenal axis such that release of cortisol in response to stress, as produced by surgery, is blunted or does not occur. It is not possible to define the precise dose of corticosteroid or duration of therapy that will produce pituitary and adrenocortical suppression in a given patient, because there is marked variation among patients. Typically, however, the larger the dose and the more prolonged the therapy, the greater is the likelihood of suppression. When appropriate, a dose of a corticosteroid administered every other day is less likely to suppress the anterior pituitary release of ACTH than is the daily administration of the drug.

CORTICOSTEROID SUPPLEMENTATION. Corticosteroid supplementation should be increased whenever the patient being treated for chronic hypoadrenocorticism undergoes a surgical procedure. This recommendation is based on the concern that these patients are susceptible to cardiovascular collapse since they cannot release additional endogenous cortisol in response to the stress of surgery. More controversial is the management of the patient who may manifest suppression of the hypothalamic–pituitary–adrenal axis because of current or previous administration of corticosteroids for treatment of a disease unrelated to pituitary or adrenocortical dysfunction.

A rational regimen for corticosteroid supplementation in the perioperative period is the intravenous administration of cortisol, 25 mg, at the induction of anesthesia followed by a continuous intravenous infusion of cortisol, 100 mg, during the following 24 hours (Symreng *et al,* 1981). This approach maintains the plasma concentration of cortisol above normal during major surgery in patients receiving chronic treatment with corticosteroids and manifesting a subnormal response to the

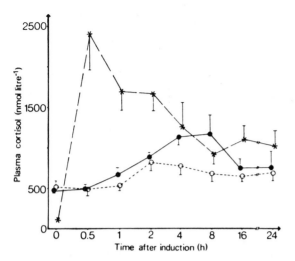

FIGURE 23-9. Intravenous administration of cortisol, 25 mg, plus a continuous infusion of 100 mg over 24 hours maintains the plasma cortisol concentration above normal in patients (*asteriks*) receiving chronic treatment with corticosteroids and manifesting a subnormal response to the preoperative infusion of ACTH. (From Symreng T, Karlberg BE, Kagedal B, Schildt B. Physiological cortisol substitution of long-term steroid-treated patients undergoing major surgery. Br J Anaesth 1981;53:949–53. Reproduced by permission of the authors and publisher.)

preoperative infusion of ACTH (Fig. 23-9) (Symreng *et al*, 1981). It is likely that patients undergoing minor operations will need minimal to no additional corticosteroid coverage during the perioperative period.

In addition to intravenous supplementation with cortisol, patients receiving daily maintenance doses of a corticosteroid should also receive this dose with the preoperative medication on the day of surgery. There is no objective evidence to support increasing the maintenance dose of corticosteroid preoperatively. In those instances in which events such as burns or sepsis could exaggerate the needs for exogenous corticosteroid supplementation, the continuous infusion of cortisol, 100 mg, every 12 hours should be sufficient. Indeed, endogenous cortisol production during stress introduced by major surgery or extensive burns is not greater than 150 mg daily (Hardy and Turner, 1957; Hume *et al*, 1962).

Electrolyte and Metabolic Changes

Hypokalemic metabolic alkalosis reflects mineralocorticoid effects of corticosteroids on distal renal tubules leading to enhanced reabsorption of sodium ions and loss of potassium ions. Edema and weight gain accompany this corticosteroid effect.

Corticosteroids inhibit utilization of glucose in peripheral tissues and promote hepatic gluconeogenesis. The resulting corticosteroid-induced hyperglycemia can usually be managed with diet and/or insulin. The dose requirement for oral hypoglycemics may be increased by corticosteroids.

There is a redistribution of body fat characterized by deposition of fat in the back of the neck (buffalo hump), supraclavicular area, and face (moon facies) and loss of fat from the extremities. The mechanism by which corticosteroids elicit this redistribution of body fat is not known.

Peripherally, corticosteroids mobilize amino acids from tissues. This catabolic effect manifests as reduced skeletal muscle mass, osteoporosis, thinning of the skin, and a negative nitrogen balance.

Osteoporosis

Osteoporosis, vertebral compression fractures, and rib fractures are frequent and serious complications of corticosteroid therapy in patients of all ages. Corticosteroids appear to inhibit the activities of osteoblasts and stimulate osteoclasts by virtue of inhibition of calcium ion absorption from the gastrointestinal tract, which causes an increased secretion of parathyroid hormone. Osteoporosis is an indication for withdrawal of corticosteroid therapy. Evidence of osteoporosis should be sought on radiographs of the spines of patients being treated chronically with corticosteroids. The presence of osteoporosis could predispose patients to fractures during positioning in the operating room.

Peptic Ulcer Disease

Although a cause-and-effect relationship has not been proved, the incidence of peptic ulcer disease seems to be increased by chronic corticosteroid therapy (Fenster, 1973). Indeed, corticosteroids may decrease the normal protective barrier provided by gastric mucus.

Skeletal Muscle Myopathy

Skeletal muscle myopathy characterized by weakness of the proximal musculature is occasionally observed in patients taking large doses of corticosteroids. In some patients, this skeletal muscle weakness is so severe that ambulation is not possible and corticosteroid therapy must be discontinued.

Central Nervous System Dysfunction

Corticosteroid therapy is associated with an increased incidence of neuroses and psychoses. Behavioral changes include manic depression and suicidal tendencies. Cataracts develop in almost all patients who receive prednisone, 20 mg daily, or its equivalent for at least 4 years (Lubkin, 1977).

Peripheral Blood Changes

Corticosteroids tend to increase the hematocrit and number of circulating leukocytes. Conversely, a single dose of cortisol reduces, by almost 70%, the number of circulating lymphocytes and, by over 90%, the number of circulating monocytes in 4 to 6 hours. This acute lymphocytopenia most likely reflects sequestration from the blood rather than destruction of cells (Fauci and Dale, 1974).

Inhibition of Normal Growth

Inhibition or arrest of growth can result from the administration of relatively small doses of glucocorticoids to children. This cannot be overcome with exogenous human growth hormone. The mechanism for this effect is presumed to be the generalized inhibitory effect of glucocorticoids on DNA synthesis and cell division.

Inhibitors of Corticosteroid Synthesis

Metyrapone

Metyrapone reduces cortisol secretion by inhibition of the 11-β-hydroxylation reaction, resulting in accumulation of 11-desoxycortisol. Metyrapone may induce acute adrenal insufficiency in patients with reduced adrenocortical function. A deficiency of mineralocorticoids does not occur, because metyrapone-induced inhibition of 11-β-hydroxylation results in increased production of the mineralocorticoid 11-desoxycorticosterone.

Metyrapone has been used to treat excessive adrenocortical function that results from adrenal neoplasms that function autonomously or as a result of ectopic production of ACTH by tumors.

Aminoglutethimide

Aminoglutethimide inhibits the conversion of cholesterol to 20-α-hydroxycholesterol. This inhibition interrupts production of both cortisol and aldosterone. As such, this drug is effective in decreasing the excessive secretion of cortisol in autonomously functioning adrenal tumors and in hypersecretion resulting from ectopic production of ACTH.

POSTERIOR PITUITARY HORMONES

Antidiuretic hormone (ADH) and oxytocin are the two principal hormones secreted by the posterior pituitary (see Chapter 52). The target sites for ADH are renal collecting ducts, where this hormone acts to increase permeability of cell membranes to water. As a result, water is passively reabsorbed from renal collecting ducts into extracellular fluid. Nonrenal actions of ADH include intense vasoconstriction, accounting for its alternative designation as vasopressin. Oxytocin elicits contractions of the uterus, which are indistinguishable from those that occur in spontaneous labor.

Antidiuretic Hormone

ADH and its congeners (desmopressin, lypressin) are used in the treatment of diabetes insipidus that results from inadequate secretion of the hormone by the posterior pituitary. Failure to secrete adequate amounts of ADH results in polyuria and hypernatremia. Trauma or surgery in the region of the pituitary and hypothalamus are recognized causes of diabetes insipidus. Nephrogenic diabetes insipidus resulting from an inability of the renal tubules to respond to adequate amounts of centrally produced ADH does not respond to exogenous administration of the hormone or its congeners.

The oral hypoglycemic chloropropamide sensitizes renal tubules to the effects of low circulating concentrations of ADH, accounting for its beneficial effects in patients with diabetes insipidus (Miller and Moses, 1976). Inhibition of prostaglandin production produced by chlorpropamide may be responsible for increased sensitivity of the renal tubules to ADH (see Chapter 24). This drug is not effective in the treatment of nephrogenic diabetes insipidus. A high incidence of hypoglycemic reactions detracts from the therapeutic value of chlorpropamide in the treatment of diabetes insipidus (Thompson *et al*, 1977). Acetaminophen and indomethacin probably enhance the effects of ADH by a similar inhibitory effect on the synthesis of prostaglandins. Clofibrate may directly stimulate secretion of ADH by the posterior pituitary, leading to a significant antidiuretic action in patients with diabetes insipidus. The combination of clofibrate with chlorpropamide may produce an additive effect, emphasizing the speculated differences in mechanism of action of these drugs. Thiazide diuretics exert a paradoxical antidiuretic action in patients with nephrogenic diabetes insipidus and serve as the only drugs effective in the treatment of this disorder (Lant and Wilson, 1971).

Inappropriate and excessive secretion of ADH with subsequent retention of water and dilutional hyponatremia may occur in patients with head injuries, intracranial tumors, meningitis, and pulmonary infections. Aberrant production of ADH is observed most commonly in patients with cancer, especially oat cell carcinoma, in which the tumor itself produces ADH. In these patients, the antibiotic demeclocycline promotes diuresis by antagonizing the effects of ADH on renal tubules (Forrest *et al*, 1978).

Vasopressin

Vasopressin is the exogenous preparation of ADH used for the (1) treatment of ADH-sensitive diabetes insipidus, (2) evaluation of the urine concentrating abilities of the kidneys as following administration of a fluorinated anesthetic, and (3) management of uncontrolled hemorrhage from esophageal varicies. This drug is not effective in the management of the patient with nephrogenic diabetes insipidus.

Intravenous vasopressin is used for the initial evaluation of patients with suspected diabetes insipidus, as may follow head trauma or hypophysectomy. Under these circumstances, polyuria may be transient, and a longer antidiuretic effect (1–3 days) as produced by intramuscular vaso-

pressin tannate in oil could produce water intoxication. Oral administration of vasopressin is followed by rapid inactivation by trypsin, which cleaves a peptide linkage. Likewise, intravenous administration results in a brief effect because of rapid enzymatic breakdown by peptides in the tissues, especially the kidneys.

Vasopressin may serve as an adjunct in the control of bleeding esophageal varicies and during abdominal surgery in patients with cirrhosis and portal hypertension. Infusion of 20 units over 5 minutes results in marked reductions in hepatic blood flow and pressure lasting about 30 minutes (Edmunds and West, 1962). Only a moderate rise in blood pressure occurs. This effect on portal circulation is attributable to marked splanchnic vasoconstriction. An alternative to systemic administration is infusion of vasopressin directly into the superior mesenteric artery. It has not been established whether selective arterial administration is safer than systemic administration with respect to cardiac and vascular side-effects (Getzen *et al*, 1978).

SIDE EFFECTS. Vasoconstriction and increased blood pressure occur only with doses of vasopressin that are much larger than those administered for the treatment of diabetes insipidus. This response is due to a direct and generalized effect on vascular smooth muscle that is not antagonized by denervation or adrenergic blocking drugs. Facial pallor owing to cutaneous vasoconstriction may also accompany large doses of vasopressin. The magnitude of elevation in blood pressure caused by vasopressin depends, to some extent, on the reactivity of the baroreceptor reflexes. For example, when baroreceptor reflexes are depressed by anesthesia, smaller amounts of vasopressin are capable of evoking a pressor response. Pulmonary artery pressures are also increased by vasopressin.

Vasopressin, even in small doses, may produce selective vasoconstriction of the coronary arteries, with reductions in coronary blood flow manifesting as angina pectoris, electrocardiographic evidence of myocardial ischemia, and, in some instances, myocardial infarction. Ventricular cardiac dysrhythmias may accompany these cardiac effects.

Large doses of vasopressin stimulate gastrointestinal smooth muscle, and the resulting increased peristalsis may manifest as abdominal pain, nausea, and vomiting. Smooth muscle of the uterus is also stimulated by large doses of vasopressin.

The circulating plasma concentration of factor VIII is increased by vasopressin (Mannucci *et al,* 1977; Sutor *et al,* 1978). As a result, these drugs may be beneficial in the management of moderately severe hemophilia, particularly to reduce bleeding associated with surgery. The mechanisms of this effect are not known.

Allergic reactions ranging from urticaria to anaphylaxis may occasionally follow the administration of vasopressin. Prolonged use of vasopressin may result in antibody formation and a shortened duration of action of the drug.

Desmopressin

Desmopressin is a synthetic analog of ADH possessing intense antidiuretic effects that last 6 to 20 hours as well as hemostatic responses (see Chapter 36). Administered intranasally, twice daily, using a calibrated catheter (rhinyle), desmopressin is the drug of choice in the treatment of diabetes insipidus owing to inadequate ADH production by the posterior pituitary (Cobb *et al,* 1978). Desmopressin, like all the ADH analogs is not effective in the treatment of nephrogenic diabetes insipidus. There are fewer side-effects produced by desmopressin than are associated with vasopressin, although nausea and increases in blood pressure can occur.

Lypressin

Lypressin is a synthetic analog of ADH that produces antidiuresis for about 4 hours following intranasal administration. Its short duration of action limits its usefulness in the treatment of diabetes insipidus.

Oxytocin

Oxytocin, along with ergot derivatives (see the section entitled Ergot Derivatives) and certain prostaglandins, is sufficiently selective in its stimulation of uterine smooth muscle to be clinically useful.

Clinical Uses

The principal clinical uses of oxytocin are (1) to induce labor at term and (2) to counter uterine hypotonicity and reduce hemorrhage in the postpartum or postabortion period.

For induction of labor, a continuous intravenous infusion is preferred, because the low dose of oxytocin needed can be precisely controlled. Indeed, the sensitivity of the uterus to oxytocin increases as pregnancy progresses. To induce labor, a dilute solution (10 milliunits ml^{-1}) is administered by a constant infusion pump beginning at 1 to 2 milliunits min^{-1}. This infusion rate is increased 1 to 2 milliunits min^{-1} every 15 to 30 minutes until an optimal response (one uterine contraction every 2 to 3 minutes) is obtained. The average dose of oxytocin to induce labor is 8 to 10 milliunits min^{-1}. Infusion rates up to 40 milliunits min^{-1} of oxytocin may be necessary to initially treat uterine atony following delivery. Intramuscular injections of oxytocin are commonly used to provide sustained uterine contraction in the postpartum period.

All preparations of oxytocin used clinically are synthetic, and their potency is described in units. These synthetic preparations are identical to the hormone normally released from the posterior pituitary but devoid of contamination by other polypeptide hormones and proteins found in natural preparations. Indeed, many of the complications previously observed when oxytocin was administered were the result of contamination with ADH, which, in high doses, is a coronary artery vasoconstrictor.

Side Effects

High doses of oxytocin produce a direct relaxant effect on vascular smooth muscle that manifests as a decrease in systolic and diastolic blood pressure and flushing. Reflex tachycardia and increased cardiac output accompany this transient reduction in blood pressure. When high doses are infused continuously, the brief reduction in blood pressure is followed by a modest but sustained increase in blood pressure. The amounts of oxytocin administered for most obstetrical purposes are inadequate to produce marked alterations in blood pressure. A marked fall in blood pressure, however, may occur if oxytocin is administered to patients with blunted compensatory reflex responses, as may be produced by anesthesia. Likewise, hypovolemic patients would be particularly susceptible to oxytocin-induced hypotension.

In the past, oxytocin preparations were often contaminated with ergot alkaloids, resulting in exaggerated blood pressure elevations when administered to patients previously treated with a sympathomimetic. Modern synthetic commercial preparations are pure oxytocin and do not introduce the risk of exaggerated vasoconstriction when administered in the presence of a sympathomimetic drug.

Oxytocin exhibits a slight ADH-like activity when administered in high doses, introducing the possibility of water intoxication if excessive volumes of fluid are administered (Saunders and Munsick, 1966). The risk of this complication can be minimized by infusion of oxytocin in an electrolyte-containing solution rather than in dextrose in water.

Ergot Derivatives

Ergot is the product of a fungus that grows on grain. Ingestion of contaminated grain results in generalized and intense vasoconstriction, reflecting the peripheral vascular effects of ergot alkaloids. The ergot alkaloids ergotamine and ergonovine are derivatives of 6-methylergoline. Hydrolysis of ergonovine yields lysergic acid and an amine. Semisynthetic derivatives of the ergot alkaloids include lysergic acid diethylamide, and methylergonovine. Methysergide is formed by the addition of a methyl group to the indole nitrogen of methylergonovine.

Clinical Uses

All the natural alkaloids of ergot produce dose-related increases in the motor activity of the uterus. The sustained elevation of resting uterine tone produced by high doses of ergots precludes their use for induction of labor but increases their value in the postpartum or postabortion period to control bleeding and maintain uterine contraction. Ergonovine is less toxic and produces a more rapid uterine response than ergotamine. For these reasons, ergonovine and its semisynthetic derivative methylergonovine have replaced other ergot derivatives. Ergonovine and methylergonovine are rapidly absorbed after oral or intramuscular (0.2 mg) administration, producing a uterotonic action within about 10 minutes that lasts 3 to 6 hours. Administered intravenously (0.2 mg), uterine contraction occurs within 30 to 45 seconds. The uterine stimulating effects of these drugs most likely reflect interactions with specific receptors.

Ergotamine is effective in relieving migraine headaches. This beneficial effect may be due to ergotamine-induced constriction of dilated cerebral blood vessels, particularly in the meningeal branches of the external carotid artery. In addition to reducing extracranial blood flow, ergotamine reduces hyperperfusion of regions supplied by the basilar artery and decreases shunting of blood via arteriovenous anastomoses. Caffeine increases by about twofold the absorption of ergotamine following oral administration. Metabolism is almost complete, as emhasized by minimal recovery of unchanged drug in the urine. Storage in the tissues probably accounts for prolonged therapeutic and toxic effects, despite an elimination half-time of about 2 hours. Other types of headache are not improved and may even be aggravated by ergotamine.

Ergoloid is the combination of three ergot alkaloids (dihydroergocristine, dihydroergocornine, and dihydroergocryptine [as the mesylates]) that may provide symptomatic relief in some elderly patients who are manifesting changes of idiopathic mental decline (*e.g.,* Alzheimer's disease) (Jarvik, 1981). Improvement in cognitive and emotional symptoms is presumed to reflect a drug-induced effect on cerebral metabolism and not a direct cerebrovascular action. Following oral administration, the elimination half-time of ergoloid is about 4 hours. Side-effects of treatment with ergoloid include nausea, vomiting, and gastric irritation. Sinus bradycardia occasionally occurs. A sublingual preparation of ergoloid may produce local tissue irritation.

Side Effects

Ergonovine and methylergonovine are weak peripheral vasoconstrictors but produce additive effects with sympathomimetics, such as ephedrine and phenylephrine (Munson, 1965). Intravenous injection of these drugs has been associated with intense vasoconstriction leading to acute hypertension, seizures, cerebrovascular accidents and retinal detachment (Abouleish, 1976). For this reason, these drugs should be used cautiously, if at all, in patients with preeclampsia, essential hypertension, or cardiac disease. Both drugs should be avoided in patients with atherosclerotic peripheral vascular disease. Nausea and vomiting most likely reflect a direct central nervous system effect.

CHYMOPAPAIN

Chymopapain is a proteolytic enzyme used in the treatment of herniated lumbar intervertebral disc disease that has not responded to conservative therapy. Injected into the intervertebral disc, chymopapain dissolves the proteoglycan portion of the nucleus pulposus but does not affect collagenous components. Evidence of dissolution of the nucleus pulposus is the appearance in the urine of glycosaminoglycans of the type known to occur in human intervertebral discs. Dissolution of the nucleus pulposus of the herniated intervertebral disc by chymopapain is known as *chemonucleolysis.* The recommended dose is 2000 to 5000 units per disc in a volume of 1 to 2 ml. The maximal dose in a single patient with multiple disc herniations is 10,000 units.

Injection of chymopapain into the intervertebral space has been associated with allergic reactions of varying severity, including cardiovascular collapse and death (Rajagopalan *et al,* 1974). The allergic potential of chymopapain appears to be greatest in females and in those with preexisting allergies. Known allergy to papaya is a contraindication to injection of chymopapain, because this enzyme is derived from the crude latex of Carica papaya. Preoperative administration of a corticosteroid (prednisone, 50 mg) plus H_1 (diphenhydramine, 50–100 mg) and H_2 (cimetidine 300–600 mg) receptor antagonists as a single dose with the preoperative medication or up to four doses every 6 hours in the 24 hours preceding the induction of anesthesia may decrease the incidence and severity of allergic reactions (Bruno *et al,* 1984). Utilizing preoperative histamine receptor antagonists and avoidance of chemonucleolysis in patients with known allergies has reduced the incidence of allergic reactions following injection of chymopapain to 0.44% (Moss *et al,* 1985).

REFERENCES

Abouleish E. Postpartum hypertension and convulsion after oxytocic drugs. Anesth Analg 1976;55:813-5.

Abram SE. Subarachnoid corticosteroid injection following inadequate response to epidural steroids for sciatica. Anesth Analg 1978;57:313–5.

Baum JK, Bookstein JJ, Holtz F, Klein EW. Possible association between benign hepatomas and oral contraceptives. Lancet 1973;2:926–9.

Bennion LJ, Ginsberg RL, Garnick MB, Bennett PH. Effects of oral contraceptives on the gallbladder bile of normal women. N Engl J Med 1976;294:189–92.

Briggs M. Biochemical effects of oral contraceptives. Adv Steroid Biochem Pharmacol 1976;5:66–160.

Bruno, LA, Smith DS, Bloom MJ, et al. Sudden hypotension with a test dose of chymopapain. Anesth Analg 1984;63:533–5.

Bullard JR, Houghton FM. Epidural steroid treatment of acute herniated nucleus pulposus. Anesth Analg 1977;56:862–3.

Cobb WE, Spare S, Reichlin S. Neurogenic diabetes insipidus: management with dDAVP (1-desamino-8-D-arginine vasopressin). Ann Intern Med 1978;88:183-8.

Cooper DS. Antithyroid drugs. N Engl J Med 1984;311:1353–62.

Downs JB, Chapman RL, Modell JH, Hood CI. An evaluation of steroid therapy in aspiration pneumonitis. Anesthesiology 1974;40:129–35.

Dudley WR, Marshall BE. Steroid treatment for acid-aspiration pneumonia. Anesthesiology 1974;40:136–41.

Edmunds R, West SP. A study of the effect of vasopressin on portal and systemic blood pressure. Surg Gynecol Obstet 1962;114:458–62.

Fauci AS, Dale DC. The effect of in vivo hydrocortisone on subpopulations of human lymphocytes. J Clin Invest 1974;53:240–6.

Feek CM, Stewart J, Sawers A, et al. Combination of potassium iodide and propranolol in preparation of patients with Graves' disease for thyroid surgery. N Engl J Med 1980;302:883–5.

Fenster LF. The ulcerogenic potential of glucocorticoids and possible prophylactic measures. Med Clin North Am 1973;57:1289–94.

Forrest JM, Cox H, Hong C, Morrison G, Bia M, Singer I. Superiority of demeclocycline over lithium in the treatment of chronic syndrome of inappropriate antidiuretic hormone. N Engl J Med 1978;298;173–7.

Frossman O, Mulder J. Hypersensitivity to different ACTH peptides. Acta Med Scand 1973;193:557–9.

Getzen LC, Brink RR, Wolfman EF. Survival following infusion of Pitressin into the superior mesenteric artery to control bleeding esophageal varices in cirrhotic patients. Ann Surg 1978;187:337–42.

Givens JR. Normal and abnormal androgen metabolism. Clin Obstet Gynecol 1978;21:115–23.

Glennon JA, Gordon ES, Sawin CT. Hypothyroidism after low dose ^{131}I treatment of hyperthyroidism. Ann Intern Med 1972;76:721–3.

Gorski DW, Rao TLK, Glisson SN, Chinthagada M, El-Etr AA. Epidural triamcinolone and adrenal response to hypoglycemic stress in dogs. Anesthesiology 1982;57:364–6.

Gralnick HR, Maisonneuve P, Sultan Y, Rick ME. Benefits of danazol treatment in patients with hemophilia A (Classic hemophilia). JAMA 1985;253:1151–3.

Hardy JD, Turner MD. Hydrocortisone secretion in man: studies of adrenal vein blood. Surgery 1957;42:194–201.

Henderson JT, Richmond J, Sumerling MD. Androgenic-anabolic steroid therapy and hepatocellular carcinoma. Lancet 1973;1:934.

Horwitz RI, Feinstein AR. Alternative analytic methods for case-control studies of estrogens and endometrial cancer. N Engl J Med 1978;299:1089–94.

Hume DM, Bell CC, Bartter FC. Direct measurement of adrenal secretion during operative trauma and convalescence. Surgery 1962;52:174–87.

Jarvik LF. Hydergine as treatment for organic brain syndrome in late life. Psychopharmacol Bull 1981;17:40–1.

Kaplan NM. Cardiovascular complications of oral contraceptives. Annu Rev Med 1978;29:31–40.

Kay CR. Oral contraceptives — the clinical perspective. In: Garattini S, Berendes HW, eds. Pharmacology of Steroid Contraceptive Drugs. New York, Raven Press, 1977;1–24.

Lant AF, Wilson GM. Long-term therapy of diabetes insipidus with oral benzothiadiazine and phthalimidine diuretics. Clin Sci 1971;40:497–511.

Laragh JH. Oral contraceptive-induced hypertension — nine years later. Am J Obstet Gynecol 1976;126:141–7.

Littenberg B, Gluck EH. A controlled trial of methylprednisolone in the emergency treatment of acute asthma. N Engl J Med 1986;314:150–2.

Lubkin VL. Steroid cataract — a review and conclusion. J Asthma Res 1977;14:55–9.

Mann JI, Inman WHW, Thorogood M. Oral contraceptive use in older woman and fatal myocardial infarction. Br Med J 1976;2:445–7.

Mannucci PM, Pareti FI, Ruggeri ZM, Capitano A. 1-desamino-8-arginine vasopressin: a new pharmacological approach to the management of haemophilia and von Willebrand's disease. Lancet 1977;1:869–72.

Miller M, Moses AM. Drug-induced states of impaired water excretion in the mammalian kidney. Kidney Int 1976;10:96–103.

Moss J, Roizen MF, Norbdy ET, et al. Decreased incidence and mortality of anaphylaxis to chymopapain. Anesth Analg 1985;64:1197–201.

Munson WM. The pressor effect of various vasopressor–oxytocic combinations: a laboratory study and a review. Anesth Analg 1965;44:114–9.

Pisarev MA, DeGroot LJ, Hati R. KI and imidazole inhibition of TSH and c-AMP–induced thyroidal iodine secretion. Endocrinology 1971;88:1217–21.

Plorn GW. Clinical considerations in the use of corticosteroids. N Engl J Med 1966;274:775–81.

Rajagopalan R, Tindal S, MacNab LT, et al. Anaphylactic reactions to chymopapain during general anesthesia: a case report. Anesth Analg 1974;53:191–3.

Saberi M, Sterling FH, Utiger RD. Reduction in extrathyroidal triiodothyronine production of propylthiouracil in man. J Clin Invest 1975;55:218–23.

Saunders WG, Munsick RA. Antidiuretic potency of oxytocin in women past partum. Am J Obstet Gynecol 1966;95:5–11.

Schumer W. Steroids in the treatment of clinical peptic shock. Ann Surg 1976;184;333–9.

Sprung CL, Caralis PV, Marcial EH, et al. The effects of high-dose corticosteroids in patients with peptic shock. A prospective, controlled study. N Engl J Med 1984;311:1137–43.

Sutor AH, Uollman H, Arends P. Intranasal application of DDAVP in severe haemophilia (letter). Lancet 1978;1:446.

Symreng T, Karlberg BE, Kagedal B, Schildt B. Physiological cortisol substitution of long-term steroid-treated patients undergoing major surgery. Br J Anaesth 1981;53:949–53.

Thompson P, Earll JM, Schaff M. Comparison of clofibrate and chlorpropamide in vasopressin-responsive diabetes insipidus. Metabolism 1977;26:749–62.

Webb–Johnson DC, Andrews JL. Bronchodilator therapy. N Engl J Med 1977;297:476–82, 758–64.

Weston WL, Claman HN, Krueger GG. Site of action of cortisol in cellular immunity. J Immunol 1973;110:880–3.

Winnie AP, Hartman JT, Meyers HL, Ramamurthy S, Barangan V. Pain clinic. II: Intradural and extradural corticosteroids for sciatica. Anesth Analg 1972;51:990–1003.

Wolfe JE, Bone RC, Ruth WE. Effects of corticosteroids in the treatment of patients with gastric aspiration. Am J Med 1977;63:719–22.

Wynne JW, DeMarco FJ, Hood CI. Physiological effects of corticosteroids in foodstuff aspiration. Arch Surg 1981;116:46–9.

CHAPTER 24

Insulin and Oral Hypoglycemics

INTRODUCTION

Insulin administered exogenously is the only effective treatment for Type I diabetes mellitus (Banting *et al,* 1922). Oral hypoglycemic drugs may serve as alternatives to exogenous administration of insulin to patients with Type II diabetes mellitus.

INSULIN

Beta cells of the islet of Langerhans of the pancreas form insulin from a single-chain precursor termed *proinsulin*. The two most important effects of insulin are to facilitate transport of glucose across cell membranes and to enhance phosphorylation of glucose within cells. For example, insulin can increase the rate of carrier-mediated diffusion of glucose seven- to tenfold. It is not known whether insulin increases the amount of carrier in cell membranes or whether it increases the rate at which chemical reactions take place between glucose and the carrier.

Structure Activity Relationships

Insulin is composed of two chains (A and B) of amino acids joined by three disulfide bonds (Fig. 24-1) (Larner, 1985). Porcine insulin most closely resembles human insulin, differing only by substitution of an alanine residue on the B chain. By using porcine insulin as the starting material, human insulin can be synthesized with relative ease (Ruttenberg, 1972). Production of human insulin by cloning of chemically synthesized deoxyribonucleic acid (DNA) in bacteria is also possible.

The activity of various mammalian insulins is similar, ranging from 22 to 26 units mg^{-1}. Proinsulin has only slight biologic activity, whereas the separated A and B amino acid chains are inactive.

Pharmacokinetics

The elimination half-time of insulin injected intravenously is 5 to 10 minutes in normal patients or in the presence of diabetes mellitus. Insulin is metabolized in the kidneys and liver by a proteolytic enzyme. About 50% of the insulin that reaches the liver by way of the portal vein is destroyed in a single passage through the liver. Nevertheless, renal dysfunction alters the rate of disappearance of circulating insulin to a greater extent than does hepatic disease. Indeed, unexpected prolonged effects of insulin may occur in patients with renal disease, reflecting impairment of both metabolism and excretion of this hormone by the kidneys. Peripheral tissues such as skeletal muscles and fat can bind and inactivate insulin, but this is of minor quantitative significance.

Despite rapid clearance from the plasma following intravenous injection of insulin, there is a sustained pharmacologic effect for 30 to 60 min-

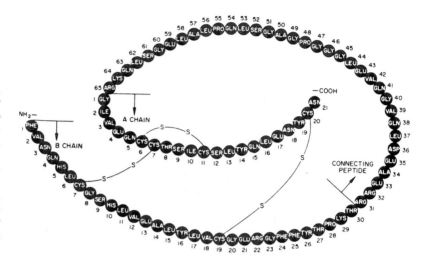

FIGURE 24-1. Proinsulin, which is converted to insulin by proteolytic cleavage of amino acids 31, 32, 64, 65, and the connecting peptide. (Reproduced by permission of Larner J. Insulin and oral hypoglycemic drugs;glucagon. In: Gilman AG, Goodman LS, Rall TW, Murad F, eds. The Pharmacological Basis of Therapeutics, 7th ed. New York. Macmillan Publishing Co., 1985;1490.)

utes, because insulin is tightly bound to tissue receptors. Insulin administered subcutaneously is released slowly into the circulation to produce a sustained biologic effect.

The majority of insulin circulates as free hormone not bound to protein. Under fasting conditions, the pancreas secretes 20 μg of insulin each hour into the portal vein, resulting in a circulating plasma concentration of 500 pg ml^{-1} (12 microunits ml^{-1}) (Devis *et al,* 1977).

Receptors

Receptors for insulin in cell membranes are characterized as insulin-binding proteins (Jacobs *et al,* 1977). It has not been proved that insulin activates adenylate cyclase to increase the intracellular concentrations of cyclic AMP (Charles *et al,* 1973). In fact, it is possible that insulin actually inhibits adenylate cyclase, leading to an increase in glycogen synthesis.

Insulin receptors become fully saturated with low circulating concentrations of insulin (Bar and Roth, 1977). For example, continuous intravenous infusion of insulin, 1 to 2 units hr^{-1}, has the same or even greater pharmacologic effect than a single larger intravenous dose that is cleared rapidly from the circulation. Large doses of insulin, however, will last longer and exert a greater net effect than small doses.

The number of insulin receptors seems to be inversely related to the plasma concentration of insulin. This relationship may reflect the ability of insulin to regulate the population of its receptors. Obesity and insulin-dependent diabetes mellitus appear to be associated with a decrease in the number of insulin receptors (Olefsky, 1976).

Preparations

Insulin preparations differ in their concentration, time to onset, duration of action, purity, and species of origin (Rosenbloom, 1974). Commercially prepared insulin is bioassayed, and its physiologic activity (potency), based on the ability to lower the blood glucose concentration, is expressed in units. The potency of insulin is 22 to 26 units mg^{-1}. Insulin U-100 (100 units ml^{-1}) is the most commonly used commercial preparation (Committee on the Use of Therapeutic Agents of the American Diabetes Association, 1972). A total daily exogenous dose of insulin for treatment of diabetes mellitus is usually in the range of 20 to 60 units. This insulin requirement, however, may be acutely increased by stress associated with sepsis or trauma.

Most commercial preparations of insulin are mixtures of porcine and bovine hormones. Pure porcine or bovine insulin is also available. Although use of purified insulin preparations is associated with lower antibody titers, the species of origin is more important to immunogenicity than is the degree of purity. Porcine insulin differs from human insulin by only one amino acid and is less immunogenic than bovine preparations. Indeed, pure porcine insulin preparations are the least antigenic. Alternatively, the risk of antigenicity is negated by bacterial synthesis of human insulin using recombinant DNA technology.

Classification

Insulin preparations are classified as fast-acting, intermediate-acting, and long-acting, based on the time to onset, duration of action, and intensity of action following subcutaneous administration (Table 24-1). These classifications are, however, artificial; a particular insulin preparation can show wide variations of activity in a group of patients and even within an individual patient, especially one with labile diabetes mellitus.

REGULAR INSULIN. Regular insulin is a fast-acting preparation and is the only one that can be administered intravenously as well as subcutaneously. This form of insulin can be mixed in the same syringe with other insulin preparations, assuming that the pH of the solutions is similar. Zinc, present in longer-acting insulin preparations, may retard full activity of regular insulin when the two are mixed together in the same syringe.

Administration of regular insulin is the preparation of choice for the treatment of the abrupt onset of hyperglycemia or the appearance of ketoacidosis. In the perioperative period, regular insulin is administered intravenously as single injections (1–5 units) or as a continuous intravenous infusion (1–2 units hr^{-1}) to treat metabolic derangements associated with diabetes mellitus.

SEMILENTE INSULIN. Semilente insulin is a rapid-acting insulin preparation that is most often used to supplement intermediate- and long-acting insulin preparations. The rapid onset and short duration of action of semilente insulin reflect its small size and amorphous structure.

Lente insulin preparations (*e.g.,* semilente insulin, lente insulin, ultralente insulin) contain methylparaben as a preservative, whereas all other insulin preparations use pheno or cresol for this purpose. Methylparaben resembles para-aminobenzoic acid and has been incriminated as a cause of allergic reactions, especially when combined with local anesthetics.

ISOPHANE INSULIN. Isophane insulin (NPH) is an intermediate-acting preparation whose absorption from its subcutaneous injection site is delayed because the insulin is conjugated with protamine. NPH designates a neutral solution (N), protamine (P), and origin in Hagedorn's laboratory (H) (Hagedorn *et al*, 1936). This insulin preparation contains less protamine (0.005 mg unit^{-1}) than protamine zinc insulin (0.028 mg unit^{-1}).

LENTE INSULIN. Lente insulin is a mixture of 30% semilente (*i.e.,* prompt onset) and 70% ultralente (*i.e.,* extended duration) insulin. Lente in-

Table 24-1
Classification of Insulin Preparations

	Protein Content	Time to Onset*	Duration of Action*
Fast-Acting			
Regular insulin	None	30–60 min	5–7 hr
Semilente insulin	None	30–60 min	5–7 hr
Intermediate-Acting			
Isophane insulin	Protamine	2 hr	24 hr
Lente insulin	None	2–4 hr	24 hr
Long-Acting			
Protamine zinc insulin	Protamine	4–6 hr	36 hr
Ultralente insulin	None	4–6 hr	36 hr

* Approximate

sulin is used interchangeably with NPH insulin in the initial treatment of diabetes mellitus. Zinc is present in lente insulin to provide stability, but proteins such as protamine are lacking.

PROTAMINE ZINC INSULIN. Protamine zinc insulin (PZI) results from letting insulin and zinc react with the basic protein protamine. Each unit of PZI is combined with 0.028 mg of protamine. Injected subcutaneously, this insulin preparation has a delayed onset and prolonged duration of action. These characteristics have led to the infrequent clinical use of this preparation.

ULTRALENTE INSULIN. Ultralente insulin is long-acting, reflecting the large particle size and crystalline form of this insulin preparation. This insulin preparation lacks protamine but, like PZI, has limited clinical usefulness because of its slow onset and prolonged duration of action.

Side Effects

Side effects of treatment with insulin may manifest as (1) hypoglycemia, (2) allergic reactions, (3) insulin resistance, (4) lipodystrophy, and (5) drug interactions.

Hypoglycemia

The most serious side effect of insulin therapy is hypoglycemia. Patients vulnerable to hypoglycemia are those who continue to receive exogenous insulin in the absence of carbohydrate intake, as may occur in the perioperative period, especially prior to surgery. Initial symptoms of hypoglycemia reflect the compensatory effects of increased epinephrine secretion manifesting as diaphoresis, tachycardia, and hypertension. Rebound hyperglycemia caused by sympathetic nervous system activity in response to hypoglycemia (Somogyi effect) may mask the correct diagnosis. Central nervous system symptoms of hypoglycemia include mental confusion progressing to seizures and coma. The intensity of central nervous system effects reflects the dependence of the brain on glucose as a selective substrate for oxidative metabolism. A prolonged period of hypoglycemia may result in irreversible brain damage.

The diagnosis of hypoglycemia during general anesthesia is made difficult, because classic signs of sympathetic nervous system stimulation are likely to be masked by the anesthetic drugs. If signs of sympathetic nervous system stimulation due to hypoglycemia occur, they are likely to be confused with responses evoked by painful stimulation in a lightly anesthetized patient. Furthermore, autonomic nervous system neuropathy associated with diabetes mellitus may attenuate the usual heart rate increase caused by hypoglycemia. Finally, nonselective beta antagonists may also mask signs and symptoms of hypoglycemia (see Chapter 14).

Severe hypoglycemia is treated with 50 to 100 ml of 50% glucose solution. Alternatively, 0.5 to 1 mg of glucagon administered intravenously or subcutaneously may be used. Nausea and vomiting are frequent side-effects of glucagon treatment. In the absence of central nervous system depression, carbohydrates may be given orally.

Allergic Reactions

Local or systemic allergic reactions to insulin may occur. Local allergic reactions are about 10 times more frequent than systemic allergic reactions. These local allergic reactions are characterized by an erythematous indurated area that develops at the site of insulin injection. The cause of local allergic reactions is likely to be noninsulin materials in the insulin preparation.

Systemic allergic reactions to insulin range from urticaria to life-threatening cardiovascular collapse. These allergic reactions have been ascribed to sensitivity to the insulin molecule, as reflected by high circulating concentrations of antibodies to insulin. Commonly, there is a history of allergy to other drugs such as penicillin. A systemic allergic reactin to insulin requires changing to insulin derived from a different species or source. In this regard, porcine insulin is less antigenic than the bovine product.

Chronic exposure to low doses of protamine in certain insulin preparations (*e.g.*, NPH insulin, PZI) may serve as an antigenic stimulus for the production of antibodies against protamine. These patients remain asymptomatic until a relatively large dose of protamine is administered intravenously to antagonize the anticoagulant effects of heparin. Indeed, patients with diabetes mellitus being treated with NPH insulin have a 50-fold increase in the likelihood of experiencing an allergic reaction to protamine (Stewart *et al,* 1984) (see Chapter 27).

Lipodystrophy

Lipodystrophy reflects atrophy of fat at the sites of subcutaneous injection of insulin. This side effect is minimized by frequently changing the site used for injection of insulin.

Insulin Resistance

Patients requiring more than 200 units of exogenous insulin daily are considered to be manifesting insulin resistance. Even this value is high, since insulin requirements for pancreatectomized adults are often as low as 30 units.

Insulin resistance may be acute or chronic. Acute insulin resistance is associated with trauma, as produced by surgery and infection. It is likely that increased circulating plasma cortisol concentrations contribute to this acute resistance. Chronic insulin resistance is often associated with circulating antibodies against insulin (Davidson and DeBra, 1978). Sulfonylureas can reduce insulin requirements in some resistant patients, presumably as a consequence of the release of endogenous insulin, which has less affinity for circulating antibodies than does exogenous porcine or bovine insulin.

Drug Interactions

Hormones administered as drugs that counter the hypoglycemic effect of insulin include adrenocorticotrophic hormone, glucocorticoids, thyroid hormones, estrogens, and glucagon. Epinephrine inhibits the secretion of insulin and stimulates glycogenolysis. Guanethidine decreases blood glucose concentrations and may reduce exogenous insulin requirements. Certain antibiotics (tetracyclines, chloramphenicol), salicylates, and phenylbutazone increase the duration of action of insulin and may also have a direct hypoglycemic effect. The hypoglycemic effect on insulin may be potentiated by monoamine oxidase inhibitors.

ORAL HYPOGLYCEMICS

Sulfonylurea compounds that function as oral hypoglycemics include tolbutamide, acetohexamide, tolazamide, chlorpropamide, glyburide, and glipizide (Fig. 24-2) (Table 24-2). The biquanide oral hypoglycemic drug phenformin causes lactic acidosis in some patients and, for this reason, is no longer commercially available (Fig. 24-3).

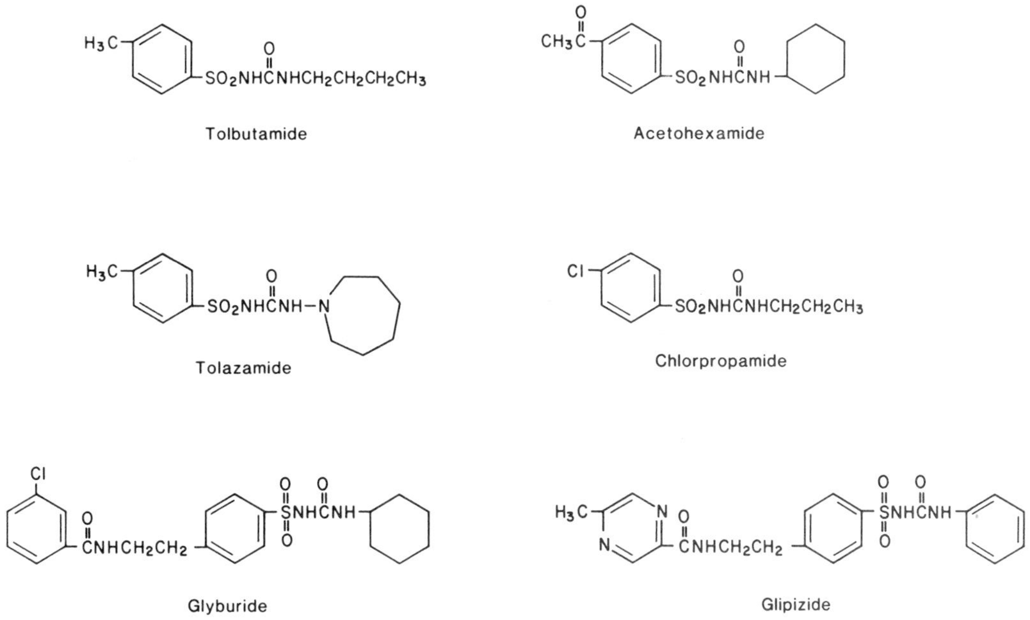

FIGURE 24-2. Oral hypoglycemics derived from sulfonylurea.

Table 24-2
Oral Hypoglycemics

	Approximate Duration of Action (hr)
Tolbutamide	6–12
Acetohexamide	12–24
Tolazamide	10–18
Chlorpropamide	24–72
Glyburide	16
Glipizide	12

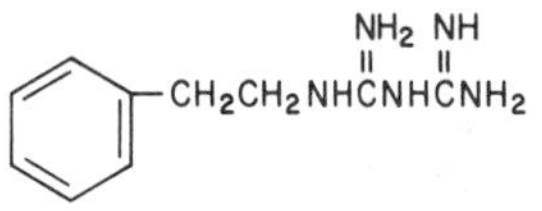

FIGURE 24-3. Phenformin.

Depending on dietary compliance, oral hypoglycemics fail to control hyperglycemia in 15% to 30% of patients. Even when initial control of blood glucose is obtained, secondary failure occurs in 5% of patients annually. Furthermore, successful control of the blood glucose concentration is unlikely if daily exogenous insulin requirements are greater than 40 units.

Mechanism of Action

Sulfonylureas stimulate pancreatic beta cells to secrete insulin in response to circulating glucose. The mechanism of this drug-induced insulin release is not known but may reflect sensitization of responsive pancreatic beta cells to the secretagogue effects of glucose (Lebovitz and Feinglos, 1978). Clearly, these drugs are not effective in patients who lack endogenous insulin stores. Although sulfonylureas are derivatives of sulfonamides, they have no antibacterial action.

Pharmacokinetics

Oral hypoglycemics are readily absorbed from the gastrointestinal tract, with the most important distinguishing features being differences in duration of action and elimination half-times (Table 24-2).

These drugs are weakly acidic and circulate bound to protein (70%–99%), principally to albumin. Metabolism in the liver is extensive, and resulting active and inactive metabolites are eliminated by renal tubular secretion.

Side Effects

Hypoglycemia, including coma, may occur with use of oral hypoglycemic drugs. This complication is more likely to occur with use of long-acting drugs in the presence of inadequate glucose intake, as may accompany the perioperative period. Advanced age and the presence of hepatic or renal dysfunction or both may increase the likelihood of drug-induced hypoglycemia. Drugs that may increase the risk of hypoglycemia from sulfonylureas include beta-adrenergic antagonists, salicylates, dicumarol, phenylbutazone, guanethidine, fenfluramine, clofibrate, monoamine oxidase inhibitors, and alcohol. Flushing of the skin, especially in the blush area, similar to that evoked by disulfiram may occur when patients being treated with oral hypoglycemics ingest alcohol. Dose requirements for oral hypoglycemics may be increased by drugs such as phenytoin, thiazide diuretics, and chlorpromazine that inhibit the endogenous release of insulin (Levin *et al,* 1970).

There is no proof that the use of oral hypoglycemic drugs is beneficial in the prevention of long-term complications associated with diabetes mellitus (Knatterud, 1971). In fact, one multiple institution study even suggested that the incidence of cardiovascular complications was greater in patients treated with oral hypoglycemics (University Group Diabetes Program, 1970).

Cutaneous rashes, photosensitivity, and pruritus may accompany treatment with oral hypoglycemics. If persistent, this side effect will necessitate discontinuation of therapy. Hematologic side effects manifesting as leukopenia, thrombocytopenia, and hemolytic anemia occur rarely. Acute intermittent porphyria has been observed in patients treated with sulfonylureas. Jaundice resulting from cholestasis occurs rarely.

Tolbutamide

Tolbutamide can be detected in the blood within 30 minutes after oral administration, with peak concentrations being reached in 3 to 5 hours. The drug is administered in a daily dose of 0.5 to 1.5 g, which must be given in two to three doses, because tolbutamide is excreted quickly. Tolbutamide is metabolized in the liver mainly to inactive substances that are excreted by the kidneys. The elimination half-time is about 6 hours. This short elimination half-time and duration of action is desirable in severely debilitated patients in whom blood – glucose concentrations and insulin needs may change unpredictably and abruptly.

Intravenous tolbutamide produces characteristic decreases in the blood glucose concentration of patients with an insulinoma serving as a diagnostic test, along with direct measurement of the plasma concentrations of insulin. Hypoglycemia may be severe, requiring careful monitoring and immediate availability of glucose.

Acetohexamide

Acetohexamide is rapidly absorbed after oral administration, and its total duration of action is 12 to 24 hours. Much of this prolonged activity is due to a metabolite, hydroxyhexamide, which has an elimination half-time of about 6 hours compared with 1.3 hours for the parent compound. This active metabolite has 2.5 times the hypoglycemic potency of the parent compound. Since the active metabolite is secreted by the kidneys, this drug should be avoided in patients with renal disease. This is the only sulfonylurea with uricosuric properties, making it an appropriate drug for the diabetic patient with gout.

Tolazamide

Tolazamide is slowly absorbed after oral administration, with an onset of hypoglycemic action after 4 to 6 hours that persists for 10 to 18 hours. It is metabolized in the liver to several different substances, some of which possess weak hypoglycemic activity. The active as well as inactive metabolites are excreted by the kidneys. For most patients, a single daily dose is sufficient. Tolazamide possesses a mild diuretic action and may be particularly useful in patients who have a tendency to retain water.

Chlorpropamide

Chlorpropamide is rapidly absorbed after oral administration and, in contrast to the other oral hypoglycemic drugs, is not significantly metabolized, being excreted unchanged in the urine. The elimination half-time is 36 hours, necessitating a single daily dose. Because of the long elimination half-time, the maximal effect of chlorpropamide may not be apparent for 7 to 14 days, and several weeks may be required for complete elimination of the drug.

Untoward reactions, especially severe hypoglycemia, have occurred more frequently with chlorpropamide than with other sulfonylureas. This drug should not be used in patients with renal insufficiency, because the duration of action may be prolonged. Facial flushing after ingestion of alcohol occurs in about one third of patients treated with chlorpropamide. Water retention and dilutional hyponatremia have been associated with the administration of chlorpropamide, especially in the presence of preexisting cardiac failure or hepatic cirrhosis. Chlorpropamide potentiates the action of antidiuretic hormone at renal tubules and augments release of hormone from the anterior pituitary, accounting for the usefulness of this oral hypoglycemic in the management of the patient with diabetes insipidus (see Chapter 23).

Glyburide

Glyburide produces a maximal hypoglycemic effect similar to other sulfonylureas. The drug is as effective as other sulfonylureas when given orally. Once-daily dosing is usually adequate. Metabolism is in the liver, with the majority of metabolites appearing in the bile and only about 25% being recovered in the urine. Following the last dose, it takes about 36 hours for this drug to be cleared from the plasma.

Glipizide

Glipizide produces a maximal hypoglycemic effect similar to other sulfonylureas. An oral dose in the morning stimulates secretion of insulin for up to 12 hours. Metabolism is in the liver, with these inactive metabolites as well as less than 10% of the unchanged drug appearing in the urine. This rapid inactivation and elimination should minimize the potential for glipizide to produce long-lasting hypoglycemia.

Phenformin

Phenformin is a biguanide oral hypoglycemic drug that can be associated with the development of life-threatening lactic acidosis (Fig. 24-3). For this reason, phenformin is available only for special circumstances, such as failure to respond to diet and for the patient who cannot tolerate sulfonylureas or to whom insulin cannot be administered.

Phenformin is not related chemically to insulin or the sulfonylureas and does not stimulate the release of insulin from pancreatic beta cells. Possible mechanisms of action include inhibition of hepatic gluconeogenesis, decreased intestinal absorption of glucose, up-regulation of insulin receptors, and increased anaerobic glycolysis, which increases glucose utilization. Phenformin alone rarely causes hypoglycemia. Large doses of phenformin appear to inhibit the conversion of alanine to glucose (*i.e.,* gluconeogenesis) and lactate to glucose.

REFERENCES

Banting FG, Best CH, Collip JB, Campbell WR, Fletcher AA. Pancreatic extracts in the treatment of diabetes mellitus. Can Med Assoc J 1922;12:141–6.

Bar RS, Roth J. Insulin receptor status in disease states in man. Arch Intern Med 1977;137:474–81.

Charles MA, Fanska R, Schmid FG, Forsham PA, Grodsky GM. Adenosine 3′,5′-monophosphate in pancreatic islets: glucose-induced insulin release. Science 1973;179:569–71.

Committee on the Use of Therapeutic Agents of the American Diabetes Association. U100 insulin: a new era in diabetes mellitus therapy. Diabetes 1972;21:832.

Davidson JK, DeBra DW. Immunologic insulin resistance. Diabetes 1978;27:307–18.

Devis G, Somers G, Malaisse WJ. Dynamics of calcium-induced insulin release. Diabetotogia 1977;13:531–6.

Hagedorn HC, Jensen BN, Krarup NB, Woodstrup I. Protamine insulinate. JAMA 1936;106:179–80.

Jacobs S, Shechter Y, Bissell K, Cuatrecasas P. Purification and properties of insulin receptors from rat liver membranes. Biochem Biophys Res Commun 1977;77:981–8.

Knatterud GL, Meinert CL, Klimt CR, Osborne RK, Martin DB. Effects of hypoglycemic agents on vascular complications in patients with adult-onset diabetes. JAMA 1971;217:777–84.

Larner J. Insulin and oral hypoglycemic drugs; glucagon. In: Gilman AG, Goodman LS, Rall TW, Murad F, eds. The Pharmacological Basis of Therapeutics, 7th ed. New York, Macmillan Publishing Co., 1985;1490.

Lebovitz HE, Feinglos MN. Sulfonylurea drugs: mechanism of antidiabetic action and therapeutic usefulness. Diabetes Care 1978;1:189–98.

Levin SR, Booker J, Smith DF, Grodsky GM. Inhibition of insulin secretion by diphenylhydantoin in the isolated perfused pancreas. J Clin Endocrinol Metab 1970;30:400–1.

Olefsky JM. The insulin receptor: its role in insulin resistance of obesity and diabetes. Diabetes 1976;25:1154–62.

Rosenbloom AL. Advances in commercial insulin preparations. Am J Dis Child 1974;128:631–3.

Ruttenberg MA. Human insulin: facile synthesis by modification of porcine insulin. Science 1972;177:623–6.

Stewart WJ, McSweeney SM, Kellett MA, Faxon DP, Ryan TJ. Increased risk of severe protamine reactions in NPH-insulin–dependent diabetics undergoing cardiac catheterization. Circulation 1984;70:788–92.

University Group Diabetes Program. A study of the effects of hypoglycemic agents on vascular complications in patients with adult-onset diabetes. Diabetes 1970;19:747–830.

CHAPTER 25

Diuretics

INTRODUCTION

Diuretics are among the most frequently prescribed drugs, with the classic pharmacologic response being diuresis. These drugs are classified according to their site of action on renal tubules and the mechanism by which they alter the excretion of solute as (1) thiazide diuretics, (2) loop diuretics, (3) osmotic diuretics, (4) potassium-sparing diuretics, (5) aldosterone antagonists, and (6) carbonic anhydrase inhibitors (Tables 25-1 and 25-2) (Merin and Bastron, 1986).

THIAZIDE DIURETICS

Thiazide diuretics are administered orally in divided daily doses for the treatment of essential hypertension and mobilization of edema fluid, as associated with renal, hepatic, or cardiac dysfunction (Fig. 25-1). Most often, a thiazide diuretic is selected as the initial treatment of essential hypertension, either as the sole drug or in combination with an antihypertensive drug (see Chapter 15). In combination with thiazide diuretics, the dose of more potent antihypertensive drugs can be reduced 25% to 50%, thus minimizing drug-induced side effects. Less common uses of thiazide diuretics are in the management of diabetes insipidus and treatment of hypercalcemia.

Mechanism of Action

Thiazide diuretics produce diuresis by virtue of inhibition of reabsorption of sodium and chloride ions, principally in the cortical portion of the ascending loops of Henle and, to a lesser extent, in the proximal renal tubules and distal renal tubules (Table 25-2) (Merin and Bastron, 1986). The result is a marked increase in the urinary excretion of sodium, chloride, and bicarbonate ions (Table 25-3) (Tonnesen, 1983). There is an associated increased secretion of potassium ions into the renal tubules that occurs whenever there is enhanced distal delivery of sodium ions and water. This emphasizes that the normal driving force for potassium ion secretion by distal renal tubules is the transtubular electrical potential difference created by sodium ion reabsorption. Thiazide diuretics, by inhibiting sodium ion reabsorption, lead to the delivery of higher concentrations of sodium ions to the distal renal tubules and the subsequent enhancement of secretion of potassium ions into the renal tubules (Goldberg, 1973). The diuretic effect of thiazide diuretics is independent of acid–base balance.

Antihypertensive Effect

The antihypertensive effect of thiazide diuretics is due initially to a reduction in extracellular fluid

Table 25-1
Classification of Diuretics

Thiazide Diuretics
  Chlorothiazide
  Hydrochlorothiazide
  Benzthiazide
  Cyclothiazide
Loop Diuretics
  Ethacrynic Acid
  Furosemide
Osmotic Diuretics
  Mannitol
  Urea
Potassium-Sparing Diuretics
  Triamterene
  Amiloride
Aldosterone Antagonists
  Spironolactone
Carbonic Anhydrase Inhibitors
  Acetazolamide

volume, often with a reduction in cardiac output (Jewkes *et al,* 1970). The sustained antihypertensive effect of thiazide diuretics, however, is due to peripheral vasodilation, which takes several weeks to develop. This peripheral vasodilation may reflect a diminished effect of sympathetic nervous system activity at peripheral vascular smooth muscle, which correlates roughly with the reduction in total body stores of sodium ions. This diuretic-induced reduction in peripheral vascular resistance is accompanied by at least partial correction of the decreased extracellular fluid volume. The importance of diuretic-induced sodium excretion is suggested by the absence of an antihypertensive effect when thiazide diuretics are administered to anephric animals (Freis, 1976).

Side Effects

Thiazide diuretic-induced hypokalemic, hypochloremic, metabolic alkalosis is a common side effect when these drugs are administered chronically, as in the treatment of essential hypertension (Table 25-4). Depletion of sodium ions and mag-

Table 25-2
Sites of Action of Diuretics

	Thiazide Diuretics	Loop Diuretics	Osmotic Diuretics	Potassium-Sparing Diuretics	Aldosterone Antagonists	Carbonic Anhydrase Inhibitors
Early proximal convoluted tubule		+	+			
Proximal convoluted tubule	+	+				+++
Medullary portion of ascending loop of Henle		+++	+++			
Cortical portion of ascending loop of Henle	+++	+	+			
Distal convoluted tubule	+	+	+	+++		+
Collecting duct					+++	

+ Minor site of action
+++ Major site of action
(Adapted from Merin RG, Bastron RD. Diuretics. In: Smith NT, Miller RD, Corbascio AN, eds. Drug Interactions in Anesthesia. Philadelphia, Lea & Febiger, 1986:206; with permission of the authors and publisher.)

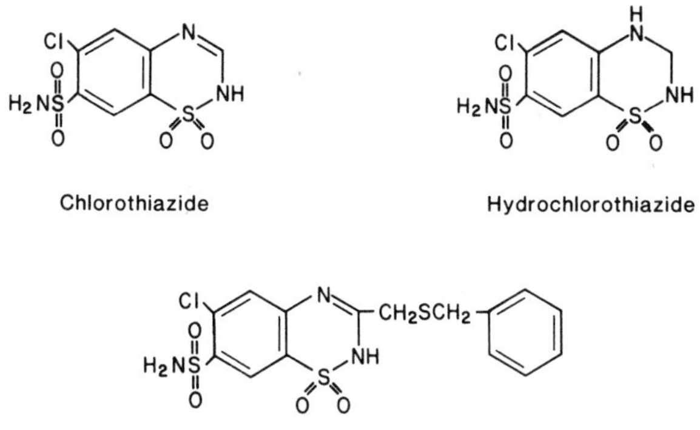

Chlorothiazide

Hydrochlorothiazide

Benzthiazide

FIGURE 25-1. Thiazide diuretics.

Table 25-3
Effect of Diuretics on Urine Composition

	Volume (ml min^{-1})	pH	Sodium (mEq L^{-1})	Potassium (mEq L^{-1})	Chloride (mEq L^{-1})	Bicarbonate (mEq L^{-1})
No drug	1	6.4	50	15	60	1
Thiazide diuretics	13	7.4	150	25	150	25
Loop diuretics	8	6.0	140	25	155	1
Osmotic diuretics	10	6.5	90	15	110	4
Potassium-sparing diuretics	3	7.2	130	10	120	15
Carbonic anhydrase inhibitors	3	8.2	70	60	15	120

(Adapted from Tonnesen AS. Clinical pharmacology and use of diuretics. In: Hershey SG, Bamforth BJ, Zauder HL, eds. Review Course in Anesthesiology, Philadelphia, JB Lippincott Co, 1983:217; with permission of the author and publisher.)

Table 25-4
Side Effects of Diuretics

	Hypokalemic Hypochloremic Metabolic Alkalosis	Hyperkalemia	Hyperglycemia	Hyperuricemia	Hyponatremia
Thiazide diuretics	Yes	No	Yes	Yes	Yes
Loop diuretics	Yes	No	Minimal	Minimal	Yes
Potassium-sparing diuretics	No	Yes	Minimal		Minimal
Aldosterone antagonists	No	Yes	No	No	Yes

nesium ions may accompany kaliuresis. Cardiac dysrhythmias may occur as the result of diuretic-induced hypokalemia or hypomagnesemia. Other important side effects of hypokalemia may include (1) skeletal muscle weakness, (2) gastrointestinal ileus, (3) nephropathy characterized by polyuria and azotemia, (4) increased likelihood of developing digitalis toxicity (see Chapter 13), and (5) potentiation of nondepolarizing neuromuscular blocking drugs (see Chapter 8).

Intravascular fluid volume should be evaluated in all patients being treated with thiazide diuretics and scheduled for surgery. The presence of orthostatic hypotension in such patients should arouse suspicion that intravascular fluid volume is reduced. Laboratory evidence of hemoconcentration (increased hematocrit, elevated blood urea nitrogen concentration) and decreased right or left atrial filling pressures are further evidence of hypovolemia.

Thiazide diuretics may cause hyperglycemia and aggravate diabetes mellitus. The mechanism of hyperglycemia is unknown but may reflect drug-induced inhibition of release of insulin from the pancreas and blockade of peripheral utilization of glucose.

Inhibition of renal tubular secretion of urate by thiazide diuretics can result in hyperuricemia. This thiazide-induced retention of uric acid can cause an exacerbation of gouty arthritis, even in patients being treated with probenecid (Ascione, 1976).

Borderline renal or hepatic function may further deteriorate during treatment with thiazide diuretics, presumably reflecting drug-induced reductions in blood flow to these organs. A maculopapular rash occurs in 1% or more of patients treated with chlorothiazide (Kirkendall, 1959).

LOOP DIURETICS

Ethacrynic acid and furosemide are examples of diuretics that inhibit reabsorption of sodium and chloride ions primarily in the medullary portion of the ascending limb of the loop of Henle (Fig. 25-2; Table 25-2) (Merin and Bastron, 1986). This site of action accounts for the designation of these drugs as loop diuretics. Intravenous administration of either ethacrynic acid or furosemide produces a diuretic response within 2 to 10 minutes that is independent of acid–base changes (Table

25-3) (Tonnesen, 1983). Indeed, responsiveness to furosemide is directly related to the glomerular filtration rate over a wide range. Conversely, responses to thiazide diuretics follow this relationship only when glomerular filtration rates are greatly reduced to levels below 20 ml min^{-1}.

Pharmacokinetics

Ethacrynic Acid

Ethacrynic acid is effective when administered orally (0.75–3 mg kg^{-1}) or intravenously (0.5–1 mg kg^{-1}). A high incidence of gastrointestinal reactions follows oral administration of this diuretic. Protein binding is extensive. Ethacrynic acid is excreted by the kidneys as unchanged drug and an unstable metabolite.

Furosemide

Furosemide is effective when administered orally (0.75–3 mg kg^{-1}) or intravenously (0.1–1 mg kg^{-1}). Protein binding to albumin is extensive, accounting for about 90% of the drug. Glomerular filtration and renal tubular secretion account for about 50% of the excretion of furosemide (Sawbney *et al,* 1981). About one third of a dose of furosemide is metabolized or excreted unchanged in the bile. The elimination half-time is less than 1 hour, accounting for the short duration of action of furosemide.

Clinical Uses

Clinically, furosemide is used far more often than ethacrynic acid. Common clinical uses of furosemide include (1) mobilization of edema fluid owing to renal, hepatic, or cardiac dysfunction, (2) treatment of increased intracranial pressure, and (3) differential diagnosis of acute oliguria. Loop diuretics have little use in the chronic treatment of essential hypertension. Indeed, the antihypertensive effect of furosemide is due entirely to its ability to reduce intravascular fluid volume, which, if it occurs rapidly, may evoke baroreceptor reflex–mediated increases in sympathetic nervous system activity. Acceleration of excretion of other drugs such as long-acting nondepolarizing neuromuscular blocking drugs by furosemide-induced diuresis is limited by the fact that this di-

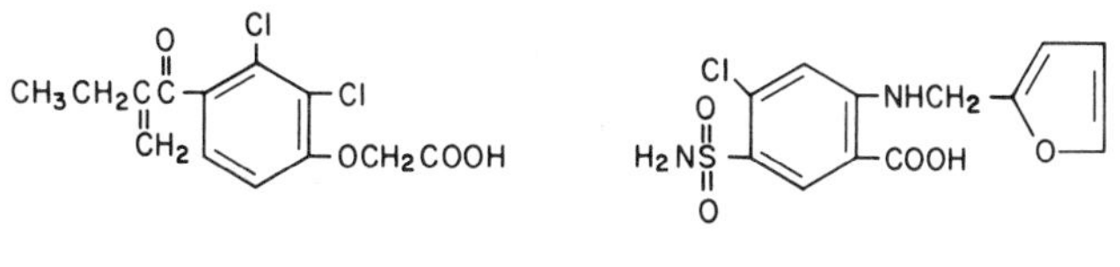

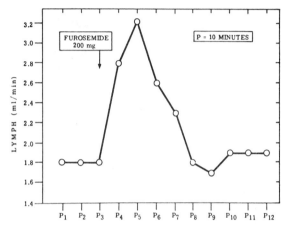

Ethacrynic Acid   Furosemide

FIGURE 25-2. Loop diuretics.

uretic does not increase glomerular filtration rate or renal tubular secretion (see Chapter 8).

Mobilization of Edema Fluid

Furosemide, administered intravenously in doses of 0.1 to 1 mg kg^{-1}, produces prompt diuresis of edema fluid owing to renal, hepatic, or cardiac dysfunction. Peripheral vasodilation precedes the onset of diuresis, and the associated reduction in venous return is consistent with the prompt and efficacious effects of furosemide in the management of acute pulmonary edema (Austin *et al,* 1976). Furosemide also increases thoracic duct lymph flow (Fig. 25-3) (Szwed *et al,* 1972).

Treatment of Increased Intracranial Pressure

Intravenous furosemide, 0.1 to 1 mg kg^{-1}, reduces intracranial pressure without producing alterations in plasma osmolarity (Cottrell *et al,* 1977). This reflects mobilization of edema fluid and intracellular dehydration. Furthermore, furosemide may decrease production of cerebrospinal fluid by interfering with sodium transport in glial tissue.

In addition, alterations in the blood–brain barrier do not influence the immediate or subsequent effects of furosemide on intracranial pressure. This contrasts with mannitol, which may produce rebound intracranial hypertension if a disrupted blood–brain barrier allows mannitol to enter the central nervous system.

Differential Diagnosis of Acute Oliguria

Furosemide administered intravenously in small doses (0.1 mg kg^{-1}) will stimulate diuresis in the presence of excessive antidiuretic hormone effect. This drug must not be used, however, to treat acute oliguria owing to decreased intravascular fluid volume, because furosemide-induced diuresis could further exaggerate hypovolemia and aggravate renal ischemic changes that result from

FIGURE 25-3. Furosemide increases flow of lymph through the thoracic duct. (From Szwed JJ, Kleit SA, Hamburger RJ. Effect of furosemide and chlorothiazide on the thoracic duct lymph flow in the dog. J Lab Clin Med 1972;79:693–700. Reproduced by permission of the authors and publisher.)

poor renal blood flow (Fink, 1982). Furthermore, continued urine output in the presence of furosemide can no longer be considered evidence of adequate intravascular fluid volume, cardiac output, and renal blood flow.

The use of furosemide to treat acute renal failure is controversial. Furosemide does not change glomerular filtration rate in normal patients or in the presence of acute renal failure (Epstein *et al,* 1975). Nevertheless, large intravenous doses of furosemide (up to 10 mg kg^{-1}) can increase renal blood flow, principally to the renal cortex (Koechel, 1981). This increase in renal blood flow, however, occurs only when intravascular fluid volume is maintained. Redistribution of renal blood flow may reflect furosemide-induced release of prostaglandins and renin. Indeed, indomethacin in doses adequate to block the synthesis of prostaglandins prevents an increase in renal blood flow following the administration of furosemide (Patak *et al*, 1975). In an animal model, furosemide, 1 to 10 mg kg^{-1}, administered intravenously during or immediately following an acute ischemic insult (*e.g.*, unilateral renal artery infusion of norepinephrine for 40 minutes) limits the extent of experimental renal failure (Cronin *et al*, 1978).

Side Effects

Side effects of loop diuretics are most often manifested as abnormalities of fluid and electrolyte balance (Jewkes *et al*, 1970). Potassium and chloride ion loss are prominent, and hypokalemia is a constant threat in the patient treated with furosemide (Table 25-4).

In animals, loop diuretics deplete myocardial potassium stores and increase the likelihood of digitalis toxicity. Hypokalemia has been associated with enhancement of the effects of nondepolarizing neuromuscular blocking drugs (see Chapter 8). Furosemide may also act on presynaptic nerve terminals to inhibit production of cyclic AMP and the subsequent release of acetylcholine, which would also potentiate nondepolarizing neuromuscular blocking drugs (Miller *et al*, 1976). As with thiazide diuretics, loop diuretics may cause hyperuricemia, but this is rarely clinically significant. Likewise, hyperglycemia, although possible, is less likely to occur than with thiazide diuretics.

Furosemide elevates renal tissue concentrations of aminoglycosides and enhances the possible nephrotoxic effect of these antibiotics. Cephalosporin nephrotoxicity may also be increased by furosemide (Dodds and Foord, 1970). Furosemide has been associated with allergic interstitial nephritis similar to that occasionally produced by penicillin. Cross-sensitivity may exist between furosemide and patients allergic to other sulfonamides. The renal clearance of lithium is decreased in the presence of diuretic-induced reductions in sodium ion reabsorption. Consequently, plasma concentrations of lithium may be acutely increased by the intravenous administration of furosemide in the perioperative period (Havdala *et al*, 1979) (see Chapter 35). In symptomatic hypercalcemia, furosemide may lower the plasma concentration of calcium by stimulating urine output.

High doses of furosemide, as may be used in the treatment of acute renal failure, may result in the accumulation of reactive intermediary metabolites. These reactive intermediary metabolites

produce hepatic necrosis in animals (Mitchell *et al*, 1974). At the usual clinical doses, however, hepatotoxicity is not observed, but this theoretical possibility should be kept in mind when massive doses of furosemide are administered to patients with renal failure (see the section entitled Clinical Uses).

Development of deafness, either transient or permanent, is a rare and unique complication produced by furosemide and ethacrynic acid. This side effect is most likely to occur with prolonged elevations of the plasma concentrations of these drugs. Drug-induced changes in the electrolyte composition of the endolymph is a possible mechanism.

OSMOTIC DIURETICS

Osmotic diuretics such as mannitol and urea are freely filterable at the glomerulus, undergo limited reabsorption from renal tubules, resist metabolism, and are pharmacologically inert. These characteristics permit administration of osmotic diuretics in sufficiently large quantities so as to alter the osmolarity of the plasma, glomerular filtrate, and renal tubular fluid, resulting in osmotic diuresis.

Mannitol

Mannitol is the most frequently used osmotic diuretic. Structurally, mannitol is a six-carbon sugar that does not undergo metabolism (Fig. 25-4). It is not absorbed from the gastrointestinal tract, thus necessitating its exclusive use by intravenous injection to achieve a diuretic effect. Mannitol does not enter cells, and its only means of clearance from the plasma is by way of the glomerular filtrate.

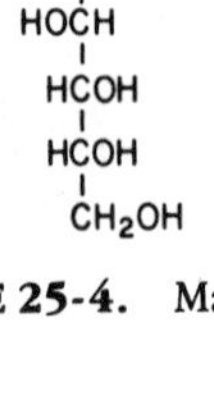

```
      CH2OH
       |
     HOCH
       |
     HOCH
       |
      HCOH
       |
      HCOH
       |
      CH2OH
```

FIGURE 25-4. Mannitol.

Mechanism of Action

Following intravenous administration, mannitol is completely filtered at the glomeruli, and none of the filtered drug is subsequently reabsorbed from the renal tubules (Table 25-2) (Merin and Bastron, 1986). As a result, mannitol raises the osmolarity of renal tubular fluid and prevents reabsorption of water. Sodium ions are diluted in this retained water in the renal tubules, leading to less reabsorption of this ion. As a result of this osmotic effect in the renal tubular fluid, there is an osmotic diuretic effect, with urinary excretion of water, sodium, chloride, and bicarbonate ions (Table 25-3) (Tonnesen, 1983). Urinary *p*H is not altered by mannitol-induced osmotic diuresis (Table 25-3) (Tonnesen, 1983).

In addition to renal tubular effects, intravenous mannitol administration also increases plasma osmolarity, which serves to draw fluid from intracellular to extracellular spaces. This may result in an acute expansion of the intravascular fluid volume. Redistribution of fluid from intracellular to extracellular sites decreases brain size and may increase renal blood flow (see the section entitled Clinical Uses). Likewise, the acute increase in intravascular fluid volume may have detrimental effects in patients with poor myocardial function (see the section entitled Side Effects).

Clinical Uses

Mannitol is administered for (1) prophylaxis against acute renal failure, (2) differential diagnosis of acute oliguria, (3) treatment of increased intracranial pressure, and (4) reduction of intraocular pressure.

PROPHYLAXIS AGAINST ACUTE RENAL FAILURE. Mannitol is used as prophylaxis against acute renal failure as may occur after (1) cardiovascular operations, (2) extensive trauma, (3) operations in the presence of jaundice, and (4) in the treatment of hemolytic transfusion reactions. In these situations, mannitol exerts an osmotic effect within the renal tubular fluid, inhibits renal tubular reabsorption of water, and maintains urine output. As a consequence, the concentration of any nephrotoxin in the renal tubular fluid does not reach the excessively high levels that would occur in the presence of more complete reabsorption of water. Maintenance of an adequate output of dilute urine

is considered an important factor in protection of the kidney. Mannitol may also increase renal blood flow and glomerular filtration rate, particularly when renal perfusion is decreased.

The protective effect of mannitol administration after the development of oliguria is not well established. Likewise, the protective effect of mannitol as used for prevention of acute renal failure following a transfusion reaction has not been proved (Goldfinger, 1977). The rationale for its use, which is relief of renal tubular obstruction by precipitated hemoglobin, has been largely discounted.

TREATMENT OF INCREASED INTRACRANIAL PRESSURE. Mannitol, 0.25 – 1 g kg^{-1} administered intravenously, acts to reduce intracranial pressure by increasing plasma osmolarity, which draws water from tissues, including the brain, along an osmotic gradient. There is little difference in the effect of this dose range on intracranial pressure, but the larger dose may last longer (Marsh *et al*, 1977). Importantly, mannitol is not associated with a high incidence of rebound increases in intracranial pressure. An intact blood – brain barrier is necessary to prevent entrance of mannitol into the central nervous system. If the blood – brain barrier is not intact, mannitol may enter the brain, drawing fluid with it and producing rebound cerebral edema. Regardless, the brain eventually adapts to sustained elevations in plasma osmolarity, such that chronic use of mannitol is likely to become less effective for lowering intracranial pressure.

DIFFERENTIAL DIAGNOSIS OF ACUTE OLIGURIA. Mannitol, 0.25 g kg^{-1} administered intravenously, is useful in the differential diagnosis of acute oliguria. For example, urine output is increased by mannitol when the cause of acute oliguria is decreased intravascular fluid volume. Conversely, when glomerular or renal tubular function are severely compromised, mannitol will not increase urine flow.

REDUCTION OF INTRAOCULAR PRESSURE. Mannitol, glycerin, and isosorbide are occasionally used for the short-term reduction of intraocular pressure in patients undergoing ophthalmologic surgery. Glycerin and isosorbide are administered orally and may contribute to an increased gastric fluid volume at the time of induction of anesthesia. In addition, glycerin is metabolized to glucose and can cause hyperglycemia and glycosuria.

Side Effects

In patients who are oliguric secondary to cardiac failure, acute mannitol-induced increases in intravascular fluid volume may precipitate pulmonary edema. Conversely, hypovolemia may follow excessive excretion of water and sodium. Nephrotoxins and prolonged renal ischemia may damage the renal tubular epithelium such that the renal tubule is no longer impermeable to mannitol and the osmotic effect of the diuretic is lost.

Diuresis secondary to mannitol does not alter the rate of elimination of long-acting nondepolarizing neuromuscular blocking drugs (see Chapter 8). This is predictable because these neuromuscular blocking drugs depend on glomerular filtration, which is not altered by mannitol. Venous thrombosis is not likely to occur after the intravenous administration of mannitol.

Urea

Urea, 1 to 1.5 g kg^{-1}, is an effective osmotic diuretic, but, unlike mannitol, its small molecular size results in reabsorption of over 60% of urea filtered at the glomerulus (Fig. 25-5). This drug eventually penetrates cells and crosses the blood–brain barrier, resulting in a greater degree of rebound increase in intracranial pressure than occurs after administration of mannitol. Another disadvantage of urea is a high incidence of venous thrombosis and the possibility of tissue necrosis if extravasation of urea-containing solutions occurs. Elevated blood urea nitrogen concentrations following administration of urea should not be confused with acute renal failure.

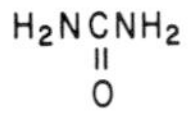

POTASSIUM-SPARING DIURETICS

Potassium-sparing diuretics such as triamterene and amiloride act directly on renal tubular transport mechanisms in the distal convoluted tubule

$$H_2NCNH_2$$
$$\overset{\|}{O}$$

FIGURE 25-5. Urea.

independent of aldosterone to produce diuresis (Fig. 25-6; Table 25-2) (Baba et al, 1964; Merin and Bastron, 1986). This diuresis is characterized by an increase in the urinary excretion of sodium, chloride, and bicarbonate ions and an elevation of the urine pH (Table 25-3) (Tonnesen, 1983). Diuresis is accompanied either by no increase or a decrease in potassium ion excretion in the urine (Table 25-3) (Tonnesen, 1983). The lack of diuretic-induced potassium ion excretion results from inhibition of the secretion of potassium ions into the distal renal tubule.

Clinical Uses

The greatest value of potassium-sparing diuretics is in combination with hydrochlorothiazide. This combination maximizes diuretic efficiency of both drugs while offsetting their opposite effects on urinary excretion of potassium.

Side Effects

Hyperkalemia is the principal side effect of therapy with potassium-sparing diuretics (Table 25-4). Unlike other diuretics, these drugs do not produce hyperuricemia.

ALDOSTERONE ANTAGONISTS

Spironolactone is the prototype of drugs that act as competitive antagonists at receptor sites on the collecting duct that otherwise respond to aldosterone (Fig. 25-7; Table 25-2) (Merin and Bastron, 1986). This drug is effective only when aldosterone is present (Covrol et al, 1981). Normally, aldosterone augments the renal tubular reabsorption of sodium and chloride ions and increases the excretion of potassium ions. Spironolactone blocks these renal tubular effects of aldosterone, as reflected by inhibition of the reabsorption of sodium and chloride ions.

Clinical Uses

Spironolactone is often prescribed for fluid overload owing to cirrhosis of the liver, on the assumption that reduced hepatic function and metabolism leads to increased plasma concentrations of

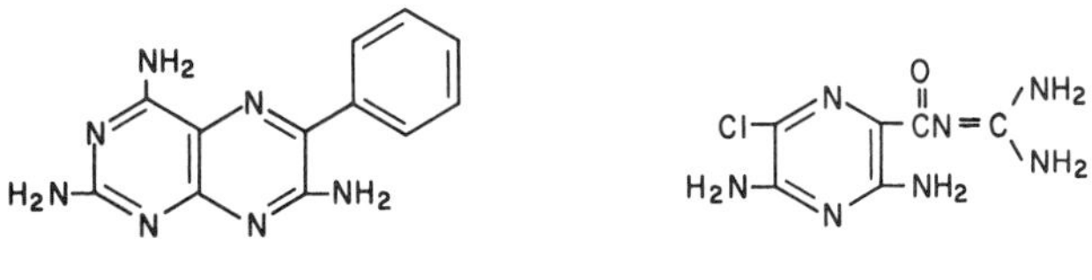

Triamterene   Amiloride

FIGURE 25-6. Potassium-sparing diuretics.

aldosterone. The antihypertensive effect of this diuretic is similar to that of thiazide diuretics, but side effects are different (see the following section). The combination of spironolactone and hydrochlorothiazide (Aldactazide) is an attempt to maximize diuretic efficiency of both drugs while offsetting their opposite effects on potassium ion secretion.

Side Effects

Hyperkalemia, especially in the presence of renal dysfunction, is the most serious side effect of treatment with spironolactone (Table 25-4). In contrast to thiazide diuretics, spironolactone does not cause hypokalemia, hyperglycemia, or hyperuricemia (Table 25-4). Gynecomastia and amenorrhea may accompany chronic treatment with spironolactone.

CARBONIC ANHYDRASE INHIBITORS

Acetazolamide is the prototype of a class of sulfonamide drugs that bind tightly to the carbonic anhydrase enzyme, producing noncompetitive inhibition of enzyme activity, principally in the proximal renal tubule (Fig. 25-8; Table 25-2) (Merin and Bastron, 1986). As a result of this enzyme inhibition, the excretion of hydrogen ions is diminished and loss of bicarbonate ions is increased (Table

25-3) (Tonnesen, 1983). Chloride ions are retained by the kidney to offset the loss of bicarbonate ions and thus maintain an ionic balance. Decreased availability of hydrogen ions in the distal renal tubule results in excretion of potassium ions in exchange for sodium ions. The net effect of all these changes is excretion of an alkaline urine in the presence of hyperchloremic metabolic acidosis. The diuretic action of acetazolamide is not altered by metabolic or respiratory acidosis. Following oral administration, acetazolamide is excreted unchanged by the kidneys in 24 hours.

Clinical Uses

The most common clinical uses of acetazolamide, 250 to 500 mg administered orally, are to reduce intraocular pressure in the treatment of glaucoma and as an adjuvant for management of petit mal and grand mal epilepsy. Decreased intraocular pressure reflects the presence of high concentrations of carbonic anhydrase enzyme in the ocular structures, and a resulting decrease in formation of aqueous humor when enzyme activity is inhibited by acetazolamide. Formation of cerebrospinal fluid is also inhibited by acetazolamide. Acetazolamide inhibits seizure activity, presumably by virtue of producing metabolic acidosis.

Beneficial effects of acetazolamide in the management of familial periodic paralysis may reflect drug-induced metabolic acidosis, which raises the local concentration of potassium ions in skeletal muscle. Acetazolamide, by producing metabolic acidosis, may stimulate ventilation in patients who are hypoventilating as a compensa-

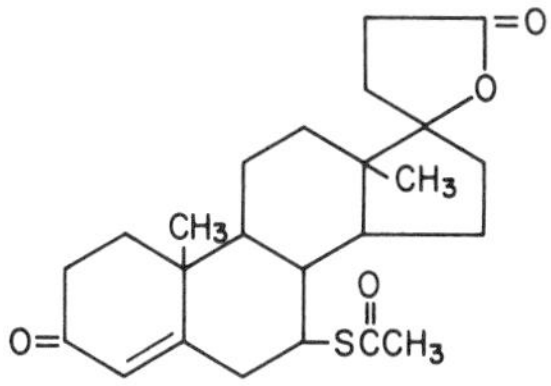

FIGURE 25-7. Spironolactone.

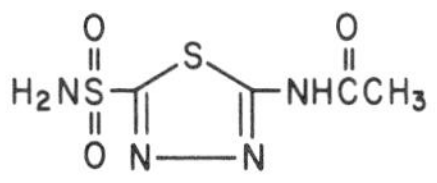

FIGURE 25-8. Acetazolamide.

tory response to metabolic alkalosis. Conversely, the loss of bicarbonate ions necessary to buffer carbon dioxide may result in exacerbation of hypercarbia in patients with chronic obstructive airways disease leading to central nervous system depression (Schwartz *et al,* 1955).

REFERENCES

Ascione FJ. Probenecid-chlorothiazide. In: Evaluations of Drug Interactions, 2nd ed. Washington DC, American Pharmaceutical Association, 1976.

Austin SM, Schreiner BF, Kramer DH, Shah PM, Yu PN. The acute hemodynamic effects of ethacrynic acid and furosemide in patients with chronic postcapillary pulmonary hypertension. Circulation 1976;53:364 – 8.

Baba WI, Tudhope GR, Wilson GM. Site and mechanism of action of the diuretic triamterene. Clin Sci 1964;27:181 – 9.

Cottrell JE, Robustelli A, Post K, Turndorf H. Furosemide and mannitol-induced changes in intracranial pressure and serum osmolality and electrolytes. Anesthesiology 1977;47:28 – 30.

Covrol P, Claire M, Oblin ME, Geering K, Rossier B. Mechanism of the antimineralocorticoid effects of spirolactones. Kidney Int 1981;20:1 – 6.

Cronin RE, McColl AL, DeTorrente A, McDonald KM, Schrier RW. Norepinephrine-induced acute renal failure. Kidney Int 1978;14:73 – 6.

Dodds MG, Foord RD. Enhancement by potent diuretics of renal tubular necrosis induced by cephaloridine. Br J Pharmacol 1970;40:227 – 36.

Epstein M, Schneider NS, Befeler B. Effect of intrarenal furosemide on renal function and intrarenal hemodynamics in acute renal failure. Am J Med 1975;58:510 – 6.

Fink M. Are diuretics useful in the treatment or prevention of acute renal failure. South Med J 1982;75:329 – 44.

Freis ED. Salt, volume, and the prevention of hypertension. Circulation 1976;53:589 – 95.

Goldberg M. The renal physiology of diuretics. In: Orloff J, Berliner RW, eds. Renal Physiology. Handbook of Physiology. Washington DC, American Physiological Society, 1973.

Goldfinger D. Acute hemolytic transfusion reactions — a fresh look at pathogenesis and considerations regarding therapy. Transfusion 1977;17:85 – 98.

Havdala HS, Borison RL, Diamond BI. Potential hazards and applications of lithium in anesthesiology. Anesthesiology 1979;50:534 – 7

Jewkes RF, Burki N, Guz A. Observations of renal function in patients undergoing therapeutic diuresis with furosemide. Clin Sci 1970;38:439 – 49.

Kirkendall WM. Clinical evaluation of chlorothiazide. Circulation 1959;19:933 – 41.

Koechel DA. Ethacrynic acid and related diuretics: Relationship of structure to beneficial and detrimental actions. Annu Rev Pharmacol Toxicol 1981;21:265 – 93.

Marsh ML, Marshall LF, Shapiro HM. Neurosurgical intensive care. Anesthesiology 1977;47:149 – 63.

Merin RG, Bastron RD. Diuretics. In: Smith NT, Miller RD, Corbascio AN, eds. Drug Interactions in Anesthesia. Philadelphia, Lea and Febiger, 1986:206.

Miller RD, Sohn YJ, Matteo RS. Enhancement of d-tubocurarine neuromuscular blockade by diuretics in man. Anesthesiology 1976;45:442 – 5.

Mitchell JR, Potter WZ, Hinson JA, Jollow DJ. Hepatic necrosis caused by furosemide. Nature 1974;251:508 – 11.

Patak R, Mookerjee BK, Bentzel CJ, Hysert PE, Babej M, Lee JB. Antagonism of the effects of furosemide by indomethacin in normal and hypertensive man. Prostaglandins 1975;10:649 – 53.

Sawbney VK, Gregory PB, Swezey SE, Blaschke TF. Furosemide disposition in cirrhotic patients. Gastroenterology 1981;81:1012 – 6.

Schwartz WB, Relman AS, Leaf A. Oral administration of a potent carbonic anhydrase inhibitor (Diamox). Its use as a diuretic in patients with severe congestive heart failure due to corpulmonale. Ann Intern Med 1955;42:79 – 89.

Szwed JJ, Kleit SA, Hamburger RJ. Effect of furosemide and chlorothiazide on the thoracic duct lymph flow in the dog. J Lab Clin Med 1972;79:693 – 700.

Tonnesen AS. Clinical pharmacology and use of diuretics. In: Hershey SG, Bamforth BJ, Zauder HL, eds. Review Courses in Anesthesiology, Philadelphia, JB Lippincott Co, 1983:217.

CHAPTER 26

Gastric Antacids, Stimulants, and Antiemetics

GASTRIC ANTACIDS

Gastric antacids are drugs that neutralize or remove acid from the gastric contents. Clinically useful antacids are aluminum, calcium, and magnesium salts that react with hydrochloric acid to form neutral, less acidic, or poorly soluble salts. Doses of antacids that increase gastric fluid pH above 5 inactivate pepsin and facilitate healing of a peptic ulcer. Neutralization of gastric fluid pH increases gastric motility via the action of gastrin (with the exception of aluminum hydroxide) and increases lower esophageal sphincter tone by a mechanism that is independent of gastrin (Hurwitz *et al*, 1976). Liquid preparations are generally more effective than tablets for neutralizing acids *in vivo*. When antacids are appropriately utilized, they are as effective as cimetidine in the treatment of peptic ulcer, reflux esophagitis, and prophylaxis against stress-induced ulceration and hemorrhage.

Side Effects

The only adverse effects shared by all antacids are those resulting from changes in gastric and urinary pH and alterations in acid–base status. Gastric alkalinization has been suggested as a cause of increased susceptibility to various acid-sensitive microbial pathogens. In the presence of renal failure, all antacids except aluminum compounds can cause metabolic alkalosis. Elevation of the urinary pH may persist for longer than 24 hours following administration of an antacid, leading to alterations in the renal elimination of drugs. Alkalinization of the urine may predispose to urinary tract infections and, if chronic, urolithiasis is possible.

Drug Interactions

Since gastric alkalinization hastens gastric emptying, antacids, other than aluminum compounds, will hasten delivery of drugs into the small intestine. This may speed absorption of drugs that are poorly absorbed, or it may shorten the time available for absorption. The rate of absorption of salicylates, indomethacin, and naproxen is increased when gastric fluid pH is elevated. Aluminum hydroxide accelerates absorption and increases bioavailability of diazepam by an unknown mechanism. Conversely, bioavailability of drugs may be decreased because of their capacity to form complexes with antacids. For example, antacids reduce bioavailability of orally administered cimetidine by about 25% (Gugler *et al*, 1981). One hour should elapse between the ingestion of an antacid and oral cimetidine to minimize this interaction. Antacids containing aluminum, and to a lesser extent calcium and magnesium, interfere with the absorption of tetracyclines and possibly digoxin from the gastrointestinal tract.

Commercial Preparations

Aluminum Hydroxide

Aluminum hydroxide is actually a mixture of aluminum hydroxide, aluminum oxide, and some fixed carbon dioxide (*e.g.*, carbonate). Systemic absorption of aluminum is minimal, but in patients with renal disease, the plasma and tissue concentrations of aluminum may become excessive (Berlyne *et al*, 1970). Encephalopathy in patients undergoing hemodialysis has been attributed to intoxication with aluminum (Alfrey *et al*, 1976). Among the compounds formed in the intestine from aluminum hydroxide are insoluble aluminum phosphates, which pass through the intestinal tract unabsorbed. Hypophosphatemia can occur and is the basis for the occasional therapeutic use of aluminum hydroxide in the treatment of phosphate nephrolithiasis. Decreased phosphate absorption is accompanied by increased calcium absorption, which sometimes causes hypercalciuria and nephrolithiasis (Cooke *et al*, 1978). Hypomagnesemia can also occur. Aluminum compounds, in contrast to other antacids, cause slowing of gastric emptying and marked constipation. These effects, plus an unpleasant taste, contribute to poor patient acceptance.

SUCRALFATE. Sucralfate is a complex of sulfated sucrose and aluminum hydroxide that is used for the short-term (up to 8 weeks) treatment of duodenal ulcer. This compound lacks antacid action but instead adheres to the ulcer to form a protective barrier against pepsin penetration (McHardy, 1981). The efficacy of sucralfate in facilitating healing of duodenal ulcers appears to be comparable to that of cimetidine (Martin *et al*, 1982).

The most common side effect of sucralfate is constipation. Simultaneous administration of antacids may interfere with the action of sucralfate.

Calcium Carbonate

Calcium carbonate produces rapid and effective neutralization of gastric acidity. Although systemic absorption is slight, sufficient absorption occurs with chronic therapy to produce a detectable metabolic alkalosis. The plasma concentration of calcium is increased transiently. Clinically, dangerous hypercalcemia may occur in patients with renal disease. The administration of calcium carbonate – containing antacids may be accompanied by hyperphosphatemia. Even small amounts of calcium carbonate – containing antacids evoke hypersecretion of hydrogen ions (*i.e.*, acid rebound) (Clayman, 1980). The chalky taste of calcium carbonate is a disadvantage. The release of carbon dioxide in the stomach may cause eructation and flatulence. Constipation is minimized by including magnesium oxide with calcium carbonate. Acute appendicitis has been produced by impacted calcium carbonate fecoliths.

MILK–ALKALI SYNDROME. The milk–alkali syndrome may occur after prolonged admnistration of calcium carbonate with sodium bicarbonate and/or homogenized milk containing vitamin D. This rare syndrome is characterized by hypercalcemic alkalosis, nausea, and occasionally renal failure. Conjunctival and episcleral suffusion accompanies the alkalosis. Calcium deposits manifest as band keratopathy. Symptoms are reversible with discontinuation of the antacid and/or milk. Magnesium and aluminum salts have not been implicated in this syndrome.

Magnesium Oxide

Magnesium hydroxide (milk of magnesia) produces prompt neutralization of gastric acid and is not associated with significant acid rebound. In contrast to aluminum hydroxide, a prominent laxative effect is characteristic of magnesium hydroxide. Systemic absorption of magnesium may be sufficient to cause neurologic, neuromuscular, and cardiovascular impairment in patients with renal dysfunction. In normal patients, absorption of magnesium is attended by little danger of systemic alkalosis. Magnesium is often combined with aluminum hydroxide.

Sodium Bicarbonate

The high solubility of sodium bicarbonate results in an immediate and rapid antacid action in the stomach. The effect, however, is short-lived, and systemic alkalosis is possible. Weight gain may be prominent with chronic therapy. Sodium bicarbonate is useful when the goal is to alkalinize the urine.

Antacid Selection

There is considerable variation in the acid neutralizing effects of different antacids (Table 26-1).

Table 26-1
Contents (mg per 5 ml) of Particulate Antacids

	Aluminum Hydroxide	Magnesium Hydroxide	Calcium Carbonate	Sodium
Aludrox	307	103		1.1
Amphogel	320			6.9
Di-Gel	282	85		10.6
Gelusil	200	200		0.7
Maalox	225	200		1.35
Mylanta	200	200		0.68
Riopan	480			0.3
Tums			500	<3
WinGel	180	160		<2.5

Poorly absorbed antacids are preferred in the treatment of peptic ulcer. Mixtures of aluminum hydroxide and magnesium hydroxide are used most frequently. Calcium carbonate has a greater neutralizing capacity, but it is infrequently used because of concern about systemic calcium absorption and calcium-induced acid rebound. There is no convincing evidence that mixtures of antacids have greater beneficial effects than those provided by the individual antacid.

Preoperative Administration of Antacids

Preoperative administration of antacids to increase gastric fluid pH prior to the induction of general anesthesia would theoretically reduce the risk of acid pneumonitis if inhalation (aspiration) of gastric fluid occurs. Indeed, about 17% of patients scheduled for elective surgery have a gastric fluid pH below 2.5 and a gastric fluid volume above 20 ml (Table 26-2) (Stoelting, 1978). Despite the predictable ability of antacids to increase gastric fluid pH and theoretically reduce the risk associated with aspiration, it has not been documented that routine use of antacids in a high-risk patient population (e.g., the parturient in labor) decreases mortality (Taylor, 1975; Tompkinson *et al*, 1982). Furthermore, antacids or other prophylactic drugs (e.g., H_2 receptor antagonists, metoclopramide) do not reduce the possibility of regurgitation and aspiration.

The duration of antacid action is highly dependent on gastric emptying time. For example, opioid-induced slowing of gastric motility prolongs the pH-elevating effects of antacids in these patients compared with the effects in patients not receiving opioids (O'Sullivan and Bullingham, 1985). Repeated administration of antacids, such as to the parturient in labor who has also received opioids, could result in a greatly increased gastric fluid volume and could predispose the parturient to regurgitation if general anesthesia is induced. In this regard, it is logical to administer an antacid as a single dose about 30 minutes before the induction of anesthesia.

Even a single dose of antacid may increase the gastric fluid volume, and it has been speculated that this effect could offset desirable effects on pH if aspiration occurs. Nevertheless, in an animal model, mortality was 90% following inhalation of only 0.3 ml kg^{-1} of gastric fluid with a pH of 1 compared with 14% mortality following inhalation of 1 to 2 ml kg^{-1} of gastric fluid with a pH above 1.8 (Table 26-3) (James *et al*, 1984). These data suggest that an increased gastric fluid volume produced by administration of an antacid would not increase the likelihood of aspiration pneumonitis as long as the gastric fluid pH is elevated.

Particulate Antacids

Occasional failure of particulate antacids to elevate gastric fluid pH may reflect inadequate mixing with stomach contents or an unusually large volume of gastric fluid such that the standard dose of antacid is inadequate. Layering is common with particulate antacids (Holdsworth *et al*, 1980). Pneumonitis associated with functional and histologic changes in the lung may reflect a foreign

Table 26-2
Percentages of Patients with Gastric Fluid pH Below 2.5 and/or Volume Above 20 ml

	pH Below 2.5	Volume Above 20 ml	pH Below 2.5 and Volume Above 20 ml
Morphine	63	27	16
Morphine-atropine (n − 75)	58	27	17
Morphine-glycopyrrolate (n − 75)	52	23	16
Morphine-atropine-Riopan (n − 25)	0*	60*	0*

* $P < 0.05$ compared with morphine
n = number of patients
(Data from Stoelting RK: Responses to atropine, glycopyrrolate, and Riopan of gastric fluid pH and volume in adult patients. Anesthesiology 1978;48:367 – 9; with permission.)

Table 26-3
Mortality Rates (%) for Rats After Aspiration of Solutions of Various pHs and Volumes

Volume (ml kg⁻¹)	Fluid pH					
	1.0	1.4	1.8	2.5	3.5	5.8
0.2	20	0				
0.3	90	0	9			
0.4	90	40	9	0		
1.0	100	90	20	0	0	0
2.0	100	100	27	30	20	10
4.0	100	100	38	20	40	30

(Data from James CF, Modell JH, Gibbs CP, Kuck EJ, Ruiz BC. Pulmonary aspiration effects of volume and pH in the rat. Anesth Analg 1984;63:665 – 8; with permission.)

body reaction to inhaled particulate antacid particles. Indeed, aspiration of a particulate antacid in a dog model produced changes comparable to those induced by acid (Gibbs *et al*, 1979). Clinical reports suggest that particulate antacids have caused or aggravated aspiration pneumonitis in humans (Bond *et al*, 1979; Heaney and Jones, 1979).

Nonparticulate Antacids

Nonparticulate (*i.e.*, clear) antacids such as sodium citrate are less likely to cause a foreign body reaction if aspirated, and their mixing with gastric fluid is more effective than is that of particulate antacids (Gibbs *et al*, 1979; Holdsworth *et al*, 1980). Furthermore, the onset of effect is more rapid with sodium citrate than with particulate antacids that require longer times for adequate mixing with gastric fluid. Sodium citrate, 15 to 30 ml of 0.3 M solution administered 15 to 30 minutes before the induction of anesthesia, is effective in reliably elevating gastric fluid pH in pregnant and nonpregnant patients (Table 26-4) (Gibbs *et al*, 1982; Viegas *et al*, 1981). The pH of 0.3 M sodium citrate is about 8.4, accounting for its unpleasant taste and frequent addition of a flavoring agent to improve its palatability.

Bicitra is a nonparticulate antacid containing sodium citrate and citric acid that provides effective buffering of gastric fluid pH (Eyler *et al*, 1982). Polycitra is a nonparticulate antacid containing sodium citrate, potassium citrate, and citric acid that has greater buffering capacity than Bicitra (Conklin and Ziadlou-Rad, 1983). Both Bicitra and Polycitra are more palatable than sodium citrate, possibly due to their lower pH's of 4.5 and 5.2, respectively.

Table 26-4
Individual Gastric pH Measurements

	Control	Sodium Citrate
	1.9	6.2
	2.2	5.8
	1.5	5.2
	1.6	6.7
	1.6	6.2
	1.5	7.1
	2.1	7.1
	1.5	6.0
	1.6	3.9
	1.9	7.1
	2.2	6.4
	6.0	6.6
	2.0	6.3
	6.3	6.0
	2.0	6.3
Mean ± SD	2.4 ± 1.5	6.2 ± 0.8*

* $P < 0.001$ compared with control
(Data from Viegas OJ, Ravindran RS, Shumacker CA. Gastric fluid pH in patients receiving sodium citrate. Anesth Analg 1981;60:521–3; with permission.)

GASTRIC STIMULANTS

Metoclopramide

Metoclopramide (methoxychloroprocainamide) is a dopamine antagonist that is structurally similar to procainamide but lacks local anesthetic activity (Fig. 26-1). Instead, this drug stimulates motility of the upper gastrointestinal tract and increases lower esophageal sphincter tone by 10 to 20 cm H_2O in normal persons and parturients (Brock-Utne *et al*, 1978) (see Chapter 44). Gastric acid secretion is not altered. The net effect is accelerated gastric clearance of liquids and solids (*i.e.*, decreased gastric emptying time) and a shortened transit time through the small intestine.

Mechanism of Action

Metoclopramide produces selective cholinergic stimulation of the gastrointestinal tract (*i.e.*, gastrokinetic effect) consisting of (1) increased smooth muscle tension in the lower esophageal sphincter and gastric fundus, (2) increased gastric and small intestinal motility, and (3) relaxation of the pylorus and duodenum during contraction of the stomach (Schulze-Delrieu, 1981). Cholinergic stimulating effects of metoclopramide are largely restricted to smooth muscle of the proximal gastrointestinal tract and require some background cholinergic activity. There is evidence that metoclopramide sensitizes gastrointestinal smooth muscle to the effects of acetylcholine, which explains why metoclopramide, unlike conventional cholinergic drugs, requires background cholinergic activity to be effective. Postsynaptic activity results from the ability of metoclopramide to cause the release of acetylcholine from cholinergic nerve endings. Indeed, atropine opposes metoclopramide-induced increases in lower esophageal sphincter tone and gastrointestinal hypermotility, indicating that metoclopramide acts on postganglionic cholinergic nerves intrinsic to the wall of the gastrointestinal tract (Brock-Utne *et al*, 1976). In the central nervous system, metoclopramide blocks dopamine receptors. As a result, metoclopramide induces secretion of prolactin, and extrapyramidal symptoms may occur.

Pharmacokinetics

Metoclopramide is rapidly absorbed after oral administration, reaching peak plasma concentrations in 40 to 120 minutes (Schulze-Delrieu, 1981). Most patients achieve therapeutic plasma concentrations of 40 to 80 ng ml^{-1} after 10 mg of metoclopramide administered orally. Intravenous doses of metoclopramide as used to speed gastric emptying are 10 to 20 mg (see the section entitled Clinical Uses). The elimination half-time is 2 to 4 hours. About 85% of an oral dose of metoclopramide appears in the urine, equally divided among unchanged drug and sulfate and glucuronide conjugates. Impairment of renal function prolongs the elimination half-time and necessitates a reduction in metoclopramide dosage.

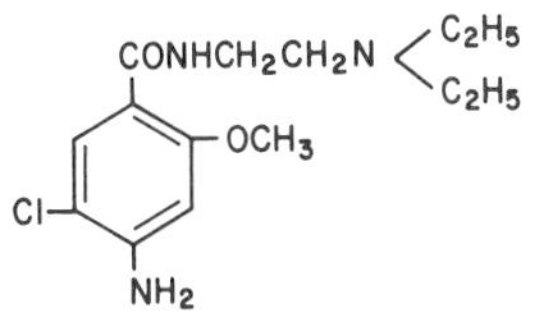

FIGURE 26-1. Metoclopramide.

Clinical Uses

Clinical uses of metoclopramide include (1) preoperative reduction of gastric fluid volume, (2) treatment of gastroparesis, and (3) production of an antiemetic effect. Increased prolactin secretion evoked by metoclopramide has been proposed as a means to test the function of the anterior pituitary or to improve lactation in the postpartum period (Schulze-Delrieu, 1981). Metoclopramide has been used to improve the effectiveness of oral medication when other drugs or the patients underlying condition slows gastric emptying (Nimmo, 1976). A possible benefit of metoclopramide in the management of patients with reflux esophagitis is suggested by the ability of this drug to increase lower esophageal sphincter tone. Indeed, metoclopramide reduces the incidence of heartburn (Johnson, 1971). Nevertheless, lower esophageal sphincter tone has probably been overrated as a factor in reflux esophagitis (Schulze-Delrieu, 1981).

PREOPERATIVE REDUCTION OF GASTRIC FLUID VOLUME. Metoclopramide, 10 to 20 mg administered intravenously over 3 to 5 minutes 15 to 30 minutes before induction of anesthesia, results in increased lower esophageal sphincter tone and a reduction in gastric fluid volume (Howard and Sharp, 1973; Wyner and Cohen, 1982). More rapid intravenous administration may produce abdominal cramping. This gastric emptying effect of metoclopramide would be of particular benefit prior to the induction of anesthesia in (1) the patient who has eaten, (2) the trauma patient, (3) the obese patient, (4) outpatients, and (5) parturients, especially those with a history of heartburn, suggesting lower esophageal sphincter dysfunction and gastric hypomotility. Nevertheless, beneficial effects of metoclopramide on gastric fluid volume may be difficult to document in otherwise normal patients with low gastric fluid volumes awaiting elective surgery (Table 26-5) (Cohen et al, 1984a). Regardless of the effect on gastric fluid volume, the administration of metoclopramide does not reliably alter gastric fluid pH. Furthermore, it is important to recognize that opioid-induced inhibition of gastric motility may not be reversible with metoclopramide (Nimmo et al, 1976). Likewise, the beneficial cholinergic stimulant effects of metoclopramide on the gastrointestinal tract may be offset by concomitant administration of atropine as in the preoperative medication.

Under no circumstances does metoclopramide or other protective drugs (e.g., antacids, H_2 receptor antagonists) replace the need for protection of the airway with a cuffed tracheal tube placed in the awake patient or following the appropriate induction of general anesthesia.

Table 26-5
Volume of Gastric Contents and pH in Study Groups

	Metoclopramide (n − 30)	Placebo (n − 28)
Gastric volume	24 ± 2 ml	30 ± 5 ml
(range)	(3–60)	(4–155)
Volume above 25 ml	16[t]	15[t]
	(53%)	(54%)
Gastric pH	2.86 ± 0.27	2.55 ± 0.24
(range)	(1–6)	(1–5.5)
pH below 2.5	12[t]	16[t]
	(40%)	(57%)

* Mean ± SEM
t = number of patients
(Data from Cohen SE, Jasson J, Talafre M–L, Chauvelot–Moachan L, Barrier G. Does metoclopramide decrease the volume of gastric contents in patients undergoing cesarean section? Anesthesiology 1984;61:604–7; with permission.)

TREATMENT OF GASTROPARESIS. Treatment of gastroparesis, as associated with diabetes mellitus, is with orally administered metoclopramide, 10 to 20 mg. Intravenous administration of metoclopramide, 10 to 20 mg, is indicated to facilitate small bowel intubation or to speed gastric emptying to improve radiographic examination of the small intestine. This dose should be administered over 3 to 5 minutes to minimize the likelihood of abdominal cramping.

PRODUCTION OF AN ANTIEMETIC EFFECT. The antiemetic properties of metoclopramide result from its antagonism of dopamine receptors in the central nervous system (*i.e.*, vomiting center and chemoreceptor trigger zone) and its selective peripheral cholinergic stimulant effects of the proximal gastrointestinal tract (Dundee and Clarke, 1973). In this regard, metoclopramide has been used for treatment of hyperemesis gravidarum and nausea due to chemotherapy. Reports of its antiemetic efficacy in the postoperative period have been inconsistent, perhaps reflecting the brief duration of action of metoclopramide (Cohen *et al*, 1984b). In ambulatory patients, despite lack of an antiemetic effect, metoclopramide is associated with a decreased incidence of postoperative dizziness (Cohen *et al*, 1984b). All factors considered, it may be more appropriate to treat only those patients who experience protracted postoperative vomiting rather than routinely administer to all patients an antiemetic with potential adverse effects.

Side Effects

Side effects of metoclopramide are mild and infrequent but include sedation, dysphoria, agitation, dry mouth, glossal or periorbital edema, hirsutism, and urticarial or maculopapular rash. These side effects, including sedation, have not been observed following single doses of metoclopramide (Cohen *et al*, 1984a). Extrapyramidal reactions are rare but have been observed when large doses (40–80 mg daily) were administered for many months. These extrapyramidal reactions are identical to the Parkinsonism syndrome evoked by antipsychotic drugs that antagonize the central nervous system actions of dopamine (Grimes *et al*, 1982) (see Chapter 19). Akathisia, a feeling of unease and restlessness of the lower limbs, seems to be related to plasma concentrations of metoclopramide that exceed 100 ng ml^{-1}. This response has been noted even with short-term use, particularly in young children or elderly patients with renal dysfunction.

Placental transfer of metoclopramide occurs rapidly, but adverse fetal effects with single doses have not been observed (Cohen *et al*, 1984a). The usual dopamine-induced inhibition of aldosterone secretion is prevented by metoclopramide. As a result, the possibility of sodium retention and hypokalemia should be considered, especially in patients who develop edema during chronic therapy (Carey *et al*, 1979). The major concern of chronic therapy with metoclopramide is stimulation of prolactin secretion and resulting galactorrhea. For this reason, patients with a history of carcinoma of the breast probably should not be treated with metoclopramide.

Metoclopramide may increase the sedative actions of central nervous system depressants and the incidence of extrapyramidal reactions caused by certain drugs. For this reason, metoclopramide should not be given in combination with phenothiazine or butyrophenone drugs or to patients with extrapyramidal symptoms or epilepsy. Patients being treated with monoamine oxidase inhibitors or tricyclic antidepressants should not receive metoclopramide. This drug reduces the bioavailability of orally administered cimetidine by 25% to 50% (Gugler *et al*, 1981). Metoclopramide is contraindicated in the presence of gastrointestinal obstruction, and pheochromocytoma.

ANTIEMETICS (See Chapters 19 and 21)

Domperidone

Domperidone, like metoclopramide, is a dopamine receptor antagonist (Fig. 26-2). Unlike metoclopramide, domperidone does not easily cross the blood–brain barrier, thus its antidopaminergic activity is limited to peripheral sites. Indeed, extrapyramidal reactions do not accompany

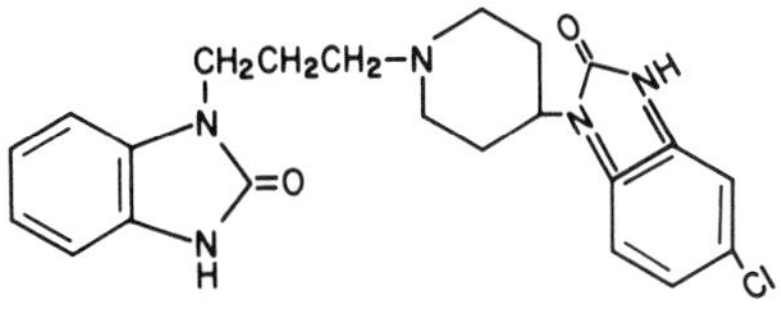

FIGURE 26-2. Domperidone.

administration of domperidone. Restriction of antidopaminergic activity to peripheral sites allows domperidone to influence the chemoreceptor trigger zone, which is outside the blood–brain barrier, without affecting the basal ganglia. Domperidone increases lower esophageal sphincter tone and speeds gastric emptying (Brock-Utne, 1980).

Domperidone appears to be particularly effective in the treatment of postprandial nausea and vomiting and nausea associated with gastroenteritis (Reyntjens, 1979). It may be useful for nausea and vomiting associated with dysmenorrhea, migraine headache, and radiation therapy. Domperidone is of no value for postoperative nausea and vomiting or that induced by opioids and is of limited value against vomiting induced by chemotherapeutic drugs (Fragen and Caldwell, 1979).

Domperidone is rapidly absorbed after oral or intramuscular administration. Metabolism occurs in the liver, and biliary excretion of inactive metabolites is the main route of elimination. The elimination half-time is about 7 hours.

Benzquinamide

Benzquinamide is a short-acting benzquinoline derivative (*i.e.*, an ataractic) that is used most often to prevent postoperative nausea and vomiting (Fig. 26-3). This drug apparently inhibits stimuli at the chemoreceptor trigger zone. The intramuscular dose is 0.5 to 1 mg kg^{-1} injected at least 15 minutes prior to administration of antineoplastic drugs or emergence from anesthesia. The intravenous dose of benzquinamide is 0.2 to 0.4 mg kg^{-1}. Elimination half-time is brief, being about 40 minutes.

Side Effects

Drowsiness is noted frequently following administration of benzquinamide. Shivering, chills, and

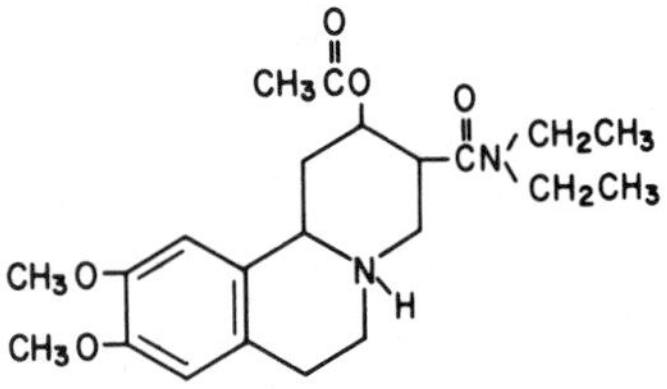

FIGURE 26-3. Benzquinamide.

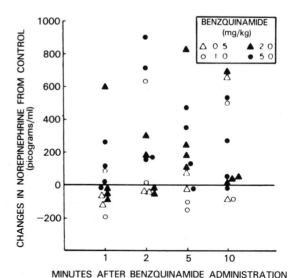

FIGURE 26-4. Intravenous administration of benzquinamide is accompanied by reflex activation of the sympathetic nervous system that often manifests as increased plasma concentrations of norepinephrine. (From Smith DJ, Rushin JM, Urquilla PR, *et al,* Cardiovascular effects of benzquinamide. Anesth Analg 1979;58:189–94. Reproduced by permission of the authors and the International Anesthesia Research Society.)

mild anticholinergic reactions have been observed. Benzquinamide directly relaxes vascular smooth muscle, producing reduction in peripheral vascular resistance and hypotension that are compensated for by reflex activation of the sympathetic nervous system that manifests as increased circulating concentrations of norepinephrine (Fig. 26-4) (Smith *et al,* 1979). Reflex increases in heart rate and cardiac output are also possible. Indeed, sudden increases in blood pressure and cardiac dysrhythmias may accompany rapid intravenous administration benzquinamide. Administration of benzquinamide to patients with moderate to severe hypertension or severe cardiovascular disease may be questionable, particularly if the drug is given intravenously during anesthesia.

The modest ventilatory stimulant effect of benzquinamide may offset opioid-induced depression of ventilation (Mull and Smith, 1974). Conversely, phenothiazine antiemetics can potentiate opioid-induced depression of ventilation.

Benzquinamide has anticholinergic properties and can induce delirium (*i.e.*, central anticholinergic syndrome) that is responsive to physostigmine (Chapin and Wingard, 1977). Conversely, in other patients, benzquinamide may produce dystonic extrapyramidal reactions (Rose and Averbuch, 1975). It is important to distinguish between these two responses, since administration of physostigmine in the presence of extrapyramidal effects produced by benzquinamide could cause the symptoms to become worse (Ambani *et al*, 1973). Likewise, treating a patient with drug-induced central anticholinergic syndrome with atropine would be deleterious. An important difference between these two reactions is the impairment of consciousness during anticholinergic excess but not during extrapyramidal responses.

Tetrahydrocannabinol

Tetrahydrocannabinol (THC) is the psychoactive component of marijuana that possesses antiemetic efficacy when given orally during cancer chemotherapy (Poster *et al*, 1981). This antiemetic effect is more effective in patients treated with methotrexate than in those treated with cyclophosphamide, doxorubicin, and cisplatin. THC may also be effective as an antiemetic in patients who develop tolerance to the phenothiazines.

The antiemetic effect of THC lasts 2 to 3 hours, which parallels its psychoactive effects. The occasional dysphoric response or hallucinations limit the usefulness of THC as an antiemetic, particularly in patients with psychiatric disorders. Administration of THC to patients with epilepsy is questionable, because the drug may enhance seizure activity. THC may produce transient tachycardia, and large doses may cause orthostatic hypotension. These effects should be considered before THC is administered to patients with coronary artery or valvular heart disease. In animals, the acute intravenous administration of THC produces a transient dose-related reduction in anesthetic requirements (*e.g.*, MAC) that parallels sedative effects (Fig. 26-5) (Stoelting *et al*, 1973; Vitez *et al*, 1973).

THC is slowly and erratically absorbed from the gastrointestinal tract. The peak plasma concentration is reached in 60 to 90 minutes. Protein binding is extensive, accounting for 97% to 99% of the drug. Following systemic absorption, THC is converted to 11-hydroxyl-THC, which possesses equivalent pharmacologic activity. Subsequent

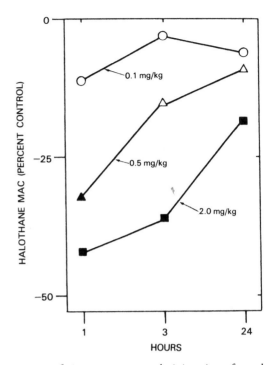

FIGURE 26-5. Intravenous administration of tetrahydrocannabinol produces a transient dose-dependent reduction in anesthetic requirements (MAC) for halothane. (From Stoelting RK, Martz RC, Gartner J, Creasser C, Brown DJ, Forney RB. Effects of delta-9-tetrahydrocannabinol on halothane MAC in dogs. Anesthesiology 1973;38:521–4. Reproduced by permission of the authors and publisher.)

metabolism results in inactive compounds that are excreted in the urine and feces. The elimination half-time for THC is about 19 hours, and that of its metabolites is about 48 hours (Anderson and McGuire, 1981).

Diphenidol

Diphenidol acts on the vestibular apparatus and is useful as an antiemetic for nausea and vomiting associated with radiation, chemotherapeutic drugs, and general anesthesia (Fig. 26-6). This drug is also effective in labyrinthine-induced vertigo following surgery on the middle and inner ear. Because of its central anticholinergic actions, diphenidol may induce visual or auditory hallucinations, disorientation, or confusion. Dryness of

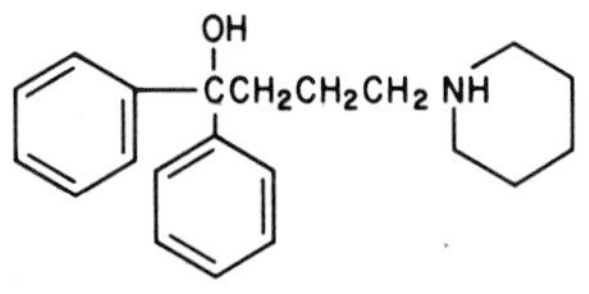

FIGURE 26-6. Diphenidol.

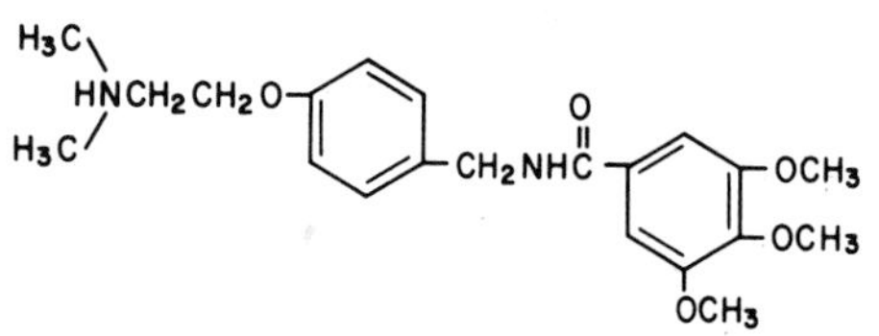

FIGURE 26-7. Trimethobenzamide.

the mouth, sedation, and tachycardia may occur. More than 90% of diphenidol is eliminated by the kidney.

Trimethobenzamide

Trimethobenzamide is useful as an antiemetic by inhibiting stimuli at the chemoreceptor trigger zone (Fig. 26-7). It is not as effective as phenothiazines in treating postoperative vomiting and has little or no value in the prevention of treatment of vertigo or motion sickness. Extrapyramidal reactions have been noted.

REFERENCES

Alfrey AC, LeGendre GR, Kaehny WS. The dialysis encephalopathy syndrome. Possible aluminum intoxication. N Engl J Med 1976;294:184–8.

Ambani CM, VanWoert MH, Bowers MB. Physostigmine effects on phenothiazine-induced extrapyrimidal reactions. Arch Neurol 1973;29:444–6.

Anderson PO, McGuire GG. Delta-9-tetrahydrocannabinol as an antiemetic. Am J Hosp Pharm 1981;38:639–46.

Berlyne GM, Ben-Ari J, Pest D, et al. Hyperaluminaemia from aluminum resins in renal failure. Lancet 1970;2:494–6.

Bond VK, Stoelting RK, Gupta CD. Pulmonary aspiration syndrome after inhalation of gastric fluid containing antacids. Anesthesiology 1979;51:452–3.

Brock-Utne JG, Dow TGB, Welman S, Dimopoulos GE, Moshal MG. The effect of metoclopramide on lower oesophageal sphincter tone in late pregnancy. Anaesth Intensive Care 1978;6:26–9.

Brock-Utne JG, Downing JW, Dimopoulos GE, Rubin J, Moshal MG. Effect of domperidone on lower esophageal sphincter tone in late pregnancy. Anesthesiology 1980;52:321–3.

Brock-Utne JG, Rubin J, Downing JW, Dimopoulos GE, Moshal MG, Naiker M. The administration of metoclopramide with atropine. Anaesthesia 1976;31:1186–90.

Carey RM, Thorner MO, Ortt EM. Effects of metoclopramide and bromocriptine on the renin-angiotensin-aldosterone system in man: dopaminergic control of aldosterone. J Clin Invest 1979;63:727–35.

Chapin JW, Wingard DW. Physostigmine reversal of benzquinamide-induced delirium. Anesthesiology 1977;46:364–5.

Clayman CB. The carbonate affair: Chalk one up (editorial). JAMA 1980;244:2554.

Cohen SE, Jasson J, Talafre M–L, Chauvelot–Moachon L, Barrier G. Does metoclopramide decrease the volume of gastric contents in patients undergoing cesarean section? Anesthesiology 1984a;61:604–7.

Cohen SE, Woods WA, Wyner J. Antiemetic efficacy of droperidol and metoclopramide. Anesthesiology 1984b;60:67–9.

Conklin KA, Ziadlou-Rad F. Buffering capacity of citrate antacids. Anesthesiology 1983;58:391–2.

Cooke N, Teitelbaum S, Avioli LV. Antacid-induced osteomalacia and nephrolithiasis. Arch Intern Med 1978;138:1007–9.

Dundee JW, Clarke RSJ. The premedicant and antiemetic action of metoclopramide. Postgrad Med 1973;48:34–7.

Eyler SW, Cullen BF, Murphy ME, Welch WD. Antacid aspiration in rabbits: a comparison of Mylanta and Bicitra. Anesth Analg 1982;61:288–92.

Fragen RJ, Caldwell N. Antiemetic effectiveness of intramuscularly administered domperidone. Anesthesiology 1979;51:460–1.

Gibbs CP, Schwartz DJ, Wynne JW, Hood CI, Kuck EJ. Antacid pulmonary aspiration in the dog. Anesthesiology 1979;51:380–5.

Gibbs CP, Spohr L, Schmidt D. The effectiveness of sodium citrate as an antacid. Anesthesiology 1982;57:44–6.

Grimes JD, Hassan MN, Preston DN. Adverse neurologic effects of metoclopramide. Can Med Assoc J 1982;126:23–5.

Gugler R, Brand M, Somogyi A. Impaired cimetidine absorption due to antacids and metoclopramide. Eur J Clin Pharmacol 1981;20:225–8.

Heaney GAH, Jones HD. Aspiration syndrome in pregnancy (correspondence). Br J Anaesth 1979;51:266–7.

Holdsworth JD, Johnson K, Mascall G, Roulston RG, Tomlinson PA. Mixing of antacids with stomach contents. Anaesthesia 1980;35:641–50.

Howard FA, Sharp DS. Effects of metoclopramide on gastric emptying during labour. Br Med J 1973;1:446 – 8.

Hurwitz A, Robinson RG, Vats TS, Whittier FC, Herrin WF. Effects of antacids on gastric emptying. Gastroenterology 1976;71:268 – 73.

James CF, Modell JH, Gibbs CP, Kuck EJ, Ruiz BC. Pulmonary aspiration effects of volume and pH in the rat. Anesth Analg 1984;63:665 – 8.

Johnson AG. Controlled trial of metoclopramide in the treatment of flatulent dyspepsia. Br Med J 1971;2:25 – 6.

Martin F, Farley A, Gagnon M, Bensemana D. Comparison of healing capacities of sucralfate and cimetidine in short-term treatment of duodenal ulcer: Double-blind randomized trial. Gastroenterology 1982;82:401 – 5.

McHardy GG. Multicenter double-blind trial of sucralfate and placebo in duodenal ulcer. J Clin Gastroenterol 1981;3:S147 – 52.

Mull TD, Smith TC. Comparison of the ventilatory effects of two antiemetics, benzquinamide and prochlorperazine. Anesthesiology 1974;40:581 – 7.

Nimmo WS. Drugs, diseases, and altered gastric emptying. Clin Pharmacokinet 1976;1:189 – 203.

O'Sullivan GM, Bullingham RE. Noninvasive assessment by radiotelemetry of antacid effect during labor. Anesth Analg 1985;64:95 – 100.

Poster DS, Penta JS, Bruno S, MacDonald JS. Delta-nine-tetrahydrocannabinol in clinical oncology. JAMA 1981;245:2047 – 51.

Reyntjens A. Domperidone as antiemetic: Summary of research reports. Postgrad Med J 1979;55:50 – 4.

Rose TE, Averbuch SD. Acute dystonic reaction to benzquinamide. Ann Intern Med 1975;83:231 – 2.

Schulze-Delrieu. Drug therapy: Metoclopramide. N Engl J Med 1981;305:28 – 33.

Smith DJ, Rushin JM, Urquilla PR, et al. Cardiovascular effects of benzquinamide. Anesth Analg 1979;58:189 – 94.

Stoelting RK. Responses to atropine, glycopyrrolate, and Riopan of gastric fluid pH and volume in adult patients. Anesthesiology 1978;48:367 – 9.

Stoelting RK, Martz RC, Gartner J, Creasser C, Brown DJ, Forney RB. Effects of delta-9-tetrahydrocannabinol on halothane MAC in dogs. Anesthesiology 1973;38:521 – 4.

Taylor G. Acid pulmonary aspiration syndrome after antacids. Br J Anaesth 1975;47:615 – 6.

Tompkinson J, Turnbull A, Robson R, et al. Report on Confidential Enquiries into Maternal Deaths in England and Wales 1976 – 1978. London, Her Majesty's Stationery Office, 1982;79 – 80.

Viegas OJ, Ravindran RS, Shumacker CA. Gastric fluid pH in patients receiving sodium citrate. Anesth Analg 1981;60:521 – 3.

Vitez TS, Way WL, Miller RD, Eger EI. Effects of delta-9-tetrahydrocannabinol on cyclopropane MAC in the rat. Anesthesiology 1973;38:525 – 7.

Wyner J, Cohen SE. Gastric volume in early pregnancy: Effect of metoclopramide. Anesthesiology 1982;57:209 – 12.

Anticoagulants

INTRODUCTION

Anticoagulants are drugs that delay or prevent the clotting of blood by direct or indirect actions on the coagulation system (see Chapter 57). These drugs, however, have no effect on the thrombus (*i.e.*, clot) after it is formed. Antithrombotic drugs usually influence the formation of thrombus by an action on platelets. Thrombolytic drugs are those that possess inherent fibrinolytic effects or enhance the body's fibrinolytic system.

HEPARIN

Heparin is a water-soluble mucopolysaccharide organic acid that is present endogenously in high concentrations in the liver and granules of mast cells and basophils. The designation, heparin, emphasizes the abundance of this substance in the liver (see Chapter 57).

Commercial Preparations

Heparin for clinical uses is most commonly prepared from bovine lung and bovine or porcine gastrointestinal mucosa. Standardization of heparin potency is based on *in vitro* comparison with a known standard. A unit of heparin is defined as the volume of heparin-containing solution that will prevent 1 ml of citrated sheep blood from clotting for 1 hour following the addition of 0.2 ml of 1:100 calcium chloride. Heparin must contain at least 120 U.S.P. units per ml. Because the potency of different commercial preparations of heparin may vary greatly, the heparin dose should always be prescribed in units.

Clinical Uses

Commercially prepared solutions of heparin are used exclusively to produce an anticoagulant effect. Associated with this anticoagulant effect is a reduction in plasma triglyceride concentrations owing to heparin-induced release of lipid-hydrolyzing enzymes, such as lipoprotein lipase, into the circulation.

The onset of anticoagulant effect is almost instantaneous following intravenous injection of heparin and occurs 20 to 30 minutes after subcutaneous injection. In addition to providing anticoagulation during specific operative procedures, low-dose heparin is efficacious as a primary prophylaxis against postoperative deep vein thrombosis and pulmonary embolism. For example, the incidence of pulmonary embolism is reduced in patients older than 40 years of age undergoing abdominal–thoracic surgery who are treated with low-dose heparin (Cerrato *et al,* 1978). Treatment is initiated with 5000 units administered subcutaneously about 2 hours before surgery and repeated every 8 to 12 hours postoperatively.

Continuous intravenous infusion of a solution containing a small amount of heparin is commonly used to maintain patency of intravascular catheters. Some catheters for intravascular use and tubing for cardiopulmonary bypass are impregnated with heparin to prevent deposition of thrombus on the surface of the material. Heparin has been recommended for use in the treatment of disseminated intravascular coagulation. The rationale is that heparin will arrest intravascular coagulation, which will allow accumulation of normal amounts of coagulation factors with subsequent cessation of bleeding. Conversely, heparin may aggravate symptoms of disseminated intravascular coagulation, making it difficult to select patients who would benefit from this unconventional therapeutic approach (Hamilton *et al,* 1978).

Mechanism of Action

The anticoagulant effect of heparin is due to its ability to accelerate the formation of antithrombin III, which is an α_2-globulin normally present in the plasma (Seegers, 1978). Antithrombin III forms a complex with activated thrombin, resulting in neutralization of thrombin activity, thus preventing the conversion of fibrinogen to fibrin (see Fig. 57-1). Antithrombin III also neutralizes activated factor X, thus preventing conversion of prothrombin to thrombin (see Fig. 57-1). Thus, heparin functions as an anticoagulant by accelerating antithrombin III – induced neutralization of activated clotting factors. Low doses of heparin seem to exert predominant effects on factor X, whereas large doses of heparin have predominant effects on antithrombin III.

Route of Administration

Heparin is a poorly lipid-soluble high – molecular weight substance that cannot cross lipid barriers in significant amounts. As a result, it is not effective when administered orally. Likewise, maternal administration of heparin does not result in passage across the placenta to the fetus.

Deep subcutaneous (intrafat) injection of heparin is recommended when low-dose therapy is being administered for a prolonged effect in ambulatory patients. Intramuscular administration of heparin is avoided because of the risk of hematoma formation.

Administration of high doses of heparin is accomplished by intermittent or continuous intrave-nous injection. Intermittent intravenous therapy is often performed by means of an indwelling, rubber-capped needle (*i.e.*, heparin lock). The size and frequency of the maintenance dose of heparin are based on the anticoagulant response to the previous dose as measured 1 hour previously (see the section entitled Laboratory Evaluation of Anticoagulation). Continuous intravenous infusion of heparin is by means of constant infusion pump that delivers about 1000 units hr^{-1}.

Duration of Action

The duration of action of heparin is dependent on body temperature and the dose of drug administered. For example, intravenous doses of 100, 200, and 400 units kg^{-1} have elimination half-times of 56, 96, and 152 minutes, respectively, and these durations are prolonged by reductions in body temperature below 37 Celsius (Bull *et al*, 1975). The duration of action of heparin is also prolonged in the presence of hepatic and renal dysfunction (Teien, 1977) (see the section entitled Clearance). Conversely, patients with pulmonary embolism require larger doses because of more rapid clearance of the drug (Simon *et al*, 1978).

Clearance

Heparin is metabolized in the liver by the enzyme heparinase, and pharmacologically inactive metabolites are eliminated by the kidneys. A portion is also metabolized by depolymerization to an inactive product known as *uroheparin*. Unchanged heparin appears in the urine only after large doses are administered intravenously.

Laboratory Evaluation of Coagulation

Heparin effect is monitored by the partial thromboplastin time (PTT) or activated coagulation (clotting) time (ACT) or both (Hattersley, 1966). Bleeding time is not altered by heparin.

Partial Thromboplastin Time

The PTT in the patient treated with heparin should be maintained at about twice the patient's predrug value of 30 to 35 seconds. An excessively prolonged PTT (greater than 120 seconds) is readily shortened by omitting a dose, since heparin has a short elimination half-time. When low-dose heparin therapy is used, laboratory tests may not be required to monitor treatment since the dosage and schedule are well known.

Activated Coagulation Time

Heparin effect and its antagonism by protamine is commonly monitored in patients undergoing surgical procedures by measurement of the ACT. A baseline value for the ACT is determined (1) prior to the intravenous administration of heparin, (2) about 3 minutes after the administration of heparin, and (3) at 30-minute intervals thereafter. A dose–response curve for heparin can be constructed with the dose of heparin in mg kg^{-1} on the vertical axis and the ACT in seconds on the horizontal axis (Fig. 27-1) (Bull *et al*, 1975). A line connecting the points before and 3 minutes after heparin is used to calculate the additional dose of heparin necessary to achieve an acceptable ACT.

The control ACT is usually 90 to 120 seconds. During cardiopulmonary bypass, the anticoagulant effect of heparin is often considered adequate when the ACT is above 300 seconds, questionable with ACT levels between 180 to 300 seconds, and inadequate at levels below 130 seconds. In animals, however, fibrin monomers may appear during cardiopulmonary bypass at ACT levels lower than 400 seconds (Young *et al*, 1978). The need for measurement of ACT is emphasized by the fourfold variation in heparin sensitivity between patients and the threefold variation in the rate at which heparin is metabolized.

Side Effects

Hemorrhage

Hemorrhage is the most serious complication associated with heparin therapy. This complication is minimized by control of dosage based on laboratory measurement of heparin effect (see the section entitled Laboratory Evaluation of Anticoagulation).

Heparin should not be administered to patients with known bleeding tendencies or to persons undergoing intraocular or intracranial surgery. Performance of a lumbar subarachnoid or epidural for injection of a drug has been questioned in the patient who is receiving, or will sub-

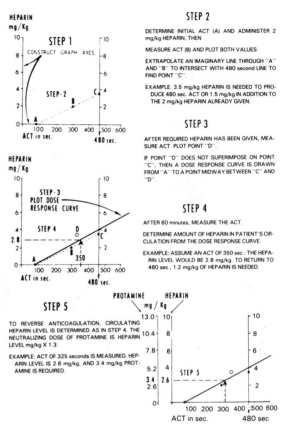

FIGURE 27-1. Calculation of heparin and protamine doses based on measurement of the activated coagulation time (ACT). (From Bull BS, Huse WM, Brauer FS, Korpman RA. Heparin therapy during extracorporeal circulation, II. The use of a dose–response curve to individualize heparin and protamine dosage. J Thorac Cardiovasc Surg 1975;69:685–9. Reproduced by permission of the authors and publisher.)

sequently receive, heparin. The concern is related to the possible occurrence of an epidural hematoma and compression of the spinal cord if a blood vessel were punctured during performance of these injections. Likewise, hematomas and compression of peripheral nerves may be more likely to occur in association with performance of a peripheral nerve block in a patient being treated with heparin. Despite these concerns, a large retrospective study did not confirm an increased incidence of epidural hematoma formation in patients receiving a spinal or epidural anesthetic followed by heparin anticoagulation (Rao and El-Etr, 1981).

Allergic Reactions

Heparin is obtained from animal tissues; thus, caution should be used in its administration to patients with a pre-existing history of allergy. Indeed, fever, urticaria, and even cardiopulmonary changes occasionally occur after administration of heparin.

Thrombocytopenia

Mild and usually clinically insignificant thrombocytopenia occurs in 30% to 40% of heparin-treated patients, reflecting drug-induced platelet aggregation (Esposito *et al,* 1983). Approximately 0.6% of patients develop severe thrombocytopenia (often less than 5000 mm^{-3}) after 7 to 10 days of heparin therapy (Esposito *et al,* 1983). This severe response is probably due to formation of heparin-dependent antiplatelet antibodies that trigger platelet aggregation and resulting thrombocytopenia. All patients treated chronically with heparin should have frequent platelet counts to provide early warning of the development of life-threatening thrombocytopenia. This drug-induced thrombocytopenia is associated with resistance to the anticoagulant effects of heparin and an increased incidence of thromboembolism. Discontinuation of heparin is necessary if excessive thrombocytopenia occurs.

Patients with a history of heparin-induced thrombocytopenia who subsequently require surgical procedures involving cardiopulmonary bypass present a therapeutic dilemma. Although experience is limited, preoperative preparation with a platelet-inhibiting drug such as dipyridamole may be efficacious in reducing platelet aggregation in these patients (Smith *et al,* 1985). Another option would be to use warfarin for anticoagulation during cardiopulmonary bypass, but the difficulty posed in rapid reversal of this drug is a major disadvantage.

Altered Protein Binding

Acute administration of heparin, as before cardiac catheterization or initiation of cardiopulmonary bypass, displaces basic drugs from protein binding sites. Evidence of this displacement is increased circulating concentrations of unbound fractions of propranolol and diazepam following the administration of heparin (Fig. 27-2) (Wood *et al,* 1980). It is conceivable that increased pharma-

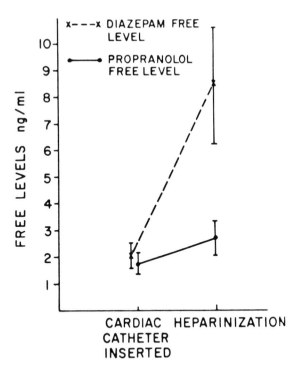

FIGURE 27-2. Administration of heparin displaces diazepam and propranolol from protein binding sites leading to an increase in unbound (free) concentration of these drugs in the plasma. (By permission, Wood AJJ, Robertson D, Robertson RM, Wilkinson GR, Wood M. Elevated plasma-free drug concentrations of propranolol and diazepam during cardiac catheterization. Circulation 1980; 62:1119–22 and the American Heart Association, Inc.)

cologic effects of propranolol and diazepam would accompany this heparin-induced reduction in protein binding. Certainly, measurement of plasma concentrations of drugs in heparinized blood must be interpreted differently than in the absence of heparin.

Cardiovascular Changes

Rapid intravenous infusion of large doses of heparin (300 units kg^{-1}) as administered prior to cardiopulmonary bypass may cause modest reductions in mean arterial pressure and pulmonary artery pressure (Konchigeri, 1984). These changes principally reflect decreases in peripheral vascular resistance, perhaps due to a direct heparin–relaxant effect on vascular smooth muscle. Ionized calcium concentrations are decreased in a dose-dependent manner by *in vitro,* but not *in vivo,* administration of heparin (Goto *et al,* 1985). These results indicate that blood pressure declines that are occasionally observed following administration of heparin are not related to changes in the plasma concentrations of ionized calcium.

Decreased Antithrombin III Concentrations

Paradoxically, patients who receive intermittent or continuous therapy with heparin manifest a progressive reduction of antithrombin III activity to values that approximate one third of normal (Marciniak and Gockerman, 1977). Thus, a heparin-induced reduction of the activity of antithrombin III may paradoxically increase the thrombotic tendency in man. Estrogen-containing contraceptives also decrease concentrations of antithrombin III, which is consistent with the clinical impression that the incidence of thromboembolic episodes are increased in patients who take these drugs. Patients with genetically determined low levels of antithrombin III have a tendency to develop thromboembolism and may manifest increased dose requirements for heparin (Anderson, 1986). When heparin resistance is secondary to a deficiency in antithrombin III, administration of fresh frozen plasma restores the levels to normal and promotes the anticoagulant effects of heparin.

Altered Cell Morphology

Heparin added to whole blood distorts the morphology of leukocytes and erythrocytes. For this reason, heparinized blood is not acceptable for tests that involve complement, isoagglutinins, or erythrocyte fragility. Hematocrit, white blood cell count, and erythrocyte sedimentation rate are not altered by the presence of heparin.

Protamine

Protamine is the specific antagonist of heparin's anticoagulant effect. Protamines are strongly basic low–molecular weight proteins found in sperm and testes of certain fish. The basic protamine combines with acidic heparin to form a stable complex that is devoid of anticoagulant activity. Despite the formation of this complex, the effect of heparin on platelet aggregation may persist and be responsible for continued bleeding, especially after cardiopulmonary bypass (Ellison *et al,* 1978). The dose of protamine required to antagonize heparin is 1 to 1.3 mg for every 100 units of heparin predicted to still be circulating. A more specific dose of protamine is calculated by *in vitro* titration of the patient's blood with protamine (Fig. 27-1) (Bull *et al,* 1975). A guideline is administration of 1.3 mg kg^{-1} of protamine for each 100 units of heparin present as calculated from the ACT.

Protamine administered intravenously in the absence of heparin interacts with platelets and proteins, including fibrinogen. These interactions may manifest as an anticoagulant effect of protamine.

Cardiovascular Effects

Rapid intravenous injection of protamine may be associated with evidence of histamine release, including facial flushing, bronchoconstriction, tachycardia, and hypotension. Indeed, protamine is a basic drug that would be expected to evoke release of histamine, particularly if the rate of intravenous injection is rapid. Infusion of protamine (3 – 5 mg kg^{-1}) over 5 minutes to reverse heparin anticoagulation at the conclusion of cardiopulmonary bypass is not, however, associated with evidence of histamine release (Stoelting *et al,* 1984). Furthermore, there is no evidence that protamine has direct negative inotropic or chronotropic effects in patients (Conahan *et al,* 1981; Sethna *et al,* 1982). Patients with poor left ventricular function, however, may be more susceptible to protamine-induced reductions in blood pressure since compensatory increases in cardiac output to offset peripheral vasodilation are limited (Michaels and Barash, 1983). Protamine has been reported to produce pulmonary vascular vasoconstriction with corresponding increases in pulmonary vascular resistance (Lowenstein *et al,* 1983).

The site of intravenous administration may influence the subsequent circulatory changes evoked by protamine. For example, administration of protamine into the right atrium of anesthetized dogs is followed by (1) elevations in the plasma concentration of histamine, (2) increases in cardiac output, and (3) decreases in blood pressure and peripheral vascular resistance (Casthely *et al,* 1986). These changes do not occur when protamine is injected into a peripheral vein or the

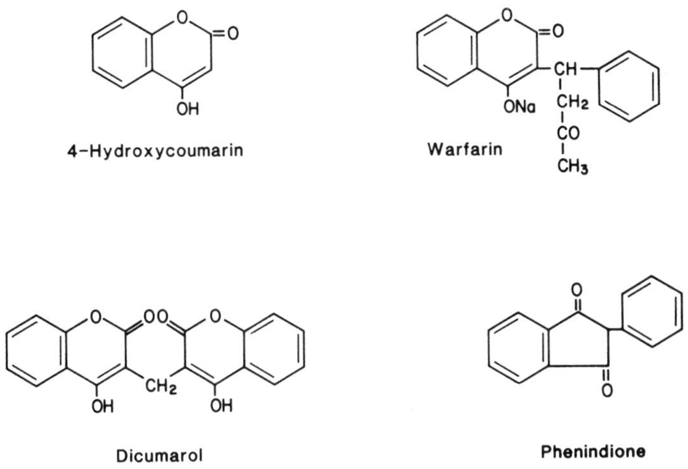

4-Hydroxycoumarin

Warfarin

Dicumarol

Phenindione

FIGURE 27-3. Oral anticoagulants are derivatives of 4-hydroxycoumarin.

left atrium. It is speculated that the heparin–protamine complex that evokes the release of histamine in the lungs is diluted before reaching the lung when protamine is injected into a peripheral vein or the left atrium. Despite these animal data, intravenous or intra-arterial injection of protamine to patients has not been documented to produce different circulatory effects (Milne *et al*, 1983).

Allergic Reactions

Allergic reactions to protamine have been described most often in patients receiving protamine-containing insulin preparations (Doolan *et al*, 1981; Lakin *et al*, 1978; Moorthy *et al*, 1980). For example, there are approximately 2.8 mg of protamine per 100 units of protamine zinc insulin and 0.5 mg per 100 units of NPH insulin. Presumably, chronic exposure to low doses of protamine in patients treated with protamine-containing insulin preparations evokes the production of antibodies against protamine (see Chapter 24). In this situation, the subsequent administration of large doses of protamine, as required to antagonize heparin-induced anticoagulation, may result in life-threatening allergic reactions. Patients allergic to fish may also be at increased risk for development of allergic reactions to protamine (Knape *et al*, 1981). The presence of circulating anti-sperm antibodies in vasectomized or infertile males does not seem sufficient to increase the likelihood of allergic reactions to protamine.

Patients known to be allergic to protamine and requiring heparin anticoagulation, as for cardiopulmonary bypass, present a unique problem (Campbell *et al*, 1984). Proposed options include (1) pretreatment with histamine receptor antagonists followed by a slow trial intravenous infusion of protamine, (2) avoidance of protamine entirely, allowing the heparin effect to dissipate spontaneously, and (3) administration of an alternate heparin antagonist, hexadimethrine. Spontaneous dissipation of heparin effect may take several hours and is likely to be associated with substantial bleeding, requiring the administration of multiple blood transfusions. Hexadimethrine is the only drug alternative to protamine. In dogs, however, hexadimethrine produces hypotension, reductions in cardiac output, and increases in pulmonary vascular resistance that are more marked than hemodynamic derangements produced by protamine (Castaneda *et al*, 1967). In addition, hexadimethrine has an inherent anticoagulant effect resulting from inhibition of factor XII activation. For this reason, hexadimethrine must be administered by careful titration to avoid an exaggeration of the existing heparin-induced anticoagulant state. Most important, however, is the fact that hexadimethrine is not commercially available in the United States.

ORAL ANTICOAGULANTS

Oral anticoagulants are derivatives of 4-hydroxycoumarin (*i.e.*, coumarin) (Fig. 27-3). The essential chemical characteristics of coumarin derivatives for anticoagulant activity are an intact

4-hydroxycoumarin residue with a carbon substitution at the number 3 position. Among the coumarin derivatives, warfarin is the most widely used drug (Table 27-1) (Hull *et al*, 1978). Warfarin may be administered orally or parenterally.

Clinical Uses

Oral anticoagulants, in combination with dipyridamole, are commonly used to reduce the incidence of thromboembolism associated with prosthetic heart valves and atrial fibrillation in the presence of rheumatic heart disease. A frequent approach is an initial oral warfarin dose of 10 to 15 mg, followed by a daily maintenance dose of 2 to 15 mg as guided by the prothrombin time.

Mechanism of Action

The anticoagulant effect of coumarin derivatives is due to interference with hepatic synthesis of vitamin K–dependent clotting factors (*i.e.,* factors II, VII, IX, and X) (see Fig. 57-1). Specifically, coumarins prevent the reduction (carboxylation) of vitamin K from its inactive oxidized form. Normally, carboxylated residues bind calcium and facilitate orientation of clotting factors on a phospholipid surface, thus accelerating their interaction and subsequent generation of thrombin.

The anticoagulant effect of oral or intravenous warfarin is delayed for 8 to 12 hours, reflecting the onset of inhibition of synthesis of clotting factors and the elimination half-times of previously formed clotting factors that are not altered by the oral anticoagulant. Peak effects of warfarin do not occur for 36 to 72 hours. Large initial doses of warfarin (about 0.75 mg kg^{-1}) hasten the onset of hypoprothrombinemia only to a limited extent.

Distribution and Clearance

Warfarin is rapidly and completely absorbed, with peak concentrations in plasma occurring within 1 hour after oral ingestion. It is 97% bound to albumin, and this contributes to its negligible urinary excretion and long elimination half-time of 24 to 36 hours after oral administration. Elimination half-time is prolonged by exposure to trace concentrations of anesthetic gases, presumably reflecting inhibition of warfarin metabolism (Ghoneim *et al*, 1975). Extensive protein binding prevents diffusion into erythrocytes, cerebrospinal fluid, and breast milk (Orme *et al,* 1977). Warfarin does, however, cross the placenta and produces exaggerated responses in the fetus who has a limited ability to synthesize clotting factors.

Warfarin is metabolized to inactive metabolites that are conjugated with glucuronic acid and are ultimately excreted in the bile (*i.e.,* enterohepatic circulation) and urine.

Laboratory Evaluation of Anticoagulation

Treatment with oral anticoagulants is best guided by the prothrombin time. The prothrombin time is particularly sensitive to three of the four vitamin K–dependent clotting factors (*i.e.,* factors II, VII, and X). Conversion of the prothrombin time in seconds to percent of normal prothrombin activity

Table 27-1
Comparative Pharmacology of Oral Anticoagulants

	Time to Peak Effect (br)	*Duration After Discontinuation*	*Initial Dose (Adult, mg)*	*Maintenance Dose (Adult, mg)*
Warfarin	36–72	2–5	15—first day 10—second day 10—third day	2.5–10
Dicumarol	36–48	2–6	200–300 first day	25–200
Phenindione	18–24	1–2	300—first day 200—second day	50–150

compensates for variations between different laboratories. Patients receiving oral anticoagulants should be maintained at a prothrombin activity of about 25% of normal, which, in seconds, is about twice the normal baseline of 12 to 15 seconds.

An excessively prolonged prothrombin time (more than 30 seconds) is not readily shortened by omitting a dose because of the long elimination half-times of oral anticoagulants. Likewise, an inadequate therapeutic effect is not readily corrected by increasing the dose because of the delayed onset of therapeutic effect. These slow responses of oral anticoagulants contrast with rapid and predictable changes that are possible by virtue of altering the dose of heparin.

Inadequate diet, disease of the small intestine, impaired delivery of bile into the gastrointestinal tract, preexisting liver disease, and advanced age are associated with enhanced effects of oral anticoagulants (Williams *et al,* 1976). Pregnancy is accompanied by increased activity of factors VII, VIII, IX, and X and a resulting decreased responsiveness to oral anticoagulants. Hereditary resistance to oral anticoagulants is an autosomal dominant trait (O'Reilly, 1971).

Management Prior to Elective Surgery

Relatively minor surgical procedures can be safely performed in patients receiving oral anticoagulants. For major surgery, discontinuation of oral anticoagulants 1 to 3 days preoperatively is recommended so as to permit the prothrombin time to return to within 20% of the normal range (Tinker and Tarhan, 1978). This approach, followed by reinstitution of the oral anticoagulant regimen 1 to 7 days postoperatively, is not accompanied by an increased incidence of thromboembolic complications in vulnerable patients, such as those with prosthetic heart valves. In emergency situations, intravenous administration of vitamin K, fresh whole blood, or fresh frozen plasma may be necessary to abruptly counter the effects of oral anticoagulants (see Chapter 34).

Drug Interactions

Drug interactions occur between oral anticoagulants and salicylates, phenylbutazone, and barbiturates. For example, it is hazardous to administer any drug containing aspirin during anticoagulant therapy. Even a single 325-mg tablet of aspirin can impair platelet aggregation, and three aspirin tablets will prolong the bleeding time of most normal patients. Impairment of platelet aggregation owing to aspirin plus inhibition of formation of fibrin by oral anticoagulants can result in catastrophic hemorrhage. Acetaminophen and sodium salicylate lack effects on platelets and therefore do not interact adversely when administered for antipyresis to patients being treated with oral anticoagulants.

Phenylbutazone impairs platelet aggregation, displaces warfarin from albumin, and inhibits the metabolism of warfarin, leading to an enhanced anticoagulant effect (Leis *et al,* 1974). Disulfiram inhibits drug metabolism and prolongs the anticoagulant effect. Cimetidine prolongs prothrombin time by an unknown mechanism (Flind, 1978). Clofibrate reduces adhesiveness of platelets and stimulates the metabolism of vitamin K–dependent clotting factors so as to enhance responsiveness to oral anticoagulants.

Side Effects

Hemorrhage is the most serious side effect of oral anticoagulant therapy. In this regard, these drugs may increase the incidence of intracranial hemorrhage following a cerebrovascular accident. Bleeding may occur, even when the prothrombin time is in the desired therapeutic range. Compression neuropathy has been observed in treated patients following brachial artery puncture to obtain a sample for blood gas analysis. Treatment of mild hemorrhage is administration of vitamin K (phytonadione), 10 to 20 mg orally, or 1 to 5 mg intravenously at a rate of 1 mg min⁻¹, which will usually return the prothrombin time to a normal range within 4 to 24 hours (see Chapter 57).

Warfarin is associated with serious teratogenic effects when administered during the first trimester of pregnancy. Indeed, about one third of infants exposed to coumarin derivatives are stillborn or born with serious abnormalities such as nasal hypoplasia, stippled epiphyses, and blindness.

ANTITHROMBOTIC DRUGS

Antithrombotic drugs suppress platelet function and are used primarily for treatment of arterial thrombotic disease. In contrast, heparin and oral anticoagulants suppress function or synthesis of clotting factors and are used to control venous thromboembolic disorders. Platelet thrombi commonly occur in arterial walls, emphasizing the logic of using drugs that inhibit platelet aggregation in the treatment of arterial thromboembolic disease, especially that which leads to myocardial infarction or cerebrovascular accident (Olsson *et al*, 1980). Nevertheless, there are no statistically significant data from large prospective studies that prove that drugs that interfere with platelet function alter the incidence of myocardial infarction (Mackie and Douglas, 1978). Oral anticoagulants have no effect on platelet function; thus, they are unlikely to be useful in the treatment of thrombotic disease in the arterial system.

Examples of antithrombotic drugs are aspirin, dipyridamole, and dextran.

Aspirin

Aspirin inhibits thromboxane synthesis and the release of adenosine diphosphate by platelets and their subsequent aggregation (see Chapters 11 and 20). Despite rapid clearance from the body, the effects of aspirin on platelets are irreversible and last for the life of the platelet. Single doses of 325 mg of aspirin may prolong bleeding time for several days (Weiss, 1978). Aspirin may also inhibit synthesis of prostacyclin in vessel walls and thus tend to offset its effectiveness as an antithrombotic drug (Moncada and Vane, 1979).

Dipyridamole

Dipyridamole, in combination with warfarin, inhibits embolization from prosthetic heart valves. This drug may interfere with platelet function by potentiating the effect of prostacyclin or inhibiting phosphodiesterase activity leading to increased intracellular concentrations of cyclic AMP. Addition of dipyridamole to the blood prime reduces microaggregate formation in the pump oxygenator (Nuutinen and Mononen, 1975).

Dextran

Dextran-70 prolongs bleeding time, and polymerization of fibrin and platelet function may be impaired. For these reasons, dextran may have some value in the prevention of postoperative thromboembolic disease.

THROMBOLYTIC DRUGS

Thrombolytic drugs, such as streptokinase and urokinase, are proteins that promote the dissolution of thrombi by stimulating the conversion of endogenous plasminogen to plasmin (fibrinolysin). Plasmin is a proteolytic enzyme that hydrolyzes fibrin. Following administration of these drugs, there is a high incidence of bleeding from sites of cutaneous trauma and surgical wounds reflecting lysis of fibrin in hemostatic plugs. This hemorrhage greatly limits the clinical usefulness of these drugs. Epsilon aminocaproic acid is a specific antidote for an overdose with a fibrinolytic drug. Fever is common, and allergic reactions resulting from formation of antibodies (*i.e.*, anaphylaxis) can occur. Urokinase may be used as an alternative drug in patients allergic to streptokinase.

REFERENCES

Anderson EF. Heparin resistance prior to cardiopulmonary bypass. Anesthesiology 1986;64:504–7.

Bull BS, Huse WM, Brauer FS, Korpman RA. Heparin therapy during extracorporeal circulation, II. The use of a dose–response curve to individualize heparin and protamine dosage. J Thorac Cardiovasc Surg 1975;69:685–9.

Campbell FW, Goldstein MF, Atkins PC. Management of the patient with protamine hypersensitivity for cardiac surgery. Anesthesiology 1984;61:761–4.

Castaneda AR, Gans H, Weber KC, Fox IJ. Heparin neutralization: Experimental and clinical studies. Surgery 1967;62:686–97.

Casthely PA, Goodman K, Fyman PN, Abrams LM, Aaron D. Hemodynamic changes after the administration of protamine. Anesth Analg 1986;65:78–80.

Cerrato D, Ariano C, Fiacchino F. Deep vein thrombosis and low-dose heparin prophylaxis in neurosurgical patients. J Neurosurg 1978;49:378–81.

Conahan TJ, Andrews RW, MacVaugh H. Cardiovascular effects of protamine sulfate in man. Anesth Analg 1981;60:33–6.

Doolan L, McKenzie L, Krafcheck J, Parsons B, Buxton B. Protamine sulfate hypersensitivity. Anaesth Intens Care 1981;9:147–9.

Ellison N, Edmunds LH, Colman RW. Platelet aggregation following heparin and protamine administration. Anesthesiology 1978;48:65–8.

Esposito RA, Culliford AT, Colvin SB, Thomas SJ, Lackner H, Spencer FC. Heparin resistance during cardiopulmonary bypass. J Thorac Cardiovasc Surg 1983;85:346 – 53.

Flind AC. Cimetidine and oral anticoagulants. Br Med J 1978;2:1367.

Ghoneim MM, Delle M, Wilson WR, Ambre JJ. Alteration of warfarin kinetics in man associated with exposure to an operating-room environment. Anesthesiology 1975;43:333 – 6.

Goto H, Kushihashi T, Benson KT, Kato H, Fox DK, Arakawa K. Heparin, protamine, and ionized calcium in vitro and in vivo. Anesth Analg 1985;64:1081 – 4.

Hamilton PJ, Stalker AL, Douglas AS. Disseminated intravascular coagulation: a review. J Clin Pathol 1978;31:609 – 19.

Hattersley PG. Activated coagulation time of whole blood. JAMA 1966;196:436 – 40.

Hull JH, Murray WJ, Brown HS, Williams BO, Chi SL, Koch GG. Potential anticoagulant interactions in ambulatory patients. Clin Pharmacol Ther 1978; 24:644 – 9.

Knape JA, Schuller JL, DeHaan P, DeJong AP, Bovill JG. An anaphylactic reaction to protamine in a patient allergic to fish. Anesthesiology 1981;55:324 – 5.

Konchigeri HN. Hemodynamic effects of heparin in patients undergoing cardiac surgery. Anesth Analg 1984;63:235.

Lakin JD, Blocker TJ, Strong DM, Yocum MW. Anaphylaxis to protamine sulfate mediated by a complement-dependent IgG antibody. J Allergy Clin Immunol 1978;61:102 – 7.

Lewis RJ, Trager WF, Chan KK, et al. Warfarin. Stereochemical aspects of its metabolism and the interaction with phenylbutazone. J Clin Invest 1974;53:1607 – 17.

Lowenstein E, Johnston WE, Lappas DG, et al. Catastrophic pulmonary vasoconstriction associated with protamine reversal of heparin. Anesthesiology 1983;59:470 – 3.

Mackie MJ, Douglas AS. Oral anticoagulants in arterial disease. Br Med Bull 1978;34:177 – 82.

Marciniak E, Gockerman JP. Heparin-induced decrease in circulating antithrombin-III. Lancet 1977;2: 581 – 4.

Michaels IAL, Barash PG. Hemodynamic changes during protamine administration. Anesth Analg 1983;62:831 – 5.

Milne B, Rogers K, Cervenko F, Salerno T. Haemodynamic effects of intra-aortic versus intravenous administration of protamine for reversal of heparin in man. Can Anaesth Soc J 1983;30:347 – 51.

Moncada S, Vane JR. Arachidonic acid metabolites and the interactions between platelets and blood vessel walls. N Engl J Med 1979;300:1142 – 7.

Moorthy SS, Pond W, Roland RG. Severe circulatory shock following protamine (an anaphylactic reaction). Anesth Analg 1980;59:77 – 8.

Nuutinen LS, Mononen P. Dipyridamole and thrombocyte count in open heart surgery. J Thorac Cardiovasc Surg 1975;70:707 – 11.

Olsson J-E, Brechter C, Backlund H, et al. Anticoagulant vs. anti-platelet therapy as prophylactic against cerebral infarction in transient ischemic attacks. Stroke 1980;11:4 – 9.

O'Reilly RA. Vitamin K in hereditary resistance to oral anticoagulant drugs. Am J Physiol 1971;221:1327 – 30.

Orme MLE, Lewis PJ, DeSwiet M, et al. May mothers given warfarin breast-feed their infants? Br Med J 1977;1:1564 – 5.

Rao TLK, El-Etr AA. Anticoagulation following placement of epidural and subarachnoid catheters: an evaluation of neurologic sequelae. Anesthesiology 1981;55:618 – 20.

Seegers WH. Antithrombin III. Theory and clinical applications. H. P. Smith Memorial Lecture. Am J Clin Pathol 1978;69:367 – 74.

Sethna DH, Moffitt E, Gray RJ, et al. Effects of protamine sulfate on myocardial oxygen supply and demand in patients following cardiopulmonary bypass. Anesth Analg 1982;61:247 – 51.

Simon TL, Hyers TM, Gaston JP, Harker LA. Heparin pharmacokinetics: increased requirements in pulmonary embolism. Br J Haematol 1978;39: 111 – 20.

Smith JP, Walls JT, Muscato MS, et al. Extracorporeal circulation in a patient with heparin-induced thrombocytopenia. Anesthesiology 1985;62: 363 – 5.

Stoelting RK, Henry DP, Verburg KM, McCammon RL, King RD, Brown JW. Haemodynamic changes and circulating histamine concentrations following protamine administration to patients and dogs. Can Anaesth Soc J 1984;31:534 – 40.

Teien AN. Heparin elimination in patients with liver cirrhosis. Thrombo Haemostas 1977;38:701 – 6.

Tinker JH, Tarhan S. Discontinuing anticoagulant therapy in surgical patients with cardiac valve prosthesis. Observations in 180 operations. JAMA 1978;239:738 – 40.

Weiss HJ. Drug therapy. Antiplatelet therapy. N Engl J Med 1978;298:1344 – 7; 1403 – 6.

Williams RL, Schary WL, Blaschke TF, Meffin PJ, Melmon KL, Rowland M. Influence of acute viral hepatitis on disposition and pharmacologic effect of warfarin. Clin Pharmacol Ther 1976;20:90 – 7.

Wood AJJ, Robertson D, Robertson RM, Wilkinson GR, Wood M. Elevated plasma free drug concentrations of propranolol and diazepam during cardiac catheterizaton. Circulation 1980;62:1119 – 22.

Young JA, Kisker CT, Doty DB: Adequate anticoagulation during cardiopulmonary bypass determined by activated clotting time and the appearance of fibrin monomer. Ann Thor Surg 1978;26:231 – 40.

Antibiotics

INTRODUCTION

The therapeutic value and associated dangers of antibiotics are particularly relevant for care of patients in the perioperative period and intensive care unit who are at high risk for hospital-acquired infections. The choice of an antibiotic is determined by both the properties of the individual drug and the nature of the infecting organism as confirmed by bacteriologic investigation. In seriously ill patients or patients with decreased immune defense mechanisms, selection of a bactericidal rather than bacteriostatic antibiotic is often recommended (Table 28-1). Narrow-spectrum antibiotics should be considered before broad-spectrum antibiotics or combination antibiotic therapy is prescribed so as to preserve normal bacterial flora of the patient (Table 28-2). These normal bacterial flora help prevent colonization by pathogens, because they will compete for nutrients and produce their own antibiotic substances. Normal bacterial flora assume special importance in the hospitalized patient, because the hospital may serve as a reservoir of resistant bacteria from previously treated patients. It is inadvisable to use less than recommended doses of antibiotics except in the presence of renal, and occasionally hepatic dysfunction.

Antibiotics can be classified according to their mode of antibacterial action. For example, penicillins are drugs that exert antibacterial effects by inhibiting synthesis of bacterial cell walls. Amphotericin is a drug that affects permeability of the bacterial cell membranes. Drugs that act by inhibiting bacterial synthesis of essential proteins include aminoglycosides, tetracyclines, erythromycin, clindamycin, and chloramphenicol. Alteration in nucleic acid production is the mechanism of action of rifampin. Sulfonamides and trimethoprim exert an antibacterial effect by virtue of an antimetabolite effect.

PROPHYLACTIC ANTIBIOTICS

Prophylactic use of antibiotics during the perioperative period should be brief (about 24 hours), beginning with administration of the antibiotic at the time of preoperative medication. A more prolonged course of therapy may predispose to suprainfection with resistant bacteria. Prophylactic use of antibiotics is used for (1) cardiac surgery, (2) urinary tract surgery, (3) biliary tract surgery, (4) joint surgery, (5) compound fractures, and (6) when the surgical incision is across a contaminated surface, such as the gastrointestinal tract or vagina. Antibiotics selected for prophylaxis should be appropriate for the organism likely to be encountered during surgery. For example, streptococci are encountered during cardiac surgery, whereas staphylococci are likely after severe trauma and orthopedic surgery.

PENICILLINS

The basic structure of penicillins is a decyclic nucleus (aminopenicillanic acid), which consists of

Table 28-1

Examples of Bactericidal and Bacteriostatic Antibiotics

Bactericidal	Bacteriostatic
Penicillins	Tetracyclines
Cephalosporins	Chloramphenicol
Aminoglycosides	Erythromycin
Colistin	Clindamycin
Vancomycin	Sulfonamides
Co-trimoxazole	

Table 28-2

Examples of Narrow-Spectrum and Broad-Spectrum Antibiotics

Narrow-Spectrum	Broad-Spectrum
Benzylpenicillin	Ampicillin
Erythromycin	Cephalosporins
Clindamycin	Aminoglycosides
	Tetracyclines
	Chloramphenicol
	Sulfonamides
	Co-trimoxazole

a thiazolidine ring connected to a beta-lactam ring (Fig. 28-1). Benzylpenicillin (penicillin G) was the first penicillin derivative discovered (Fig. 28-2). This penicillin and its closely related cogener, phenoxymethylpenicillin (penicillin K) are highly active against gram-positive bacteria (*e.g.,* streptococci) but are readily hydrolyzed by penicillinase (beta-lactamase), rendering them ineffective against most strains of *Staphylococcus aureus* (Figs. 28-1 and 28-2). Benzylpenicillin is five to ten times more active against gram-negative bacteria, especially Neisseria, than is phenoxymethyl penicillin.

The bacteriocidal action of penicillins reflects the ability of these antibiotics to interfere with the synthesis of peptidoglycan, which is an essential component of cell walls of susceptible bacteria. Penicillins also decrease the availability of an inhibitor of murein hydrolase such that the uninhibited enzyme can then destroy (lyse) the structural integrity of bacterial cell walls. Cell membranes of resistant gram-negative bacteria prevent penicillins from gaining access to sites where synthesis of peptidoglycan is taking place (Benveniste and Davies, 1973).

Benzylpenicillin

Benzylpenicillin is the drug of choice for treatment of pneumococcal, streptococcal, and meningococcal infections. The majority of staphylococcal infections (60%–80%) are caused by bacteria that produce penicillinase and are thus resistant to treatment with most penicillins. Gonococci have gradually become more resistant to benzylpenicillin, requiring higher doses for adequate treatment. Treatment of syphilis with benzylpenicillin is highly effective. Benzylpenicillin is the drug of choice for the treatment of all forms of actinomycosis and clostridial infections causing gas gangrene.

Prophylactic administration of penicillin is highly effective against streptococcal infections, accounting for its value in patients with rheumatic fever. Transient bacteremia occurs in the majority of patients undergoing dental extractions, emphasizing the importance of prophylactic penicillin in patients with congenital or acquired heart disease.

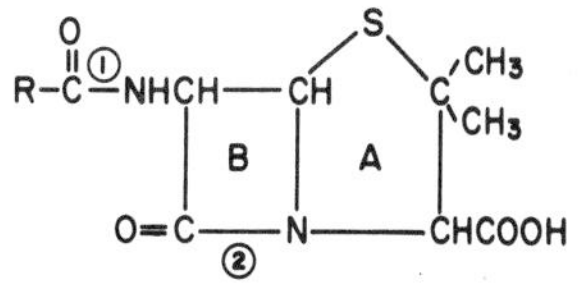

FIGURE 28-1. The basic structure of penicillins is a thiazolidine ring *(A)* connected to a beta-lactam ring *(B)*. Breakdown of penicillin occurs at sites (1) and (2) by the actions of amidase and penicillinase, respectively.

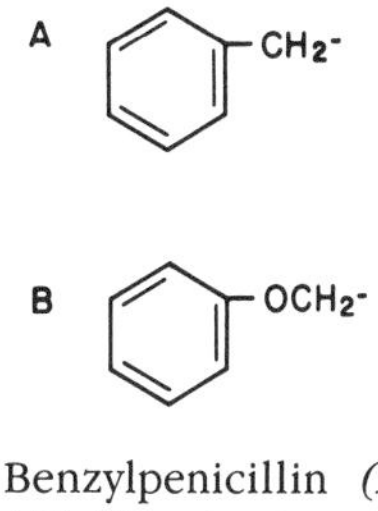

FIGURE 28-2. Benzylpenicillin *(A)* and phenoxymethylpenicillin *(B)*. The structures shown are equivalent to R in Figure 28-1.

Transient bacteremia may also accompany surgical procedures, such as tonsillectomy and operations on the genitourinary and gastrointestinal tracts, and vaginal delivery.

Route of Administration

Benzylpenicillin is more stable in an acidic medium than is phenoxymethylpenicillin following oral administration. Absorption after intramuscular injection is rapid but may result in sterile inflammatory responses at the site of injection. Benzylpenicillin can be administered intravenously or as a continuous infusion (6–20 million units daily). Thrombophlebitis may occur along the vein used for intravenous administration. Potassium salts of penicillin are most commonly administered intravenously, with 1.7 mEq of potassium being present in every 1 million units of penicillin. This amount of potassium may result in hyperkalemia in patients who are in renal failure. Stability of benzylpenicillin is greatest at a pH of 6 to 7.2, which is important when considering a fluid diluent for continuous infusion. Other drugs should not be mixed with penicillin, because the combination may inactivate the antibiotic. Intrathecal administration of penicillins is not recommended, because these drugs are potent convulsants when administered by this route. Furthermore, arachnoiditis and encephalopathy may follow intrathecal penicillin administration.

Excretion

Renal elimination of penicillin is rapid (60%–90% of an intramuscular dose in the first hour), such that the concentration in plasma declines to half its peak value within 1 hour after injection. About 10% is eliminated by glomerular filtration, and 90% is eliminated by renal tubular secretion. Anuria increases the elimination half-time of benzylpenicillin about tenfold.

Duration of Action

Methods to prolong the duration of action of penicillin include the simultaneous administration of probenecid, which blocks renal tubular secretion of penicillin. Alternatively, the intramuscular injection of poorly soluble salts of penicillin, such as procaine or benzathine, will delay absorption and thus prolong the duration of action. Procaine penicillin contains 120 mg of the local anesthetic for every 300,000 units of the antibiotic. Possible hypersensitivity to procaine must be considered when selecting this form of the antibiotic for administration.

PENICILLINASE-RESISTANT PENICILLINS

Penicillinase-resistant penicillins are not susceptible to hydrolysis by staphylococcal penicillinase. Specific indications for these drugs are infections caused by staphylococci known or suspected to produce this enzyme. These antibiotics are less effective than benzylpenicillin against infections caused by bacteria that do not produce penicillinase, including nonpenicillinase-producing staphylococci.

Methicillin

Methicillin (demethyoxybenzylpenicillin) is bactericidal for nearly all strains of *S. aureus* that produce penicillinase. Oral administration is not effective because the drug is readily destroyed by acidic gastric fluid. Renal excretion, as with benzylpenicillin, is rapid.

Oxacillin and Cloxacillin

Oxacilln and cloxacillin, like methicillin are markedly resistant to hydrolysis by penicillinase, but unlike methicillin, they are relatively stable in an acidic medium, resulting in adequate systemic absorption after oral administration. Nevertheless, variability of absorption from the gastrointestinal tract often dictates a parenteral route of administration for treatment of serious infections caused by penicillinase-producing staphylococci. Renal excretion is rapid, with up to 50% of the drug eliminated unchanged in the urine in the first 6 hours. Significant hepatic elimination into the bile also occurs. Hepatitis has been associated with high-dose oxacillin therapy (Pollack *et al,* 1978).

Nafcillin

Nafcillin is highly resistant to penicillinase, being more active than oxacillin against benzylpenicillin resistant *S. aureus.* Oral absorption of nafcillin is irregular because of variable inactivation by acidic gastric fluid. The usual parenteral dose is 8 to 12 g daily, given in divided doses every 4 hours. There is selective sequestration of the drug in the liver, with peak concentrations in the bile exceeding those in the blood. Only about 10% of the drug appears unchanged in the urine. Penetration of nafcillin into the central nervous system is sufficient to treat staphylococcal meningitis.

BROAD-SPECTRUM PENICILLINS

Broad-spectrum penicillins, such as ampicillin, have a wider range of activity than other penicillins, being bactericidal against gram-positive and gram-negative bacteria. They are, nevertheless, all destroyed by penicillinase produced by certain gram-negative and gram-positive bacteria. Therefore, these drugs are ineffective against most staphylococcal infections.

Ampicillin

Ampicillin (alpha-aminobenzylpenicillin) is considered the drug of choice for initial treatment of gonococcal urethritis. Upper respiratory tract infections owing to *Haemophilus influenzae* and streptococcal organisms and most urinary tract infections caused by enterococci respond to ampicillin. Acute bacterial meningitis in children is often treated with ampicillin, but since 5% to 30% of strains of *H. influenzae* may be resistant to ampicillin, it is recommended that chloramphenicol be administered concurrently until sensitivities of the infecting bacteria are determined.

Route of Administration

Ampicillin is stable in acid and is thus well absorbed after oral administration. Nevertheless, considerably higher blood levels can be obtained with intramuscular injections.

Among the penicillins, ampicillin is associated with the highest incidence (9%) of skin rash (Levine, 1972). This reaction is delayed, appearing 7 to 10 days after initiation of therapy. It is likely that a mechanism different from true penicillin hypersensitivity is responsible for this ampicillin-induced skin rash. Many ampicillin rashes are due to protein impurities that may be reduced by refinements in the manufacturing process.

Excretion

About 50% of an oral dose of ampicillin is excreted unchanged by the kidney in the first 6 hours following administration, compared with approximately 70% of an intramuscular or intravenous dose in this same period of time. This emphasizes that renal function greatly influences the duration of action of ampicillin as well as the dose administered. Ampicillin also appears in the bile and undergoes enterohepatic circulation.

Carbenicillin

Carbenicillin (alpha-carboxybenzylpenicillin) is active against most infections owing to *Pseudomonas aeruginosa* and certain Proteus strains tht are resistant to ampicillin. It is penicillinase susceptible and, therefore, ineffective against most strains of *S. aureus*.

Carbenicillin is not absorbed from the gastrointestinal tract; therefore, it must be given parenterally, often in large doses. The elimination half-time of carbenicillin in the presence of normal renal function is about 1 hour, and this time is prolonged to almost 2 hours when there is hepatic dysfunction. About 85% of the unchanged drug is recovered in the urine over 9 hours. Probenecid, by delaying renal excretion of the drug, increases the plasma concentration of carbenicillin by about 50%.

Cardiac failure may occur in patients treated with carbenicillin and receiving excessive sodium. Hypokalemia may occur because of obligatory excretion with the large amount of nonreabsorbable carbenicillin. Carbenicillin interferes with normal platelet aggregation such that bleeding is prolonged but platelet count remains normal.

ALLERGY TO PENICILLINS

Allergic reactions are noted in up to 10% of patients treated with penicillin, making these drugs one of the most common causes of drug allergy (Green *et al,* 1977). This high incidence of allergy reflects the action of penicillins and their metabolites as haptens. The most common manifestations of allergy to penicillins is a maculopapular or urticarial rash and fever. In a few patients, life-threatening bronchospasm and angioedema manifesting as marked swelling of the face, lips, and tongue with or without laryngeal edema occurs. Fatal allergic reactions have occurred in patients receiving as little as 1 unit of penicillin for skin testing.

There seems to be no difference between the individual penicillins with respect to the potential for causing allergic reactions. Allergic reactions can occur with any dose or route of administration, although severe anaphylactic reactions are more often associated with parenteral than with oral administration. The presence of a common nucleus in the structure of all penicillins means that allergy to one penicillin increases the likelihood of an allergic reaction to another penicillin. Conversely, the occurrence of an allergic reaction does not necessarily imply repetition on subsequent exposures. For example, some patients who experience cutaneous reactions may later receive the same penicillin without experiencing a similar response. Patients with life-threatening infections, such as endocarditis or meningitis, may continue to receive penicillin despite the development of a skin rash. Indeed, the skin rash often clears as therapy is continued, presumably reflecting development of immunoglobulin G-blocking antibodies.

Allergic reactions may occur in the absence of previous known exposure to a penicillin antibiotic. This may reflect prior unknown exposure to penicillin, presumably in ingested foods. Antipenicillin antibodies are detectable in virtually all patients who have received penicillin (Klaus and Fellner, 1973). The incidence of positive skin reactions is four times greater in atopic than in nonatopic patients.

The vast majority of patients who give a history of allergy to penicillin should be treated with a different type of antibiotic. Skin tests may be helpful when treatment with penicillin is considered essential. For example, lack of response to benzylpenicilloyl-polylysine makes it unlikely that a patient will develop an immediate or accelerated allergic reaction to penicillin. Furthermore, this preparation is not allergenic nor is it likely to provoke severe reactions. Patients with a positive response to benzylpenicilloyl-polylysine are at high risk for developing a serious allergic reaction if they receive penicillin.

CEPHALOSPORINS

Cephalosporins are derived from 7-aminocephalosporanic acid (Fig. 28-3). These antibiotics in-

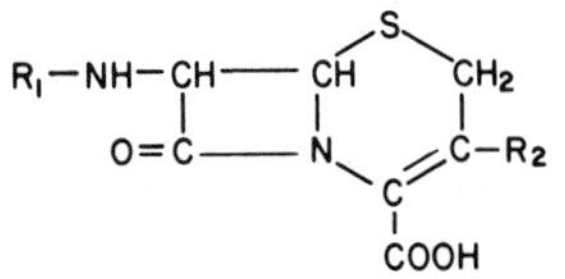

FIGURE 28-3. Basic structural formula of cephalosporins.

hibit bacterial cell wall synthesis in a manner similar to the penicillins. Resistance to cephalosporins, as to penicillins, may be due to an inability of the antibiotic to penetrate to its site of action. Bacteria can also produce cephalosporinases (*i.e.,* beta-lactamases) that disrupt the beta-lactam structure of cephalosporins and thus inhibit their antibacterial activity.

All cephalosporins have a similar antibacterial spectrum, being effective for the treatment of infections of the respiratory tract, skin, and joints. Effectiveness, in the treatment of joint infections reflects rapid penetration of cephalosporins into synovial fluids. Conversely, penetration of cephalosporins into the eye is poor, and the concentration achieved in the cerebrospinal fluid is insufficient to treat meningitis. Despite these limitations, cephalosporins readily cross the placenta. Aminoglycosides can be avoided if gramnegative bacteria are susceptible to cephalosporins. Cephalosporins are commonly used for perioperative prophylaxis against infections caused by *S. aureus* and *S. epidermidis.*

Individual cephalosporins differ significantly with respect to extent of absorption following oral absorption, severity of pain produced by intramuscular injection, and protein binding. Intravenous administration of any of the cephalosporins can cause thrombophlebitis (Berger *et al,* 1976). Excretion of cephalosporins is principally by glomerular filtration and renal tubular secretion, emphasizing the need to reduce dosage of these drugs in the presence of renal dysfunction. Deacetyl metabolites of cephalosporins can occur, being associated with reduced antibiotic activity.

A positive Coombs' reaction frequently occurs in patients who receive large doses of cephalosporins. Hemolysis, however, is rarely associated with this response. Nephrotoxicity with cephalosporins, with the exception of cephaloridine, is less frequent than that following administration of aminoglycosides or polymyxins (Barza, 1978).

Allergy to Cephalosporins

Allergy to cephalosporins, as with penicillins, is the most common adverse response associated with administration of these antibiotics. Indeed, an estimated 3% to 5% of patients experience allergic reactions following administration of cephalosporins. These allergic reactions may be life-threatening and manifest as hypotension, arterial hypoxemia, and bronchospasm following intravenous administration of the drug (Beaupre *et al,* 1984).

The beta-lactam structure present in both penicillins and cephalosporins results in potential cross-sensitivity between these two classes of antibiotics (Scholand *et al,* 1968). Indeed, patients with a history of an anaphylactic reaction to penicillin should probably not receive a cephalosporin. Nevertheless, the incidence of documented cross-sensitivity between penicillins and cephalosporins is low, being estimated to occur in 10% of patients. Indeed, a common indication for use of a cephalosporin is the prior history of an allergic reaction to a penicillin antibiotic.

Cephalothin

Cephalothin is the most resistant of the cephalosporins to attack by staphylococcal cephalosporinases and is considered an ideal drug for treatment of severe staphylococcal infections (Fig. 28-4). Oral absorption is poor, and intramuscular injection is painful, accounting for its common administration by the intravenous route. The usual intravenous dose is 1 g infused over 20 to 30 minutes. Although cephalothin is found in many tissues and fluids, it does not enter the cerebrospinal fluid in significant amounts and should not be used for treatment of meningitis.

About 50% of a dose of cephalothin is eliminated unchanged by the kidneys. Up to 30% is metabolized to a weakly antibacterial deacetyl metabolite, which is also excreted by the kidneys.

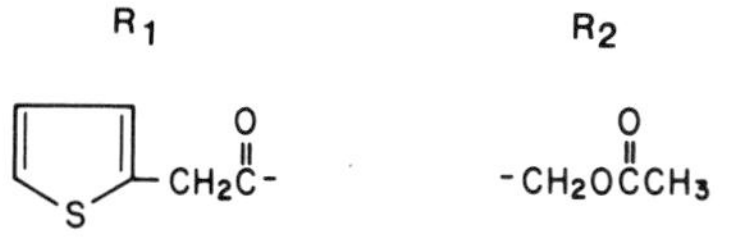

FIGURE 28-4. Cephalothin. R_1 and R_2 correspond to Figure 28-3.

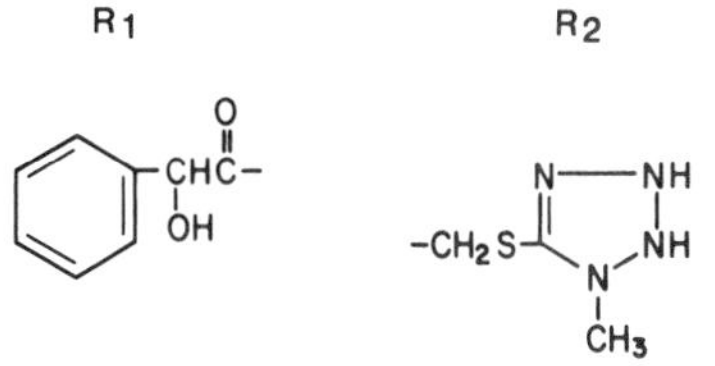

FIGURE 28-5. Cefamandole. R_1 and R_2 correspond to Figure 28-3.

Excretion of cephalothin is delayed when there is renal dysfunction, requiring consideration of a decreased dosage or greater dosing intervals. Concurrent administration of cephalothin and gentamicin or tobramycin may cause nephrotoxicity (Wade *et al,* 1978).

Cefazolin

Cefazolin has an antibacterial spectrum similar to cephalothin and is more active against *Escherichia coli* and Klebsiella. Cefazolin is highly (about 80%) bound to plasma proteins. The elimination half-time is nearly 2 hours, compared with 1 to 1.5 hours for cephaloridine and 30 to 40 minutes for cephalothin (Bergeron *et al,* 1973). Cefazolin is primarily eliminated by glomerular filtration, with renal tubular secretion being less important than with cephalothin. Cefazolin is relatively well tolerated after intramuscular or intravenous injection.

Cefamandole

Cefamandole is more active than cephalothin against certain gram-negative bacteria (Fig. 28-5). Conversely, this drug is less active than cephalothin against gram-positive bacteria. The elimination half-time is 40 to 50 minutes, and the drug is excreted unchanged by the kidneys. The activity of cefamandole against *H. influenzae* in addition to activity against streptococci and staphylococci renders this antibiotic suitable for the majority of cases of bacterial pneumonia.

Cefoxitin

Cefoxitin is highly resistant to cephalosporinases produced by gram-negative bacteria. It is effective in the treatment of urethritis due to penicillinase-producing strains of *Neisseria gonorrhoeae* (Berg *et al,* 1979). The drug is eliminated unchanged by the kidneys.

Cephalexin

Cephalexin has an antibacterial spectrum similar to cephalothin. It is well absorbed from the gastrointestinal tract. Less than 15% is bound to plasma proteins. The elimination half-time is about 50 minutes, with more than 90% of the drug excreted unchanged in the urine within 6 hours, primarily by renal tubular secretion. As such, probenecid is effective in slowing renal elimination of cephalexin and enhancing the duration of systemic antibiotic activity.

AMINOGLYCOSIDES

Aminoglycosides are poorly lipid-soluble drugs that are rapidly bactericidal for aerobic gram-negative bacteria by virtue of their ability to inhibit protein synthesis in bacterial ribosomes. To reach ribosomes, the antibiotic must be transported across bacterial cell membranes by an active process, since poor lipid solubility limits passive diffusion. This is an oxygen-dependent active transport system that is absent in anaerobic bacteria, explaining the resistance of these bacteria to the effects of aminoglycosides. Most of the acquired resistance to aminoglycosides results from inactivation of the antibiotic by enzymes located in bacterial cell membranes. Structurally, aminoglycosides contain three separate ring structures, two of which are substituted amino sugars with a glycosidic linkage.

Route of Administration

Less than 1% of an orally administered aminoglycoside is absorbed into the systemic circulation, reflecting the poor lipid solubility of these drugs. Orally administered drug is thus eliminated unchanged in the bile. Rapid systemic absorption occurs after intramuscular injection, with peak plasma concentrations occurring in 30 to 90 minutes. Negligible binding to plasma proteins takes place, which is consistent with poor lipid solubility.

As would be predicted from poor lipid solubility, concentrations of aminoglycosides in secretions, eye, and central nervous system are poor. The principal exception is the renal cortex, where high concentrations of aminoglycosides accumulate, which very likely contributes to adverse effects on the kidney (see the section entitled Nephrotoxicity). Inflammation improves penetration of aminoglycosides into peritoneal and pericardial cavities and the cerebrospinal fluid. For example, concentrations of aminoglycosides in the cerebrospinal fluid are less than 10% of those in plasma in the absence of inflammation. This value may approach 20% in the presence of meningitis (Strausbaugh *et al,* 1977). Nevertheless, these concentrations are usually inadequate, and intrathecal or intraventricular administration of the aminoglycoside is necessary.

Excretion

Aminoglycosides, because of their poor lipid solubility, have a volume of distribution similar to the extracellular fluid volume and undergo extensive renal excretion owing almost exclusively to glomerular filtration. Probenecid has no detectable effect on the rate of elimination, suggesting that renal tubular secretion mechanisms are not important. About 60% of an aminoglycoside is eliminated unchanged by the kidneys during the first 24 hours, and, eventually, all the drug is eliminated by the kidneys.

There is a linear relationship between the plasma creatinine concentration and the elimination half-time of aminoglycosides. In the presence of normal renal function, the elimination half-time of all aminoglycosides is 2 to 3 hours, and this is prolonged 20- to 40-fold in the presence of renal failure. Determination of the plasma concentration of aminoglycodies is an essential guide to the safe administration of these antibiotics.

Side Effects

Side effects of aminoglycosides that limit their clinical usefulness include ototoxicity, nephrotoxicity, skeletal muscle weakness, and potentiation of nondepolarizing neuromuscular blocking drugs. These side effects parallel the plasma concentration of aminoglycoside, emphasizing the need to reduce the dose of these drugs in patients with renal dysfunction.

Ototoxicity

Ototoxicity manifests as vestibular or auditory dysfunction or both and parallels the accumulation of aminoglycosides in the perilymph of the inner ear (Federspil, 1977). This accumulation of drug in the inner ear parallels the plasma concentration. The incidence of ototoxicity is 1% to 3% for patients treated with an aminoglycoside for less than 14 days. Prolonged administration, high doses, and advanced age that is likely to be associated with preexisting auditory defects and renal disease increase the incidence of ototoxicity. Furosemide, mannitol, and probably other diuretics seem to accentuate the ototoxic effects of aminoglycosides.

Aminoglycoside-induced ototoxicity reflects progressive destruction of vestibular or cochlear sensory hair cells in a dose-dependent manner by the antibiotic. Streptomycin and gentamicin predominantly produce vestibular toxicity manifesting as nystagmus, vertigo, nausea, and acute onset of Meniere's syndrome. Neomycin, kanamycin and amikacin predominantly produce auditory dysfunction manifesting as tinnitus or a sensation of pressure or fullness in the ears. Deafness may develop suddenly. Tobramycin adversely affects vestibular and cochlear function equally.

Nephrotoxicity

Aminoglycosides accumulate in the renal cortex; this correlates with the potential for these drugs to cause nephrotoxicity. As with ototoxicity, the incidence of nephrotoxicity depends on the specific drug, duration of treatment, total dosage, and presence of predisposing factors such as advanced age and preexisting renal disease. Neomycin is the most nephrotoxic of the aminoglycosides and, for this reason, is not administered by the parenteral route. The incidence of nephrotoxicity with gentamicin is about 4% (Gary *et al*, 1976). Nephrotoxicity is estimated to occur in 3% to 8% of patients treated with kanamycin and amikacin and 1% or less with tobramycin and streptomycin.

Nephrotoxicity induced by aminoglycosides is a form of acute renal tubular necrosis that initially manifests as an inability to concentrate urine and the appearance of proteinuria and red cell casts. This damage rarely manifests before 5 to 7 days of treatment. These changes are usually reversible if the drug is discontinued.

Skeletal Muscle Weakness

Skeletal muscle weakness can occur with intrapleural or intraperitoneal instillation of large doses of aminoglycosides (Holtzman, 1976). Patients with myasthenia gravis are particularly susceptible to this aminoglycoside effect with any route of administration. Patients with chronic obstructive airways disease may be susceptible to the skeletal muscle–weakening effects of aminoglycosides. Nevertheless, single doses of tobramycin or gentamicin lack clinically significant neuromuscular blocking effects when administered to otherwise healthy patients (Lippmann *et al*, 1982).

The neuromuscular effects of aminoglycosides most likely reflect the ability of these drugs to inhibit the prejunctional release of acetylcholine while also reducing postsynaptic sensitivity to the neurotransmitter (Pittinger and Adamson, 1972). Intravenous administration of calcium overcomes the effect of aminoglycosides at the neuromuscular junction.

Potentiation of Nondepolarizing Neuromuscular Blocking Drugs

Intravenous administration of aminoglycosides and associated high plasma concentrations are most likely to potentiate nondepolarizing neuromuscular blocking drugs (Sokoll and Gergis, 1981). Likewise, irrigation of the peritoneal or pleural cavities with large volumes of aminoglycoside-containing solution can result in substantial systemic absorption and potentiation of previously administered neuromuscular blocking drugs. Reappearance of neuromuscular blockade is a possibility if aminoglycosides are administered systemically in the early postoperative period to a patient who has been judged to have adequately recovered from neuromuscular blocking drugs administered during anesthesia. Furthermore, the neuromuscular blocking effects of lidocaine are enhanced in the presence of neuromuscular blocking drugs and aminoglycosides. Conceivably, administration of lidocaine in the early postoperative period could produce skeletal muscle weakness in a patient having previously received a neuromuscular blocking drug and an aminoglycoside (Bruckner *et al*, 1980).

Neostigmine or calcium-induced antagonism of aminoglycoside-potentiated neuromuscular blockade may be incomplete or transient (Sokoll and Gergis, 1981). Speculation that reversal of antibiotic-induced neuromuscular blockade would also antagonize antibiotic effects, however, has not been demonstrated (Booij *et al,* 1980). Clinical evaluation, as well as electrophysiologic criteria, are necessary to evaluate aminoglycoside-potentiated neuromuscular blockade. The importance of clinical observation is the fact that neuromuscular blockade in the presence of neomycin can be characterized by a sustained response to continuous electrical stimulation and a train-of-four ratio near 1, despite a greatly decreased single twitch response (Lee *et al,* 1976).

Effects of antibiotics at the neuromuscular junction probably involve multiple sites of action (Fig. 28-6) (Sokoll and Gergis, 1981). In terms of producing clinically significant skeletal muscle effects with therapeutic doses, the penicillins, cephalosporins, tetracyclines, and erythromycin are devoid of effects at the neuromuscular junction. The mechanism of the neuromuscular block-

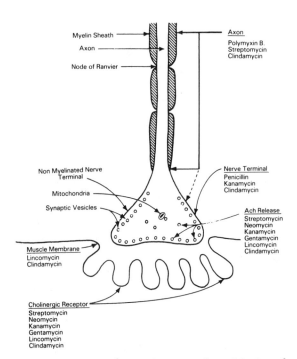

FIGURE 28-6. Schematic depiction of possible sites of action of antibiotics at the neuromuscular junction. (From Sokoll MD, Gergis SD. Antibiotics and neuromuscular function. Anesthesiology 1981;55:148–59. Reproduced by permission of the authors and publisher.)

ing effects of polymyxins is complex but is most likely postsynaptic. Neomycin and gentamicin reduce the amount of acetylcholine released by presynaptic motor nerves and decrease the sensitivity of the postsynaptic motor end-plate to the depolarizing action of acetylcholine. Oral neomycin, as used to reduce the bacterial population of the gastrointestinal tract prior to abdominal surgery, is unlikely to produce effects at the neuromuscular junction, since this antibiotic is not absorbed into the systemic circulation. Nevertheless, prolonged oral administration of neomycin has been associated with antibiotic-induced neuromuscular blockade (Pittinger *et al,* 1970).

Streptomycin

Streptomycin is most often used in combination with other antibiotics to treat specific but unusual infections. For example, streptomycin and penicillin produce a synergistic bactericidal effect in the treatment of bacterial endocarditis. Brucellosis is treated with the combination of streptomycin and tetracycline. Tularemia and all forms of plague are treated with streptomycin. Streptomycin is occasionally administered for treatment of tuberculosis. Diffusion of streptomycin occurs readily into most tissues, but the drug does not enter the cerebrospinal fluid.

Deep intramuscular injection of streptomycin, 15 to 25 mg kg^{-1} daily in two divided doses, is the most common method of parenteral administration. Intramuscular injection is painful and may be associated with tender masses in the injected area. Skin eruptions occur in about 5% of patients. Neutropenia occurs in less than 1% of patients. Streptomycin is the least likely of all the aminoglycosides to produce nephrotoxicity, although excretion occurs primarily by glomerular filtration. Up to 15% of patients receiving the drug for more than 1 week, however, manifest a measurable decrease in hearing.

Gentamicin

Gentamicin, because of its potential to cause ototoxicity, is used for the treatment of only life-threatening gram-negative infections. For example, this antibiotic administered alone or in combination with ampicillin provides effective initial treatment of the critically ill patient with a gram-negative urinary tract infection. Patients with impaired immune defense mechanisms and requiring mechanical ventilation of the lungs have an increased incidence of gram-negative pneumonia. In these patients, gentamicin in combination with a penicillin or cephalosporin antibiotic is effective, especially if the invading bacteria is Klebsiella or *P. aeruginosa*. Intrathecal administration of gentamicin is necessary for the treatment of meningitis caused by bacteria sensitive to this antibiotic. Resistance to the antibiotic effects of gentamicin is likely to develop in critically ill patients in burn units and in intensive care units.

Intramuscular administration of gentamicin in three divided doses is the recommended route of administration. Periodic determination of the plasma concentration of gentamicin is necessary to guide therapy, especially in the presence of preexisting renal disease.

Tobramycin

Tobramycin closely resembles the antibiotic effects of gentamicin. Ototoxicity and nephrotoxicity, however, are less likely following the administration of tobramycin as compared to gentamicin. Tobramycin can be administered intramuscularly or intravenously. Indications for the use of tobramycin are similar to those of gentamicin. In contrast to other aminoglycosides, tobramycin is not effective against mycobacteria (Gangadharam *et al*, 1977).

Amikacin

Amikacin is uniquely resistant to hydrolysis by aminoglycoside-inactivating enzymes, making it a useful drug in hospitalized patients where gentamicin-resistant bacteria are prevalent. This antibiotic may be administered intramuscularly or intravenously.

Kanamycin

Kanamycin has a limited spectrum of activity compared with other aminoglycosides and, as a result, is not frequently used. Oral administration of kanamycin, 6 to 8 g daily, is used as an adjunct to the treatment of hepatic coma and to suppress intestinal flora prior to surgery on the gastrointestinal tract.

Neomycin

Neomycin is commonly used for topical application to treat infections of the skin (as after burn injury), cornea, and mucous membranes. Continuous irrigation of the bladder with neomycin solution is used to prevent bacteriuria and bacteremia associated with the use of indwelling bladder catheters. Oral neomycin, 4 to 8 g daily, does not undergo systemic absorption and is thus administered to decrease bacterial flora in the intestine prior to gastrointestinal surgery and as an adjunct to the therapy of hepatic coma. Indeed, blood ammonia concentrations in the presence of hepatic failure are reduced by oral therapy with neomycin. Nephrotoxicity and ototoxicity associated with plasma concentrations of neomycin that occur after parenteral administration have led to the abandonment of administration of the drug by this route.

Allergic reactions occur in 6% to 8% of patients treated with topical neomycin. Oral administration of neomycin may result in suprainfection and intestinal malabsorption. Oral, but not parenteral, administration of neomycin produces a marked decrease in the plasma concentration of cholesterol. Neuromuscular blockade produced by neomycin is similar to that produced by hypermagnesemia (Corrado and Nicolette, 1961) (see the section entitled Skeletal Muscle Weakness). Delayed awakening from anesthesia has been reported in a single patient in association with irrigation of the bladder with neomycin (Yao *et al*, 1980). It was speculated that neomycin decreased the release of acetylcholine in the central nervous system by competing with calcium ions necessary for release of neurotransmitter. Indeed, neomycin has been shown to bind calcium, but the serum-ionized calcium concentration is not altered by this antibiotic (Wright and Collier, 1977).

TETRACYCLINES

Tetracyclines consist of four interconnected carbon rings with side chains on which various substitutions are made (Fig. 28-7). These drugs possess a wide range of antibiotic activity against gram-positive and gram-negative bacteria. For example, tetracycline antibiotics are frequently administered in the treatment of chronic bronchitis. Prophylactic administration of tetracyclines may

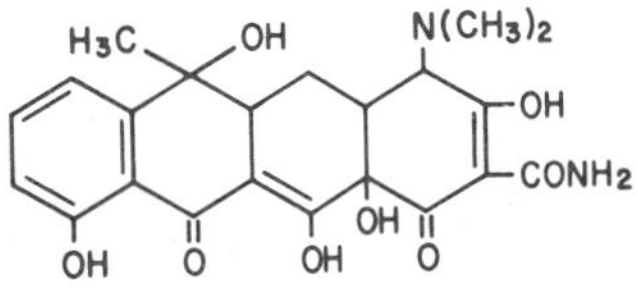

FIGURE 28-7. Tetracyclines consist of four interconnected carbon rings with side chains.

reduce the number of acute pulmonary infections in patients with chronic obstructive airways disease (Reynolds, 1979). These drugs are effective against mycoplasma that cause mycoplasma pneumonia, chlamydia causing nonspecific urethritis, Rickettsia causing Rocky Mountain spotted fever and lymphogranuloma venereum. Tetracyclines have been administered in small oral doses to treat acne, presumably producing a beneficial effect by reducing the fatty acid content of sebum (Fry and Ramsay, 1966).

Mechanism of Action

Therapeutic concentrations of tetracyclines are bacteriostatic, affecting only multiplying bacteria. Nevertheless, high plasma concentrations may be bacteriocidal. The site of action of tetracyclines is the bacterial ribosome where the antibiotic acts by inhibiting protein synthesis. Both passive diffusion and an energy-dependent active transport system are necessary for tetracyclines to cross bacterial cell membranes and reach ribosomes. Resistance to tetracyclines can develop by way of genetic changes in bacteria that affect active transport of the drug into bacterial cells.

Route of Administration

Tetracyclines are adequately but incompletely absorbed from the gastrointestinal tract. The percentage of an oral dose that is absorbed when the stomach is empty is 30% for chlortetracycline; 60% to 80% for oxytetracycline, demeclocycline, and tetracycline; and almost 100% for doxycycline and minocycline (Barza and Scheife, 1977). Most absorption takes place from the stomach and upper small intestine. Absorption is impaired by the presence of milk and particulate antacids, presumably reflecting chelation and an increase in gastric pH (Barr et al, 1971).

Indications for intravenous administration for tetracyclines are few since more acceptable alternatives exist. Thrombophlebitis is likely to occur following intravenous injection of these drugs. The advantage of intravenous injection is rapid penetration of these lipid-soluble antibiotics into tissues and fluids. The greater lipid solubility of minocycline compared with other tetracyclines results in unique penetration into the central nervous system so as to eradicate the meningococcal carrier state. Local irritation and poor absorption generally make intramuscular administration of tetracyclines unacceptable. Topical administration, except for use in the eye, is not recommended because of a high incidence of sensitization.

Excretion

All tetracyclines are concentrated in the liver and excreted by way of bile into the small intestine from which they are partially reabsorbed. Chlortetracycline is more dependent on biliary excretion for its elimination from the body than are the other tetracyclines. Decreased hepatic function or obstruction of the common bile duct results in reduced biliary excretion and persistence in the blood. Enterohepatic circulation of the tetracyclines ensures the presence of antibiotic in the blood for prolonged periods following the cessation of therapy. Elimination half-times are prolonged, averaging 6 to 9 hours for chlortetracycline, oxytetracycline, and tetracycline; 16 hours for demeclocycline; and 17 to 20 hours for doxycycline and minocycline.

Glomerular filtration and renal tubular secretion are also important for the excretion of tetracyclines. Minocycline is an exception in that renal clearance is low and hepatic metabolism seems to be extensive. Doxycycline is unique in that it does not accumulate significantly in the plasma of patients in renal failure, making it an attractive drug for treatment of extrarenal infections in patients with renal dysfunction. This drug is excreted in the bile largely as an inactive conjugate or possibly as a chelate, accounting for its modest impact on intestinal bacterial flora.

Side Effects

Gastrointestinal distress and the possibility of tetracycline-resistant bacterial enteritis limit the oral dose of these antibiotics. Tetracyclines evoke a catabolic effect, presumably owing to a generalized inhibition of amino acid utilization for protein synthesis. This catabolic effect may contribute to additional weight loss in critically ill patients, and the associated increase in urea excretion is undesirable in the presence of renal dysfunction. Phototoxicity characterized by increased sensitivity of the skin to sunlight occurs in patients treated with tetracyclines. Fatty liver infiltration has been observed, and parturients seem to be uniquely susceptible (Schultz *et al,* 1963). Cross-sensitization occurs between tetracyclines, requiring the use of a different class of antibiotics if an allergic reaction occurs following administration of a tetracycline. Tetracyclines may cause increased intracranial pressure (pseudotumor cerebri), especially when administered to infants (Stuart and Litt, 1978). Outdated tetracyclines have been associated with a form of Fanconi's syndrome (nausea, polyuria, polydipsia, proteinuria), emphasizing the importance of discarding unused supplies of the drug (Fulop and Drapkin, 1965).

Tetracycline is deposited in enamel of teeth, including unerupted teeth, when given to children between the ages of 2 months and 5 years, resulting in hypoplasia and brown discoloration of the tooth (Grossman *et al,* 1971). Even treatment of parturients with tetracyclines can produce discoloration in the offspring's teeth. Deposition of tetracycline in teeth and bones is probably due to its chelating property and the formation of a tetracycline – calcium – orthophosphate complex.

CHLORAMPHENICOL

Chloramphenicol is unique among antibiotics in that it contains a nitrobenzene moiety and is a derivative of dichloroacetic acid (Fig. 28-8). The drug is actively transported into bacterial cells, where it inhibits protein synthesis. Chloramphenicol possesses a wide range of antibacterial activity, including all anaerobic bacteria and gram-negative rods. It is primarily bacteriostatic, although it is bactericidal to certain bacterial strains such as *H. influenzae.* The risk of aplastic anemia dictates that use of chloramphenicol be reserved for treatment of diseases unresponsive to other antibiotics (Kucers, 1980) (see the section entitled Side Effects). For example, ampicillin-resistant strains of *H. influenzae* causing meningitis may be an indication for treatment with chloramphenicol (Feldman, 1978). Chloramphenicol is the drug of choice for treatment of typhoid fever. Resistance to chloramphenicol develops when a specific bacterial acetyltransferase acetylates the drug to a form that cannot bind to bacterial ribosomes.

Route of Administration

Chloramphenicol is rapidly absorbed from the gastrointestinal tract. The preparation of chloramphenicol for intravenous administration is the inactive succinate ester, which is rapidly hydrolyzed *in vivo* to the biologically active drug. Absorption after intramuscular administration is unpredictable. Chloramphenicol is distributed in body fluids and achieves therapeutic concentrations in the cerebrospinal fluid. This drug readily crosses the placenta.

Excretion

Chloramphenicol is inactivated primarily in the liver by glucuronyl transferase. Elimination halftime is 1.5 to 3.5 hours, and this is prolonged in the presence of liver disease. Over a 24-hour period, 75% to 90% of an orally administered dose of chloramphenicol is excreted in the urine, of which 5% to 10% is the unchanged drug. The unchanged drug is eliminated mainly by glomerular filtration, whereas inactive metabolites undergo renal tubular secretion. The elimination half-time of the active drug is only slightly prolonged by renal failure, necessitating the administration of usual doses to maintain a therapeutic concentration. Conversely, inactive metabolites accumulate in anuric patients.

Side Effects

The most important side effect of chloramphenicol is bone marrow depression, which occurs in

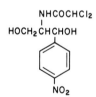

FIGURE 28-8.   Chloramphenicol.

approximately 1 of every 30,000 treated patients and, manifests as leukopenia, thrombocytopenia, and ultimately, fatal aplastic anemia (Best, 1967; Yunis, 1973). The incidence of this adverse response is not related to the dose of chloramphenicol but does seem to occur more commonly in patients who undergo prolonged therapy or who are exposed more than one time to chloramphenicol. An allergic reaction or genetically determined idiosyncratic response to the drug may be responsible for bone marrow depression (Nagao and Mauer, 1969).

Chloramphenicol can inhibit hepatic microsomal enzymes and prolong the duration of action of drugs such as dicumarol, phenytoin, and tolbutamide (Adams *et al,* 1977). This hepatic microsomal enzyme inhibitory effect may protect the liver from toxic effects of known hepatotoxins, such as carbon tetrachloride, by inhibiting metabolism (Dolci and Brabec, 1978).

ERYTHROMYCIN

Erythromycin is an orally effective antibiotic that may be bacteriostatic or bactericidal for gram-positive bacteria depending on the microorganism and concentration. It has moderate activity against *H. influenzae* and excellent activity against most strains of *N. gonorrhoeae.* Erythromycin, administered orally, reduces the duration of fever caused by *Mycoplasma pneumoniae.* Legionnaires' disease is effectively treated with erythromycin. The diphtheria carrier state is predictably eradicated by erythromycin. Streptococcal infections, including pharyngitis and scarlet fever, and pneumococcal pneumonia respond promptly to erythromycin.

Erythromycin diffuses readily into intracellular fluids, and antibiotic activity can be achieved at essentially all sites except the brain and cerebrospinal fluid. This is one of the few antibiotics that penetrates into prostatic fluid, achieving concentrations that are about one half those present in the circulation. An important use of oral erythromycin (250 mg every 6 hours) is an alternative to benzylpenicillin in patients who are allergic to penicillin antibiotics. Intramuscular injections of erythromycin are painful, and intravenous administration often results in thrombophlebitis.

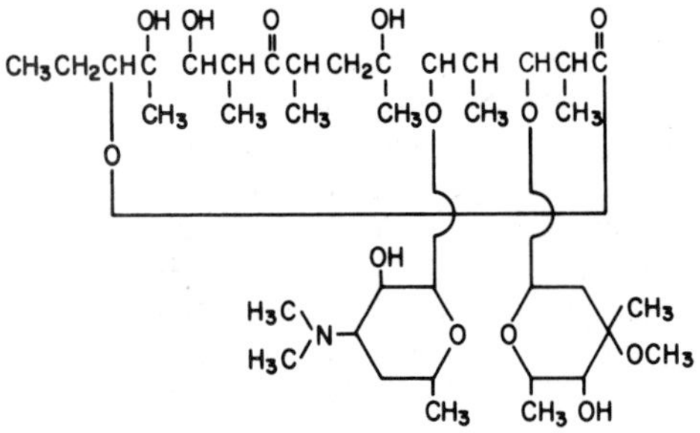

FIGURE 28-9. Erythromycin.

Mechanism of Action

Erythromycin is a structually complex macrolide antibiotic containing a many-membered lactone ring to which are attached one or more deoxysugars (Fig. 28-9). Erythromycin inhibits protein synthesis by bacterial ribosomes.

Route of Administration and Excretion

Erythromycin is absorbed from the upper part of the small intestine but is inactivated by gastric juice, requiring its administration as an enteric-coated tablet that dissolves in the duodenum. Only 2% to 5% of orally administered drug is excreted unchanged by the kidneys. The antibiotic is concentrated in the liver and bile. Some drug may be inactivated by demethylation in the liver. The elimination half-time is about 1.4 hours.

Side Effects

Erythromycin is one of the safest antibiotics, having minimal side effects (Griffith and Black, 1970). Cholestatic hepatitis with jaundice is the most serious side effect and is caused primarily by erythromycin estolate and only rarely by other preparations (Cooksley and Powell, 1977; McCormack *et al,* 1977). Indeed, the syndrome may represent an allergic reaction to the estolate ester. Pain associated with onset of hepatic dysfunction may mimic acute cholecystitis. Hepatic dysfunction is reversible when erythromycin is discontinued.

CLINDAMYCIN

Clindamycin resembles erythromycin in antibacterial activity except that it is more active against many anaerobic bacteria (Fig. 28-10). A number of gram-positive cocci are sensitive to clindamycin, but a high incidence of gastrointestinal side effects limit its use to infections in which it is clearly superior to other antibiotics (Fass *et al*, 1973). Intravenous administration is useful in the treatment of staphylococcal osteomyelitus.

Antibiotic activity of clindamycin is due to suppression of protein synthesis by bacterial ribosomes. Oral absorption of the drug is nearly complete, and the elimination half-time is about 24 hours. Significant concentrations of clindamycin are not achieved in the cerebrospinal fluid.

Clindamycin is occasionally associated with pseudomembranous colitis, which is presumably caused by elaboration of an exotoxin by clindamycin-resistant bacteria (Barlett *et al*, 1978). If diarrhea occurs, clindamycin should be discontinued and oral vancomycin should be administered. Skin rashes occur in about 10% of patients treated with clindamycin.

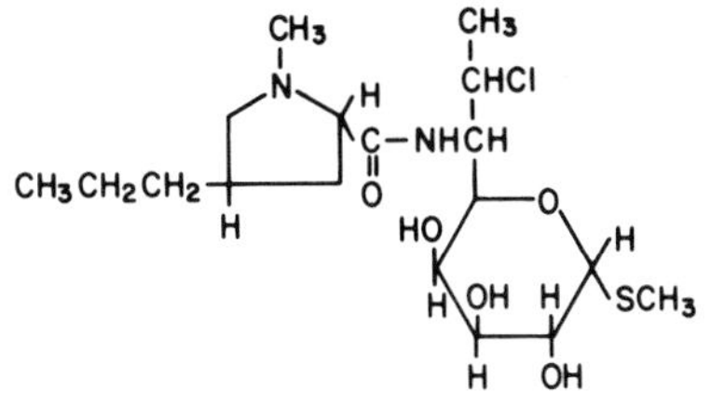

POLYMYXIN AND COLISTIN

Polymyxin B and colistin are basic peptides with molecular weights near 1000 that are effective against gram-negative bacteria, including *E. coli*, *Klebsiella*, and *P. aeruginosa*. Proteus and most strains of Neisseria are resistant to these drugs. Polymyxin B and colistin are used primarily to treat severe urinary tract infections caused by *P. aeruginosa* and other gram-negative bacteria that are not susceptible to other antibiotics. Meningeal infections caused by similar organisms are treated with intrathecal polymyxin B, since systemically administered drug does not enter the cerebrospinal fluid. Infections of the skin, mucous membranes, eye, and ear can be effectively treated with topical application. Indeed, *P. aeruginosa* is a common cause of corneal ulcers.

Polymyxin B and colistin are surface-active antibiotics that interact with phospholipids and penetrate into and disrupt the structure of bacterial cell membranes. Oral or mucous membrane absorption is inadequate such that these drugs are administered intramuscularly. Pain after intramuscular injection is common and may follow the distribution of a nearby peripheral nerve. Elimination is predominantly by the kidney, and these drugs accumulate in patients with renal failure.

Side Effects

Polymyxin applied to intact or denuded skin is not absorbed systemically and, therefore, allergic reactions are unlikely to occur. Like aminoglycosides, polymyxin B can produce skeletal muscle weakness resembling nondepolarizing neuromuscular blockade, particularly in the presence of high plasma concentrations of drug as are likely to occur in patients with renal dysfunction (Lindersmith *et al*, 1968). Neostigmine or calcium does not antagonize this drug-induced effect at the neuromuscular junction, which contrasts with the ability of these drugs to reverse aminoglycoside-induced skeletal muscle weakness (Sokoll and Gergis, 1981). This antibiotic-induced neuromuscular effect may also manifest as marked potentiation of nondepolarizing neuromuscular blocking drugs.

The most significant side effect of these antibiotics is nephrotoxicity, with polymyxin B being more toxic than colistin (Appel and Neu, 1977). For this reason, these antibiotics should not be used in patients with renal disease if alternative drugs are available.

VANCOMYCIN

Vancomycin is a glycopeptide antibiotic that is bactericidal for gram-positive cocci, including strains of *S. aureus* that are resistant to methicillin. This drug is also useful in the treatment of severe staphylococcal infections in patients who are allergic to penicillin and cephalosporin antibi-

FIGURE 28-10.   Clindamycin.

otics (Geraci, 1977). Oral vancomycin is used to treat colitis associated with the overgrowth of exotoxin-producing bacteria in patients being treated with other antibiotics. Penetration into the cerebrospinal fluid is substantial.

Vancomycin acts by inhibiting synthesis of cell walls of sensitive bacteria. Oral absorption of the drug is poor, with large amounts being excreted in the feces. Intravenous infusion of 500 mg over 30 minutes produces therapeutic plasma concentrations for up to 12 hours. Thrombophlebitis is rare following intravenous injection.

Vancomycin is principally excreted by the kidneys, with 90% of a dose being recovered unchanged in the urine. The elimination half-time is about 6 hours, and this may be greatly prolonged in the presence of renal failure.

Side Effects

Skin rashes and allergic reactions with profound hypotension caused by drug-induced histamine release may accompany the rapid intravenous administration of vancomycin (Miller and Tausk, 1977). The occurrence of hypotension during intravenous administration of vancomycin may also reflect a direct myocardial depressant effect of this drug (Cohen *et al,* 1970). Ototoxicity is likely when excessively high plasma concentrations (greater than 30 μg ml^{-1}) are present. The incidence of nephrotoxicity is low.

BACITRACIN

Bacitracins are a group of polypeptide antibiotics effective against a variety of gram-positive bacteria. Bacitracin inhibits bacterial cell wall synthesis. Its use is limited to topical application in ophthalmic and dermatologic ointments. An advantage of bacitracin compared with other antibiotics is that topical application of it rarely results in allergic reactions. Established topical uses of bacitracin include treatment of furunculosis, carbuncle, impetigo, suppurative conjunctivitis, and infected corneal ulcer.

SULFONAMIDES

Sulfonamides are drugs that are derivatives of sulfanilamide. These drugs were the first antibiotics

that exhibited a wide range of bacteriostatic activity against gram-positive and gram-negative bacteria (Weinstein *et al,* 1960). The important structural features for antibacterial activity are the benzene ring and the para-amino group (Fig. 28-11). The para-amino group can be replaced only by radicals capable of being converted in the tissues to a free amino group.

Mechanism of Action

Antibiotic activity of sulfonamides is due to the ability of these drugs to prevent normal utilization of para-aminobenzoic acid by bacteria to synthesize folic acid (pteroylglutamic acid). Specifically, sulfonamides act as competitive inhibitors of the bacterial enzyme responsible for the incorporation of para-aminobenzoic acid into the immediate precursor of folic acid. Bacteria that do not require folic acid or normal mammalian cells that can utilize preformed folic acid that is absorbed from the gastrointestinal tract are not affected by sulfonamides. Bacteriostatic effects of sulfonamides are counteracted by para-aminobenzoic acid. For example, ester local anesthetics that are hydrolyzed to para-aminobenzoic acid antagonize the *in vivo* antibacterial effects of sulfonamides. Indeed, resistance that develops to the antibacterial effects of sulfonamides may reflect the development of the ability of bacteria to synthesize para-aminobenzoic acid (White and Woods, 1965).

Route of Administration

Except for sulfonamides that are especially designed for their local effects in the bowel, these antibiotics are rapidly and highly absorbed (70% – 100%) from the gastrointestinal tract, primarily from the small intestine. Sulfonamides readily enter pleural, peritoneal, synovial, ocular, and cerebrospinal fluid, reaching concentrations similar to those in the blood. Passage across the placenta is prompt.

Excretion

Metabolism of sulfonamides is predominantly acetylation in the liver to pharmacologically inactive compounds. Acetyl metabolites, however, are

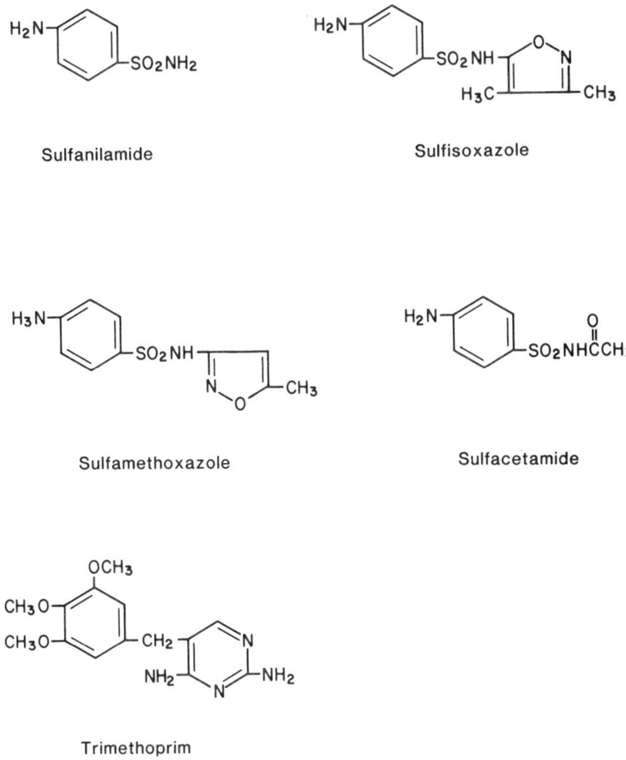

Sulfanilamide

Sulfisoxazole

Sulfamethoxazole

Sulfacetamide

Trimethoprim

FIGURE 28-11. Sulfonamides are derivatives of sulfanilamide.

often less soluble, which increases the likelihood of crystalluria. The magnitude of acetylation varies greatly among the various sulfonamides. Elimination of unchanged and acetylated drug is primarily by glomerular filtration, with renal tubular secretion being of variable importance. The elimination half-time of sulfonamides is dependent on renal function.

Side Effects

Side effects that may follow administration of sulfonamides are numerous and varied (Weinstein *et al*, 1960). Allergic reactions ranging from skin rash to anaphylaxis are possible with any of the sulfonamides, and cross-sensitivity may or may not occur. Drug fever is a common side effect of sulfonamide treatment. Hepatotoxicity resulting from direct toxicity or sensitization occurs in less than 0.1% of patients. Acute hemolytic anemia and agranulocytosis are rare but possible adverse effects of treatment with sulfonamides. Formation

and deposition of crystalline aggregates in the kidneys and ureter are infrequent with the use of highly soluble sulfonamides. Administration of sulfonamides may increase the effect of oral anticoagulants, methotrexate, sulfonylurea hypoglycemic drugs, and thiazide diuretics, probably by displacement of these drugs from binding sites on plasma albumin. Likewise, sulfonamides can compete for the same protein binding sites as albumin, enhancing the risk of jaundice in premature infants. Conversely, indomethacin, probenecid, and salicylates may displace sulfonamides from plasma albumin and increase the concentration of free drug in the plasma. Hemolytic anemia may occur in patients with glucose-6-phosphate deficiency who receive sulfonamides.

Sulfisoxazole

Sulfisoxazole administered orally is rapidly absorbed from the gastrointestinal tract (Fig. 28-11). The usual adult oral dose is 2 to 4 g initially, followed by 1 g every 4 to 6 hours. Sulfisoxazole is primarily used as a treatment for urinary tract infections. In susceptible patients who are allergic to penicillin antibiotics, sulfisoxazole can be used as prophylaxis against streptococcal infections and recurrences of rheumatic fever. Its high water solubility minimizes the hazards of renal toxicity such as crystalluria. About 95% of a single oral dose is excreted by the kidneys in 24 hours. Concentrations of sulfisoxazole in the urine greatly exceed those in the blood and may be bactericidal. The cerebrospinal fluid concentration averages about one third of that in the plasma.

Sulfamethoxazole

Sulfamethoxazole is a congener of sulfisoxazole, but its rate of absorption and urinary excretion are slower (Fig. 28-11). Crystalluria is a risk with sulfamethoxazole, and anuria may occur as a result of precipitation of crystals of the acetylated drug in the renal tubules and ureter. Alkalinization of the urine or increased fluid intake is effective in preventing such precipitation.

Sulfasalazine

Sulfasalazine is poorly absorbed from the gastrointestinal tract. For this reason, it is used in the treatment of ulcerative colitis and regional enteritis (Summers *et al*, 1979).

Sulfacetamide

Sulfacetamide is frequently used for topical application as an ointment or solution for treatment of ophthalmic infections (Fig. 28-11). The preparation has a *p*H of 7.4, is nonirritating, and penetrates into ocular fluid in high concentrations.

Co-trimoxazole

Co-trimoxazole is a combination of trimethoprim with sulfamethoxazole that results in a synergistic antibacterial action (Fig. 28-11) (Nolte and Buttner, 1973). The usual combination is 800 mg sulfamethoxazole plus 16 mg of trimethoprim (*i.e.,* 5:1 ratio). Chronic and recurrent urinary tract infections are particularly responsive to treatment

with this combination (Gleckman, 1975). In females, this may be related to the presence of therapeutic concentrations of trimethoprim in vaginal secretions. Trimethoprim is also found in prostatic secretions and is often effective for treatment of bacterial prostatitis. Acute exacerbations of chronic bronchitis are effectively treated with this combination. Infection by *Pneumocystis carinii* is eradicated by high doses, whereas low doses provide protection against this infection in immunosuppressed hosts. Acute gonococcal urethritis, but not syphilis, is effectively treated. In fact, this combination appears to be as effective as 4.8 million units of benzylpenicillin plus 1 g of probenecid for the treatment of gonorrhea.

Mechanism of Action

The antimicrobial activity of this drug combination results from its actions on two sequential steps of the enzymatic pathway for the synthesis of tetrahydrofolic acid. Sulfamethoxazole inhibits the incorporation of para-aminobenzoic acid into folic acid, and trimethoprim prevents the reduction of dihydrofolate to tetrahydrofolate by selective inhibition of dihydrofolate reductase. The dihydrofolate reductase of the host is many thousands of times less sensitive to trimethoprim than are the bacterial enzymes, accounting for the selectivity of this drug. Development of resistance to the combination is lower than if either of the drugs were used alone. This is predictable, since bacteria that have acquired resistance to one of the components may still be destroyed by the other.

Excretion

After a single oral dose of the combined preparation, trimethoprim is absorbed more rapidly than sulfamethoxazole. The elimination half-times of both trimethoprim and sulfamethoxazole are approximately 9.5 hours. Trimethoprim is rapidly distributed and concentrated in tissues, achieving a volume of distribution that is about six times that of sulfamethoxazole. It enters cerebrospinal fluid and sputum readily. Up to 60% of administered trimethoprim and from 25% to 50% of sulfamethoxazole are excreted in the urine as metabolites and unchanged drug.

Side Effects

The most common side effects of this combined preparation are skin rashes, glossitis, and stomatitis (Arndt and Jick, 1976). Mild and transient jaundice with histologic features resembling allergic cholestatic hepatitis have been observed. Impairment of renal function may follow administration of this drug combination to patients with renal disease, and a reversible decrease in creatinine clearance has been noted in patients with normal renal function (Shouval *et al*, 1978).

There is no evidence that co-trimoxazole induces folate deficiency in normal persons, but the margin between toxicity for bacteria and patients may be narrow when the cells of the patient are already deficient in folate. In this situation, the drug combination may cause or precipitate megaloblastic anemia, leukopenia, or thrombocytopenia. Accordingly, complete blood counts should be followed in patients being treated longer than 2 weeks. Previous or simultaneous administration of diuretics may increase the likelihood of thrombocytopenia, particularly in elderly patients.

URINARY TRACT ANTISEPTICS

Urinary tract antiseptics are drugs that are concentrated in the renal tubules, making them effective for the treatment of infections in the kidney and bladder. Because these drugs are selectively concentrated in the renal tubules, their plasma concentrations do not reach adequate levels to be effective against systemic infections.

Methenamine

Methenamine is a urinary tract antiseptic that decomposes in water at a pH below 7.4 to formaldehyde (Fig. 28-12). Formaldehyde is responsible for the antibacterial action. Proteus organisms, as urea-splitting bacteria, often raise the pH of urine above 5.5 and thus inhibit the release of formaldehyde. Bacteria do not develop resistance to formaldehyde. Methenamine is not used as a treatment of acute urinary tract infections but is of value for chronic suppressive treatment (Gerstein *et al*, 1968).

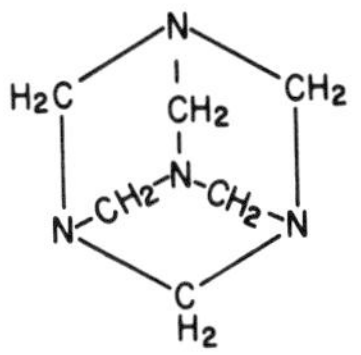

Nalidixic Acid

Nalidixic acid is bactericidal to most of the common gram-negative bacteria that cause urinary tract infections (Fig. 28-13). It appears to act by inhibiting DNA synthesis (Brumfitt and Pursell, 1971). Therapeutic concentrations do not occur in prostatic fluid, which may account for reinfection of the urinary tract. Resistance may develop rapidly.

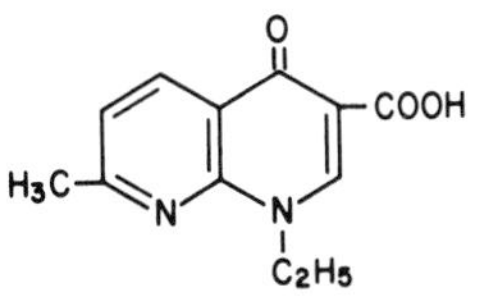

Nitrofurantoin

Nitrofurantoin is active against many strains of *E. coli* in the urine, and its antibacterial activity is higher in acidic urine (Fig. 28-14). In addition to use for treatment of urinary tract infections, this drug is used for the prevention of bacteriuria after prostatectomy.

Chronic active hepatitis is a rare complication (Tolman, 1980). Acute pneumonitis with fever, chills, dyspnea, and chest pain may accompany administration of this drug. Elderly patients are especially susceptible to the pulmonary toxicity of nitrofurantoin (Hailey *et al*, 1969). Neuropathies are most likely to occur in patients with impaired renal function (Lindholm, 1967).

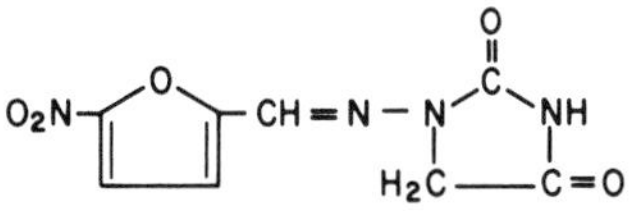

FIGURE 28-13. Nalidixic acid.

FIGURE 28-14. Nitrofurantoin.

FIGURE 28-12. Methenamine.

Phenazopyridine

Phenazopyridine is not a urinary antiseptic but provides an analgesic action on the urinary tract that alleviates symptoms of dysuria, frequency, and urgency. The compound is an azo dye, and the urine is colored orange or red. Overdose may result in methemoglobinemia. This drug may be marketed in combination with sulfisoxazole or sulfamethoxazole.

DRUGS FOR TREATMENT OF TUBERCULOSIS

The majority of patients with tuberculosis can be successfully treated with drugs such as isoniazid, rifampin, ethambutol, and streptomycin. Administration of isoniazid in combination with rifampin or ethambutol represents optimal therapy for all forms of disease caused by sensitive strains of *Mycobacterium tuberculosis.* Treatment must include at least two drugs to which the mycobacteria are sensitive to offset the impact of development of resistance that commonly occurs during therapy. Isoniazid alone is used for prophylaxis. For example, patients without apparent disease but whose skin test has changed from negative to positive should be treated with isoniazid for 12 months.

Isoniazid

Isoniazid is the hydrazide derivative of isonicotinic acid and is considered the primary drug for the chemotherapy of tuberculosis (Fig. 28-15). A congener of isoniazid is the isopropyl derivative, iproniazid, which markedly inhibits the multiplication of the tubercle bacillus and is also a potent inhibitor of monoamine oxidase (see Chapter 19). Isoniazid is both tuberculostatic and tuberculocidal. Resistance during therapy can occur, presumably as a result of emergence of strains that do not take up the drug. Cross-resistance, however, between isoniazid and other tuberculostatic drugs

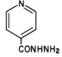

FIGURE 28-15. Isoniazid.

does not occur. The mechanism of action of isoniazid is not known but may reflect drug-induced inhibition of synthesis of mycolic acids, which are important constituents of the myobacterial cell wall (Takayama *et al,* 1975).

Excretion

Isoniazid is readily absorbed when administered orally or parenterally. The drug diffuses into all body fluids and cells. Up to 95% of a dose of isoniazid is excreted in the urine over 24 hours entirely as metabolites. The primary route of metabolism is hepatic acetylation to acetylisoniazid. There is a genetic determination of the rate of acetylation of isoniazid, with patients being categorized as slow and rapid acetylators (Ellard, 1978). Rapid acetylation is inherited as an autosomal dominant trait. Rapid acetylators are homozygous. The average concentration of active isoniazid in the plasma of rapid acetylators is 30 to 50 times less than that present in the plasma of slow acetylators. The elimination half-time of isoniazid averages about 1.5 hours in rapid acetylators and 3 hours in patients who are slow acetylators.

The clearance of isoniazid is dependent to only a small degree on the status of renal function, but patients who are slow acetylators may be susceptible to accumulation of toxic concentrations if renal function is impaired.

Side Effects

Side effects can be minimized by prophylactic therapy with pyridoxine and careful surveillance of the patient. For example, pyridoxine, 10 mg daily, is administered with isoniazid to minimize the occurrence of peripheral neuritis and anemia. The protective effect of pyridoxine is based on the fact that isoniazid increases the excretion of pyridoxine, resulting in a deficiency of this vitamin. Isoniazid may precipitate seizures in patients with epilepsy and rarely in patients with no prior history of seizures. Optic neuritis has occurred during therapy with this drug. Mental changes during treatment with isoniazid include euphoria, impairment of memory, and occasionally psychoses. Excessive sedation may occur in slow acetylators given isoniazid who are also receiving phenytoin, reflecting isoniazid-induced inhibition of the metabolism of the anticonvulsant (Kutt *et al,* 1966).

Severe hepatic injury characterized pathologically by bridging and multilobular necrosis (*i.e.,* similar to the changes associated with halothane) can occur (Garibaldi *et al,* 1972). The mechanism for hepatotoxicity is not known, although a metabolite of isoniazid, acetylisoniazid, is a known hepatotoxin (Mitchell *et al,* 1976). Rapid acetylators who produce more acetylhydrazine may be more vulnerable to isoniazid-induced hepatotoxicity than those who do not. Age seems to be an important determinant in the incidence of isoniazid-induced hepatic dysfunction, with an incidence of 0.3% in patients 20 to 34 years old, 1.2% in patients 35 to 49 years old, and 2.3% in patients older than 50 years of age. Up to 12% of patients treated with isoniazid manifest elevated plasma transaminase enzyme levels. A greater than threefold elevation in the serum glutamic oxalacetic transaminase activity is cause for discontinuation of isoniazid (Byrd *et al,* 1977).

Isoniazid treatment significantly enhances defluorination of volatile anesthetics, presumably by inducing the necessary hepatic microsomal enzymes (Mazze *et al,* 1982). Indeed, in patients treated with isoniazid, the serum fluoride concentration increases after enflurane anesthesia. The magnitude of this increase is variable, presumably reflecting different levels of enzyme induction among rapid and slow acetylators (Fig. 28-16)

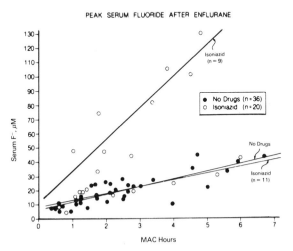

PEAK SERUM FLUORIDE AFTER ENFLURANE

FIGURE 28-16. Isoniazid enhances defluorination of enflurane in patients who are rapid acetylators. (From Mazze RI, Woodruff RE, Heerdt ME. Isoniazid-induced enflurane defluorination in humans. Anesthesiology 1982;57:5 – 8. Reproduced by permission of the authors and publisher.)

(Mazze *et al,* 1982). Serum fluoride concentrations may be in a nephrotoxic range in those patients presumed to be rapid acetylators.

Rifampin

Rifampin is a complex macrocyclic antibiotic that inhibits the growth of most gram-positive bacteria as well as many gram-negative bacteria. This antibiotic is the drug of choice for prophylaxis against meningococcal disease in household contacts of patients with such infections. Resistance to the antibacterial effects of rifampin develop rapidly (within 48 hours), emphasizing that it must not be used alone in the chemotherapy of tuberculosis (Devine *et al,* 1971). Rifampin is effective by virtue of its ability to inhibit ribonucleic acid synthesis in bacteria at concentrations far below those that produce this effect in normal cells.

Route of Administration

Oral absorption of rifampin is adequate but often highly variable. Salicylates may delay absorption and prevent achievement of therapeutic plasma concentrations. Rifampin penetrates tissues and body fluids, including cerebrospinal fluid, imparting a red color to the urine and saliva of patients treated with this drug.

Excretion

Rifampin undergoes hepatic deacetylation, and the resulting metabolite, which has antibacterial activity similar to the parent compound, enters bile where enterohepatic circulation occurs. The elimination half-time of rifampin varies from 1.5 to 5 hours and is prolonged in patients with hepatic dysfunction.

Side Effects

Side effects of rifampin are infrequent but with high doses may include thrombocytopenia, anemia, hepatic dysfunction with jaundice, and occasionally hepatorenal syndrome (Flynn *et al,* 1974). Elevations of the serum glutamic oxalacetic transaminase activity and alkaline phosphatase concentrations may occur. Hepatic dysfunction rarely occurs in patients with normal hepatic function; it is more likely to occur in elderly patients with preexisting liver disease, especially that related to alcohol abuse.

Biliary excretion of rifampin competes with that of contrast media used for the study of the gallbladder. Rifampin, by an unknown mechanism, interferes with the anticoagulant effect of coumarin drugs (Romankiewicz and Ehrman, 1975). Methadone metabolism is accelerated by rifampin, and the likelihood of an opioid withdrawal syndrome may be increased. Rifampin appears to speed the breakdown of glucocorticoids and estrogens, which may decrease the reliability of oral contraceptives (Skolnik *et al,* 1976). Central and peripheral nervous system effects associated with rifampin administration include fatigue, generalized numbness, skeletal muscle weakness, and pain in the extremities.

Ethambutol

Ethambutol is tuberculostatic to mycobacteria but not to other bacteria (Fig. 28-17). It is used in combination with isoniazid for the treatment of active tuberculosis. Absorption after oral administration approaches 85% of the drug. Ethambutol is concentrated in erythrocytes, which may serve as a depot of drug to maintain a therapeutic concentration as the plasma level declines.

Excretion

About 50% of an ingested dose of ethambutol is excreted unchanged by the kidneys in 24 hours. The high renal clearance of ethambutol confirms that the drug is excreted by renal tubular secretion as well as by glomerular filtration. The elimination half-time is 3 to 4 hours. Accumulation of ethambutol is likely in patients with renal dysfunction.

Side Effects

The most important side effect of therapy with ethambutol is optic neuritis, resulting in a decrease in visual acuity and loss of ability to perceive the color green (Place and Thomas, 1963). The incidence of this complication is dose-related, occurring in about 5% of patients treated

with 25 mg kg^{-1} daily and in less than 1% of patients receiving daily doses less than 15 mg kg^{-1}. There is decreased renal excretion of uric acid, resulting in increased blood concentrations of urate in approximately 50% of patients.

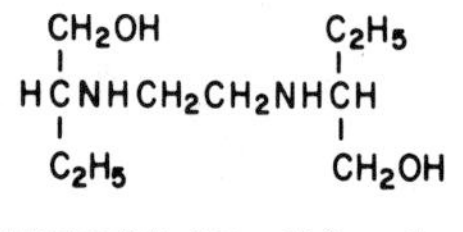

ANTIFUNGAL DRUGS

Nystatin

Nystatin is a polyene antibiotic that is both fungistatic and fungicidal but lacks effects on bacteria (Hamilton-Miller, 1974). This drug increases the permeability of the membrane of sensitive fungi such that small molecules escape. Absorption of nystatin via the skin, mucous membranes, or gastrointestinal tract is negligible. Nystatin is used primarily to treat Candida infections and is available as oral tablets, vaginal tablets, and ointments. Paronychia, vaginitis, and stomatitis (thrush) caused by Candida organisms usually respond to topical therapy. Oral, esophageal, and gastric Candida infections are common in patients receiving immunosuppressive therapy and certain antibiotics such as the tetracyclines. These infections usually respond to oral nystatin. Side effects are rare. For example, allergic reactions have not been reported. Since nystatin has no effect on bacteria, suprainfections do not occur.

Amphotericin B

Amphotericin B, like nystatin, is a polyene antibiotic that exerts maximal antifungal effects between pH 6 and 7.5 (Andrioli and Kravetz, 1962). This is the most effective antifungal drug for the management of infections due to yeasts and fungi. Cryptococcal infection of the lungs or meninges, histoplasmosis, coccidioidomycosis, blastomycosis, sporotrichosis, and disseminated candidiasis are treated with amphotericin B.

Oral absorption is poor, accounting for the need to administer amphotericin B intravenously if therapeutic concentrations in infected tissues are to be achieved. The drug does not penetrate into the cerebrospinal fluid or vitreous humor. Intrathecal injection may be necessary for treatment of Coccidioides meningitis. Renal excretion is slow, with detectable drug being present for up to 8 weeks after discontinuation of therapy.

$$\begin{array}{cc} CH_2OH & C_2H_5 \\ | & | \\ HCNHCH_2CH_2NHCH \\ | & | \\ C_2H_5 & CH_2OH \end{array}$$

FIGURE 28-17. Ethambutol.

Side Effects

Side effects are common with the use of amphotericin B. For example, renal function is impaired in more than 80% of treated patients, and some permanent reduction in glomerular filtration rate is likely (Butler *et al,* 1964). During therapy, plasma creatinine should be monitored, and the dose of amphotericin B should be reduced when the creatinine level exceeds 3.5 mg dl^{-1} (Bennett *et al,* 1979). Hypokalemia and hypomagnesemia may occur. Fever, chills, dyspnea, and hypotension are common during intravenous infusion of amphotericin B. Allergic reactions, seizures, anemia, and thrombocytopenia may occur. Hepatotoxicity is not documented to occur as a side effect of treatment with amphotericin B (Bennett *et al,* 1979).

Flucytosine

Flucytosine is converted to fluorouracil exclusively in fungal cells by the enzyme cytosine deaminase (Fig. 28-18). This selective effect avoids cytotoxicity of fluorouracil on normal cells. The drug is well absorbed from the gastrointestinal tract. Penetration into the cerebrospinal fluid and aqueous humor is excellent. Approximately 80% of flucytosine is excreted unchanged in the urine by glomerular filtration. The elimination half-time is 3 to 6 hours, but this is greatly prolonged in the presence of renal failure. In about 5% of patients, liver transaminase enzymes are increased and hepatomegaly occurs (Steer *et al,* 1972).

Flucytosine is available only for oral administration. It is used predominantly in combination with amphotericin B, because rapid emergence of resistant strains limits the use of flucytosine as a single drug.

Griseofulvin

Griseofulvin inhibits mitosis in certain fungi, accounting for its fungistatic effects, especially in

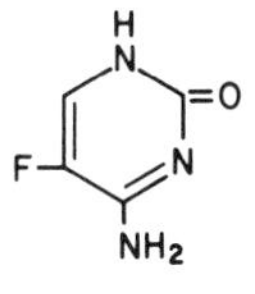

FIGURE 28-18. Flucytosine.

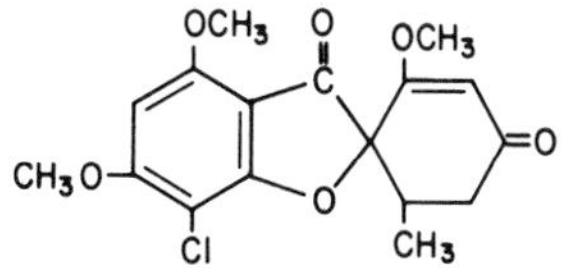

FIGURE 28-19. Griseofulvin.

dermatophytes (Fig. 28-19). Mycotic diseases of the skin, hair, and nails respond to griseofulvin. Symptomatic relief of skin infections usually occurs in 48 to 96 hours. There is no effect on bacteria.

Oral absorption of griseofulvin is adequate but highly variable. About 50% of an oral dose appears in the urine, mostly in the form of metabolites (Lin *et al,* 1973). The drug has greater affinity for cells of diseased skin than of normal skin, accounting for the prompt appearance of new growth of hair or nails.

Side Effects

Headache, which may be severe, occurs in as many as 15% of patients. Other nervous system manifestations include peripheral neuritis, fatigue, blurred vision, and syncope. Hepatotoxicity has been observed. Renal effects include proteinuria without evidence of renal insufficiency. Griseofulvin appears to reduce the activity of warfarin-like anticoagulants.

ANTIVIRAL DRUGS

Development of antiviral drugs has been hampered by the fact that viruses, in contrast to bacteria, are obligate intracellular parasites that require the active participation of the metabolic process of invaded cells. As a result, drugs that inhibit growth or destroy the virus may have similar effects on the cell.

Idoxuridine

Idoxuridine is a halogenated pyrimidine that resembles thymidine. Following phosphorylation in the cells, the triphosphate derivative is incorporated into both viral and mammalian deoxyribonucleic acid (DNA) (Prusoff and Goz, 1973). As such, the antiviral activity of idoxuridine is mainly limited to DNA viruses, usually of the herpes simplex group. The primary clinical use of this drug is topical treatment of herpes simplex keratitis lesions of the skin, conjunctiva, and mucous membranes. Rapid inactivation by nucleotidases precludes its use by routes other than intravenous or topical administration. After intravenous injection, most of the drug disappears from the blood in about 30 minutes.

Amantadine

Amantadine is a synthetic tricyclic amine antiviral drug that inhibits replication of strains of influenza A virus. It is almost completely absorbed after oral administration, with 90% of the dose appearing unchanged in the urine. Amantadine has prophylactic value when administered to persons who have had contact with an active case of influenza A virus. This drug also has therapeutic value in the treatment of patients with Parkinson's disease (see Chapter 31).

Amantadine accumulates in patients with impaired renal function. Excessive plasma concentrations are associated with central nervous system toxicity, including seizures and coma.

Vidarabine

Vidarabine is an analog of adenosine that is effective in the treatment of herpes simplex encephalitis and keratoconjunctivitis (Fig. 28-20) (Whitley *et al*, 1986). Severe infections with herpes simplex virus in neonates may also respond to vidarabine. It is ineffective in varicella, cytomegalovirus infections, and recurrent or primary genital

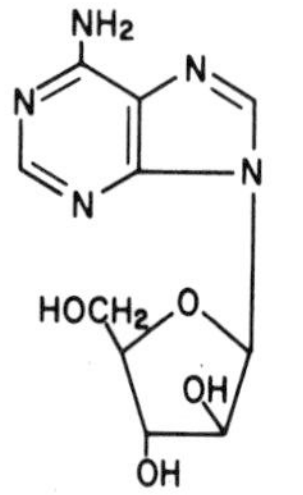

FIGURE 28-20. Vidarabine.

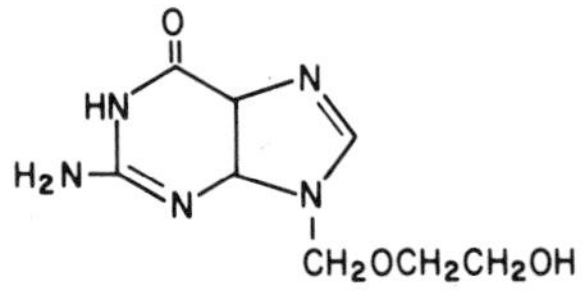

FIGURE 28-21. Acyclovir.

herpes. The drug acts by inhibiting viral DNA polymerase, while DNA synthesis in noninfected cells is inhibited less. Since vidarabine is poorly soluble in water, large volumes (*i.e.*, 2.5 L) are needed to dissolve the drug for intravenous infusion and treatment of encephalitis. Topical ointment is used for treatment of conjunctivitis. Vidarabine may be both mutagenic and carcinogenic.

Interferon

Interferon is a general term used to designate glycoproteins produced by cells infected with viruses. Binding of interferons by specific receptors on cell membranes is the first step in establishing their antiviral effect, which may include degradation of viral ribonucleic acid. In addition to antiviral effects, interferons inhibit cell proliferation and enhance tumoricidal activities of macrophages. Recombinant interferons administered as a nasal spray are particularly effective against rhinovirus infections (Hayden *et al*, 1986). Treatment with interferons may be associated with fever, headache, malaise, myalgia, and transient leukopenia, especially following intravenous or intramuscular administration. Nasal irritation may accompany intranasal administration.

Acyclovir

Acyclovir is effective orally in the initial and recurrent treatment of genital herpes (Fig. 28-21) (Corey *et al*, 1982). The drug is widely distributed in tissues and body fluids, attaining concentrations in the cerebrospinal fluid that are about 50% of those in plasma. Excretion is by glomerular filtration and renal tubular secretion, principally of unchanged drug. The elimination half-time is about 2.5 hours in the presence of normal renal function.

Side Effects

Elevations in blood urea nitrogen and serum creatinine have occurred following rapid intravenous administration. This may reflect crystallization of acyclovir in renal tubules. Thrombophlebitis may occur at the site of intravenous administration. A frequent nonspecific complaint in patients treated with oral acyclovir is headache.

REFERENCES

Adams HR, Isaacson EL, Masters BS. Inhibition of hepatic microsomal enzymes by chloramphenicol. J Pharmacol Exp Ther 1977;203:388–96.

Andrioli VT, Kravetz HM. The use of amphotericin B in man. JAMA 1962;180:269–72.

Appel GB, New HC. Nephrotoxicity of antimicrobial agents. N Engl J Med 1977;286:722–8.

Arndt KA, Jick H. Rates of cutaneous reactions to drugs. JAMA 1976;235:918–23.

Barr WH, Adir J, Garnetson L. Decrease of tetracycline absorption in man by sodium bicarbonate. Clin Pharmacol Ther 1971;12:779–84.

Bartlett JG, Chang TW, Gurwith M, Gorbach SL, Onderdonk AB. Antibiotic-associated pseudomembranous colitis due to toxin-producing clostridia. N Engl J Med 1978;298:531–4.

Barza M, Scheife RT. Antimicrobial spectrum, pharmacology, and therapeutic use of antibiotics. J Maine Med Assoc 1977;68:194–210.

Barza M. The nephrotoxicity of cephalosporins: an overview. J Infect Dis 1978;137:560–73.

Beaupre PN, Roizen MF, Cahalan MK, Alpert RA, Cassorla L, Schiller NB. Hemodynamic and two-dimensional tranesophageal echocardiographic analysis of an anaphylactic reaction in a human. Anesthesiology 1984;60:482–4.

Bennett JE, Dismules WE, Duma RJ, et al. A collaborative study. Amphotericin B–flucytosine in cryptococcal meningitis. N Engl J Med 1979;301:126–31.

Benveniste R, Davies J. Mechanisms of antibiotic resistance in bacteria. Annu Rev Biochem 1973;42:471–506.

Berg SW, Kilpatrick ME, Harrison WO, McCutchan JA. Cefoxitin as a single-dose treatment for urethritis caused by penicillinase-producing Neisseria gonorrhoeae. N Engl J Med 1979;301:509–11.

Berger S, Ernest E, Baraza M. Comparative incidence of phlebitis due to buffered cephalothin, cephapirin, and cefamandole. Antimicrob Agents Chemother 1976;9:575–9.

Bergeron MD, Brusch JL, Barza M, Weinstein L. Bactericidal activity and pharmacology of cefazolin. Antimicrob Agents Chemother 1973;4:396–401.

Best WR. Chloramphenicol-associated blood dyscrasias

—a review of cases submitted to American Medical Association Registry. JAMA 1967;201:181–8.

Booij LHDJ, VanderPloeg GCJ, Crul JF, Muytijens HL. Do neostigmine and 4-aminopyridine inhibit the antibacterial activity of antibiotics? Br J Anaesth 1980;52:1097–9.

Bruckner J, Thomas KC, Bikhazi GB, Foldes FF. Neuromuscular drug interactions of clinical importance. Anesth Analg 1980;59:678–82.

Brumfitt W, Pursell R. Observations on bacterial sensitivities to nalidixic acid and critical comments on the 6-centre survey. Postgrad Med 1971;47:16-8.

Butler WT, Bennett JE, Alling DW, Wertlake PT, Utz JP, Hill GJ. Nephrotoxicity of amphotericin B. Early and late effects in 81 patients. Ann Intern Med 1964;61:175–87.

Byrd RB, Horn BR, Griggs GA, Solomon DA. Isoniazid chemoprophylaxis. Arch Intern Med 1977;137:1130–3.

Cohen LS, Wechsler AS, Mitchell H, Glock G. Depression of cardiac function by streptomycin and other antimicrobial agents. Am J Cardio 1970;26:505–11.

Cooksley WGE, Powell LW. Erythromycin jaundice: diagnosis by an in vitro challenge test. Aust NZ J Med 1977;7:291–3.

Corey L, Nahmias AJ, Guinan ME, Benedetti JK, Critchlow CW, Holmes KK. Trial of topical acyclovir in genital herpes simplex virus infections. N Engl J Med 1982;306:1313–9.

Corrado AP, Nicolette RL. Mechanism of neuromuscular block produced by streptomycin, dihydrostreptomycin, neomycin, and kanamycin. Acta Physiol Lat Am 1961;12:212–6.

Devine LF, Johnson DP, Rhode SL, Hagerman CR, Pierce WE, Peckinpaugh RD. Rifampin-effect of two-day treatment on the meningococcal carrier state and the relationship to the level of drug in the sera and saliva. Am J Med Sci 1971;26:74–83.

Dolci ED, Brabec MJ. Antagonism by chloramphenicol of carbon tetrachloride hepatotoxicity. Examination of microsomal cytochrome P-450 and lipid peroxidation. Exp Mol Pathol 1978;28:96–106.

Ellard GA. Variations between individuals and populations in the acetylation of isoniazid and its significance for the treatment of pulmonary tuberculosis. Clin Pharmacol Ther 1978;19:610–25.

Fass RJ, Scholand JF, Hodges GR, Saslaw S. Clindamycin in the treatment of serious anaerobic infections. Ann Intern Med 1973;78:853–9.

Federspil P. Pharmacokinetics and ototoxicity of gentamicin, tobramycin, and amikacin. Arch Otolaryngol 1977;217:147–66.

Feldman WE. Effect of ampicillin and chloramphenicol against Haemophilus influenzae. Pediatrics 1978;61:406–9.

Flynn CT, Rainford DJ, Hope E. Acute renal failure and rifampicin: danger of unsuspected intermittent dosage. Br Med J 1974;2:482.

Fry L, Ramsay CA. Tetracycline in acne vulgaris: clinical evaluation and the effect on sebum production. Br J Dermatol 1966;78:653–60.

Fulop M, Drapkin A. Potassium depletion syndrome secondary to nephropathy caused by "outdated tetracycline." N Engl J Med 1965;272:986–9.

Gangadharam PRJ, Candler ER, Ramakrishna PV. In vitro anti-mycobacterial activity of some new aminoglycoside antibiotics. J Antimicrob Chemother 1977;3:285–6.

Garibaldi RA, Drusin RE, Ferebee SH, Gregg MB. Isoniazid-associated hepatitis. Report of an outbreak. Am Rev Respir Dis 1972;106:357–65.

Gary NE, Buzzeo L, Solaki RP, Eisinger RP. Gentamicin-associated acute renal failure. Arch Intern Med 1976;126:1101–4.

Geraci JE. Vancomycin. Mayo Clin Proc 1977;52:631–4.

Gerstein AR, Okun R, Gonick HC, Howard IW, Kleeman CR, Maxwell MH. The prolonged use of methenamine hippurate in the treatment of chronic urinary tract infections. J Urol 1968;100:767–71.

Gleckman RA. Trimethoprim–sulfamethoxazole vs. ampicillin in chronic urinary tract infections. JAMA 1975;233:427–31.

Green GR, Rosenblum AH, Sweet LC. Evaluation of penicillin hypersensitivity. J Allergy Clin Immunol 1977;60:339–45.

Griffith RS, Black HR. Erythromycin. Med Clin North Am 1970;54:1199–1215.

Grossman ER, Walcheck A, Freedman H. Tetracycline and permanent teeth: the relationship between doses and tooth color. Pediatrics 1971;47:567–70.

Hailey FJ, Glascock HW, Hewitt WF. Pleuropneumonic reactions to nitrofurantoin. N Engl J Med 1969;281:1087–90.

Hamilton-Miller JMT. Fungal sterols and the mode of action of the polyene antibiotics. Adv Appl Microbiol 1974;17:109–34.

Hayden FG, Albrecht JK, Kaiser DL, Gwaltney JM. Prevention of natural colds by contact prophylaxis with intranasal alpha$_2$-interferon. N Engl J Med 1986;314:71–5.

Holtzman JL. Gentamicin neuromuscular blockade (letter). Ann Intern Med 1976;84:55.

Klaus MV, Fellner MJ. Penicilloyl-specific serum antibodies in man. Analysis in 592 individuals from the newborn to old age. J Gerontol 1973;28:312–6.

Kucers A. Current position of chloramphenicol in chemotherapy. J Antimicrob Chemother 1980;6:1–9.

Kutt H, Winters W, McDowell FH. Depression of parahydroxylation of diphenylhydantoin by antituberculosis chemotherapy. Neurology 1966;16:594–602.

Lee C, Chen D, Barnes A, Katz RL. Neuromuscular block by neomycin in the cat. Can Anaesth Soc J 1976;23:527–33.

Levine BB. Skin rashes with penicillin therapy: current management. N Engl J Med 1972;286:42–3.

Lin C, Magat J, Chang R, McGlotten J, Symchowicz S. Absorption, metabolism and excretion of ^{14}C-griseofulvin in man. J Pharmacol Exp Ther 1973;187:415–22.

Lindersmith LA, Baines RD, Bigelow DB, Petty TL. Reversible respiratory paralysis associated with polymyxin therapy. Ann Intern Med 1968;68:318–27.

Lindholm T. Electromyographic changes after nitrofurantoin (Furadantin) therapy in nonuremic patients. Neurology 1967;17:1017–20.

Lippmann M, Yang E, Au E, Lee C. Neuromuscular blocking effects of tobramycin, gentamicin, and cefazolin. Anesth Analg 1982;61:767–70.

Mazze RI, Woodruff RE, Heerdt ME. Isoniazid-induced enflurane defluorination in humans. Anesthesiology 1982;57:5–8.

McCormack WM, Donner GH, Kodgis LF, Alpert S, Lower EW, Kass EH. Hepatotoxicity of erythromycin estolate during pregnancy. Antimicrob Agents Chemother 1977;12:630–5.

Miller R, Tausk HC. Anaphylactoid reaction to vancomycin during anesthesia. Anesth Analg 1977;56:870–2.

Mitchell JR, Zimmerman HJ, Ishak KG, et al. Isoniazid liver injury: clinical spectrum, pathology, and probable pathogenesis. Ann Intern Med 1976;84:181–92.

Nagao L, Mauer AM. Concordance of drug-induced aplastic anemia in identical twins. N Engl J Med 1969;281:7–11.

Nolte H, Buttner H. Pharmacokinetics of trimethoprim and its combination with sulfamethoxazole in man after single and chronic oral administration. Chemotherapy 1973;18:274–84.

Pittinger C, Adamson R. Antibiotic blockade of neuromuscular function. Annu Rev Pharmacol 1972;12:169–84.

Pittinger CP, Eryasa T, Adamson R. Antibiotic-induced paralysis. Anesth Analg 1970;49:487–501.

Place VA, Thomas JP. Clinical pharmacology of ethambutol. Am Rev Respir Dis 1963;87:901–4.

Pollack AA, Berger SA, Simberkoff MS, Rahal JJ. Hepatitis associated with high-dose oxacillin therapy. Arch Intern Med 1978;138:915–7.

Prusoff WH, Goz B. Potential mechanisms of action of antiviral agents. Fed Proc 1973;32:1679–87.

Reynolds HY. Chronic bronchitis in acute infectious exacerbations. In: Principles and Practice of Infectious Diseases. Mandell GL, Douglas RG, Bennett JE, eds. John Wiley and Sons, Inc., New York, 1979:484.

Romankiewicz JA, Ehrman M. Rifampin and warfarin: a drug interaction. Ann Intern Med 1975;82:224–5.

Scholand JF, Tennenbaum JI, Cerilli GJ. Anaphylaxis to cephalothin in a patient allergic to penicillin. JAMA 1968;206:130–2.

Schultz JC, Adamson JS, Workman WW, Norman TD. Fatal liver disease after intravenous administration of tetracycline in high dosage. N Engl J Med 1963;269:999–1004.

Shouval D, Ligumsky M, Ben-Ishay D. Effect of co-trimoxazole on normal creatinine clearance. Lancet 1978;2:244–5.

Skolnick JL, Stoler BS, Katz DB, Anderson WH. Rifampin, oral contraceptives, and pregnancy. JAMA 1976;236:1382.

Sokoll MD, Gergis SD. Antibiotics and neuromuscular function. Anesthesiology 1981;55:148–59.

Steer PO, Marks MI, Klite PD, Eickhoff TC. 5-Fluorocytosine: an oral antifungal compound. A report on clinical and laboratory experience. Ann Intern Med 1972;76:15–22.

Strausbaugh LJ, Mandaleris CD, Sande MA. Comparison of four aminoglycoside antibiotics in the therapy of experimental *E. coli* meningitis. J Lab Clin Med 1977;89:692–701.

Stuart BH, Litt TF. Tetracycline-associated intracranial hypertension in an adolescent: a complication of systemic acne therapy. J Pediatr 1978;92:679–80.

Summers RW, Switz DM, Sessions JT, et al. National cooperative Crohn's disease study—results of drug treatment. Gastroenterology 1979;77:847–69.

Takayama K, Schnoes HK, Armstrong EL, Boyle RW. Site of inhibitory action of isoniazid in the synthesis of mycolic acids in Mycobacterium tuberculosis. J Lipid Res 1975;16:308–17.

Tolman KG. Nitrofurantoin and chronic active hepatitis. Ann Intern Med 1980;92:119–20.

Wade JC, Petty BG, Conrad G. Cephalothin plus an aminoglycoside is more nephrotoxic than methicillin plus an aminoglycoside. Lancet 1978;2:604–6.

Weinstein L, Madoff MA, Samet CA. The sulfonamides. N Engl J Med 1960;263:793–800, 842–9, 900–7.

White PJ, Woods DD. The synthesis of p-aminobenzoic acid and folic acid by staphylococci sensitive and resistant to sulfonamides. J Gen Microbiol 1965;40:243–53.

Whitley RJ, Alford C, Hirsch MS, et al. Vidarabine versus acyclovir therapy in herpes simplex encephalitis. N Engl J Med 1986;314:144–9.

Wright JM, Collier B. The effects of neomycin upon transmitter release and action. J Pharmacol Exp Ther 1977;200:576–87.

Yao F-S, Seidman SF, Artusio JF. Disturbance of consciousness and hypocalcemia after neomycin irrigation, and reversal by calcium and physostigmine. Anesthesiology 1980;53:69–71.

Yunis AA. Chloramphenicol-induced bone marrow suppression. Semin Hematol 1973;10:225–34.

CHAPTER 29

Chemotherapeutic Drugs

INTRODUCTION

Chemotherapy is the best available therapeutic approach for the eradication of malignant cells that can occur anywhere in the body. Effectiveness of chemotherapy requires that there be complete destruction (total cell-kill) of all cancer cells, since a single surviving clonogenic cell can give rise to sufficient progeny to ultimately kill the host. The logical outgrowth of the recognition for the need of total cell-kill is use of several chemotherapeutic (antineoplastic) drugs concurrently or in a planned sequence. The goal of combination chemotherapy is the administration of the largest possible doses of chemotherapeutic drugs, each working by different mechanisms and not sharing similar toxic effects. Using a combination of chemotherapeutic drugs with different mechanisms of action also reduces the chances that drug-resistant tumor cell populations will emerge. Chemotherapeutic drugs used in combination are usually administered over short periods of time at specific treatment intervals rather than as continuous therapy. This approach is based on the empiric observation that normal cells usually recover more rapidly from a pulse of maximal chemotherapy than do malignant cells. Furthermore, immunosuppression is less with intermittent chemotherapy.

Malignant cells are often characterized by rapid division and synthesis of deoxyribonucleic acid (DNA). Most chemotherapeutic drugs exert their antineoplastic effects on those cells that are actively undergoing division (i.e., mitosis) or DNA synthesis. Slow growing malignant cells with a slow rate of division, such as carcinoma of the lung and colon, are often unresponsive to chemotherapeutic drugs. Conversely, rapidly dividing normal cells as in the bone marrow, gastrointestinal mucosa, skin, and hair follicles are vulnerable to the toxic effects of chemotherapeutic drugs. It is predictable, therefore, that clinical manifestations of toxicity as a result of chemotherapeutic drugs may include myelosuppression (leukopenia, thrombocytopenia, anemia), nausea, vomiting, diarrhea, mucosal ulceration, dermatitis, and alopecia. Often, myelosuppression is the dose-limiting factor for chemotherapeutic drugs and is the indication for temporary or permanent withdrawal of therapy. Fortunately, this drug-induced myelosuppression is usually reversible with discontinuation of chemotherapeutic drug therapy (Selvin, 1981).

CLASSIFICATION

Chemotherapeutic drugs are classified as (1) alkylating drugs, (2) antimetabolites, (3) vinca alkaloids, (4) antibiotics, (5) enzymes, (6) synthetics, and (7) hormones (Table 29-1).

Knowledge of drug-induced adverse effects and evaluation of appropriate laboratory tests (hemoglobin, platelet count, white blood cell count, coagulation profile, arterial blood gases, blood glucose, plasma electrolytes, liver and renal function tests, electrocardiogram, and radiograph of the chest) are essential in the preoperative evaluation of patients being treated with chemotherapeutic drugs (Table 29-1) (McCammon, 1983; Selvin, 1981). Attention to asepsis is essential, because immunosuppression makes these patients susceptible to iatrogenic infection. A history of severe diarrhea may be associated with electrolyte disturbances and decreased intravascular fluid volume. The existence of stomatitis makes placement of pharyngeal airways and esophageal catheters questionable. The response to inhaled and injected drugs may be altered by drug-induced cardiac, hepatic, or renal dysfunction. The response to nondepolarizing neuromuscular blocking drugs may be altered by impaired renal function. Furthermore, effects of succinylcholine may be prolonged if plasma cholinesterase activity is decreased by chemotherapeutic drugs. An increased incidence of spontaneous abortions has been reported in female personnel who handle certain chemotherapeutic drugs during the first trimester of pregnancy (Selevan *et al*, 1985).

ALKYLATING DRUGS

Alkylating drugs include nitrogen mustards, alkyl sulfonates, and nitrosoureas (Table 29-1). These chemotherapeutic drugs have the common property of undergoing electrophilic chemical reactions that result in the formation of covalent linkages (alkylation) with various nucleophilic substances, principally DNA. The 7-nitrogen atom of guanine residues in DNA is particularly susceptible to formation of a covalent bond. The result is a miscoding of DNA information or opening of the purine ring with damage to the DNA molecule (Shapiro, 1968). Although alkylating drugs are dependent on cell division, they are not cycle-specific, acting on the DNA molecule at any stage of the division. Acquired resistance to alkylating drugs is a common occurrence and may reflect decreased cell membrane permeability to the drugs and increased production of nucleophilic substances that can compete with target DNA for alkylation.

Side Effects

Bone marrow suppression is the most important dose-limiting factor in the clinical use of alkylat-

ing drugs. Cessation of mitosis is evident within 6 to 8 hours. Lymphocytopenia is usually present within 24 hours. Variable degrees of depression of platelet and erythrocyte counts may occur. Hemolytic anemia is predictably present.

Gastrointestinal mucosa is sensitive to the effects of alkylating drugs, manifesting as mitotic arrest, cellular hypertrophy, and desquamation of the epithelium. Nevertheless, mucosal irritation is less common than with antimetabolites. Damage to hair follicles, often leading to alopecia, is a common side effect. Increased skin pigmentation is frequent. All alkylating drugs are powerful central nervous system stimulants, manifesting most often as nausea and vomiting. Skeletal muscle weakness and seizures may be present. Pneumonitis and pulmonary fibrosis are potential adverse effects of alkylating drugs (Mark *et al*, 1972; Rosenow, 1972). Inhibition of plasma cholinesterase activity may be responsible for prolonged skeletal muscle paralysis following administration of succinylcholine (Zsigmond and Robins, 1972).

Rapid drug-induced destruction of malignant cells can produce increased purine and pyrimidine breakdown leading to uric acid nephropathy (Rundles *et al*, 1969). To minimize the likelihood of this complication, it is recommended that adequate fluid intake, alkalinization of the urine, and administration of allopurinol be established prior to drug treatment.

Nitrogen Mustards

The most commonly used nitrogen mustards are mechlorethamine, cyclophosphamide, melphalan, and chlorambucil (Fig. 29-1).

Mechlorethamine

Mechlorethamine is a rapidly acting mustard administered intravenously to minimize local tissue irritation. This drug must be freshly prepared before each administration. Mechlorethamine and other nitrogen mustards are intensely powerful vesicants, requiring that gloves be worn by personnel handling the drug. A course of therapy with mechlorethamine consists of the injection of a total dose of 0.4 mg kg^{-1}. The drug undergoes rapid chemical transformation in tissues such that active drug is no longer present after a few minutes. For this reason, it is possible to prevent tissue toxicity from the drug by isolating the blood sup-

(Text continues on p. 484.)

Table 29-1.
Classification of Chemotherapeutic Drugs and Associated Side Effects

	Immuno-suppres-sion	Thrombo-cytopenia	Leukopenia	Anemia	Cardiac Toxicity	Pulmonary Toxicity	Renal Toxicity	Hepatic Toxicity	Nervous System Toxicity	Stomatitis	Plasma Cholinesterase Inhibition
Alkylating Drugs											
Nitrogen Mustards											
Mechlorethamine	+	+++	+++			+			++		++
Cyclophosphamide	+++	+	++	+			+	+		+	++
Melphalan	+	++	++	+		++					+
Chlorambucil	+	++	++	++		+		+	+		+
Alkyl Sulfonates											
Busulfan	+	+++	+++	+++		++	++		+	+	+
Nitrosoureas											
Carmustine		+++	+++	++		+	+	+		+	
Lomustine		++	++	++				++		++	
Semustine		++	++	++				++		++	
Streptozocin		+	+	+			+++	+++			
Antimetabolites											
Folic Acid Analogs											
Methotrexate	+++	+++	+++	+++		+	++	+		+++	
Pyrimidine Analogs											
Fluorouracil	+++	+++	+++	++					+	+++	
Cytarabine	+++	+++	+++			+		+		+	

Purine Analogs							
Mercaptopurine	+++	++	++				+
Azathioprine	+++	++	++		++		+
Thioguanine	+++	+	++		++		+
Vinca Alkaloids							
Vinblastine	++	+	+	+	++	+	
Vincristine	++	+	+	+	+++	++	
Antibiotics							
Dactinomycin	+	+++	+++	+++	++		+++
Daunorubicin	+	+++	+++	+++	++		++
Doxorubicin		+	++	++	+		+++
Bleomycin	+	+++	+	+++	++		+++
Mithramycin		+++	+++	+	++	++	+++
Mitomycin		+++	+++		+	+	+++
Enzymes							
Asparaginase	++	+	+		+++	+	+
Synbetics							
Cisplatin	+	++	++		++	++	
Hydroxyurea	+	+++	++		++	+	+
Procarbazine	+	+++	++	+	++	+	+
Mitotane							
Hormones							
Corticosteroids	+++	+++	+++				
Progestins							
Estrogens/Androgens							

+ = minimal, ++ = mild, +++ = moderate, ++++ = marked

(Adapted from Selvin BF. Cancer chemotherapy: Implications for the anesthesiologist. Anesth Analg 1981;60:425–34; and McCammon RL. Cancer. In: Stoelting RK, Dierdorf SF, eds. Anesthesia and Co-Existing Disease. New York, Churchill Livingstone, 1983;631; with permission of the authors and publishers.)

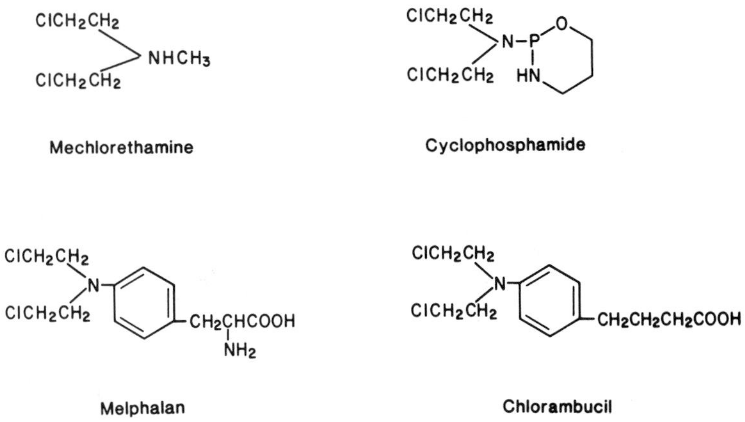

FIGURE 29-1. Nitrogen mustards.

ply to that tissue. Alternatively, it is theoretically possible to localize the action of mechloretha-mine in a specific tissue by injecting the drug into the arterial blood supply to the tissue.

CLINICAL USES. Mechlorethamine produces beneficial effects in the treatment of Hodgkin's disease and, less predictably, in other lymphomas. The drug is most often used in combination with vincristine, procarbazine, and prednisone (MOPP regimen) for treatment of Hodgkin's disease (De-Vita *et al,* 1972).

SIDE EFFECTS. The major side effects of mechlorethamine include nausea, vomiting, and myelosuppression. Leukopenia and thrombocyto-penia constitute the principal limitation on the amount of drug that can be given. Herpes zoster is a type of skin lesion frequently associated with nitrogen mustard therapy. Latent viral infections may be unmasked by treatment with mechloretha-mine. Thrombophlebitis is a potential complica-tion, and extravasation of the drug results in se-vere local tissue reaction with brawny and tender induration that may persist for prolonged periods of time.

Cyclophosphamide

Cyclophosphamide is well absorbed after oral ad-ministration and is subsequently activated in the liver to aldophosphamide for transport to target tissues. Parenteral administration is also effective. Target cells are able to convert aldophosphamide to highly cytotoxic metabolites, phosphoramide,

and acrolein that then alkylate DNA (Bagley *et al,* 1973). Maximal concentrations of cyclophospha-mide in plasma are achieved 1 hour after oral ad-ministration, and the elimination half-time is 6 to 7 hours. Urinary elimination accounts for about 14% of this drug in an unchanged form.

CLINICAL USES. The clinical spectrum of ac-tivity of cyclophosphamide is broad, making it one of the most frequently used chemotherapeutic drugs. Its versatility is improved because of its ef-fectiveness after oral as well as parenteral adminis-tration. Given in combination with other drugs, favorable responses have been shown in patients with Hodgkin's disease, lymphosarcoma, Bur-kitt's lymphoma, and acute lymphoblastic leuke-mia of childhood. Cyclophosphamide is fre-quently used in combination with methotrexate and fluorouracil as adjuvant therapy after surgery for carcinoma of the breast when there is involve-ment of axillary nodes. Cyclophosphamide has potent immunosuppressive properties, leading to its use in non-neoplastic disorders associated with altered immune reactivity, including Wegener's granulomatosis and rheumatoid arthritis (Fauci *et al,* 1978). There may also be a role for this drug in control of organ rejection after organ transplanta-tion.

SIDE EFFECTS. Cyclophosphamide differs from other nitrogen mustards in that significant degrees of thrombocytopenia are less common but alopecia is more frequent. Nausea and vomit-ing occur with equal frequency regardless of the route of administration. Mucosal ulcerations, in-creased skin pigmentation, interstitial pulmonary fibrosis, and hepatotoxicity have been reported (Bagley *et al,* 1973).

Sterile hemorrhagic cystitis occurs in 5% to 10% of patients, presumably reflecting chemical irritation produced by reactive metabolites of cyclophosphamide. Dysuria or hematuria are indications to discontinue the drug.

Inappropriate secretion of antidiuretic hormone has been observed in patients receiving cyclophosphamide, usually with doses greater than 50 mg kg^{-1} (DeFronzo *et al,* 1973). It is important to consider the possibility of water intoxication since these patients are usually being hydrated to minimize the likelihood of the development of hemorrhagic cystitis.

Extravasation of the drug does not produce local reactions, and thrombophlebitis does not complicate intravenous administration.

Melphalan

Melphalan is a phenylalanine derivative of nitrogen mustard with a range of activity similar to other alkylating drugs. It is not a vesicant. Oral absorption is excellent, resulting in drug concentrations similar to those achieved by the intravenous route of administration. Elimination halftime is about 1.5 hours, and up to 15% of the drug is eliminated unchanged in the urine (Alberts *et al,* 1979a).

It is usually necessary to maintain a significant degree of bone marrow depression (leukocyte count 3000 – 3500 cells mm^{-3}) in order to achieve optimal therapeutic effects. Beneficial effects of melphalan therapy have been observed in the treatment of multiple myeloma, malignant melanoma, and carcinoma of the breast and ovary.

Side effects of melphalan are primarily hematologic and are similar to other alkylating drugs. Nausea and vomiting are infrequent. Alopecia does not occur, and changes in renal or hepatic function have not been reported.

Chlorambucil

Chlorambucil is the aromatic derivative of mechlorethamine. Oral absorption is adequate. The drug has an elimination half-time of about 1.5 hours and is almost completely metabolized (Alberts *et al,* 1979b).

Chlorambucil is the slowest-acting nitrogen mustard in clinical use. It is the treatment of choice in chronic lymphocytic leukemia and in primary (Waldenström's) macroglobulinemia. A marked increase in the incidence of leukemia and other tumors has been noted with the use of this drug for the treatment of polycythemia vera (Lerner, 1978).

Cytotoxic effects of chlorambucil on the bone marrow, lymphoid organs, and epithelial tissues are similar to those observed with the other alkylating drugs. Its myelosuppressive action is usually moderate, gradual, and rapidly reversible. Nausea and vomiting are frequent. Central nervous system stimulation can occur but has been observed only with large doses. Hepatotoxicity may rarely occur.

Alkyl Sulfonates

Busulfan

Busulfan is well absorbed after oral administration (Fig. 29-2). Intravenous administration is also effective. Almost all of the drug is eliminated by the kidneys as methanesulfonic acid.

Busulfan produces remissions in up to 90% of patients with chronic granulocytic leukemia. The drug is of no value in the treatment of acute leukemia.

Myelosuppression and thrombocytopenia are the major toxic effects of busulfan. Nausea, vomiting, and diarrhea occur. Hyperuricemia resulting from extensive purine catabolism accompanying the rapid cellular destruction and renal damage from precipitation of urates have been noted. Allopurinol is recommended to avoid this complication.

Nitrosoureas

Nitrosoureas, represented by carmustine, lomustine, semustine, and streptozocin, possess a wide spectrum of activity for human malignancies (Fig. 29-3) (Wasserman *et al,* 1975). These drugs appear to act by alkylation of nucleic acids and carboxylation (Cheng *et al,* 1972). Their high lipid

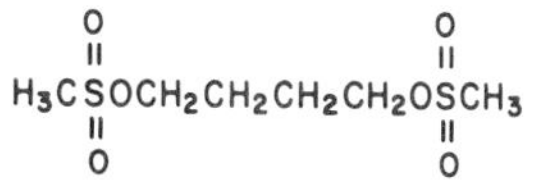

$$
\begin{array}{ccc}
\text{O} & & \text{O} \\
\parallel & & \parallel \\
\text{H}_3\text{C S OCH}_2\text{CH}_2\text{CH}_2\text{CH}_2\text{OSCH}_3 \\
\parallel & & \parallel \\
\text{O} & & \text{O}
\end{array}
$$

FIGURE 29-2. Busulfan.

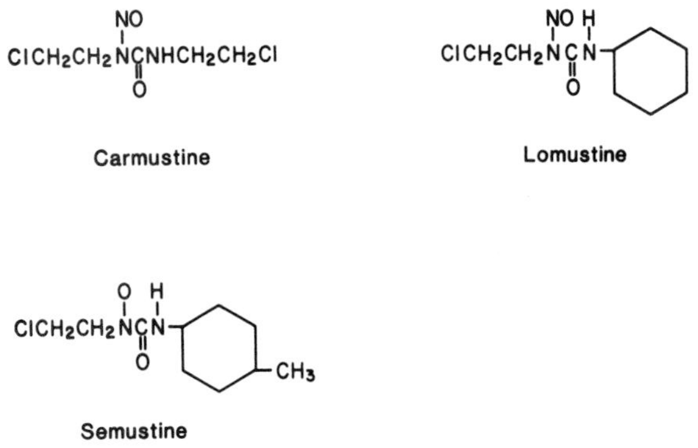

NO
|
$CICH_2CH_2NCNHCH_2CH_2CI$
‖
O

Carmustine

NO H
| |
$CICH_2CH_2NCN$
‖
O

Lomustine

O H
‖ |
$CICH_2CH_2NCN$
‖
O
—CH₃

Semustine

FIGURE 29-3. Nitrosoureas.

solubility results in passage across the blood–brain barrier and efficacy in the treatment of meningeal leukemias and brain tumors (Walker, 1973). With the exception of streptozocin, the clinical use of nitrosoureas is limited by profound drug-induced myelosuppression.

Carmustine

Carmustine is capable of inhibiting synthesis of both ribonucleic acid (RNA) and DNA. Although oral absorption is rapid, the drug is injected intravenously since tissue uptake and metabolism occur quickly. Local burning may accompany intravenous infusion. Carmustine disappears from plasma in 5 to 15 minutes. Because of its ability to rapidly cross the blood–brain barrier, carmustine is used to treat meningeal leukemia and primary as well as metastatic brain tumors (Levin *et al,* 1978).

A unique side effect of carmustine is a delayed onset (after about 6 weeks of treatment) of leukopenia and thrombocytopenia. Active metabolites may be responsible for this toxicity. Central nervous system toxicity, nausea and vomiting, flushing of the skin and conjunctiva, interstitial pulmonary fibrosis, nephrotoxicity, and hepatotoxicity have been reported (Durant *et al,* 1979).

Lomustine and Semustine

Lomustine and its methylated analog semustine possess similar clinical toxicity to carmustine, including delayed bone marrow depression manifesting as leukopenia and thrombocytopenia (Wasserman, 1976). Lomustine appears to be more effective than carmustine in the treatment of Hodgkin's disease.

Streptozocin

Streptozocin has a methylnitrosourea moiety attached to the number 2 carbon of glucose. It has a unique affinity for beta cells of the islets of Langerhans and has proved useful in the treatment of human pancreatic islet cell carcinoma and malignant carcinoid (Schein *et al,* 1973). In animals, the drug is used to produce experimental diabetes mellitus.

Almost 70% of patients receiving this drug develop hepatic or renal toxicity. Renal toxicity may manifest as tubular damage and progress to renal failure and death (Broder and Carter, 1973). Hyperglycemia can occur as a result of selective destruction of pancreatic beta cells and resultant hypoinsulinism (Selvin, 1981). Myelosuppression is not produced by this drug.

ANTIMETABOLITES

Antimetabolites include folic acid analogs, pyrimidine analogs, and purine analogs (Table 29-1). Typically, these chemotherapeutic drugs are structural analogs of normal metabolites required for cell function and replication. These drugs interact directly with specific enzymes, leading to inhibition of that enzyme and a subsequent synthesis of an aberrant molecule that cannot function normally. The principal targets for the antimetabolite chemotherapeutic drugs are the proliferating bone marrow cells and gastrointestinal epithelial cells. The majority of these drugs are also potent immunosuppressants.

Folic Acid Analogs

Methotrexate

Methotrexate is a poorly lipid soluble folic acid analog and is classified as an antimetabolite (*i.e.,* folic acid antagonist) (Fig. 29-4). Folic acid is an essential dietary factory that is the source of tetrahydrofolic acid (see Chapter 34), which is an essential co-enzyme necessary for the transfer of 1-carbon units. The enzyme dihydrofolate reductase seems to be the primary site of action of most folic acid analogs. Inhibition of dihydrofolate reductase by methotrexate prevents the formation of tetrahydrofolic acid and causes disruption of cellular metabolism by producing an acute intracellular deficiency of folate enzymes. As a result, 1-carbon transfer reactions necessary for the eventual synthesis of DNA and RNA cease.

Methotrexate is readily absorbed after oral administration. Significant metabolism of methotrexate does not seem to occur, with more than 50% of the drug appearing unchanged in the urine. Renal excretion reflects glomerular filtration and tubular secretion. Toxic concentrations of methotrexate may occur in patients with renal insufficiency. Methotrexate remains in tissues for weeks, suggesting binding of the drug to dihydrofolate reductase.

CLINICAL USES. Methotrexate is a useful drug in the management of acute lymphoblastic leukemia in children but not in adults. It is of established value in choriocarcinoma. Improvement in the treatment of psoriasis reflects the effect of methotrexate on rapidly dividing epidermal cells characteristic of this disease.

Methotrexate is poorly transported across the blood–brain barrier, and neoplastic cells that have entered the central nervous system probably are not affected by usual concentrations of drug in the plasma. Intrathecal injection is used to treat cerebral involvement with either leukemia or choriocarcinoma.

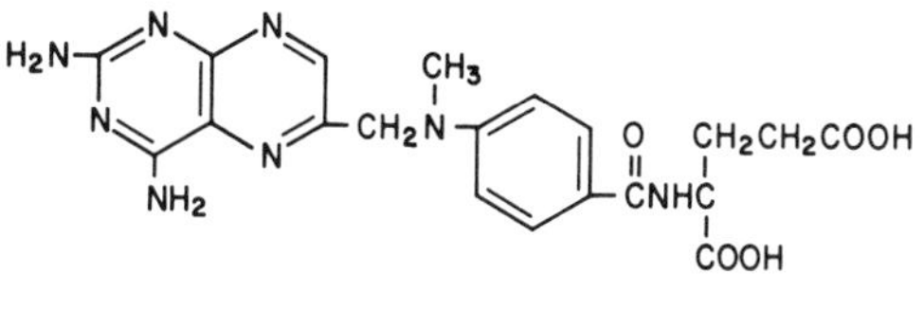

FIGURE 29-4. Methotrexate.

Acquired resistance to methotrexate develops as a result of (1) impaired transport of methotrexate into cells, (2) production of altered forms of dihydrofolate reductase that have decreased affinity for the drug, and (3) increased concentrations of intracellular dihydrofolate reductase.

SIDE EFFECTS. The most important side effects of methotrexate occur in the gastrointestinal tract and bone marrow. Leukopenia and thrombocytopenia reflect bone marrow depression. Ulcerative stomatitis and diarrhea are frequent side effects and require interruption of treatment. Hemorrhagic enteritis and death from intestinal perforation may occur (Selvin, 1981). Other toxic manifestations include alopecia, dermatitis, pneumonitis, nephrotoxicity, and hepatic dysfunction (Whitcomb *et al,* 1972). Hepatic dysfunction is usually reversible but may sometimes lead to cirrhosis.

Normal cells can be protected from lethal damage by folate antagonists with concomitant administration of leucovorin (see Chapter 34) or thymidine or both. This approach has been termed *rescue* technique. Folic acid antagonists also interfere with embryogenesis, emphasizing the risk in administering these drugs to pregnant patients.

Pyrimidine Analogs

Pyrimidine analogs have in common the ability to prevent the biosynthesis of pyrimidine nucleotides or to mimic these natural metabolites to such an extent that they interfere with vital cellular activities such as the synthesis and functioning of nucleic acids. Examples of antimetabolite chemotherapeutic drugs that function as pyrimidine analogs are fluorouracil and cytarabine (Fig. 29-5).

Fluorouracil

Fluorouracil lacks significant inhibitory activity on cells and must be converted enzymatically to 5'-monophosphate nucleotide. Administration of fluorouracil is usually by intravenous injection, since absorption after oral ingestion is unpredictable and incomplete. Metabolic degradation occurs primarily in the liver, with an important metabolite being urea. Only about 10% of fluorouracil appears unchanged in the urine. Fluorouracil readily enters the cerebrospinal fluid, with thera-

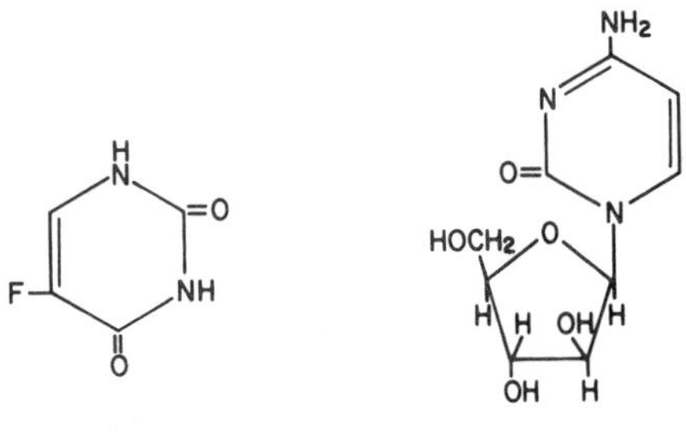

Fluorouracil   Cytarabine

FIGURE 29-5. Pyrimidine analogs.

peutic concentrations being present within 30 minutes after intravenous administration.

CLINICAL USES. Fluorouracil may be of palliative value in certain types of carcinoma, particularly of the breast and gastrointestinal tract. The drug is often used for the topical treatment of premalignant keratoses of the skin and superficial basal cell carcinomas.

SIDE EFFECTS. Side effects caused by fluorouracil are difficult to anticipate because of their delayed appearance. Stomatitis manifesting as a white patchy membrane that ulcerates and becomes necrotic is an early sign of toxicity and a warning of the possibility that similar lesions may be developing in the esophagus and gastrointestinal tract. Myelosuppression, most frequently manifesting as leukopenia between 9 and 14 days of therapy, is a serious side effect. Thrombocytopenia and anemia may complicate treatment with fluorouracil. Loss of hair progressing to total alopecia, nail changes, dermatitis, and increased pigmentation and atrophy of the skin may occur. Neurologic manifestations, including an acute cerebellar syndrome, have been reported (Boileau *et al,* 1971).

Cytarabine

Cytarabine, like other pyrimidine antimetabolites, must be activated by conversion to the 5'-monophosphate nucleotide before inhibition of DNA synthesis can occur. Both natural and acquired resistance to cytarabine develop, reflecting the activity of cytidine diaminase, an enzyme capable of converting cytarabine to the inactive metabolite arabinosyl uracil.

In addition to its chemotherapeutic activity, particularly in acute leukemia in children or adults, cytarabine has potent immunosuppressive properties (Mitchell *et al,* 1969). The drug is particularly useful in chemotherapy of acute granulocytic leukemia in adults. Intravenous administration of cytarabine is recommended, since oral absorption is poor and unpredictable. Thrombophlebitis at the site of intravenous infusion is common.

Cytarabine is a potent myelosuppressive drug capable of producing severe leukopenia, thrombocytopenia, and anemia. Other side effects include gastrointestinal disturbances, stomatitis, and hepatic dysfunction.

Purine Analogs

Antimetabolite chemotherapeutic drugs that function as purine analogs include mercaptopurine, azathioprine, and thioguanine (Fig. 29-6). Mercaptopurine and thioguanine are analogs of the natural purines hypoxanthine and guanine, respectively.

It seems likely that this class of drugs acts by multiple mechanisms, including effects on purine nucleotide synthesis and metabolism as well as alterations in the synthesis and function of RNA and DNA. As with other antimetabolites, the occurrence of acquired resistance represents a major obstacle in the successful use of purine analogs.

Mercaptopurine

Mercaptopurine is most useful in the treatment of acute leukemia in children. This drug has not been of value in the treatment of chronic lymphocytic leukemia and Hodgkin's disease. Although active as an immunosuppressant, its use has been largely superseded by azathioprine.

Mercaptopurine is readily absorbed after oral ingestion, and the gastrointestinal epithelium is not damaged. The elimination half-time is brief (about 90 minutes) owing to rapid tissue uptake, renal excretion, and hepatic metabolism. One pathway of metabolism is methylation and subsequent oxidation of the methylated derivatives. A second pathway involves the enzyme xanthine oxidase, which oxidizes mercaptopurine to 6-thiouric acid. Allopurinol, as an inhibitor of xanthine oxidase, prevents conversion of mercaptopurine to 6-thiouric acid and thus increases the exposure of cells to mercaptopurine.

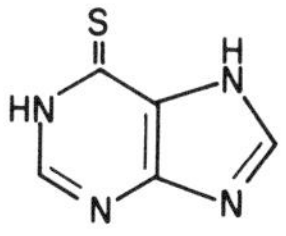

Mercaptopurine 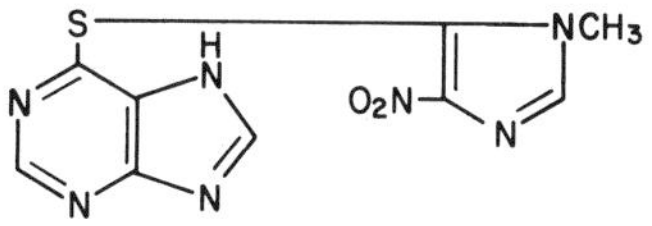   Azothioprine 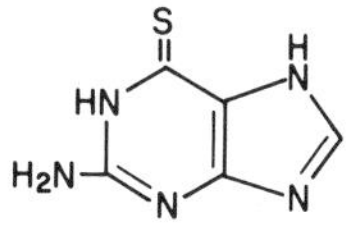   Thioguanine

FIGURE 29-6.   Purine analogs.

The principal side effect of mercaptopurine is a gradual development of bone marrow depression manifesting as thrombocytopenia, granulocytopenia, or anemia several weeks after initiation of therapy. Anorexia, nausea, and vomiting are common side effects; stomatitis and diarrhea rarely occur. Jaundice occurs in approximately one third of patients and is associated with bile stasis and occasional hepatic necrosis (Schein and Winokur, 1975). Hyperuricemia and hyperuricosuria may occur during treatment with mercaptopurine, presumably reflecting destruction of cells. This effect may require the use of allopurinol.

Azathioprine

Azathioprine is a derivative of mercaptopurine. It is a potent immunosuppressant and is used as an adjunct (often with corticosteroids) to prevent rejection following organ transplantation. The oral dose may need to be reduced in patients with impaired renal function to prevent dangerous accumulation of the drug. If allopurinol is administered concurrently, the dose of azathioprine should be reduced, since inhibition of xanthine oxidase impairs the conversion of azathioprine to 6-thiouric acid and may greatly increase tissue exposure to the drug.

Leukopenia as a manifestation of bone marrow depression is the most common side effect of azathioprine therapy. Infection is a predictable complication of any form of immunosuppressive therapy. Biliary stasis and hepatic necrosis have been described. Infrequent complications include stomatitis, dermatitis, fever, alopecia, and diarrhea.

Thioguanine

Thioguanine is of particular value in the treatment of acute granulocytic leukemia, especially when given with cytarabine. Following oral administration, thioguanine appears in the urine as a methy-lated metabolite and inorganic sulfate. Minimal amounts of 6-thiouric acid are formed, suggesting that deamination is not important in the metabolic inactivation of thioguanine. For this reason, thioguanine may be administered concurrently with allopurinol without a reduction in dosage, unlike mercaptopurine and azathioprine. Toxic manifestations of thioguanine treatment include bone marrow depression and, occasionally, gastrointestinal effects.

VINCA ALKALOIDS

Useful vinca alkaloids derived from the periwinkle plant are vinblastine and vincristine (Table 29-1). These drugs block mitosis in rapidly dividing cells. Nevertheless, most of the biological activity of vinca alkaloids is due to their ability to bind with an essential protein component of microtubules (Bucher, 1972). Disruption of microtubules of the mitotic apparatus arrests cell division in metaphase. Despite their structural similarity, there is a remarkable lack of cross-tolerance between individual vinca alkaloids.

Oral absorption of vinblastine is unpredictable; thus, intravenous infusion is recommended. Subcutaneous extravasation can cause painful inflammatory changes. Vincristine and vinblastine can be infused into the arterial blood supply of tumors in doses far greater than permissible by way of the intravenous route, suggesting that local tissue uptake or metabolism is rapid. Excretion of the vinca alkaloids appears to be primarily into the bile, with minimal amounts of drug appearing in the urine. Indeed, toxicity is increased when vincristine is administered to patients with obstructive jaundice.

Clinical Uses

The most important clinical use of vinblastine is with bleomycin and cisplatin in the treatment of metastatic testicular tumors (Einhorn and Dona-hue, 1977). Lymphomas, including Hodgkin's disease, are responsive, even when the disease is refractory to alkylating drugs. Vincristine combined with corticosteroids is an effective treatment to induce remissions in childhood leukemia. An important feature of vinca alkaloids is the lack of cross-resistance between these drugs. The rapidity of action of vincristine and its reduced tendency for myelosuppression render it a more desirable drug for therapy in the presence of pancytopenia or in conjunction with other myelotoxic drugs. Vincristine apparently does not cross the blood–brain barrier as evidenced by persistence of central nervous system leukemia despite hematopoietic remission. Intrathecal administration of vincristine is not used. The rapid onset of action of vinca alkaloids often necessitates the concomitant administration of allopurinol to prevent the complications of hyperuricemia.

Side Effects

Myelosuppression manifesting as leukopenia, thrombocytopenia, and anemia are the most prominent side effects of vinca alkaloids, appearing 7 to 10 days after initiation of treatment. Vincristine is less likely than vinblastine to cause bone marrow depression. Alopecia appears to occur more frequently with vincristine than with vinblastine.

Neuromuscular abnormalities, including skeletal muscle weakness, ataxia, and tremors, are frequently observed during treatment with vincristine. Peripheral neuropathy manifesting as tingling and weakness of the extremities, foot drop, and neuritic pains occur frequently (Rosenthal and Kaufman, 1974). Weakness of the extraocular muscles and larynx manifesting as hoarseness have been observed. The syndrome of hyponatremia associated with high urinary sodium and inappropriate secretion of antidiuretic hormone has occasionally been observed during vincristine therapy. An effect on the autonomic nervous system may be responsible for paralytic ileus and abdominal pain that frequently develops during vincristine, but only rarely during vinblastine, therapy. Urinary retention, tenderness of the parotid glands, dryness of the mouth, and sinus tachycardia are other occasionally experienced manifestations of altered autonomic nervous system activity. Transient mental depression is most

likely to occur on the second or third day of treatment with vinblastine.

ANTIBIOTICS

Clinically useful chemotherapeutic antibiotics are natural products of certain soil fungi (Table 29-1). Chemotherapeutic effects are produced by formation of relatively stable complexes with DNA, thereby inhibiting DNA or RNA synthesis or both (Umezawa, 1973).

Dactinomycin

Dactinomycin (actinomycin D) is an antibiotic with chemotherapeutic activity by virtue of its ability to bind to DNA, especially in rapidly proliferating cells. As a result of this binding, the function of RNA polymerase and thus the transcription of the DNA molecule are blocked. Following intravenous injection, dactinomycin rapidly leaves the circulation. In animals, about 50% of an injected dose is excreted unchanged in the bile, and 10% in the urine. There is no evidence that the drug undergoes metabolism. Dactinomycin does not cross the blood–brain barrier in amounts sufficient to produce a pharmacologic effect.

Clinical Uses

The most important clinical use of dactinomycin is in the treatment of Wilms' tumor in children and rhabdoymyosarcoma. It may be effective in some women with methotrexate-resistant choriocarcinoma. Occasionally, this drug is used to inhibit immunologic responses associated with organ transplantation.

Side Effects

Toxic effects of dactinomycin include the early onset of nausea and vomiting, often followed by myelosuppression manifesting as pancytopenia 1 to 7 days after completion of therapy. Pancytopenia may be preceded by thrombocytopenia as the first manifestation of bone marrow suppression. Glossitis, ulcerations of the oral mucosa, diarrhea, alopecia, and cutaneous erythema are commonly associated with dactinomycin therapy.

Daunorubicin and Doxorubicin

Daunorubicin and doxorubicin are anthracycline antibiotics. Structurally, these anthracycline antibiotics contain a tetracycline ring attached to the sugar daunosamine by a glycosidic linkage (Fig. 29-7). These drugs most likely act by binding to DNA, which results in changes in the DNA helix that inhibit the template activity of the nucleic acid (Pigram *et al*, 1972). Evidence also shows that anthracyclines cause disruptive effects on cellular membranes (Tritton *et al*, 1978). Free radicals that attack unsaturated free fatty acids in the heart may play a role in cardiotoxicity. Evidence for a role of free radicals is the protective effect of free radical scavengers such as vitamin E (Myers *et al*, 1977).

Daunorubicin and doxorubicin are administered intravenously, with care taken to prevent extravasation, since local vesicant action may result. There is rapid clearance from the plasma into the heart, kidneys, lungs, and liver. These drugs do not cross the blood–brain barrier to any significant extent. The urine may become red for 1 to 2 days after administration of these drugs.

Daunorubicin is metabolized primarily to daunorubiconol, whereas doxorubicin is excreted unchanged and as metabolites, including adriamycinol in the urine (Ahmed *et al*, 1978). Ultimately, about 40% of the drugs are metabolized. Indeed, clinical toxicity may result in patients with hepatic dysfunction.

Clinical Uses

Daunorubicin is used primarily in the treatment of acute lymphocytic and granulocytic leukemia.

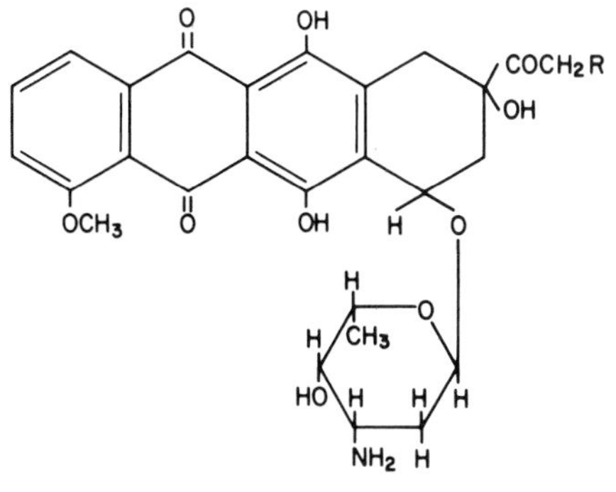

FIGURE 29-7. Anthracycline antibiotics contain a tetracycline ring attached to a sugar by a glycosidic linkage.

Doxorubicin, which differs from daunorubicin only by a single hydroxyl group on the number 14 carbon, is also effective against a wide range of solid tumors (Fig. 29-7). For example, doxorubicin is one of the most active single drugs for the treatment of metastatic adenocarcinoma of the breast, carcinoma of the bladder, bronchogenic carcinoma, metastatic thyroid carcinoma, oat cell carcinoma, and osteogenic carcinoma.

Resistance is observed to the anthracycline antibiotics, as with other chemotherapeutic drugs. Furthermore, cross-tolerance occurs between daunorubicin and doxorubicin. Cross-resistance also occurs between these antibiotics and the vinca alkaloids, suggesting that an alteration of cellular permeability may be involved.

Side Effects

Cardiomyopathy is a unique dose-related and often irreversible side effect of the anthracycline antibiotics. Two types of cardiomyopathies may occur (Selvin, 1981). An acute form occurs in about 10% of patients and is characterized by relatively benign changes on the electrocardiogram that include nonspecific ST-T changes and decreased QRS voltage (Ainger *et al*, 1971; Minow *et al*, 1975). Other cardiac changes include premature ventricular contractions, supraventricular tachydysrhythmias, cardiac conduction abnormalities, and left axis deviation. These abnormalities occur during therapy at all dose levels and, except for decreased QRS voltage on the electrocardiogram, resolve 1 to 2 months after discontinuation of therapy (Lefrak *et al*, 1975). There is an associated acute reversible reduction in the ejection fraction within 24 hours after a single dose.

The second form of cardiomyopathy is characterized by the insidious onset of symptoms such as dry nonproductive cough, suggesting bronchitis, that is followed by rapidly progressive cardiac heart failure that is unresponsive to inotropic drugs and mechanical ventricular assistance (Cortes *et al*, 1975; Selvin, 1981). This severe form of cardiomyopathy occurs in almost 2% of treated patients and is fatal approximately 3 weeks after the onset of symptoms in nearly 60% of affected patients (Gottlieb *et al*, 1973). Predictive tests are not available to permit early recognition of impending cardiomyopathy, although dimunition in QRS voltage on the electrocardiogram is consistent with the diffuse character of the myocardial damage (Minow *et al*, 1975). Serum enzyme elevations occur late in the course of cardiac failure and are of limited value in achieving an early diagnosis. Systolic time intervals and echocardiograms have been used to detect cardiotoxicity before the occurrence of clinically significant damage (Jones *et al*, 1975; Rinehart *et al*, 1974).

The incidence of cardiomyopathy is negligible when the total dose of these drugs is less than 500 mg m^{-2} of body surface area. Prior mediastinal irradiation or previous treatment with cyclophosphamide increases the subsequent risk of cardiomyopathy in response to administration of an anthracycline antibiotic (Bristow *et al*, 1978). Marked impairment of a left ventricular function for as long as 3 years after discontinuing doxorubicin has been observed (Mason *et al*, 1978).

Myelosuppression is another serious side effect of chemotherapeutic antibiotics, with leukopenia typically manifesting during the second week of therapy. Thrombocytopenia and anemia occur but are usually less pronounced. Stomatitis, gastrointestinal disturbances, and alopecia are common side effects.

Bleomycin

Bleomycins are water-soluble glycopeptides that differ from one another (there are more than 200 congeners) in their terminal amine moiety (Blum *et al*, 1973). The terminal amine is coupled through amide linkage to a carboxylic acid. The mechanism of action is most likely related to the ability of these drugs to cause fragmentation of DNA by interacting with oxygen and ferrous iron.

Bleomycin is administered intravenously, and high concentrations occur in skin and the lungs. The drug accumulates in tumors, suggesting the presence of a lower level of inactivating enzyme. About two thirds of the unchanged drug is excreted by the kidneys, probably by glomerular filtration. Indeed, excessive concentrations of drug occur if usual doses are given to patients with impaired renal function (Broughton *et al*, 1977).

Clinical Uses

Bleomycin is effective in the treatment of testicular carcinoma, particularly when administered in combination with vinblastine (Einhorn and Donahue, 1977). It is also useful in the palliative treatment of squamous cell carcinomas of the head, neck, esophagus, skin, and genitourinary tract.

Side Effects

The most commonly encountered side effects of bleomycin are mucocutaneous reactions, including stomatitis, alopecia, pruritic erythema, and hyperpigmentation that occur in about 45% of patients (Blum *et al*, 1973). In contrast to other chemotherapeutic drugs, bleomycin causes minimal myelosuppression. Unexplained exacerbations of rheumatoid arthritis have occurred.

Patients with lymphomas who are receiving bleomycin may develop an acute reaction characterized by hyperpyrexia, hypotension, and hypoventilation. The likely mechanism is release of an endogenous pyrogen, presumably from destroyed tumor cells. An initial small test dose of bleomycin is recommended to minimize the occurrence of this syndrome.

PULMONARY TOXICITY. The most serious side effect of bleomycin is pulmonary toxicity. It is estimated that 5% to 10% of patients treated with bleomycin develop pulmonary toxicity, and 1% to 2% of all patients receiving bleomycin die from this complication (Crooke and Bradner, 1976; Rudders and Mensley, 1973).

The first signs of pulmonary toxicity are cough, dyspnea, and basilar rales, which progress in one of two directions. A mild form of pulmonary toxicity is characterized by exertional dyspnea and a normal resting PaO_2. A more severe form of arterial hypoxemia at rest is associated with radiographic findings of interstitial pneumonitis and fibrosis (Luna *et al*, 1972). Lesions are found more frequently in lower lobes and subpleural areas, and radiographs of the chest often reveal bilateral basilar and perihilar infiltrates. The alveolar-to-arterial difference for oxygen is increased, and pulmonary diffusion capacity may be reduced.

Pulmonary function studies have been of no greater value than clinical signs in detecting the onset of pulmonary toxicity. The likelihood of developing pulmonary toxicity is greater when the total dose of bleomycin exceeds 400 units administered to patients older than 70 years of age with underlying pulmonary disease. Prior radiotherapy may also predispose the patient to pulmonary toxicity (Samuels *et al*, 1976). Skin toxicity may parallel the more serious pulmonary toxicity. Patients who develop pulmonary toxicity despite low-dose therapy may be manifesting an idiosyncratic or immune response in contrast to the more predictable reaction noted with higher doses (Iocovina *et al,* 1976).

Patients treated with bleomycin who have undergone anesthesia and surgery appear to be at increased risk for developing adult respiratory distress syndrome in the postoperative period (Goldiner *et al,* 1978). One speculation is that acutely increased inhaled concentrations of oxygen facilitate production of superoxide and other free radicals in the presence of bleomycin. For this reason, it has been recommended that inhaled concentrations of oxygen during surgery be maintained below 30% in bleomycin-treated patients. Nevertheless, data from animals and patients do not demonstrate enhanced pulmonary toxicity in the presence of bleomycin therapy and high concentrations of oxygen (Douglas and Coppin, 1980; LaMantia *et al,* 1984; Matalon *et al,* 1986). Another recommendation is replacement of fluids with colloids rather than crystalloids so as to decrease or prevent pulmonary interstitial edema in bleomycin-treated patients undergoing surgery (Goldiner *et al,* 1978). Accumulation of interstitial fluid may reflect impaired lymphatic function caused by bleomycin-induced fibrotic changes in the lung.

Mithramycin

Mithramycin is a highly toxic antibiotic that acts by inhibiting the synthesis of RNA without altering the synthesis of DNA (Yarbro *et al,* 1966). The drug has a specific effect on osteoclasts and lowers the plasma concentration of calcium in patients who are hypercalcemic as a result of metastatic bone tumors or tumors that produce parathyroid hormone – like substances (Robins and Jowsey, 1973). In patients with Paget's disease treated with mithramycin, the plasma alkaline phosphatase activity is decreased and pain is reduced.

Mithramycin is administered by slow intravenous infusion over 4 to 6 hours. Extravasation can cause local irritation and cellulitis.

Side Effects

Mithramycin is extremely toxic to the gastrointestinal tract and bone marrow. A fatal hemorrhagic diathesis occurs in 1% to 5% of treated patients (Monto *et al,* 1969). This hemorrhagic diathesis may reflect impaired synthesis of clotting factors in addition to thrombocytopenia. Prolongation of the prothrombin time and an increase in fibrinolytic activity are likely. Epistaxis may be the first manifestation of the presence of a drug-induced coagulopathy. Adverse neurologic and cutaneous side effects are frequently observed. Irreversible hepatic or renal toxicity may occur, especially in patients with preexisting disease (Kennedy, 1970).

Mitomycin

Mitomycin inhibits synthesis of DNA and is of value in the palliative treatment of gastric adenocarcinoma in combination with fluorouracil and doxorubicin. The drug is administered intravenously and is widely distributed in tissues but does not readily enter the central nervous system. Metabolism is in the liver, with less than 10% of mitomycin excreted unchanged in the bile or urine.

Side Effects

Myelosuppression is a prominent side effect of mitomycin and is characterized by severe leukopenia and thrombocytopenia, which may be delayed in appearance. Interstitial pneumonia and glomerular damage resulting in renal failure are rare but well-recognized complications (Orwoll *et al,* 1978).

ENZYMES

Asparaginase

Asparaginase is an enzyme with chemotherapeutic activity that is effective in the treatment of acute lymphoblastic leukemia (Table 29-1). This drug acts by catalyzing the conversion of asparagine to asparatic acid and ammonia, thus depriving malignant cells of necessary extracellular supplies of asparagine (Brome, 1961). Malignant cells that lack the enzyme necessary to form this amino acid cannot survive in the absence of exogenous sources.

Side Effects

In contrast to other chemotherapeutic drugs, asparaginase has minimal effects on the bone marrow, and it does not damage oral or gastrointesti-

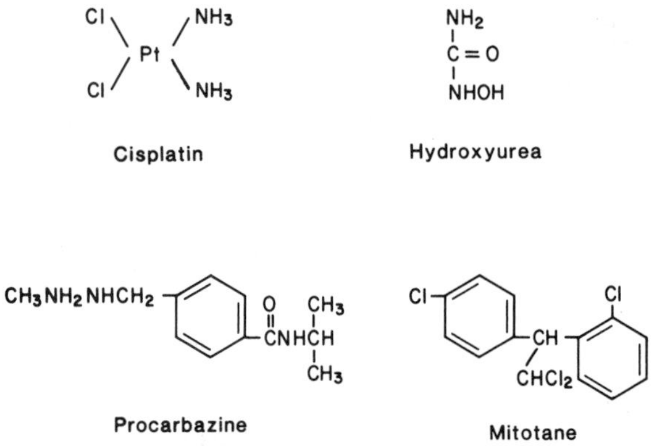

FIGURE 29-8.   Synthetic chemotherapeutic drugs.

nal mucosa or hair follicles. Conversely, severe toxicity manifests at the liver, kidneys, pancreas, central nervous system, and on clotting mechanisms (Haskell *et al,* 1969). For example, hepatic dysfunction associated with elevated blood concentrations of ammonia occurs, and approximately 5% of treated patients develop overt hemorrhagic pancreatitis. Impaired sensorium and coma may develop. Presumably, all these side effects result from widespread inhibition of protein synthesis in various tissues of the body. Since asparaginase is a relatively large foreign protein, it is antigenic, and hypersensitivity phenomena ranging from mild allergic reactions to anaphylactic shock occur in as many as 20% of treated patients.

SYNTHETICS

Examples of synthetic chemotherapeutic drugs include cisplatin, hydroxyurea, procarbazine, and mitotane (Table 29-1; Fig. 29-8).

Cisplatin

Cisplatin is an inorganic platinum-containing complex that enters cells by diffusion and disrupts the DNA helix. The drug must be administered intravenously, because oral ingestion is ineffective. High concentrations of cisplatin are found in the kidney, liver, intestines, and testes, but there is poor penetration into the central nervous system. Cisplatin is frequently used with other drugs, especially in chemotherapy of metastatic testicular and ovarian carcinoma (Bruckner *et al,* 1976; Einhorn and Donahue, 1977).

Side Effects

Renal toxicity is prominent, and hydration prior to and following administration of cisplatin is indicated. Decreased renal tubular function produced by cisplatin is dose-related and typically occurs during the second week of treatment (Dentino *et al,* 1978). Ototoxicity caused by cisplatin is manifested by tinnitus and hearing loss in the high-frequency range (Merrin *et al,* 1978). Marked nausea and vomiting occurs in almost all patients. Mild to moderate myelosuppression may develop with transient leukopenia and thrombocytopenia. Hyperuricemia, peripheral neuropathies, seizures, and cardiac dysrhythmias have been observed. Allergic reactions characterized by facial edema, bronchoconstriction, tachycardia, and hypotension may occur minutes after injection of the drug.

Hydroxyurea

Hydroxyurea acts on the enzyme ribonucleoside disphosphate reductase to interfere with the synthesis of DNA. Oral absorption is excellent, and about 80% of the drug appears in the urine within 12 hours after oral or intravenous administration. The primary use of hydroxyurea is in the treatment of chronic granulocytic leukemia. Temporary remissions in patients with metastatic malignant melanoma have been reported (Ariel, 1970).

Myelosuppression manifesting as leukopenia, megaloblastic anemia, and occasionally thrombocytopenia is the major side effect produced by hydroxyurea. Stomatitis and alopecia occur infrequently.

Procarbazine

Procarbazine inhibits DNA synthesis and is of greatest efficacy in the treatment of Hodgkin's disease, particularly when given in combination with other drugs. Oral absorption is excellent, and the drug is widely distributed, including the cerebrospinal fluid. Oxidative metabolism is extensive, with less than 5% of procarbazine excreted unchanged in the urine.

Side Effects

The most common side effects of procarbazine include nausea, vomiting, leukopenia, and thrombocytopenia, which occur in more than 50% of treated patients. Sedative effects are prominent. Synergism occurs with phenothiazine derivatives, barbiturates, opioids, and sedative-producing antihypertensive drugs. Ingestion of alcohol may cause intense warmth and reddening of the face, resembling the acetaldehyde syndrome as produced by disulfiram.

Procarbazine is a weak monoamine oxidase inhibitor. For this reason, administration of sympathomimetic drugs and tricyclic antidepressants or ingestion of foods containing tyramine may evoke hypertensive reactions. Hypersensitivity reactions, including pleural and pulmonary changes, can occur (Jones *et al,* 1972).

Mitotane

Mitotane is chemically similar to insecticides such as DDT. This drug produces selective destruction of normal or malignant adrenocortical cells, leading to a prompt reduction in the circulating concentration of corticosteroids (Hogan *et al,* 1978). The specific effect on the adrenal cortex is the basis for the use of this drug in the palliative treatment of inoperable adrenocortical carcinoma. After discontinuation of treatment, plasma concentrations of mitotane are present for up to 9 weeks, reflecting storage in fat.

Damage to the bone marrow, kidneys, or liver has not been observed. Anorexia and nausea occur in the majority of treated patients. Somnolence and lethargy are present in about one third of patients. The need for supplemental administration of corticosteroids is obvious when these patients are undergoing surgical stress.

HORMONES

Hormones, including corticosteroids, progestins, estrogens, and androgens, may have use in the treatment of neoplastic disease (Table 29-1).

Corticosteroids

Corticosteroids, because of their lympholytic effects and their ability to suppress mitosis in lymphocytes, have value in the treatment of acute leukemia in children (not adults) and malignant lymphoma. These hormones are particularly effective in the management of hemolytic anemia and thrombocytopenia that frequently accompany leukemia and lymphoma. Prednisone is commonly administered orally in high doses (0.5–1.5 mg kg^{-1}) which are then gradually reduced to maintenance levels.

Progestins

Progestational agents are useful in the management of patients with endometrial carcinoma. Presumably, unopposed overstimulation of the endometrium is responsible for neoplastic changes, and progesterone offsets this effect.

Estrogens and Androgens

Malignant changes in the prostate and breast are often dependent on hormones for their continued growth. For example, prostatic cancer is stimulated by androgens, whereas orchiectomy or estrogens (*e.g.,* diethylstilbestrol) slow growth of the tumor. Eventually, prostatic tumors become insensitive to lack of androgen or the presence of estrogen, presumably because of the survival of progressively undifferentiated cells that favor the emergence of cell types that are no longer dependent on androgen.

Estrogens and androgens have value in the treatment of advanced breast carcinoma. Malignant tissues that are responsive to estrogens contain receptors for the hormone, whereas malignant tissues lacking these receptors are unlikely to respond to hormonal manipulation. The onset of action of hormone therapy is slow, requiring 8 to 12 weeks.

Hypercalcemia may be associated with androgen or estrogen therapy, requiring adequate hydration in an attempt to facilitate renal excretion of calcium. Plasma calcium concentrations should be determined routinely in patients receiving treatment with these hormones.

Antiestrogens

Tamoxifen binds to estrogen receptors and inhibits continued growth of estrogen-dependent tumors (Legha *et al,* 1978). As such, this drug is useful in the palliative treatment of advanced carcinoma of the breast in postmenopausal women. Toxicity is minimal, and side effects include hot flashes, nausea, and vomiting. Hypercalcemia is an infrequent complication.

REFERENCES

Ahmed NK, Felsted RL, Bacher NR. Heterogeneity of antracycline antibiotic carbonylreductases in mammalian livers. Biochem Pharmacol 1978;27:2713 – 20.

Ainger LE, Bushore J, Johnson WW, et al. Daunomycin —a cardiotoxic agent. J Natl Med Assoc 1971;63: 261 – 7.

Alberts DS, Chang SY, Chen H-SG, et al. Kinetics of intravenous melphalan. Clin Pharmacol Ther 1979a;26: 73 – 80.

Alberts DS, Chang SY, Chen H-SG, Larcom BJ, Jones SE. Pharmacokinetics and metabolism of chlorambucil in man: a preliminary report. Cancer Treat Rev 1979b;6:9 – 17.

Ariel I. Therapeutic effects of hydroxyurea. Experience with 118 patients with inoperable solid tumors. Cancer 1970;25:75 – 84.

Bagley CM, Bostick FW, DeVita VT. Clinical pharmacology of cyclophosphamide. Cancer Res 1973;33: 226 – 33.

Blum RH, Carter SK, Agre KA. A clinical review of bleomycin—a new antineoplastic agent. CA 1973;31:903 – 14.

Boileau G, Piro AJ, Lahiri SR, Hall TC. Cerebellar ataxia during 5-fluorouracil (NSC-19893) therapy. Cancer Chemother Rep 1971;55:595 – 8.

Bristow MR, Billingham ME, Mason JW, Daniels JR. Clinical spectrum of anthracycline antibiotic cardiotoxicity. Cancer Treat Rep 1978;62:873 – 9.

Broder LE, Carter SK. Pancreatic islet cell carcinoma. II Results of therapy with streptozotocin in 52 patients. Ann Intern Med 1973;79:108 – 18.

Brome JD. Evidence that the L-asparaginase activity of guinea pig serum is responsible for its antilymphoma effects. Nature 1961;191:1114 – 5.

Broughton A, Strong JE, Hoyle PY, Bedrossian CWM. Clinical pharmacology of bleomycin following intravenous infusion as determined by radioimmunoassay. Cancer 1977;40:2772 – 8.

Bucher NLR. Microtubules. N Engl J Med 1972;287: 195 – 6.

Bruckner HW, Cohen CC, Deppe G, et al. Chemotherapy of gynecological tumors with platinum II. J Clin Hematol Oncol 1976;3:121 – 39.

Cheng CJ, Fujimura S, Grunberger D, Weinstein IB. Interaction of 1-(2-chloroethyl)-3-cyclohexyl-1-nitrosourea (NSC 79037) with nucleic acids and proteins in vivo and in vitro. Cancer Res 1972;32:22 – 7.

Cortes EP, Lutman G, Wanka J, et al. Adriamycin (NSC-123127) cardiotoxicity: a clinicopathologic correlation. Cancer Chemother Rep 1975;6:215 – 25.

Crooke ST, Bradner WT. Bleomycin:a review. J Med 1976;7:333 – 428.

DeFronzo RA, Braine H, Colvin OM. Water intoxication in man after cyclophosphamide therapy. Time course and relation activation. Ann Intern Med 1973;78:861 – 9.

Dentino M, Luft FC, Yum MN, Williams SD, Einhorn LH. Long-term effect of cis-diamminedichloride platinum (CDDP) on renal function and structure in man. Cancer 1978;4:1274 – 81.

DeVita VT, Canellos GP, Moxley JH. A decade of combination chemotherapy of advanced Hodgkin's disease. Cancer 1972;30:1495 – 1504.

Douglas MJ, Coppin CML. Bleomycin and subsequent anaesthesia: a retrospective study at Vancouver General Hospital. Can Anaesth Soc J 1980;27:449 – 52.

Durant JR, Norgard MJ, Murad TM, Bartolucci AA, Langford KH. Pulmonary toxicity associated with bischloroethylnitrosourea (BCNU). Ann Intern Med 1979;90:190 – 4.

Einhorn LH, Donahue J. Cis-diamminedichloroplatinum, vinblastine, and bleomycin: combination chemotherapy in disseminated testicular cancer. Ann Intern Med 1977;87:293 – 8.

Fauci AS, Haynes BF, Katz P. Treatment of granulomatous vasculitis. The spectrum of vasculitis: clinical, pathologic, immunologic, and therapeutic consideration. Ann Intern Med 1978;89:660 – 76.

Goldiner PL, Carlon G, Cvitkovic E, Schweizer O, Howland WS. Factors influencing postoperative morbidity and mortality in patients treated with bleomycin. Br Med J 1978;1:1664 – 7.

Gottlieb JA, Lefrak EA, O'Bryan RM, *et al.* Fatal adriamycin cardiomyopathy (CMY): prevention by dose limitation. Proc Am Assoc Cancer Res 1973;14:88.

Haskell CM, Canellos GP, Leventhal BG, et al. L-Asparaginase — therapeutic and toxic effects in patients with neoplastic disease. N Engl J Med 1969;281:1028 – 34.

Hogan TF, Citrin DL, Johnson BM, Nakamura S, Davis TE, Borden EC. o,p'-DDD (nitotane) therapy of adrenal cortical carcinoma. Cancer 1978;42:2177–81.

Iacovino JR, Leitner J, Abbas AK, et al. Fatal pulmonary reaction from low doses of bleomycin: an idiosyncratic tissue response. JAMA 1976;235:1253–5.

Jones SE, Moore M, Blank N, Castellino RA. Hypersensitivity to procarbazine (Matulane) manifested by fever and pleuropulmonary reaction. Cancer 1972;29:498–500.

Jones SE, Ewy GA, Groves BM. Echocardiographic detection of adriamycin heart disease. Proc Am Assoc Cancer Res 175;16:228.

Kennedy BJ. Metabolic and toxic effects of mithramycin during tumor therapy. Am J Med 1970;49:494–503.

LaMantia KR, Glick JH, Marshall BE. Supplemental oxygen does not cause respiratory failure in bleomycin-treated surgical patients. Anesthesiology 1984;60:65–7.

Lefrak EA, Pitha J, Rosenheim S, et al. Adriamycin (NSC-123127) cardiomyopathy. Cancer Chemother Rep 1975;6:203–8.

Legha SS, Davis HL, Muggia FM. Hormonal therapy of breast cancer: new approaches and concepts. Ann Intern Med 1978;88:69–77.

Lerner HJ. Acute myelogenous leukemia patients receiving chlorambucil as long-term adjuvant chemotherapy for stage II breast cancer. Cancer Treat Rep 1978;62:1135–43.

Levin VA, Hoffman W, Weinkam RJ. Pharmacokinetics of BCNU in man: a preliminary study of 20 patients. Cancer Treat Rep 1978;62:1305–12.

Luna MA, Bedrossian CW, Lichtiger B, et al. Interstitial pneumonitis associated with bleomycin therapy. Am J Clin Pathol 1972;58:501–10.

Mark GJ, Lehimgar–Zadeh A, Radsdale BD. Cyclophosphamide pneumonitis. Thorax 1978;33:89–93.

Mason JW, Bristow MR, Billingham ME, Daniels JR. Invasive and noninvasive methods of assessing adriamycin cardiotoxic effects in man: superiority of histopathologic assessment using endomyocardial biopsy. Cancer Treat Rep 1978;62:857–64.

Matalon S, Harper WV, Nickerson PA, Olszowka J. Intravenous bleomycin does not alter the toxic effects of hyperoxia in rabbits. Anesthesiology 1986; 64:614–9.

McCammon RL. Cancer. In: Stoelting RK, Dierdorf SF, eds. Anesthesia and Co-Existing Disease. New York, Churchill-Livingstone, 1983;631.

Merrin C, Beckley S, Takita H. Multimodal treatment of advanced testicular tumor with radical reductive surgery and multisequential chemotherapy with cis platinum, bleomycin, vinblastine, vincristine and actinomycin D. J Urol 1978;120:73–6.

Minow RA, Gottlieb JA, Freireich EJ. Electrocardiogram QRS voltage changes in adriamycin cardiomyopathy. Proc Am Assoc Cancer Res 1975;16:87.

Mitchell MS, Wade ME, DeConti RC, Bertino JR, Calabresi P. Immunosuppressive effects of cytosine arabinoside and methotrexate in man. Ann Intern Med 1969;70:535–47.

Monto RW, Talley RW, Caldwell MJ, Levin WC, Guest MM. Observations on the mechanism of hemorrhagic toxicity in mithramycin (NSC-24559) therapy. Cancer Res 1969;29:697–703.

Myers CE, McGuire WP, Liss RH, Ifrim E, Grotzinger K, Young RC. Adriamycin—the role of lipid peroxidation in cardiac toxicity and tumor response. Science 1977;197:165–7.

Orwoll ES, Kiessling PJ, Patterson JR. Interstitial pneumonia from mitomycin. Ann Intern Med 1978;89:352–5.

Pigram WJ, Fuller W, Hamilton LD. Sterochemistry of intercolation: interaction of daunomycin with DNA. Nature 1972;235:17–9.

Rinehart JJ, Lewis RP, Balcerzak SP. Adriamycin cardiotoxicity in man. Ann Intern Med 1974;81:475–8.

Robins PR, Jowsey J. Effect of mithramycin on normal and abnormal bone turnover. J Lab Clin Med 1973;82:576–86.

Rosenow EC III. The spectrum of drug-induced pulmonary disease. Ann Intern Med 1972;77:977–91.

Rosenthal S, Kaufman S. Vincristine neurotoxicity. Ann Intern Med 174;80:733–7.

Rudders RA, Mensley GT. Bleomycin pulmonary toxicity. Chest 1973;63:626–8.

Rundles RW, Wyngaarden JB, Hitchings GH, Elion GB III. Drugs and uric acid. Annu Rev Pharmacol Toxicol 1969;9:345–62.

Samuels ML, Johnson DE, Holoye PY, Lanzotti VJ. Pulmonary toxicity following large-dosage bleomycin: a possible role for prior radiotherapy. JAMA 1976;235:1117–20.

Schein P, Kahn R, Gorden P, Wells S, DeVita VT. Streptozotocin for malignant insulinomas and carcinoid tumor. Arch Intern Med 1973;132:555–61.

Schein PS, Winokur SH. Immunosuppressive and cytotoxic chemotherapy: long-term complications. Ann Intern Med 1975;82:84–95.

Selevan SG, Lindbohm M-L, CandPolSci, Hornung RW, Hemminki K. A study of occupational exposure to antineoplastic drugs and fetal loss in nurses. N Engl J Med 1985;313:1173–8.

Selvin BF. Cancer chemotherapy: Implications for the anesthesiologist. Anesth Analg 1981;60:425–34.

Shapiro R. Chemistry of guanine and its biologically significant derivatives. Prog Nucleic Acid Res Mol Biol 1968;8:73–112.

Tritton TR, Murphee SA, Sartorelli AC. Adriamycin: a proposal on the specificity of drug action. Biochem Biophys Res Commun 1978;84:802–8.

Umezawa H. Principles of antitumor antibiotic therapy. In: Holland JF, Frei E, eds. Cancer Medicine. Philadelphia. Lea and Febiger, 1973:817–26.

Walker MD. Nitrosureas in central nervous system tumors. Cancer Chemother Rep 1973;4:21 – 6.

Wasserman TH, Slavik M, Carter SH. Clinical comparison of the nitrosoureas. Cancer 1975;36:1258 – 68.

Wasserman TH. The nitrosoureas: an outline of clinical schedules and toxic effects. Cancer Treat Rep 1976;60:709 – 11.

Whitcomb ME, Schwarz MI, Tormey DC. Methotrexate pneumonitis: case report and review of the literature. Thorax 1972;27:636 – 9.

Yarbro JW, Kennedy BJ, Barnum CP. Mithramycin inhibition of ribonucleic acid synthesis. Cancer Res 1966;26:36 – 9.

Zsigmond EK, Robins G. The effect of a series of anticancer drugs on plasma cholinesterase activity. Can Anaesth Soc J 1972;19:75 – 82.

C H A P T E R   30

Antiepileptic Drugs

INTRODUCTION

Epilepsy is a collective term used to designate a group of chronic central nervous system disorders characterized by the onset of sudden disturbances of sensory, motor, autonomic, or psychic origin (see Chapter 41). These disturbances are usually transient and are almost always associated with abnormal discharges of the electroencephalogram. The incidence of epilepsy is between 0.3% and 0.6% of the population (Hauser, 1978). The antiepileptic drug selected to treat epilepsy is determined by the characteristics of the seizure experienced by the patient (Gastaut, 1970). Epilepsy is classified as (1) grand mal epilepsy, (2) petit mal epilepsy, (3) focal epilepsy, (4) psychomotor epilepsy, and (5) myoclonic or infantile myoclonic epilepsy (see Chapter 41). Febrile seizures typically occur between 3 months and 5 years of age in the absence of any known cause other than an association with fever. Daily administration of antiepileptic drugs prevents recurrence of febrile seizures. Seizures are sometimes a result of withdrawal from drugs such as barbiturates and alcohol.

MECHANISM OF SEIZURE ACTIVITY

Seizure activity in most patients with epilepsy has a localized or focal origin. The reason for the high frequency and synchronous firing in a seizure focus is unknown. Possible explanations include

(1) local biochemical changes, (2) ischemia, (3) loss of cellular inhibitory systems, (4) infections, and (5) head trauma.

Neurons in a chronic seizure focus exhibit a type of denervation hypersensitivity with regard to excitatory stimuli. The spread of seizure activity to neighboring normal cells is presumably restrained by normal inhibitory mechanisms (see Chapter 41). Factors such as changes in blood glucose concentration, PaO_2, $PaCO_2$, pH, electrolyte balance, endocrine function, stress, and fatigue may result in spread of a seizure focus into areas of normal brain. If the spread is sufficiently extensive, the entire brain is activated and a tonic-clonic seizure with unconsciousness ensues. Conversely, if the spread is localized, the seizure produces signs and symptoms characteristic of the anatomic focus. Once initiated, a seizure is most likely maintained by reentry of excitatory impulses in a closed feedback pathway that may not even include the original seizure focus.

MECHANISM OF DRUG ACTION

Most antiepileptic drugs act by reducing the spread of excitation from a seizure focus to normal neurons. The mechanism by which these drugs prevent spread of abnormal activity is unknown but may involve (1) post-tetanic potentiation, (2) reductions in movement of sodium or calcium ions, (3) potentiation of presynaptic or postsynaptic inhibition, and (4) reduction of responsiveness

500 SECTION I : PHARMACOLOGY

of various monosynaptic or polysynaptic pathways.

It is stated that complete drug-induced control of seizures can be achieved in up to 50% of patients, plus significant improvement in 25% of patients (Meinardi *et al,* 1977). Petit mal epilepsy responds well to one group of antiepileptic drugs, and grand mal epilepsy and focal epilepsy are usually adequately controlled by another group of drugs. Psychomotor epilepsy tends to be refractory, responding only to certain antiepileptic drugs. Infantile myoclonus and the types of epilepsy that occur in young children are frequently unresponsive to drug therapy. Multiple drug therapy is often required, because two or more seizure types may occur in the same patient.

PLASMA CONCENTRATIONS

Measurement of plasma concentrations of antiepileptic drugs greatly facilitates treatment of seizure disorders, especially when multiple drug therapy is used (Table 30-1). Nevertheless, interpretation of plasma concentrations must be cautious, because clinical effects do not always parallel these levels. Furthermore, the method of measurement may not distinguish protein bound drug from the free and pharmacologically active fraction.

HYDANTOINS

Hydantoin derivatives used as antiepileptic drugs include phenytoin, mephenytoin, and phenacemide.

Phenytoin

Phenytoin is the prototype of hydantoins and is the primary drug administered for treatment of all types of epilepsy except for petit mal epilepsy (Fig. 30-1). Phenytoin can induce complete suppression of grand mal epilepsy and focal epilepsy but does not completely eliminate the sensory aura or other prodromal signs. The antiepileptic activity of phenytoin is not accompanied by sedation.

Table 30-1
Pharmacokinetics of Antiepileptic Drugs

	Plasma Therapeutic Concentration ($\mu g\ ml^{-1}$)	Protein Binding (%)	Volume of Distribution ($L\ kg^{-1}$)	Elimination Half-Time (hr)	Clearance ($ml\ kg^{-1}\ min^{-1}$)	Site of Clearance and Percent
Phenytoin	10–20	90	0.64	24	dose dependent	hepatic, 98%
Phenobarbital	10–20	40–60	0.8	90	0.09	hepatic, 75% renal, 25%
Primidone	5–10	20	0.8	8	0.78	hepatic, 60% renal, 40%
Carbamazepine	4–12	80	1.4	13–17	0.58	hepatic, 98%
Ethosuximide	40–100	Insignificant	0.72	60	0.26	hepatic, 80% renal, 20%
Valproic Acid	50–100	80–90	0.13	12	0.12	hepatic, > 70%
Clonazepam	0.02–0.08	50	3.2	24–36	0.92	hepatic, 98%

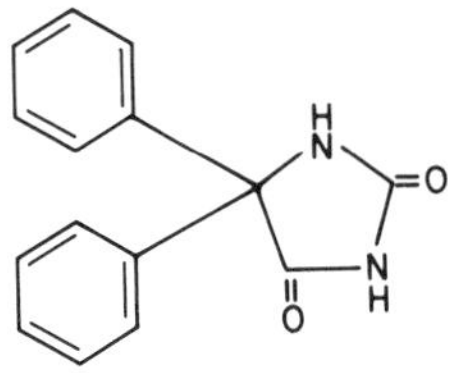

FIGURE 30-1. Phenytoin.

Mechanism of Action

Phenytoin limits the development and spread of activity from a seizure focus. Elevation of seizure threshold is relatively selective for the cerebral cortex. A stabilizing effect of phenytoin is apparent on all neuron cell membranes, including peripheral nerves. This stabilizing effect is most likely a result of drug-induced alterations in the movement of ions across cell membranes. For example, phenytoin decreases fluxes of sodium ions that occur during action potentials. In addition, influx of calcium ions during depolarization is decreased, possibly due to reduced intracellular concentrations of sodium ions (Woodbury, 1980). Phenytoin can also delay the activation of outward potassium current during an action potential, leading to an increased refractory period and a decrease in repetitive firing (Ayala and Johnston, 1977).

Pharmacokinetics

Phenytoin is a weak acid with a pKa of about 8.3 (Table 30-1). Its poor water solubility may result in slow and sometimes variable absorption from the gastrointestinal tract (30%–97%). Initial daily adult dosage is 3 to 4 mg kg^{-1}. Doses greater than 500 mg daily are rarely tolerated. The long duration of action of phenytoin allows a single daily dosage, but gastric intolerance may necessitate divided dosage. Following intramuscular injection, the drug precipitates at the injection site and is only slowly absorbed. For this reason, intramuscular administration is not recommended. Intravenous infusion of phenytoin should probably not exceed 5 mg min^{-1}.

PLASMA CONCENTRATIONS. Control of seizures is usually obtained with plasma concentrations of phenytoin between 10 and 20 μg ml^{-1}. In the control of digitalis-induced cardiac dysrhythmias, 0.5 to 1 mg kg^{-1} of phenytoin is administered intravenously every 15 to 30 minutes until a satisfactory response is achieved or a maximum dose of 15 mg kg^{-1} is administered. A plasma phenytoin concentration of 8 to 16 μg ml^{-1} is usually sufficient to suppress cardiac dysrhythmias. Adverse side effects of phenytoin such as nystagmus and ataxia are likely when the plasma concentration of drug exceeds 20 μg ml^{-1} (see the section entitled Side Effects).

PROTEIN BINDING. Phenytoin is bound approximately 90% to plasma albumin. A greater fraction of phenytoin remains unbound in neonates, in patients with hypoalbuminemia, and in uremic patients (Reidenberg et al, 1971).

METABOLISM. Metabolism of phenytoin is by hepatic microsomal enzymes that are susceptible to stimulation or inhibition by other drugs (Glazko, 1973). Below a plasma concentration of 10 μg ml^{-1}, metabolism of phenytoin follows first-order kinetics, and the elimination half-time averages 24 hours. At plasma concentrations of phenytoin above 10 μg ml^{-1}, the enzymes necessary for metabolism become saturated, and the elimination half-time becomes dose-dependent (i.e., zero-order kinetics). Zero-order kinetics resemble the metabolism of alcohol.

An estimated 98% of phenytoin is metabolized principally to the inactive derivative parahydroxyphenyl. This metabolite appears in the urine as a glucuronide. About 2% of phenytoin is recovered unchanged in the urine. A genetically determined inability to metabolize phenytoin may be present (Glazko, 1973).

Side Effects

Side effects associated with chronic phenytoin therapy include (1) cerebeller-vestibular dysfunction, (2) peripheral neuropathy, (3) gingival hyperplasia, (4) allergic reactions, (5) megaloblastic anemia, and (6) gastrointestinal irritation. Central nervous system toxicity is the most consistent effect of phenytoin overdosage. Administration of phenytoin during pregnancy may result in the fetal hydantoin syndrome, which manifests as wide-set eyes, broad mandible, and finger deformities. Phenytoin-induced hepatotoxicity, although rare, may occur in genetically susceptible persons who lack the enzyme phenytoin epoxide (Spielberg et al, 1981). This enzyme is necessary to convert an electrophilic intermediate formed after the oxidative metabolism of phenytoin to an inert and nontoxic product.

Nystagmus, ataxia, diplopia, and vertigo are likely when the plasma concentration of phenytoin exceeds 20 μg ml^{-1}. These are symptoms of cerebellar-vestibular dysfunction. Peripheral neuropathy has been reported in up to 30% of patients. Gingival hyperplasia occurs in about 20% of patients and is probably the most common manifestation of phenytoin toxicity in children and young adolescents. This complication is minimized by improved oral hygiene and does not necessarily require discontinuation of phenytoin therapy. Hyperglycemia and glycosuria appear to be due to phenytoin-induced inhibition of insulin secretion (Kiser *et al,* 1970). Allergic reactions include morbilliform rash in 2% to 5% of patients. Megaloblastic anemia is rare and has been attributed to altered folic acid absorption but probably also involves altered folic acid metabolism. Gastric irritation is due to alkalinity of the drug; this may be minimized by taking phenytoin after meals.

Mephenytoin

Mephenytoin is a hydantoin derivative, which, unlike phenytoin, is rapidly absorbed after oral administration. Its antiepileptic spectrum is the same as that of phenytoin, and it may exacerbate petit mal epilepsy. Ataxia, gingival hyperplasia, and gastric distress are less likely than with phenytoin therapy. Conversely, serious toxicity, including morbilliform rash, fever, pancytopenia, aplastic anemia, and hepatotoxicity, are more likely and greatly limit the use of this drug.

Phenacemide

Phenacemide is the straight chain analog of 5-phenylhydantoin, which is used in the treatment of psychomotor epilepsy only when other less toxic drugs are ineffective. Toxicity may manifest as hepatic, renal, and bone marrow dysfunction.

BARBITURATES

Phenobarbital, mephobarbital, and metharbital are the barbiturates used as antiepileptic drugs.

Phenobarbital

Phenobarbital is an effective antiepileptic drug for suppression of grand mal epilepsy and focal epilepsy and is the drug used most frequently for prophylaxis against the recurrence of febrile seizures (see Fig. 4-2). Although most barbiturates have antiepileptic activity, phenobarbital is unique in producing this effect at doses less than those that usually produce sedation. Phenobarbital limits the spread of seizure activity and also elevates seizure threshold. The ability to reduce the spread of seizures may depend on the potentiation of inhibitory pathways. Sedation, when it occurs, may be due to stimulation of gamma-aminobutyric acid (GABA) activity.

Pharmacokinetics

Oral absorption of phenobarbital is slow but nearly complete, with peak concentrations occurring 12 to 18 hours after a single dose (Table 30-1). Plasma protein binding is 40% to 60%. About 25% of phenobarbital is eliminated by pH-dependent renal excretion, with the remainder inactivated by hepatic microsomal enzymes. The major metabolite is an inactive parahydroxyphenyl derivative that is excreted in the urine as a sulfate conjugate. The elimination half-time is about 90 hours.

The usual daily dose of phenobarbital is 1 to 5 mg kg^{-1}. During chronic therapy, the plasma concentration of phenobarbital averages 10 μg ml^{-1} for every 1 mg kg^{-1} dose. Plasma phenobarbital concentrations of 10 to 20 μg ml^{-1} are usually necessary for control of seizures.

Side Effects

Sedation is the most common undesired side effect resulting from phenobarbital therapy. Tolerance to sedation develops, however, with chronic therapy. Phenobarbital sometimes produces irritability and hyperactivity in children and confusion in the elderly. Scarlatiniform or morbilliform rash occurs in up to 2% of patients. Megaloblastic anemia that responds to folic acid administration and osteomalacia that responds to vitamin D therapy may occur during chronic phenobarbital therapy as well as during treatment with phenytoin. Nystagmus and ataxia are likely when the plasma phenobarbital concentration exceeds 30 μg ml^{-1}.

Congenital malformations may occur when phenobarbital is administered chronically during pregnancy. A coagulation defect and hemorrhage in the newborn must be considered. Interactions between phenobarbital and other drugs usually involve induction of the hepatic microsomal enzymes by phenobarbital.

Mephobarbital

Mephobarbital undergoes N-demethylation to phenobarbital (Fig. 30-2). Consequently, the pharmacologic properties, clinical uses, and side effects of mephobarbital are identical to those of phenobarbital. Oral absorption of mephobarbital, however, is often incomplete, and the dose is about twice that of phenobarbital.

Metharbital

Metharbital undergoes N-demethylation to barbital, which is responsible for its pharmacologic activity. This drug has greater sedative and less antiepileptic activity than does phenobarbital.

PRIMIDONE

Primidone is a deoxybarbiturate that is effective against grand mal epilepsy, focal epilepsy, and psychomotor epilepsy. It is ineffective against petit mal epilepsy but is sometimes effective in the management of myoclonic seizures in children. Primidone may be administered alone but seems to be more effective when combined with phenytoin. Structurally, primidone is a congener of phenobarbital in which the carbonyl oxygen of the urea moiety is replaced by two hydrogen atoms (Fig. 30-3).

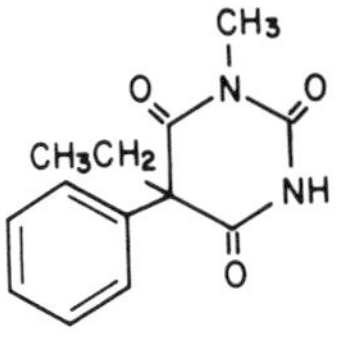

FIGURE 30-2. Mephobarbital.

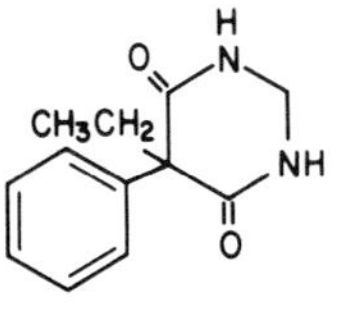

FIGURE 30-3. Primidone.

Pharmacokinetics

Primidone is rapidly and almost completely absorbed after oral administration, with peak plasma concentrations occurring in about 3 hours. The plasma elimination half-time is about 8 hours. Active metabolites of primidone are phenobarbital (elimination half-time 48 – 120 hours) and phenylethylmalonamide (elimination half-time 24 – 48 hours). Both these metabolites accumulate with chronic therapy. About 40% of the drug is excreted unchanged in the urine.

Side Effects

Sedation, nystagmus, vertigo, nausea, and vomiting are common side effects of primidone. Maculopapular rash, leukopenia, thrombocytopenia, megagloblastic anemia, and osteomalicia have been described, although these responses are rare. Ataxia and sedation usually occur when the plasma primidone concentration exceeds 12 μg ml^{-1}.

The dose of primidone is adjusted on the basis of the plasma concentrations of primidone and phenobarbital. Therapeutic plasma concentrations of primidone are 5 to 10 μg ml^{-1} and a phenobarbital concentration of 2 μg ml^{-1} for every mg kg^{-1} of the daily dose of primidone.

CARBAMAZEPINE

Carbamazepine is useful in the treatment of psychomotor epilepsy. In addition, this drug is effective in the management of patients with trigeminal and glossopharyngeal neuralgias (Crill, 1973). Structurally, carbamazepine is related to the tricyclic antidepressant imipramine (Fig. 30-4).

Pharmacokinetics

Oral absorption is rapid, with peak concentrations in plasma occurring 2 to 6 hours after ingestion

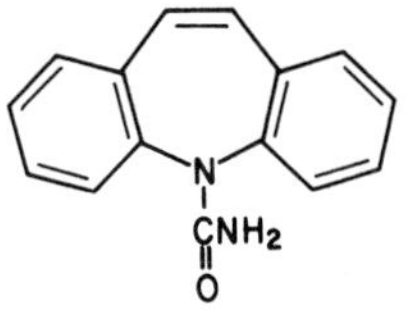

FIGURE 30-4. Carbamazepine.

(Table 30-1). Plasma protein binding approximates 80%. The plasma elimination half-time is 13 to 17 hours. An active metabolite has a shorter elimination half-time. The relatively short elimination half-time necessitates dosing intervals every 6 to 8 hours to minimize fluctuations in plasma concentrations. The usual therapeutic plasma concentration of carbamazepine is 4 to 12 μg ml^{-1}.

Side Effects

Sedation, vertigo, diplopia, nausea, vomiting, and ataxia are the most frequent side effects of carbamazepine therapy. Aplastic anemia, thrombocytopenia, hepatocellular and cholestatic jaundice, oliguria, hypertension, and acute left ventricular failure are potential life-threatening complications. For these reasons, bone marrow, hepatic, renal, and cardiac function must be monitored in patients treated with this drug. Skin rash, often with other manifestations of drug allergy, occurs in about 3% of patients. Carbamazepine may enhance the rate of metabolism of phenytoin, whereas phenobarbital may enhance the metabolism of carbamazepine.

SUCCINIMIDES

Ethosuximide, methsuximide, and phensuximide are examples of succinimides that are uniquely effective in the treatment of petit mal epilepsy.

Ethosuximide

Ethosuximide with alkyl substituents resembles other antiepileptic drugs (Fig. 30-5). This drug has a characteristic effect on thalamocortical excitation when compared with phenytoin. This is consistent with the speculated importance of the thalamocortical system in the etiology of petit mal epilepsy.

Pharmacokinetics

Oral absorption of ethosuximide is adequate, with peak concentrations occurring in 1 to 7 hours (Table 30-1). Ethosuximide is not significantly bound to albumin. About 20% of the drug is excreted unchanged in the urine, and the remainder is metabolized to inactive metabolites by the hepatic microsomal enzymes. The elimination half-time is about 60 hours. The usual maintenance dose of ethosuximide is 20 to 40 mg kg^{-1}. A plasma concentration of 40 to 100 μg ml^{-1} is required for satisfactory suppression of petit mal epilepsy.

Side Effects

The most common side effects of ethosuximide are nausea, vomiting, sedation, headache, and hiccough. Parkinson-like symptoms and photophobia have been reported. Urticaria, thrombocytopenia, and aplastic anemia have been described. Renal or hepatic toxicity has not been a problem with this drug.

Methsuximide

Methsuximide is effective in the treatment of petit mal epilepsy but less so than ethosuximide. Combined with other drugs, methsuximide may also be useful in the treatment of psychomotor epilepsy. An N-demethyl metabolite has been implicated in the production of coma following an overdose (Karch, 1973). The usual daily dose is 600 to 1200 mg. Side effects are similar to those described for ethosuximide.

Phensuximide

Phensuximide has a low efficacy and is seldom used. A dreamlike state, skin rash, fever, leukopenia, and reversible nephropathy have been reported.

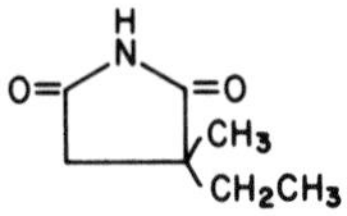

FIGURE 30-5. Ethosuximide.

VALPROIC ACID

Valproic acid is a branched chain carboxylic acid that is effective in the treatment of petit mal epilepsy (Fig. 30-6). Its mechanism of action is unknown but may involve an interaction with the metabolism of GABA (Browne, 1980).

Pharmacokinetics

Valproic acid is rapidly absorbed, with peak concentrations in plasma observed after 1 to 4 hours. Binding to plasma proteins exceeds 80%. More than 70% of the drug can be recovered as inactive glucuronide conjugates. The elimination half-time is about 12 hours. The usual daily dose of valproic acid is 1 to 3 g to achieve a therapeutic plasma concentration of 50 to 100 μg ml^{-1}.

Side Effects

Side effects produced by valproic acid are infrequent, but nausea and vomiting do occur (Browne, 1980). Sedation and ataxia are less frequent than after administration of other antiepileptic drugs. Valproic acid may affect platelet aggregation, and bleeding time should be determined prior to initiating therapy as well as preoperatively. Since valproic acid is partly eliminated as a ketone-containing metabolite, the urine ketone test may show false-positive results. The most serious side effect is hepatotoxicity, emphasizing the need to monitor liver function during chronic therapy with this drug.

Valproic acid can displace phenytoin and diazepam from protein binding sites, resulting in increased pharmacologic effects produced by these drugs. The metabolism of phenytoin is also inhibited by valproic acid. Finally, this drug causes the plasma concentration of phenobarbital to increase almost 50%, presumably owing to inhibition of hepatic microsomal enzymes (Bruni and Wilder, 1979).

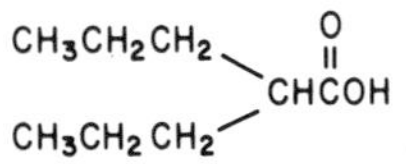

OXAZOLIDINEDIONES

Trimethadione and paramethadione are examples of oxazolidinediones that are effective in the treatment of petit mal epilepsy. Thalamic nuclei are particularly sensitive to these drugs, which is consistent with the speculated importance of the thal-

FIGURE 30-6. Valproic acid.

amocortical system in the etiology of petit mal epilepsy.

Trimethadione

Trimethadione contains structural characteristics common to other classes of antiepileptic drugs, including alkyl substitutes on the 5 carbon atom (Fig. 30-7).

Pharmacokinetics

Trimethadione is rapidly absorbed from the gastrointestinal tract, producing peak plasma concentrations in 1 to 2 hours. Plasma protein binding is insignificant. Hepatic microsomal enzymes are responsible for demethylation of trimethadione to its active metabolite dimethadione (Butler *et al*, 1965). Dimethadione is not further metabolized but is excreted unchanged in the urine, with an elimination half-time of 6 to 13 days. During chronic therapy, dimethadione accumulates and is responsible for the pharmacologic activity of the parent drug.

The usual daily dose of trimethadione is 0.9 to 2.1 g. Plasma concentrations of the active metabolite dimethadione are used to guide therapy and adjust the maintenance dose of trimethadione. The plasma concentration of dimethadione must usually be maintained above 700 μg ml^{-1} to control petit mal epilepsy.

Side Effects

The most common side effects of trimethadione therapy are sedation and blurring of vision in bright light (hemeralopia). Sedation tends to diminish with chronic therapy. Less common, but more serious, side effects include exfoliative der-

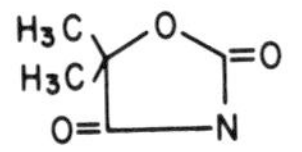

FIGURE 30-7. Trimethadione.

matitis, neutropenia, aplastic anemia, hepatitis, and nephrosis. A myasthenic syndrome has also been reported (Booker *et al,* 1968).

Paramethadione

Paramethadione differs from trimethadione only in replacement of one of the methyl groups on the 5 carbon atom with an ethyl substituent. An active metabolite results from N-demethylation and is likely to be responsible for the antiepileptic activity of the drug. The pharmacologic properties, therapeutic uses, dosage, and toxicity are similar to those of trimethadione. Nevertheless, patients who do not tolerate trimethadione may tolerate paramethadione and vice versa.

BENZODIAZEPINES

A large number of benzodiazepines have broad antiepileptic properties, but only clonazepam and diazepam are commonly used (see Fig. 5-1). The antiepileptic actions of benzodiazepines as well as barbiturates and valproic acid may involve drug-induced increases in the activity of inhibitory neurotransmitters such as GABA (Hammond *et al,* 1981). In low doses, benzodiazepines suppress polysynaptic activity in the spinal cord and decrease neuronal activity in the mesencephalic reticular system.

Clonazepam

Clonazepam is useful in the therapy of petit mal epilepsy as well as myoclonic seizures in children (Browne, 1978).

Pharmacokinetics

Absorption of clonazepam after oral administration is rapid, with peak plasma concentrations occurring within 2 to 4 hours (Table 30-1). Intravenous administration of clonazepam results in rapid central nervous system effects. About 50% of the drug is bound to plasma proteins. Clonazepam is extensively metabolized to inactive products, with less than 2% of an injected dose appearing unchanged in the urine. The elimination half-time is 24 to 36 hours. The maintenance dose of clonazepam should not exceed about 0.25 mg kg^{-1}.

Therapeutic plasma concentrations of clonazepam are 0.02 to 0.08 μg ml^{-1}.

Side Effects

Side effects are infrequent after oral administration. Sedation is present in approximately 50% of patients but tends to subside with chronic administration. Skeletal muscle incoordination and ataxia occur in about 30% of patients. Hypotonia, dysarthria, and dizziness have been described. Personality changes occur in 25% of patients, manifesting as behavioral disturbances, including hyperactivity, irritability, and difficulty in concentration. Increased salivary and bronchial secretions may be particularly prominent in children. Seizures are exacerbated in some patients, and status epilepticus may be precipitated if the drug is discontinued abruptly (Browne, 1978). Cardiovascular and respiratory depression have occurred after intravenous administration.

Diazepam

Diazepam is effective in the treatment of status epilepticus and local anesthetic-induced seizures. The usual approach is the intravenous administration of 0.1 mg kg^{-1} every 10 to 15 minutes until seizure activity has been suppressed or a maximum dose of 30 mg has been administered (see Chapter 7).

ACETAZOLAMIDE

Acetazolamide is a carbonic anhydrase inhibitor that may be effective in the treatment of petit mal epilepsy. Its effectiveness, however, is limited by the rapid development of tolerance.

REFERENCES

Ayala GF, Johnston D. The influences of phenytoin on the fundamental electrical properties of simple neural systems. Epilepsia 1977;18:299–307.

Booker HE, Chun RWM, Sanguino M. Myasthenia syndrome associated with trimethadione. Neurology 1968;18:274.

Browne TR. Clonazepam. N Engl J Med 1978;299:812–6.

Browne TR. Valproic acid. N Engl J Med 1980;302:661–6.

Bruni J, Wilder BJ. Valproic acid: Review of new antiepileptic drug. Arch Neurol 1979;36:393–98.

Butler TC, Waddell WJ, Poole DT. Demethylation of trimethadione and metharbital by rat liver macrosomal enzymes: substrate concentration-yield relationships and competition between substrates. Biochem Pharmacol 1965;14:937–42.

Crill WE. Carbamazepine. Ann Intern Med 1973;79: 844–7.

Gastaut H. Clinical and electroencephalographical classification of epileptic seizures. Epilepsia 1970;11:102–13.

Glazko AJ. Diphenylhydantoin metabolism: a prospective review. Drug Metab Dispos 1973;1:711–4.

Hammond EJ, Wilder BJ, Bruni J. Central actions of valproic acid in man and experimental models of epilepsy. Life Sci 1981;29:2561–74.

Hauser WA. Epidemiology of epilepsy. Adv Neurol 1978;19:313–39.

Karch SB. Methsuximide overdose: delayed onset of profound coma. JAMA 1973;223:1463–5.

Kiser JS, Vargas-Cordon M, Brendel K, Bressler R. The in vitro inhibition of insulin secretion by diphenylhydantoin. J Clin Invest 1970;49:1942–8.

Meinardi H, VanHeycop ten Ham MW, Meijer JWA, Bongers E. Long-term control of seizures. In: Penry JK, ed. Epilepsy: The Eighth International Symposium. New York, Raven Press, 1977;17.

Reidenberg MM, Odar-Cedarlof, VonBahr C Borga O, Sjoqvist F. Protein binding of diphenylhydantoin and desmethylimipramine in plasma from patients with poor renal function. N Engl J Med 1971;285:264–7.

Spielberg SP, Gordon GB, Blake DA, Goldstein DA, Herlong HF. Predisposition to phenytoin hepatotoxicity assessed in vitro. N Engl J Med 1981;305:722–7.

Woodbury DM. Convulsant drugs: Mechanisms of action. In: Glaser GH, ed. Antiepileptic Drugs: Mechanisms of Action. New York, Raven Press, 1980;249.

C H A P T E R   31

Drugs Used for Treatment of Parkinson's Disease

INTRODUCTION

Parkinson's disease is a manifestation of an imbalance between dopaminergic and cholinergic activity transmitted by the extrapyramidal nervous system (see Chapter 41). Conceptually, dopamine is believed to act principally as an inhibitory neurotransmitter and acetylcholine as an excitatory neurotransmitter in the extrapyramidal system. Although dopamine is more important, a proper balance with the cholinergic neurotransmitter is also necessary for normal function. The goal of treatment of Parkinson's disease is to enhance the inhibitory effect of dopamine or reduce the stimulatory effect of acetylcholine by the administration of centrally acting drugs. Often combinations of drugs with effects on the dopaminergic and cholinergic components of the extrapyramidal nervous systems are also used. Regardless of the drug or drugs selected, treatment of Parkinson's disease is always palliative and never curative.

The most common causes of Parkinson's disease are cerebral atherosclerosis, viral encephalitis, and drugs that prevent the action of dopamine in the basal ganglia (*i.e.,* butyrophenones, phenothiazines) (Calne, 1977). About 80% of the dopamine in the brain is concentrated in the basal ganglia, mostly in the caudate nucleus and putamen. In patients with Parkinson's disease, the basal ganglia content of dopamine is only about 10% of normal. As a result, there is an excess of excitatory cholinergic activity manifesting as tremor, skeletal muscle rigidity, bradykinesia, and disturbances of posture. In addition to these classic peripheral manifestations of Parkinson's disease, approximately one fifth of afflicted patients become mentally depressed and one third of patients develop cognitive and memory deficits that may progress to delirium (Lieberman, 1979). Alzheimer's disease is six times more frequent in patients with Parkinson's disease (Boller *et al,* 1980).

LEVODOPA

Levodopa, as the immediate metabolic precursor of dopamine, acts by replenishing the depleted stores of dopamine in the basal ganglia (Fig. 31-1). Indeed, about 75% of patients with Parkinson's disease respond favorably to treatment with levodopa. An optimal therapeutic response, however, may not occur in some patients until the completion of 1 to 6 months of therapy. The beneficial therapeutic response to levodopa typically diminishes after 2 to 5 years of treatment, presumably reflecting progression of the disease process and continuing loss of nigrostriatal neurons with a capacity to store dopamine.

The usual daily maintenance dose of levodopa is 3 to 8 g administered orally in at least four divided doses. Absorption from the gastrointestinal tract is efficient using an active transport system. Maximal plasma concentrations of levodopa occur 0.5 to 2 hours after administration, but the brief elimination half-time of 1 to 3 hours requires frequent dosing intervals to maintain a therapeutic

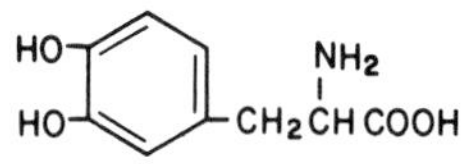

FIGURE 31-1. Levodopa.

tissue concentration. Slowed gastric emptying as caused by opioids or anticholinergics and increased gastric acidity reduce absorption of levodopa from the gastrointestinal tract.

Abrupt discontinuation of levodopa therapy may result in a precipitous return of symptoms of Parkinson's disease. For this reason, levodopa should be continued throughout the perioperative period, being included in the preoperative medication.

Metabolism

Approximately 95% of orally administered levodopa is rapidly decarboxylated to dopamine by the widely distributed enzyme dopa decarboxylase. The resulting dopamine cannot easily cross the blood–brain barrier to exert a beneficial therapeutic effect, whereas increased plasma concentrations of dopamine often lead to undesirable side effects (see the section entitled Side Effects). Inhibition of the peripheral activity of dopa decarboxylase enzyme greatly increases the fraction of administered levodopa that remains unmetabolized and available to cross the blood–brain barrier (see the section entitled Carbidopa).

At least 30 metabolites of levodopa have been identified. Most are converted to dopamine, small amounts of which are subsequently metabolized to norepinephrine and epinephrine. Metabolism of dopamine yields 3,4-dihydroxyphenylacetic acid and 3 methoxy-4-hydroxyphenylacetic acid (homovanillic acid). Dietary methionine is necessary as a source of methyl donors to permit continued activity of catechol-o-methyl transferase, which is necessary for the metabolism of the excess amounts of dopamine that result from high doses of levodopa. Most of the metabolites of dopamine are excreted by the kidneys.

Side Effects

Most patients with Parkinson's disease who are treated with levodopa experience side effects.

These side effects are typically dose-dependent and reversible. Presumably, increased formation of catecholamines, particularly dopamine, both in the central nervous system and periphery are responsible for these side effects.

Gastrointestinal Dysfunction

The most common side effects early in therapy with levodopa are anorexia, nausea, and vomiting occurring in about 80% of patients. These responses are caused primarily by stimulation of the medullary emetic center. Antiemetic drugs are not indicated, because they may interfere with the action of dopamine at basal ganglia (Stern, 1975). Gastrointestinal side effects tend to disappear with continuing therapy as tolerance develops.

Abnormal Involuntary Movements

Abnormal involuntary movements are the most common side effect of levodopa therapy, appearing in about 50% of patients within 1 to 4 months after initiation of treatment. This incidence increases to about 80% of patients on therapeutic doses of levodopa for longer than 1 year (Shaw *et al,* 1980). These involuntary movements may include faciolingual tics, grimacing, and rocking movements of the arms, legs, or trunk. Rarely, exaggerated respiratory movements can produce an irregular gasping pattern of breathing, presumably reflecting dyskinesias of the diaphragm and intercostal muscles. Tolerance does not develop to this side effect. Abnormal voluntary movements are reduced or abolished by a decrease in the dose of levodopa or administration of pyridoxine, both of which also reduce the efficacy of levodopa. The goal is to titrate the dose of levodopa to maximize the therapeutic benefit while minimizing this side effect.

Behaviorial Disturbances

Serious behavioral disturbances characterized by confusion and even delirium occur in about 15% of patients treated with levodopa (Malitz, 1972). Excessive sexual behavior may reflect actions of levodopa on the hypothalamus. Elderly patients receiving combinations of levodopa and anticholinergic drugs are particularly vulnerable to the development of psychiatric disturbances.

Cardiovascular Changes

Cardiovascular changes associated with levodopa most likely reflect alpha- and beta-adrenergic responses evoked by increased plasma concentrations of dopamine. Furthermore, large doses of levodopa cause hypokalemia associated with increased plasma concentrations of aldosterone.

CARDIAC DYSRHYTHMIAS. Cardiac dysrhythmias, including sinus tachycardia, atrial and ventricular premature contractions, atrial fibrillation, and ventricular tachycardia, although rare, have been associated with levodopa therapy. Presumably, the potential beta-adrenergic effects of dopamine on the heart contribute to cardiac dysrhythmias, although a cause-and-effect relationship has not been documented. Patients with preexisting disturbances of cardiac conduction or coronary artery disease are most likely to develop cardiac dysrhythmias in association with levodopa therapy. Propranolol is an effective treatment when cardiac dysrhythmias occur in these patients.

ORTHOSTATIC HYPOTENSION. For unknown reasons, about 30% of patients develop orthostatic hypotension early in therapy. As a result, some patients experience vertigo and rarely syncope. Orthostatic hypotension becomes less prominent with continued therapy. It is of interest that dopamine resulting from levodopa may displace norepinephrine from peripheral sympathetic nerve endings and interfere with adrenergic transmission (Liu et al, 1971). Transient flushing of the skin is common during levodopa therapy.

Endocrine Effects

Dopamine inhibits the secretion of prolactin, presumably by stimulating the release of a prolactin inhibitory factor. The release of growth hormone that occurs in response to the administration of levodopa to normal patients is minimal or absent when levodopa is administered to patients with Parkinson's disease (Eddy et al, 1971). Indeed, signs of acromegaly or diabetes mellitus do not occur in patients treated chronically with levodopa.

Laboratory Measurements

Urinary metabolites of levodopa cause false-positive tests for ketoacidosis. These metabolites also color the urine red and then black on exposure to air.

Reduced Anesthetic Requirements

Intravenous administration of levodopa to animals reduces halothane anesthetic requirements (Johnston et al, 1975). It is speculated that dopamine derived from levodopa in the central nervous system acts as an inhibitory neurotransmitter. Conversely, chronic treatment of animals with levodopa does not consistently alter anesthetic requirements.

Drug Interactions

Drug interactions may occur in patients being treated with levodopa, resulting in enhanced or reduced therapeutic effects.

Antipsychotic Drugs

Antipsychotic drugs such as butyrophenones and phenothiazines can antagonize the effects of dopamine. For this reason, these drugs should not be administered to patients with known or suspected Parkinson's disease. Indeed, administration of droperidol to patients being treated with levodopa has produced severe skeletal muscle rigidity and even pulmonary edema, presumably reflecting sudden antagonism of dopamine (Ngai, 1972). Droperidol has even produced a Parkinson-like syndrome in otherwise healthy patients (Rivera et al, 1975).

Monoamine Oxidase Inhibitors

Nonspecific monoamine oxidase inhibitors interfere with the inactivation of catecholamines, including dopamine. As a result, these drugs can exaggerate the peripheral and central nervous system effects of levodopa. Hypertension and hyperpyrexia are side effects associated with the concurrent administration of these drugs.

Anticholinergic Drugs

Anticholinergic drugs act synergistically with levodopa to improve certain symptoms of Parkinson's disease, especially tremor. Large doses, however, of anticholinergics can slow gastric emptying time such that absorption of levodopa from the gastrointestinal tract is reduced (Stern, 1975).

Methyldopa

Methyldopa is a weak dopa decarboxylase inhibitor manifesting as potentiation of the central nervous system actions of levodopa, including antiparkinson, emetic, and hypotensive effects.

Pyridoxine

Pyridoxine, in doses as low as 5 mg as present in multivitamin preparations, can abolish the therapeutic efficacy of levodopa by enhancing the activity of pyridoxine-dependent dopa decarboxylase and thus increasing the peripheral metabolism of levodopa (Yahr, 1975). As a result, even less dopamine is available to enter the central nervous system.

CARBIDOPA

Carbidopa is an effective inhibitor of the peripheral enzyme activity of dopa decarboxylase (Fig. 31-2) (Hoehn, 1980). Enzyme activity is not altered in the brain, because carbidopa does not cross the blood–brain barrier.

Concurrent administration of carbidopa with levodopa results in increased peripheral availability of levodopa to enter the central nervous system. This increased availability reflects reduced metabolism owing to carbidopa-induced inhibition of dopa decarboxylase activity. Indeed, plasma concentrations of levodopa are higher and the elimination half-time is prolonged following concurrent administration of carbidopa and levodopa compared to levodopa alone (Bianchine and Shaw, 1976). As a result of this combination therapy, the dose of levodopa can be reduced up to 75% while maintaining beneficial central nervous system effects and, at the same time, reducing the likelihood of dose-dependent side effects resulting from too high plasma concentrations of dopa-

mine. For example, nausea, vomiting, and cardiac dysrhythmias are diminished or absent compared with the incidence of these side effects in patients treated only with levodopa. Antagonism of the therapeutic effect of levodopa by pyridoxine therapy does not occur during combination therapy. The incidence of abnormal involuntary movements and behavioral disturbances, however, is not influenced by carbidopa. Administered alone, carbidopa lacks pharmacologic activity.

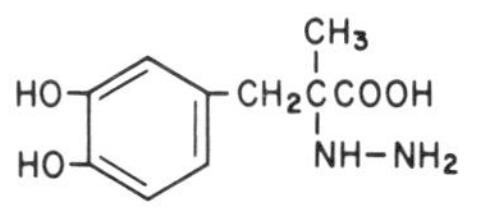

AMANTADINE

Amantadine is an antiviral drug used for prophylaxis against infection with influenza A_2. This drug also produces symptomatic improvement in patients with Parkinson's disease, presumably by facilitating the release of dopamine from intact dopaminergic terminals that remain in the nigrostriatum of patients with this disease (Schwab *et al,* 1971). In addition, amantadine delays uptake of dopamine back into nerve endings.

Amantadine is well absorbed after oral administration, and the plasma elimination half-time is about 12 hours. More than 90% of the drug is excreted unchanged by the kidneys, necessitating dosage adjustments in patients with renal dysfunction.

Side Effects

Side effects of amantadine therapy, such as nausea and vomiting, are mild and infrequent. Large doses of amantadine, particularly in combination with anticholinergic drugs, result in acute psychotic reactions (*e.g.,* hallucinations, confusion) in about 5% of patients. Long-term use of amantadine may be associated with erythromelalgia (red, tender, and edematous lower extremities) with or without cardiac failure (Pearce *et al,* 1974).

BROMOCRIPTINE

Bromocriptine is a dopaminergic agonist effective in the treatment of galactorrhea, hyperprolactinemia, and acromegaly (Fig. 31-3). The effectiveness of bromocriptine in the treatment of acromegaly reflects the paradoxical inhibitory effect of dopamine agonists on secretion of growth hor-

FIGURE 31-2. Carbidopa.

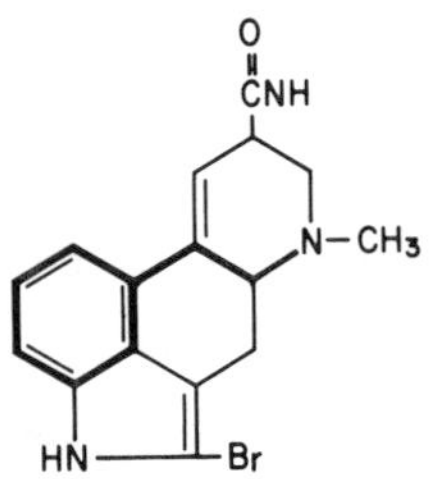

FIGURE 31-3. Bromocriptine. The darkened portion corresponds to the structure of dopamine.

mone (Goldfine, 1978). Bromocriptine also suppresses excess prolactin secretion that is often associated with growth hormone secretion. Large doses of bromocriptine are necessary to control the symptoms of Parkinson's disease. As a result, bromocriptine, in small doses, may be used to supplement treatment regimens that depend primarily on levodopa (Hoehn, 1981).

Absorption of bromocriptine from the gastrointestinal tract is rapid but incomplete. Extensive first-pass metabolism occurs in the liver, and more than 70% of the metabolites are excreted in the bile. Less than 10% of the drug is excreted unchanged or as metabolites in the urine.

Side Effects

Visual and auditory hallucinations, hypotension, dyskinesia, and erythromelalgia (red, tender, and edematous lower extremities) occur more frequently with bromocriptine than with levodopa therapy (Hoehn, 1981). Asymptomatic elevations of serum transaminase and alkaline phosphatase concentrations have been reported. Vertigo and nausea are occasionally associated with bromocriptine therapy.

DEPRENYL

Deprenyl is a highly selective inhibitor of monoamine oxidase-B enzyme (Fig. 31-4) (Lees *et al,* 1977) (see Chapter 19). In contrast to nonspecific monoamine oxidase inhibitors, deprenyl does not result in life-threatening potentiation of the effects of catecholamines when administered concurrently with a centrally active amine (Knoll, 1978). Deprenyl is effective in the treatment of Parkinson's disease because it inhibits the intrace-

rebral metabolism of dopamine, thus maximizing the therapeutic efficacy of concomitantly administered levodopa. The most common side effect of combined therapy, including deprenyl, is an increased incidence of dyskinesia. Mental depression and paranoid ideation are also common side effects.

ANTICHOLINERGIC DRUGS

Centrally active anticholinergic drugs, such as benztropine, cycrimine, and trihexyphenidyl, are useful in patients with minimal symptoms due to Parkinson's disease and in those who do not tolerate or respond to levodopa. More than 50% of patients who respond to levodopa manifest additional beneficial effects when therapy is supplemented with anticholinergic drugs. Anticholinergic drugs are also useful in the treatment of Parkinsonism-like symptoms induced by antipsychotic drugs that presumably act by blocking dopaminergic receptors (see Chapter 19). In this regard, levodopa would not be effective in reversing drug-induced Parkinsonism symptoms, because the increase in brain dopamine concentrations produced by levodopa is insufficient to overcome receptor blockade. The presumed mechanism of action of anticholinergic drugs is the ability of these drugs to blunt the effects of the excitatory neurotransmitter acetylcholine.

Certain antihistamines that are structurally related to diphenhydramine possess modest central anticholinergic properties. These drugs are less effective than anticholinergic drugs in the treatment of Parkinson's disease but are well-tolerated, especially by elderly patients. Sedative effects of these drugs may be useful in countering the insomnia produced by levodopa and potent anticholinergic drugs.

Trihexyphenidyl

Trihexyphenidyl is the prototype of anticholinergic drugs that are particularly useful in reducing the tremor and excess salivation associated with

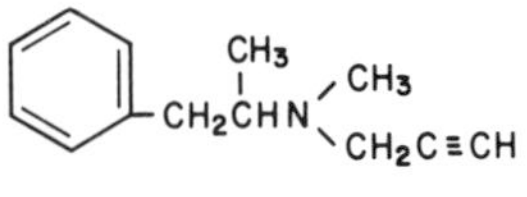

FIGURE 31-4. Deprenyl.

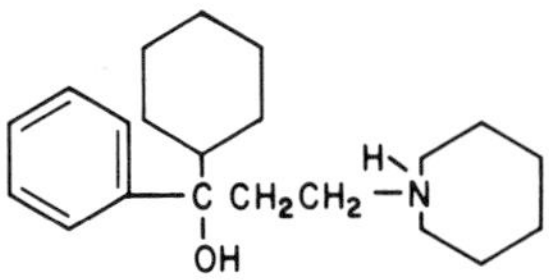

FIGURE 31-5. Trihexyphenidyl.

Parkinson's disease (Fig. 31-5). Rigidity and bradykinesia are less effectively blunted. Although the peripheral and central nervous system actions of this synthetic drug are less prominent than those of atropine, side effects such as mydriasis, cycloplegia, dry mouth, tachycardia, adynamic ileus and urinary retention, sedation, hallucinations, confusion, and delirium may still occur. Because of the mydriatic effect, trihexyphenidyl could precipitate acute glaucoma in a susceptible patient.

REFERENCES

Bianchine JR, Shaw GM. Clinical pharmacokinetics of levodopa in Parkinson's disease. Clin Pharmacokinet 1976;1:313–58.

Boller F, Mizatani T, Roessmann U, Gambetti P. Parkinson disease, dementia and Alzheimer's disease: Clinicopathological correlations. Ann Neurol 1980;7:329–35.

Calne DB. Developments in pharmacology and therapeutics of parkinsonism. Ann Neurol 1977;1:111–9.

Eddy RL, Jones AL, Chakmakjian ZH, Silverthorne MC. Effect of levodopa (L-dopa) on human hypophyseal trophic hormone release. J Clin Endocrinol Metab 1971;33:709–12.

Goldfine ID. Medical treatment of acromegaly. Annu Rev Med 1978;29:407–15.

Hoehn MM. Increased dosage of carbidopa in patients with Parkinson's disease receiving low doses of levodopa: Pilot study. Arch Neurol 1980;37:146–9.

Hoehn MM. Bromocriptine and its use in parkinsonism. J Am Geriatr Soc 1981;24:251–8.

Johnston RR, White PF, Way WL, Miller RD. The effect of levodopa on halothane anesthetic requirement. Anesth Analg 1975;54:178–81.

Knoll J. The possible mechanisms of action of deprenyl in Parkinson's disease. J Neural Trans 1978;43:177–98.

Lees AJ, Shaw KM, Kohout L, et al. Deprenyl in Parkinson's disease. Lancet 1977;2:791–5.

Lieberman AN. Dementia in Parkinson disease. Ann Neurol 1979;6:355–9.

Liu PL, Krenis LJ, Ngai SH. The effect of levodopa on the norepinephrine stores in rat heart. Anesthesiology 1971;34:4–8.

Malitz S (ed). L-Dopa and Behavior. New York, Raven Press, 1972.

Ngai SH. Parkinsonism, levodopa, and anesthesia. Anesthesiology 1972;37:344–51.

Pearce LA, Waterbury LD, Green HD. Amantadine hydrochloride: alteration in peripheral circulation. Neurology 1974;24:46–8.

Rivera VM, Keichian AH, Oliver RE. Persistent parkinsonism following neuroleptanalgesia. Anesthesiology 1975;43:635–7.

Schwab RS, Poskanzer DC, England AC, Young RR. Amantadine in Parkinson's disease. Review of more than two years' experience. JAMA 1971;222:792–5.

Shaw KM, Lees AJ, Stern GM. Impact of treatment with levodopa on Parkinson's disease. Q J Med 1980;49:283–93.

Stern G (ed). The Clinical Uses of Levodopa. University Park Press, Baltimore, 1975.

Yahr MD. Levodopa. Ann Intern Med 1975;83:677–82.

Drugs Used to Treat Hyperlipoproteinemia

INTRODUCTION

Lipoproteins are grouped as (1) chylomicrons, (2) very low-density lipoproteins (VLDL), (3) intermediate-density lipoproteins (IDL), (4) low-density lipoproteins (LDL), and (5) high-density lipoproteins (HDL). Hyperlipoproteinemia is classified according to the type of lipoprotein that is increased (Table 32-1) (Fredrickson *et al,* 1967). Hypercholesterolemia can occur from elevation in the plasma concentration of any of these lipoproteins. Hypertriglyceridemia can result from increased concentrations of chylomicrons, VLDL, or IDL, either alone or in various combinations.

There is an undeniable association between the concentration of lipids and the development of coronary atherosclerosis (Stamler, 1978; Levy 1981). For example, the risk of coronary artery disease is directly related to the plasma concentration of cholesterol, especially in persons younger than 65 years of age. Concentrations of LDL in plasma correlate closely with concentrations of cholesterol, since about 75% of total plasma cholesterol is transported in association with this lipoprotein. Therefore, elevated plasma concentrations of cholesterol or LDL carry a similar predictive power for assessment of risk for developing coronary atherosclerosis. Conversely, only about 25% of total plasma cholesterol is transported with HDL, which is consistent with the negative correlation between the plasma concentration of HDL and the risk of developing coronary

atherosclerosis or experiencing cerebral vascular accidents (Glueck *et al,* 1982). Likewise, a correlation between elevated plasma triglyceride concentrations and development of coronary atherosclerosis has not been documented.

Plasma concentrations of HDL are positively correlated with exercise and moderate ingestion of alcohol and inversely correlated with obesity, smoking, hypertension, poor control of diabetes mellitus, and the use of oral contraceptives that contain progestins (Levy, 1981). Both males and females have approximately the same levels of HDL until puberty; after that, plasma concentrations in males are about 20% lower than those in females. Familial excess of HDL or deficiency of LDL is associated with a reduced risk of developing coronary atherosclerosis. These observations emphasize the importance of identifying factors or drugs that increase the plasma concentrations of HDL.

DRUGS THAT AFFECT PLASMA CONCENTRATIONS OF LIPOPROTEINS

Drugs used to reduce the plasma concentrations of lipoproteins can be categorized as (1) those that alter the production of lipoproteins (nicotinic acid), (2) those that alter the intravascular metabolism of lipoproteins (clofibrate), and (3) those that alter clearance of lipoproteins from the circulation (cholestyramine). Dietary manipulation and weight reduction should always be attempted

Table 32-1
Classification of Hyperlipoproteinemia

Plasma Concentration of Lipoprotein That is Increased	Type
Chylomicrons	I
Low-density lipoproteins	IIa
Low-density lipoproteins and very low-density lipoproteins	IIb
Intermediate-density lipoproteins	III
Very low-density lipoproteins	IV
Chylomicrons and very low-density lipoproteins	V

before a drug is used for its effects on plasma concentrations of lipoproteins. Dietary regulation must continue during drug therapy, because the effects of diet and drugs are additive.

NICOTINIC ACID

Nicotinic acid is a water-soluble vitamin that may reduce the plasma concentration of cholesterol 20% to 80% (Altschul *et al,* 1955) (see Chapter 34). This reduction in plasma cholesterol reflects the ability of nicotinic acid to inhibit the production of VLDL, which is the immediate precursor of LDL. In addition to this effect, nicotinic acid also acts by inhibition of lipolysis in adipose tissue, decreased esterification of triglycerides, and increased activity of lipoprotein lipase.

Nicotinic acid is efficiently absorbed following oral administration. It is concentrated in the liver, where extensive metabolism takes place.

Side Effects

Hepatic dysfunction manifesting as increased plasma transaminase activity and cholestatic jaundice may be associated with large doses of nicotinic acid. Hyperglycemia and abnormal glucose tolerance occur in nondiabetic patients receiving nicotinic acid. Plasma concentrations of uric acid are elevated, and the incidence of gouty arthritis is increased. For these reasons, nicotinic acid should be used with caution, if at all, in patients with liver disease, diabetes mellitus, or gout. Finally, nicotinic acid may also exaggerate vasodilation and orthostatic hypotension caused by gan-

glionic blocking and antihypertensive drugs. Intense cutaneous flushing and pruritus occur initially in almost all treated patients and persist in 10% to 15% of patients. This effect can be ameliorated by concomitant administration of aspirin. Peptic ulcer disease may be reactivated by nicotinic acid therapy of hyperlipoproteinemia.

CLOFIBRATE

Clofibrate characteristically reduces the plasma concentration of triglyceride by enhancing the intravascular breakdown of VLDL and IDL as well as accelerating the rate of removal of these lipoproteins from the circulation (Fig. 32-1) (Berman *et al,* 1978). In addition, the plasma concentration of cholesterol and LDL often decline, although the decrease in cholesterol concentration may be minimal. Clofibrate has no effect on chylomicronemia nor does it alter plasma concentrations of HDL.

Pharmacokinetics

Clofibrate is completely absorbed from the gastrointestinal tract following oral administration. Following absorption, clofibrate rapidly undergoes hydrolysis, with peak plasma concentrations appearing as the active metabolite chlorophenoxyisobutyric acid within 4 hours. Urinary excretion accounts for excretion of about 60% of the drug as a glucuronide conjugate. The elimination halftime of clofibrate is about 15 hours.

Side Effects

Clofibrate therapy may be associated with a flulike syndrome, including skeletal muscle myalgia and weakness. Often, this syndrome is accompanied by elevations in the plasma concentrations of creatine phosphokinase and glutamic oxalacetic transaminase (Langer and Levy, 1968). The litho-

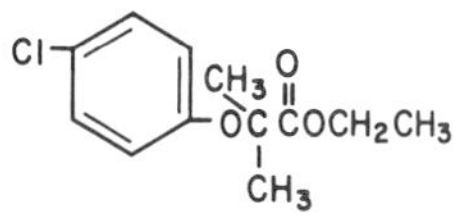

FIGURE 32-1. Clofibrate.

genicity of bile is enhanced, and there is an increased incidence of cholelithiasis and cholecystitis (Hall *et al,* 1981). Patients with coronary artery disease may be at increased risk for drug-induced cardiac dysrhythmias and exaggerated angina pectoris (LaRosa *et al,* 1969). Clofibrate enhances the pharmacologic effect of other acidic drugs such as phenytoin, tolbutamide, and oral anticoagulants, presumably by displacing these drugs from binding sites on albumin (Bjornsson *et al,* 1977). Other less serious side effects of clofibrate include nausea, diarrhea, skin rashes, alopecia, and decreased libido.

GEMFIBROZIL

Gemfibrozil is a homologue of clofibrate that reduces synthesis of VLDL by reducing incorporation of long-chain fatty acids into newly formed triglycerides (Fig. 32-2) (Hall *et al,* 1981). Effects on the plasma concentrations of triglycerides, cholesterol, and LDL are similar to those produced by clofibrate. Conversely, gemfibrozil elevates HDL.

The elimination half-time of gemfibrozil is about 1.5 hours, with about 70% of a single dose appearing unchanged in the urine. Side effects associated with gemfibrozil are similar to those observed during treatment with clofibrate.

CHOLESTYRAMINE

Cholestyramine is the chloride salt of an ion exchange resin originally used to control pruritus in patients with elevated plasma concentrations of bile acids resulting from cholestasis (Fig. 32-3) (Levy *et al,* 1973). In addition, cholestyramine, by binding bile acids in the small intestine, reduces the circulating level of bile acids, which, in turn, increases the rate of conversion of cholesterol to bile acids in the liver (Mosbach, 1969). The result is a decrease in the circulating plasma concentration of cholesterol. Cholestyramine also increases

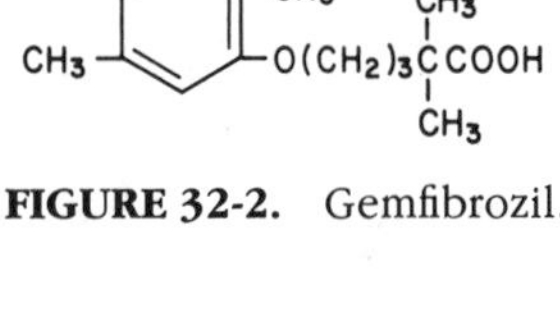

FIGURE 32-2. Gemfibrozil.

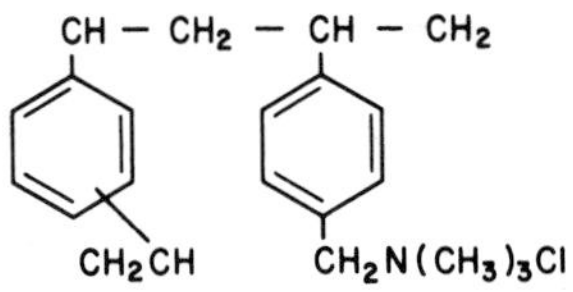

FIGURE 32-3. Cholestyramine.

the rate of LDL clearance by increasing LDL receptor activity.

Side Effects

Nausea, abdominal pain, and constipation are frequent side effects of cholestyramine therapy. A high fluid intake is useful in minimizing constipation. There may be transient increases in the plasma concentrations of alkaline phosphatase and transaminases. Since cholestyramine is a chloride form of an ion exchange resin, hyperchloremic acidosis can occur, especially in younger and smaller patients in whom the relative dose is larger. Absorption of fat-soluble vitamins may be impaired, and hypoprothrombinemia has been observed. Cholestyramine may bind other drugs in the gastrointestinal tract and impair their absorption. For this reason, other drugs should be given at least 1 hour before or 4 hours after administration of cholestyramine. Cholestyramine has a gritty quality that may reduce patient compliance.

COLESTIPOL

Colestipol is a bile-sequestering drug with pharmacologic effects similar to those of cholestyramine.

PROBUCOL

Probucol lowers plasma concentrations of cholesterol by decreasing LDL levels (Fig. 32-4) (Murphy, 1977). Therefore, like cholestyramine, this drug is useful in the management of patients with elevated LDL levels. HDL levels are also reduced. Despite its lipid solubility, less than 10% of an oral dose of probucol is absorbed from the gastrointestinal tract. Elimination is by way of the bile, with renal excretion being minimal. Nausea and diarrhea are occasional side effects. Transient

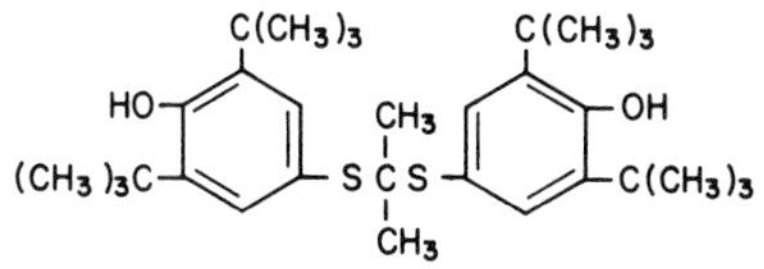

FIGURE 32-4. Probucol.

elevations of serum transaminases, alkaline phosphatase, uric acid, blood urea nitrogen, and blood glucose have been observed.

DEXTROTHYROXINE

Dextrothyroxine reduces plasma concentrations of LDL by up to 50% by increasing LDL receptor activity in euthyroid and hypothyroid patients (Boyd and Oliver, 1960). Mortality, however, is increased in patients with coronary atherosclerosis who are treated with this drug. Adverse side effects reflect metabolic stimulation.

REFERENCES

Altschul R, Hoffer A, Stephen JD. Influence of nicotinic acid on serum cholesterol in man. Arch Biochem Biophys 1955;54:558 – 9.

Berman M, Hall M, Levy RI, et al. Metabolism of apo B and apo C lipoproteins in man: Kinetic studies in normal and hyperlipoproteinemic subjects. J Lipid Res 1978;19:38 – 56.

Bjornsson TD, Mellin PJ, Blaschke TF. Interaction of clofibrate with warfarin I. Effect of clofibrate on the disposition of the optical enantiomorphs of warfarin. J Pharmacokinet Biopharm 1977;5:495 – 505.

Boyd GS, Oliver MF. Thyroid hormones and plasma lipids. Br Med Bull 1960;16:138 – 42.

Fredrickson DS, Levy RI, Lees RS. Fat transport in lipoproteins — an integrated approach to mechanisms and disorders. N Engl J Med 1967;276:32 – 44.

Glueck CJ, Daniels SR, Bates S, Benton C, Tracy T, Third JLHC. Pediatric victims of unexplained stroke and their families. Familial lipid and lipoprotein abnormalities. Pediatrics 1982;69:308 – 16.

Hall MJ, Nelson LM, Russell RI, Howard AN. Gemfibrozil: Effect on biliary cholesterol saturation of new lipid-lowering agent and comparison with clofibrate. Atherosclerosis 1981;39:511 – 6.

Langer T, Levy RI. Acute muscular syndrome associated with administration of clofibrate. N Engl J Med 1968;279:856 – 8.

LaRosa JC, Brown WV, Frommer PL, Levy RI. Clofibrate-induced ventricular arrhythmia. Am J Cardiol 1969;23:266 – 9.

Levy RI, Fredrickson DS, Stone NJ, et al. Cholestyramine in type II hyperlipoproteinemia. Ann Intern Med 1973;79:51 – 8.

Levy RI. Cholesterol, lipoproteins, apoproteins, and heart disease: Present status and future prospects. Clin Chem 1981;27:653 – 62.

Mosbach EH. Effect of drugs on bile acid metabolism. Adv Exp Med Biol 1969;4:421 – 41.

Murphy BF. Probucol (Lorelco) in treatment of hyperlipemia. JAMA 1977;238:2537 – 8.

Stamler J. Lifestyles, major risk factors, proof and public policy. Circulation 1978;58:3 – 19.

CHAPTER 33

Central Nervous System Stimulants and Muscle Relaxants

CENTRAL NERVOUS SYSTEM STIMULANTS

Drugs that produce stimulation of the central nervous system as their primary action are classified as analeptics or convulsants (Wang and Ward, 1977). Analeptics were previously used in the treatment of generalized central nervous system depression as accompanies deliberate drug overdoses. This practice, however, has been abandoned, because these drugs lack specific antagonist properties and their margin of safety is narrow (Mark, 1967).

The excitability of the central nervous system reflects a balance between excitatory and inhibitory influences that is normally maintained within relatively narrow limits. Analeptics can increase excitability either by blocking inhibition or by enhancing excitation. Strychnine and picrotoxin selectively block inhibition in the central nervous system. As such, these drugs lack clinical value, but rather, are useful as research tools to study inhibitory neurotransmitters and receptors.

Doxapram

Doxapram is a centrally acting analeptic that selectively increases minute ventilation by activating the carotid bodies (Fig. 33-1) (Mitchell and Herbert, 1975). Lack of a direct stimulant effect on the medullary respiratory center is emphasized by the lack of effect of doxapram on ventilation when carotid body activity is absent. The stimulus to

ventilation produced by 1 mg kg^{-1} of doxapram administered intravenously is similar to that produced by an arterial PO_2 of 38 mmHg acting on the carotid bodies (Hirsh and Wang, 1974). An increase in tidal volume more so than an increase in respiratory rate is responsible for the doxapram-induced increase in minute ventilation. Oxygen consumption is increased concomitantly with the increase in minute ventilation.

Doxapram has a large margin of safety as reflected by a 20- to 40-fold difference in the dose that stimulates ventilation (*i.e.*, 1 mg kg^{-1}) and that which produces seizures (Sebel *et al*, 1980). Nevertheless, continuous intravenous infusion of doxapram, as required to produce a sustained effect on ventilation, often results in evidence of subconclusive central nervous system stimulation (*e.g.*, hypertension, tachycardia, cardiac dysrhythmias, vomiting, and increased body temperature). These changes are consistent with increased sympathetic nervous system outflow from the brain.

Doxapram is extensively metabolized, with less than 5% of an intravenous dose being excreted unchanged in the urine. A single intravenous dose produces an effect on ventilation that lasts only 5 to 10 minutes (Robson and Prescott, 1978).

Clinical Uses

Doxapram administered as a continuous intravenous infusion (2–3 mg min^{-1}) has been used as a temporary measure to maintain ventilation during

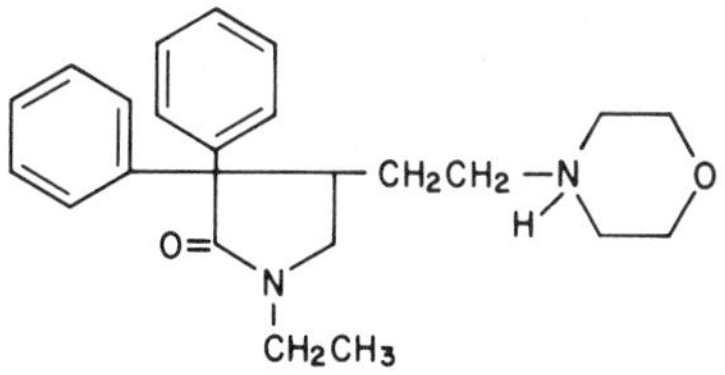

FIGURE 33-1. Doxapram.

administration of supplemental oxygen to patients with chronic obstructive airways disease who are otherwise dependent on an hypoxic drive to maintain an adequate minute ventilation (Fig. 33-2) (Moser *et al,* 1973). Administered concomitantly with intramuscular meperidine, doxapram prevents the respiratory depression produced by the opioid without altering analgesia, suggesting a possible benefit in the early postoperative period (Ramamurthy *et al,* 1975). Because controlled ventilation of the lungs and standard supportive therapy are effective in the management of ventilatory failure, doxapram should not be used in patients with drug-induced coma or exacerbation of chronic lung disease. More specific tests (peripheral nerve stimulator, airway pressures, head-lift) renders the diagnostic use of doxapram in postanesthetic apnea or hypoventilation of minimal clinical value. Arousal from residual effects of inhaled anesthetics follows administration of doxapram, but the effect is transient, nonselective, and not recommended.

Methylphenidate

Methylphenidate is structurally related to amphetamine (Fig. 33-3). This drug is a mild central nervous system stimulant, with more prominent effects on mental than on motor activities. Large doses, however, produce generalized central nervous system stimulation and seizures. Absorption after oral administration is rapid, and concentrations of methylphenidate in the brain exceed those in the plasma. The abuse potential of methylphenidate is the same as that of amphetamine.

Clinical Uses

Methylphenidate is useful in the treatment of hyperkinetic syndromes in children characterized as having minimal brain dysfunction. There have, however, been reports of bradycardia, hallucina-

tions, and growth suppression in patients treated with methylphenidate (Knights and Hinton, 1969; Safer *et al,* 1972). Methylphenidate may also be effective in the treatment of narcolepsy, either alone or in combination with a tricyclic antidepressant.

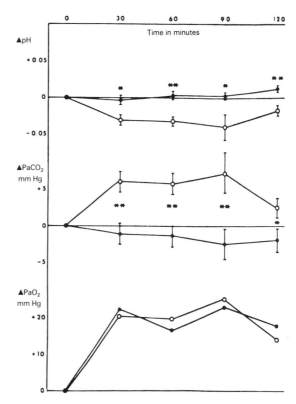

FIGURE 33-2. Doxapram, as a continuous intravenous infusion, may be used to maintain alveolar ventilation *(solid circles)* during administration of supplemental oxygen to patients with chronic obstructive airways disease. (From Moser KM, Luchsinger PC, Adamson JS, *et al.* Respiratory stimulation with intravenous doxapram in respiratory failure. N Engl J Med 1973;288:428–31. Reprinted by permission of the New England Journal of Medicine 1973;288:428–31).

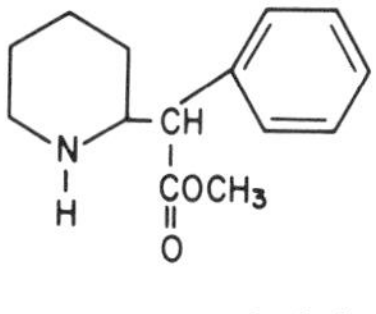

FIGURE 33-3. Methylphenidate.

Methylxanthines

Methylxanthines, theophylline and caffeine, are effective analeptics in the treatment of primary apnea of prematurity (Aranda *et al*, 1981). Unlike adults, premature infants metabolize theophylline in part to caffeine. Furthermore, the clearance of methylxanthines is greatly prolonged in the neonate compared with that in the adult.

The therapeutic plasma concentration for theophylline or caffeine in the neonate is 5 to 12 μg ml^{-1}. Seizures may occur when the plasma concentration exceeds 20 μg ml^{-1}. The plasma concentration is the best monitor of the adequacy of the oral dose. Likewise, a heart rate greater than 180 beats min^{-1} in the treated neonate is an indication to decrease the oral dose of methylxanthines.

Nicotine

Nicotine has no therapeutic action, but its toxicity and presence in tobacco lend to its medical importance. It is a natural liquid alkaloid that turns brown and acquires the odor of tobacco on exposure to air. Nicotine is readily absorbed from the respiratory tract and buccal mucous membranes and through the skin. As an alkaloid, absorption of nicotine from the acidic environment of the stomach is minimal. About 90% of nicotine is metabolized in the liver, kidneys, and lungs, with a significant portion of this metabolism occurring in the lungs (Turner *et al*, 1975). The elimination half-time of nicotine is 30 to 60 minutes.

Effects on Organ Systems

The complex and often unpredictable pharmacologic effects of nicotine may reflect the stimulant and depressant actions of nicotine. The primary action of nicotine is an initial stimulation quickly followed by persistent depression of autonomic ganglia. Nicotine markedly stimulates the central nervous system, manifesting initially as tremor. Stimulation of ventilation by small doses reflects nicotine-induced excitation of aortic and carotid body chemoreceptors. Nicotine characteristically increases heart rate and blood pressure and evokes vasoconstriction. These responses most likely reflect stimulation of sympathetic ganglia and the adrenal medulla.

In contrast to the cardiovascular system, the effects of nicotine on the gastrointestinal tract are largely due to parasympathetic nervous system stimulation leading to vomiting and diarrhea. Nicotine causes an initial stimulation of salivary and bronchial secretions that is followed by inhibition. Salivation caused by smoking is reflexively produced by irritant smoke rather than by a systemic effect of nicotine.

Overdose

Overdose from nicotine may occur from ingestion of insecticide sprays containing nicotine or from ingestion of tobacco products. The acutely fatal dose of nicotine in adults is about 60 mg. Individual cigarettes deliver up to 2.5 mg of nicotine. Gastric absorption of nicotine is minimized by vomiting caused by the central emetic effect of the initially absorbed material.

The onset of symptoms of nicotine overdose is rapid and characterized by nausea, salivation, abdominal cramps, vertigo, mental confusion, and prominent skeletal muscle weakness. Hypotension and difficulty in breathing ensue, the heart rate is rapid, and terminal seizures may occur. Paralysis of the intercostal muscles may cause apnea. Treatment is supportive, including attempts to remove any residual nicotine from the stomach.

CENTRALLY ACTING MUSCLE RELAXANTS

Centrally acting muscle relaxants act in the central nervous system or directly on skeletal muscle to relieve spasticity. Spasticity of skeletal muscle occurs when there is an abnormal increase in resistance to passive movement of a muscle group as a result of hyperactive proprioceptive or stretch reflexes. Spasticity occurs in a wide variety of neurologic conditions and is highly variable in its etiology and presentation.

Mephenesin

The relative efficacy of centrally acting muscle relaxants that are related to mephenesin has not been determined (Fig. 33-4). As a result, selection of one of these drugs over another remains highly empirical and subjective. These drugs produce skeletal muscle relaxation by an unknown mechanism in the central nervous system (Davidoff, 1978). A prominent effect of centrally acting muscle relaxants is depression of spinal polysynaptic

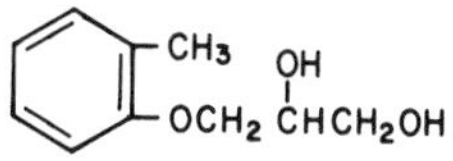

FIGURE 33-4. Mephenesin.

reflexes. Nevertheless, the importance of this effect in the mechanism of skeletal muscle relaxation is not documented. Sedation is not a prominent side effect of these drugs.

Benzodiazepines

Benzodiazepines are widely used as centrally acting skeletal muscle relaxants. These drugs appear to have a more selective action on reticular neuronal mechanisms that control skeletal muscle tone than on spinal interneuronal activity (Tseng and Wang, 1971). Sedation may limit the efficacy of diazepam as a muscle relaxant.

Baclofen

Baclofen is a gamma-aminobutyric acid (GABA) analogue that is often administered for treatment of spasticity resulting from disease or injury of the spinal cord (Fig. 33-5) (Potashner, 1978). It is particularly effective in the treatment of flexor spasms and skeletal muscle rigidity associated with multiple sclerosis. Analgesia produced by baclofen may reflect activation of receptors in the central nervous system that coexist with an independent opioid-sensitive system.

Baclofen is rapidly and almost completely absorbed from the gastrointestinal tract. Elimination half-time is 3 to 6 hours, with about 80% of the drug excreted unchanged in the urine, emphasizing the need to modify the dose in patients with renal dysfunction. Therapeutic plasma concentrations are 80 to 400 ng ml^{-1} (Young and Delwaide, 1981).

Use of baclofen is limited by its side effects, which include sedation, skeletal muscle weakness, and confusion. Sudden discontinuation of chronic baclofen therapy may result in tachycardia and both auditory and visual hallucinations. Coma, depression of ventilation, and seizures may accompany an overdose of baclofen. The threshold for initiation of seizures may be lowered in patients with epilepsy. Mild hypotension may

occur in awake patients, while bradycardia and hypotension have been observed when general anesthesia is induced in patients being treated with baclofen (Sill *et al*, 1986). A decrease in sympathetic outflow from the central nervous system mediated by a GABA, baclofen-sensitive system might contribute to this hemodynamic response.

Cyclobenzaprine

Cyclobenzaprine is related structurally and pharmacologically to tricyclic antidepressants (Fig. 33-6). Anticholinergic effects are similar to those of tricyclic antidepressants and can include dry mouth, tachycardia, blurred vision, and sedation (Ashby *et al*, 1972). The mechanism of skeletal muscle relaxant effects produced by cyclobenzaprine is unknown.

Cyclobenzaprine must not be administered in the presence of monoamine oxidase inhibitors. In view of the potential adverse side effects of tricyclic antidepressants on the heart, the use of cyclobenzaprine should be avoided in patients with cardiac dysrhythmias or altered conduction of the cardiac impulse.

Dantrolene

Dantrolene produces skeletal muscle relaxation by a direct action on excitation–contraction coupling, presumably by decreasing the amount of calcium released from the sarcoplasmic reticulum (Fig. 33-7). Neuromuscular transmission and electrical properties of the skeletal muscle mem-

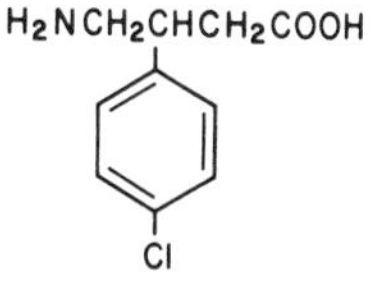

FIGURE 33-5. Baclofen.

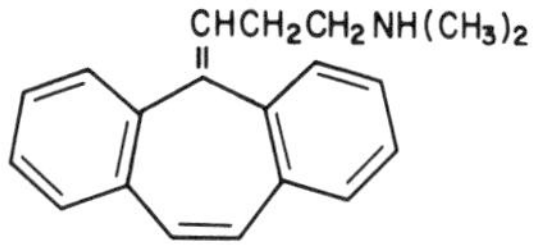

FIGURE 33-6. Cyclobenzaprine.

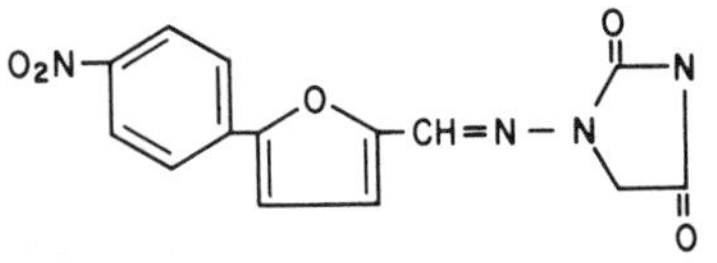

FIGURE 33-7. Dantrolene.

branes are not altered (Davidoff, 1978). Unlike centrally acting skeletal muscle relaxants, dantrolene does not impair polysynaptic reflexes.

Pharmacokinetics

Absorption of dantrolene from the gastrointestinal tract is slow but sufficient to provide consistent dose-related concentrations of drug in the plasma. Metabolism in the liver is slow, with urinary excretion of metabolites and unchanged drug occurring. The elimination half-time is about 9 hours.

Clinical Uses

Dantrolene is useful in the management of patients with skeletal muscle spasticity owing to upper motor neuron lesions. The maximum oral dose is 400 mg administered in four divided doses. Associated dantrolene-induced skeletal muscle weakness, however, often negates any significant improvement, despite reductions in skeletal muscle spasticity.

Dantrolene is effective in the prevention and treatment of malignant hyperthermia (Friesen *et al,* 1979; Pandit *et al,* 1979). Prophylaxis in malignant hyperthermia-susceptible patients is with oral dantrolene, 4 to 8 mg kg^{-1} given in divided doses for 1 to 3 days, with the last dose being administered 1 to 5 hours before the induction of anesthesia. The intravenous dose of dantrolene for treatment of malignant hyperthermia is 1 to 2 mg kg^{-1}, repeated every 5 to 10 minutes to a maximal dose of 10 mg kg^{-1}. Typically, 2 to 5 mg kg^{-1} of dantrolene is required for treatment of an acute episode of malignant hyperthermia.

Side Effects

The most common side effect of dantrolene administration is skeletal muscle weakness. Skeletal muscle weakness may be sufficient to interfere with adequate ventilation or protection of the lungs from aspiration of gastric fluid (Watson *et al.,* 1986). Large doses of dantrolene administered acutely as for prophylaxis against malignant hyperthermia may cause nausea, diarrhea, and blurred vision as well as skeletal muscle weakness.

Dantrolene produces hepatitis in 0.5% of patients treated for more than 60 days (Davidoff, 1978). Fatal hepatitis occurs in 0.1% to 0.2% of patients treated chronically. For this reason, hepatic function should be monitored when dantrolene therapy exceeds 45 days. Pleural effusion may also occur with chronic therapy.

REFERENCES

Aranda JV, Grondin D, Sasyniuk BI. Pharmacologic considerations in therapy of neonatal apnea. Pediatr Clin North Am 1981;28:113–33.

Ashby P, Burke D, Rao S. Assessment of cyclobenzaprine in the treatment of spasticity. J Neurol Neurosurg Psychiatry 1972;35:599–605.

Davidoff RA. Pharmacology of spasticity. Neurology 1978;28:46–51.

Friesen CM, Brodsky JB, Dillingham MF. Successful use of dantrolene sodium in human malignant hyperthermia syndrome. A case report. Can Anaesth Soc J 1979;26:319–21.

Hirsh WH, Wang SC. Selective respiratory stimulating action of doxapram compared to pentylenetetrazol. J Pharmacol Exp Ther 1974;189:1–11.

Knights RM, Hinton GS. The effects of methylphenidate (Ritalin) on the motor skills and behavior of children with learning problems. J Nerv Ment Dis 1969;148:643–53.

Mark LC. Analeptics: changing concepts, declining status. Am J Med Sci 1967;254:196–302.

Mitchell RM, Herbert DA. Potencies of doxapram and hypoxia in stimulating carotid-body chemoreceptors and ventilation in anesthetized cats. Anesthesiology 1975;42:559–66.

Moser KM, Luchsinger PC, Adamson JS, et al. Respiratory stimulation with intravenous doxapram in respiratory failure. N Engl J Med 1973;288:428–31.

Pandit SK, Kothary SP, Cohen PJ. Orally administered dantrolene for prophylaxis of malignant hyperthermia. Anesthesiology 1979;50:156–8.

Potashner SJ. Baclofen: effects of amino acid release. Can J Physiol Pharmacol 1978;56:150–4.

Ramamurthy S, Steen SN, Winnie AP. Doxapram antagonism of meperidine-induced respiratory depression. Anesth Analg 1975;54:352–6.

Robson RH, Prescott LF. Pharmacokinetics study of doxapram in patients and volunteers. Br J Clin Pharmacol 1978;7:81 – 7.

Safer D, Allen R, Barr E. Depression of growth in hyperactive children on stimulant drugs. N Engl J Med 1972;287:217 – 20.

Sebel PS, Kershaw EJ, Rao WS. Effects of doxapram on postoperative pulmonary complications following thoracotomy. Br J Anaesth 1980;52:81 – 4.

Sill JC, Schumacher K. Southorn PA, Reuter J, Yaksh TL. Bradycardia and hypotension associated with baclofen used during general anesthesia. Anesthesiology 1986;64:255 – 8.

Tseng TC, Wang SC. Locus of action of centrally acting muscle relaxants, diazepam and tybamate. J Pharmacol Exp Ther 1971;178:350 – 60.

Turner DM, Armitage AK, Briant RH, Dollery CT. Metabolism of nicotine by the isolated perfused dog lung. Xenobiotica 1975;5:539 – 51.

Want SC, Ward JW. Analeptics. Pharmacol Ther 1977;3: 123 – 65.

Watson CB, Reierson N, Norfleet EA. Clinically significant muscle weakness induced by oral dantrolene sodium prophylaxis for malignant hyperthermia. Anesthesiology 1986;65:312 – 4.

Young RR, Delwaide PJ. Drug therapy-spasticity. N Engl J Med 1981;304:96 – 9.

C H A P T E R 34

Vitamins

INTRODUCTION

Vitamins are a group of structurally diverse organic substances that must be provided in small amounts in the diet for the subsequent synthesis of cofactors that are essential for various metabolic reactions. Food is the best source of vitamins, and healthy persons consuming an adequate balanced diet will not benefit from additional vitamins. Nevertheless, many otherwise healthy persons take supplemental vitamins, despite the absence of scientific evidence that these substances are necessary or useful (Herbert, 1980). Often, the patient's intake of vitamins remains undiscovered when a preoperative drug history is elicited. Excessive intake of fat-soluble vitamins, particularly vitamins A or D, is more likely to cause toxicity than are water-soluble vitamins (Lewis, 1980). For example, unrecognized vitamin A–induced hydrocephalus may result in unnecessary neurosurgery. Excessive intake of vitamin D leads to hypercalcinosis. High intake of water-soluble vitamins can elevate circulating plasma concentrations of administered salicylates and interfere with the anticoagulant action of warfarin.

The use of dietary vitamin supplements is medically indicated in situations associated with inadequate intake, malabsorption, increased tissue needs, or inborn errors of metabolism. Inadequate vitamin intake may reflect socioeconomic conditions, self-imposed dieting, or food faddism. Disturbances of vitamin absorption may occur in diseases of the liver and biliary tract, diarrhea, hy-

perthyroidism, small bowel bypass surgery for treatment of obesity, and alcoholism (Leevy and Baker, 1968). Antibiotic therapy may alter the usual bacterial flora of the gastrointestinal tract necessary for the synthesis of vitamin K. Loss of vitamins may occur during hemodialysis or hyperalimentation. Indeed, multivitamin preparations for parenteral administration are essential during long-term hyperalimentation (Nichoalds *et al,* 1977). Infants require vitamins to support normal growth. Vitamin supplementation is also indicated for people who are on low-calorie diets. Healthy adults, however, require no vitamin supplementation except during pregnancy and lactation.

WATER-SOLUBLE VITAMINS

Water-soluble vitamins include members of the vitamin B complex (*i.e.,* thiamine, riboflavin, nicotinic acid, pyridoxine, pantothenic acid, biotin, cyanocobalamin, folic acid) and ascorbic acid (Fig. 34-1).

Thiamine (Vitamin B$_1$)

Thiamine is converted to a physiologically active coenzyme known as thiamine pyrophosphate. This coenzyme is essential for the decarboxylation of alpha-keto acids such as pyruvate and in the utilization of pentose in the hexose-monophos-

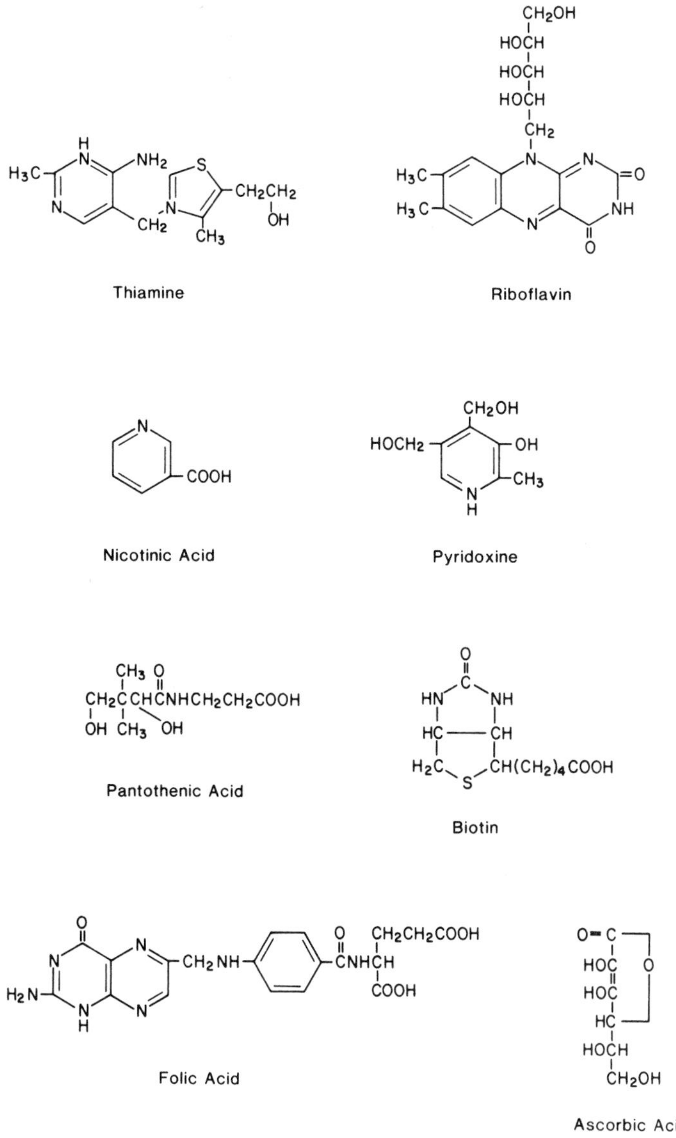

Thiamine

Riboflavin

Nicotinic Acid

Pyridoxine

Pantothenic Acid

Biotin

Folic Acid

Ascorbic Acid **FIGURE 34-1.** Water-soluble vitamins.

phate shunt pathway. Indeed, increased plasma concentrations of pyruvate are a diagnostic sign of thiamine deficiency.

Causes of Deficiency

The requirement for thiamine is related to the metabolic rate and is greatest when carbohydrate is the source of energy. This is important in patients maintained by hyperalimentation in which the majority of calories are provided in the form of glucose. Such patients should receive supplemental amounts of thiamine. Thiamine requirements are also increased during pregnancy and lactation.

Symptoms of Deficiency

Symptoms of mild thiamine deficiency (beriberi) include loss of appetite, skeletal muscle weakness, a tendency to develop peripheral edema, decreased blood pressure, and low body temperature. Severe thiamine deficiency (Korsakoff's syndrome), as often occurs in alcoholics, may be associated with peripheral polyneuritis, including areas of hyperesthesia and anesthesia of the legs, impairment of memory, and encephalopathy (McIntyre and Stanley, 1971). High output cardiac failure with extensive peripheral edema reflecting hypoproteinemia is often prominent. There is flattening or inversion of the T wave and prolongation of the Q-T interval on the electrocardiogram.

Treatment of Deficiency

Severe thiamine deficiency is treated with the intravenous administration of the vitamin. Once severe thiamine deficiency has been corrected, oral supplementation is acceptable.

Riboflavin (Vitamin B₂)

Riboflavin is converted in the body to one of two physiologically active coenzymes: flavin mononucleotide, or flavin adenine dinucleotide. These coenzymes primarily influence hydrogen transport in oxidative enzyme systems, including cytochrome C reductase, succinic dehydrogenase, and xanthine oxidase (Rivlin, 1970). Chlorpromazine and tricyclic antidepressants interfere with the flavokinase reaction necessary to convert riboflavin to its active coenzymes, thus increasing requirements (Rivlin, 1979). Tissue storage of this water-soluble vitamin is not extensive.

Symptoms of Deficiency

Pharyngitis and angular stomatitis are typically the first signs of riboflavin deficiency. Later, glossitis, red denuded lips, seborrheic dermatitis of the face, and dermatitis over the trunk and extremities occur. Anemia and neuropathy may be prominent. Corneal vascularization and cataract formation occur in some subjects. Treatment is with oral vitamin supplements that contain riboflavin.

Nicotinic Acid (Niacin)

Nicotinic acid is converted to the physiologically active coenzyme nicotinamide adenine dinucleotide (NAD) and nicotinamide adenine dinucleotide phosphate (NADP). These coenzymes are necessary to catalyze oxidation–reduction reactions essential for tissue respiration.

Symptoms of Deficiency

Nicotinic acid is an essential dietary constituent, the lack of which leads to dermatitis, diarrhea, and dementia. Pellagra is the all inclusive term for the symptoms of nicotinic acid deficiency. The skin characteristically becomes erythematous and rough in texture, especially in areas exposed to sun, friction, or pressure. The chief symptoms referable to the digestive tract are stomatitis, enteritis, and diarrhea. The tongue becomes very red and swollen. Salivary secretions are excessive, and nausea and vomiting are common. In addition to dementia, motor and sensory disturbances of the peripheral nerves also occur, mimicking changes that accompany a deficiency of thiamine.

The dietary requirement for this vitamin can be satisfied not only by nicotinic acid but also by nicotinamide and the amino acid tryptophan. The relationship between nicotinic acid requirement and the intake of tryptophan explains the association of pellagra with tryptophan-deficient corn diets. Carcinoid syndrome is associated with diversion of tryptophan from the synthesis of nicotinic acid to the production of serotonin, leading to symptoms of pellagra. Isoniazid inhibits incorporation of nicotinic acid into NAD and may produce pellagra.

Pellagra is uncommon in the United States, reflecting the supplementation of flour with nicotinic acid. Common causes of pellagra include chronic gastrointestinal disease and alcoholism, which are characteristically associated with multiple nutritional deficiencies. When pellagra is severe, intravenous nicotinic acid is indicated. In less severe cases, oral administration of nicotinic acid is adequate. The response to nicotinic acid is dramatic, with symptoms waning within 24 hours after initiation of therapy.

Toxic effects of nicotinic acid include flushing, pruritus, hepatotoxicity, hyperuricemia, and activation of peptic ulcer disease (Mosher, 1970). Nicotinic acid has also been used to lower the plasma concentration of cholesterol.

Pyridoxine (Vitamin B₆)

Pyridoxine is converted to its physiologically active form, pyridoxal phosphate, by the enzyme pyridoxal kinase. Pyridoxal phosphate serves an important role in metabolism as a coenzyme for conversion of tryptophan to serotonin and methionine to cysteine (Sturman, 1978).

Symptoms of Deficiency

Pyridoxine deficiency is frequent in the alcoholic (estimated incidence 30%) manifesting as alterations in the skin, central nervous system dysfunction, and anemia (Li, 1978). Seborrhea-like skin lesions about the eyes, nose, and mouth accompanied by glossitis and stomatitis occur. Seizures accompany deficiency of pyridoxine, and peripheral neuritis such as carpal tunnel syndrome is common. The lowered seizure threshold may reflect decreased concentration of the inhibitory neurotransmitter gamma-aminobutyric acid (GABA), the synthesis of which requires a pyridoxal phosphate – requiring enzyme (Roberts, 1963).

It is presumed that a person with a deficiency of other B vitamins may also have a relative deficiency of pyridoxine. For this reason, pyridoxine is incorporated into many multivitamin preparations for prophylactic use. Pyridoxine is unpredictably effective in the treatment of sideroblastic anemias (*i.e.,* deficiency of the synthesis of hemoglobin and accumulation of iron in the mitochondria.).

Drug Interactions

Isoniazid and hydralazine act as potent inhibitors of pyridoxal kinase, thus preventing synthesis of the active coenzyme form of the vitamin. Indeed, administration of pyridoxine reduces the incidence of the neurologic side effects associated with the administration of these drugs. Pyridoxine enhances the peripheral decarboxylation of levodopa and reduces its effectiveness for the treatment of Parkinson's disease. There is a decrease in the plasma concentration of pyridoxal phosphate in patients taking oral contraceptives (Donald and Bosse, 1979).

Pantothenic Acid

Pantothenic acid is converted to its physiologically active form, coenzyme A, which serves as a cofactor for enzyme-catalyzed reactions involving transfer of two carbon (acetyl) groups. Such reactions are important in the oxidative metabolism of carbohydrates, gluconeogenesis, and the synthesis and degradation of fatty acids (Wright, 1976).

Pantothenic acid deficiency in humans is rare, reflecting the ubiquitous presence of the vitamin in ordinary foods as well as its production by intestinal bacteria. No clearly defined uses for pantothenic acid exist, although it is commonly included in multivitamin preparations and in products for hyperalimentation.

Biotin

Biotin is an organic acid that functions as a coenzyme for enzyme-catalyzed carboxylation reactions and fatty acid synthesis. In adults, a deficiency of biotin manifests as glossitis, anorexia, dermatitis, and mental depression (Bonjour, 1977). Seborrheic dermatitis of infancy is most likely a form of biotin deficiency. For this reason, it is recommended that formulas contain supplemental biotin. Prolonged hyperalimentation may result in a deficiency of biotin.

Cyanocobalamin (Vitamin B_{12})

Cyanocobalamin and vitamin B_{12} are generic terms that are used interchangeably to designate several cobalt-containing compounds (*i.e.,* cobalamins). Dietary vitamin B_{12} in the presence of hydrogen ions in the stomach is released from proteins and subsequently binds to a glycoprotein intrinsic factor. This vitamin – intrinsic factor complex travels to the ileum, where it interacts with a specific receptor and is transported into the circulation. Following absorption, vitamin B_{12} binds to a beta globulin, transcobalamin II, for transport to tissues, especially the liver, which serves as a storage depot.

Causes of Deficiency

Although humans depend on exogenous sources of vitamin B_{12}, a deficient diet is rarely the cause of a deficiency state. Instead, gastric achlorhydria and decreased gastric secretion of intrinsic factor are more likely to be causes of vitamin B_{12} deficiency in adults. Antibodies to intrinsic factor may interfere with attachment of the complex to gastrin receptors in the ileum (DeAizpurua *et al,* 1985). Bacterial overgrowth may prevent an adequate amount of vitamin B_{12} from reaching the ileum. Surgical resection or disease of the ileum predictably interferes with the absorption of vitamin B_{12}. Finally, nitrous oxide irreversibly oxidizes the cobalt atom of vitamin B_{12} such that the activity of two vitamin B_{12}–dependent enzymes, methionine synthetase and thymidylate synthetase, are reduced (see Chapter 2).

Diagnosis of Deficiency

The plasma concentration of vitamin B_{12} is below 200 pg ml^{-1} when there is a deficiency state. Measurements of gastric acidity may provide indirect evidence of a defect in gastric parietal cell function, whereas the Schilling test can be used to quantitate ileal absorption of vitamin B_{12} (radioactivity in urine measured after oral administration of labeled vitamin B_{12}). Finally, observation of reticulocytosis following a therapeutic trial of vitamin B_{12} confirms the diagnosis.

Symptoms of Deficiency

Deficiency of vitamin B_{12} results in defective synthesis of DNA, especially in tissues with the greatest rate of cell turnover. In this regard, symptoms of vitamin B_{12} deficiency manifest most often on the hematopoietic and nervous systems. Changes in the hematopoietic system are most apparent in erythrocytes, but when deficiency of vitamin B_{12} is severe, a pronounced cytopenia may occur. Clinically, the earliest sign of vitamin B_{12} deficiency is megaloblastic (pernicious) anemia. Anemia may be so severe that cardiac failure occurs, especially in elderly patients with limited cardiac reserves. Damage to the myelin sheath is the most obvious symptom of nervous system dysfunction associated with vitamin B_{12} deficiency. Demyelination and cell death occur in the spinal cord and cerebral cortex, manifesting as paresthesias of the hands and feet and diminution of sensation of vibration and proprioception with resultant unsteadiness of gait. Deep tendon reflexes are decreased, and, in advanced stages, there is loss of memory and mental confusion. Indeed, vitamin B_{12} deficiency should be considered as a possibility in elderly patients with psychosis. Folic acid therapy will correct the hematopoietic but not nervous system effects produced by vitamin B_{12} deficiency.

Treatment of Deficiency

Vitamin B_{12} is available in a pure form for oral or parenteral use or in combination with other vitamins for oral administration. These preparations are of little value in the treatment of patients with deficiency of intrinsic factor or ileal disease. In the presence of clinically apparent vitamin B_{12} deficiency, oral absorption cannot be relied upon; the preparation of choice is cyanocobalamin administered intramuscularly. For example, in the patient with (1) neurologic changes, (2) leukopenia, or, (3) thrombocytopenia, treatment must be aggressive. Initial treatment is with intramuscular vitamin B_{12}, 100 μg, and folic acid, 1 to 5 mg. For the next 7 to 14 days, the patient should receive 100 μg vitamin B_{12} intramuscularly and folic acid, 1 to 2 mg orally. An increase in hematocrit does not occur for 10 to 20 days. The plasma concentration of iron, however, usually declines within 48 hours, because iron is now used in the formation of hemoglobin. Platelet counts can be expected to reach normal levels within 10 days of treatment; the granulocyte count requires a longer period of time to normalize. Memory and sense of well-being may improve within 24 hours after initiation of therapy. Neurologic signs and symptoms that have been present for prolonged periods, however, often regress slowly and may never return to complete normal function. Indeed, neurologic damage from pernicious anemia that is not reversed after 12 to 18 months of treatment is likely to be permanent.

Once initiated, vitamin B_{12} therapy must be continued indefinitely at monthly intervals. It is important to monitor plasma concentrations of vitamin B_{12} and examine the peripheral blood cells every 3 to 6 months to confirm the adequacy of therapy.

Hydroxocobalamin has hematopoietic activity similar to that of vitamin B_{12} but appears to offer no advantage despite its somewhat longer duration of action. Furthermore, some patients develop antibodies to the complex of hydroxocobalamin and transcobalamin II. Large doses of hydroxocobalamin have been proposed for treatment of cyanide poisoning owing to nitroprusside (Cottrell *et al*, 1979). Conceptually, cyanide reacts with hydroxocobalamin to form cyanocobalamin.

Folic Acid

Folic acid is transported and stored as 5-methylhydrofolate following absorption from the small intestine, principally the jejunum. Conversion to the metabolically active form, tetrahydrofolate, is dependent on activity of vitamin B_{12}. Tetrahydrofolate acts as an acceptor of one-carbon units necessary for the (1) conversion of homocysteine to methionine, (2) conversion of serine to glycine, (3) synthesis of DNA, and (4) synthesis of purines. Supplies of folic acid are maintained by ingestion in food and by enterohepatic circulation of the vitamin. Virtually, all foods contain folic acid, but protracted cooking can destroy up to 90% of the vitamin.

Causes of Deficiency

Folic acid deficiency is a common complication of diseases of the small intestine, such as sprue, that interfere with absorption of the vitamin and its enterohepatic recirculation. Alcoholism reduces intake of folic acid in food, and enterohepatic recirculation may be damaged by the toxic effect of alcohol on hepatocytes. Indeed, alcoholism is the most common cause of folic acid deficiency, with reductions in the plasma concentration of folic acid manifesting within 24 to 48 hours of steady alcohol ingestion. Drugs that inhibit dehydrofolate reductase (*e.g.,* methotrexate, trimethoprim) or interfere with absorption and storage of folic acid in tissues (*e.g.,* phenytoin) may cause folic acid deficiency (Stebbins and Bertino, 1976).

Symptoms of Deficiency

Megaloblastic anemia is the most common manifestation of folic acid deficiency. This anemia cannot be distinguished from that caused by a deficiency of vitamin B_{12}. Folic acid deficiency, however, is confirmed by the presence of a folic acid concentration in the plasma of less than 4 ng ml^{-1}. Furthermore, the rapid onset of megaloblastic anemia produced by folic acid deficiency (1–4 weeks) reflects the limited *in vivo* stores of this vitamin and contrasts with the slower onset (2–3 years) of symptoms of vitamin B_{12} deficiency.

Treatment of Deficiency

Folic acid is available as an oral preparation alone or in combination with other vitamins and as a parenteral injection. The therapeutic uses of folic acid are limited to the prevention and treatment of deficiencies of the vitamin. For example, pregnancy is associated with increased folic acid requirements, and oral supplementation, usually in a multivitamin preparation, is indicated. In the presence of megaloblastic anemia as a result of folic acid deficiency, the administration of the vitamin is associated with a decline in the plasma concentration of iron within 48 hours, reflecting new erythropoiesis. Likewise, the reticulocyte count begins to rise within 48 to 72 hours, and the hematocrit begins to increase during the second week of therapy.

LEUCOVORIN. Leucovorin (citrovorum factor) is a metabolically active, reduced form of folic acid. Following treatment with folic acid antagonists, such as methotrexate, patients may receive leucovorin (rescue therapy), which serves as a source for tetrahydrofolate that cannot be formed owing to drug-induced inhibition of dihydrofolate reductase (see Chapter 29). In children, leucovorin may be administered during general anesthesia that may include nitrous oxide. It is possible that nitrous oxide, by inhibiting vitamin B_{12}–dependent enzymes, would impair the efficacy of leucovorin as a source for tetrahydrofolate (see Chapter 2) (Ueland *et al,* 1986).

Ascorbic Acid (Vitamin C)

Ascorbic acid is a six-carbon compound structurally related to glucose. This vitamin acts as a coenzyme and is important in a number of biochemical reactions, mostly involving oxidation. For example, ascorbic acid is necessary for the synthesis of collagen, cornitine, and corticosteroids. Ascorbic acid is readily absorbed from the gastrointestinal tract. Many foods have a high content of ascorbic acid; for example, orange juice and lemon juice contain about 0.5 mg ml^{-1} of ascorbic acid. When gastrointestinal absorption is impaired, ascorbic acid can be administered intramuscularly or intravenously. Apart from its role in nutrition, ascorbic acid is commonly used as an antioxidant to protect the natural flavor and color of many foods.

Despite contrary claims, controlled studies do not support the efficacy of even large doses of ascorbic acid in the treatment of cancer of the colon or viral respiratory tract infections (Moertel *et al,* 1985; Pit and Costrini, 1979). A risk of large doses of ascorbic acid is formation of kidney stones resulting from the excessive excretion of oxalate (Anderson, 1977). Excessive doses of ascorbic acid can also enhance the absorption of iron and interfere with anticoagulant therapy (Cook and Monsen, 1977).

Symptoms of Deficiency

A deficiency of ascorbic acid is known as scurvy. Humans, in contrast to many other mammals, are unable to synthesize ascorbic acid, emphasizing the need for dietary sources of the vitamin to prevent scurvy. Specifically, humans lack the hepatic enzyme necessary to produce ascorbic acid from gluconate (Crandon *et al,* 1940). Manifestations of scurvy include gingivitis, rupture of capillaries with formation of numerous petechiae, defects in tooth formation, and failure of wounds to heal. An associated anemia may reflect a specific function of ascorbic acid on hemoglobin synthesis. Scurvy is evident when the plasma concentrations of ascorbic acid decline below 0.15 mg dl^{-1}.

Scurvy is encountered among the elderly, alcoholics, and drug addicts. Ascorbic acid requirements are increased during pregnancy, lactation, and stresses such as infection or following surgery. Infants receiving formula diets with inadequate concentrations of ascorbic acid can develop scurvy. Patients receiving hyperalimentation should receive supplemental ascorbic acid. Urinary loss of infused ascorbic acid is large, necessitating daily doses of 200 mg to maintain normal concentrations in plasma of 1 mg dl^{-1} (Nichoalds *et al,* 1977). Increased urinary excretion of ascorbic acid is caused by salicylates, tetracyclines, and barbiturates.

FAT-SOLUBLE VITAMINS

Fat-soluble vitamins are vitamins A, D, E, and K (Fig. 34-2). They are absorbed from the gastrointestinal tract by complex processes that parallel absorption of fat. Thus, any condition that causes malabsorption of fat, such as obstructive jaundice, may result in deficiency of one or all these vitamins. Fat-soluble vitamins are stored principally in the liver and excreted in the feces. Since these vitamins are metabolized very slowly, overdose may produce toxic effects. Vitamin D, despite its name, functions as a hormone.

Vitamin A

Vitamin A exists in a variety of forms, including retinol and 3-dehydroretinol. This vitamin is im-

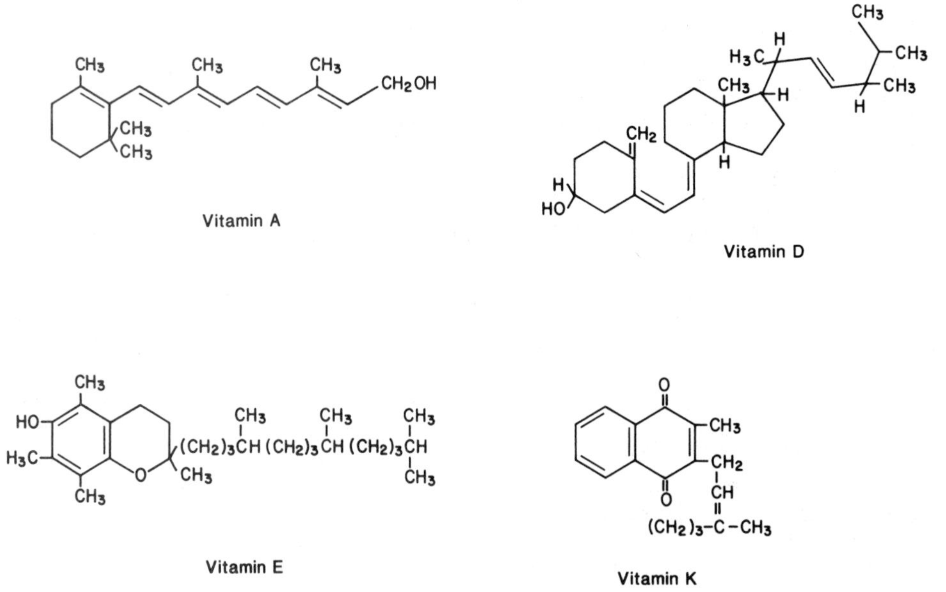

Vitamin A

Vitamin D

Vitamin E

Vitamin K

FIGURE 34-2. Fat-soluble vitamins.

portant in the function of the retina, integrity of mucosal and epithelial surfaces, bone develoment and growth, reproduction, and embryonic development (see Chapter 41). It also has a stabilizing effect on various membranes and acts to regulate membrane permeability (Wasserman and Taylor, 1972). Vitamin A may exert transcriptional control of the production of specific proteins, a process that has important implications with respect to regulation of cellular differentiation and development of malignancies. Limitations in the therapeutic use of vitamin A for antineoplastic uses are the associated hepatotoxicity and its failure to distribute to specific organs (Smith and Goodman, 1976).

Major dietary sources of vitamin A are liver, butter, cheese, milk, certain fish, and various yellow or green fruits and vegetables. Fish liver oils contain large amounts of vitamin A. Sufficient vitamin A is stored in the liver of well-nourished persons to satisfy requirements for several months. Plasma concentrations of vitamin A are maintained at the expense of hepatic reserves and thus do not always reflect a person's vitamin A status. Vitamin A may interact with cellular proteins, which function analogously to receptors for estrogens and other steroids.

Symptoms of Deficiency

In the United States, it is estimated that about 15% of the population has concentrations of vitamin A in the plasma below 20 μg dl^{-1}, indicating a risk of deficiency (Roels, 1970). Most of these people are infants or children. Signs and symptoms of mild vitamin A deficiency are easily overlooked. Skin lesions such as follicular hyperkeratosis and infections are often the earliest signs of deficiency. Nevertheless, the most recognizable manifestation of vitamin A deficiency is night blindness (nyctalopia), which occurs only when depletion is severe (see Chapter 41). Respiratory infections are increased as bronchial epithelium for mucous secretion undergoes keratinization. Keratinization and drying of the epidermis occur. Urinary calculi are frequently associated with vitamin A deficiency, which may reflect epithelial changes that provide a nidus around which a calculus is formed. Abnormalities of reproduction include impairment of spermatogenesis and spontaneous abortion. Impairment of taste and smell is common in patients with vitamin A deficiency, presumably reflecting a keratinizing effect. De-

creased erythropoiesis may be masked by abnormal losses of fluids.

Hypervitaminosis A

Hypervitaminosis A is the toxic syndrome that results from excessive ingestion of vitamin A, particularly in children (James *et al,* 1982). Typically, high vitamin A intakes have resulted from overzealous prophylactic vitamin therapy. Plasma concentrations of vitamin A above 300 μg dl^{-1} are diagnostic of hypervitaminosis A. Treatment consists of withdrawal of the vitamin source, which is usually followed within 7 days by disappearance of the manifestations of excess vitamin activity.

Early signs and symptoms of vitamin A toxicity include irritability, vomiting, headache, and dermatitis. Fatigue, myalgia, loss of body hair, diplopia, nystagmus, gingivitis, stomatitis, and lymphadenopathy have been observed. Hepatosplenomegaly is accompanied by cirrhosis, portal vein hypertension, and ascites. Intracranial pressure may be increased, and neurologic symptoms, including papilledema, may mimic those of a brain tumor (*i.e.,* pseudotumor cerebri) (Vollbracht and Gilroy, 1976). The diagnosis is confirmed by radiologic demonstration of hyperostoses underlying tender hard swellings on the extremities and the occipital region of the head. The activity of plasma alkaline phosphatase is increased, reflecting osteoblastic activity. Hypercalcemia may occur as a result of bone destruction. Bones continue to grow in length but not in thickness, with increased susceptibility to fractures. Congenital abnormalities may occur in infants whose mothers have consumed excessive amounts of vitamin A during pregnancy (Strange *et al,* 1978). Psychiatric disturbances may mimic depression or schizophrenia.

Vitamin D

Vitamin D is the generic designation for several sterols and their metabolites that act as hormones to maintain plasma concentrations of calcium and phosphate ions in an optimal range for normal neuromuscular function, mineralization of bone, and other calcium-dependent functions (DeLuca, 1976) (see Chapter 52). This regulation of plasma concentrations of calcium and phosphate ions reflects the ability of vitamin D to facilitate absorption of these ions from the gastrointestinal tract and enhance the mobilization of calcium from bone. In addition, there may be a direct effect of vitamin D on proximal renal tubules that results in increased retention of calcium and phosphate ions.

The principal provitamin of vitamin D in tissues, 7-dehydrocholesterol, is synthesized in the skin and converted to vitamin D on exposure of the skin to sunlight. Vitamin D is also absorbed from the gastrointestinal tract following oral administration. Bile salts are necessary for this absorption, emphasizing that hepatic or biliary dysfunction may impair passage of vitamin D into the circulation. Absorbed vitamin D is hydroxylated in the liver to calcifediol, which is further hydroxylated in the kidneys to calcitriol, the active form of vitamin D. This conversion to calcitriol is regulated in a negative feedback manner by the plasma calcium concentration. The elimination half-time of calcitriol is 3 to 5 days.

Symptoms of Deficiency

A deficiency of vitamin D results in reduced concentrations of calcium and phosphate ions, with the subsequent stimulation of parathyroid hormone secretion. Parathyroid hormone acts to restore the plasma calcium concentrations of calcium ions at the expense of bone calcium. In infants and children, this results in failure to mineralize newly formed osteoid tissue and cartilage, causing the formation of soft bone, which, with weightbearing, results in deformities known as rickets. In adults, vitamin D deficiency results in osteomalacia. Anticonvulsant therapy with phenytoin increases target organ resistance to vitamin D, resulting in an increased incidence of rickets and osteomalacia (Hunter *et al*, 1971; Jubiz *et al*, 1977).

Hypervitaminosis D

Administration of excessive amounts of vitamin D results in hypervitaminosis manifesting as hypercalcemia, skeletal muscle weakness, fatigue, headache, and vomiting. Early impairment of renal function from hypercalcemia manifests as polyuria, polydipsia, proteinuria, and decreased urine concentrating ability. In addition to withdrawal of the vitamin, treatment includes increased fluid intake and administration of glucocorticoids.

Vitamin E (Tocopherol)

Vitamin E is a group of fat-soluble substances occurring in plants. There is little persuasive evidence that vitamin E is of nutritional significance in humans or of any value in therapy (Roberts, 1981). Alpha-tocopherol is the most abundant and important of the eight naturally occuring tocopherols that constitute vitamin E. An important chemical feature of the tocopherols is that they are antioxidants. In acting as an antioxidant, vitamin E presumably prevents oxidation of essential cellular constituents or prevents the formation of toxic oxidation products. There seems to be a relationship between vitamins A and E in which vitamin E facilitates the absorption, hepatic storage, and utilization of vitamin A. In addition, vitamin E seems to protect against the development of hypervitaminosis A by enhancing utilization of the vitamin (Bauernfeind *et al*, 1974). Vitamin E is stored in adipose tissue and is thought to stabilize the lipid portions of cell membranes. Other functions attributed to vitamin E are inhibition of prostaglandin production and stimulation of an essential cofactor in steroid metabolism.

Vitamin E requirements may be increased in people exposed to high oxygen environments or in those taking therapeutic doses of iron or large doses of thyroid replacement. The severity of retrolental fibroplasia is alleged to be less in premature infants given large daily doses of vitamin E (Hittner *et al*, 1981). Vitamin E may be important in hematopoiesis, with occasional forms of anemia responding favorably to the administration of alpha-tocopherol.

Despite absence of conclusive supportive evidence, vitamin E has been used in females for treatment of recurrent abortion and for sterility in both sexes. In animals, vitamin E deficiency leads to the development of muscular dystrophy, but there is no evidence that similar events occur in humans (Berneske *et al*, 1960). Similar changes to those observed in skeletal muscle have occurred in cardiac muscle of animals. Nevertheless, carefully controlled studies have failed to show any value in the treatment of cardiac failure in patients.

Vitamin K

Vitamin K is a lipid-soluble dietary principal essential for the biosynthesis of several factors required for the normal clotting of blood (see Chapter 57). Phytonadione (vitamin K_1) is present in a variety of foods and is the only natural form of vitamin K available for therapeutic use. Vitamin K_2 represents a series of compounds that are synthesized by gram-positive bacteria in the gastrointestinal tract. Synthesis of vitamin K provides about 50% of the estimated daily requirement of vitamin K; the rest is supplied by the diet. Vitamin K is absorbed from the gastrointestinal tract only in the presence of adequate quantities of bile salts. Vitamin K accumulates in the liver, spleen, and lungs, but, despite its lipid solubility, significant amounts are not stored in the body for prolonged periods of time.

Mechanism of Action

Vitamin K functions as an essential cofactor for the hepatic microsomal enzyme system that converts glutamic acid residues to gamma-carboxyglutamic acid residues in factors II (prothrombin), VII, IX, and X. The gamma-carboxyglutamic acid residues make it possible for these coagulation factors to bind calcium and attach to phospholipid surfaces, leading to clot formation (Nelsestuen, 1978). If vitamin K deficiency occurs, the plasma concentrations of these coagulation factors decrease and a hemorrhagic disorder develops, which is characterized by ecchymoses, epistaxis, hematuria, gastrointestinal bleeding, and postoperative hemorrhage. Intracranial hemorrhage is also a possibility. Prothrombin time is used to monitor vitamin K activity.

Clinical Uses

Vitamin K is administered to treat its deficiency and attendant reduction in plasma concentrations of prothrombin and related clotting factors. Deficiency of vitamin K may be due to (1) inadequate dietary intake, (2) decreased bacterial synthesis owing to antibiotic therapy, (3) impaired gastrointestinal absorption resulting from obstructive biliary tract disease and absence of bile salts, or (4) hepatocellular disease (Frick *et al*, 1967). Newborn infants have hypoprothrombinemia owing to vitamin K deficiency until adequate dietary intake of the vitamin occurs and a normal intestinal bacterial flora is established. Indeed, at birth, the normal infant has only 20% to 40% of the adult plasma concentrations of clotting factors II, VII, IX, and X. These plasma concentrations decline even further during the first 2 to 3 days after birth; they

begin to rise toward adult values after about 6 days. In premature infants, plasma concentrations of clotting factors are even lower. Human breast milk has low concentrations of vitamin K. Administration of vitamin K to the normal newborn infant (0.5 – 1 mg intramuscularly at birth) prevents the decline in concentration of vitamin K – dependent clotting factors on the first days following birth but does not increase these concentrations to adult levels.

Vitamin K replacement therapy will not be effective when severe hepatocellular disease is responsible for decreased production of clotting factors. In the absence of severe hepatocellular disease and the presence of adequate bile salts, the administration of oral vitamin K preparations is effective in reversing hypoprothrombinemia. Phytonadione and menadione are the vitamin K preparations most often used to treat hypoprothrombinemia.

PHYTONADIONE. Phytonadione (vitamin K_1) is the preferred drug to treat hypoprothrombinemia, particularly when large doses or prolonged therapy is necessary. Hypoprothrombinemia of the newborn is treated with phytonadione, 0.5 to 1 mg administered intramuscularly within 24 hours of birth. A frequent indication for phytonadione is to reverse the effects of oral anticoagulants. For example, phytonadione, 10 to 20 mg orally or administered intravenously at a rate of 1 mg min^{-1}, is usually adequate to reverse the effects of oral anticoagulants (see Chapter 27). The oral and intramuscular routes of administration are less likely than intravenous injections of phytonadione to cause side effects and are thus preferred for nonemergency reversal of oral anticoagulants. Even large doses of phytonadione are ineffective against heparin-induced anticoagulation. Vitamin K supplementation is also indicated for patients receiving prolonged parenteral hyperalimentation, especially if antibiotics are concomitantly administered.

Intravenous injection of phytonadione may cause life-threatening allergic reactions characterized by hypotension and bronchospasm. Intramuscular administration may produce local hemorrhage at the injection site in hypoprothrombinemic patients. In newborns, doses of phytonadione in excess of 1 mg may cause hemolytic anemia and increase plasma concentrations of unbound bilirubin, thus increasing the risk of kernicterus (Machin, 1980). The occurrence of

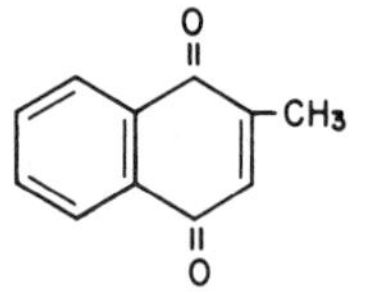

FIGURE 34-3. Menadione.

hemolytic anemia reflects a deficiency of glycolytic enzymes in some newborns.

MENADIONE. Menadione has the same actions and uses as phytonadione (Fig 34-3). Water-soluble salts of menadione do not require the presence of bile salts for their systemic absorption following oral administration. This characteristic becomes important when malabsorption of vitamin K is due to biliary obstruction.

Menadione hemolyzes erythrocytes in patients genetically deficient in glucose-6-phosphate dehydrogenase as well as in newborn infants, particularly the premature infant (Zinkham and Childs, 1957). This hemolysis and occasionally hepatic toxicity reflects combination of menadione with sulfhydral groups in tissues. Kernicterus has occurred following menadione administration to neonates. For this reason, menadione is not recommended for treatment of hemorrhagic disease of the newborn. Administration of large doses of menadione or phytonadione may depress liver function, particularly in the presence of preexisting liver disease.

REFERENCES

Anderson TW. Large scale studies with vitamin C. Acta Vitaminol Enzymol 1977;31:43–50.

Bauernfeind JC, Newmark H, Brin M. Vitamin A and E nutrition via intramuscular or oral route. Am J Clin Nutr 1974;27:234–53.

Berneske GM, Butson ARC, Gauld EN, Levy D. Clinical trial of high dose vitamin E in human muscular dystrophy. Can Med Assoc J 1960;80:418–21.

Bonjour JP. Biotin in man's nutrition and therapy—a review. Int J Vitam Nutr Res 1977;47:107–18.

Cook JD, Monsen ER. Vitamin C, the common cold and iron absorption. Am J Clin Nutr 1977;30:235–41.

Cottrell JE, Casthely P, Brodie JD, Patel K, Klein A, Turndorf H. Prevention of nitroprusside-induced cyanide toxicity with hydroxocobalamin. N Engl J Med 1979;298:809–11.

Crandon JH, Lund CC, Dill DB. Experimental human scurvy. N Engl J Med 1940;223:353–69.

DeAizpurua HJ, Ungar B, Toh B-H. Autoantibody to the gastrin receptor in pernicious anemia. N Engl J Med 1985;313:479–83.

DeLuca HF. Vitamin D endocrinology. Ann Intern Med 1976;85:367–77.

Donald EA, Bosse TR. The vitamin B_6 requirement in oral contraceptive users. II. Assessment by tryptophan metabolites, vitamin B_6, and pyridoxic acid levels in urine. Am J Clin Nutr 1979;32:1024–32.

Frick PG, Riedler G, Brogli H. Dose response and minimal daily requirement for vitamin K in man. J Appl Physiol 1967;23:387–9.

Herbert V. The vitamin craze. Arch Intern Med 1980;140:173–80.

Hittner HM, Godio LB, Rudolph AJ, et al. Retrolental fibroplasia: Efficacy of vitamin E in double-blind clinical study of preterm infants. N Engl J Med 1981;305:1365–71.

Hunter J, Maxwell JD, Stewart DA, Parsons V, Williams R. Altered calcium metabolism in epileptic children on anticonvulsants. Br Med J 1971;4:202–4.

James MB, Leonard JC, Fraser JJ, Stuemby JH. Hypervitaminosis A: Case report. Pediatrics 1982;69:112–5.

Jubiz W, Haussler MR, McCain TA, Tolman KG. Plasma 1, 25-dihydroxyvitamin D levels in patients receiving anticonvulsant drugs. J Clin Endocrinol Metab 1977;44:617–21.

Leevy CM, Baker H. Vitamins and alcoholism: introduction. Am J Clin Nutr 1968;21:1325–8.

Lewis JG. Adverse reactions to vitamins. Adverse Drug React Bull 1980;82:296–9.

Li T. Factors influencing vitamin B_6 requirement in alcoholism. In, Human B_6 Requirements. Washington, DC, National Academy of Sciences, 1978;210–25.

Machin SJ. The bleeding patient. Br J Hosp Med 1980;24:152–8.

McIntyre N, Stanley NN. Cardiac beriberi: Two modes of presentation. Br Med J 1971;4:567–9.

Moertel CG, Fleming TR, Creagan ET, Rubin J, O'Connell MJ, Ames MM. High-dose vitamin C versus placebo in the treatment of patients with advanced cancer who have had no prior chemotherapy. N Engl J Med 1985;312:137–41.

Mosher LR. Nicotinic acid side effects and toxicity: a review. Am J Psychiatry 1970;126:1290–6.

Nelsestuen GL. Interaction of vitamin K–dependent proteins with calcium ions and phospholipid membranes. Fed Proc 1978;37:2621–5.

Nicholalds GE, Meng HC, Caldwell MD. Vitamin requirements in patients receiving total parenteral nutrition. Arch Surg 1977;112:1061–4.

Pitt HA, Costrini AM. Vitamin C prophylaxis in marine recruits. JAMA 1979;241:908–11.

Rivlin RS. Riboflavin metabolism. N Engl J Med 1970;283:463–72.

Rivlin RS. Hormones, drugs and riboflavin. Nutr Rev 1979;37:241–6.

Roberts E. Some thoughts about the gamma-aminobutyric acid system in nervous tissue. Nutr Rev 1963;21:161 – 5.

Roberts HJ. Perspective on vitamin E as therapy. JAMA 1981;246:129 – 31.

Roels OA. Vitamin A physiology. JAMA 1970;214:1097 – 1102.

Smith FR, Goodman DS. Vitamin A transport in human vitamin A toxicity. N Engl J Med 1976;294:805 – 8.

Stebbens R, Bertino JR. Megaloblastic anemia produced by drugs. Clin Haematol 1976;5:619 – 30.

Strange L, Carlstrom, Ericksson M. Hypervitaminosis A in early human pregnancy and malformations of the central nervous system. Acta Obstet Gynecol Scand 1978;57:289 – 91.

Sturman JA. Vitamin B_6 and the metabolism of sulfur amino acids. In, Human Vitamin B_6 Requirements. Washington DC, National Academy of Sciences, 1978;37 – 60.

Ueland PM, Refsum H, Wesenberg F, Kvinnsland S. Methotrexate therapy and nitrous oxide anesthesia. N Engl J Med 1986;314:1514.

Vollbracht R, Gilroy J. Vitamin A – induced benign intracranial hypertension. Can J Neurol Sci 1976;3:59 – 61.

Wasserman RH, Taylor AN. Metabolic roles of fat-soluble vitamins D, E, and K. Annu Rev Biochem 1972;41:179 – 201.

Wright LD. Pantothenic acid. In, Present Knowledge in Nutrition. Eds. Hegsted DM, Chichester CO, Darby WJ, McNutt KW, Stalvey RM, Stotz EH. Washington DC, The Nutrition Foundation, 1976;226:31.

Zinkham WH, Childs B. Effect of vitamin K and naphthalene metabolites on glutathione metabolism of erythrocytes from normal newborns and patients with naphthalene hemolytic anemia. Am J Dis Child 1957;94:420 – 3.

C H A P T E R 35

Minerals

INTRODUCTION

Many minerals function as essential constituents of enzymes and regulate a variety of physiologic functions including (1) maintenance of osmotic pressure, (2) transport of oxygen, (3) skeletal muscle contraction, (4) integrity of the central nervous system, (5) growth and maintenance of tissues and bones, and (6) hematoporesis. Elements present in the body in large amounts include calcium, phosphorus, sodium, potassium, magnesium, sulfur and chloride. Iron, cobalt in vitamin B_{12}, copper, zinc, chromium, selenium, manganese, and molybdenum are present in trace amounts (Ulmer, 1977). Nickel, tin, silicon, and arsenic also are considered essential elements.

In the absence of absorption abnormalities, severe mineral deficiency is unlikely as most minerals, with the exception of zinc, are present in foods. Nevertheless, iron deficiency is common especially in infants and women consuming inadequate diets. Modest zinc and copper deficiencies also occur frequently.

A balanced, varied diet supplies adequate amounts of trace elements and dietary supplements containing minerals should be used only when evidence of deficiency exists or when demands are known to be increased as during pregnancy and lactation. Mineral deficiencies may develop during prolonged hyperalimentation emphasizing the importance of monitoring plasma concentrations of trace metals in these patients.

CALCIUM

Calcium is present in the body in greater amounts than any other mineral. The plasma concentration of calcium is maintained between 4.5 and 5.5 mEq L^{-1} (*i.e.,* 8.5 to 10.5 mg dl^{-1}) by an endocrine control system that includes vitamin D, parathyroid hormone, and calcitonin (see Chapter 52). Total plasma calcium consists of (1) calcium bound to albumin, (2) calcium complexed with citrate and phosphate ions, and (3) freely diffusible ionized calcium. It is the ionized fraction of calcium that produces physiological effects.

The ionized fraction of calcium represents about 45% of the total plasma concentration. Therefore, a normal plasma ionized calcium concentration is 2 to 2.5 mEq L^{-1}. Symptoms due to altered concentrations of calcium reflect changes in the plasma level of ionized calcium. This emphasizes the need to evaluate disturbances in calcium homeostasis by measurement of ionized calcium. It must be remembered that the concentration of ionized calcium is dependent on arterial pH with acidosis increasing and alkalosis decreasing the concentration. Likewise, the plasma albumin concentration must be considered when interpreting plasma calcium measurements. For example, albumin in plasma binds nonionized calcium. When the serum albumin concentration is decreased, there will be less calcium bound to protein. As a result, nonionized calcium is free to return to storage sites such as bone. Therefore, the total plasma calcium concentration can be reduced in the presence of hypoalbuminemia, but symptoms of hypocalcemia do not occur unless the ionized calcium concentration is also reduced. For example, hypocalcemia due to hypoproteinemia is not accompanied by signs of hypocalcemia unless the ionized fraction of calcium in the plasma is also decreased. For this reason, accurate interpretation of the plasma concentration of calcium is not possible without knowledge of the plasma albumin concentration.

Role of Calcium

Calcium ions are important for (1) neuromuscular transmission, (2) skeletal muscle contraction, (3) cardiac muscle contractility, (4) blood coagulation, and (5) exocytosis necessary for release of neurotransmitters and autocoids. In addition, calcium is a principal component of bone (see the section entitled Bone Composition). The cytoplasmic concentration of ionized calcium is maintained at low levels by extrusion from the cell and sequestration of the ion within cellular organelles, particularly mitochondria, and in skeletal muscle, the sarcoplasmic reticulum. The large gradient for calcium ions across cell membranes contributes to the utilization of this ion for transmembrane signaling in response to various electrical or chemical stimuli.

Cardiovascular Effects

Calcium chloride 7 mg kg^{-1} administered intravenously transiently increases myocardial contractility and cardiac output in halothane-anesthetized volunteers (Denlinger *et al*, 1975). At the same time, heart rate decreases while mean arterial pressure and central venous pressure are unchanged. The net effect of these changes is a decrease in calculated peripheral vascular resistance. Calcium administered in the presence of an artificial mechanical heart (*e.g.,* myocardial contractility constant) also produces transient dose-related reductions in peripheral vascular resistance (Stanley *et al*, 1976). Heart rate slowing may reflect a calcium-mediated increase in vagal activity or a delay in transmission of the cardiac impulse through the atrioventricular node (Sialer *et al*, 1967). Absence of an effect of calcium on pulmonary blood flow is suggested by the lack of

change in shunt fraction following the intravenous injection of calcium (Gallagher *et al*, 1984).

It is possible that anesthetics could alter the effect of calcium ions on the heart (Pitt *et al*, 1969). For example, anesthetics that produce peripheral vasoconstriction or vasodilation could augment or diminish the peripheral vascular effects of calcium. Volatile anesthetics may induce myocardial depression by inhibiting calcium uptake by the sarcoplasmic reticulum (Su and Kerrick, 1980). The direct dilating effect of ketamine on cerebral arteries may be in part due to interference with the transmembrane influx of calcium ions (Fukuda *et al*, 1983).

Hypocalcemia

The most common cause of hypocalcemia (plasma concentration of calcium below 4.5 mEq L^{-1}) is a reduced plasma concentration of albumin. Other causes of hypocalcemia include hypoparathyroidism, acute pancreatitis, vitamin D deficiency, and chronic renal failure associated with hyperphosphatemia. Malabsorption states resulting in deprivation of calcium and vitamin D readily lead to hypocalcemia.

Citrate binding of calcium can result in hypocalcemia, but this is unlikely in adults as the rate of whole blood infusion must exceed 50 ml min^{-1} before a reduction in the plasma concentration of ionized calcium occurs (Fig. 35-1) (Delinger *et al*, 1976). This reflects mobilization of calcium from bone and the ability of the liver to metabolize rapidly citrate to bicarbonate ions. Therefore, the arbitrary administration of supplemental intravenous calcium to adults receiving stored blood, is not indicated in the absence of objective evidence of hypocalcemia. Supplemental administration of calcium, however, is indicated to prevent citrate-induced hypocalcemia in the neonate receiving stored blood. Furthermore, in the presence of hypothermia or severe liver dysfunction, the ability to metabolize citrate to bicarbonate may be reduced and the administration of supplemental calcium indicated.

Symptoms

Symptoms of hypocalcemia include (1) tetany, (2) circumoral paresthesias, (3) increased neuromuscular excitability, (4) laryngospasm, and (5) seizures. Abrupt reductions in the ionized por-

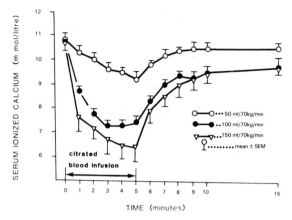

FIGURE 35-1. Citrate-induced reductions in serum ionized calcium concentrations do not occur unless the rate of whole blood infusion exceeds 50 ml 70 kg^{-1} min^{-1}. (From Denlinger JK, Nahrwold ML, Gibbs PS, Lecky JH. Hypocalcemia during rapid blood transfusion in anesthetized man. Br J Anaesth 1976;48:995–1000. Reproduced by permission of the authors and publisher.)

tions of the total plasma concentration of calcium are associated with hypotension and increased left ventricular end-diastolic pressure (Fig. 35-2) (Denlinger and Nahrwold, 1976; Scheidegger and Drop, 1979). The Q–T interval on the electrocardiogram may be prolonged, but this is not a consistent observation. For this reason, monitoring the Q–T interval on the electrocardiogram may not be a clinically reliable guide to the presence or absence of hypocalcemia.

Treatment

Treatment of hypocalcemia is with a commercially available preparation of calcium (*e.g.,* calcium chloride, calcium gluconate, calcium gluceptate) administered intravenously. For example, calcium chloride contains 27% calcium and is given intravenously (5%–10% solution; 1.4–2.8 mEq ml^{-1}) in a dose of 3 to 6 mg kg^{-1} over 5 to 15 minutes. Each mmol of calcium is equivalent to 20 mg. This injection is irritating to veins and may cause discomfort in an awake patient. Vasodilation and a moderate decrease in blood pressure may occur. Since calcium chloride is an acidifying salt, it is not recommended for the treatment of hypocalcemia caused by chronic renal failure. Conversely, calcium chloride administered intra-

venously produces the most rapid increase in the plasma concentration of ionized calcium favoring its use during cardiopulmonary resuscitation.

Calcium gluconate contains 9% calcium and is administered intravenously (10% solution; 0.9 mEq ml^{-1}) in doses of 7 to 14 mg kg^{-1} to treat hypocalcemia. Mild symptoms of hypocalcemia may be treated with orally administered calcium gluconate. Calcium gluceptate is a 23% solution of calcium that may be injected intramuscularly as well as intravenously.

HYPERKALEMIA. Life-threatening hyperkalemia is initially treated by intravenous administration of calcium. Calcium counteracts the effects of hyperkalemia by activation of calcium channels

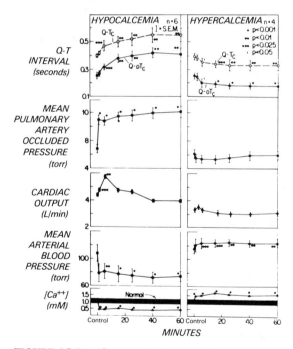

FIGURE 35-2. Abrupt reductions in the plasma concentration of calcium result in an increased Q–T interval on the electrocardiogram, increased mean pulmonary artery occlusion pressure, and decreased mean arterial pressure. Hypercalcemia results in a decreased Q–T interval on the electrocardiogram. (From Scheidegger D, Drop LJ. The relationship between duration of Q–T interval and plasma ionized calcium concentration: Experiments with acute, steady-state (CA^{++}) changes in the dog. Anesthesiology 1979;51:143–8. Reproduced by permission of the authors and publisher.)

such that ion flux through these channels generates an action potential and restores myocardial contractility. For example, intravenous administration of 10 to 20 ml of a 10% calcium chloride solution restores myocardial contractility in 1 to 2 minutes. This effect lasts 15 to 20 minutes. Serum potassium concentrations are not significantly changed by intravenous administration of calcium.

Other measures to treat hyperkalemia include intravenous infusion of sodium bicarbonate and glucose-insulin mixtures. Sodium bicarbonate (0.5 – 1 mEq kg^{-1}) causes a shift of potassium into cells in about 5 minutes. Serum potassium will be decreased as long as pH is increased. Glucose-insulin infusion (50 ml of 50% glucose plus 10 units of regular insulin) produce a sustained transfer of potassium into cells resulting in a 1.5 to 2.5 mEq L^{-1} decrease in serum potassium concentration after about 30 minutes.

Hypercalcemia

Neoplasms are the most common cause of life-threatening hypercalcemia (plasma calcium concentration above 5.5 mEq L^{-1}) presumably reflecting secretion by tumors of a substance that stimulates resorption of bone. The most common cause of mild hypercalcemia is hyperparathyroidism. Hyperparathyroidism due to chronic renal failure may manifest as hypercalcemia following successful renal transplantation. Sarcoidosis is associated with hypercalcemia in about 20% of patients.

Symptoms

Early symptoms of hypercalcemia include sedation and vomiting. When the plasma concentration of calcium exceeds about 10 mEq L^{-1}, cardiac conduction disturbances, characterized on the electrocardiogram as prolonged P – R interval, wide QRS complex, and shortened Q – T interval, occur. The most serious adverse effect of persistent hypercalcemia is renal damage.

Treatment

Asymptomatic patients with mild hypercalcemia are managed with intravenous administration of saline and furosemide to speed the renal excretion of calcium. When the plasma concentration of calcium exceeds about 10 mEq L^{-1}, aggressive therapy is necessary. In this situation, administration of mithramycin, a cytotoxic antibiotic, lowers plasma concentrations of calcium in 24 to 48 hours at doses one-tenth those used for chemotherapy. This calcium-lowering property reflects the ability of mithramycin to reduce the responsiveness of osteoclasts to parathyroid hormone. Calcitonin is also potentially useful for lowering the plasma concentration of calcium. Corticosteroids, such as prednisone, reduce the absorption of calcium from the gastrointestinal tract by antagonizing the actions of vitamin D. The onset of calcium-lowering effects by this mechanism, however, is often slow (7 to 14 days) and unpredictable. Edetate disodium (EDTA) is a chelating agent that forms soluble complexes with calcium in the blood and results in a rapid decrease in the plasma concentration of ionized calcium. Hypocalcemia may be so abrupt, however, that seizures occur. For this reason, EDTA is rarely utilized except as a slow intravenous infusion.

Bone Composition

Bone is composed of an organic matrix that is strengthened by deposits of calcium salts. The organic matrix is over 90% collagen fibers, and the remainder is a homogenous material called *ground substance*. Ground substance is composed of proteoglycans that include chondroitin sulfate and hyaluronic acid.

Salts deposited in the organic matrix of bone are composed principally of calcium and phosphate ions in a combination known as *hydroxyapatites*. Many different ions can conjugate to these bone crystals explaining deposition of radioactive substances in bone that may lead to an osteogenic sarcoma from prolonged irradiation.

The initial stage of bone production is the secretion of collagen and ground substance of osteoblasts. Calcium salts precipitate on the surfaces of collagen fibers forming nidi that develop into hydroxyapatite crystals. Bone is continually being deposited by osteoblasts and is constantly being absorbed where osteoclasts are active. Parathyroid hormone controls the bone absorptive activity of osteoclasts. Except in growing bones, the rates of bone deposition and absorption are equal so the total mass of bone remains constant.

Bone is deposited in proportion to the compressional load that the bone must carry. For example, continual physical stress stimulates new bone formation. The deposition of bone at points of compression may be caused by a piezoelectric effect. Indeed, small amounts of electrical current flowing in bone cause osteoblastic activity at the negative end of the current flow. Fracture of a bone maximally activates osteoblasts involved in the break. The resulting bulge of osteoblastic tissue and new bone matrix is known as the *callus*.

Osteoblasts secrete large amounts of alkaline phosphatase when they are actively depositing bone matrix. As a result, the rate of new bone formation is mirrored by measurement of the plasma concentration of alkaline phosphatase. Alkaline phosphatase is also elevated by any disease process that causes destruction of bone (osteomalacia, rickets).

Other than bone, calcium salts almost never precipitate in normal tissues. A notable exception, however, is atherosclerosis in which calcium precipitates in the walls of large arteries. Calcium salts are also frequently deposited in degenerating tissues or in old blood clots.

Exchangeable Calcium

Exchangeable calcium is that calcium in the body which is in equilibrium with calcium ions in the extracellular fluids. Most of this exchangeable calcium is in bone providing a rapid buffering mechanism to keep the calcium ion concentration in the extracellular fluids from changing excessively in either direction. The movement of exchangeable calcium in either direction is so rapid that a single passage of blood containing excess calcium through bone will remove almost all the excess calcium. It is estimated that about 5% of the cardiac output flows through bone.

Teeth

The major functional parts of teeth are the enamel, dentine, cementum, and pulp (Fig. 35-3) (Guyton, 1986). The tooth can also be divided into (1) the crown which is the portion that protrudes above the gum, (2) the root which protrudes into the bony sockets of the jaw, and (3) the neck which separates the crown from the root.

STRUCTURE. Dentine is the main body of the tooth and is composed principally of hydroxyapatite crystals similar to those in bone. In contrast to

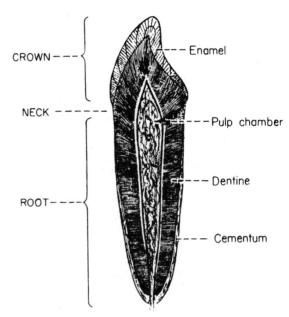

FIGURE 35-3. Schematic depiction of the functional parts of a tooth. (From Guyton AC. Textbook of Medical Physiology. 6th ed. Philadelphia, WB Saunders, 1986:937. Reproduced by permission of the author and publisher.)

bone, dentine lacks osteoblasts, osteoclasts, or spaces for nerves or blood vessels.

The outer surface of the tooth is covered by a layer of enamel that is formed prior to eruption of the tooth by special epithelial cells. Once the tooth has erupted, no more enamel is formed. Enamel is a protein that is extremely hard and resistant to corrosive agents such as acids or enzymes.

Cementum is a body substance secreted by cells that line the socket of the tooth. This substance is important in holding the tooth in place in the bony socket. Cementum has characteristics similar to normal bone including the presence of osteoblasts and osteoclasts.

The inside of each tooth is filled with pulp containing nerves, blood vessels, and lymphatics.

DENTITION. Each human forms two sets of teeth. The first set of 20 teeth are known as deciduous teeth. These deciduous teeth erupt between the ages of 7 and 24 months and remain in place until 6 to 13 years of age. After each deciduous tooth is lost, a permanent tooth replaces it. An additional 8 to 12 molars appear posteriorly in the mandible and maxilla making a total of 28 to 32 permanent teeth.

DENTAL CARIES. Dental caries result from the action of bacteria, the most common of which are streptococci. The first event in the development of caries is deposit of plaque which is a film of precipitated products of saliva and food. Bacteria inhabit this plaque setting the stage for the development of caries. Formation of acids by bacteria is the most important event leading to the development of caries. Enamel is very resistant to demineralization by acids and thus serves as a primary barrier to the development of caries. Once the carious process has penetrated through enamel of dentine, it proceeds rapidly reflecting the high solubility of the dentine salts.

Bacteria depend on carbohydrates for survival explaining the association between caries and the frequent ingestion of food containing glucose. If carbohydrates are eaten in small amounts through the day, such as in the form of candy, bacteria are supplied with their preferential metabolic substrate for many hours of the day. Conversely, ingestion of carbohydrates only at meals followed by brushing of the teeth limits availability of metabolic substrate to the bacteria and thus reduces the likelihood of caries formation.

Teeth formed in children who drink fluorinated water develop enamel that is about three times more resistant than normal to the formation of caries. Fluorine does not make the enamel harder than usual but instead it displaces hydroxyl ions in the hydroxyapatite crystals which, in turn, makes the enamel less soluble.

PHOSPHATE

Inorganic phosphate exists in two forms in the plasma. Since it is difficult to measure the exact amounts of each ion, it is common to express the total quantity of phosphate as mg dl^{-1} of phosphorus. The total quantity of inorganic phosphorus represented by both phosphate ions is 3.0 to 4.5 mg dl^{-1}.

Phosphate is important in energy metabolism and maintenance of acid – base balance. For example, phosphate ions are the most abundant buffer in the distal renal tubule allowing excretion of large quantities of hydrogen ions. These ions are also important intracellular buffers.

Vitamin D stimulates the systemic absorption of phosphate ions from the gastrointestinal tract. This absorbed phosphate is almost entirely excreted by the kidneys with parathyroid hormone acting to block reabsorption from the renal tubules. Conversely, vitamin D facilitates reabsorption of phosphate ions from the proximal renal tubules.

A decrease in the plasma concentration of phosphate permits the presence of a greater plasma concentration of calcium ions and inhibits deposition of new bone salts. Hypophosphatemia (phosphorus concentration below 1.5 mg dl^{-1}) causes a decrease in the concentration of adenosine triphosphate and 2,3-diphosphoglycerate in erythrocytes. Profound skeletal muscle weakness sufficient to contribute to respiratory failure may be a manifestation of hypophosphatemia (Aubier *et al*, 1985). Central nervous system dysfunction and peripheral neuropathy may accompany hypophosphatemia. Ethanol abuse and prolonged parenteral nutrition are causes of phosphorus deficiency.

MAGNESIUM

The most important physiologic effect of magnesium is regulation of the presynaptic release of acetylcholine from nerve endings. Magnesium activates enzyme systems such as alkaline phosphatase and is an essential cofactor in oxidative phosphorylation. Magnesium is distributed principally in intracellular spaces. Therapeutically, magnesium is most often used to treat toxemia of pregnancy. Typically, intravenous administration of 4 g of magnesium is followed by deep intramuscular injection of 5 g every 4 hours if a hyperreactive patellar reflex persists (Pritchard and Pritchard, 1975).

Hypomagnesemia

Hypomagnesemia is present when the serum magnesium concentration is less than 1.6 mEq L^{-1}. Causes of hypomagnesemia include malabsorption syndromes, chronic alcoholism, hyperalimentation, and protracted vomiting or diarrhea. Manifestations of hypomagnesemia mimic hypocalcemia and include central nervous system irritability, skeletal muscle spasm, and cardiac dysrhythmias. Treatment is intravenous administration of magnesium 10 to 15 mg kg^{-1} administered over 15 to 20 minutes.

Hypermagnesemia

Hypermagnesemia is present when the plasma concentration of magnesium exceeds 2.6 mEq L^{-1}. The most common cause is administration of magnesium to treat toxemia of pregnancy. Therapeutic plasma concentrations of magnesium for the treatment of toxemia of pregnancy are 4 to 6 mEq L^{-1}. Patients with chronic renal dysfunction are at an increased risk for developing hypermagnesemia since excretion of magnesium is dependent on glomerular filtration rate.

Hypermagnesemia is associated with sedation, cardiac depression, and suppression of peripheral neuromuscular function due to reduction in acetylcholine release from motor nerve endings as well as decreased responsiveness of the postjunctional membrane to acetylcholine. Furthermore, magnesium exerts a direct relaxant effect on skeletal muscle. Deep tendon reflexes diminish when the plasma concentration of magnesium exceeds 10 mEq L^{-1}. Paralysis of respiratory muscles and heart block may appear at concentrations that exceed 12 mEq L^{-1}. Treatment of life-threatening hypermagnesemia is with the intravenous administration of calcium followed by fluid loading and drug-induced diuresis.

Magnesium enhances neuromuscular blockade produced by both depolarizing and nondepolarizing neuromuscular blocking drugs (Ghoneim and Long, 1970) (see Chapter 8). The prolongation of neuromuscular blockade is greater for d-tubocurarine than for succinylcholine. Intravenous calcium is not predictably effective in antagonizing magnesium-enhanced neuromuscular blockade.

IRON

Iron present in food is absorbed from the proximal small intestine, especially the duodenum, into the circulation where it is bound to transferrin. Transferrin is a glycoprotein which serves to deliver iron to specific receptors on cell membranes. About 80% of the iron in plasma enters the bone marrow to be incorporated into new erythrocytes. In addition to bone marrow, iron is incorporated into reticuloendothelial cells of the liver and spleen. Iron is also an essential component of many enzymes necessary for energy transfer. A normal range for the plasma iron concentration is 50 to 150 μg dl^{-1}.

Iron that is stored in tissues is bound to protein as ferritin or in an aggregated form known as hemosiderin. Hemoglobin synthesis is the principal determinant of the rate of plasma iron turnover. When blood loss occurs, hemoglobin concentration is maintained by mobilization of tissue iron stores. Indeed, hemoglobin concentration becomes chronically reduced only after these iron reserves are depleted. For this reason, the presence of a normal hemoglobin concentration is not a sensitive indicator of tissue iron stores. The infant, parturient, and menstruating female may have iron requirements that exceed amounts available in the diet (Finch *et al,* 1977). Absorption of iron from the gastrointestinal tract is increased by ascorbic acid or the presence of iron deficiency. Antacids bind iron and impair its absorption.

Iron Deficiency

Iron deficiency is estimated to be present in 20% to 40% of menstruating females and in less than 5% of adult males and postmenopausal females (Cook *et al,* 1976). Attempts to achieve better iron balance in large parts of the population are evidenced by addition of iron to flour, use of iron-fortified formulas for infants, and by the prescription of iron-containing vitamin supplements during pregnancy.

Causes

Causes of iron deficiency anemia include inadequate dietary intake of iron (*e.g.,* nutritional) or increased iron requirements due to pregnancy, blood loss, or interference with absorption from the gastrointestinal tract. Most nutritional iron deficiency in the United States is mild. Severe iron deficiency is usually the result of blood loss, either from the gastrointestinal tract or in the female from the uterus. Partial gastrectomy and sprue are causes of inadequate absorption of iron.

Diagnosis

Iron deficiency initially results in a reduction of iron stores and a parallel decrease in erythrocyte content of iron. Depleted iron stores are recognized by a decreased plasma concentration of ferritin and the absence of reticuloendothelial hemosiderin in the bone marrow aspirate. A plasma ferritin concentration less than 12 μg dl^{-1} is diagnostic of iron deficiency (Cook, 1982). Iron deficiency anemia is present when depletion of total body iron is associated with a recognizable decrease in the blood concentration of hemoglobin. The large physiological variation in hemoglobin concentration, however, makes it difficult to reliably identify all individuals with iron deficiency anemia.

The frequency of iron deficiency anemia in infancy and in the menstruating or parturient female makes an exhaustive search for the cause of mild anemia less important. Conversely, in the male and postmenopausal female, in whom iron balance should be favorable, it becomes more important to pursue the search for a site of bleeding whenever anemia is present.

Treatment

Prophylactic use of iron preparations should be reserved for individuals at high risk for developing iron deficiency, such as pregnant and lactating women, low-birth-weight infants, and women with heavy menses. The inappropriate prophylactic use of iron should be avoided in adults because of excessive accumulation of iron which may damage tissues (Olsson *et al*, 1978).

Administration of medicinal iron is followed by an increased rate of erythrocyte production that manifests as an improved hemoglobin concentration within 72 hours. If the concentration of hemoglobin before treatment is reduced by more than 3 g dl^{-1}, an average daily incremental increase of 0.2 g dl^{-1} of hemoglobin is achieved with the usual therapeutic doses of oral or parenteral iron. An increase of 2 g dl^{-1} or more in the plasma concentration of hemoglobin within 3 weeks is evidence of a positive response to iron. If a positive response does not occur within this time, the presence of (1) continuous bleeding, (2) an infectious process, or (3) impaired gastrointestinal absorption of iron should be considered.

There is no justification for continuation of iron therapy beyond 3 weeks if a favorable response in the hemoglobin concentration has not occurred. Once a response to iron therapy is demonstrated, the medication should be continued until the hemoglobin concentration is normal. Iron therapy may be continued beyond this point for 4 to 6 weeks if it is desired to reestablish tissue iron stores. The creation of tissue iron stores requires several months of therapy.

ORAL IRON. Ferrous sulfate administered orally is the most frequently utilized approach for the treatment of iron deficiency anemia. Ferric salts are less efficiently absorbed than ferrous salts from the gastrointestinal tract. Ferrous sulfate is available as syrup, pills, or tablets. Although other salts of the ferrous form of iron are available, they offer little, or no advantage, over sulfate preparations. The usual therapeutic dose of iron for adults to treat iron deficiency anemia is 2 to 3 mg kg^{-1} (*e.g.*, 200 mg daily) in three divided doses. Prophylaxis and mild nutritional iron deficiency can be treated with modest doses of iron such as 15 to 30 mg daily if the object is the prevention of iron deficiency in pregnant patients.

Nausea and upper abdominal pain are the most frequent side effects of oral iron therapy particularly if the dose exceeds 200 mg. Hemochromatosis is unlikely to result from oral iron therapy that is administered to treat nutritional anemia. Fatal poisoning from overdoses of iron is rare but children 1 to 2 years of age are most vulnerable. Symptoms of severe iron poisoning may manifest within 30 minutes as vomiting, abdominal pain, and diarrhea. In addition, there may be sedation, hyperventilation due to acidosis, and cardiovascular collapse. Hemorrhagic gastroenteritis and hepatic damage are often prominent at autopsy. When iron overdose is suspected, a plasma concentration above 0.5 mg dl^{-1} confirms the presence of a life-threatening situation that should be treated with deferoxamine.

PARENTERAL IRON. Parenteral iron acts similarly to oral iron but should be used only when patients cannot tolerate or do not respond to oral therapy (*e.g.*, continuing loss is greater than can be replaced because of limitations to oral absorption). For example, parenteral iron therapy is necessary when disease processes, such as sprue, impair gastrointestinal absorption of iron. In addition, tissue iron stores may be rapidly restored by administration of parenteral iron in contrast to the slow response with oral therapy (Strickland *et al,* 1977). There is no evidence, however, that the therapeutic response to parenteral iron is more prompt than achieved with oral iron.

Iron dextran injection contains 50 mg ml^{-1} of iron and is available for intramuscular or intravenous use. After absorption, the iron must be split from the glucose molecule of the dextran before it becomes available to tissue. Intramuscular injection is painful for prolonged periods, and there is concern about malignant changes at the injection site (Weinbren *et al,* 1978). For these reasons, the intravenous administration of iron is preferred over intramuscular injections. A dose of 500 mg of iron can be infused over 5 to 10 minutes.

The principal side effect of parenteral iron therapy is the rare occurrence of a severe allergic reaction, presumably due to the presence of dextran. Less severe reactions include headache, fever, generalized lymphadenopathy, and arthralgias. Hemosiderosis is more likely to occur with parenteral iron therapy that bypasses gastrointestinal regulatory mechanisms.

COPPER

Copper is present in ceruloplasmin and is a constituent of other enzymes including dopamine beta-hydroxylase and cytochrome C oxidase. It is bound to albumin and is an essential component of several proteins. Copper is thought to act as a catalyst in the storage and release of iron to form hemoglobin. It is believed to be essential for the formation of connective tissues, hematopoiesis, and function of the central nervous system.

Copper deficiency is rare in the presence of an adequate diet. Supplements of copper should be given during prolonged hyperalimentation.

ZINC

Zinc is a cofactor of enzymes and is essential for cell growth and synthesis of nucleic acid, carbohydrates, and proteins. Adequate zinc is provided by a diet containing sufficient animal protein. Diets in which protein is obtained primarily from vegetable sources may not supply adequate zinc.

Zinc deficiency may occur in elderly or debilitated patients ingesting an inadequate diet or during periods of increased requirements as in growing children, pregnancy, lactation, or infection. Severe zinc deficiency is most likely in the presence of malabsorption syndromes. Based on animal evidence, it has been suggested that maternal zinc deficiency during pregnancy may have teratogenic effects. Cutaneous manifestations of zinc deficiency may occur during prolonged hyperalimentation emphasizing the need for zinc supplements in these patients. During hemodialysis, zinc chloride may be added to the dialysis bath. Symptoms of zinc deficiency include disturbances in taste and smell, suboptimal growth in children, hepatosplenomegaly, alopecia, cutaneous rashes, glossitis, and stomatitis.

CHROMIUM

Chromium is important in a cofactor complex with insulin and thus is involved in normal glucose utilization. Deficiency has been accompanied by a diabetes-like syndrome, peripheral neuropathy, and encephalopathy.

SELENIUM

Selenium is a constituent of several metabolically important enzymes. A selenium-dependent glutathione peroxidase is present in human erythrocytes. There seems to be a close relationship between vitamin E and selenium. Deficiency of selenium has been associated with cardiomyopathy suggesting the need to add this trace element to supplements administered during prolonged hyperalimentation.

MANGANESE

Manganese is concentrated in mitochondria especially in the liver, pancreas, kidney, and pituitary. It influences the synthesis of mucopolysaccharides and stimulates hepatic synthesis of cholesterol and fatty acids and is a cofactor in many enzymes. Deficiency is unknown clinically, but supplementation is recommended during prolonged hyperalimentation.

MOLYBDENUM

Molybdenum is an essential constituent of many enzymes. It is well absorbed from the gastrointestinal tract and is present in bones, liver, and kidneys. Deficiency is rare while excessive ingestion has been associated with a gout-like syndrome.

REFERENCES

Aubier M, Murciano D, Lecocguic Y, *et al.* Effect of hypophosphatemia on diaphragmatic contractility in patients with acute respiratory failure. N Engl J Med 1985;313:420 – 4.

Cook JD, Finch CA, Smith N. Evaluation of the iron status of a population. Blood 1976;48:449 – 55.

Cook JD. Clinical evaluation of iron deficiency. Semin Hematol 1982;19:6 – 18.

Denlinger JK, Kaplan JA, Lecky JH, Wollman H. Cardiovascular responses to calcium administered intravenously to man during halothane anesthesia. Anesthesiology 1975;42:390 – 7.

Denlinger JK, Nahrwold ML. Cardiac failure associated with hypocalcemia. Anesth Analg 1976;55:34 – 6.

Denlinger JK, Nahrwold ML, Gibbs PS, Lecky JH. Hypocalcemia during rapid blood transfusion in anesthetized man. Br J Anaesth 1976;48:995 – 1000.

Finch CA, Cook JD, Labbe RF, Culala M. Effect of blood donation on iron stores as evaluated by serum ferritin. Blood 1977;50:441 – 7.

Fukada S, Murakawa T, Takeshita H, Toda N. Direct effects of ketamine on isolated canine cerebral and mesenteric arteries. Anesth Analg 1983;62:553 – 8.

Gallagher JD, Geller EA, Moore RA, Botros SB, Jose AB, Clark DL. Hemodynamic effects of calcium chloride in adults with regurgitant valve lesions. Anesth Analg 1984;63:723 – 8.

Ghoneim MM, Long JP. The interaction between magnesium and other neuromuscular blocking agents. Anesthesiology 1970;32:23 – 7.

Guyton AC. Textbook of Medical Physiology. 6th ed. Philadelphia, WB Saunders, 1986:937.

Olsson KS, Heedman PA, Staugard F. Preclinical hemochromatosis in a population on high – iron-fortified diet. JAMA 1978;239:1999 – 2000.

Pitt B, Sugishita Y, Gregg DE. Coronary hemodynamic effects of calcium in the unanesthetized dog. Am J Physiol 1969;216:1456 – 9.

Pritchard JA, Pritchard SA. Standardized treatment of 154 consecutive cases of eclampsia. Am J Obstet Gynecol 1975;123:543 – 52.

Scheidegger D, Drop LJ. The relationship between duration of Q – T interval and plasma ionized calcium concentration: Experiments with acute, steady-state (CA^{++}) changes in the dog. Anesthesiology 1979;51:143 – 8.

Sialer S, McKenna DH, Corliss RJ, Rowe GR. Systemic and coronary hemodynamic effects of intravenous administration of calcium chloride. Arch Int Pharmacodyn Ther 1967;169:177 – 84.

Stanley TH, Isern-Amaral J, Liu W-S, Lunn JK, Gentry S. Peripheral vascular versus direct cardiac effects of calcium. Anesthesiology 1976;45:46 – 58.

Strickland ID, DeSaintouge C, Boulton FE, Francis B, Ronbikova J, Waters JI. The therapeutic equivalence of oral and intravenous iron in renal dialysis patients. Clin Nephrol 1977;7:55 – 7.

Su JY, Kerrick WGL. Effects of enflurane and functionally skinned myocardial fibers from rabbits. Anesthesiology 1980;52:385 – 9.

Ulmer DD. Trace elements. N Engl J Med 1977;297:318 – 21.

Weinbren K, Salm R, Greenberg G. Intramuscular injections of iron compounds and oncogenesis in man. Br Med J 1978;1:683 – 5.

Blood Components and Substitutes

INTRODUCTION

Blood components and certain drugs are most often administered systemically to overcome specific coagulation defects. Topical application of hemostatics is used to control surface bleeding and capillary oozing. Blood substitutes lack coagulation activity but are administered systemically to replace and maintain intravascular fluid volume.

BLOOD COMPONENTS

The advantages of blood components include (1) replacement of only the deficient blood procoagulant, cell, or protein, (2) minimization of the likelihood of circulatory overload, and (3) avoidance of transfusion of unnecessary donor plasma which may contain undesirable antigens or antibodies (Blajchman *et al,* 1979). Administration of specific components is recommended in all circumstances other than acute hemorrhage. In the presence of acute hemorrhage, whole blood is indicated to both replace oxygen-carrying capacity and intravascular fluid volume. A unit of whole blood can be divided into several components (Table 36-1).

Packed Erythrocytes

Packed erythrocytes are prepared by removing most of the plasma from whole blood at any time during the dating period. The resulting volume is about 300 ml and the hematocrit is 70% to 80%. Preparation of packed erythrocytes from whole blood just prior to transfusion results in the infusion of less sodium, potassium, ammonia, citrate, and lactic acid. As a result, packed erythrocytes so prepared are ideal for administration to patients with renal or hepatic dysfunction. The decreased amount of plasma infused with packed erythrocytes reduces the likelihood of allergic transfusion reactions as compared with whole blood.

Packed erythrocytes are stored at 1 to 6 Celsius. The expiration date for these cells is not different than that of the whole blood from which they are derived. The expiration date for frozen erythrocytes stored at −65 Celsius is 3 years. Once the unit has been thawed and deglycerolized or saline washed, however, it is outdated in 24 hours. The normal function of frozen packed erythrocytes after prolonged storage reflects the maintenance of concentrations of 2,3-diphosphoglycerate and adenosine triphosphate in the erythrocyte at levels near those present at the time the cells were frozen. At present, the major indication for frozen erythrocytes is a source of rare blood types (Chaplin, 1984). Otherwise, the cost of frozen erythrocytes is too great to justify their more frequent use. Furthermore, transmission of viral hepatitis still can occur following administration of frozen erythrocytes (Alter *et al,* 1978).

Packed erythrocytes are the product of choice when the goal is to increase oxygen-carrying capacity in the absence of preexisting hypovolemia.

Table 36-1

Components Available from Whole Blood

Component	Content	Approximate Volume	Shelf Life
Packed erythrocytes	Erythrocytes Leukocytes Plasma	300 ml	35 days in CPD-A
Fresh frozen plasma	Clotting factors	225 ml	Frozen — 1 year Thawed — 6 hours
Cryoprecipitated antihemophiliac factor	Factor VIII	Lyophilized powder	Determined by manufacturer
Factor IX concentrate	Factor IX Some factors II, VII, and X	Lyophilized powder	Determined by manufacturer
Fibrinogen			
Platelet concentrates	Platelets Few leukocytes Some plasma Few erythrocytes	50 ml	1–5 days
Granulocyte concentrates	Leukocytes Platelets Few erythrocytes	50–300 ml	24 hours
Albumin	5% albumin or 25% albumin	250 or 500 ml 50 or 100 ml	3 years
Plasma protein fraction	Albumin Alpha and beta Globulins	500 ml	3 years
Immune globulin	Gamma globulin	1–2 ml	3 years

One unit of packed erythrocytes typically elevates the hemoglobin concentration 1 g dl^{-1} (*i.e,* hematocrit 3%) in a 70-kg adult. Mixing of packed erythrocytes with 50 to 100 ml of saline decreases the viscosity of the blood product and allows more rapid infusion. Glucose solutions, in the absence of sufficient sodium to prevent osmotic lysis, cause hemolysis when mixed with packed erythrocytes. Calcium in lactated Ringer's solution may cause clotting if mixed with packed erythrocytes.

Fresh Frozen Plasma

Fresh frozen plasma is the liquid portion of a single unit of whole blood that has been separated from the erythrocytes within 6 hours and frozen promptly. It may be stored at −18 Celsius for up to 1 year. After thawing in a water bath at 37 Celsius the unit must be administered within a few hours.

Fresh frozen plasma contains all procoagulants except platelets in a concentration of 1 unit ml^{-1} and is specifically indicated for patients with documented deficiencies of labile plasma coagulation factors. Fresh frozen plasma is also effective for the rapid reversal of oral anticoagulants. Less frequent uses of fresh frozen plasma include treatment of antithrombin III deficiency and replacement of proteins as in infants with protein-losing enteropathy. There is no documentation that fresh frozen plasma has a beneficial effect when used as part of the transfusion management of patients with massive hemorrhage (Bove, 1985; Mannucci *et al,* 1982).

A substantial sodium load is associated with the administration of fresh frozen plasma. Dosage is determined by clinical response and, when possible, by laboratory measurements of plasma concentrations of appropriate coagulation factors. Compatibility for ABO antigens is desirable, but cross-matching is not necessary. Life-threatening allergic reactions may occur and transmission of diseases including hepatitis and acquired immunodeficiency syndrome is possible (Bove, 1985).

Plasma

Plasma is the liquid portion of a single unit of citrated whole blood separated during the dating period. Storage is at 1 to 6 Celsius for no more than 5 days beyond the maximum storage period of the whole blood from which it was derived. Plasma is used as a volume expander in treatment of burns and occasionally as a source of stable clotting factors II, VII, IX, and X. Cross-matching is desirable but not mandatory. Dosage is determined by clinical response and, when possible, by measurement of the plasma concentration of appropriate coagulation factors.

Cryoprecipitated Antihemophiliac Factor

Cryoprecipitated antihemophiliac factor (*i.e.,* factor VIII) is that fraction of plasma that precipitates when fresh frozen plasma is thawed (Ratnoff, 1978). This fraction can then be stored for future use. Cryoprecipitate is useful for treating hemophilia A since it contains high concentrations of factor VIII (80 – 120 units) in a volume of only about 10 ml. This preparation does not contain factor IX, and the content of factor VIII varies from donor to donor. Cryoprecipitate should be kept at room temperature after thawing and used within 3 hours.

Commercial factor VIII concentrates, in contrast to single donor cryoprecipitate, contain a standardized amount of antihemophiliac factor (Hoyer, 1981). These preparations, however, are more expensive than cryoprecipitated antihemophiliac factor and have a potentially greater risk for transmitting viral diseases since they are prepared from pooled plasma derived from a large number of donors. Indeed, hepatitis is the most common adverse side effect of pooled plasma products reflecting the multiple donor sources of fibrinogen that are present.

Hemolytic anemia may occur when cryoprecipitated antihemophiliac factor is given to individuals with group A, B, or AB erythrocyte antigens. These patients should be treated with cryoprecipitate from type specific or type O donors who have low titers of antibodies. About 10% to 15% of patients with hemophilia develop an immunoglobulin inhibitor that inactivates infused antihemophiliac factor. Assay for this inhibitor should be performed in all hemophiliacs prior to cryoprecipitate infusion, especially preoperatively. Multiple transfusions of cryoprecipitate may result in hyperfibrinogenemia emphasizing the substantial fibrinogen content of these preparations.

The major portion of transfused cryoprecipitate remains in the intravascular space with an elimination half-time of about 12 hours. Hemophilia A patients with factor VIII levels that are 5% of normal usually do not experience spontaneous bleeding. Effective hemostasis during and after major surgery, however, requires maintenance of a factor VIII level of at least 40% of normal for 7 to 10 days (Ellison, 1977).

Desmopressin

Desmopressin, a synthetic analogue of antidiuretic hormone, greatly increases factor VIII activity in patients with mild to moderate hemophilia and von Willebrand's disease (see Chapter 23) (Mannuci *et al,* 1977). Doses of 0.3 to 0.5 μg kg^{-1} given before and soon after dental surgery have prevented abnormal bleeding. Even cholecystectomy, thoracotomy, and tonsillectomy have been performed successfully in hemophiliac patients treated with desmopressin. This drug also improves hemostasis following cardiopulmonary bypass perhaps reflecting desmopressin-induced release of von Willebrand factor necessary for adequate activity of factor VIII and optimal function of platelets (Salzman *et al,* 1986). Desmopressin causes few adverse side effects although nausea and increases in blood pressure can occur. In contrast to blood components, desmopressin administration does not introduce the risk of transmission of viral diseases.

Factor IX Concentrate

Factor IX concentrate (*e.g.,* prothrombin complex, plasma thromboplastin component) is prepared from pooled plasma (Lusher *et al,* 1980). Cryoprecipitated antihemophiliac factor preparations do not contain factor IX. Factor IX concentrates can be infused without typing or cross-matching. Hypervolemic reactions do not occur because of the concentrated nature of these products and the small amount of fluid needed for administration. Factor IX concentrates are stable for at least 12 hours at room temperature following reconstitution.

Factor IX concentrates have a significant potential to cause hepatitis because of the pooled origin of these products. In addition, there is a high risk of thrombotic complications associated with infusion presumably reflecting the high concentrations of prothrombin and factor X that result from factor IX (Fuerth and Mahrer, 1981). This complication seems particularly likely and severe in patients with coexisting liver disease.

Fibrinogen

Fibrinogen preparations carry a high risk of hepatitis, and for this reason, are no longer commercially available. If fibrinogen is required, cryoprecipitated antihemophiliac factor may be administered. More important than administration of cryoprecipitate is control of the underlying defect leading to hypofibrinogenemia. Hypofibrinogenemia is most often due to decreased synthesis by a diseased liver or increased consumption associated with disseminated intravascular coagulation.

Aminocaproic Acid

Aminocaproic acid may be of benefit in the control of hemorrhage associated with excessive fibrinolysis caused by increased plasminogen activation. This drug is a monoaminocarboxylic acid that acts as a competitive inhibitor of plasminogen activators and to a lesser degree inhibits plasmin (Fig. 36-1). As a result, aminocaproic acid prevents formation of excessive plasmin which could destroy fibrinogen.

PHARMACOKINETICS. Aminocaproic acid is efficiently absorbed following oral administration and may also be administered intravenously. The usual adult dose administered slowly intravenously is 5 to 6 g every 6 hours. This dosage

$$\overset{\displaystyle O}{\underset{\displaystyle \parallel}{}}$$
$$H_2NCH_2(CH_2)_3CH_2COH$$

FIGURE 36-1. Aminocaproic acid.

produces therapeutic plasma concentrations of about 13 mg dl^{-1}. After prostatic surgery a dose of 6 g over 24 hours is effective because the drug is concentrated in the urine. Indeed, unchanged aminocaproic acid is rapidly excreted by the kidneys.

CLINICAL USES. Aminocaproic acid is useful for the treatment of hypofibrinogenemia that is due to primary fibrinolysis and not secondary fibrinolysis (*e.g.,* disseminated intravascular coagulation). A normal platelet count in the presence of hypofibrinogenemia supports the diagnosis of primary fibrinolysis. Nevertheless, isolated primary fibrinolysis is rare, and administration of aminocaproic acid in the presence of disseminated intravascular coagulation may cause fatal side effects (see the section entitled Side Effects).

Aminocaproic acid is useful in surgical and nonsurgical hematuria arising from the bladder, prostate, or urethra. For example, postoperative hematuria following transurethral and suprapubic prostatectomy is reduced by aminocaproic acid. This drug, however, is recommended only when hemorrhage is severe and correctable causes have been eliminated.

Aminocaproic acid has been used to treat hemorrhage in patients with hereditary angioedema or subarachnoid hemorrhage. This drug has also been administered before and during surgery for ruptured intracranial aneurysms, although the value in this situation and in patients following a subarachnoid hemorrhage is not convincingly documented. Aminocaproic acid does not control hemorrhage caused by thrombocytopenia or most other coagulation defects. Nevertheless, aminocaproic acid has been useful in hemophiliacs prior to and following dental extractions.

SIDE EFFECTS. Aminocaproic acid administered to a patient with disseminated intravascular coagulation may cause serious or even fatal thrombus formation. Nausea, vomiting, and diarrhea are frequent side effects of aminocaproic acid therapy. When aminocaproic acid is given during surgery, it is important to eliminate blood clots from the bladder because the drug accumulates in these clots and inhibits their dissolution. Administration of aminocaproic acid in the presence of renal or ureteral bleeding is not recommended since ureteral clot formation and possibly obstruction may result.

Platelet Concentrates

Platelet concentrates are prepared by centrifugation of citrated whole blood at room temperature within 4 hours after collection (Aisner, 1977). An average single unit of platelets contains more than 5.5 million platelets. Multiple units of platelets may be obtained from a single donor by plateletpheresis. The dating period of donor platelets stored at room temperature is 3 days except when placed in polyolefin plastic containers the dating period is 5 days. Platelets stored at 1 to 6 Celsius have a dating period of only 2 days. Single donor platelets obtained by plateletpheresis must be used within 24 hours after collection.

Ideally ABO-compatible platelets are used but, when unavailable, platelets from non–ABO-compatible donors may be administered if the preparations are not grossly contaminated with erythrocytes. Rh-compatible platelets should be used in females of childbearing age. Platelets possess HLA antigens on the cell membrane, and patients sensitized to these antigens will destroy infused platelets which manifests as the absence of a therapeutic response. In these patients, the administration of type-specific HLA platelets is the only effective treatment.

One unit of platelet concentrate will increase the platelet count 5000 to 10,000 mm³ (Aisner, 1977). Platelets stored at room temperature and infused within 24 hours of collection remain viable for as long as 8 days but require 8 to 24 hours following their administration to exert a hemostatic effect (Barrer and Ellison, 1977). In contrast, platelets that have been stored at 1 to 6 Celsius are viable for only 2 to 3 days, but the onset of hemostatic function is sooner than with cells stored at room temperature. Therefore, administration of platelets stored at 1 to 6 Celsius is more likely to shorten bleeding time in the presence of acute hemorrhage in the perioperative period due to thrombocytopenia. Platelets stored at 22 Celsius are appropriate for administration to the nonsurgical patient at risk for spontaneous hemorrhage due to thrombocytopenia (*e.g.*, platelet count less than 30,000 mm³).

Granulocyte Concentrates

Leukapheresis is continuous or intermittent flow centrifugation to obtain granulocytes for infusion to treat infection (Higby and Burnett, 1980; Schiffer, 1977). Granulocytes have been beneficial in patients recovering from bone marrow transplants. Phagocytic and microbicidal functions of collected granulocytes persist for about 48 hours.

Fever often accompanies granulocyte transfusion and can be ameliorated by administration of an antihistamine and an antipyretic. Granulocytes should be administered slowly to avoid pulmonary insufficiency which may be caused by sequestration of granulocytes in the pulmonary capillaries. Acute dyspnea, arterial hypoxemia, and interstitial infiltrates may be more likely when patients treated with amphotericin B receive granulocyte transfusions (Wright *et al,* 1981). Cytomegalovirus infections frequently are observed following granulocyte transfusions because the virus is concentrated in granulocytes.

Albumin

Albumin is obtained by fractionating human plasma that is nonreactive for hepatitis B surface antigen (Tullis, 1977). Coagulation factors and blood group antibodies are not present. In fact, an albumin-induced increase in the intravascular fluid volume may actually dilute the plasma concentrations of coagulant factors. Albumin is heated for 10 hours at 60 Celsius, which appears to remove the hazard of viral hepatitis. Albumin preparations contain sodium capylate and/or acetyltryptophanate as stabilizers allowing storage for about 3 years.

Albumin, 25 g, is equivalent osmotically to about 500 ml of plasma but contains only about one seventh the amount of sodium present in the same volume of plasma. Hypoalbuminemia is the most frequent indication for the administration of albumin. Albumin also binds bilirubin and has been used during exchange transfusions to treat hyperbilirubinemia. Administration of hypertonic 25% albumin will draw 3 to 4 ml of fluid from the interstitial space into the intravascular fluid space for every 1 ml of albumin administered. This is the reason 25% albumin is not recommended for administration to patients in cardiac failure or in the presence of anemia. The 5% solution of albumin is isotonic with plasma and is most often administered undiluted at a rate of 2 to 4 ml min⁻¹.

Plasma Protein Fraction

Plasma protein fraction is a 5% pooled solution of stabilized human plasma proteins in saline containing at least 83% albumin and no more than 17% globulins of which less than 1% are gamma globulins. Each 100 ml of solution provides 5 g of proteins. The preparation is equivalent osmotically to an equal volume of plasma. Although plasma protein fraction is prepared from large pools of normal human plasma, viral hepatitis is not a hazard because of heating to 60 Celsius for 10 hours. It must be recognized that plasma protein fraction does not contain any coagulation factors and may even dilute the plasma concentration of existing coagulants.

Plasma protein fraction is used to treat hypovolemic shock and provide protein to patients with hypoproteinemia. It is also effective for the initial treatment of shock in infants and small children with dehydration, hemoconcentration, and electrolyte deficiency caused by diarrhea. Although dose is guided by individual response, the usual treatment of hypovolemia or hypoproteinemia is with 20 to 30 ml kg^{-1} of plasma protein fraction (*i.e.,* 75 to 100 g of protein).

Hypotension accompanying rapid infusion of plasma protein fraction has been attributed to the presence of a prekallikrein activator that leads to production of bradykinin with resultant peripheral vasodilatation (Bland *et al,* 1973; Isbister and Fisher, 1980) (see Chapter 22). The level of prekallikrein activator in plasma protein fraction has subsequently been reduced and hypotension no longer seems to occur.

Signs of hypervolemia may occur when plasma protein fraction is administered to patients with increased intravascular fluid volumes. Administration of large quantities of plasma protein fraction to patients with impaired renal function has been reported to cause electrolyte imbalances resulting in metabolic alkalosis (Rahilly and Berl, 1979).

Immune Globulin

Immune globulin is a concentrated solution of globulins, primarily immunoglobulins, prepared from large pools of human plasma. This preparation protects against clinical manifestations of hepatitis A when administered before or within 2 weeks after exposure. Replacement therapy for patients with hypogammaglobulinemia is another use of immune globulin. Immune globulin prevents or modifies rubeola, rubella, and varicella. Low concentrations of immunoglobulin A are present in immune globulin emphasizing the need to avoid administration of this preparation to patients with anti-immunoglobulin A.

Hepatitis B immune globulin is a special preparation with a high antibody titer that delays the onset of hepatitis B and ameliorates the severity of the disease (Prince, 1978).

TOPICAL HEMOSTATICS

Topical hemostatics include absorbable gelatin sponge or film, oxidized cellulose, microfibrillar collagen hemostat, and thrombin. These substances may help to control surface bleeding and capillary oozing as associated with biliary tract surgery, partial hepatectomy, resections or injuries of the pancreas, spleen or kidneys, oral surgery, neurologic surgery, and otolaryngologic surgery. Although usually innocuous, the presence of bacterial contamination at the site of application of topical hemostatics may exacerbate infections.

Absorbable Gelatin Sponge (Gelfoam)

This sterile gelatin-base surgical sponge controls bleeding in highly vascular areas that are difficult to suture. The preparation may be left in place following closure of a surgical wound. Absorption is complete in 4 to 6 weeks, and scar formation or cellular reaction is minimal. When this material is placed into closed tissue spaces, it must be remembered that the material absorbs fluid and expands, which could press on neighboring structures.

Absorbable Gelatin Film (Gelfilm)

This sterile thin film is used primarily in neurologic and thoracic surgery for nonhemostatic purposes to repair defects in the dura and pleural membranes. It is also used in ocular surgery. Absorption is complete within 6 months of implantation.

Oxidized Cellulose (Oxycel) and Oxidized Regenerated Cellulose (Surgicel)

These celluloses do not enter into the normal clotting cascade, but when exposed to blood they expand and are converted to a reddish-brown or black gelatinous mass that forms an artificial clot. Oxidized cellulose has a low *p*H which contributes to a local cauterizing action. The hemostatic action of these celluloses is not enhanced by other hemostatic agents, and thrombin is destroyed by the low *p*H. Absorption of these products may require 6 weeks or longer. Some stenosis of arterial anastomoses may occur apparently from cicatricial contraction. These products should not be used for permanent packing or implantation in fractures because they may interfere with bone regeneration and cause cyst formation.

Microfibrillar Collagen Hemostat (Avitene)

When applied directly onto a bleeding surface this water-insoluble fibrous material attracts and entraps platelets to initiate formation of a platelet plug and development of a natural clot. Absorption without cellular reaction occurs in about 7 weeks. This topical hemostatic appears to retain its effectiveness in heparinized patients, in those receiving oral anticoagulants, and in the presence of moderate thrombocytopenia. Microfibrillar collagen hemostat is a useful adjunct to therapy in the oral cavity of patients with hemophilia. This material can be used on skin graft donor sites, around a vascular anastomosis where only minimal suturing is possible, and to control oozing from cancellous bone. It should not, however, be used on bone surfaces to which prosthetic materials are to be attached with methylmethacrylate adhesives.

As a foreign protein, microfibrillar collagen hemostat may exacerbate infection, abscess formation, and dehiscence of cutaneous incisions. Use of this hemostatic is not recommended for skin incisions because healing of the wound edges is impaired. Despite its protein structure, allergic reactions have not been described.

Thrombin

Thrombin is a sterile protein derived from bovine prothrombin. It is applied topically as a powder or in a solution to control capillary oozing in operative procedures and has also been effective in shortening the duration of bleeding from puncture sites in heparinized patients. Thrombin may be combined with gelatin sponge but should not be used to moisten microfibrillar collagen hemostat. Thrombin alone does not control arterial bleeding.

When applied to denuded tissue, thrombin is inactivated by antithrombins and by absorption onto fibrin. A *p*H below 5 also inactivates thrombin. Systemic absorption is unlikely and direct intravenous injection is contraindicated because resulting thrombosis could be fatal. Allergic reactions are a theoretical possibility when thrombin is used.

BLOOD SUBSTITUTES

Blood substitutes are useful to temporarily restore intravascular fluid volume until definitive treatment can be established. Commonly used blood substitutes tend to be inexpensive, have prolonged storage times, and lack the risk of transmitting viral diseases. It must be recognized that blood substitutes lack coagulation activity.

Dextran

Dextran 70 is a water-soluble glucose polymer (*i.e.*, polysaccharide) synthesized by certain bacteria from sucrose. The mean molecular weight of dextran 70 is about 70,000. This high molecular weight dextran is treated to yield low molecular weight dextran (*i.e.*, dextran 40) with a molecular weight of about 40,000. The renal threshold for dextran is at a molecular weight of about 55,000. Therefore, more dextran 40 than dextran 70 is filtered by the glomeruli. Dextran 70 is ultimately degraded enzymatically to glucose.

Clinical Uses

High molecular weight dextrans remain in the intravascular space for 12 hours. For this reason, they may be suitable alternatives to blood or plasma for expansion of intravascular fluid volume. For replacement of intravascular fluid volume, the recommended maximum dose during the first 24 hours is 20 ml kg^{-1} and 10 ml kg^{-1} on subsequent days. Therapy should not be continued for more than 5 days. Dextran 70 with 10% glucose is used in hysteroscopy to help distend and irrigate the uterine cavity and to prevent tubal adhesions after reconstructive tubal surgery for infertility. Because this dextran may be absorbed, adverse reactions are the same as those encountered after intravenous administration (Reisner, 1984) (see the section entitled Side Effects). Dextran 40 remains intravascular for only 2 to 4 hours and is used most often to prevent thromboembolism by reducing blood viscosity.

Low molecular weight dextran injected concomitantly with epinephrine slows intravascular absorption of the catecholamine (Ueda *et al*, 1985). Likewise, intercostal nerve blocks performed with bupivacaine plus low molecular weight dextran provide postoperative analgesia lasting an average of 40 hours compared with less than 12 hours following bupivacaine alone (Chinn and Wirjoatmadja, 1967; Kaplan *et al*, 1975). Presumably, dextran prolongs local anesthetic effects by delaying systemic absorption of the drug by an unknown mechanism.

Side Effects

The potential side effects of dextran must be considered before this blood substitute is selected in lieu of safer, although more expensive, products such as albumin or plasma protein fraction.

ALLERGIC REACTIONS. The incidence of allergic reactions following infusion of high or low molecular weight dextrans appears to be approximately 1 in every 3300 administrations (Isbister and Fisher, 1980). Nevertheless, low molecular weight dextran probably has considerably less antigenic potential than high molecular weight dextran. Histamine release may manifest as urticaria, angioedema, hypotension, and bronchospasm. Discontinuation of the dextran infusion is usually sufficient treatment but in rare cases, life-threatening allergic reactions require aggressive therapy. Indeed, fatal allergic reactions have occurred after intravenous administration of as little as 10 ml of dextran 70 (Isbister and Fisher, 1980).

INCREASED BLEEDING TIME. Increased bleeding time caused by interference with platelet function occurs especially when high molecular weight dextran is infused and the dose exceeds 1500 ml. This impairment of coagulation may not appear for 6 to 9 hours after the infusion.

ROULEAUX FORMATION. Dextran solutions, regardless of their molecular weight, may induce rouleaux formation and, therefore, interfere with subsequent cross-matching of blood. For this reason, blood for cross-matching should be obtained prior to dextran infusion. Dextrans may also interfere with certain tests of renal and hepatic function.

Hetastarch

Hetastarch (hydroxyethyl starch) is a synthetic colloid solution in which the molecular weight of at least 80% of the polymers ranges from 10,000 to 2,000,000. A 6% solution of hetastarch is as effective as 5% albumin as a plasma expander. The *p*H of hetastarch is about 5.5, and the osmolarity is near 310 mOsm L^{-1}. The larger molecules (molecular weight above 50,000) are removed from the circulation and stored temporarily in tissues, principally the liver and spleen. These larger molecules are degraded enzymatically by amylase. The average elimination half-time of hetastarch is 17 days with 90% being eliminated by the kidneys in about 42 days.

Clinical Uses

Hetastarch is used to expand intravascular fluid volume in the treatment of hypovolemia due to burns or hemorrhage (Puri *et al*, 1983). The usual total daily dose is 20 ml kg^{-1} but 40 to 60 ml kg^{-1} have been administered to patients with severe hypovolemia.

Side Effects

The hemodynamic effects of hetastarch are similar to albumin. Hetastarch probably has the same risk as dextran for producing allergic reactions (Porter and Goldberg, 1986). Excessive doses of hetastarch decrease the hematocrit, dilute plasma proteins, and interfere with the normal coagulation mechanism by diluting platelets and procoagulants (Straus, 1981). Thus, hetastarch is contraindicated in patients with bleeding disorders. Unlike dextrans, hetastarch does not cause rouleaux formation and cross-matching of blood is not impaired. Hypervolemia is a potential danger particularly in patients with impaired renal function because hetastarch is excreted primarily by the kidneys.

Stroma-Free Hemoglobin

Stroma-free solutions of hemoglobin may be useful as plasma volume expanders with the potential capacity for delivering oxygen to tissues and carrying carbon dioxide away from these same tissues (Rabiner *et al*, 1967). The value of stroma-free solutions for expanding the intravascular fluid volume is related to the high molecular weight (68,000) of hemoglobin. There is no need for cross-matching, and prolonged storage is possible. Renal dysfunction does not accompany administration of stroma-free hemoglobin solutions.

REFERENCES

Aisner J. Platelet transfusion therapy. Med Clin North Am 1977;61:1133 – 45.

Alter HJ, Tabor E, Meryman HT, *et al*. Transmission of hepatitis B virus infection by transfusion of frozen-deglycerolized red blood cells. N Engl J Med 1978;298:637 – 42.

Barrer MJ, Ellison N. Platelet function. Anesthesiology 1977;46:202 – 11.

Blajchman MA, Shepherd FA, Perrault RA. Clinical use of blood, blood components and blood products. Can Med Assoc J 1979;121:33 – 42.

Bland JHL, Laver MB, Lowenstein E. Vasodilator effect of commercial 5% plasma protein fraction solutions. JAMA 1973;224:1721 – 4.

Bove JR. Fresh frozen plasma: Too few indications — too much use (editorial). Anesth Analg 1985; 64:849 – 50.

Chaplin H. Frozen red cells revisited. N Engl J Med 1984;311:1696 – 8.

Chinn MA, Wirjoatmadja K. Prolonging local anesthesia. Lancet 1967;2:834 – 5.

Ellison N. Diagnosis and management of bleeding disorders. Anesthesiology 1977;47:171 – 80.

Fuerth JH, Mahrer P. Myocardial infarction after factor IX therapy. JAMA 1981;245:1455 – 6.

Higby DJ, Burnett D. Granulocyte transfusions: Current status. Blood 1980;55:2 – 8.

Hoyer LW. Factor VIII complex: Structure and function. Blood 1981;58:1 – 13.

Isbister JP, Fisher MM. Adverse effects of plasma volume expanders. Anaesth Intensive Care 1980;8:145 – 51.

Kaplan JA, Miller ED, Gallagher EG. Postoperative analgesia for thoracotomy patients. Anesth Analg 1975;54:773 – 7.

Lusher JM, Shapiro SS, Palascak JE, *et al*. Prothrombin complex concentrates in hemophilia with inhibitors: Multicenter therapeutic trial. N Engl J Med 1980;303:421 – 5.

Mannucci PM, Ruggeri ZM, Pareti FI, Capitanio A. 1-Deamino-8-D-arginine vasopressin: New pharmacological approach to management of hemophilia and von Willebrand's disease. Lancet 1977;1:869 – 72.

Mannucci PM, Frederici AB, Serchia G. Hemostasis testing during massive blood replacement. A study of 172 cases. Vox Sang 1982;42:113 – 23.

Porter SS, Goldberg RJ. Intraoperative allergic reactions to hydroxyethyl starch: A report of two cases. Can Anaesth Soc J 1986;33:394 – 8.

Prince AM. Use of hepatitis B immune globulin. Reassessment needed. N Engl J Med 1978;299:198 – 9.

Puri VK, Howard M, Paidipaty BB, Singh S. Resuscitation in hypovolemia and shock: A prospective study of hydroxyethyl starch and albumin. Crit Care Med 1983;11:518 – 23.

Rabiner SF, Helbert JR, Lopas H, Friedman LH. Evaluation of a stroma-free hemoglobin solution for use as a plasma expander. J Exp Med 1967;126:1127 – 41.

Rahilly GT, Berl T. Severe metabolic alkalosis caused by administration of plasma protein fraction in end-stage renal failure. N Engl J Med 1979;301:824 – 6.

Ratnoff OD. Antihemophilic factor (factor VIII). Ann Intern Med 1978;88:403 – 9.

Reisner LS. Anaphylaxis to intraperitoneal dextran. Anesthesiology 1984;60:259 – 60.

Salzman EW, Weinstein MJ, Weintraub RM, *et al*. Treatment with desmopressin acetate to reduce blood loss after cardiac surgery. A double-blind randomized trial. N Engl J Med 1986;314:1402 – 6.

Schiffer CA. Principles of granulocyte transfusion therapy. Med Clin North Am 1977;61:1119 – 31.

Straus RG. Review of the effects of hydroxyethyl starch on the blood coagulation system. Transfusion 1981;21:299 – 302.

Tullis JL. Albumin. 1. Background and use, 2. Guidelines for clinical use. JAMA 1977;237:355 – 63, 460 – 3.

Ueda W, Hirakawa M, Mori K. Inhibition of epinephrine absorption by dextran. Anesthesiology 1985; 62:72 – 5.

Wright DG, Robichaud KJ, Rizzo PA, Deisseroth AB. Lethal pulmonary reactions associated with combined use of amphotericin B and leukocyte transfusion. N Engl J Med 1981;304:1185 – 9.

C H A P T E R   37

Hyperalimentation Solutions

INTRODUCTION

Hyperalimentation is designed to supply all the essential inorganic and organic nutritional elements necessary to maintain optimal body composition as well as positive nitrogen balance. Alimentation by the gastrointestinal tract (*i.e.,* enteral nutrition) is preferred to intravenous alimentation (*i.e.,* parenteral nutrition) so as to avoid catheter-induced sepsis and to maintain the absorptive activity of the small intestine.

Hyperalimentation is indicated to prevent malnutrition in patients with (1) intestinal obstruction, (2) major burns, (3) trauma, (4) prolonged hypermetabolic states as associated with infection and malabsorption syndromes, and (5) serious gastrointestinal symptoms that occur during chemotherapy or radiotherapy. It is recommended that debilitated patients who have lost more than 20% of their body weight be treated with supplemental nutrients before operation (Powell-Tuck and Goode, 1981).

Hyperalimentation increases survival and improves recovery from many diseases (Mullen *et al,* 1979). Caloric needs should be individualized. Mildly catabolic patients usually gain weight with a daily provision of 35 to 45 calories kg^{-1} while patients in severe catabolic states may require up to 80 calories kg^{-1} (Harden, 1981). Adequate ca-

loric intake is essential for efficient utilization of amino acids.

ENTERAL NUTRITION

The ingredients and nutritional value of enteral alimentation solutions vary greatly. Some solutions contain minimally altered foods and others provide nutrients in the form of processed or chemically isolated food derivatives. Carbohydrates are the source of up to 90% of the calories emphasizing the increased osmolarity of these solutions. Fat has a higher caloric density than carbohydrates, does not increase the osmolarity of the formula as much as carbohydrates, and improves palatability. The amount of fat in enteral solutions varies. Unless the patient has maldigestion or malabsorption of fat, formulas with a normal range of fat content are preferred. In patients with hepatic cirrhosis or portacaval shunts, excessive plasma concentrations of fatty acids may act synergistically with high levels of ammonia and other toxins to exacerbate or cause hepatic encephalopathy. Selection of a formula that provides sufficient total nitrogen as protein or amino acids is essential for all patients. Low-protein formulations, however, are indicated for patients with severe renal dysfunction. Specialized crystalline amino acid supplements are available for nutritional deficiencies associated with liver or renal disease. Increased amounts of protein or amino acids are indicated when the nitrogen requirement is increased, as in those with trauma, burns, or sepsis. The efficient utilization of amino acids for tissue synthesis depends on adequate caloric intake.

Enteral Tube Feeding

Enteral tube feeding may be necessary when patients are unable to consume nutritionally complete liquefied food orally. Commercial formulations of natural foods can be so finely suspended that they pass through small bore tubes. Defined formula diets are necessary when luminal hydrolysis or absorption is impaired as in malabsorption syndromes. The tip of the 4 to 8 French nasogastric tube used to deliver enteral nutrition must be properly positioned in the stomach, duodenum, or jejunum. Dislodgement of the tip can result in pulmonary aspiration. Surgical placement of an esophagostomy or gastrostomy tube may be indicated for long-term feeding. For slow drip feeding, use of an automated infusion pump to control the rate of administration is useful. Indeed, absorption and tolerance are improved, and the incidence of side effects is reduced by slow constant feeding over several hours. The rate of infusion is typically 100 to 120 ml hr^{-1}. This slow rate of infusion prevents the dumping syndrome which may occur when hyperosmolar solutions are introduced rapidly into the small intestine (Kaminski, 1976).

Side Effects

Complications of enteral tube feedings are infrequent. Most side effects related to enteral nutrition are due to osmolar load. Too rapid administration of the more concentrated solutions may produce nausea and delayed gastric emptying as well as hypovolemia due to osmotic diuresis induced by glycosuria. Hyperosmolar dehydration progressing to nonketotic coma results from administration of a high glucose load. Caution is necessary if enteral nutrition is administered to patients prone to develop hyperglycemia (e.g., diabetes mellitus, treatment with glucocorticoids or adrenergic drugs). Excessive carbohydrates can also cause significant hypophosphatemia. Cutane-

ous rashes that occur after prolonged enteral nutrition are thought to be caused by fatty acid deficiency.

Pulmonary aspiration is always a danger when enteral tube feeding is utilized. Patients should be maintained in a semisitting position (head of bed elevated 30 degrees) during and for 1 hour after feeding. Preparations containing large amounts of electrolytes should be given cautiously to patients with cardiovascular, renal, or hepatic disease. Many commercial formulas contain large amounts of sodium. Dry preparations mixed with water become excellent culture media unless they are kept sterile and refrigerated.

PARENTERAL NUTRITION

Parenteral nutrition is indicated for patients who are unable to ingest, digest, or absorb nutrients from the gastrointestinal tract. Parenteral nutrition using isotonic solutions delivered through a peripheral vein is acceptable when the patient requires less than 2000 calories day^{-1} and the anticipated need for nutritional support is brief. When caloric requirements exceed 2000 calories day^{-1} or prolonged nutritional support is required, a catheter is placed in the central venous system to permit infusion of a hypertonic (1900 mOsm L^{-1}) nutrition solution.

Short-Term Parenteral Therapy

Short-term parenteral therapy (e.g., 3–5 days in patients without nutritional deficits) after uncomplicated surgical procedures is most often provided by a hypocaloric, non-nitrogen glucose-electrolyte solution. For example, glucose solutions, 5% to 10%, with supplemental sodium, chloride, and other electrolytes are commonly administered for short-term therapy (Table 37-1) (Stoelting and Miller, 1984). These solutions provide total fluid and electrolyte needs and sufficient calories to reduce protein catabolism and prevent ketosis. For example, daily infusion of approximately 150 g of glucose maintains brain and erythrocyte metabolism and decreases protein catabolism from skeletal muscle and viscera.

Amino acids may have a greater protein-sparing effect than glucose, but amino acids without glucose do not prevent negative nitrogen balance completely following major surgery. The higher

Table 37-1
Comparison of Crystalloid Solutions

Solutions	Glucose (mg dl⁻¹)	Na*	Cl*	K*	Mg*	Ca*	Lactate*	pH	mOsm L⁻¹
Extracellular fluid	90–110	140	108	4.5	2.0	5.0	5.0	7.4	290
5% Glucose/water	50							5.0	253
5% Glucose/ 0.45% NaCl	50	77	77					4.2	407
5% Glucose/ 0.9% NaCl	50	154	154					4.2	561
0.9% NaCl		154	154					5.7	308
Lactated Ringer's		130	109	4.0		3.0	28	6.7	273
5% Glucose/lactated Ringer's	50	130	109	4.0		3.0	28	5.3	527
Normosol-R		140	98	5.0	3.0		†	7.4	295

* mmol L⁻¹
† –contains acetate 27 mmol L⁻¹ and gluconate 23 mmol L⁻¹
(Adapted from Stoelting RK, Miller RD, eds. Basics of Anesthesia. New York, Churchill Livingstone, 1984; by permission of the authors and publisher.)

cost of amino acid solutions relative to potential benefit has prevented their popularity for use in place of glucose for short-term therapy (Craig *et al*, 1977; Greenberg *et al*, 1976).

Peripheral infusion of fat emulsions may be administered as a nonprotein source of calories to augment those supplied by glucose. Thrombosis of the peripheral vein used for infusion of the fat emulsion is a common problem.

Long-Term (Total) Parenteral Nutrition

Total parenteral nutrition (*i.e.*, intravenous hyperalimentation) is the technique of providing total nutrition needs by intravenous infusion of amino acids combined with glucose and varying amounts of fat emulsion (Fleming *et al*, 1976). Lean body mass is preserved, wound healing may be enhanced, and there may even be an improvement of an impaired immune response mechanism.

Total parenteral nutrition solutions contain a large proportion of calories from glucose and thus are hypertonic. For this reason, these solutions must be infused into a central vein with a high blood flow to provide rapid dilution. A catheter is often placed percutaneously into the subclavian vein and guided into the right atrium. The parenteral nutrition solution may be infused contin-

uously or intermittently over a 12- to 16-hour period. When intermittent administration is utilized, the infusion must be reduced gradually during the 1 to 1.5 hours preceding discontinuation to avoid hypoglycemia (see the section entitled Side Effects). The daily volume of infusion is about 40 ml kg⁻¹.

The efficacy of nutritional support is reflected by body weight measurements that confirm a maintenance or increase in lean body mass. Daily weight gains that exceed 0.5 kg, however, may signify fluid retention. Serum electrolytes, blood glucose concentration, and blood urea nitrogen should be measured frequently during total parenteral nutrition. Tests of hepatic and renal function are also recommended but at less frequent intervals.

Side Effects

The side effects of total parenteral nutrition are numerous and include catheter-related sepsis and metabolic abnormalities resulting from the administered nutrients (Table 37-2) (Michel *et al*, 1981).

SEPSIS. Total parenteral nutrition solutions infused through the intravenous catheter can support the growth of bacteria and fungi. Indeed, infection at the infusion site as well as systemic in-

Table 37-2
Side Effects Associated with Total Parenteral Nutrition

Sepsis
Fatty acid deficiency
Hyperglycemia
Nonketotic hyperosmolar hyperglycemic coma
Hypoglycemia
Metabolic acidosis
Hypercarbia
Fluid overload
Renal dysfunction
Hepatic dysfunction
Thrombosis of central veins

fection is a serious side effect of parenteral nutrition therapy.

A spiking temperature most likely reflects contamination via the delivery system or catheter. The catheter should be removed and the tip cultured to determine the appropriate antibiotic therapy. In view of the hazard of contamination, the use of the central venous hyperalimentation catheter for administration of medications, as during the perioperative period, or for sampling of blood, is not recommended.

FATTY ACID DEFICIENCY. Fatty acid deficiency may develop during prolonged total parenteral nutrition. Administration of 3% to 5% of the total caloric input as linoleic acid prevents or corrects this deficiency.

HYPERGLYCEMIA. The blood glucose concentration should be monitored until glucose tolerance is demonstrated, which usually occurs after 2 to 3 days as endogenous insulin production increases. In addition, blood glucose concentration should be carefully monitored during the perioperative period. Persistent hyperglycemia may lead to osmotic diuresis with resulting hypovolemia. Nonketotic hyperosmolar hyperglycemic coma is a potential complication of total parenteral nutrition. For these reasons, it may be necessary to add insulin to total parenteral nutrition solutions.

HYPOGLYCEMIA. Accidental sudden discontinuation of the infusion of total parenteral nutrition solution (*e.g.,* catheter kink or disconnect) may cause hypoglycemia. Indeed, total parenteral

nutrition infusion should be discontinued gradually over 60 to 90 minutes. Hypoglycemia occurs because the pancreatic insulin response does not always cease in unison with discontinuation of the parenteral nutrition solution. As a result, a high plasma concentration of insulin may persist in the absence of continued infusion of glucose. If total parenteral nutrition must be stopped suddenly, exogenous glucose should be infused for up to 90 minutes to prevent hypoglycemia.

METABOLIC ACIDOSIS. Hyperchloremic metabolic acidosis may occur because of the liberation of hydrochloric acid during the metabolism of amino acids in the parenteral nutrition solution.

HYPERCARBIA. Increased production of carbon dioxide resulting from the metabolism of large quantities of glucose may result in the need to initiate artificial ventilation of the lungs or in failure to wean from long-term ventilation support (Askanazi *et al,* 1981).

Preparation of Total Parenteral Nutrition Solutions

Total parenteral nutrition solutions are prepared from commercially available solutions by mixing hypertonic glucose with an amino acid solution. Sodium, potassium, phosphorus, calcium, magnesium, and chloride ions are added to total parenteral nutrition solutions. Trace elements including zinc, copper, manganese, and chromium must also be added if the need for parenteral therapy is prolonged (see Chapter 35). Requirements for vitamins may be increased emphasizing the need to add a multivitamin preparation to total parenteral nutrition solutions (see Chapter 34). Vitamin B_{12} and folic acid may be administered as components of a multivitamin preparation or separately. Vitamin D should be used sparingly because metabolic bone diseases may be associated with use of this vitamin in some patients on long-term total parenteral nutrition (Shike *et al,* 1980). Vitamin K is administered separately once every week. The serum albumin concentration will usually increase in patients receiving total parenteral nutrition if adequate amino acids and calories are given. Therefore, the routine administration of supplemental albumin is not necessary in the absence of signs or symptoms of hypoalbuminemia.

Fat emulsions are not mixed with the total parenteral nutrition solutions. Instead, these isotonic emulsions are administered intravenously through a separate peripheral vein or by a Y-connector into the same vein. Drugs should not be added to total parenteral nutrition solutions unless compatibility has been determined. To reduce the possibility of bacterial contamination, total parenteral nutrition solutions are prepared aseptically under a lamina air-flow hood, refrigerated, and administered within 24 to 48 hours.

Crystalline Amino Acid Solutions

Amino acid solutions contain a mixture of essential and nonessential amino acids but no peptides. Mild thrombophlebitis occurs infrequently during and after infusion of amino acid solutions. Flushing, fever, and nausea have been reported. Because amino acids increase the blood urea nitrogen concentration, they should be given cautiously to patients with impaired renal function. In patients with severe liver disease, hepatic coma may be precipitated by accumulation of nitrogenous substances in the blood.

Intralipid

Intralipid is a fat emulsion that is stabilized with egg yolk phospholipids and made isotonic by the addition of glycerol (Bryan *et al,* 1976). The major component fatty acids are linoleic acid (50%), oleic acid, and palmitic acid. This emulsion is metabolized in the same manner as natural chylomicrons, and a transient increase in the plasma concentration of triglycerides often occurs (see the section entitled Side Effects). These triglycerides are hydrolyzed to free fatty acids and glycerol.

Intralipid is used to prevent or correct essential fatty acid deficiency and to provide calories in high-density form on a regular basis during prolonged total parenteral nutrition (Meng and Wilmore, 1976). Because intralipid is isotonic with plasma, it is suitable for peripheral infusion and, if sufficient calories can be provided by this method, the use of hypertonic (greater than 10%) glucose by way of a central vein catheter may be avoided. Intralipid should comprise no more than 60% of the total caloric intake with the remainder supplied by glucose and amino acids.

Intralipid should not be mixed with other solutions, and electrolytes or vitamins are not added.

The emulsion may be infused into the same vein as glucose-amino acid solutions by means of a Y-connector. The emulsion contains particles that are too large to pass through a bacterial or particulate filter.

Side Effects

Increased plasma concentrations of triglycerides occur predictably when Intralipid is infused too rapidly or the emulsion is administered to patients with impaired fat metabolism. Excessive accumulation of lipids can be recognized by visual inspection of the plasma 6 to 8 hours after the infusion is completed. Because free fatty acids compete with bilirubin for albumin binding sites, Intralipid may increase the risk of kernicterus in infants with hyperbilirubinemia and may interfere with estimation of serum bilirubin concentrations (Andrew *et al,* 1976).

The fat particles in Intralipid do not aggregate, and there appears to be no risk of fat embolism. Hepatomegaly, altered liver function tests, decreased pulmonary diffusing capacity, thrombocytopenia, and anemia may occasionally occur (Postuma and Trevenen, 1979). Indeed, periodic liver function tests and platelet counts should be performed during long-term total parenteral nutrition. Vomiting, chest pain, allergic reactions, and thrombophlebitis have occurred during the infusion of Intralipid.

Liposyn

Liposyn is an intravenous fat emulsion that is 77% linoleic acid. Osmolarity is 300 to 340 mOsm L^{-1}. Liposyn, like Intralipid, is used to prevent essential fatty acid deficiency and as a source of calories during total parenteral nutrition.

Travamulsion

Travamulsion is an intravenous fat emulsion that is 56% linoleic acid. Osmolarity is about 270 mOsm L^{-1}.

REFERENCES

Andrew G, Chan G, Schiff D. Lipid metabolism in neonate: I. Effects of Intralipid infusion on plasma triglyceride and free fatty acid concentrations in neonate, II. Effect of Intralipid on bilirubin binding in vitro and in vivo. J Pediatr 1976;88:273 – 78, 279 – 84.

Askanazi J, Nordenstrom J, Rosenbaum SH, *et al.* Nutrition for the patient with respiratory failure: Glucose vs. fat. Anesthesiology 1981;54:373 – 7.

Bryan H, Shennan A, Griffin E, Angel A. Intralipid: Its rational use in parenteral nutrition of newborn. Pediatrics 1976;58:787 – 90.

Craig RP, Davidson HA, Tweedle D, Johnston IDA. Intravenous glucose, aminoacids, and fat in postoperative period. Controlled evaluation of each substrate. Lancet 1977;2:8 – 11.

Fleming CR, McGill DB, Hoffman HN, Nelson RA. Total parenteral nutrition. Mayo Clin Proc 1976;51:187 – 99.

Greenberg GR, Marliss EB, Anderson GH, *et al.* Protein-sparing therapy in postoperative patients. Effects of added hypocaloric glucose or lipid. N Engl J Med 1976;294:1411 – 6.

Harden WB. Clinical parenteral nutrition. Contin Educat 1981;14:43 – 53.

Kaminski MV. Enteral hyperalimentation. Surg Gynecol Obstet 1976;143:12 – 6.

Meng HC, Wilmore DW, eds. Fat Emulsions in Parenteral Nutrition. Chicago, American Medical Association, 1976.

Michel L, Serrano A, Malt RA. Nutritional support of hospitalized patients. N Engl J Med 1981;304:1147 – 52.

Mullen JL, Gertner MH, Buzby GP, Goodhart GL, Rasati EF. Implications of malnutrition in surgical patients. Arch Surg 1979;114:121 – 5.

Postuma R, Trevenen CL. Liver disease in infants receiving total parenteral nutrition. Pediatrics 1979;63:110 – 5.

Powell-Tuck J, Goode AW. Principles of enteral and parenteral nutrition. Br J Anaesth 1981;53:169 – 80.

Shike M, Harrison JE, Sturtridge WC, *et al.* Metabolic bone disease in patients receiving long-term total parenteral nutrition. Ann Intern Med 1980;92:343 – 50.

Stoelting RK, Miller RD, eds. Basics of Anesthesia. 1st edition. New York, Churchill Livingstone, 1984: 247.

Antiseptics
and Disinfectants

INTRODUCTION

Antiseptics and disinfectants are of obvious importance in the preoperative preparation of both patient and surgeon. Substances that are applied topically to living tissues to kill or prevent the growth of microorganisms are antiseptics. A disinfectant is an agent that is applied topically to an inanimate object to destroy pathogenic microorganisms and thus prevent infection. Antiseptics most often employed include (1) ethyl and isopropyl alcohols, (2) cationic surface active quaternary ammonium compounds, (3) the biguanide, chlorhexidine, (4) iodine compounds, and (5) hexachlorophene. Disinfectants most often employed are (1) the two aldehydes, formaldehyde and glutaraldehyde, (2) the phenolic compound, cresol, and (3) elemental chlorine.

Sterilization is the complete and total destruction of all microbial life including vegetative bacteria, spores, fungi, and viruses. Ethylene oxide is the only chemical available that is approved for sterilization of objects that cannot be heated or sterilized by other physical methods such as radiation.

ALCOHOLS

Alcohols are applied topically to reduce local cutaneous bacterial flora prior to penetration of the skin with needles. Their antiseptic action can be enhanced by prior mechanical cleansing of the skin with water and a detergent and gentle rubbing with sterile gauze during application.

Ethyl alcohol is an antiseptic of low potency but moderate efficacy being bactericidal to many bacteria (Lowbury et al, 1974). On the skin, 70% ethyl alcohol kills nearly 90% of the cutaneous bacteria within 2 minutes provided the area is kept moist. Greater than a 75% reduction in cutaneous bacterial count is unlikely with a single wipe of an ethyl alcohol wetted sponge and allowing the residual solution to evaporate. Isopropyl alcohol has a slightly greater bactericidal activity than ethyl alcohol due to its greater depression of surface tension. Neither alcohol, however, is fungicidal or virucidal.

QUATERNARY AMMONIUM COMPOUNDS

Quaternary ammonium compounds are bactericidal in vitro to a wide variety of gram-positive and gram-negative bacteria. Mycobacterium tuberculosis, however, is relatively resistant. Many fungi and viruses are also susceptible. Alcohol enhances the germicidal activity of quaternary ammonium compounds so that tinctures are more effective than aqueous solutions. The major site of action of quaternary ammonium compounds appears to be the cell membrane where these solutions cause a change in permeability.

Benzalkonium and cetylpyridinium (mouthwash) are examples of quaternary ammonium compounds. These compounds may be used preoperatively to diminish the number of organisms on intact skin. There is a rapid onset of action, but the availability of superior agents has reduced their frequency of use. Quaternary ammonium compounds have been widely used for the sterilization of instruments (Frank and Schaffner, 1976). Endoscopes and other instruments made of polyethylene or polypropylene, however, absorb quaternary ammonium compounds which may reduce the concentration of the active agent below the bactericidal concentration.

CHLORHEXIDINE

Chlorhexidine is a chlorophenyl biguanide that disrupts the cell membrane of the bacterial cell and is effective against both gram-positive and gram-negative bacteria (Fig. 38-1). As a handwash or surgical scrub, 4% chlorhexidine causes a greater initial decrease in the number of normal cutaneous bacteria than does povidone-iodine or hexachlorophene, and it has a persistent effect equal to or greater than hexachlorophene (Peterson et al, 1978). A 0.5% solution of chlorhexidine in 95% alcohol exerts a greater effect than 4% chlorhexidine alone.

Chlorhexidine is mainly used for the preoperative preparation of the surgeon and patient. It is also used to treat superficial infections caused by gram-positive bacteria and to disinfect wounds. As an antiseptic, chlorhexidine is rapid acting, has considerable residual adherence to the skin, has a low potential for producing contact sensitivity and photosensitivity, and is poorly absorbed even after many daily hand washings.

IODINE

Iodine is a rapid-acting antiseptic, that, in the absence of organic material kills bacteria, viruses, and spores. For example, on the skin a 1% tincture of iodine will kill 90% of the bacteria in 90 seconds while a 5% solution achieves this response in 60 seconds. In the presence of organic matter,

some iodine is bound covalently diminishing the immediate but not the eventual effect. Nevertheless, commercial preparations contain iodine in such excess that organic matter usually does not adversely influence immediate efficacy. The local toxicity of iodine is low with cutaneous burns occurring only with concentrations greater than 7%. In rare instances, an individual may be allergic to iodine and react to topical application. Symptoms of an allergic reaction usually manifest as fever and generalized skin eruption.

The most important use of iodine is disinfection of the skin for which it is probably superior to any other antiseptic. For this use, it is best employed in the form of a tincture of iodine because the alcohol vehicle facilitates spreading and penetration. Iodine may also be used in the treatment of wounds and abrasions. Applied to abraded tissue, 0.5% to 1% iodine aqueous solutions are less irritating than the tincture.

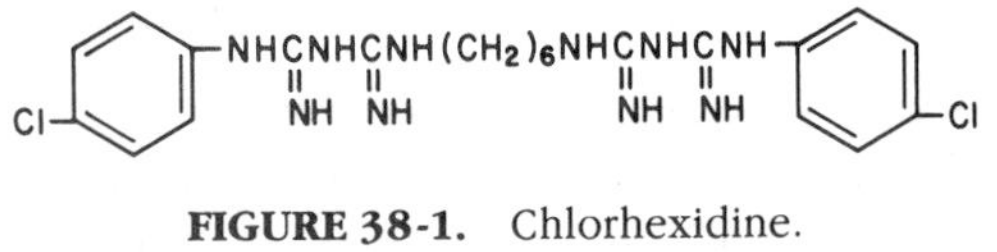

Iodophors

An iodophor is a loose complex of elemental iodine with an organic carrier that serves not only to increase the solubility of iodine but also to provide a reservoir for sustained release. The most widely used iodophor is povidone-iodine in which the carrier molecule is polyvinylpyrrolidone. A 10% solution contains 1% available iodine, but the free iodine concentration is less than 1 ppm. This is sufficiently low that little, if any, staining of the skin occurs. Because of the low concentration, the immediate bactericidal action is only moderate compared to that of iodine solutions.

Clinical Uses

The iodophors have a broad antimicrobial spectrum and are widely used as handwashes, including surgical scrubs, preparation of the skin prior to surgery or needle puncture, and to treat minor cuts, abrasions, and burns. A standard surgical scrub with a 10% solution will decrease the usual cutaneous bacterial population by over 90% with a return to normal in about 6 to 8 hours (Michaud, 1976; Dineen, 1978). As a vaginal disinfectant, iodophors may be absorbed introducing the risk of fetal hypothyroidism if used in a parturient (Vorherr et al, 1980). For the disinfection of endoscopes and other instruments, povidone-iodine is

FIGURE 38-1. Chlorhexidine.

superior to 3% hexachlorophene (Dunkerley *et al,* 1977).

HEXACHLOROPHENE

Hexachlorophene is a polychlorinated *bis*-phenol that exhibits bacteriostatic activity especially against gram-positive organisms (Fig. 38-2). Immediately after a hand scrub with hexachlorophene, the cutaneous bacterial population may be decreased by only 30% to 50% compared to over 90% following use of an iodophor (Michaud *et al,* 1976; Dineen, 1978). Nevertheless, 60 minutes later, the bacterial population surviving a hexachlorophene scrub will have decreased further to about 4%, while with the iodophor scrub the bacterial population will have recovered to about 16% of normal.

Since most of the potentially pathogenic bacteria on the skin are gram-positive, hexachlorophene is commonly used by physicians and nurses to reduce spread of contaminants from hands. This antiseptic is also used to cleanse the skin of patients scheduled for certain surgical procedures. Daily bathing of newborns with hexachlorophene, however, as a prophylactic measure against staphylococcal infections has been associated with brain damage (Cooperman, 1977; Check, 1978). Indeed, hexachlorophene is absorbed through intact skin in amounts sufficient to produce neurotoxic effects including cerebral irritability. In this regard, the routine use of hexachlorophene by pregnant nurses may be questionable.

FORMALDEHYDE

Formaldehyde is a potential volatile wide-spectrum disinfectant that is effective against bacteria, fungi, and viruses by virtue of precipitating proteins. A 0.5% concentration requires 6 to 12 hours to kill bacteria and 2 to 4 days to kill spores. A 2% to 8% concentration is used to disinfect inanimate objects such as surgical instruments.

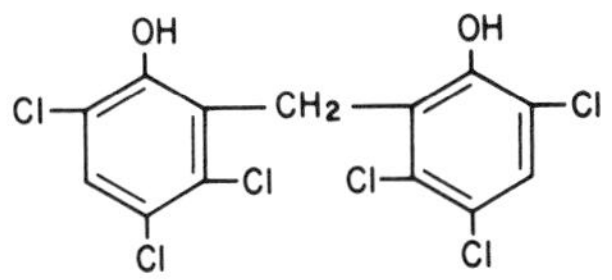

FIGURE 38-2. Hexachlorophene.

GLUTARALDEHYDE

Glutaraldehyde is superior to formaldehyde as a disinfectant because it is rapidly effective against all microorganisms including viruses and spores (Bovallius and Anas, 1977). This disinfectant also possesses tuberculocidal activity. Glutaraldehyde is less volatile than formaldehyde and hence causes minimal odor and irritant fumes. A period of 10 hours is necessary to sterilize dried spores while an acid-stabilized solution kills dried spores in 20 minutes. Neither alkaline nor acidic solutions are damaging to most surgical instruments and endoscopes. As a sterilizing agent for endoscopes, glutaraldehyde is superior to iodophors and hexachlorophene.

CRESOL

Cresol is bactericidal against common pathogenic organisms including *Mycobacterium tuberculosis.* It is widely used for disinfecting inanimate objects. Cresol should not be used to disinfect materials that can absorb this agent because burns could result upon subsequent tissue contact.

SILVER NITRATE

Silver nitrate is used as a caustic, antiseptic, and astringent. A solid form is used for the cauterization of wounds and for removing granulation tissue. It is conveniently dispensed in pencils that should be moistened before use. Solutions of silver nitrate are strongly bactericidal especially for gonococci accounting for its frequent use as prophylaxis of ophthalmia neonatorum.

Silver sulfadiazine or nitrate is used in the treatment of burns (Kucan *et al,* 1981). In this regard, hypochloremia may occur reflecting combination of the silver ion with chloride. Hyponatremia also results because the cations are attracted by chloride ions into the exudate. Furthermore, absorbed nitrate can cause methemoglobinemia.

MERCURY

Organic mercurial compounds are nonirritating but lack bactericidal activity. In fact, these compounds possess only weak bacteriostatic activity and are less effective than ethyl alcohol. Serum and tissue proteins reduce antimicrobial activity, and skin sensitization is common.

ETHYLENE OXIDE

Ethylene oxide is readily diffusible, noncorrosive, and antimicrobial to all organisms at room temperature. This gaseous alkylating agent is widely used as an alternative to heat sterilization. It reacts with chloride and water to produce two additional active germicides, ethylene chlorohydrin and ethylene glycol. Special sterilizing chambers are required because the gas must remain in contact with the objects for several hours. Adequate airing of sterilized materials, such as tracheal tubes, is essential to ensure removal of residual ethylene oxide and thus minimize tissue irritation (Stetson *et al,* 1976).

REFERENCES

Bovallius A, Anas A. Surface-decontaminating action of glutaraldehyde in the gas-aerosol phase. Appl Environ Microbiol 1977;34:129–34.

Check W. New study shows hexachlorophene is teratogenic in humans (Editorial). JAMA 1978;240:513–4.

Cooperman EM. Hexachlorophene in the nursery. Can Med Assoc J 1977;117:205–6.

Dineen P. Hand-washing degerming: A comparison of povidone-iodine and chlorhexidine. Clin Pharmacol Ther 1978;23:63–7.

Dunkerley RC, Cromer MD, Edmiston CE, Dunn GD. Practical technique for adequate cleansing of endoscopes: A bacteriological study of pHisoHex and Betadine. Gastrointest Endosc 1977;23:148–9.

Frank MJ, Schaffner W. Contaminated aqueous benzalkonium chloride. An unnecessary hospital infection hazard. JAMA 1976;236:2418–9.

Kucan JO, Robson MC, Heggers JP, Ko F. Comparison of silver sulfadiazine, povidone-iodine, and physiological saline in treatment of chronic pressure ulcers. J Am Geriatr Soc 1981;29:232–5.

Lowbury EJL, Lilly HA, Ayliffe GAJ. Preoperative disinfection of surgeon's hands: Use of alcohol solutions and effects of gloves on skin flora. Br Med J 1974;4:369–72.

Michaud RN. Application of a gloved-hand model for multiparameter measurements of skin-degerming activity. J Clin Microbiol 1976;3:406–13.

Peterson AF, Rosenberg A, Alatery SD. Comparative evaluation of surgical scrub. Surg Gynecol Obstet 1978;146:63–5.

Stetson JB, Whitbourne BS, Eastman C. Ethylene oxide degassing of rubber and plastic materials. Anesthesiology 1976;44:174–80.

Vorherr H, Mehta P, Ulrich JA, Messer RH. Vaginal absorption of povidone-iodine. JAMA 1980;244:2628–9.

SECTION II

Physiology

C H A P T E R   39

Cell Structure
and Function

INTRODUCTION

The basic living unit of the body is the cell. Each organ is a mass of cells held together by intercellular supporting structures. The entire body consists of an estimated 75 trillion cells of which about 25 trillion are erythrocytes (Guyton, 1986a). A common characteristic of all cells is dependence on oxygen to combine with nutrients (carbohydrates, lipids, proteins) to release energy that is necessary for cellular function (see Chapter 58). The end-products of these chemical reactions are delivered into the surrounding fluids. Most cells have the ability to reproduce especially when injury reduces the number of a specific cell type.

FLUID ENVIRONMENT OF CELLS

All cells exist in nearly the same environment of extracellular fluid (see Chapter 40). This is the reason extracellular fluid is referred to as the internal environment (*milieu intérieur*) of the body. The various organs of the body function to maintain a constant composition of extracellular fluid (*i.e.,* homeostasis) (Soderberg, 1964). For example, the lungs provide oxygen to extracellular fluid, the kidneys maintain optimal concentrations of ions, and the gastrointestinal tract provides nutrient sources. The liver contributes to homeostasis by changing the chemical composition of many of the nutrients absorbed from the gastrointestinal tract to more usable materials. The nervous system, especially the autonomic nervous system, and hormones from the endocrine glands produce responses essential to maintenance of extracellular fluid composition. Furthermore, the lungs and kidneys are of critical importance for removing metabolic end-products that result from cellular activity. Almost every cell is within 25 to 50 microns of a capillary assuring diffusion of substances from plasma to cells within seconds.

ANATOMY OF A CELL

The two principal components of cells are the nucleus and the cytoplasm (Fig. 39-1). The nucleus is separated from the cytoplasm by a nuclear membrane, and the cytoplasm is separated from the surrounding fluids by a cell membrane. Organelles of the cell include the cell membrane, nuclear membrane, mitochondria, endoplasmic reticulum, and lysosomes.

Protoplasm

Protoplasm is a collective term for the substances that make up the cell. The five basic components of protoplasm are (1) water, (2) electrolytes, (3) proteins including enzymes, (4) lipids, and (5) carbohydrates.

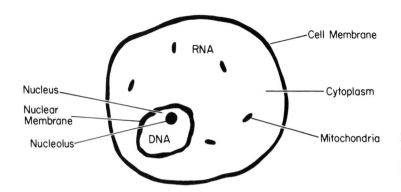

FIGURE 39-1. The principal components of cells are the nucleus and cytoplasm and their corresponding membranes.

Water

About 70% to 85% of the cell substance is water. Cellular chemicals are dissolved in this water, and these substances can diffuse to all parts of the cell in this fluid medium.

Electrolytes

The most important electrolytes in the cell are potassium, magnesium, phosphate, sulfate, bicarbonate, and small amounts of sodium, chloride, and calcium ions. These ions are dissolved in water and provide inorganic chemicals for cellular reactions. Ions acting at the cell membrane allow transmission of electrochemical impulses in skeletal muscle fibers and nerve fibers. Furthermore, intracellular electrolytes determine the activity of different enzymatically catalyzed reactions that are necessary for cellular metabolism.

Proteins

Proteins, next to water, are the most abundant substances in most cells accounting for 10% to 20% of the cell mass. These proteins are categorized as structural proteins and globular proteins (see Chapter 58).

STRUCTURAL PROTEINS. Conjugated or structural proteins are present in the cell as long thin filaments. In skeletal muscle, these proteins provide the contractile mechanism. Microtubules are structural proteins that provide the basis of cilia (Stephens and Edds, 1976).

GLOBULAR PROTEINS. Globular proteins function as enzymes that catalyze chemical reactions. Nucleoproteins of the cell contain deoxyribonucleic acid (DNA) which constitutes the genes. Genes control the overall function of the cell and the transmission of hereditary characteristics from cell to cell.

Lipids

Important lipids in most cells are phospholipids and cholesterol. These lipids constitute about 2% of total cell mass. A special feature of phospholipids and cholesterol is their poor or absent solubility in water. Lipids are major components of membranes present in cells including the nuclear membrane, cell membrane, and membranes surrounding intracytoplasmic organelles such as the endoplasmic reticulum and mitochondria.

In addition to phospholipids and cholesterol, certain cells contain large amounts (up to 95% of cell mass) of triglycerides. The fat stored in these adipose cells is an important reserve for energy whenever it is required.

Carbohydrates

Typically, about 1% of the total mass of cells is carbohydrates. Nevertheless, carbohydrate in the form of glucose is present in the surrounding extracellular fluid and readily available to supply nutrient needs of the cell. Furthermore, a small amount of carbohydrate is often stored in the cells as glycogen, which can rapidly supply the cells' energy requirements.

Membranes

Membranes of cells include the cell membrane, nuclear membranes, membranes of the endoplasmic reticulum, and membranes of the mitochondria, lysosomes, and Golgi complex. These membranes are composed primarily of lipids and proteins (Lodish and Rothman, 1979). Lipids provide a barrier to the movement between cells of water and substances dissolved in water.

Cell Membranes

Cell membranes completely envelop every cell. These membranes typically consist of proteins (55%), phospholipids (25%), cholesterol (13%), and other lipids and carbohydrates. Continuous over the entire cell membrane surface is a lipid bilayer (*i.e.,* two molecules thick) that is interspersed with large globular proteins (Fig. 39-2) (Lodish and Rothman, 1979). The lipid bilayer of the cell membrane is nearly impermeable to water and water-soluble substances such as ions, glucose, and urea. Conversely, fat-soluble substances such as oxygen and carbon dioxide readily cross the cell membrane. Because the lipid bilayer is fluid, it can flow to other areas of the cell membrane carrying proteins or other dissolved substances with it (Capaldi, 1974).

Proteins in cell membranes function as enzymes and provide the structural framework for passageways (channels or pores) that allow movement of ions and other water-soluble substances between the extracellular and intracellular fluid. In the cytoplasm immediately below the cell membranes are proteins which provide a semisolid support for the cell membrane (Goldman *et al,* 1979). These fibrillar proteins may also be organized in tubular structures known as microtubules which likewise provide a rigid physical skeleton for certain parts of the cell (Stephens and Edds, 1976).

Carbohydrate components of cell membranes are the glyco portion of glycoprotein molecules. This is the portion of cell membranes that enters into immune reactions. Furthermore, these glycoproteins often serve as receptor substances for binding hormones which evoke activity in the cells.

Nuclear Membranes

Nuclear membranes are actually two membranes separated by a wide space. Constituents of these membranes are similar to cell membranes including the bilayer of lipid molecules and channels through which dissolved or suspended substances, including large ribosomes, can freely pass between fluids of the nucleus and cytoplasm.

Endoplasmic Reticulum Membranes

The endoplasmic reticulum is a series of lipid bilayer protein membranes present in the membranes of cells. The total surface area of these endoplasmic reticulum membranes is great and combined with the presence of many enzyme systems provides the machinery for a major portion of the metabolic functions of the cell. For example, the surface area of the endoplasmic reticulum membranes in hepatocytes is 30 to 40 times the surface area of the cell membrane (Guyton, 1986b).

Ribosomes, composed mainly of ribonucleic acid (RNA), are attached to the outer portions of many parts of the endoplasmic reticulum mem-

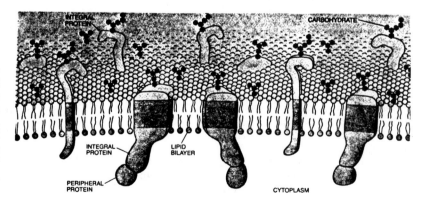

FIGURE 39-2. The cell membrane is a two-molecule-thick lipid bilayer containing protein molecules that extend through the bilayer. (From Lodish HF, Rothman JE. The assembly of cell membranes. Sci Am 1979; 240:48–63. Copyright 1979 by Scientific American, Inc. All rights reserved.)

branes. These ribosomes function in the synthesis of proteins in the cells. The portion of the membrane containing these ribosomes is known as the rough endoplasmic reticulum. The part of the membrane that lacks ribosomes is the smooth endoplasmic reticulum. This smooth portion of the endoplasmic reticulum membrane functions in the synthesis of lipid substances and many enzymatic processes.

Golgi Complex Membranes

The membranes of the Golgi complex resemble the smooth endoplasmic reticulum. Golgi complexes are particularly prominent in secretory cells.

Proteins synthesized in the endoplasmic reticulum are transported to the Golgi complex where they are stored in highly concentrated packets (secretory vesicles) for subsequent release into the cell cytoplasm. The vesicles may also diffuse to the surface of the cell membrane and discharge their contents to the exterior by the process of exocytosis. Exocytosis is often stimulated by the entrance of calcium ions into the cell.

Specialized portions of the Golgi complex form lysosomes and other portions form peroxisomes. Peroxisomes can both form and destroy hydrogen peroxide (Masters and Holmes, 1977). Destruction of hydrogen peroxide, which is formed by many metabolic reactions, is essential as accumulation of high concentrations has a toxic effect on important enzyme systems.

Organelles

Organelles are large particles in the cytoplasm as represented by the mitochondria and lysosomes.

Mitochondria

The mitochondria are composed principally of an inner and outer lipid bilayer protein membrane (Williamson, 1979). Infoldings of the inner membrane form shelves onto which the oxidative enzymes of the cell are attached. The inner portions of the mitochondria are filled with a gel matrix containing large amounts of dissolved enzymes that are necessary for extracting energy from nutrients in the cell. These enzymes operate in association with oxidative enzymes on the shelves to cause oxidation of nutrients leading to formation of carbon dioxide and water. The liberated energy from the nutrients is used to synthesize adenosine triphosphate (ATP). This ATP leaves the mitochondria and diffuses throughout the cell providing energy for cellular functions. Increased needs for ATP in the cell lead to an increase in the number of mitochondria. In the absence of mitochondria, the cell is unable to extract sufficient energy from nutrients and oxygen leading to a cessation of cellular function. The major portion of ATP formed in the cell is synthesized in the mitochondria via the Krebs' cycle (see Chapter 58).

Lysosomes

Lysosomes are scattered throughout the cytoplasm providing an intracellular digestive system (DeDuve and Williams, 1966). This system permits the cell to remove damaged structures or foreign particles, especially bacteria. Structurally lysosomes are surrounded by bilayer lipid membranes and filled with digestive (hydrolytic) enzymes. These enzymes are capable of splitting organic compounds including proteins, nucleic acids, lipids, glycogen, and polysaccharides. Bactericidal substances in the lysosome kill phagocytized bacteria before they can cause cellular damage. These bactericidal substances include (1) lysozyme that dissolves the cell membrane of bacteria, (2) lysoferrin that binds iron and other metals that are essential for bacterial growth, (3) acid that has a *p*H below 4, and (4) hydrogen peroxide that can disrupt some bacterial metabolic systems.

Disruption of lysosome membranes permits digestive enzymes to escape from lysosomes into the cytoplasm of the cell where they split substances such as amino acids and glucose. Indeed, damage to cells causes lysosomes to rupture releasing digestive enzymes that begin immediately to digest and remove components of the damaged cell (*i.e.,* autolysis) making room for its replacement by a new cell from mitotic reproduction of an adjacent cell.

Nucleus

The nucleus contains large amounts of deoxyribonucleic acid (DNA) (*i.e.,* genes) that determines the characteristics of the protein enzymes present in the cytoplasm. As such, the nucleus controls the chemical reactions that occur in the cell and the reproduction of the cell by mitosis. During mitosis, the chromatin material in the nucleus becomes readily identifiable even under the light microscope as highly structured chromosomes (Fig. 39-1).

The nucleus may contain nucleoli which, unlike most organelles, lack a limiting membrane. Nucleoli are proteins that contain large amounts of RNA similar to that present in ribosomes. RNA can diffuse through channels in the nuclear membrane and attach to the endoplasmic reticulum in the cytoplasm where it plays an important role in the synthesis of proteins.

INGESTION BY CELLS

Cells may obtain essential nutrients and other substances by (1) diffusion through the matrix or channels in cell membranes, (2) active transport through cell membranes mediated by enzymes and specialized carrier substances, and (3) endocytosis by which cell membranes engulf particulate matter or extracellular fluid and its contents. Endocytosis is dependent on energy derived from ATP within the cell and the presence of calcium ions in extracellular fluid (Allison and Davies, 1974). Phagocytosis and pinocytosis are forms of endocytosis.

Phagocytosis

Phagocytosis is the ingestion of particulate matter (*e.g.,* bacteria, damaged cells) by a cell. The process of phagocytosis is initiated when certain objects contact the cell membrane. Typically, objects that have an electronegative charge are repelled by cell membranes. Most normal particulate matter in extracellular fluid is also negatively charged and thus not vulnerable to phagocytosis. Conversely, most damaged tissue and foreign substances have been prepared for phagocytosis by attachment of antibodies. This process is referred to as opsonization and results in acquirement of a positive charge that renders the substance vulnerable to phagocytosis.

Pinocytosis

Pinocytosis refers to ingestion of small amounts of extracellular fluid and dissolved substances in the form of minute vesicles. Contact of the cell membrane by strong electrolyte solutions or proteins initiates pinocytosis. Indeed, pinocytosis is the only mechanism by which proteins can pass through cell membranes.

CONTROL OF CELL FUNCTION

A specific nucleic acid in the nucleus of the cell known as DNA functions as a gene which controls the formation of another specific nucleic acid known as RNA (Fig. 39-3). This RNA leaves the nucleus and enters the cytoplasm of the cell where it controls the formation of a specific protein (Friedman, 1976; Rich and Kim, 1978). The majority of formed proteins are enzymes that catalyze the different cellular reactions including oxidative reactions that supply energy to the cell. The ultimate importance of DNA lies in its ability to control the formation of other substances in the cell by means of the so-called genetic code.

Cell Reproduction

Cell reproduction (*i.e.,* mitosis) is determined by the DNA-genetic system. The first stage of mitosis is prophase during which the DNA becomes shortened into well-defined chromosomes. This stage is followed by prometaphase, metaphase, and anaphase. During anaphase, there is complete separation of the chromosomes to form chromatids. During the subsequent telophase, a new nuclear membrane develops around each set of chromosomes. The period between mitosis is called interphase. This interphase may be as brief as 10 hours

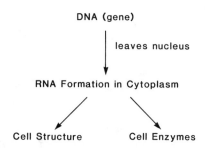

FIGURE 39-3. Deoxyribonucleic acid (DNA) functions as a gene and is responsible for initiating the events that control cell function.

for rapidly dividing bone marrow cells or germinal layers of the skin and epithelium of the gastrointestinal tract. Conversely, interphase lasts a lifetime for nerve and striated muscle cells.

If there is an insufficient number of some types of cells in the body, these insufficient cells will grow and reproduce rapidly until appropriate numbers are again available. For example, nearly all the liver can be removed surgically and the remaining cells will reproduce until liver mass is returned to almost normal. Similar reproduction occurs for glandular cells, cells of the bone marrow, and gastrointestinal epithelium. Highly differentiated cells, however, such as nerve and muscle cells are not capable of reproduction to replace lost cells.

Chromosomes

Chromosomes consist of DNA and proteins. Histones are major portions of the protein component. These proteins are presumed to keep the DNA strands arranged in a double helix that is folded and sufficiently compact to fit in the nucleus. Each human cell contains 46 chromosomes arranged in 23 pairs. Chalones are substances that are secreted by cells to initiate a negative feedback mechanism to stop cell growth and mitosis when the number of cells present is adequate.

CELL MEMBRANE TRANSPORT

Extracellular fluid is the source of nutrients and other substances needed for cellular function. Transport of substances from extracellular fluid to intracellular fluid of the cell occurs by diffusion and/or active transport across cell membranes. Diffusion reflects free movement of substances in a random fashion due to normal kinetic motion of molecules. Active transport reflects movement of substances in chemical combination with carrier systems in the cell membrane. Furthermore, active transport occurs from a site of low concentration of a substance to one of high concentration requiring chemical energy.

Diffusion

All molecules and ions in body fluids are in constant and random motion. Motion of these particles is reflected as heat. This continual movement of molecules or ions in liquids or gases is called diffusion. The rate of diffusion is increased by a (1) large concentration gradient, (2) small molecular weight, (3) short diffusion distance, (4) large cross-sectional areas, and (5) elevated temperature. Substances can diffuse through cell membranes by (1) becoming dissolved in the lipid bilayer or by (2) passing through special channels.

Lipid Bilayer

The primary factor that determines how rapidly a substance can diffuse through the lipid bilayer of cell membranes is its solubility in lipids. For example, highly lipid-soluble carbon dioxide and oxygen diffuse readily. Conversely, water, glucose, and electrolytes are poorly lipid-soluble and cannot diffuse freely through the lipid bilayer.

Carrier-Mediated Diffusion

Some poorly lipid-soluble substances, such as glucose and amino acids, pass through the lipid bilayer by carrier-mediated or facilitated diffusion. In this mechanism, glucose combines with a carrier substance to form a complex that is lipid soluble. This lipid-soluble complex can diffuse to the interior of the cell membrane where glucose is released to the interior of the cell and the carrier moves back to the exterior of the cell membrane where it becomes available to transport more glucose (Fig. 39-4) (Guyton, 1986a). As such, the carrier renders glucose soluble in a cell membrane that otherwise would prevent its passage. Insulin greatly speeds carrier-mediated diffusion of glucose and some amino acids (see Chapter 24). An important difference between carrier-mediated diffusion and active transport (see the section entitled Active Transport) is that carrier-mediated diffusion can move substances only from a high concentration toward a low concentration. Conversely, active transport can move substances across cell membranes against concentration, electrical, or pressure gradients.

Channels

Water and many dissolved ions such as sodium and potassium ions are believed to pass through channels in the cell membranes to gain access to the interior of the cell. These channels are likely to be intermolecular spaces in large proteins that extend through the entire cell membrane

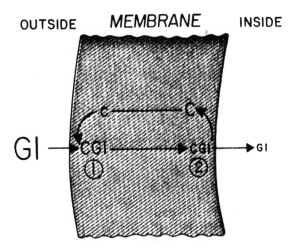

OUTSIDE   MEMBRANE   INSIDE

FIGURE 39-4. Glucose (Gl) can combine with a carrier substance (C) at the outside surface of the cell membrane to facilitate passage (*i.e.,* carrier-mediated diffusion) of glucose across the cell membrane. At the inside surface of the cell membrane, glucose is released to the interior of the cell and the carrier becomes available for reuse. (From Guyton AC. Textbook of Medical Physiology. 6th ed. Philadelphia: WB Saunders, 1981:41. Reproduced by permission of the author and publisher.)

(Keynes, 1979). The diameter of these channels is about 0.8 nm, which is larger than the diameter of water and hydrated ions (Table 39-1). Water diffuses in either direction to maintain optimal cell size. The rates of diffusion of ions through the channels are less than water which is in keeping with the fact that their diameters are slightly greater than that of water. Most of the carbohydrates including glucose have diameters slightly greater than the channels preventing their passage to the interior of cells by this route and emphasizing their dependence on carrier-mediated diffusion (Table 39-1).

The electrical charges of ions often influence the ability of these substances to diffuse through channels, sometimes impeding and sometimes enhancing their diffusion. It is speculated that different channels are lined by either negative or positive charges. For example, some channels are particularly able to permit rapid diffusion of sodium ions (*e.g.,* sodium channels). It is believed that these sodium channels are lined by negative charges that attract sodium ions into the channels and then transfer the sodium ions from one nega-

tive charge to the next, thus allowing rapid movement through the channels.

In another variation, one end of the sodium channel may become blocked by the presence of a positive charge at its external opening. This charge is designated as a gate because it repels the sodium ions and interferes with the passage of these ions through the channel.

Another factor that influences diffusion through channels is the state of hydration of the ion. Most ions are loosely bound with water and these water molecules usually must be removed before the particle size is small enough to allow passage through the channels (Table 39-1). Water molecules can be broken away from potassium ions more easily than sodium ions such that flow of sodium ions through some channels is impeded more than for potassium ions. Such channels are referred to as potassium channels.

Many cell membranes have different electrical potentials in the fluid on each side of the membrane. Negative ions are attracted through channels toward positive fluid while positive ions pass toward the negative fluid. In addition to the electrical difference, a pressure difference also contributes to the diffusion of substances. The pressure difference is particularly important for diffusion at the capillary which has a pressure about 23 mm Hg higher inside the capillary than outside.

Permeability of nerve membranes to sodium and potassium ions may change as much as 50- to 5000-fold during the course of nerve impulse transmission. These changes most likely reflect

Table 39-1
Diameters of Ions, Molecules, and Channels

	Diameter (nm*)
Channel (average)	0.80
Water	0.30
Sodium ion (hydrated)	0.51
Potassium ion (hydrated)	0.40
Chloride ion (hydrated)	0.39
Lactate ion	0.52
Glucose	0.86
Mannitol	0.86

* 1 nm = 10 Angstroms

rapid alterations in the electrical charges lining the channels or guarding their entrances.

Permeability of channels is influenced by the extracellular fluid concentration of calcium ions and the presence of antidiuretic hormone. For example, decreased calcium ion concentrations greatly increase channel permeability manifesting as exaggerated activity of nerves throughout the body. Conversely, excess calcium ions in extracellular fluid diminish channel permeability, and activity of nerve tissue is greatly reduced. In the kidneys, the presence of antidiuretic hormone enlarges pores in cells lining the collecting ducts allowing water and other substances to diffuse from the renal tubules back into the blood (see Chapter 53).

Active Transport

Active transport is movement of substances across cell membranes against concentration, electrical, or pressure gradients. Substances that are actively transported through cell membranes include sodium ions, potassium ions, calcium ions, hydrogen ions, chloride ions, carbohydrates, and amino acids. The mechanism of active transport is speculated to depend on carriers that combine with the material to be transported at the outside (exterior) surface of cell membranes (Fig. 39-4) (Guyton, 1981a) (see the section entitled Carrier-Mediated Diffusion). At the inside (interior) surface of the cell membranes, the carrier releases its material and moves back to the outside to pick up more material. The only difference between carrier-mediated diffusion and active transport is that energy is imparted to the system in the course of active transport so that transport can occur against a concentration, electrical, or pressure gradient.

A specific enzyme and energy from adenosine triphosphate (ATP) is required for active transport. The mechanism for active transport becomes saturated when the concentration of the substance to be transported is high. This saturation results from limitation of either (1) carrier available to transport the substance or (2) enzymes to promote the chemical reactions that release the substance from the carrier. Carrier substances are believed to be proteins.

Sodium – Potassium Pump

A mechanism for active transport of sodium and potassium ions across cell membranes, known as

the sodium–potassium pump ("sodium pump"), exists in all cells (Wallick *et al*, 1979). The carrier for this mechanism transports sodium ions from inside the cell to the outside and potassium ions from the outside to the inside of the cell (Fig. 39-5) (Guyton, 1981b). Because this carrier has the capability of splitting ATP from molecules and utilizing the energy from this source to promote sodium and potassium ion transport, it is known as sodium–potassium ATPase. Magnesium ATP binds with the sodium–potassium ATPase at the inside surface of the cell membrane. The energy released from the ATP causes potassium ions to split away from the sodium–potassium ATPase carrier molecule and simultaneously causes sodium ions to bind. Then, at the outside surface of the cell membrane, the sodium ions split away from the carrier while potassium ions bind. The sodium–potassium pump is powerful enough to transport sodium ions against concentration gradients as great as 20 to 1 and potassium ions against concentration gradients as great as 30 to 1.

A unique feature of the sodium–potassium transport system is the transfer of three sodium

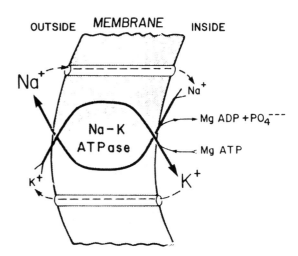

FIGURE 39-5. The active transport of sodium and potassium ions across cell membranes (*e.g.,* sodium ions inside to outside and potassium ions outside to inside) uses a carrier mechanism that derives energy by splitting adenosine triphosphate (ATP) from molecules (*i.e.,* Na-K ATPase). (From Guyton AC. Textbook of Medical Physiology. 6th ed. Philadelphia: WB Saunders, 1981:101. Reproduced by permission of the author and publisher.)

ions to the exterior of the cell membrane for every two potassium ions transported into the cell. This net positive transfer of sodium ions outward creates a potential difference across the cell membrane with the interior of the cell being negative with respect to the exterior. Maintenance of this electrical potential difference is essential to nerve conduction and skeletal muscle contraction (see the section entitled Electrical Potentials Across Cell Membranes). Furthermore, the sodium–potassium pump opposes the tendency of the cell to swell by continually transporting sodium ions to the exterior which initiates an opposite osmotic tendency to move water out of the cell (Macknight and Leaf, 1977). Whenever the metabolism of the cell ceases so that energy from ATP is not available to keep the sodium–potassium pump operating, the cell begins to swell.

Calcium and magnesium ions are most likely transported across cell membranes in a manner similar to sodium and potassium ions. Furthermore, certain cells have a unique ability to transport other ions as emphasized by transport of large amounts of iodide ions into thyroid gland cells.

Sodium Co-transport of Glucose

Sodium co-transport of glucose is an active transport system that supplements carrier-mediated diffusion of glucose into the cell (see the section entitled Carrier-Mediated Diffusion) (Ullrich, 1979). This active transport system is prominent in the gastrointestinal tract and renal tubules acting to transport even minute concentrations of glucose back into the circulation, thus preventing its excretion.

The carrier system involved in sodium co-transport is unique in that it will not transport sodium ions by itself but must also transport a glucose molecule at the same time. It is the sodium ion gradient across the brush border of gastrointestinal and renal tubular epithelial cells that provides the energy to promote the active transport of both sodium ions and glucose.

Sodium Co-transport of Amino Acids

Sodium co-transport of amino acids is an active transport mechanism that supplements carrier-mediated diffusion of amino acids into the cell (Ullrich, 1979). Epithelial cells lining the gastrointestinal tract and renal tubules are able to reabsorb amino acids into the circulation by this mech-

anism, thus preventing their excretion. This active transport system, in addition to being dependent on sodium ions, is also dependent on pyridoxine for the transport of some amino acids. Furthermore, hormones including insulin, growth hormone, glucocorticoids, and estradiol influence amino acid transport by the sodium co-transport mechanism. For example, estradiol facilitates transport of amino acids into the musculature of the uterus thus promoting the development of this organ.

ELECTRICAL POTENTIALS ACROSS CELL MEMBRANES

Electrical potentials exist across essentially all cell membranes. These electrical potentials make possible self-generation of electrochemical impulses at the cell membranes of nerves and skeletal muscles (Ehrenstein and Lecar, 1972).

Fluids inside and outside the cells are electrolyte solutions containing 150 to 160 meq L^{-1} of positive ions and the same concentration of negative ions. Usually, a small excess of negative ions accumulate along the inner surface of the cell membrane opposite an equal number of positive ions just outside the cell membrane. This uneven distribution of positive and negative ions results in electrical potential differences between the inside and outside of the cell.

The two means by which electrical potential differences across cell membranes can develop are (1) active transport of ions through the cell membrane thus creating an imbalance of negative and positive charges on the two sides of the membrane, and (2) diffusion of ions through the membrane as a result of ion concentration differences between the two sides of the membrane, thus also creating an imbalance of charges (Guyton, 1981b).

Active Transport

Active transport results in an excess of negative ions inside the cell and an excess of positively charged sodium ions outside the cell. A pump that results in such a distribution of ions to create a membrane potential is an electrogenic pump. The sodium–potassium pump is an example of such a pump being responsible for establishing the electrical potential across cell membranes of nearly all cells in the body (see the section entitled Sodium–Potassium Pump).

Diffusion

A concentration difference of ions across a semipermeable membrane can result in movement of ions such that an electrical potential develops. Under resting conditions, the electrical potential across the cell membrane is about −90 mv reflecting the high permeability of the cell membrane to potassium ions and only limited permeability to sodium ions. When a nerve impulse is transmitted, the cell membrane becomes much more permeable to sodium ions than potassium ions and the electrical potential across the cell membrane rises to about −45 mv. These electrical membrane potentials due to diffusion of ions are calculated using the Nernst equation.

Chloride ions are not pumped through the nerve membrane in either direction although they readily diffuse through the membrane. Because there is no pump to cause a buildup of a concentration difference of chloride ions across the cell membrane, the distribution of chloride ions on the two sides of the membrane is determined entirely by the degree and polarity of the electrical membrane potential. For example, the negativity that develops in the cell repels chloride ions causing the intracellular concentration to fall to about 4 mEq L^{-1} in comparison with an extracellular fluid concentration of about 103 mEq L^{-1}. During an action potential, chloride ions move rapidly but passively through the cell membrane to alter the duration and magnitude of the action potential.

Distribution of other ions across cell membranes is determined in much the same way as occurs for sodium, potassium, and chloride ions. For example, distribution of calcium ions is determined in the same manner as sodium ions while magnesium ions resemble potassium ions. Both magnesium ions and calcium ions also influence membrane potentials by altering permeability of the cell membrane to other ions.

ACTION POTENTIALS

Action potentials are abrupt pulse-like changes from the resting membrane potential that result in

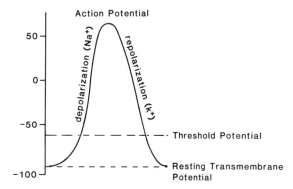

FIGURE 39-6. Action potentials are abrupt pulse-like changes of the transmembrane potentials, which result in transmission of nerve impulses. Acetylcholine-induced changes in cell membrane permeability lead to the initial decrease in transmembrane potential known as depolarization. This phase is followed by a return of sodium ion permeability to normal and an increase in permeability of the cell membrane to potassium ions resulting in repolarization, which is characterized by a decrease of the transmembrane potential toward the resting transmembrane potential.

transmission of nerve impulses (Fig. 39-6). An action potential can be elicited in a nerve fiber by any factor (electrical, mechanical, chemical) that abruptly increases the permeability of the cell membrane to sodium ions. Indeed, it is the opening and closing of sodium and potassium channels that is responsible for the depolarization and repolarization phases of the action potential. Acetylcholine, as an endogenous neurotransmitter, is the most important chemical substance that is capable of enlarging sodium channels and increasing cell membrane permeability to these ions up to 5000-fold. The action potential results from this initial increase in permeability of the cell membrane to sodium ions followed by return of sodium ion permeability to normal and an increase in permeability of the membrane to potassium ions. The initial sudden inward rush of sodium ions leads to a positive charge inside the cell corresponding to the phase of the action potential known as depolarization. Subsequent increased permeability of the cell membrane to potassium ions allows loss of this positive ion tending to return the electrical charge inside the cell towards the resting membrane potential of −90 mv. This phase of the action potential is known as repolarization. Once the negative resting membrane potential is reestablished, it remains at this level until the cell membrane is disturbed once again. The negative resting membrane potential is sustained by the continued diffusion of potassium ions to the exterior via partially open potassium channels.

A deficiency of calcium ions in the extracellular fluid prevents the sodium gates from closing between action potentials. The resulting continuous leak of sodium ions contributes to sustained depolarization or repetitive firing of the cell membrane (*e.g.,* tetany). Conversely, high calcium ion concentrations decrease membrane permeability to sodium ions and thus reduce excitability of the nerve membrane. Low potassium ion concentrations in extracellular fluid increase the negativity of the resting membrane potential resulting in hyperpolarization and decreased membrane excitability. Skeletal muscle weakness that accompanies hypokalemia presumably reflects hyperpolarization of the skeletal muscle membrane. Local anesthetics decrease the permeability of the nerve membrane to sodium ions preventing achievement of a threshold potential that is necessary for generation of an action potential.

Tetrodotoxin is a drug, which, when applied to the exterior of a cell membrane, blocks sodium channels. Conversely, application of tetraethylammonium ion to the inside of the cell membrane blocks potassium channels. These drugs allow selective blockade and study of each type of channel (Ritchie, 1979).

Propagation of the Action Potential

An action potential excites adjacent portions of the cell membrane resulting in propagation of the action potential. Propagation of the action potential occurs when flow of electrical current increases the permeability of the adjacent cell membranes to sodium ions resulting in successive portions of the cell membrane becoming depolarized. These propagated action potentials travel in both directions along the entire extent of the fiber (*e.g.,* all-or-nothing principle). The transmission of the depolarization process along a nerve or muscle fiber is called a nerve or muscle impulse. The entire action potential usually occurs in less than 1 millisecond.

REFERENCES

Allison AC, Davies P. Mechanisms of endocytosis and exocytosis. Symp Soc Exp Biol 1974;28:419–46.

Capaldi RA. A dynamic model of cell membranes. Sci Am 1974;230:26–33.

DeDuve C, Williams R. Functions of lysosomes. Annu Rev Physiol 1966;28:435–92.

Ehrenstein G, Lecar H. The mechanism of signal transmission in nerve axons. Annu Rev Biophys Bioeng 1972;1:347–68.

Friedman DL. Role of cyclic nucleotides in cell growth and differentiation. Physiol Rev 1976;56:652–708.

Goldman RD, Milstad A, Schloss JA, Starger J, Yerna MJ. Cytoplasmic fibers in mammalian cells: Cytoskeletal and contractile elements. Annu Rev Physiol 1979;41:703–22.

Guyton AC. Textbook of Medical Physiology. 7th ed. Philadelphia: WB Saunders, 1986a:2.

Guyton AC. Textbook of Medical Physiology. 7th ed. Philadelphia: WB Saunders, 1986b:11.

Guyton AC. Textbook of Medical Physiology. 6th ed. Philadelphia: WB Saunders, 1981a:41.

Guyton AC. Textbook of Medical Physiology. 6th ed. Philadelphia: WB Saunders, 1981b:101.

Keynes RD. Ion channels in the nerve-cell membrane. Sci Am 1979;240:126–35.

Lodish HF, Rothman JE. The assembly of cell membranes. Sci Am 1979;240:48–63.

Macknight ADC, Leaf A. Regulation of cellular volume. Physiol Rev 1977;57:510–73.

Masters C, Holmes R. Peroxisomes: New aspects of cell physiology and biochemistry. Physiol Rev 1977;57:816–82.

Rich A, Kim SH. The three-dimensional structure of transfer RNA. Sci Am 1978;238:52–63.

Ritchie JM. A pharmacological approach to the structure of sodium channels in myelinated axons. Annu Rev Neurosci 1979;2:341–62.

Soderberg U. Neurophysiological aspects of homeostasis. Annu Rev Physiol 1964;26:271–88.

Stephens RE, Edds KT. Microtubules: Structure, chemistry and function. Physiol Rev 1976;56:709–29.

Ullrich KL. Sugar, amino acid, and Na+ cotransport in the proximal tubule. Annu Rev Physiol 1979;41:181–95.

Wallick ET, Lane LK, Schwartz A. Biochemical mechanism of the sodium pump. Annu Rev Physiol 1979;41:397–411.

Williamson JR. Mitochondrial function in the heart. Annu Rev Physiol 1979;41:485–506.

C H A P T E R   40

Body Fluids

INTRODUCTION

Total body fluids can be divided into intracellular and extracellular fluids depending on their location relative to the cell membrane (Fig. 40-1). About 25 liters of the 40 liters of total body fluid present in a 70-kg adult are within the confines of the estimated 75 trillion cells of the body. The fluid in these cells, despite individual differences in constituents, is collectively designated *intracellular fluid*. The 15 liters of fluid outside the cells is collectively referred to as *extracellular fluid*. Extracellular fluid is divided into interstitial fluid and plasma (intravascular fluid) by the capillary membrane (Fig. 40-1).

The interstitial fluid is that fluid present in the spaces between the cells. An estimated 99% of this fluid is held in the gel structure of the interstitial space. Plasma is the noncellular portion of blood. The average plasma volume is 3 liters. Plasma communicates continually with the interstitial fluid through pores in the capillaries. Likewise, interstitial fluid is in dynamic equilibrium, with the plasma serving as an available reservoir from which water and electrolytes can be mobilized into the circulation. Loss of plasma from the circulatory system through the capillary pores is minimized by the colloid osmotic pressure exerted by the plasma proteins. Nevertheless, the capillaries are sufficiently porous to allow constant mixing between the constituents of plasma and interstitial fluid with the exception of proteins.

Other extracellular fluids which are often considered as part of the interstitial fluid include cerebrospinal fluid, intraocular fluid, fluids of the gastrointestinal tract, and fluids in potential spaces (*e.g.*, pleural space, pericardial space, peritoneal cavity, synovial cavities). Excess amounts of fluid in the interstitial space manifest as peripheral edema.

TOTAL BODY WATER

Water is the most abundant single constituent of the body and is the medium in which all metabolic reactions occur. The total amount of water in a 70-kg male adult is about 40 liters accounting for nearly 60% of total body weight (Fig. 40-2) (Hilgenberg, 1983). In a newborn, total body water may represent 70% of body weight (Fig. 40-2) (Hilgenberg, 1983). Total body water is less in females and in the presence of obesity reflecting the reduced water content of adipose tissue (Bradbury, 1973). For example, total body water represents about 50% of the body weight in females (Fig. 40-2) (Hilgenberg, 1983).

The normal daily intake of water by an adult averages 2300 ml of which only 150 to 250 ml is derived from oxidation of hydrogen in food. About 1400 ml of the normal daily intake of water is excreted as urine, 100 ml is lost in the sweat, and 100 ml is present in the feces. The remaining 700 ml is lost by evaporation from the respiratory tract or by diffusion. Loss of water by evaporation from the respiratory tract and diffusion through the skin

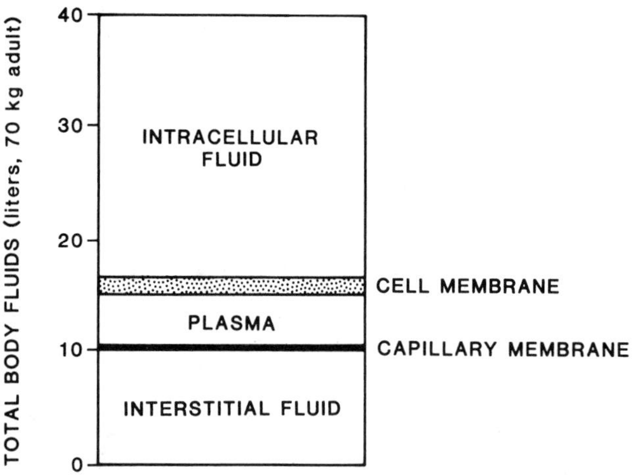

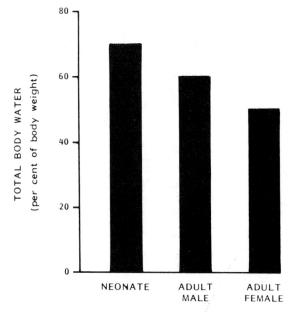

FIGURE 40-1. Total body fluids can be divided into intracellular and extracellular fluids depending on their location relative to the cell membrane. Extracellular fluid is divided into plasma and interstitial fluid by the capillary membrane.

FIGURE 40-2. Total body water varies with age and sex. (By permission, Hilgenberg JC. Renal Disease, In Stoelting RK, Dierdorf SF, eds.: Anesthesia and Co-Existing Disease. Churchill Livingstone Inc., New York, 1983.)

is known as insensible water loss because it is not perceived by the individual. The average daily loss of water by diffusion through the skin is 300 to 400 ml. This loss occurs in the absence of diaphoresis as water molecules are capable of diffusing through the cells of the skin. The cholesterol-filled, cornified layer of the skin acts as a protector against a greater insensible water loss through the skin. Indeed, when the cornified layer becomes denuded, as after burn injury, the outward diffusion of water is greatly increased.

All gases that are inhaled become saturated with water vapor (*i.e.*, 47 mmHg). This water vapor is subsequently exhaled, accounting for an average water loss through the lungs of 300 to 400 ml every 24 hours. The water content of inhaled gases decreases with temperature such that more endogenous water is required to achieve a water vapor pressure of 47 mmHg. As a result, insensible water loss from the lungs is greatest in cold environments and least in warm temperatures. This is consistent with the dry feeling perceived in the respiratory passages in cold weather.

BLOOD VOLUME

Blood contains both extracellular fluid (*i.e.*, plasma) and intracellular fluid represented by the fluid in erythrocytes. The main priority of the body is to maintain the intravascular fluid (*i.e.*, blood) volume. Acute reductions in blood volume, as occur with (1) fluid deprivation in the preoperative period, (2) blood loss, or (3) surgical trauma that results in tissue edema, elicit the release of renin and antidiuretic hormone. These hormones evoke changes at the renal tubules that lead to restoration of the intravascular fluid volume (see Chapter 53).

The average blood volume of an adult is 5 liters, of which about 3 liters are plasma and 2 liters are erythrocytes. These volumes, however, vary greatly with age, weight, and sex. For example, in nonobese persons, the blood volume varies in direct proportion to body weight averaging 70 ml kg^{-1} for both lean males and females. The greater the ratio of fat to body weight, however, the less is the blood volume in ml kg^{-1} because adipose tissue has a reduced vascular supply.

Hematocrit

The true hematocrit is about 96% of the measured value because 3% to 8% of plasma remains entrapped among the erythrocytes even after centrifugation. The measured hematocrit is approximately 40% for normal males and 36% for normal females. The hematocrit of blood in arterioles and capillaries is less than that in large arteries and veins. This reflects axial streaming of erythrocytes in small vessels. Specifically, erythrocytes tend to migrate to the center of vessels while a large portion of the plasma remains near the walls. In large vessels, the ratio of wall surface to total volume is slight so that the accumulation of plasma near the walls does not significantly affect the hematocrit. In small vessels, however, this ratio of wall surface to volume is great causing the ratio of plasma to cells to be greater than in large vessels.

MEASUREMENT OF COMPARTMENTAL FLUID VOLUMES

The volume of a fluid compartment can be measured by the indicator dilution principle in which a known amount of a substance is placed in the compartment and the resulting concentration of this material is then determined after complete mixing has occurred. Using this principle, blood volume, extracellular fluid volume, and total body water can be measured while interstitial fluid volume can be calculated (Guyton, 1986).

Blood Volume

Substances used for measuring blood volume must be capable of dispersing throughout the blood with ease. Furthermore, these substances must remain in the circulation long enough for measurements to be completed. Any substance that attaches to erythrocytes or plasma proteins will remain in the circulation. Examples of substances that combine with erythrocytes and that are used for determining blood volume are radioactive iron, radioactive chromium, and radioactive phosphate. Examples of substances that combine with proteins are dyes (Evans blue) and radioactive iodine.

Most often, a small amount of the patient's blood is removed and mixed with radioactive chromium. After determining the total content of chromium with a scintillation counter, the tagged blood sample is injected into the patient. After mixing for about 10 minutes in the systemic circulation, the chromium content of blood is determined. Using the dilution principle, the total blood volume is calculated.

Extracellular Fluid Volume

Substances used to measure extracellular fluid volume must be capable of rapid diffusion through capillaries into extracellular fluid and at the same time incapable of crossing cell membranes to gain access to intracellular fluid. Radioactive sodium, radioactive chloride, radioactive bromide, thiosulfate ions, thiocynate ions, and sucrose are examples of substances that have been used to measure extracellular fluid volume. None of these substances, however, is ideal or measures reliably only the extracellular fluid volume. The average extracellular fluid volume in adults using these techniques is 15 liters.

Total Body Water

Total body water is most often measured using tritiated water or heavy water, either of which is capable of diffusing into extracellular fluid and across cell membranes into the intracellular fluid. Several hours are required for adequate mixing. The average measured total body water in adults is 40 liters or about 60% of body weight.

Interstitial Fluid Volume

Interstitial fluid volume cannot be measured separately from the entire extracellular fluid volume.

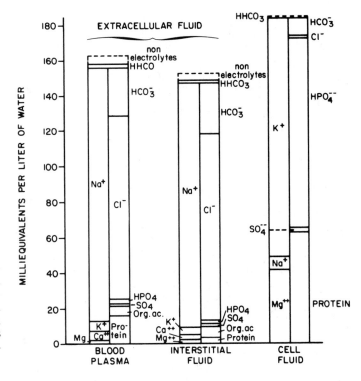

FIGURE 40-3. The concentration of substances that make up plasma, interstitial fluid, and intracellular fluid (cell fluid) varies substantially among compartments. (From Guyton, AC. Textbook of Medical Physiology. 7th ed. Philadelphia: WB Saunders, 1986:382. Reproduced by permission of the author and publisher.)

The interstitial fluid volume, however, can be calculated as the extracellular fluid volume (15 liters) minus the plasma volume (3 liters).

CONSTITUENTS OF BODY FLUID COMPARTMENTS

The constituents of plasma, interstitial fluid, and intracellular fluid are identical, but the actual quantity of each substance varies greatly among the compartments (Fig. 40-3) (Guyton, 1986).

Extracellular Fluid

Plasma and interstitial fluid contain large quantities of sodium and chloride ions, but only small quantities of potassium, calcium, and magnesium ions. Plasma contains far more protein than does interstitial fluid. The constituents of the extracellular fluid are carefully regulated by the kidneys so that the cells remain bathed continually in a fluid containing the proper concentrations of electro-

lytes and nutrients for continued optimal function of the cells (see Chapter 53).

Intracellular Fluid

In contrast to extracellular fluid, intracellular fluid contains only small quantities of sodium and chloride ions and almost no calcium ions. Potassium ions, however, are present in large quantities in the intracellular fluid along with moderate quantities of magnesium ions. The unequal distribution of ions results in establishment of a potential difference across cell membranes. The protein content of intracellular fluid is about four times that present in plasma. The intracellular pH is more acidic than extracellular fluid ranging from 6.8 to 7.2 (Waddell and Bates, 1969).

Trauma is associated with progressive loss of potassium ions through the kidneys. For example, a patient undergoing surgery excretes about 100 mEq of potassium in the first 48 hours and after this about 25 mEq daily. If the 24-hour urinary excretion of potassium exceeds more than 20 to 30 mEq L^{-1}, the resulting hypokalemia is renal in origin (Harrington and Cohen, 1975). Conversely, patients with hypokalemia due to potassium loss by the gastrointestinal tract excrete lesser amounts of potassium in the urine.

OSMOSIS

Osmosis is the net movement of water caused by a concentration difference across cell membranes. Membranes are semipermeable when water can diffuse freely but certain ions such as sodium and chloride cannot diffuse. In this instance, water crosses semipermeable membranes in the direction of the highest concentration of nondiffusible ions. This diffusion of water can be stopped by pressure. The amount of pressure required to stop diffusion of water (*i.e.,* osmosis) is called the *osmotic pressure.*

Osmotic Pressure

The osmotic pressure exerted by nondiffusible particles in a solution, whether they are molecules or ions, is determined by the numbers of particles per unit volume of fluid and not the mass of the particles. Osmole rather than grams is used to express the concentration of solute in terms of numbers of particles (*e.g.,* molecules or ions) capable of exerting osmotic pressure. The osmole is too large a unit for expressing osmotic activity of solutes in the body. Therefore, the term milliosmole (*i.e.,* 1/1000 osmole) is commonly used.

One osmole is the number of particles in 1 gram molecular weight of undissociated solute. For example, one molecule of albumin with a molecular weight of 70,000 has the same osmotic effect as a molecule of glucose with a molecular weight of 180. Conversely, if 1 gram molecular weight of a solute such as sodium chloride (58.5 g) dissociates into two ions, this 1 gram molecular weight of solute equals 2 osmoles because the number of osmotically active particles is now twice as great as when sodium chloride was not dissociated.

The osmole concentration of a solution is called its *osmolality* when the concentration is expressed in osmoles per kilogram of water. *Osmolarity* is the correct terminology when osmole concentration is expressed in liters. In the dilute solutions of the body, these terms are frequently used interchangeably. Furthermore, because it is much easier to express body fluids in liters rather than in kilograms almost all physiologic calculations are based on osmolarity rather than osmolality.

Osmolarity of Body Fluids

Normal plasma osmolarity is about 280 mOsm L^{-1}, which is about 1.3 mOsm greater than that of the interstitial and intracellular fluids. This slight difference between plasma and interstitial fluid is due to the osmotic effect of the plasma proteins which act to maintain a higher pressure in the capillaries than in the surrounding interstitial fluid spaces. About 90% of the osmolarity of plasma and interstitial fluid is due to sodium ions and chloride ions while about 50% of the intracellular osmolarity is due to potassium ions. The transfer of water through cell membranes by osmosis occurs so rapidly that any lack of osmotic equilibrium between two fluid compartments in a given tissue is corrected usually within seconds.

Tonicity of Fluids

A fluid into which a cell can be placed without transfer of fluid into or out of the cell occurring is said to be *isotonic*. An isotonic solution exerts the same osmotic pressure as plasma. A 0.9% solution of sodium chloride is isotonic. Solutions less than 0.9% sodium chloride are *hypotonic* (cells swell) and greater than 0.9% sodium chloride are *hypertonic* (cells shrink). Indeed, packed erythrocytes must be suspended in isotonic solutions to avoid damage to the cells prior to infusion. Glucose in a solution is metabolized rendering a hypertonic solution less hypertonic or converting an isotonic solution to a hypotonic solution. For example, a solution of 5% glucose in lactated Ringer's solution is initially hypertonic (about 560 mOsm L^{-1}), but as glucose is metabolized, the solution becomes less hypertonic.

CHANGES IN VOLUMES OF BODY FLUID COMPARTMENTS

Factors that may alter significantly extracellular or intracellular fluid volumes include (1) intravenous infusion of fluids and (2) dehydration from gastrointestinal fluid loss, diaphoresis, and fluid loss by the kidneys (Gauer *et al,* 1970). As a rule, chronic diseases are characterized by a decline in intracellular fluid volume and concomitant expansion of extracellular fluid volume.

Intravenous Fluids

Intravenous fluids that do not remain in the circulation (*e.g.,* 5% glucose) can dilute extracellular fluid causing it to become hypotonic with respect to intracellular fluid. When this occurs, osmosis begins instantly at cell membranes with large amounts of water entering the cells. Within a few minutes, this water becomes distributed almost evenly among all the body fluid compartments. Increased intracellular fluid volume is particularly undesirable in patients with intracranial masses or elevated intracranial pressure.

Dehydration

Loss of water by gastrointestinal or renal routes or by diaphoresis is associated with an initial deficit in extracellular fluid volume. At the same instant, intracellular water passes to the extracellular fluid compartment by osmosis thus keeping the osmolarities in both compartments equal despite reduced absolute volume (*e.g.,* dehydration) of both compartments.

REFERENCES

Bradbury MW. Physiology of body fluids and electrolytes. Br J Anaesth 1973;45:937–44.

Gauer OH, Henry JP, Behn C. The regulation of extracellular fluid volume. Annu Rev Physiol 1970; 32:547–95.

Guyton AC. Textbook of Medical Physiology. 7th ed. Philadelphia, WB Saunders, 1986:382.

Harrington JT, Cohen JJ. Measurement of urinary electrolytes. Indications and limitations. N Engl J Med 1975;293:1241–3.

Hilgenberg JC. Renal Disease. In Stoelting RK, Dierdorf SF. Anesthesia and Co-Existing Disease. New York, Churchill Livingstone, 1983:379.

Waddell WN, Bates RG. Intracellular pH. Physiol Rev 1969;49:285–329.

C H A P T E R 41

Central
Nervous System

INTRODUCTION

The three principal components of the nervous system are the cerebral cortex, brain stem, and spinal cord. The activity of the central nervous system reflects a balance between excitatory and inhibitory influences that are normally maintained within relatively narrow limits.

CEREBRAL CORTEX

The cerebral cortex functions primarily as a site for storage of information that is often characterized as memory. For each area of the cerebral cortex there is a corresponding and connecting area to the thalamus such that stimulation of a small portion of the thalamus activates the corresponding and much larger portion of the cerebral cortex. Indeed, the cerebral cortex is actually an outgrowth of the lower regions of the nervous system, especially the thalamus.

The functional part of the cerebral cortex is comprised mainly of a 2- to 5-mm layer of neurons covering the surface of all the convolutions. It is estimated the cerebral cortex contains about 100 billion neurons (Hubel, 1979). Histologically, there are six layers of the cerebral cortex that include granular, fusiform, and pyramidal cells.

Anatomy of Motor Areas

The sensorimotor cortex is that area of the cerebral cortex that is responsible for receiving sensa-

tion from somatic areas of the body or with control of body movement (Fig. 41-1) (Guyton, 1986a). The somesthetic cortex is the posterior portion of the sensorimotor cortex and is important in controlling the functions of the motor cortex. The motor cortex lies anterior to the central sulcus. Its posterior portion is characterized by the presence of large pyramid-shaped (pyramidal or Betz) cells.

Pyramidal and Extrapyramidal Tracts

A major pathway for transmission of motor signals from the cerebral cortex to the anterior motorneurons of the spinal cord is through the pyramidal tract which is also known as the corticospinal tract (Fig. 41-2) (Guyton, 1986a). About 3% of the pyramidal tract fibers are large diameter myelinated fibers that originate from giant pyramidal cells. The remaining fibers are smaller than 4 microns in diameter. A unique feature of the giant pyramidal cells in the motor cortex is the ability of even a weak electrical signal to stimulate these cells. As a result, motor responses can be evoked with minimal stimulation applied to specific areas of the motor cortex.

All pyramidal tract fibers pass downward through the brain stem and then cross to the opposite side to form the pyramids of the medulla (Fig. 41-2) (Guyton, 1986a). These fibers descend in the lateral corticospinal tracts of the spinal cord and terminate on interneurons at the bases of the dorsal horns of the spinal cord gray matter. A few

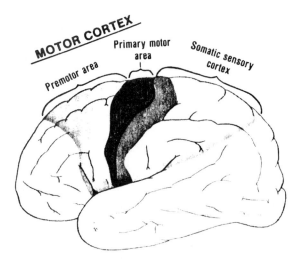

FIGURE 41-1. The sensorimotor cortex consists of the motor cortex, pyramidal (Betz) cells, and the somesthetic cortex. (From Guyton AC. Textbook of Medical Physiology. 7th ed. Philadelphia: WB Saunders, 1986:382. Reproduced by permission of the author and publisher.)

fibers do not cross to the opposite side at the medulla but rather descend in the ventral corticospinal tracts to decussate to the opposite side farther down the spinal cord. In addition to these pyramidal fibers, a large number of collateral fibers pass from the motor cortex into the basal ganglia forming the extrapyramidal tracts. The extrapyramidal tracts are, collectively, all the tracts besides the pyramidal tracts, that transmit motor signals from the cerebral cortex to the spinal cord. Other fibers from the pyramidal area pass to the cerebellum.

The pyramidal and extrapyramidal tracts have opposing effects on the tone of skeletal muscles. For example, the pyramidal tract causes continuous facilitation and, therefore, a tendency to produce increases in skeletal muscle tone. Conversely, the extrapyramidal system transmits inhibitory signals through the basal ganglia with resultant inhibition of skeletal muscle tone. Selective or predominant damage to one of these tracts manifests as spasticity or flaccidity.

Thalamocortical System

The thalamus serves as entryway to the cerebral cortex for nearly all sensory signals from peripheral receptors (Singer, 1977). For example, sig-

nals from the cerebellum, basal ganglia, visual, auditory, pain, and taste receptors pass through the thalamus on the way to the cerebral cortex. Signals from olfactory receptors are the only peripheral sensory signals that do not pass through the thalamus. Overall, the thalamocortical system controls the level of activity of the cerebral cortex.

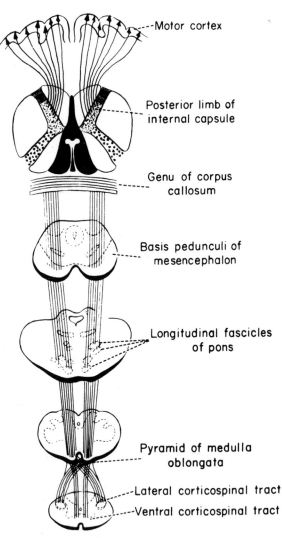

FIGURE 41-2. The pyramidal tract is a major pathway for transmission of motor signals from the cerebral cortex to the spinal cord. (From Guyton AC. Textbook of Medical Physiology. 7th ed. Philadelphia: WB Saunders, 1986:382. Reproduced by permission of the author and publisher.)

At times, this system facilitates activity in regional areas of the cerebral cortex distinct from the remainder of the cortex. Collateral signals from the thalamus also control the level of activity in the specific nuclei of the thalamus, basal ganglia, and hypothalamus.

Topographical Areas

In the motor cortex, there are various topographical areas from which skeletal muscles in different parts of the body can be activated. In general, the size of the area in the motor cortex is proportional to the discreteness of the skeletal muscle movement required. As such, the digits, lips, tongue, and vocal cords have large representations in humans. The spatial organization of the somatic motor cortex is similar to the somatic sensory cortex.

The various topographical areas in the motor cortex were originally determined by electrical stimulation of the brain during local anesthesia and observing the evoked skeletal muscle response. Such stimulation can be used intraoperatively to identify the location of the motor cortex and avoidance of damage to this area. The motor cortex is frequently damaged by loss of blood supply as occurs during a stroke.

Corpus Callosum

The two hemispheres of the cerebral cortex, with the exception of the anterior portions of the temporal lobes, are connected by fibers in the corpus callosum (Nebes, 1974). The anterior portions of the temporal lobes including the amygdala are connected by fibers that pass through the anterior commissure. One of the functions of the corpus callosum and anterior commissure is to make information stored in the cerebral cortex of one hemisphere available to the corresponding hemisphere.

Babinski's Sign

A positive Babinski's sign is characterized by upward extension of the first toe and outward fanning of the other toes in response to a firm tactile stimulus applied to the dorsum of the foot. A normal response to the same tactile stimulus is downward motion of all the toes. A positive Babinski's sign reflects damage to the pyramidal tracts. Damage to the extrapyramidal system does not cause a positive Babinski's sign.

Stimulation of Spinal Motorneurons

The pyramidal tracts terminate mainly on small interneurons on the base of the dorsal horns of the spinal cord although nearly 10% may also terminate directly on the anterior motorneurons. Most signals, however, pass from the primary interneurons through several other neurons before exciting the anterior motorneurons. Other signals reach the anterior motorneurons by numerous extrapyramidal tracts that include the rubrospinal tract, reticulospinal tracts, tectospinal tract, and vestibulospinal tract. Extrapyramidal fibers are more likely than pyramidal fibers to terminate directly on the anterior motorneurons. Furthermore, some extrapyramidal fibers terminate on inhibitory neurons which cause inhibition of the anterior motorneurons, an effect opposite to the excitatory effects of the pyramidal fibers.

Specific Functions of the Cerebral Cortex

Specific functions of the cerebral cortex are localized to general areas of the cortex as determined by electrical stimulation (see the section entitled Topographical Areas). It is believed that complicated memory patterns are stored at least partially in the temporal lobe (see the section entitled Memory). The general interpretative functions including speech and motor functions are commonly more highly developed in one cerebral hemisphere. At birth, the interpretative area of the cerebral cortex (*i.e.,* posterior temporal lobe and angular gyrus where the temporal, parietal, and occipital lobes meet) is often as much as 50% larger in the left than right hemisphere. Indeed, more than 90% of individuals are right-handed emphasizing the presence of a dominant left cerebral hemisphere. Destruction of this interpretative area results in loss of nearly all intellectual function while destruction of the prefrontal areas of the frontal lobes is less harmful.

Failure to document an important role of prefrontal lobes in intellectual function is surprising because the main difference between the brain of monkeys and humans is the prominence of human prefrontal areas. It seems that the importance of the prefrontal areas in the human is to provide additional cortical area in which cerebration can occur. Furthermore, selection of behavior patterns for different situations may be an important role of the prefrontal areas that transmit signals to the limbic areas of the brain. The person without prefrontal areas may react precipitously in response to incoming sensory signals, manifesting undue anger to slight provocations. The same person is likely to lose most of the behavior associated with morals. Ability to maintain a sustained level of concentration is lost in the absence of the prefrontal lobes.

Memory

The mechanism for short-term and long-term memory is not known (Olton, 1977).

SHORT-TERM MEMORY. Short-term memory may involve the presence of reverberating circuits. As the reverberating circuit fatigues or as new signals interfere with the reverberations, the short-term memory fades. Evidence in favor of a reverberating theory of short-term memory is the ability of a general disturbance of brain function (e.g., fright, loud noise) to immediately erase the short-term memory.

Another possible mechanism for short-term memory is the phenomenon of post-tetanic potentiation. For example, tetanic stimulation of a synapse for a few seconds causes increased excitability of the synapse that lasts for seconds to hours. This change in excitability of the synapse could function as short-term memory. Another change that often occurs in neurons following a prolonged period of excitation is a sustained decrease in the resting transmembrane potential of the neuron. This change in excitability of the neuron could also result in short-term memory.

LONG-TERM MEMORY. Long-term memory does not depend on continued activity of the nervous system as evidenced by total inactivation of the brain by hypoxia, cooling, or anesthesia without the loss of long-term memory. For this reason, it is assumed that long-term memory results from physical or chemical alterations of the synapses. Anatomically, repeated use of a neuronal circuit may result in changes in the number of presynaptic terminals or alterations in the size and conductivities of the dendrites. These anatomical changes could cause permanent or semipermanent increases in the degree of facilitation of spe-

cific neuronal circuits. The entire facilitated circuit is called a *memory engram* or *memory trace.* If memory is to last, these synapses must become permanently facilitated (*i.e.,* consolidated). Maximal consolidation requires at least 1 hour. For example, if a strong sensory impression is made on the brain but is followed within a few seconds to minutes by a disruptive signal such as an electrically induced convulsion or institution of deep general anesthesia, the sensory experience is erased. An obvious analogy is the lightly anesthetized patient who reacts purposefully to a painful stimulus but later has no recall if the depth of anesthesia is adjusted following the purposeful movement. Conversely, the same sensory stimulus allowed to persist for 5 to 10 minutes may result in at least partial establishment of the memory trace. If the sensory stimulus is unopposed for 60 minutes, it is likely the memory will have become fully consolidated. Indeed, intraoperative awareness with or without associated pain is a recognized phenomenon especially when minimal amounts of anesthetic drugs are combined with drugs producing neuromuscular blockade (Bennett *et al,* 1985; Bogetz and Katz, 1984; Saucier *et al,* 1983).

Rehearsal of the same information accelerates and potentiates the process of consolidation (*e.g.,* short-term memory is converted to long-term memory). This explains why a person can remember small amounts of information studied in depth far better than large amounts of information studied only superficially. Each time a memory is recalled, a more indelible memory trace develops which may last a lifetime.

An important feature of consolidation is that long-term memories are coded into different categories. Thus, during consolidation, new memories are not stored randomly in the brain, but rather stored in association with previously stored similar information. This form of storage is necessary if one is to be able to scan the memory store at a later date to retrieve the required information.

Removal of the hippocampus does not alter previously stored memory but prevents subsequent consolidation of short-term memory into long-term memory (*i.e.,* anterograde amnesia occurs) (DeSilva and Arnolds, 1978). Retrograde amnesia is inability to recall memories from the long-term storage areas even though the memory persists. The presence of hippocampal lesions produces some element of retrograde amnesia, but damage to the thalamus also results in this phenomenon. This suggests the thalamus may be important in coding, storing, and recalling memories.

New sensory experiences are immediately compared with previous experiences of the same type. Recognition of an individual face is an example of this phenomenon. It is possible this new sensory pattern of stimulation matches a previous memory trace resulting in the sense of recognition.

CEREBRAL BLOOD FLOW

Cerebral blood flow averages 50 ml min^{-1} for each 100 g of brain tissue. For an adult, this is equivalent to 750 ml min^{-1} or about 15% of the resting cardiac output delivered to an organ that represents about 2% of the body's mass. The gray matter of the brain has a higher flow rate (80 ml 100 g^{-1} min^{-1}) than white matter (20 ml 100 g^{-1} min^{-1}).

Regulation of Cerebral Blood Flow

As in most other tissues of the body, cerebral blood flow is closely related to the metabolism of cerebral tissue (Lassen, 1974). Carbon dioxide concentration and oxygen concentration influence cerebral blood flow (Fig. 41-3). Sympathetic and parasympathetic nerves play little or no role in the regulation of cerebral blood flow.

Autoregulation

Cerebral blood flow is closely autoregulated between mean arterial pressures of about 60 to 140 mmHg (Fig. 41-3). As a result, changes in blood pressure within this range will not significantly alter cerebral blood flow. Chronic hypertension shifts the autoregulation curve to the right such that reductions in cerebral blood flow occur at mean arterial pressures greater than 60 mmHg. Autoregulation of cerebral blood flow is reduced or abolished by hypercapnia, severe arterial hypoxemia, and volatile anesthetics (Smith *et al,* 1970). Furthermore, autoregulation is often abolished in the area surrounding an acute cerebral infarction. For example, reactivity of blood vessels in areas surrounding cerebral infarcts and tumors is abolished. These blood vessels are maximally vasodilated, presumably reflecting accumulation of acidic metabolic products. As a result, cerebral

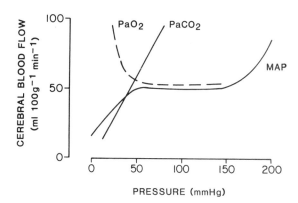

FIGURE 41-3. Cerebral blood flow is influenced by arterial oxygenation (PaO$_2$), alveolar ventilation (PaCO$_2$), and mean arterial pressure (MAP).

blood flow to this area is already maximal (*e.g.,* luxury perfusion) and changes in PaCO$_2$ will have no effect on its blood flow. If PaCO$_2$ should increase, however, it is theoretically possible that resulting vasodilation in normal blood vessels would act to shunt blood flow away from the diseased area (*i.e.,* intracerebral steal syndrome). Conversely, a decrease in PaCO$_2$ that constricts normal cerebral vessels could divert blood flow to diseased areas (*i.e.,* Robin Hood phenomenon). Elevations in mean arterial pressure above the limits of autoregulation can so increase cerebral blood flow that cerebral blood vessels become overdistended resulting in cerebral edema. Because the brain is enclosed in a solid vault, the accumulation of edema fluid increases intracranial pressure and compresses blood vessels which decreases cerebral blood flow and leads to destruction of brain tissue.

Carbon Dioxide

Changes in the arterial PaCO$_2$ between about 20 and 80 mmHg produce corresponding changes in the cerebral blood flow. For example, in this range, a 1 mmHg increase in the PaCO$_2$ evokes a 2 ml 100 g^{-1} min^{-1} increase in cerebral blood flow (Grubb *et al,* 1974). Carbon dioxide increases cerebral blood flow by combining with water in body fluids to form carbonic acid with subsequent dissociation to form hydrogen ions. Hydrogen ions produce vasodilation of cerebral vessels that is proportional to the increase in hydrogen ion concentration. Any other acid that increases hydrogen ion concentration, such as lactic acid, also increases cerebral blood flow.

Increased brain concentrations of hydrogen ions greatly depress neuronal activity. Therefore, it is essential that an increase in hydrogen ion concentration as produced by an accumulation of carbon dioxide causes an increase in cerebral blood flow to carry away carbon dioxide and dissolved acids from the brain tissues.

Oxygen

Except during periods of intense brain activity, the cerebral utilization of oxygen remains constant near 3.5 ml 100 g^{-1} min^{-1}. If cerebral blood flow is unable to supply this amount of oxygen, local factors result in vasodilation to return blood flow and oxygen delivery to acceptable levels. If the $PaCO_2$ is maintained constant, the cerebral blood flow begins to increase when the PaO_2 declines below 50 mmHg or the cerebral venous PO_2 decreases from its normal value of 35 mmHg to about 30 mmHg (Severinghaus and Lassen, 1967). Thus, unlike the continuous response of cerebral blood flow to changes in $PaCO_2$, the response to decreased PaO_2 is a threshold phenomenon.

Measurement of Cerebral Blood Flow

Cerebral blood flow can be measured by injecting a radioactive substance, usually xenon, into the carotid artery and measuring the rate of decay of the radioactivity in each tissue segment as reflected by as many as 256 radioactive scintillation detectors (Beta, 1972). Using this technique, it can be demonstrated that cerebral blood flow changes within seconds in response to changes in local neuronal activity. For example, clasping the hand can be shown to cause an immediate increase in blood flow in the motor cortex of the opposite side of the brain. Reading increases blood flow in the occipital cortex and language areas of the temporal cortex. This measuring procedure can also be used to localize the origin of epileptic attacks because the blood flow increases acutely at the site of origin of the attack.

CEREBROSPINAL FLUID

Cerebrospinal fluid (CSF) is present in the (1) ventricles of the brain, (2) cisterns around the brain, and (3) subarachnoid space around both the brain and spinal cord (Fig. 41•4). The total volume of CSF is about 150 ml, and the specific gravity is 1.002 to 1.009. A major function of CSF is to cushion the brain in the cranial cavity. The brain and the CSF have about the same specific gravity, so the brain floats in CSF. For this reason, a blow on the head moves the entire brain simultaneously causing no one portion of the brain to be selectively contorted by the blow. When a blow of the head is particularly severe, it usually does not damage the brain on the ipsilateral side, but instead damage manifests on the opposite side. This phenomenon is known as *contrecoup* and reflects the creation of a vacuum between the brain and skull opposite the blow caused by sudden movement of the skull at this site away from the brain. When the skull is no longer being accelerated by the blow, the vacuum suddenly collapses and the brain strikes the interior surface of the skull.

Formation

The choroid plexuses in the four cerebral ventricles are the major site of formation of CSF, although by far the greatest amount of CSF is formed by the two lateral ventricles (Cutler *et al*, 1968). The choroid plexus is a cauliflowerlike growth of blood vessels covered by a thin layer of epithelial cells. CSF continually exudes from the surface of the choroid plexus. In comparison with other extracellular fluids, the concentration of sodium and chloride ions in CSF is 7% greater, and the concentration of glucose and potassium ions 30% and 40% less, respectively. This difference in composition from other extracellular fluids emphasizes that CSF is a choroid secretion and not a simple filtrate from the capillaries. The rate of choroidal secretion is estimated to be about 800 ml daily, which is about 5 times the total volume of CSF present at any one time. The rate of CSF production is increased by enflurane but not isoflurane, halothane, or fentanyl (see Chapter 2).

The *p*H of CSF is closely regulated and maintained at 7.32. Changes in $PaCO_2$, but not *p*H, promptly alter the CSF *p*H (see Chapter 49). This reflects the ability of carbon dioxide, but not hydrogen ions, to easily cross the blood–brain barrier. As a result, acute respiratory acidosis or alkalosis produce corresponding changes in the CSF *p*H. Active transport of bicarbonate ions in an appropriate direction eventually returns the CSF *p*H

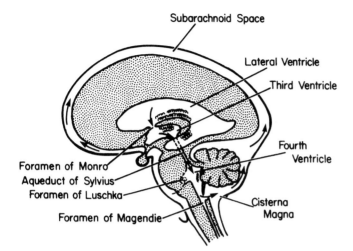

FIGURE 41-4. Circulation of cerebrospinal fluid.

to 7.32 despite persistence of alterations in the arterial pH (see Chapter 51).

Diffusion

The surfaces of cerebral ventricles are lined with epithelial cells called the *ependyma* which are in constant contact with CSF. In addition, CSF fills the subarachnoid space between the pia mater that covers the brain and the arachnoid membrane. The CSF, therefore, is in contact with large surface areas of ependyma and meninges. Diffusion of CSF occurs continually between the CSF and brain tissue beneath the ependyma and also between the CSF and the blood vessels of the meninges.

Reabsorption

Almost all the CSF formed each day is reabsorbed into the venous circulation through special structures known as *arachnoid villi* or *granulations.* These villi project from the subarachnoid spaces into the venous sinuses of the brain and occasionally into the veins of the spinal cord. Arachnoid villi are actually trabeculae that protrude through the venous walls, resulting in highly permeable areas that permit relatively free flow of CSF into the circulation. The magnitude of reabsorption depends upon the pressure gradient between CSF and the venous circulation. Enflurane, but not isoflurane, increases the resistance to the reabsorption of CSF (see Chapter 2).

Circulation

CSF formed in the lateral cerebral ventricle passes into the third ventricle through the foramen of Monro (Fig. 41-4). In the third ventricle, the CSF mixes with that secreted in the lateral ventricle, and then passes along the aqueduct of Sylvius into the fourth cerebral ventricle where still more CSF is formed. The CSF then passes into the cisterna magna through the lateral foramen of Luschka and via a midline foramen of Magendie. From this point, CSF flows through the subarachnoid spaces upward toward the cerebrum where the majority of arachnoid villi are located.

Cerebrospinal Fluid Pressure

Normal CSF pressure is less than 15 mmHg. The CSF pressure is regulated by the rate of its formation and resistance to reabsorption through the arachnoid villi (*e.g.,* venous pressure). In addition, increases in cerebral blood flow as during inhalation of volatile anesthetics can cause the CSF pressure to rise because of the concomitant increase in cerebral blood volume. Arterial blood pressure does not alter CSF pressure within the range of normal autoregulation. Phasic variations in blood pressure, however, are transmitted to CSF pressure.

Papilledema

Anatomically, the dura of the brain extends as a sheath around the optic nerve and then connects with the sclera of the eye. When the pressure rises in the CSF system, it also increases in the optic nerve sheath. The increased pressure in the optic sheath impedes blood flow in the retinal veins leading to elevations in retinal capillary pressure and retinal edema. The tissues of the optic disc are more distensible than the rest of the retina so the disc becomes more edematous than the remainder of the retina and swells into the cavity of the eye. The swelling of the optic disc is termed *papilledema* and is a reflection of increased CSF pressure.

Hydrocephalus

Obstruction to free flow of CSF in the newborn results in hydrocephalus. For example, block of the aqueduct of Sylvius results in expansion of the lateral and third ventricles and compression of the brain (Fig. 41-4). This type of obstruction producing a noncommunicating type of hydrocephalus is treated by surgical creation of an artificial pathway for flow of CSF between the ventricular system and the subarachnoid space.

Blood – Brain Barrier

Just as the choroid plexus is selective in secreting substances into the CSF, there exists a barrier between blood and brain tissue (Oldendorf, 1974). The exception to the existence of a blood – brain barrier is the region of the hypothalamus which is uniquely sensitive to alterations in extracellular fluid constituents. The blood – CSF and blood – brain barriers are highly permeable to water, carbon dioxide, and oxygen, less permeable to electrolytes, and almost totally impermeable to other materials such as injected drugs. The cause of the low permeability of the blood – CSF barrier is the almost total impermeability of the secretory cells of the choroid plexus. All substances entering the CSF must be transported through the secretory cells in addition to passing through the capillary membranes of the choroid plexus. The cause of the blood – brain barrier is not known but may reflect tight junctions between the endothelial cells of the capillaries and envelopment of brain capillaries by glial cells that further reduce permeability of the vessels.

ELECTROENCEPHALOGRAM

The electroencephalogram is a recording of the brain waves that result from the continuous electrical activity in the brain. The intensity of the electrical activity recorded from the surface of the scalp ranges from 0 to 300 μv, and the frequency may exceed 50 cycles sec^{-1}. The character of the waves is greatly dependent on the level of activity of the cerebral cortex and the degree of wakefulness. There is a direct relationship between the degree of cerebral activity and the frequency of brain waves. Furthermore, during periods of increased mental activity, brain waves usually become asynchronous rather than synchronous so the voltage decreases despite increased cortical activity.

Classification of Brain Waves

Brain waves are classified as alpha, beta, theta, and delta waves depending on their frequency and amplitude (Fig. 41-5). The classic electroencephalogram is a plot of voltage against time usually recorded by 16 channels on paper running at 30 mm sec^{-1}. One page of recording is 10 seconds of data.

Alpha Waves

Alpha waves occur at a frequency of 8 to 12 cycles sec^{-1} and a voltage of about 50 μv. These waves are typical of an awake resting state of cerebration with the eyes closed. During sleep, alpha waves disappear. Because alpha waves do not occur

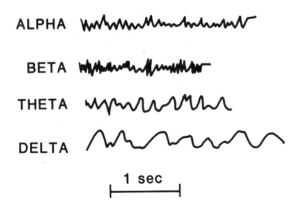

FIGURE 41-5. The electroencephalogram consists of alpha, beta, theta, and delta waves.

when the cerebral cortex is not connected to the thalamus, it is assumed these waves result from spontaneous activity in the thalamocortical system.

Beta Waves

Beta waves occur at a frequency of 13 to 30 cycles sec^{-1} and a voltage usually less than 50 μv. These high frequency and low voltage asynchronous waves replace alpha waves in the presence of increased mental activity or visual stimulation.

Theta Waves

Theta waves occur at a frequency of 4 to 7 cycles sec^{-1}. These waves occur in healthy children during sleep and also during general anesthesia.

Delta Waves

Delta waves include all the brain waves with a frequency less than 4 cycles sec^{-1}. These waves occur (1) in deep sleep, (2) during general anesthesia, and (3) in the presence of serious organic brain disease. Delta waves occur even when the connections of the cerebral cortex to the reticular activating system are severed. This indicates that delta waves originate in the cerebral cortex independent of lower brain structures. Occurrence of delta waves during sleep suggests that the cerebral cortex is released from the activating influences of the reticular activating system.

Clinical Uses

The electroencephalogram is useful in diagnosing different types of epilepsy and for determining the focus in the brain causing epilepsy. Brain tumors, which compress surrounding neurons and cause abnormal electrical activity, may be localized using the electroencephalogram. Monitoring the electroencephalogram during carotid endarterectomy, cardiopulmonary bypass, or deliberate hypotension may provide an early warning of inadequate cerebral blood flow. In this regard the electroencephalogram may be influenced by anesthetic drugs, depth of anesthesia, and hyperventilation (see Chapter 2).

Epilepsy

Epilepsy is characterized by excessive activity of either a part or all of the central nervous system

(Prince, 1978) (see Chapter 30). About 1 in every 50 persons manifests a hereditary predisposition for epilepsy. In these individuals, alkalosis, fever, loud noises, or flashing lights may precipitate an attack. Even in persons not genetically predisposed, traumatic lesions in the brain can cause excess excitability of local brain areas which can transmit signals to the reticular activating system to elicit grand mal seizures.

GRAND MAL EPILEPSY. Grand mal epilepsy is characterized by intense neuronal discharges in multiple areas of the cerebral cortex and reticular activating system. These impulses are transmitted to the spinal cord resulting in alternating skeletal muscle contractions known as *tonic-clonic seizures*. Signals to the viscera often result in defecation or urination. The grand mal seizure lasts from a few seconds to several minutes and is followed by generalized depression of the entire central nervous system.

The electroencephalogram reveals high voltage synchronous brain wave discharges over the entire cerebral cortex during a grand mal seizure. Similar discharges can be recorded from the reticular activating system. Presumably, grand mal epilepsy is caused by abnormal activation of the reticular activating system leading to massive activation of reverberating pathways throughout the brain.

Synaptic fatigue is a likely mechanism that contributes to cessation of a grand mal seizure (see the section entitled Synaptic Fatigue). The generalized feeling of fatigue that occurs after a grand mal seizure is believed to reflect intense synaptic fatigue. In addition to synaptic fatigue there may be active inhibition from feedback circuits through inhibitory areas of the brain that act to stop the grand mal seizure. Conceivably, the grand mal seizure excites areas such as the basal ganglia which in turn emit inhibitory impulses into the reticular activating system.

PETIT MAL EPILEPSY. Petit mal epilepsy most likely involves the thalamocortical portion of the reticular activating system. This contrasts with activation of the mesencephalic portion characteristic of grand mal epilepsy. A period of unconsciousness lasting less than 30 seconds and associated with twitching contractions of some skeletal muscles particularly in the face is the usual manifestation of petit mal epilepsy. The brain waves on the electroencephalogram manifest as a spike and dome pattern which can be recorded over most of the cerebral cortex confirming that the seizure usually involves the reticular activating system. Occasionally, petit mal attacks are more localized suggesting an origin in focal regions of specific thalamic nuclei.

FOCAL EPILEPSY. Focal epilepsy can involve nearly any part of the brain and almost always results from a localized lesion such as a (1) scar that pulls on neuronal tissue, (2) tumor that compresses an area of the brain, or (3) congenital abnormality in neuronal circuitry. Lesions such as these can promote rapid discharges in local neurons presumably by creating reverberating circuits that gradually recruit adjacent areas of the cerebral cortex into the discharge zone. As a result, there is a progressive spread ("march") of skeletal muscular contractions most often beginning in the mouth region and spreading eventually to the legs. A focal epileptic seizure may remain confined to a single area of the cerebral cortex but often strong impulses excite the mesencephalic portion of the reticular activating system leading to a grand mal seizure.

PSYCHOMOTOR EPILEPSY. Psychomotor epilepsy is a form of focal epilepsy that characteristically involves the limbic portion of the brain that includes the temporal cortex. The electroencephalogram may be used to localize the site of origin of the abnormal activity. Anesthetic drugs, such as methohexital or etomidate may be used to activate focal seizure sites thus facilitating their identification and subsequent surgical resection (Gancher et al, 1984; Rockoff and Goudsouzian, 1981).

EVOKED POTENTIALS

Evoked potentials are the electrophysiologic responses of the nervous system to sensory stimulation. The waveforms resulting from sensory stimulation reflect transmission of impulses through specific sensory pathways. The modes of sensory stimulation utilized in the operating room are somatosensory, auditory, and visual. *Poststimulus latency* is the time in milliseconds from application of the stimulus to a peak in the recorded waveform. Volatile anesthetics may influence poststimulus amplitude and latency of evoked potentials (see Chapter 2). Although less than volatile anesthetics, morphine and fentanyl also produce de-

pressant effects on somatosensory evoked potentials with low-dose continuous infusions of these opioids producing less depression than intermittent injections (Pathak *et al,* 1984). Conversely, acute hyperventilation of the lungs to produce a $PaCO_2$ near 20 mmHg does not significantly alter amplitude or latencies of somatosensory evoked potentials (Schubert and Drummond, 1986). Evoked potentials are used to monitor (1) spinal cord function during operations near or on the spinal cord, (2) auditory nerve and brain stem function during posterior fossa craniotomies, and (3) visual function during operations on pituitary tumors or other lesions that impinge on the optic nerves or optic chiasm.

Somatosensory Evoked Potentials

Somatosensory evoked potentials are produced by application of a small electrical current that stimulates a peripheral nerve such as the median nerve at the wrist or posterior tibial nerve at the ankle. The resulting evoked potentials reflect the intactness of neural pathways from the peripheral nerve to the somatosensory cortex.

Auditory Evoked Potentials

Auditory evoked potentials arise from brain stem auditory pathways. Volatile anesthetics produce dose-dependent depression of auditory evoked potentials.

Visual Evoked Potentials

Visual evoked potentials are produced by flashes from light-emitting diodes that are mounted on goggles over the patient's closed eyes. During neurosurgical procedures involving visual pathways (transsphenoidal or anterior fossa surgery), the monitoring of visual evoked potentials has been used. Volatile anesthetics produce dose-dependent depression of visual evoked potentials especially above concentrations equivalent to about 0.8 MAC (Chi and Field, 1986).

BRAIN STEM

Subconscious activities of the body (*e.g.,* intrinsic life processes) are controlled in the brain stem.

The brain stem includes the medulla, pons, thalamus, hypothalamus, limbic system, basal ganglia, reticular activating system, and cerebellum. Examples of subconscious activities of the body regulated by the brain stem include control of blood pressure and ventilation in the medulla (see Chapters 44, 47, and 49). The thalamus serves as a relay station for all afferent impulses. The hypothalamus receives fibers from the thalamus and is also closely associated with the cerebral cortex.

Limbic System

Behavior associated with emotions is primarily a function of subcortical structures known as the limbic system located in the basal regions of the brain (Bentley and Konishi, 1978; Norrsel, 1980). The hypothalamus functions with the limbic system in this role. Indeed, some consider the hypothalamus a part of the limbic system rather than a separate structure. In addition, the hypothalamus controls many internal conditions of the body such as body temperature, thirst, and appetite. These internal functions represent functions of the body whose control is closely related to behavior. The reticular activating system is also an important component in the control of behavior. The hypothalamus indirectly affects cerebral function and thus behavior by activation or inhibition of the reticular activating system.

Amygdala

The amygdala is a complex of nuclei located immediately beneath the medial surface of the cerebral cortex in the pole of each temporal lobe. There are numerous connections between the amygdala, hypothalamus, and limbic system. Stimulation of the amygdala produces effects similar to stimulation of the hypothalamus.

Basal Ganglia

Basal ganglia include the caudate nucleus, putamen, globus pallidus, substantia nigra, and the subthalamus. Numerous nerve pathways pass from the motor portion of the cerebral cortex to the caudate nucleus and putamen. Many of the impulses from basal ganglia are inhibitory, and the neurotransmitters are dopamine and gamma-aminobutyric acid (GABA) (Baldessarini and Tarsey, 1980). Basal ganglia can originate motor signals and provide long-term continuous signals to the motor control pathway. The balance between agonist and antagonist skeletal muscle contractions is an important role of the basal ganglia. A general effect of diffuse excitation of basal ganglia is inhibition of skeletal muscles reflecting transmission of inhibitory signals from the basal ganglia to both the motor cortex and the lower brain stem. Therefore, whenever widespread destruction of the basal ganglia occurs, there is associated skeletal muscle rigidity.

Chorea

Chorea is a disease in which random uncontrolled movement patterns occur continuously. This pattern results from damage in the caudate and putamen nuclei. Neurons that secrete the inhibitory neurotransmitter, GABA, are reduced in number.

Hemiballismus

Hemiballismus is an uncontrollable succession of violent movements of large areas of the body such as the lower limb that occur at short intervals. The lesion is in the opposite side of the subthalamus.

Parkinson's Disease

Parkinson's disease is due to widespread destruction of the substantia nigra and corresponding nigrostriatal fibers. As a result, dopamine is no longer present in adequate amounts. Remaining fibers are excitatory and secrete acetylcholine leading to skeletal muscle rigidity characteristic of Parkinson's disease. Dopamine from the nigrostriatal pathway normally acts to inhibit these excitatory acetylcholine-evoked impulses. Dopamine precursors or anticholinergic drugs are used in the treatment of Parkinson's disease in an attempt to restore the balance between excitatory and inhibitory impulses traveling from the basal ganglia (see Chapter 31).

Reticular Activating System

The reticular activating system (also known as the reticular formation) consists of cells and nuclei that are present throughout the brain stem. This system is important in numerous visceral and somatic activities. The neurons of the reticular activating system are both excitatory and inhibitory and the presumed neurotransmitter is acetylcholine. The reticular activating system determines the overall level of central nervous system activity including control of sleep and wakefulness (Gillin *et al*, 1978). The cerebral cortex exerts its influence on spinal cord activities through the cells of the reticular activating system. Electrical stimulation of the mesencephalic portion of the reticular activating system causes generalized activation of the entire nervous system (*e.g.*, cerebral cortex, basal ganglia, hypothalamus, and spinal cord). Presumably, this is the portion of the reticular activating system that is responsible for normal wakefulness. Hemorrhage or a brain tumor involving this area of the reticular activating system causes a person to lapse into coma.

Stimulation of the thalamic portion of the reticular activating system activates specific regions of the cerebral cortex more than others. This is distinctly different from generalized activation of the entire nervous system that accompanies stimulation of the mesencephalic portion of the reticular activating system. Selective activation of certain areas of the cerebral cortex by the thalamic portion of the reticular activating system is crucial for the direction of the attention to certain aspects of mental activity.

Anatomy

Anatomically, the reticular activating system is optimally constructed to provide an arousal mechanism. For example, the reticular activating system receives numerous signals from multiple sites including pain, proprioception, visual and auditory receptors. In turn, this area can transmit signals both upward into the brain and downward into the spinal cord. A large number of nerve fibers pass from the motor cortex to the reticular activating system which is consistent with the importance of movement to keep a person awake. Likewise, any intense activity in the cerebral cortex maintains a high level of activity of the reticular activating system and consequently a high degree of wakefulness.

Drug Effects

It is likely that many of the clinically used anesthetics exert depressant effects on the reticular activating system contributing to their role as general anesthetics (Roth, 1979). Barbiturates have a specific depressant effect on the brain stem portion of the reticular activating system. Nevertheless, barbiturates do not entirely block function of the thalamic portion of the reticular activating system.

Sleep and Wakefulness

Sleep is a state of unconsciousness from which an individual can be aroused by sensory stimulation. Therefore, total inactivity of the reticular activating system, as produced by anesthesia or as present in the comatose individual cannot be defined as sleep. Sleep can occur from decreased activity of the reticular activating system (*i.e.*, slow wave sleep) or it can result from abnormal channeling of signals in the brain even though activity of the reticular activating system may not be depressed (*i.e.*, desynchronized sleep). Discrete lesions placed bilaterally in the locus ceruleus will cause sleep that resembles natural sleep. Lesions in the mesencephalic portion of the reticular activating system lead to coma. Sleep deprivation is associated with the appearance in the blood and cerebrospinal fluid of a low molecular weight polypeptide (Pappenheimer, 1976). Injection of this polypeptide into the third ventricle produces sleep.

Wakefulness is maintained by continued activity of the reticular activating system. Stimulation of an area in the pons immediately beneath the floor of the fourth ventricle is especially important in maintaining activity in the reticular activating system. This area is known as the *locus ceruleus* and is a collection of neurons that secrete norepinephrine. For this reason, it is presumed that norepinephrine and the closely related neurotransmitters, epinephrine and dopamine, play an important role in wakefulness (Moore and Bloom, 1979). Indeed, depletion of central nervous system catecholamine stores by antihypertensive drugs is associated with sedation and reductions in anesthetic requirements (*e.g.*, MAC) for inhaled drugs (Miller *et al*, 1968).

SLOW WAVE SLEEP. Most of the sleep that occurs each night is slow wave sleep. The electroencephalogram is characterized by high voltage delta waves occurring at a rate of 1 to 2 cycles sec^{-1}. Delta waves are generated intrinsically in the cerebral cortex independent of the reticular activating system (see the section entitled Electroencephalogram). Presumably, decreased activity of the reticular activating system that accompanies sleep permits an unmasking of this inherent rhythm in the cerebral cortex. Slow wave sleep is exceedingly restful and dreamless. During slow wave sleep, sympathetic nervous system activity declines, parasympathetic nervous system activity increases, and skeletal muscle tone is greatly reduced. As a result, there is a 10% to 30% decrease in blood pressure, heart rate, breathing rate, and basal metabolic rate.

DESYNCHRONIZED SLEEP. Periods of desynchronized sleep typically occur for 5 to 20 minutes during each 90 minutes of sleep. These periods tend to be shortest when the person is extremely tired. As the person becomes more rested through the night, the duration of desynchronized sleep increases. This form of sleep is characterized by active dreaming, irregular heart rate and breathing, and a desynchronized pattern of low voltage beta waves on the electroencephalogram similar to those that occur during wakefulness. This brain wave pattern emphasizes that desynchronized sleep is associated with an active brain, but this activity is not channeled in a direction that permits persons to be aware of their surroundings and thus be awake. Despite the inhibition of skeletal muscle activity, the eyes are an exception exhibiting rapid movements. For this reason, desynchronized sleep is also referred to as *paradoxical sleep* or *rapid eye movement sleep*.

Cerebellum

The cerebellum operates subconsciously to monitor and elicit corrective responses in motor activities caused by stimulation of other parts of the brain and spinal cord. Rapid skeletal muscle activities such as typing, playing musical instruments, and running require intact function of the cerebellum. Loss of function of the cerebellum causes incoordination of fine skeletal muscle activities even though paralysis of the muscles does not occur. The cerebellum is also important in maintenance of equilibrium and postural adjustments of the body.

An important afferent pathway to the cerebellum is the corticocerebellar pathway which originates mainly in the motor area of the cerebral cortex. The cerebellum also receives sensory impulses from the peripheral parts of the body via the dorsal and ventral spinocerebellar tracts. Signals transmitted in these tracts originate in muscle spindles, Golgi tendon organs, and receptors in skin and joints. The spinocerebellar pathways can transmit impulses at velocities greater than 100 m sec^{-1} which is the most rapid conduction of any pathway in the central nervous system. This extremely rapid conduction is important for the instantaneous appraisal by the cerebellum of changes that take place in the positional status of the body. A special feature of the cerebellum is the absence of reverberatory pathways. For this reason, the input–output signals of the cerebellum are always transient.

Dysfunction of the Cerebellum

In the absence of cerebellar function, a person cannot predict prospectively how far movements will go, thus resulting in overshoot of the intended mark (*e.g.,* past-pointing). This overshoot is known as *dysmetria,* and the resulting incoordinate movements are called *ataxia. Dysarthria* is present when rapid and orderly succession of individual skeletal muscle movements of the larynx, mouth, and respiratory system do not occur. Failure of the cerebellum to damp skeletal muscle movements results in *intention tremor* when a person performs a voluntary act. *Cerebellar nystagmus* is associated with loss of equilibrium presumably because of dysfunction of the pathways that pass through the cerebellum from the semicircular canals. In the presence of cerebellar disease, a person is unable to activate antagonist muscles that will prevent a certain portion of the body from moving unexpectedly in an unwanted direction. For example, a person's arm that was previously contracted but restrained by another person will move back rapidly when it is released rather than automatically remain in place.

SPINAL CORD

The spinal cord extends from the medulla oblongata to the lower border of the first and occasionally the second lumbar vertebra. Below the spinal cord, the vertebral canal is filled by the roots of the lumbar and sacral nerves which are collectively known as the *cauda equina.* The spinal cord is composed of gray and white matter, spinal nerves, and covering membranes.

Gray Matter

The gray matter of the spinal cord has been divided into nine separate laminae and has the shape of the letter H when viewed in cross-section (Fig. 41-6). This gray matter is divided into anterior, lateral, and posterior horns. The anterior horn is the location of (1) alpha motorneurons that supply axons that leave the spinal cord via the anterior roots and innervate skeletal muscles, (2) gamma motorneurons that leave the spinal cord via the anterior roots to innervate muscle spindles, and (3) cells of Renshaw. Cells of Renshaw are intermediary neurons that provide axons that synapse in the gray matter with anterior motorneurons. These cells inhibit the action of anterior motorneurons to limit excessive activity.

Cells of the preganglionic neurons of the sympathetic nervous system are located in the lateral horns of the thoracolumbar portions of the spinal cord. Cells of the intermediate neurons located in the portion of the posterior horns known as the *substantia gelatinosa* transmit tactile, pain, and temperature impulses to the spinothalamic tract.

White Matter

The white matter of the spinal cord is formed by axons of intermediate neurons and the ascending and descending tracts. This area of the spinal cord is divided into dorsal, lateral, and ventral columns (Fig. 41-6).

The dorsal column of the spinal cord is composed of tracts that transmit touch and pressure sensations with precise gradation and localization, vibratory sensations, and kinesthetic sensations. The spinothalamic tract is composed of small and usually unmyelinated nerve fibers that are less precise than the fibers in the dorsal column for the transmission of sensory impulses. The velocity of conduction of impulses in the spinothalamic tract is slow, and the fibers have poor spatial orientation. Specific sensations such as pain and temperature are transmitted selectively by the spinothalamic tract.

Spinal Nerves

A pair of spinal nerves arise from each of the 31 segments of the spinal cord. Spinal nerves are made up of fibers of the anterior and posterior

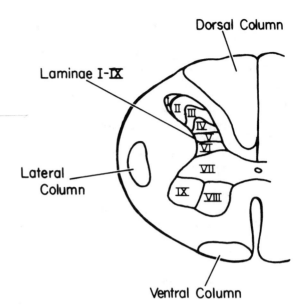

FIGURE 41-6. Schematic diagram of a cross-section of the spinal cord depicting anatomical laminae I–IX of the spinal cord gray matter and the ascending dorsal, lateral, and ventral sensory columns of the spinal cord white matter.

roots. Efferent motor fibers travel in the anterior roots. The cell bodies of the axons forming the anterior roots lie in the gray matter of the anterior and lateral horns of the spinal cord. Sensory fibers travel in the posterior roots. The posterior roots are formed by axons that originate from cell bodies in the spinal cord ganglia. These cell bodies send a branch to the spinal cord and to the periphery. Both the anterior and posterior roots leave the spinal cord through the intervertebral foramina enclosed in a common dural sheath that extends just past the spinal cord ganglia where the spinal nerve originates.

Dermatomes and Myotomes

Each spinal nerve innervates a segmental area of skin designated as a *dermatome* and skeletal muscles known as a *myotome*. Despite common depiction of dermatomes as having distinct borders, there is extensive overlap between segments. For example, three consecutive posterior nerve roots need to be interrupted to produce complete denervation of a dermatome. Segmental innervation of myotomes is even less well defined than dermatomes emphasizing that skeletal muscle groups receive innervation from several anterior nerve roots.

The anal region lies in the dermatome of the most distal cord segment corresponding to the tail region in the embryo. The legs develop from the lumbar and upper sacral segments rather than from the distal sacral segments. A dermatome map is useful in determining the level of spinal cord injury or the height of sensory blockade produced by a regional anesthetic (Fig. 41-7) (Guyton, 1986b).

Impulse Transmission

Sensory signals from the periphery are transmitted through the spinal nerves into each segment of the spinal cord. These signals can cause localized motor responses either in the segment of the body from which the sensory information is received or in adjacent segments. Spinal cord motor responses are automatic and characterized as reflex responses that occur almost instantly in response to the sensory signal. Examples of spinal cord reflex responses are the (1) muscle stretch reflex which causes a skeletal muscle to contract, and (2) withdrawal reflex. Spinal cord reflexes are important in causing emptying of the bladder and rectum. Segmental temperature reflexes allow localized cutaneous vasodilatation or vasoconstriction in response to changes in skin temperature. The function of the spinal cord component of the nervous system and spinal cord reflexes is particularly apparent in the patient with spinal cord transection.

Covering Membranes

The spinal cord is enveloped by membranes (dura, arachnoid, and pia) which are direct continuations of the same membranes surrounding the brain. The dura consists of an inner and outer layer. The outer periosteal layer in the cranial cavity is the periosteum of the skull. In the spine, this periosteal layer acts as the periosteal lining of the spinal canal. The epidural space is located between inner and outer layers of the dura. The fact that the inner layer of the dura adheres to the margin of the foramen magnum and blends with the periosteal layer means the epidural space does not extend beyond this point. As a result, drugs, such

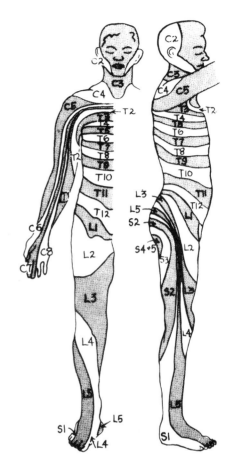

FIGURE 41-7. Dermatome map used to evaluate the level of sensory anesthesia produced by a regional anesthetic. (From Guyton AC. Textbook of Medical Physiology. 7th ed. Philadelphia: WB Saunders, 1986:580. Reproduced by permission of the author and publisher.)

as local anesthetics or opioids placed in the epidural space cannot extend beyond the first cervical nerves into the cranial cavity.

The inner layer of the dura extends as dural cuffs that blend with the perineurium of spinal nerves. The cerebral arachnoid extends as the spinal arachnoid ending at the second sacral vertebra. The pia is in close contact with the spinal cord.

ANATOMY OF NERVE FIBERS

Nerve fibers are *afferent* if they transmit impulses from peripheral receptors to the spinal cord and *efferent* if they relay signals from the spinal cord and central nervous system to the periphery.

Neuron

The neuron consists of a (1) cell body or soma, (2) dendrites, and (3) nerve fiber or axon (Fig. 41-8). Dendrites are extensions of the cell body. The axon of one neuron terminates near (*i.e.,* synapses) the cell body or dendrites of another neuron. The end areas of an axon are called the *presynaptic terminals.* The space between the presynaptic terminals and the cell body or dendrites of the next neuron is known as the *synaptic cleft.* Transmission of an impulse between two excitable neurons at a synapse is mediated by the release of a neurotransmitter such as norepinephrine or acetylcholine. This chemically mediated response differs from the electrical transmission of the impulse along the axon. The main function of the neuron is to relay information between the central nervous system and periphery.

Nerve fibers derive their nutrition from the cell body. Interruption of the nerve fiber causes

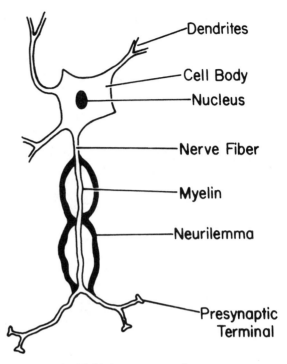

FIGURE 41-8. Anatomy of a neuron.

Table 41-1
Classification of Peripheral Nerve Fibers

	Myelinated	Fiber Diameter (microns)	Conduction Velocity (m sec^{-1})	Function	Sensitivity to Local Anesthetic (subarachnoid, procaine)
A-alpha	yes	6–22	30–120	Innervation of skeletal muscles Proprioception	1%
-beta	yes	6–22	30–120	Tactile sensory receptors (touch, pressure)	1%
-gamma	yes	3–6	15–35	Skeletal muscle tone	1%
-delta	yes	1–4	6–25	Stabbing pain Touch Temperature	0.5%
B	yes	3	3–15	Preganglionic autonomic fibers	0.25%
C	no	0.3–1.3	0.5–2	Burning and aching pain Touch Temperature Pruritus	0.5%

the peripheral portion to degenerate (*i.e.,* Wallerian degeneration). The central part of the neuron, however, is able to regenerate as does the myelin sheath. Nevertheless, lack of neurilemma prevents this type of regeneration from occurring in the brain or spinal cord.

Functionally, the nerve membrane is the most important part of the nerve fiber for impulse conduction. Indeed, removal of the axoplasm from the axon does not alter impulse conduction.

Classification of Nerve Fibers

Nerve fibers are classified as A, B, and C fibers on the basis of their diameters and velocity of conduction of nerve impulses (Table 41-1). The largest diameter A fibers are subdivided into alpha, beta, gamma, and delta. Type A-alpha fibers innervate skeletal muscles. Almost all the specialized tactile sensory receptors, such as Meissner's corpuscles, hair receptors, and Pacinian corpuscles transmit signals in type A-beta fibers. Type A-gamma fibers are distributed to skeletal muscle spindles. Touch and stabbing pain are transmitted by type A-delta fibers (see Chapter 43). Type C fibers transmit burning and aching pain, pruritus, and temperature impulses at low velocities (see Chapter 43). Type A and B fibers are myelinated while type C fibers are unmyelinated.

Myelin that covers type A and B nerve fibers acts as an insulator that prevents flow of ions across the nerve membrane. The myelin sheath, however, is interrupted approximately every millimeter by nodes of Ranvier. Ions can flow freely between the nerve fiber and extracellular fluid at the nodes of Ranvier. Action potentials are conducted from node to node by the myelinated nerve rather than continuously along the entire fiber as occurs in the unmyelinated nerve. This successive excitation of nodes of Ranvier by an impulse that jumps between successive nodes is termed *saltatory conduction* (Fig. 41-9) (Guyton, 1986c). Saltatory conduction greatly increases the velocity of nerve transmission in myelinated fibers and also conserves energy because only the nodes of Ranvier depolarize, resulting in less loss of ions than would otherwise occur. Furthermore, since depolarization is limited to only the nodes of Ranvier little extra metabolism for re-establishing the sodium and potassium ion concentration differences across nerve membranes is necessary.

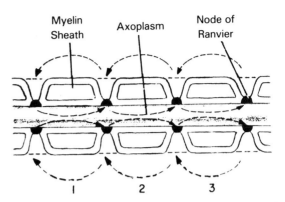

FIGURE 41-9. Saltatory conduction is transmission of nerve impulses that jump between successive nodes of Ranvier of a myelinated nerve. (From Guyton AC. Textbook of Medical Physiology. 7th ed. Philadelphia: WB Saunders, 1986:101. Reproduced by permission of the author and publisher.)

Synapse

A synapse is the junction between neurons and serves as an important control mechanism for transmission of impulses (Lynch and Schubert, 1980). Some synapses transmit signals with ease while others transmit impulses only with great difficulty. Strong signals may be transmitted while weak signals are suppressed. Furthermore, facilitatory and inhibitory signals can act at synapses thus controlling transmission of information between neurons. Inhaled anesthetics may interfere with transmission of impulses at synapses contributing to the state characterized as anesthesia (Koblin and Eger, 1979).

Synaptic Varicosities

The cell body of the neuron and associated dendrites contain structures known as *synaptic varicosities*. These synaptic varicosities are filled with vesicles that contain neurotransmitters such as norepinephrine and acetylcholine. Synaptic varicosities at excitatory synapses secrete an excitatory neurotransmitter while an inhibitory neurotransmitter is secreted at inhibitory synapses (Iversen, 1979). An action potential causes the release of neurotransmitter, the amount of which is often proportional to the extracellular concentration of calcium, magnesium, and sodium ions

(Kelly *et al*, 1979). Synaptic varicosities have the capability of continually synthesizing new neurotransmitter. Otherwise, synaptic transmission would become completely ineffective in a few minutes.

Postsynaptic Membrane and Receptors

The nerve membrane of the postsynaptic neuron is speculated to contain receptors that bind the neurotransmitter released by the presynaptic nerve terminal. These receptors are probably proteins that change their configuration when combined with neurotransmitter. This change in protein configuration alters permeability to ions. Specifically, permeability to most ions is increased if the neuron is excitatory, and permeability to chloride and potassium ions is increased if the neuron is inhibitory (Snyder and Bennett, 1976).

TRANSMISSION OF NEURONAL INFORMATION

Information derived from peripheral receptors (*e.g.,* pain, temperature, pressure, position, visual, auditory, factual) is transmitted to the brain in the form of impulses. Specific areas of the brain process these impulses, and new impulses are then transmitted either to other sites in the brain or into peripheral nerves to evoke a motor response. The overall pattern of several impulses relaying similar information is termed a *signal*. The intensity of a signal such as pain that is transmitted to the brain can be increased by increasing the number of parallel fibers participating (spatial summation) or increasing the frequency of impulses traveling along a single fiber (temporal summation) (Guyton, 1986d). The increase in number of participating fibers as the intensity of the signal increases is termed *recruitment*.

A stimulus to a neuron that exceeds the threshold for stimulation is an excitatory stimulus at an excitatory synapse. A subthreshold stimulus fails to excite the neuron but does make the neuron more excitable to impulses from other sources. The neuron that becomes more excitable by virtue of a subthreshold stimulus is said to be facilitated. Subthreshold stimuli can converge from several sources and summate at a neuron to evoke an excitatory stimulus at the responding synapse. The stimulus to a neuron may terminate

at an inhibitory synapse rather than excitatory synapse. Likewise, subthreshold inhibitory impulses may summate to produce an exaggerated inhibitory signal.

Information from one part of the nervous system is transmitted to another part through successive neuronal pools. For example, a painful cutaneous stimulus such as a surgical incision passes initially through peripheral nerve fibers to neurons in the spinal cord and then to neurons originating in the thalamus for transmission to the cerebral cortex. When a single point of the skin is stimulated, not only is a single fiber excited but a number of fringe fibers are simultaneously stimulated with less intensity. The blurring effect that stimulation of these fringe fibers would have on spatial recognition of the site of stimulation is offset by lateral inhibitory circuits that inhibit the fringe neurons and re-establish a truer spatial pattern.

Spatial Organization

All the different nerve tracts in peripheral nerves and in the fiber tracts of the central nervous system are spatially organized. For example, sensory fibers from the feet lie toward the midline of the dorsal columns of the spinal cord while those fibers entering the dorsal columns at higher levels of the body are located toward the lateral sides of the dorsal columns. This spatial organization is precisely maintained all the way to the sensory area of the cerebral cortex. Likewise, the fiber tracts within the brain and those extending into motor nerves are spatially oriented in the same way. This spatial organization allows the brain to recognize the origin of a peripheral sensory signal and subsequently transmit signals to individual skeletal muscles.

Reverbatory Circuit

A reverbatory or oscillatory circuit in the central nervous system occurs when an impulse returns to again excite the same neuron. This means a single input stimulus can produce output signals for prolonged periods ranging from milliseconds to even hours. This phenomenon is known as *after-discharge*. The duration of after-discharge due to a reverbatory circuit is dependent on the rapidity with which fatigue develops in the involved synapses (see the section entitled Synaptic Fatigue). Inhibitory circuits and synaptic fatigue are the mechanisms by which the brain prevents reverbatory circuits from producing generalized stimulation of the central nervous system.

An example of a repetitive and rhythmic reverbatory circuit may be the continuous stimulation of the inspiratory neuronal pool in the medullary respiratory center which typically lasts about 2 seconds (see Chapter 49). Wakefulness may reflect a continuous reverbatory circuit in the brain stem (Friesen and Stent, 1978). Inhibitory circuits and synaptic fatigue are the mechanisms by which the brain prevents reverbatory circuits from producing generalized stimulation of the central nervous system.

Sensory Receptors

Sensory receptors are responsible for converting sensory stimuli such as pain, temperature, and vision into signals that can be received by the brain. The five basic types of sensory receptors are (1) nociceptors which detect painful stimuli due to physical or chemical damage in tissue (see Chapter 43), (2) mechanoreceptors which detect tissue deformation, (3) thermoreceptors for cold and warmth, (4) electromagnetic receptors which detect light on the retina of the eye, and (5) chemoreceptors which detect taste, smell, arterial partial pressure of oxygen and carbon dioxide, and serum osmolarity. The type of sensation perceived when a fiber is stimulated is determined by the specific area in the brain to which the fiber leads. For example, stimulation of a pain fiber causes the patient to perceive pain regardless of the type of stimulus that excites the cutaneous receptor. Likewise, stimulation of a touch receptor, regardless of the stimulus, causes perception of touch because these fibers lead to specific touch areas in the brain. Sensory receptors, with the exception of nocieptors, adapt either partially or completely to stimuli after a period of time. The longest time for complete adaptation of a mechanoreceptor is about 2 days for the carotid and aortic baroreceptors (Catton, 1970).

Pathways for Sensory Impulses

Sensory information from somatic segments of the body enters the spinal cord through the posterior

roots. After entering the spinal cord, these nerve fibers divide into (1) the dorsal-lemniscal system that includes the dorsal column pathways and spinocervical tracts, and (2) anterolateral spinothalamic system. The dorsal-lemniscal system is comprised mainly of large myelinated nerve fibers that transmit signals to the brain at velocities of 30 to 120 m sec^{-1}, while the anterolateral spinothalamic system is comprised of small myelinated nerve fibers with conduction velocities of 10 to 60 m sec^{-1}. Sensations that are discretely localized to exact points in the body are transmitted in the dorsal-lemniscal system; those transmitted in the anterolateral spinothalamic system are localized much less precisely. The dorsal-lemniscal system, however, is limited to transmission of mechanoreceptive sensations (touch, position, pressure), while the anterolateral spinothalamic system has the capability for transmitting a broad spectrum of sensory modalities including pain, temperature, nondiscrete touch, pressure, pruritus, and sexual sensations.

Role of Spinal Cord

The gray matter of the spinal cord functions as the initial processor of incoming sensory signals from peripheral somatic receptors and as a relay station to send these signals to the brain. In addition, this area of the spinal cord is the site for final processing of motor signals that are being transmitted downward from the brain to skeletal muscles.

Upon entering the spinal cord through the posterior roots, the terminals of large sensory nerve fibers synapse with (1) local neurons that play an intricate role in the control of spinal cord reflexes, and (2) neurons that give rise to long ascending fiber tracts that transmit sensory information to the brain. Most of the sensory fibers for these long ascending tracts ascend in the spinocervical tract. Smaller sensory fibers entering the spinal cord from the posterior roots typically enter the anterolateral spinothalamic tract that crosses to the opposite side of the spinal cord before ascending to the brain.

Dorsal-Lemniscal System

Sensory signals are transmitted to the brain by dorsal column pathways and spinocervical tracts of the dorsal-lemniscal system (Fig. 41-10) (Guyton,

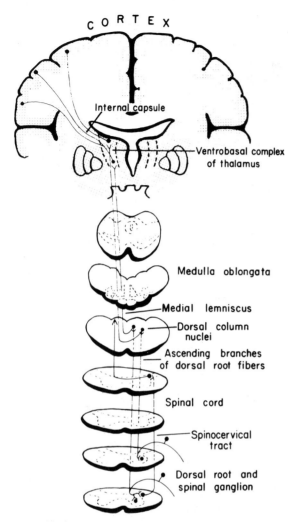

FIGURE 41-10. Sensory signals are transmitted to the brain by the dorsal column pathways and spinocervical tracts of the dorsal-lemniscal system. (From Guyton AC. Textbook of Medical Physiology. 7th ed. Philadelphia: WB Saunders, 1986:580. Reproduced by permission of the author and publisher.)

1986b). Impulses in the dorsal column pathways cross in the spinal cord to the opposite side before passing upward to the thalamus in pathways called the *medial lemnisci*. The crossing of these pathways is the reason the left side of the body is represented by the right side of the thalamus and cerebral cortex. Synapses in the thalamus are followed by neurons that extend to the somatic sensory area of the cerebral cortex.

Anterolateral Spinothalamic System

The anterolateral spinothalamic system transmits sensory signals that do not require highly discrete localization of the signal source or discrimination of fine gradations of intensity. Fibers for this system cross in the anterior commissure to the opposite side of the spinal cord where they turn upward toward the brain (Fig. 41-11) (Guyton, 1986b). Fibers of this system are divided into the ventral spinothalamic tract and lateral spinothalamic tract.

Signals from the anterolateral spinothalamic system are relayed from the thalamus to the somesthetic cortex in association with impulses from the dorsal-lemniscal system. These relayed signals seem to be concerned primarily with tactile sensation and very little with pain sensation. Pain signals seem to be relayed into other areas of the thalamus and hypothalamus. Indeed, loss of the somesthetic cortex has little effect on perception of pain and only a moderate effect on the perception of temperature. Therefore, it is likely the thalamus and other associated basal regions of the brain are dominant in discrimination of pain and temperature. This is consistent with the presumed early phylogenetic development of these sensibilities while critical tactile sensibilities were a late development.

Somesthetic Cortex

The area of the cerebral cortex to which the peripheral sensory signals are projected from the thalamus is designated the *somesthetic cortex* (Fig. 41-1) (Guyton, 1986a). This area is principally the anterior portions of the parietal lobes which receive afferent nerve fibers from relay nuclei of the thalamus (Darian-Smith *et al,* 1979). Each side of the cerebral cortex receives sensory information exclusively from the opposite side of the body. The size of these areas is directly proportional to the number of specialized sensory receptors in each respective area of the body. For example, a large number of specialized nerve endings are present in the lips and thumbs while only a few are present in the skin of the trunk. All sensory information that enters the cerebral cortex, with the exception of the olfactory system, passes through one of the several thalamic nuclei.

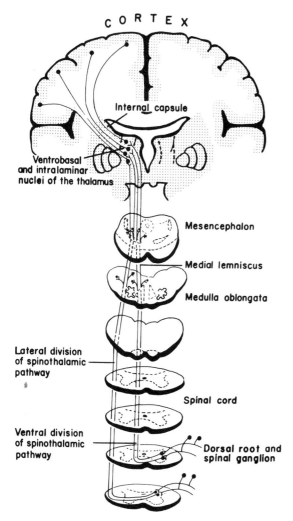

FIGURE 41-11. The anterolateral spinothalamic system fibers cross in the anterior commissure of the spinal cord before ascending to the brain. The fibers of this system transmit sensory signals by the ventral spinothalamic tract and lateral spinothalamic tract. (From Guyton AC. Textbook of Medical Physiology. 7th ed. Philadelphia: WB Saunders, 1986:580. Reproduced by permission of the author and publisher.)

NEUROTRANSMITTERS

Excitation or inhibition that occurs in response to the release of a neurotransmitter from varicosities of nerve endings is determined by the nature of the neurotransmitter and the type of postsynaptic receptor. For example, norepinephrine causes inhibition at some receptor sites in the central nervous system while at other sites excitation occurs. This is due to the presence of an inhibitory or excitatory receptor for the same neurotransmitter. A postsynaptic receptor may be excited by one neurotransmitter (acetylcholine) but inhibited by a different neurotransmitter (glycine). This reflects the existence of both an excitatory and inhibitory receptor on the same postsynaptic neuron. The onset and duration of effect of either inhibitory or excitatory neurotransmitters are variable. Some neurotransmitters function as modulators in that they influence the sensitivity of neurons to other neurotransmitters (Kupfermann, 1979).

Types of Neurotransmitters

A single neuron releases only one type of neurotransmitter. Therefore, release of the estimated 30 or more different types of neurotransmitters in the central nervous system requires different types of neurons. Neurotransmitters may include acetylcholine, norepinephrine, epinephrine, dopamine, glycine, GABA, glutamic acid, substance P, endorphins, serotonin, histamine, prostaglandins, and cyclic AMP (Nicoll *et al,* 1980). Acetylcholine and norepinephrine are widely and unevenly distributed suggesting these substances may be the principal neurotransmitters in the central nervous system.

Acetylcholine

Acetylcholine is a widely distributed excitatory neurotransmitter that interacts with muscarinic and nicotinic receptors in the central nervous system. This excitatory effect in the central nervous system contrasts with inhibitory effects (*e.g.,* hyperpolarization of the postsynaptic membrane) of acetylcholine in the peripheral parasympathetic nervous system.

Norepinephrine

Norepinephrine is secreted in large amounts in the reticular activating system of the brain stem and also the hypothalamus. These neurons send predominantly inhibitory impulses to widespread areas of the brain.

Dopamine

Distributions of dopamine and norepinephrine in the central nervous system are markedly different. More than one half of the central nervous system content of catecholamines is dopamine. High concentrations of dopamine are found in the basal ganglia, especially the caudate nucleus, and the amygdala. Most observations suggest dopamine is an inhibitory neurotransmitter perhaps by acting on dopamine-sensitive adenylate cyclase.

Epinephrine

Epinephrine-containing neurons are present in the reticular activating system. The presumed effects of this neurotransmitter are inhibitory.

Glycine

Glycine is secreted mainly at synapses in the spinal cord where it functions predominantly as an inhibitory neurotransmitter. Glycine also appears to be the most likely neurotransmitter for inhibitory neurons in the reticular activating system.

Gamma-Aminobutyric Acid (GABA)

GABA is an inhibitory neurotransmitter secreted by neurons in diverse areas of the nervous system including the spinal cord, cerebellum, and basal ganglia. Nonselective central nervous system stimulants may be acting as selective antagonists of GABA (see Chapter 33).

Glutamic Acid

Glutamic acid is an excitatory neurotransmitter secreted by many of the sensory pathways of the central nervous system. It causes depolarization of cell membranes primarily by increasing their permeability to sodium ions.

Substance P

Substance P is an excitatory neurotransmitter presumed to be released by terminals of pain fibers in the substantia gelatinosa of the spinal cord (see Chapter 43).

Endorphins

Endorphins are secreted by the nerve terminals in the spinal cord, brain stem, thalamus, and hypothalamus where they most likely act as excitatory neurotransmitters for systems that inhibit the transmission of pain (see Chapter 43).

Serotonin

Serotonin is secreted by neurons with wide distribution in the spinal cord and brain where it is believed to act as an inhibitory neurotransmitter at spinal cord pathways. In the brain, serotonin influences mood and may even cause sleep.

Histamine

Histamine is present in high concentrations in the hypothalamus and reticular activating system where it is presumed to act as an inhibitory neurotransmitter. Cyclic AMP may serve as a second messenger to mediate the actions of histamine in the central nervous system.

ELECTRICAL EVENTS DURING NEURONAL EXCITATION

Resting transmembrane potential of neurons in the central nervous system is about -70 mv which is less than the -90 mv in large peripheral nerve fibers and in skeletal muscle. This reduced magnitude of the resting transmembrane potential is important for controlling the responsiveness of the neuron. Threshold potential usually occurs when the transmembrane potential decreases about 11 mv to -59 mv.

At inhibitory synapses, neurotransmitter increases permeability of postsynaptic receptors only to potassium and chloride ions. The open channels of inhibitory neurons are too small to allow passage of larger hydrated sodium ions. The predominant outward diffusion of potassium ions increases the negativity of the resting transmembrane potential, and the neuron is hyperpolarized (e.g., functions as an inhibitory neuron). This is the way that permeability changes caused by an inhibitory neurotransmitter cause a neuron to function in the inhibitory mode. Conversely, permeability changes evoked by an excitatory neurotransmitter decrease the resting transmembrane potential bringing it nearer threshold potential. As a result, these neurons function in the excitatory mode.

In addition to postsynaptic inhibition due to inhibitory synapses at the neuron cell membrane, there is also presynaptic inhibition. Postsynaptic inhibition reflects release of neurotransmitters that suppress the action potential that normally occurs at the synaptic varicosity. GABA may be the presynaptic inhibitory neurotransmitter in the brain while glycine may be the presynaptic inhibitory neurotransmitter in the spinal cord.

Synaptic Delay

Synaptic delay is the 0.3 to 0.5 second necessary for the transmission of an impulse from the synaptic varicosity to the postsynaptic neuron. This synaptic delay reflects the time for release of neurotransmitter from the synaptic varicosity, diffusion of neurotransmitter to the postsynaptic receptor and the subsequent change in permeability of the postsynaptic membrane to various ions. This is followed by inward diffusion of sodium ions in sufficient amounts to decrease intracellular negativity to the point that threshold potential is reached and an action potential occurs.

Synaptic Fatigue

Synaptic fatigue is the decrease in number of discharges by the postsynaptic membrane when excitatory synapses are repetitively and rapidly stimulated. The function of the synaptic fatigue mechanism is to automatically adjust the sensitivity of the neuron to a lower level. For example, synaptic fatigue decreases excessive excitability of the brain as may accompany a seizure, thus acting as a protective mechanism against excess neuronal activity. The mechanism of synaptic fatigue is presumed to be exhaustion of the stores of neurotransmitter in the synaptic varicosities.

Post-tetanic Facilitation

Post-tetanic facilitation is increased responsiveness of the postsynaptic neuron to stimulation after a rest period that was preceded by repetitive stimulation of an excitatory synapse. This phenomenon may reflect increased release of neurotransmitter due to enhanced permeability of synaptic varicosities to calcium ions. Post-tetanic facilitation may be a mechanism for short-term memory (see the section entitled Memory).

Factors that Influence Neuron Responsiveness

Neurons are highly responsive to changes in pH of the surrounding interstitial fluids. For example, alkalosis enhances neuron excitability. Indeed, voluntary hyperventilation can often evoke a seizure in a vulnerable person. Conversely, acidosis depresses neuron excitability with a decline in arterial pH to 7.0 causing coma. Lack of oxygen can cause total inexcitability of neurons within 3 to 5 seconds as reflected by the onset of unconsciousness in this period of time when cerebral blood flow is interrupted.

Inhaled anesthetics may increase the membrane threshold for excitation and thus decrease neuron activity throughout the body. This concept is based on the speculation that most lipid-soluble volatile anesthetics may change the physical characteristics of neuron cell membranes making the membrane less responsive to excitatory neurotransmitters (Koblin and Eger, 1979).

MOTOR RESPONSES

Sensory information is integrated at all levels of the nervous system and causes appropriate motor responses beginning in the spinal cord with relatively simple reflex responses. Motor responses originating in the brain stem are more complex while the most complicated and precise motor responses originate from the cerebral cortex.

Spinal Cord

The spinal cord gray matter is the integrative area for spinal cord reflexes and other motor functions (Fig. 41-6). After entering the spinal cord, sensory signals either terminate in the gray matter of the spinal cord and elicit local segmental responses or the signals travel to higher levels in the nervous system. Neurons in each segment of the spinal cord are classified as (1) sensory relay neurons to transmit signals upward to the brain, (2) anterior motorneurons, and (3) interneurons.

Anterior Motorneurons

Anterior motorneurons are located in the anterior horns of the spinal cord gray matter. These motorneurons give rise to nerve fibers that leave the spinal cord by way of the anterior nerve roots and innervate skeletal muscle fibers. Nerve fibers arising from anterior motorneurons are designated as alpha motorneurons and gamma motorneurons.

ALPHA MOTORNEURONS. Alpha motorneurons give rise to large A-alpha fibers that pass through spinal nerves to innervate skeletal muscles. Stimulation of a single A-alpha fiber excites a motor unit which consists of up to 3000 skeletal muscle fibers.

GAMMA MOTORNEURONS. Gamma motorneurons located in the anterior horns of the spinal cord give rise to small A-gamma fibers. These A-gamma fibers are distributed to special skeletal muscle fibers designated intrafusal fibers which are part of the muscle spindle.

Interneurons

Interneurons are more numerous and more widely distributed than anterior motorneurons in the gray matter of the spinal cord (Kostyuk and Vasilenko, 1979). Interneurons are small and highly excitable, often exhibiting spontaneous activity being capable of firing as rapidly as 1500 times sec^{-1}. These neurons have many interconnections with other interneurons and often directly innervate anterior motorneurons. Indeed, many of the integrative functions of the spinal cord reflect interconnections between interneurons and anterior motorneurons.

Most of the incoming signals to the spinal cord from the periphery or brain are initially processed in interneurons before stimulating anterior motorneurons. For example, the corticospinal tract terminates almost entirely on interneurons and it is through these neurons that the brain transmits most of its signals for control of skeletal muscle function.

RENSHAW CELLS. Renshaw cells are interneurons located in the anterior horns of the spinal cord in close association with anterior motorneurons. These are inhibitory neurons that transmit inhibitory signals to nearby anterior motorneurons. This arrangement of lateral inhibition allows transmission of the primary signal from anterior motorneurons while suppressing the tendency for signals to spread to adjacent neurons.

Spinal Cord Synapses

Most sensory fibers entering each segment of the spinal cord terminate on interneurons, but a small number of large sensory fibers from muscle spindles terminate directly on the anterior motorneurons. Direct termination on anterior motorneurons represents a monosynaptic pathway which provides an extremely rapid reflex feedback system and is the basis for the muscle stretch reflex. Those sensory fibers that initially terminate on interneurons become polysynaptic pathways that can modify incoming signals to produce complex protective reflex patterns such as the withdrawal reflex.

Control of Skeletal Muscle Function

Skeletal muscles and tendons contain two special types of receptors known as *muscle spindles* and *Golgi tendon organs* that operate at a subconscious level to relay information to the spinal cord and brain relative to skeletal muscle contraction (Stein, 1978). Muscle spindles detect changes in the length of skeletal muscle fibers. Golgi tendon organs detect tension applied to the muscle tendon during contraction of the skeletal muscle.

Muscle Spindles

Muscle spindles are innervated by small type A-gamma fibers. Stretch is responsible for stimulation of the muscle spindle resulting in an increased rate of sensory impulse discharge. Conversely, shortening of the spindle decreases this rate of firing.

STRETCH REFLEX. The stretch reflex is reflex contraction of the skeletal muscle whenever stretch of the skeletal muscle results in stimulation of the muscle spindle. In this reflex circuit, a nerve fiber originating in the muscle spindle enters the dorsal root of the spinal cord where it synapses directly with an anterior motorneuron. A motor nerve fiber from the anterior motorneuron transmits an appropriate reflex signal with almost no delay back to the same skeletal muscle containing the muscle spindle. More delayed impulses result from collaterals that leave the fiber before it synapses with the anterior motorneuron. These collateral fibers pass to interneurons resulting in a polysynaptic rather than the more rapidly responsive monosynaptic reflex.

The stretch reflex is also important in preventing jerking and oscillation movements of the body. Muscle spindles have the ability to dampen and smooth out muscle contractions even though the input signals to the muscle system may themselves be jerky. This has been called a signal averaging effect of the muscle spindle reflex.

VOLUNTARY MOTOR CONTROL. The importance of the gamma efferent system is emphasized by the fact that nearly one third of all motor nerve fibers are small type A-gamma rather than large type A-alpha fibers. Whenever signals are transmitted from motor areas of the cerebral cortex to anterior motorneurons, there is invariably simultaneous activation of type A-alpha and A-gamma fibers.

CONTROL OF THE GAMMA EFFERENT SYSTEM. The gamma efferent system is excited primarily by the bulboreticular facilitory region of the brain stem and secondarily by impulses transmitted into this area from the cerebellum, basal ganglia, and cerebral cortex. The bulboreticular facilitory area is especially important for postural contractions (Pearson, 1976).

EVALUATION OF STRETCH REFLEX. The knee jerk reflects the functional integrity of stretch reflexes. The striking of the patellar tendon with a reflex hammer stretches the quadriceps and stimulates a stretch reflex. Transmission of large numbers of facilitory impulses from upper regions of the central nervous system to the spinal cord results in an exaggerated knee jerk response. Large lesions in the contralateral motor areas of the cerebral cortex, as caused by cerebral vascular accidents or brain tumors, cause greatly enhanced knee jerks.

Clonus is when the evoked muscle jerks oscillate. This phenomenon typically occurs when the stretch reflex is sensitized by facilitory impulses from the brain resulting in exaggerated facilitation of the spinal cord. The decerebrate state is classically associated with clonus. Decerebrate rigidity results mainly from hyperactivity of the muscle spindle system.

Golgi Tendon Organs

Golgi tendon organs are present within muscle tendons immediately beyond their attachments to skeletal muscle fibers. Typically, 10 to 15 skeletal muscle fibers are connected in series with each Golgi tendon organ and the organ is stimulated by the tension produced by this small bundle of muscle fibers. As such, Golgi tendon organs detect skeletal muscle tension while the muscle spindle detects skeletal muscle length.

Signals from Golgi tendon organs are transmitted to local areas of the spinal cord as well as through the spinocerebellar tracts into the cerebellum and by other pathways to the cerebral cortex. The reflex elicited in the spinal cord by impulses from the Golgi tendon organ is entirely inhibitory which is opposite of the muscle spindle reflex. As such, this reflex provides a negative feedback mechanism that prevents development of too much tension on the skeletal muscle. This prevents damage of the tendon from excessive stretch and provides a servomechanism to maintain proper tension in the skeletal muscle.

Withdrawal Reflexes

Withdrawal flexor reflexes are most often elicited by a painful stimulus. Pathways for eliciting the withdrawal reflex do not pass directly to the anterior motorneurons but instead pass first through several interneurons. Associated with withdrawal of the stimulated limb is extension of the opposite limb (*i.e.,* cross-extensor reflex) which occurs 0.2 to 0.5 second later and serves to push the body away from the object causing the painful stimulus. The delayed onset of the cross-extensor reflex is due to the time necessary for the signal to pass through additional interneurons to reach the opposite side of the spinal cord.

Reflex Skeletal Muscle Spasm

Spasm of skeletal muscles surrounding a broken bone seems to result from pain impulses initiated from the broken edges of bone. Relief of pain and skeletal muscle spasm is provided by infiltration of a local anesthetic. In some instances, general anesthesia may be necessary to relieve skeletal muscle spasm and permit proper alignment of the two ends of the bone.

Abdominal muscle spasm caused by irritation of the parietal peritoneum by peritonitis is an example of local skeletal muscle spasm caused by a spinal cord reflex. Relief of pain allows the spastic skeletal muscles to relax. Similar spasm of the abdominal skeletal muscles occurs during surgical operations in which stimulation of the parietal peritoneum causes the abdominal muscles to contract and cause extrusion of intestines through the surgical wound. During surgical operations in the abdomen, this skeletal muscle spasm is attenuated by volatile anesthetics and abolished by regional anesthesia or neuromuscular blocking drugs.

Autonomic Reflexes

Segmental autonomic reflexes occur in the spinal cord and include changes in vascular tone resulting from heat and cold, diaphoresis, and evacuation reflexes from the bladder and colon. Simultaneous elicitation of all the segmental reflexes is the mass reflex.

Mass Reflex

The mass reflex (also referred to as denervation hypersensitivity or autonomic hyperreflexia) typically occurs in the presence of a spinal cord transection when a painful stimulus to the skin below the level of spinal cord transection or distention of a hollow viscus such as the bladder or gastrointestinal tract occurs (see Chapter 42). The mass reflex is analogous to epileptic attacks that involve the central nervous system. The sustained duration of the mass reflex suggests activation of large numbers of reverberating circuits that simultaneously excite large areas of the spinal cord. The principal manifestation of the mass reflex is hypertension due to intense peripheral vasoconstriction reflecting inability of vasodilating inhibitory impulses from the central nervous system to pass beyond the site of cord transection. Baroreceptor-mediated reflex bradycardia accompanies the hypertension associated with the mass reflex.

Spinal Shock

Spinal shock is a manifestation of the abrupt loss of spinal cord reflexes that immediately follows transection of the spinal cord. This emphasizes the dependence of spinal cord reflexes on continual tonic discharges from higher centers, particularly discharges transmitted through the reticulospinal tracts and corticospinal tracts (Peterson, 1979). The immediate manifestations of spinal shock are hypotension, due to loss of vasocon-

strictor tone, and absence of all skeletal muscle reflexes. Within a few days to weeks, the spinal cord neurons gradually regain their intrinsic excitability. In some instances, recovery is associated with hyperexcitability of spinal cord reflexes. Sacral reflexes for control of bladder and colon evacuation are completely suppressed for the first few weeks following spinal cord transection, but these spinal cord reflexes also eventually return.

VISION

The eye is optically equivalent to a photographic camera in that it contains a lens system, a variable aperture system (*i.e.*, the pupil), and a retina that corresponds to the film. If all the refractive surfaces of the eye are algebraically added together and considered as a single lens, this single lens may be considered to exist with its central point 17 mm in front of the retina and to have a total refractive power of about 59 diopters when the lens is accommodated for distant vision. One diopter is equivalent to the ability of a lens to converge parallel light rays to a focal point 1 meter beyond the lens. The anterior surface of the cornea provides about 48 diopters of the eye's total diopter strength.

The lens system of the eye acts to focus an image on the retina. The image is inverted and reversed with respect to the object. The individual, however, perceives objects in the upright position despite the upside-down orientation of the retina because the brain is trained to consider an inverted image as the normal.

Lens

The refractive power of the crystalline lens of the eye can be voluntarily increased from 15 diopters to about 29 diopters in young children (Toates, 1972). Relaxation and contraction of the ciliary muscle are responsible for altering the tension of ligaments attached to the lens causing its refractive power to change. The ciliary muscle is controlled primarily by the parasympathetic nervous system. Stimulation of parasympathetic nervous system fibers to the ciliary muscle causes this muscle to relax, which in turn relaxes the ligaments of the lens and increases its refractive power. This increased refractive power allows the eye to focus on objects that are nearby. Interference with this process of accommodation may be noted by patients in the postoperative period who have received an anticholinergic drug in the preoperative medication.

The lens loses its elastic nature with aging probably because of progressive denaturation of the lens proteins. As a result, the ability to accommodate is almost totally absent by 45 to 50 years of age. This lack of ability of the lens to accommodate is known as *presbyopia*.

Progressive denaturation of the proteins in the lens leads to the formation of a cataract (Van-Heyningen, 1975). In later stages, calcium is often deposited in the coagulated proteins, thus further increasing the opacity. When the cataract impairs vision, the lens is surgically removed and replaced by an artificial convex lens that compensates for the loss of refractive power caused by removal of the lens.

Errors of Refraction

The clinical method for describing visual acuity uses a mathematical fraction that expresses the ratio of two distances. For example, if a person can see the size of letters at 20 feet that corresponds to a normal individual's visual acuity, the vision is said to be 20/20. Conversely, if the individual can see at 20 feet only letters that should be clearly visible at 100 feet, the visual acuity is 20/100.

A normal eye (emmetropia) can sharply focus parallel light rays from distant objects on the retina (Fig. 41-12) (Guyton, 1986e). Hypermetropia ("far-sighted") is usually due to an eyeball that is too short such that light rays do not converge by the time they reach the retina (Fig. 41-12) (Guyton, 1986e). Addition of refractive power by placing a convex lens in front of the eye is the treatment. Myopia ("near-sighted") is present when the light rays coming from distant objects are focused in front of the retina which usually is due to an eyeball that is too long (Fig. 41-12) (Guyton, 1986e). This excess refractive power of the lens can be offset by placing a concave lens in front of the eye.

Astigmatism is a refractive error of the lens system which is most often caused by an oblong shape of the cornea. Because the curvature of the astigmatic lens along one plane is less than the curvature along the other plane, light rays striking the peripheral portions of the lens in one plane are not bent as much as are rays striking the peripheral portions of the other plane. As a result, light rays

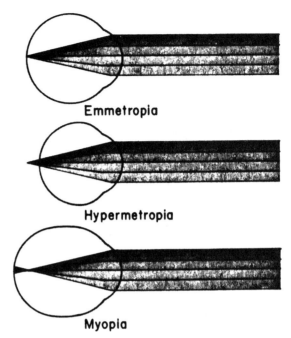

FIGURE 41-12.   Parallel light rays focus on the retina in emmetropia, behind the retina in hypermetropia, and in front of the retina in myopia. (From Guyton AC. Textbook of Medical Physiology. 7th ed. Philadelphia: WB Saunders, 1986:700. Reproduced by permission of the author and publisher.)

passing through an astigmatic lens do not all converge on a point. Placing an appropriate spherical lens in front of an astigmatic eye can only partially correct the refractive error.

A special feature of a contact lens is that this lens nullifies almost entirely the refraction that normally occurs at the anterior surface of the cornea. Thus, the refraction of the contact lens substitutes for the cornea's usual refraction. This is particularly important in persons whose refractive errors are caused by an abnormally shaped cornea.

Pupil

A major function of the iris is to increase or decrease the amount of light that enters the eye. The pupil of the human eye may vary from 1.5 to 8 mm in diameter permitting a 30-fold variation in the amount of light that enters the eye.

Intraocular Fluid

Intraocular fluid consists of aqueous humor, which lies in front and at the sides of the lens, and vitreous humor, which lies between the lens and retina. Aqueous humor is a freely flowing fluid which is continuously formed ($2-3$ ml min^{-1}) and reabsorbed. This fluid is secreted by ciliary processes of the ciliary body in a manner similar to formation of CSF by the choroid plexus. After flowing into the anterior chamber, aqueous humor enters Schlemm's canal which is a thin-walled vein that extends circumferentially around the eye. Schlemm's canal also reabsorbs proteins and thus serves the function of a lymphatic vessel. Vitreous humor is a gelatinous mass into which substances can diffuse slowly but there is little flow of fluid.

Intraocular Pressure

Intraocular pressure is normally 15 to 25 mmHg. This pressure is measured clinically by tonometry in which the amount of displacement of the cornea produced by placement of the tonometer is calibrated in terms of intraocular pressure. It is believed that intraocular pressure is regulated primarily by resistance to outflow of aqueous humor from the anterior chamber into Schlemm's canal.

Glaucoma

Glaucoma is a disease of the eye in which elevated intraocular pressure compresses retinal artery inflow to the eye leading to ischemic pain and eventually atrophy of the retina and blindness. Abnormally high intraocular pressure is almost always due to increased resistance to outflow of aqueous humor. When medical control of intraocular pressure fails, it may be necessary to surgically create an artificial outflow tract for aqueous humor.

Retina

The retina is the light-sensitive portion of the eye containing the cones, which are responsible for color vision, and the rods, which are mainly responsible for vision in the dark (Kaneko, 1979). Together, the cones and rods are classified as photoreceptors. When the cones and rods are stimulated, impulses are transmitted through successive neurons in the retina and optic nerve before reaching the cerebral cortex.

The presence of melanin in the pigment layer of the retina prevents reflection of light throughout the globe of the eyeball. Without this pigment, light rays would be reflected in all directions within the eyeball causing visual acuity to be impaired. Indeed, albinos who lack melanin have greatly diminished visual acuity.

The nutrient blood supply for the retina is largely derived from the central retinal artery which accompanies the optic nerve. This independent retinal blood supply prevents rapid degeneration of the retina should it become detached from the pigment epithelium and allows time for surgical correction.

Photochemicals

The light-sensitive photochemical continuously synthesized in rods is rhodopsin. Rhodopsin is a combination of the protein scotopsin and the carotenoid pigment, retinal. Cones contain several photochemicals that differ from rhodopsin only in that the protein portions, called photopsins, differ from scotopsin present in rhodopsin. Cones also have a different spectral sensitivity than rods being selectively sensitive to the different colors of blue, green, and red. Vitamin A is an important precursor of photosensitive pigments.

Photochemicals in rods and cones decompose on exposure to light and in the process stimulate fibers of the optic nerve. The decomposition of rhodopsin decreases conductance of the membranes of rods for sodium ions (Cervetto and Fuortes, 1978). This decreases the leakage of sodium ions to the interior of rods and creates increased negativity inside the membranes. The resulting hyperpolarization in rods is opposite to the effect that occurs in almost all other sensory receptors in which the degree of negativity is generally reduced during stimulation producing a state of depolarization. The intensity of the hyperpolarization signal is proportional to the logarithm of light energy, in contrast to the more linear response of most other receptors. This logarithmic response is important to vision because it allows the eyes to detect contrasts on the image even when light intensities vary several thousandfold. This effect would not be possible if there was a linear transduction of the signal.

Receptor potentials are transmitted unchanged through the bodies of the rods and cones. Neither the rods nor the cones generate action potentials. Instead, the receptor potentials, acting at synapses, induce signals in the adjoining neurons. An unknown neurotransmitter substance is most likely secreted by rods and cones to stimulate adjoining neurons. Neurotransmitter substances found in the retina include acetylcholine, dopamine, GABA, and glycine. Glycine probably acts as an inhibitory neurotransmitter in the retina (Kennedy *et al*, 1977). Indeed, transient visual disturbances and even blindness have been associated with elevated plasma concentrations of glycine following transurethral resection of the prostate using glycine-containing irrigating solutions (Ovassapian *et al*, 1982). Amplitude and latency of visual evoked responses are altered by intravenous infusions of glycine (Wang *et al*, 1985).

ADAPTATION. The retinal component of rhodopsin is in dynamic equilibrium with vitamin A. Most of the vitamin A of the retina is stored in the pigment layer of the retina rather than in the rods themselves, but this vitamin A is readily available to the rods. During total darkness, essentially all the photochemicals already in the rods are converted into rhodopsin within minutes (*i.e., dark adaptation*). For example, within 1 minute of entering darkness, the sensitivity of the retina is increased 10-fold, and by 20 minutes, the sensitivity has increased 6000-fold (Guyton, 1986f). The early response phase of dark adaptation is due to the adaptation of cones which resynthesize their photochemicals more rapidly than rods. Nevertheless, cones do not achieve the degree of sensitivity as the rods which continue to adapt for several minutes increasing their sensitivity tremendously.

If a person is in bright light for a prolonged period, large proportions of the photochemicals in both the rods and cones are depleted. This results in reduced sensitivity of the eye to light (*i.e., light adaptation*).

In addition to adaptation caused by changes in concentrations of rhodopsin or color photochemicals, the eye can adapt by changing the size of the pupillary opening and by the mechanism of neural adaptation. The change in pupillary size can cause a maximum 30-fold change in the degree of adaptation by virtue of altering the amount of light that reaches the retina. Neural adaptation is even less responsive but does occur in less than a second.

Below a certain light level, vision is capable of discriminating only between shades of black and white (*i.e.,* vision is scotopic). This occurs because only rods are capable of becoming dark-adapted to the sensitivity level required for detection of light. Conversely, in bright light, the function of rods is reduced and cones function optimally (*i.e.,* vision is photopic).

NIGHT BLINDNESS. The formation of rhodopsin permits much of the vitamin A to be converted into additional retinal. This is the reason night blindness occurs in the presence of severe vitamin A deficiency. Depletion of vitamin A, however, requires several months because large quantities of the vitamin are normally stored in the liver.

Color Blindness

Red-green color blindness is present when either the red or green types of cones are absent (Rushton, 1975). Rarely, an individual has "blue weakness" which results from diminished or absent blue receptor cones. Color blindness is sex-linked and results from absence of appropriate color genes in the X chromosomes. The lack of color genes is a recessive trait such that color blindness will not appear as long as another X chromosome carries the genes necessary for the development of color-receptor cones. Since the male has only one X chromosome, all three color genes must be present in this single chromosome to prevent color blindness. In about 1 of every 50 times, the X chromosome lacks the red gene and in about 1 of every 16 times the gene for the green cone is absent. As a result, about 2% of males are green color blind (deuteranopes). Color blindness is rare in females because they possess two X chromosomes. Spot charts are used to diagnose color blindness.

Visual Pathway

Impulses from the retina pass backward through the optic nerve (Fig. 41-13) (Guyton, 1986g; Rodieck, 1979). At the optic chiasm, all the fibers from the nasal halves of the retina cross to the opposite side to join fibers from the opposite temporal retina to form the optic tracts. The fibers of the optic tract synapse in the lateral geniculate body before passing to the visual area of the cerebral cortex. It is estimated that each retina contains about 125 million rods and 5.5 million cones, but only 1 million optic nerve fibers lead from each retina to the brain (Guyton, 1986g). As a result, about 125 rods and 5 cones converge on

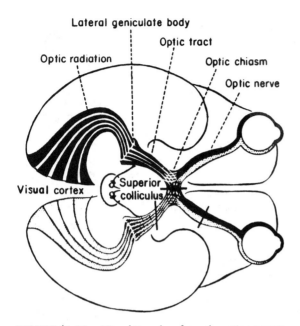

FIGURE 41-13. Visual impulses from the retina pass to the optic chiasm where fibers from the nasal halves of the retina cross to the opposite side to join temporal fibers and form the optic tract. These fibers synapse in the lateral geniculate body before passing to the visual (occipital) area of the cerebral cortex. (From Guyton AC. Textbook of Medical Physiology. 7th ed. Philadelphia: WB Saunders, 1986:724. Reproduced by permission of the author and publisher.)

each optic nerve fiber. There are, however, differences in the central and peripheral retina with fewer rods and cones converging on each optic nerve fiber in the central retina. For this reason, visual acuity increases toward the central retina. The macula is a small area in the center of the retina that is uniquely capable of detailed vision. It is composed entirely of cones. The central portion of the macula is called the *fovea* and is the site of the most clear vision. This largely explains the high level of visual acuity in the central portion of the retina in comparison with the poor acuity of vision in the peripheral portions.

Each geniculate body is composed of six layers of cells which relay visual information to the primary visual cortex through the geniculocalcarine tract. Specific points of the retina connect with specific points of the visual cortex. This vi-

sual cortex is located bilaterally on the medial aspect of each occipital cortex. The macula is represented by a large area at the occipital pole of the visual cortex. Based on this area, the fovea has 35 times as much representation in the primary visual cortex as do the peripheral portions of the retina (Guyton, 1986g).

A pattern of contrasts in the visual scene is impressed upon the neurons of the visual cortex, and this pattern has a spatial orientation roughly the same as that of the retinal image (Hubel and Wiesel, 1979). In addition to detecting the existence of lines and borders in the different areas of the retinal image, the visual cortex also detects the orientation of each line or border. Detection and deciphering of color are other important roles of the visual cortex.

Field of Vision

Field of vision is the area seen by an eye at a given instant. The area seen to the nasal side is called the *nasal field of vision* and the area seen to the lateral side is called the *temporal field of vision*. A blind spot caused by the lack of rods and cones in the retina over the optic disc is found about 15 degrees lateral to the central point of vision. Blind spots found in other portions of the visual field are called *scotomata* and reflect toxic or allergic reactions in the retina. Retinitis pigmentosa is degeneration of peripheral portions of the retina with subsequent deposition of melanin in the degenerated areas.

An important use of visual fields is for localization of lesions in the visual neural pathway. For example, destruction of the optic chiasm prevents the passage of impulses from the nasal halves of the two retinas to the opposite optic tracts. As a result, the individual is blind in both temporal fields of vision (*i.e.*, bitemporal hemianopia). Such lesions frequently result from tumors of the anterior pituitary pressing upward on the optic chiasm. Interruption of the optic tract denervates the corresponding half of each retina on the same side as the lesion, and, as a result neither eye can see objects to the opposite side (*i.e.*, homonymous hemianopia). Thrombosis of the posterior cerebral artery is a common cause of infarction of the visual cortex. The fovea area, however, is frequently spared, thus preserving central vision.

Muscular Control of Eye Movements

The cerebral control system for directing the eyes toward the object to be viewed is as important as the cerebral system for interpretation of the visual signals (Bizzi, 1974). Movements of the eyes are controlled by three pairs of muscles designated the (1) medial and lateral recti, (2) superior and inferior recti, and (3) superior and inferior obliques. The medial and lateral recti contract reciprocally to move the eyes from side to side, the superior and inferior recti move the eyes upward or downward, and rotation of the eyeball is accomplished by the superior and inferior obliques. Each of the three sets of eye muscles is reciprocally innervated by cranial nerves III, IV, and VI so that one muscle of the pair contracts while the other relaxes.

Simultaneous movement of both eyes in the same direction is called *conjugate movement* of the eyes. Occasionally, abnormalities occur in the control system for eye movements that cause continuous nystagmus. Nystagmus is likely to occur when one of the vestibular apparatuses is damaged or when deep nuclei in the cerebellum are damaged.

Innervation of the Eye

The eyes are innervated by the parasympathetic and sympathetic nervous system. The preganglionic fibers of the parasympathetic nervous system arise in the Edinger-Westphal nucleus of cranial nerve III and then pass to the ciliary ganglion. In this ganglion, the preganglionic fibers synapse with postganglionic neurons that innervate the ciliary muscle and sphincter of the iris. Innervation of the eye by the sympathetic nervous system involves fibers that originate in the first segment of the spinal cord and pass upward to the superior cervical ganglion where they synapse with postganglionic neurons. These postganglionic neurons innervate the radial fibers of the iris as well as several extraocular structures.

Transmission of motor signals to the ciliary muscle through the Edinger-Westphal nucleus is important in the accommodation mechanism that focuses the lens system of the eye (Toates, 1972). Stimulation of the parasympathetic nervous system fibers to the eye excites the ciliary sphincter thereby decreasing the pupillary aperture (*i.e.,*

miosis). Conversely, stimulation of sympathetic nervous system fibers to the eye excites the radial fibers of the iris and causes pupillary dilatation (*i.e.,* mydriasis).

Horner's Syndrome

Interruption in the superior cervical chain of the sympathetic nervous system innervation to the eye results in miosis, ptosis, vasodilation on the ipsilateral side of the face, and absence of sweating on this same side. These findings are known as Horner's syndrome and characteristically occur following a stellate ganglion block. Miosis occurs because of interruption of sympathetic nervous system innervation to the radial fibers of the iris. Ptosis reflects the normal innervation of the superior palpebral muscle by the sympathetic nervous system.

HEARING

The ear responds to the mechanical vibration of sound waves in the air. Transmission of sound from the tympanic membrane to the cochlea (inner ear) utilizes an ossicle system.

Ossicle System

The ossicle system of the middle ear is composed of the malleus, incus, and stapes. The handle of the malleus is attached to the tympanic membrane while the other end is bound by ligaments to the incus. The opposite end of the incus articulates with the stapes which lies against the membranous labyrinth in the opening of the oval window where sound waves are transmitted to the cochlea. The handle of the malleus is constantly pulled inward by ligaments and by the tensor tympani muscle, which keeps the tympanic membrane tensed. This allows vibrations on any portion of the tympanic membrane to be transmitted to the malleus.

Cochlea

The cochlea is embedded in a bony cavity in the temporal bone. For this reason, vibrations of the skull can cause fluid vibrations in the cochlea. The cochlea is a system of coiled tubes that are separated from each other by the vestibular membrane and basilar membrane. The organ of Corti, which contains a series of mechanically sensitive hair cells, lies on the basilar membrane. These hair cells are the receptive end-organs that generate nerve impulses in response to sound vibrations. The bases and sides of the hair cells synapse with a network of cochlear nerve endings which then enter the central nervous system at the level of the upper medulla. Several important pathways also exit from the auditory system into the cerebellum. The auditory cerebral cortex lies principally on the supratemporal plane of the superior temporal gyrus (Aitkin, 1976).

Deafness

Nerve deafness is due to an abnormality of the cochlear or auditory nerve. Conversely, conduction deafness is present when an abnormality exists in the middle ear mechanisms for transmitting sound into the cochlea. Certain drugs such as streptomycin, kanamycin, and chloramphenicol damage the organ of Corti causing nerve deafness. Conduction deafness is often caused by fibrosis of structures in the middle ear following repeated infection in the middle ear or by the hereditary disease known as osteosclerosis.

EQUILIBRIUM

The vestibular apparatus is a sensory organ that detects sensations necessary for the maintenance of equilibrium (Precht, 1979). It is composed of a bony labyrinth which contains the functional part of the vestibular apparatus known as the membranous labyrinth. The membranous labyrinth consists of the cochlear duct, three semicircular canals, and chambers known as the utricle and saccule. The cochlear duct is the major sensory area for hearing and plays no role in the maintenance of equilibrium.

The utricle and saccule contain cilia that transmit nerve impulses to the brain necessary for maintenance of orientation of the head in space. The three semicircular canals are filled with endolymph. Flow of endolymph in response to changes in head position causes signals to be transmitted to the brain by the vestibular nerve. Most of the fibers of the vestibular nerve end in the vestibular nuclei, but some fibers also pass directly to the cerebellum.

The semicircular canals predict, ahead of time, that loss of equilibrium is going to occur leading to the initiation of preventive adjustments. For this reason, a person need not fall off balance before corrective responses begin to occur. Each time the head is suddenly angulated, signals from the semicircular canals cause the eyes to angulate in an equal and opposite direction to the angulation of the head. Nystagmus occurs when the semicircular canals are stimulated.

Tests of Vestibular Function

A simple test of the integrity of the equilibrium mechanism is to have the individual stand motionless with the eyes closed. In the absence of a functioning static equilibrium system of the utricles, the person will tend to fall to one side. Nevertheless, proprioceptive mechanisms of equilibrium may be sufficiently developed to maintain balance even with the eyes closed. Separate testing of the vestibular apparatus depends on placing ice water in one ear. The external semicircular canal is adjacent to the tympanic membrane such that selective cooling of the endolymph occurs. This causes nystagmus in the presence of normal functioning of the semicircular canals.

Other Factors in Control of Equilibrium

The vestibular apparatus detects movements and orientation of the head only. The orientation of the head with respect to the rest of the body is provided by proprioceptive joint receptors. Vision may also effectively maintain equilibrium even in the absence of proprioceptive information and function of the vestibular apparatus.

CHEMICAL SENSES

Chemical senses are manifest as taste and smell.

Taste

Taste is mainly a function of taste buds located principally in the papillae of the tongue (Dastoli, 1974). Sweet, sour, salty, and bitter are the four primary sensations of taste. Adults have about 10,000 taste buds, but after age 45, many taste buds degenerate causing taste discrimination to be less. There is a tendency for specific taste buds to be localized to selected areas. For example, taste buds responsive to sweet sensations are localized principally on the anterior surface and tip of the tongue. Salty and sour sensations are detected by taste buds on the lateral sides of the tongue, and bitter taste buds are present on the posterior aspect of the tongue. Adaptation to taste sensations is almost complete within 1 to 5 minutes of continuous stimulation. Persons with upper respiratory tract infections complain of loss of taste sensation when, in fact, taste bud function is normal, emphasizing the fact that most of what is considered taste is actually smell.

The multitudes of different tastes, like color vision, are combinations of the four primary taste sensations. Sour taste is caused by acids, and the taste sensation is approximately proportional to the logarithm of the hydrogen ion concentration. Bitter taste of alkaloids causes the individual to reject the substance. This is probably protective because many toxins in poisonous plants are alkaloids. Indeed, the threshold for stimulation of a bitter taste is much lower than for other primary taste sensations.

Mechanism of Stimulation

The interior of the membrane of the epithelial cell of the taste bud is normally negatively charged. Application of a taste substance causes partial loss of the negative potential in proportion to the logarithm of concentration of the stimulating substances. This change in potential in the taste cell is the receptor potential for taste. Presumably, the taste substance causes the cell membrane to become more permeable to sodium ions and thus depolarize. The taste substance is gradually washed away from the taste bud by saliva thus removing the taste stimulus.

Transmission of Taste Signals

Taste signals travel via cranial nerves V, IX, and X to synapse in the tractus solitarius. From the tractus solitarius neurons pass to the thalamus and then to an area in the parietal cerebral cortex. These pathways closely parallel the somatic pathways from the tongue. Taste preference is pre-

sumed to be a central nervous system phenomenon.

Smell

The olfactory membrane is located in the superior part of each nostril (Moulton and Beidler, 1967). Olfactory receptor cells are bipolar nerve cells derived originally from the central nervous system. Olfactory hairs or cilia are believed to sense odors in the air causing stimulation of the olfactory cells. Compared with lower animals, the sense of smell in humans is almost rudimentary.

A substance must be volatile and lipid soluble to stimulate olfactory cells. Olfactory cells are stimulated only when air moves rapidly upward into the superior portion of the nose. As a result, smell occurs in cycles along with inspiration emphasizing that olfactory receptors respond within seconds. The importance of upward air movement in smell acuity is the reason sniffing improves the sense of smell while holding one's breath prevents the sensation of an adverse smell. There may be more than 50 primary smell sensations in contrast to only three primary sensations of color detected by the eyes and only four primary sensations of taste detected by the tongue.

Transmission of Smell Signals

It is presumed that olfactory stimuli cause a receptor potential in olfactory cells which in turn initiates nerve impulses in the olfactory nerve fibers (Oakley and Benjamin, 1966). The intensity of the olfactory nerve impulses is approximately proportional to the logarithm of the stimulus strength which illustrates that olfactory receptors obey principles of transduction similar to those of other sensory receptors. Olfactory receptors adapt about 50% in the first few seconds of stimulation. Within about 1 minute, smell sensations adapt almost to extinction presumably reflecting adaptation in the central nervous system. The threshold for smell is low. For example, methyl mercaptan can be detected when the concentration in 1 ml of air is 2.5×10^{-10} mg (Guyton, 1986h). Because of this low threshold, methyl mercaptan is mixed with natural gas to give it an odor that can be detected when gas leaks occur.

Olfactory signals travel in the olfactory tract and terminate in the medial and lateral olfactory areas of the brain. Secondary olfactory tracts from these areas pass to other areas including the thalamus, hypothalamus, and hippocampus.

BODY TEMPERATURE

Heat is continually being produced in the body as a by-product of metabolism. At the same time, heat is continually being lost to the environment. The net effect is regulation of body temperature within a narrow range with a normal core body temperature being considered 37 Celsius. Regulation of body temperature is by nervous system feedback mechanisms that operate principally through preoptic areas in the hypothalamus (Benzinger, 1969; Cabanac, 1975).

Metabolism

Metabolism refers to all the chemical reactions of the body while the metabolic rate is expressed in terms of the rate of heat liberation during these chemical reactions. Basal metabolic rate is the rate of energy utilization during absolute rest but when the person is awake. The average basal metabolic rate varies in proportion to body surface area which parallels body weight. Metabolic rate declines with increasing age and is reduced 10% to 15% during physiologic sleep presumably reflecting decreased activity of skeletal muscles and the sympathetic nervous system. Factors that increase metabolic rate include fever, sympathetic nervous system stimulation, growth hormone, and thyroid hormone.

The normal metabolic rate of the newborn in relation to body weight is about two times that of the adult. This accounts for the fact that cardiac output and minute ventilation are about twice as great in the infant. Nevertheless, the body surface area of the infant relative to body mass is great making the infant vulnerable to excessive heat loss.

An estimated 55% of the energy in nutrients becomes heat during the formation of adenosine triphosphate (ATP) (see Chapter 58). The calorie is the unit for expressing the quantity of energy released from different nutrients. Average daily caloric requirements for basal function are about 2000 calories (Table 41-2) (Guyton, 1986i).

Table 41-2
Energy Expenditure for Various Forms of Physical Activity

	Calories per Hour
Physiologic sleep	65
Awake but no activity	77–100
Typing	140
Walking slowly (2.6 mph)	200
Swimming	500
Running (5.3 mph)	570
Walking slowly (2.6 mph)	200
Walking up stairs	1100

(Adapted from Guyton AC. Textbook of Medical Physiology. 7th ed. Philadelphia, WB Saunders, 1986:841; by permission of the author and publisher.)

Heat Loss

Heat loss occurs as radiation, conduction, and convection. Evaporation and diaphoresis are additional mechanisms for heat loss.

Radiation

Loss of heat by radiation is in the form of infrared heat rays. All objects that are not at absolute zero temperature radiate infrared heat rays. If the temperature of the body is greater than the temperature of the surroundings, a greater quantity of heat is radiated from the body than is radiated to the body.

INSULATION SYSTEM. Skin, subcutaneous tissues, and the fat of subcutaneous tissues are effective insulation systems. Fat is particularly important because it conducts heat only one-third as readily as other tissues. As a result, the degree of insulation varies among individuals depending on the quantity of adipose tissue.

Blood vessels penetrate subcutaneous insulator tissues. Variations in blood flow permit about an eightfold increase in heat conductance between the fully vasoconstricted state and the fully vasodilated state. Blood flow through the skin is the most effective mechanism of heat transfer from the interior (core) of the body to the skin (see the section entitled Cutaneous Blood Flow).

Conduction

Only minute amounts of heat are lost from the body by contact with other objects (*i.e.,* conduction). Conversely, loss of heat by conduction to air represents a significant amount of total heat loss from the body. Once the temperature of the air immediately adjacent to the skin equals the temperature of the skin, no further loss of heat from the body to the air can occur. As a result, conduction of heat from the body to the air is self-limited unless new unheated air is continually brought into contact with the skin (*i.e.,* convection).

Convection

After heat is conducted to air, this heat is carried away by air currents designated as convection. Wind accelerates the rate of change of the air to which the skin is exposed. The rate of heat loss to water, however, is much greater than the rate of heat loss to air of the same temperature. This occurs because water has a greater specific heat (*i.e.,* can absorb more heat) than air. The effectiveness of clothing in preventing heat loss is almost completely lost when it becomes wet because the high conductivity of water increases the rate of heat transmission.

Evaporation

Heat is lost for each gram of water that evaporates from the body surface. Water evaporates insensibly from the skin and lungs at a rate of about 700 ml each day. This evaporation occurs regardless of body temperature. When the temperature of the surroundings is greater than that of the skin, the body gains heat by radiation and conduction. In these instances, evaporation is the only mechanism by which the body can eliminate excess heat.

Diaphoresis

Diaphoresis occurs in response to stimulation of the preoptic area in the anterior hypothalamus. Impulses from this area are transmitted by the autonomic nervous system to the spinal cord and then through the sympathetic outflow to the skin. Sweat glands are innervated by sympathetic cholinergic fibers. It is also possible that sweat glands of certain areas, such as the hands and feet, have sympathetic adrenergic innervation as reflected by responses to emotional stimulation.

Large amounts of sodium and chloride ions as well as potassium and lactic acid are lost in sweat. A normal unacclimatized person can produce maximally about 700 ml of sweat each hour but with continued exposure to a warm environment, sweat production may increase to 1500 ml each hour (Guyton, 1986j). Evaporation of this much sweat can remove heat from the body at a rate more than ten times the normal basal rate of heat production. Associated with acclimatization is increased secretion of aldosterone to prevent excessive loss of sodium and chloride ions in the sweat.

Regulation of Body Temperature

Regulation of body temperature is by nervous system feedback mechanisms that operate principally through the preoptic area in the hypothalamus. The preoptic area of the hypothalamus contains large numbers of heat-sensitive neurons that function as temperature sensors for controlling body temperature. The overall heat controlling mechanism of the hypothalamus is that of a hypothalamic thermostat (Guyton, 1986j). When the hypothalamic thermostat detects that body temperature is above or below 37 Celsius, it initiates appropriate heat-decreasing or heat-increasing responses.

Mechanisms to Reduce Body Temperature

The hypothalamic thermostat utilizes three primary mechanisms to decrease body temperature. First, inhibition of sympathetic nervous system centers in the posterior hypothalamus that cause vasoconstriction results in vasodilation of cutaneous blood vessels. Maximum vasodilation can increase the rate of heat transfer to the skin as much as eightfold. Second, sweating is stimulated. Finally, heat production by such mechanisms as shivering and chemical thermogenesis is inhibited.

Mechanisms to Increase Body Temperature

Body temperature is increased by generalized vasoconstriction of cutaneous blood vessels caused by stimulation of the posterior hypothalamic sympathetic centers. Shivering reflects stimulation of the motor center for shivering located in the dorsomedial portion of the posterior hypothalamus. During maximum shivering, body heat production can rise five times above normal.

CHEMICAL THERMOGENESIS. Chemical thermogenesis is an increase in the rate of cellular metabolism evoked by sympathetic nervous system stimulation or by circulating catecholamines (Himms-Hagen, 1976). In adults, who have almost no brown fat, it is rare that chemical thermogenesis increases the rate of heat production more than 10% to 15%. In infants, however, chemical thermogenesis in brown fat located in the interscapular space, can increase the rate of heat production as much as 100%. This probably is an important factor in maintaining normal body temperature in the neonate. Brown fat contains large numbers of mitochondria, and these cells are innervated by the sympathetic nervous system.

THYROID. Stimulation of the preoptic area of the hypothalamus increases the release of thyrotropin-releasing hormone from the hypothalamus. This hormone stimulates the release of thyroid-stimulating hormone and subsequent release of thyroxine from the thyroid gland. Thyroxine increases the rate of cellular metabolism throughout the body. The continuous stimulatory effect of cold on the thyroid gland is consistent with the higher incidence of thyroid goiters in persons living in colder climates.

FEVER. Many proteins, breakdown products of proteins, and polysaccharide toxins secreted by bacteria can cause the set point of the hypothalamic thermostat to rise. Substances that cause this effect are called *pyrogens*. It is pyrogens secreted by bacteria or released from degenerating tissues that cause fever. Presumably, pyrogens interact with polymorphonuclear leukocytes to form endogenous pyrogens that have intense direct effects on the heat-sensitive neurons of the hypothalamus.

Dehydration can cause fever which in part reflects lack of available fluid for sweating. In addition, dehydration in some way stimulates the hypothalamus.

CHILLS. Sudden resetting of the hypothalamic thermostat to a higher level as a result of tissue destruction, pyrogenic substances, or dehydration results in a lag between blood temperature and the setting of the hypothalamus. During this period, the person experiences chills and feels cold even though body temperature may already be elevated. The skin is cold because of vasoconstriction of cutaneous blood vessels. Chills continue until the body temperature rises to the new setting of the hypothalamic thermostat. As long as the factor that is causing the hypothalamic thermostat to be set at a higher level is present, the body temperature remains elevated above 37 Celsius. Sudden removal of the factor that is causing temperature to remain elevated is accompanied by intense sweating and sudden development of a hot skin because of generalized vasodilatation of the cutaneous blood vessels.

Cutaneous Blood Flow

Cutaneous blood flow supplies nutrients to the skin and conducts heat from the internal structures of the body for dissipation to the environment (Nicoll and Cortese, 1972). Vascular structures concerned with heat loss from skin consist of subcutaneous venous plexuses which can hold large quantities of blood. Furthermore, in some areas of the skin, direct arteriovenous anastomoses facilitate heat loss. Arteriovenous anastomoses are most prominent in the volar surfaces of the hands and feet, the lips, nose, and ears. These are areas of the body most often exposed to extremes of temperature. Sympathetic nervous system stimulation produces intense vasoconstriction and reduces blood flow into the venous plexuses to almost zero.

RATE OF CUTANEOUS BLOOD FLOW. Cutaneous blood flow is among the most variable in the body reflecting changes required to regulate body temperature in response to alterations in the rate of metabolism and the temperature of the external surroundings. Nutritional requirements are so low for skin that this need does not significantly influence cutaneous blood flow. For example, at ordinary skin temperatures, cutaneous blood flow is about ten times that needed to supply nutritive needs of the skin.

Cutaneous blood flow in an adult is about 400 ml min^{-1}. This flow can decrease to as little as 50 ml min^{-1} in severe cold and to as much as 2800 ml min^{-1} in extreme heat. Indeed, patients with borderline cardiac function may become symptomatic in hot environments emphasizing the increase in cardiac output necessitated by marked elevations in cutaneous blood flow.

REGULATION OF CUTANEOUS BLOOD FLOW. Cutaneous blood flow is largely regulated by the sympathetic nervous system and not local regulatory mechanisms as is true in most other parts of the body (Heistad and Abboud, 1974). This emphasizes that the principal role of cutaneous blood flow is heat regulation of the body and not nutrition of the skin. Nevertheless, no vasodilator fibers have been identified to the cutaneous blood vessels. Vasodilation is achieved either by decreasing vasoconstrictor tone or by activating cholinergic pathways to sweat glands which apparently release bradykinin formed by enzymes in the sweat glands. Reactive hyperemia can be demonstrated as a reflection of increased blood flow to an area of skin that has been rendered ischemic by prolonged external pressure and compression of cutaneous blood vessels. Inhaled anesthetics increase cutaneous blood flow, perhaps by inhibiting the temperature-regulating center of the hypothalamus (Heistad and Abboud, 1974).

When cold is applied directly to the skin, cutaneous blood vessels constrict until a maximum effect is reached at about 15 Celsius. Below 15 Celsius cutaneous blood vessels begin to dilate presumably due to a direct effect of cold on the contractile mechanism. Maximum vasodilation is reached at about 0 Celsius. This vasodilation in severe cold serves a purposeful role in preventing freezing of the exposed portions of the body, especially the hands and ears.

During exercise or acute hemorrhage, or even in states of anxiety, the sympathetic nervous system can produce sufficient vasoconstriction to transfer large amounts of blood into the central circulation. As such, the cutaneous veins act as an important blood reservoir which can supply 5% to 10% of the blood volume in times of need.

SKIN COLOR. Skin color is primarily due to the color of blood in the cutaneous capillaries and veins. The skin is red when the skin is hot and arterial blood is flowing rapidly through these tissues. Conversely, when the skin is cold and blood is flowing slowly, the removal of oxygen for nutritive purposes gives the skin the bluish hue (*i.e.,* cyanosis) of deoxygenated blood. Severe vasoconstriction of the skin forces most of the blood into the central circulation, and skin takes on the whitish hue (*i.e.,* pallor) of underlying connective tissue which is composed primarily of collagen fibers.

NAUSEA AND VOMITING

Nausea is the conscious recognition of excitation of an area in the medulla that is associated with the vomiting center (Fig. 41-14) (Swenson and Orkin, 1983). Impulses are transmitted by afferent fibers of the parasympathetic and sympathetic nervous system to the vomiting center in the medulla which is at the approximate level of the dorsal motor nucleus of the vagus. Appropriate motor reactions are then instituted to cause the act of vomiting. These motor impulses are transmitted through cranial nerves V, VII, IX, X, and XII to the upper gastrointestinal tract and through the spinal nerves to the diaphragm and abdominal muscles.

Vomiting can also be caused by impulses that arise in areas of the brain outside the vomiting center. For example, stimulation of a small area located bilaterally on the floor of the fourth ventricle known as the chemoreceptor trigger zone initiates vomiting. Drugs such as morphine and

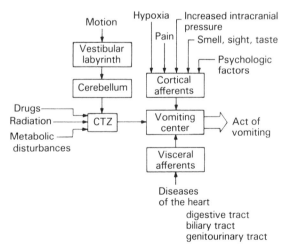

FIGURE 41-14. Schematic diagram of stimuli causing nausea and vomiting. Chemoreceptor trigger zone (CTZ). (From Swenson EJ, Orkin FK. Postoperative nausea and vomiting. In: Complications in Anesthesiology. Orkin FK, Cooperman LH, eds. Philadelphia, J.B. Lippincott, 1983:429. Reproduced by permission of the authors and publisher.)

digitalis derivatives can directly stimulate the chemoreceptor trigger zone to cause vomiting. Blockade of impulses from this area, however, does not prevent vomiting resulting from irritative stimuli arising in the gastrointestinal tract.

Motion can stimulate receptors of the vestibular labyrinth, and impulses are transmitted mainly by way of the vestibular nuclei to the cerebellum. After passing through the cerebellum, these signals are presumed to be transmitted to the chemoreceptor trigger zone and then to the vomiting center to initiate vomiting.

Various psychic stimuli including unpleasant visual input or odors can cause vomiting. It is likely these impulses directly stimulate the vomiting center.

REFERENCES

Aitkin LM. Tonotopic organization at higher levels of the auditory pathway. Int Rev Physiol 1976;10:249 – 79.

Baldessarini RJ, Tarsey D. Dopamine and the pathophysiology of dyskinesias induced by antipsychotic drugs. Annu Rev Neurosci 1980;3:23 – 41.

Bennett HL, Davis HS, Giannini JA. Non-verbal response to intraoperative conversation. Br J Anaesth 1985;57:174 – 9.

Bentley D, Konishi M. Neural control of behavior. Annu Rev Neurosci 1978;1:35 – 59.

Benzinger TH. Heat regulation: Homeostasis of central temperature in man. Physiol Rev 1969;49:671 – 759.

Betz E. Cerebral blood flow: Its measurement and regulation. Physiol Rev 1972;52:595 – 630.

Bizzi E. The coordination of eye-head movements. Sci Am 1974;231:100 – 6.

Bogetz MS, Katz JA. Recall of surgery for major trauma. Anesthesiology 1984;61:6 – 9.

Cabanac M. Temperature regulation. Annu Rev Physiol 1975;37:415 – 39.

Catton WT. Mechanoreceptor function. Physiol Rev 1970;50:297 – 318.

Cervetto L, Fuortes MGF. Excitation and interactions in the retina. Annu Rev Biophys Bioeng 1978;7:229 – 51.

Chi OZ, Field C. Effects of isoflurane on visual evoked potentials in humans. Anesthesiology 1986;65:328 – 30.

Cutler RWP, Page L, Galichich J, Watters GV. Formation and absorption of cerebrospinal fluid in man. Brain 1968;91:707 – 20.

Darian-Smith I, Johnson O, Goodwin AW. Posterior parietal cortex: Relations of unit activity to sensorimotor function. Annu Rev Physiol 1979;41:141 – 57.

Dastoli FR. Taste receptor proteins. Life Sci 1974;14:1417 – 26.

DeSilva FHL, Arnolds DEAT. Physiology of the hippocampus and related structures. Annu Rev Physiol 1978;40:185 – 216.

Friesen WO, Stent GS. Neural circuits for generating rhythmic movements. Annu Rev Biophys Bioeng 1978;7:37 – 61.

Gancher S, Laxer KD, Krieger W. Activation of epileptogenic activity by etomidate. Anesthesiology 1984;61:616 – 8.

Gillin JC, Mendelson WB, Sitaram N, Wyatt RJ. The neuropharmacology of sleep and wakefulness. Annu Rev Pharmacol Toxicol 1978;18:563 – 79.

Grubb RL, Raichle ME, Eichling JO, Ter-Pogossian MM. The effects of changes in $PaCO_2$ on cerebral blood volume, blood flow, and vascular mean transit time. Stroke 1974;5:630 – 9.

Guyton AC. Textbook of Medical Physiology. 7th ed. Philadelphia: WB Saunders, 1986a:632.

Guyton AC. Textbook of Medical Physiology. 7th ed. Philadelphia: WB Saunders, 1986b:580.

Guyton AC. Textbook of Medical Physiology. 7th ed. Philadelphia: WB Saunders, 1986c:101.

Guyton AC. Textbook of Medical Physiology. 7th ed. Philadelphia: WB Saunders, 1986d:562.

Guyton AC. Textbook of Medical Physiology. 7th ed. Philadelphia: WB Saunders, 1986e:700.

Guyton AC. Textbook of Medical Physiology. 7th ed. Philadelphia: WB Saunders, 1986f:711.

Guyton AC. Textbook of Medical Physiology. 7th ed. Philadelphia: WB Saunders, 1986g:724.

Guyton AC. Textbook of Medical Physiology. 7th ed. Philadelphia: WB Saunders, 1986h:745.

Guyton AC. Textbook of Medical Physiology. 7th ed. Philadelphia: WB Saunders, 1986i:841.

Guyton AC. Textbook of Medical Physiology. 7th ed. Philadelphia: WB Saunders, 1986j:849.

Heistad DD, Abboud FM. Factors that influence blood flow in skeletal muscle and skin. Anesthesiology 1974;41:139 – 56.

Himms-Hagen J. Cellular thermogenesis. Annu Rev Physiol 1976;38:315 – 51.

Hubel DH. The brain. Sci Am 1979;241:44 – 53.

Hubel DH, Wiesel TN. Brain mechanisms of vision. Sci Am 1979;241:150 – 62.

Iversen LL. The chemistry of the brain. Sci Am 1979;241:3:134 – 49.

Kaneko A. Physiology of the retina. Annu Rev Neurosci 1979;2:169 – 91.

Kelly RB, Deutsch JW, Carlson SS, Wagner JA. Biochemistry of neurotransmitter release. Annu Rev Neurosci 1979;2:399 – 446.

Kennedy AJ, Neal MJ, Lolly RN. The distribution of amino acids within the rat retina. J Neurochem 1977;29:157 – 9.

Koblin DD, Eger EI. Theories of narcosis. N Engl J Med 1979;301:1224 – 6.

Kostyuk PG, Vasilenko D. Spinal interneurons. Annu Rev Physiol 1979;41:115 – 26.

Kupfermann I. Modulatory actions of neurotransmitters. Annu Rev Neurosci 1979;2:447 – 65.

Lassen NA. Control of the cerebral circulation in health and disease. Circ Res 1974;34:749 – 60.

Lynch G, Schubert P. The use of in vitro brain slices for multidisciplinary studies of synaptic function. Annu Rev Neurosci 1980;3:1 – 22.

Miller RD, Way WL, Eger EI. The effects of alpha-methyldopa, reserpine, guanethidine, and iproniazid on minimum alveolar anesthetic requirement (MAC). Anesthesiology 1968;29:1153 – 8.

Moore RY, Bloom FE. Central catecholamine neuron systems: Anatomy and physiology of the norepinephrine and epinephrine systems. Annu Rev Neurosci 1979;2:113 – 68.

Moulton DG, Beidler LM. Structure and function in the peripheral olfactory system. Physiol Rev 1967;47:1 – 52.

Nebes RD. Hemispheric specialization in commissurotomized man. Psychol Bull 1974;81:1 – 14.

Nicoll PA, Cortese TA. The physiology of skin. Annu Rev Physiol 1972;34:177 – 203.

Nicoll RA, Schenker C, Leeman SE. Substance P as a transmitter candidate. Annu Rev Neurosci 1980;3:227 – 68.

Norrsel U. Behavioral studies of the somatosensory system. Physiol Rev 1980;60:327 – 54.

Oakley B, Benjamin RM. Neural mechanisms of taste. Physiol Rev 1966;46:173 – 211.

Oldendorf WH. Blood – brain barrier permeability to drugs. Annu Rev Pharmacol 1974;14:239 – 47.

Olton DS. Spatial memory. Sci Am 1977;236:82 – 107.

Ovassapian A, Joshi CW, Brunner EA. Visual disturbances: An unusual symptom of transurethral prostatic resection reaction. Anesthesiology 1982;57:332 – 4.

Pappenheimer JR. The sleep factor. Sci Am 1976;235:24 – 9.

Pathak KS, Brown RH, Cascorbi HF, Nash CL. Effects of fentanyl and morphine on intraoperative somatosensory cortical-evoked potentials. Anesth Analg 1984;63:833 – 7.

Pearson K. The control of walking. Sci Am 1976;235:72 – 86.

Peterson BW. Reticulospinal projections to spinal motor nuclei. Annu Rev Physiol 1979;41:127 – 40.

Precht W. Vestibular mechanisms. Annu Rev Neurosci 1979;2:265 – 89.

Prince DA. Neurophysiology of epilepsy. Annu Rev Neurosci 1978;1:395 – 415.

Rockoff MA, Goudsouzian NG. Seizures induced by methohexital. Anesthesiology 1981;54:333 – 5.

Rodieck RW. Visual pathways. Annu Rev Neurosci 1979;2:193 – 225.

Roth SH. Physical mechanisms of anesthesia. Annu Rev Pharmacol Toxicol 1979;19:159 – 78.

Rushton WAH. Visual pigments and color blindness. Sci Am 1975;232:64 – 75.

Saucier N, Walts LF, Moreland JR. Patient awareness during nitrous oxide, oxygen, and halothane anesthesia. Anesth Analg 1983;62:293 – 340.

Schubert A, Drummond JC. The effect of acute hypocapnia on human median nerve somatosensory evoked responses. Anesth Analg 1986;65:240 – 4.

Severinghaus JW, Lassen NA. Step hypocapnia to separate arterial from tissue PCO_2 in the regulation of cerebral blood flow. Circ Res 1967;20:272 – 8.

Singer W. Control of thalamic transmission by corticofugal and ascending reticular pathways in the visual system. Physiol Rev 1977;57:386 – 420.

Smith AL, Neigh JL, Hoffman JC, Wollman H. Effects of general anesthesia on autoregulation of cerebral blood flow in man. J Appl Physiol 1970;29:665 – 9.

Snyder SH, Bennett JP. Neurotransmitter receptors in the brain. Biochemical identification. Annu Rev Physiol 1976;38:153 – 75.

Stein PSG. Motor systems with specific reference to the control of locomotion. Annu Rev Neurosci 1978;1:61 – 81.

Swenson EJ, Orkin FK. Postoperative nausea and vomiting. In: Complications in Anesthesiology. Orkin FK, Cooperman LH, eds. Philadelphia, J.B. Lippincott. 1983:429.

Toates FM. Accommodation function of the human eye. Physiol Rev 1972;52:828 – 63.

VanHeyningen R. What happens to the human lens in cataract. Sci Am 1975;233:70 – 81.

Wang JM, Wong KC, Creel DJ, Clark WM, Shahangian S. Effects of glycine on hemodynamic responses and visual evoked potentials in the dog. Anesth Analg 1985;64:1071 – 7.

CHAPTER 42

Autonomic
Nervous System

INTRODUCTION

The autonomic nervous system controls the visceral functions of the body. In addition, the autonomic nervous system exerts partial control of blood pressure, gastrointestinal motility and secretion, urinary bladder emptying, sweating, and body temperature. Activation of the autonomic nervous system occurs mainly by centers located in the spinal cord, brain stem, and hypothalamus (see Chapter 41). Impulses are conducted over the sympathetic nervous system (SNS) and parasympathetic nervous system (PNS) divisions of the autonomic nervous system.

The SNS and PNS usually function as physiologic antagonists such that activity of organs innervated by both divisions of the autonomic nervous system represents a balance of the influence of each component (Table 42-1) (Guyton, 1986; Weiner and Taylor, 1985). An understanding of the anatomy and physiology of the autonomic nervous system is essential for predicting the pharmacologic effects of drugs that act on either the SNS or PNS (Table 42-2) (Weiner and Taylor, 1985).

ANATOMY OF THE SYMPATHETIC NERVOUS SYSTEM

Nerves of the SNS arise from the thoracolumbar (T1 to L2) segments of the spinal cord (Fig. 42-1) (Guyton, 1986). These nerve fibers pass to the paravertebral sympathetic chains located lateral to

the spinal cord. From the paravertebral chain, the nerve fibers pass to tissues and organs that are innervated by the SNS.

Each nerve of the SNS consists of a preganglionic neuron and a postganglionic neuron (Fig. 42-2) (Guyton, 1986). Cell bodies of preganglionic neurons are in the intermediolateral horn of the spinal cord. Fibers from these preganglionic cell bodies pass from spinal nerves by way of white rami into one of 22 pairs of ganglia comprising the paravertebral sympathetic chain. In the ganglia of the paravertebral sympathetic chain the preganglionic fibers can synapse with postganglionic neurons or pass upwards or downwards in the chain to synapse with postganglionic neurons in ganglia. Postganglionic neurons then exit from paravertebral ganglia to travel to various peripheral organs. Other postganglionic neurons return to spinal nerves by way of gray rami and subsequently travel in skeletal muscle nerves to control blood vessels, sweat glands, and piloerector muscles. Indeed, about 8% of the fibers in the average skeletal muscle nerve are fibers of the SNS.

Fibers of the SNS are not necessarily distributed to the same part of the body as the spinal nerve fibers from the same segments. For example, fibers from T1 usually ascend in the paravertebral sympathetic chain into the head, T2 into the neck, T3–T6 into the chest, T7–T11 into the abdomen, and T12 and L1–L2 into the legs (Guyton, 1986). The distribution of these SNS fibers to each organ is determined in part by the position in the embryo from which the organ originates. In this

Table 42-1

Responses Evoked by Autonomic Nervous System Stimulation

	Sympathetic Nervous System Stimulation	Parasympathetic Nervous System Stimulation
Heart		
Sinoatrial node	Increase heart rate	Decrease heart rate
Atrioventricular node	Increase conduction velocity	Decrease conduction velocity
His-Purkinje system	Increase automaticity and conduction velocity	Minimal effect
Ventricles	Increase contractility, conduction velocity, automaticity	Minimal effect, slight decrease in contractility?
Bronchial Smooth Muscle	Relaxation	Contraction
Gastrointestinal Tract		
Motility	Decrease	Increase
Secretion	Decrease	Increase
Sphincters	Contraction	Relaxation
Gallbladder	Relaxation	Contraction
Urinary Bladder		
Smooth muscle	Relaxation	Contraction
Sphincter	Contraction	Relaxation
Eye		
Radial muscle	Mydriasis	
Sphincter muscle		Miosis
Ciliary muscle	Relaxation for far vision	Contraction for near vision
Liver	Glycogenolysis Gluconeogenesis	Glycogen synthesis
Pancreatic beta cell secretion	Decrease	
Salivary gland secretion	Increase	Marked increase
Arterioles		
Coronary	Constriction (alpha) Relaxation (beta)	Relaxation? Relaxation
Skin and mucosa	Constriction	Relaxation
Skeletal muscle	Constriction (alpha) Relaxation (beta)	Relaxation
Pulmonary	Constriction	Relaxation

Table 42-2
Mechanism of Action of Drugs that Act on the Autonomic Nervous System

Mechanism	Site	Drug
Inhibition of neurotransmitter synthesis	SNS	alpha-methyltyrosine
False neurotransmitter	SNS	methyldopa
Inhibition of uptake of neurotransmitter	SNS	tricyclic antidepressants cocaine
Displacement of neurotransmitter from storage sites	SNS	amphetamines, guanethidine
	PNS	carbachol
Prevention of neurotransmitter release	SNS	bretylium
	PNS	botulinum toxin
Mimic action of neurotransmitter at receptor	SNS	
alpha		phenylephrine, methoxamine
beta-1		dobutamine
beta-2		terbutaline
Inhibition of action of neurotransmitter	SNS	
on postsynaptic receptor	alpha	phenoxybenzamine, phentolamine
	beta-1, beta-2	propranolol
	beta-1	metoprolol
	PNS	
	muscarinic	atropine
	nicotinic	d-tubocurarine
Inhibition of metabolism of neurotransmitter	SNS	monoamine oxidase inhibitors
	PNS	neostigmine, pyridostigmine, edrophonium

SNS—sympathetic nervous system
PNS—parasympathetic nervous system

regard, the heart receives many SNS fibers from the neck portion of the paravertebral sympathetic chain because the heart originates in the neck of the embryo. Abdominal organs receive their SNS innervation from lower thoracic segments reflecting the origin of the gastrointestinal tract from this area.

ANATOMY OF THE PARASYMPATHETIC NERVOUS SYSTEM

Nerves of the PNS leave the central nervous system through cranial nerves III, V, VII, IX, and X (vagus) and from the sacral portions of the spinal cord (Fig. 42-3) (Guyton, 1986). About 75% of all PNS fibers are in the vagus nerves passing to the entire thoracic and abdominal regions of the body. As such, the vagus nerves supply PNS innervation to the heart, lungs, esophagus, stomach, small intestine, proximal portion of the large intestine, liver, gallbladder, pancreas, and upper portions of the ureters. Fibers of the PNS in cranial nerve III pass to the eye. The lacrimal, nasal, and submaxillary glands receive PNS fibers via cranial nerve VII while the parotid gland receives PNS innervation via cranial nerve IX.

The sacral part of the PNS consists of the second and third sacral nerves, and, occasionally, the first and the fourth sacral nerves. Sacral nerves form the sacral plexus on each side of the spinal cord. These nerves distribute fibers to the distal colon, rectum, bladder, and lower portions of the ureters. In addition, PNS fibers to the external genitalia cause various sexual responses.

In contrast to the SNS, preganglionic fibers of the PNS pass uninterrupted to the innervated organ (Fig. 42-3) (Guyton, 1986). Postganglionic

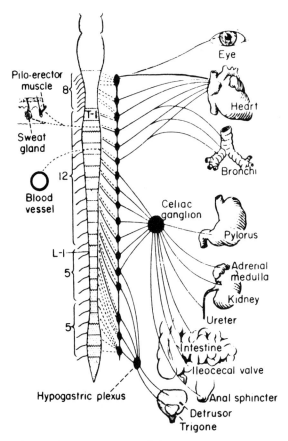

FIGURE 42-1. Anatomy of the sympathetic nervous system. Dashed lines represent postganglionic fibers in gray rami leading into spinal nerves for subsequent distribution to blood vessels and sweat glands. (From Guyton AC. Textbook of Medical Physiology. 7th ed. Philadelphia: WB Saunders, 1986:686. Reproduced by permission of the author and publisher.)

neurons of the PNS are short being located in the wall of the innervated organ. This contrasts with the SNS in which postganglionic neurons almost always originate in ganglia of the paravertebral sympathetic chain.

PHYSIOLOGY OF THE AUTONOMIC NERVOUS SYSTEM

Postganglionic fibers of the SNS secrete norepinephrine as the neurotransmitter (Fig. 42-4) (Langer and Hicks, 1984). These norepinephrine-

secreting neurons are classified as adrenergic fibers. Postganglionic fibers of the PNS secrete acetylcholine as the neurotransmitter (Fig. 42-4). These acetylcholine-secreting fibers are classified as cholinergic fibers. In addition, innervation of sweat glands and some blood vessels is by postganglionic sympathetic nerve fibers that release acetylcholine as the neurotransmitter. All preganglionic neurons of the SNS and PNS release acetylcholine as the neurotransmitter and are thus classified as cholinergic fibers. For this reason, acetylcholine released at preganglionic fibers will activate both sympathetic and parasympathetic postganglionic neurons.

Norepinephrine as a Neurotransmitter

Synthesis

Synthesis of norepinephrine involves a series of enzyme-controlled steps that begin in the cytoplasm of postganglionic sympathetic nerve endings (*e.g.*, the varicosities) and are completed in the synaptic vesicles (Fig. 42-5). For example, the initial enzyme-mediated steps leading to the formation of dopamine take place in the cytoplasm. Dopamine then enters the synaptic vesicle where

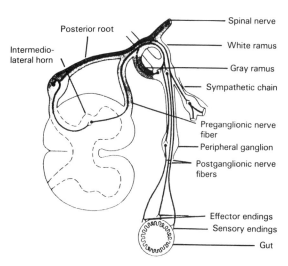

FIGURE 42-2. Anatomy of a sympathetic nervous system nerve. (From Guyton AC. Textbook of Medical Physiology. 7th ed. Philadelphia: WB Saunders, 1986:686. Reproduced by permission of the author and publisher.)

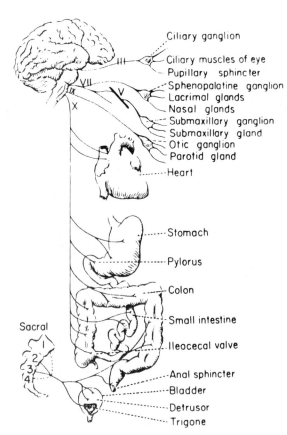

FIGURE 42-3. Anatomy of the parasympathetic nervous system. (From Guyton AC. Textbook of Medical Physiology. 7th ed. Philadelphia: WB Saunders, 1986:686. Reproduced by permission of the author and publisher.)

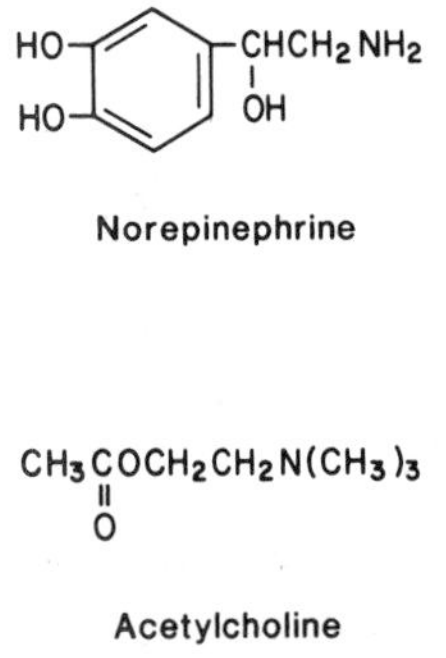

Norepinephrine

Acetylcholine

FIGURE 42-4. Neurotransmitters of the autonomic nervous system.

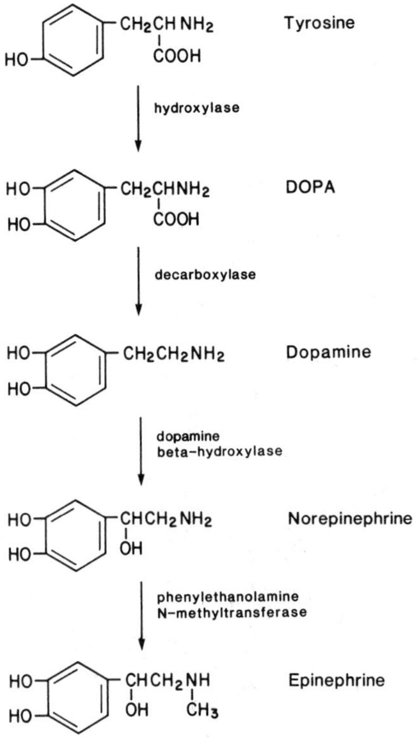

FIGURE 42-5. Steps in enzymatic synthesis of endogenous catecholamines and neurotransmitters.

it is converted to norepinephrine by dopamine beta-hydroxylase. It is likely that the enzymes that participate in the synthesis of norepinephrine are produced in postganglionic sympathetic nerve endings. These enzymes are not highly specific and other endogenous substances, as well as certain drugs, may be acted upon by the same enzymes. For example, dopa-decarboxylase can convert methyldopa to alpha-methyldopamine which is subsequently converted by dopamine beta-hydroxylase to the weakly active (*i.e.,* false) neurotransmitter, alpha-methylnorepinephrine (see Chapter 15).

Storage and Release

Norepinephrine is stored in synaptic vesicles for subsequent release in response to an action potential. Calcium ions are important in coupling the nerve impulse to the subsequent release of norepinephrine from postganglionic sympathetic nerve endings into the extracellular fluid. Evidence that exocytosis is the primary event in the release of norepinephrine from synaptic vesicles in the nerve terminals is the observation that increased activity of the SNS is accompanied by elevated circulating concentrations of dopamine beta-oxidase and norepinephrine. This should occur only if the entire contents of the synaptic vesicles are released.

Adrenergic fibers can sustain output of norepinephrine during prolonged periods of stimulation. Tachyphylaxis, which accompanies ephedrine and other indirect-acting sympathomimetics, may reflect depletion of the limited pool of neurotransmitter at these binding sites in contrast to the large total amount of norepinephrine stored in the sympathetic nerve ending (see Chapter 12).

ACETYLCHOLINE AND NOREPINEPHRINE RELEASE. It has been proposed that activation of SNS fibers initially results in the release of acetylcholine which in turn causes the release of norepinephrine to act on receptors (Burns and Rand, 1959). Although this theory is not generally accepted, there is evidence that acetylcholine can cause the release of norepinephrine by effects at nicotinic cholinergic receptors (Westfall, 1977).

Termination of Action

Termination of the action of norepinephrine is by (1) uptake (*i.e.,* reuptake) back into postganglionic sympathetic nerve endings, (2) dilution by diffusion from receptors, and (3) metabolism by the enzymes, monoamine oxidase (MAO) and catechol-O-methyltransferase (COMT). Norepinephrine released in response to an action potential exerts its effect at receptors for only a brief period reflecting the efficiency of these termination mechanisms.

UPTAKE. Uptake of previously released norepinephrine back into postganglionic sympathetic nerve endings is probably the most important mechanism for the termination of the action of this neurotransmitter on receptors. Indeed, it is estimated that as much as 80% of released norepinephrine undergoes uptake. Furthermore, this uptake provides a second important source of norepinephrine (*e.g.,* reuse) in addition to synthesis.

It is likely that two active transport systems are involved in uptake of norepinephrine with one system responsible for uptake into the cytoplasm

of the varicosity and a second system for passage of norepinephrine into the synaptic vesicle for storage and reuse. The active transport systems for norepinephrine uptake can concentrate the neurotransmitter 10,000-fold in the postganglionic sympathetic nerve ending. Magnesium and adenosine triphosphate (ATP) are essential for function of the transport system necessary for the transfer of norepinephrine from cytoplasm into the synaptic vesicle. The transport system for uptake of norepinephrine into cytoplasm is blocked by numerous drugs including cocaine and tricyclic antidepressants (see Chapter 19).

METABOLISM. Metabolism of norepinephrine is of relatively minor significance in terminating the action of endogenously released norepinephrine. The exception may be at some blood vessels where enzymatic breakdown and diffusion account for the termination of the action of norepinephrine. Norepinephrine that undergoes uptake is vulnerable to metabolism in the cytoplasm of the varicosity by MAO. Neurotransmitter that escapes uptake is vulnerable to metabolism by COMT, principally in the liver. Inhibitors of MAO cause an increase in tissue levels of norepinephrine and are accompanied by a variety of pharmacological effects (see Chapter 19). Conversely, no striking pharmacological change accompanies inhibition of COMT.

The primary urinary metabolite resulting from metabolism of norepinephrine by MAO or COMT is 3-methoxy-4-hydroxymandelic acid (Fig. 42-6). This metabolite is also referred to as vanillylmandelic acid (VMA). Normally, the 24-hour urinary excretion of 3-methoxy, 4-hydroxymandelic acid is 2 to 4 mg representing primarily norepinephrine that is deaminated by MAO in the cytoplasm of the varicosity of the postganglionic sympathetic nerve endings.

Acetylcholine as a Neurotransmitter

Synthesis

Synthesis of acetylcholine occurs in the cytoplasm of varicosities of the preganglionic and postganglionic parasympathetic nerve endings. The enzyme, choline acetyltransferase, is responsible for catalyzing the combination of choline with acetyl coenzyme A to form acetylcholine. Choline enters parasympathetic nerve endings from the extracel-

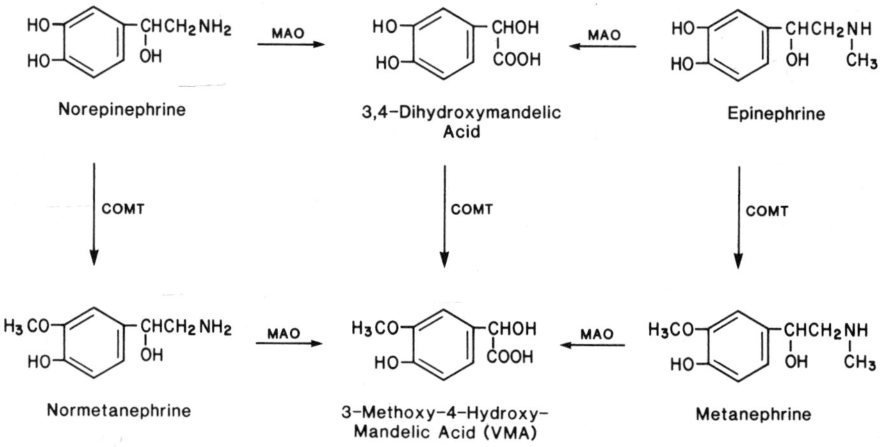

FIGURE 42-6. Norepinephrine and epinephrine are initially deaminated by monoamine oxidase (MAO) or alternatively they are first methylated by catechol-O-methyltransferase. The resulting metabolites are then further metabolized by the other enzyme to form the principal end-metabolite, 3-methoxy-4-hydroxymandelic acid (vanillylmandelic acid or VMA).

lular fluid by virtue of an active transport system. Acetyl coenzyme A is synthesized in mitochondria present in high concentrations in parasympathetic nerve endings.

Storage and Release

Acetylcholine is stored in synaptic vesicles for release in response to an action potential. Arrival of an action potential at the parasympathetic nerve ending results in the release of 100 or more vesicles of acetylcholine (Weiner and Taylor, 1985). It is estimated that a single nerve ending contains 300,000 or more synaptic vesicles.

Preceding arrival of the action potential is the initial depolarization which permits the influx of calcium ions. Conceptually, calcium ions bind to sites on axonal and vesicular membranes resulting in the extrusion of the contents of the synaptic vesicles. Thus, the presence of calcium ions in the extracellular fluid is essential for the subsequent release of acetylcholine in response to an action potential. The effect of calcium is antagonized by magnesium ions.

Metabolism

Acetylcholine has a brief effect at receptors (1 msec or less) because of its rapid hydrolysis by acetylcholinesterase (true cholinesterase) to cho-

line and acetate. Choline is transported back into the parasympathetic nerve ending where it is reused for synthesis of new acetylcholine.

Plasma cholinesterase (pseudocholinesterase) is an enzyme found in only low concentrations around receptors being present in the greatest amounts in plasma. The physiologic significance of plasma cholinesterase is unknown. Indeed, this enzyme hydrolyzes acetylcholine too slowly to be physiologically important. Furthermore, absence of plasma cholinesterase produces no detectable signs or symptoms.

INTERACTIONS OF NEUROTRANSMITTERS WITH RECEPTORS

Norepinephrine and acetylcholine acting as neurotransmitters interact with receptors (e.g., protein molecules) in cell membranes (Kunos, 1978). This interaction may (1) activate the enzyme adenylate cyclase which results in the formation of cyclic AMP or (2) alter permeability of cell membranes to various ions.

Norepinephrine Receptors

The pharmacologic effects of catecholamines led to the original concept of alpha- and beta-adrenergic receptors (Ahlquist, 1948). Subdivision of these receptors into alpha-1 (postsynaptic), alpha-2 (presynaptic), beta-1 (cardiac), and beta-2 (noncardiac) allows an understanding of drugs that act as either agonists or antagonists at these sites (Table 42-3) (Lands *et al*, 1967) (see Chapter 12). Dopamine receptors are also subdivided as dopamine-1 (postsynaptic) and dopamine-2 (presynaptic). Activation of dopamine-1 receptors is responsible for vasodilation in the splanchnic and renal circulations. Presynaptic alpha-2 and dopamine-2 receptors function as a negative feedback loop such that their activation inhibits subsequent release of neurotransmitter (Table 42-3). Postsynaptic alpha-2 receptors are also present on platelets where they mediate platelet aggregation by influencing platelet adenylate cyclase concentration (Steer and Wood, 1979).

The key substance that is involved in the mediation of responses evoked by activation of beta-

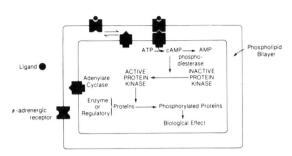

FIGURE 42-7. The beta-adrenergic receptor is speculated to exist in the phospholipid bilayer of the cell membrane as a recognition site and catalytic site (adenylate cyclase). Activation of the recognition site by the neurotransmitter, norepinephrine, causes coupling with the catalytic site leading to the formation of intracellular cyclic AMP (second messenger). (From Maze M. Clinical implications of membrane receptor function in anesthesia. Anesthesiology 1981;55:160–71. Reproduced by permission of the author and publisher.)

adrenergic receptors is cyclic AMP (Fig. 42-7) (Maze, 1981). Specifically, norepinephrine is speculated to interact with the enzyme, adenylate cyclase (*e.g.,* the beta-adrenergic receptor) in the cell membrane. The catecholamine-binding portion (recognition site) of the beta-adrenergic receptor is oriented externally in the cell membrane such that poorly lipid-soluble norepinephrine does not have to traverse a lipid barrier to activate the receptor. Activation of adenylate cyclase (first messenger) catalyzes the conversion of ATP to cyclic AMP (second messenger). Cyclic AMP then initiates a series of intracellular events (cascading protein phosphorylation reactions) resulting in the metabolic and pharmacologic effects considered typical of beta-adrenergic receptor stimulation by norepinephrine, epinephrine, or agonist drugs.

Acetylcholine Receptors

Acetylcholine interacts with cholinergic receptors leading to the opening of channels in the cell membrane. As a result of this channel opening, sodium and potassium ions flow along electrochemical gradients. Depending on the direction of ion flow, acetylcholine is associated with excitatory or inhibitory effects.

Table 42-3

Responses Evoked by Selective Stimulation of Adrenergic Receptors

---

Alpha-1 (postsynaptic) Receptors
  Vasoconstriction
  Mydriasis
  Relaxation of gastrointestinal tract
  Contraction of gastrointestinal sphincters
  Contraction of bladder sphincter

Alpha-2 (presynaptic) Receptors
  Inhibition of norepinephrine release

Alpha-2 (postsynaptic) Receptors
  Platelet aggregation

Beta-1 (postsynaptic) Receptors
  Increased conduction velocity
  Increased automaticity
  Increased contractility

Beta-2 (postsynaptic) Receptors
  Vasodilation
  Bronchodilation
  Gastrointestinal relaxation
  Uterine relaxation
  Bladder relaxation
  Glycogenolysis
  Lipolysis

Dopamine-1 (postsynaptic) Receptors
  Vasodilation

Dopamine-2 (presynaptic) Receptors
  Inhibition of norepinephrine release

Cholinergic receptors are designated as muscarinic and nicotinic. This classification is based on the fact that muscarine activates muscarinic but not nicotinic receptors while the opposite response is produced by nicotine (Lester, 1977). By convention, effects produced at cardiac receptors by acetylcholine are muscarinic. Effects produced by acetylcholine at autonomic ganglia or the neuromuscular junction are nicotinic. Nicotinic receptors at autonomic ganglia and the neuromuscular junction, however, are not identical. For example, hexamethonium blocks receptors at the autonomic ganglia but not neuromuscular junction. d-Tubocurarine blocks nicotinic receptors at autonomic ganglia and the neuromuscular junction, but blockade at the neuromuscular junction predominates. Atropine selectively blocks all muscarinic responses produced by acetylcholine, but the intensity of blockade at various receptors depends on dose. For example, low doses of atropine block cardiac muscarinic response while blockade of smooth muscle responses to acetylcholine requires large doses suggesting that all muscarinic receptors, like nicotinic receptors, are not identical. A possible molecular basis for the difference between nicotinic and muscarinic receptors is a different distance between atoms of the receptors necessary to interact with acetylcholine or drugs.

EFFECTS OF AUTONOMIC NERVOUS SYSTEM INNERVATION

It is not possible to develop a scheme that will predict whether SNS or PNS stimulation will cause excitation or inhibition of a particular organ (Table 42-1) (Guyton, 1986; Weiner and Taylor, 1985).

Eye

The autonomic nervous system controls the pupillary opening of the eye and the focus of the lens. Stimulation of the SNS, as by excitement, contracts the meridional fibers of the iris which dilate the pupil. Conversely, PNS stimulation, as by excess light, contracts the circular muscle of the iris which constricts the pupil.

Focus of the lens is controlled by the PNS. For example, stimulation of the PNS contracts the ciliary muscle which releases the tension on the lens allowing it to become more convex. This allows the eye to focus on near objects as for reading. Inhibition of PNS activity, as produced by an anticholinergic drug included in the preoperative medication, may interfere with focusing on near objects.

Glands

Nasal, lacrimal, and salivary glands produce copious secretions in response to PNS stimulation. Sweat glands secrete large quantities of perspiration when the SNS is stimulated. Nevertheless, postganglionic sympathetic fibers to most sweat glands are cholinergic. Apocrine glands are innervated by adrenergic fibers and produce an odoriferous secretion in response to SNS stimulation.

Gastrointestinal Tract

Stimulation of the PNS promotes peristalsis and relaxes the sphincters of the gastrointestinal tract thus allowing rapid movement of contents. The reverse response accompanies SNS stimulation.

Cardiovascular System

Stimulation of the SNS increases the rate and force of myocardial contraction which is accompanied by a concomitant increase in oxygen requirements. The reverse responses accompany PNS stimulation.

Most blood vessels, particularly in the skin and abdominal viscera, are constricted by SNS stimulation. Stimulation of the PNS has minimal effects on blood vessel tone but does dilate blood vessels in certain areas such as the blush area of the face.

RESIDUAL AUTONOMIC NERVOUS SYSTEM TONE

The SNS and PNS are continually active, and this basal rate of activity is referred to as sympathetic or parasympathetic tone. The value of this tone is that it permits alterations in SNS or PNS activity to either increase or decrease responses at innervated organs. For example, SNS tone normally keeps blood vessels about 50% constricted. As a result, increased or decreased SNS activity produces corresponding changes in peripheral vascular resistance. If sympathetic tone did not exist, the SNS could only cause vasoconstriction.

In addition to continual direct sympathetic stimulation, a portion of the overall SNS tone reflects basal secretion of norepinephrine and epinephrine by the adrenal medulla. The normal resting rate of secretion of norepinephrine is about $0.05 \mu g \ kg^{-1} \ min^{-1}$ and of epinephrine is about $0.2 \mu g \ kg^{-1} \ min^{-1}$. These secretion rates are nearly sufficient to maintain normal blood pressure even if all direct SNS innervation to the cardiovascular system is removed.

Acute Denervation

Acute removal of SNS tone, as produced by a regional anesthetic or spinal cord transection, results in immediate maximal vasodilatation of blood vessels. Over several days, however, intrinsic tone of the vascular smooth muscle increases, usually restoring almost normal vasoconstriction. Similar intrinsic PNS compensation occurs, but return of an organ to basal function may require several months.

Denervation Hypersensitivity

Denervation hypersensitivity (also referred to as autonomic hyperreflexia or mass reflex) is the increased responsiveness (*i.e.,* decreased threshold) of the innervated organ to either acetylcholine or norepinephrine that develops during the first week or so after acute interruption of autonomic nervous system innervation (see Chapter 41). The presumed mechanism for denervation hypersensitivity is the proliferation of receptors on postsynaptic membranes that occurs when acetylcholine or norepinephrine are no longer released at synapses. As a result, more receptor sites become available to produce an exaggerated response when circulating neurotransmitter does become available.

ADRENAL MEDULLA

The adrenal medulla is innervated by preganglionic fibers that bypass the paravertebral ganglia. As a result, these fibers pass directly from the spinal cord to the adrenal medulla. Cells of the adrenal medulla are derived embryologically from neural tissue and are analogous to postganglionic neurons. Stimulation of the SNS causes release of epinephrine (80%) and norepinephrine from the adrenal medulla. Epinephrine and norepinephrine released by the adrenal medulla function as hormones and not neurotransmitters.

Synthesis

In the adrenal medulla, the majority of formed norepinephrine is converted to the hormone, epinephrine, by the action of phenylethanolamine-N-methyltransferase (Fig. 42-5). Activity of this enzyme is enhanced by cortisol which is carried by the intra-adrenal portal vascular system, directly to the adrenal medulla cells. For this reason, any stress that releases glucocorticoids also results in increased synthesis and release of epinephrine (Wurtman *et al,* 1972).

Release

The triggering event in the release of epinephrine and norepinephrine from the adrenal medulla is the liberation of acetylcholine by preganglionic cholinergic fibers. Acetylcholine acts on specific receptors resulting in a change in permeability (*e.g.,* localized depolarization) that permits entrance of calcium ions. Calcium ions result in extrusion, by exocytosis, of synaptic vesicles containing epinephrine (Kirshner, 1974).

Norepinephrine and epinephrine released from the adrenal medulla evoke responses similar to direct SNS stimulation. The difference, however, is that effects are greatly prolonged (10 – 30 seconds) compared with the brief action on receptors produced by norepinephrine released as a neurotransmitter from postganglionic sympathetic nerve endings. The prolonged effect of circulating epinephrine and norepinephrine released by the adrenal medulla reflects the time necessary for metabolism of these substances by COMT.

Circulating norepinephrine from the adrenal medulla causes vasoconstriction of blood vessels, inhibition of the gastrointestinal tract, increased cardiac activity, and dilatation of the pupils. Effects of circulating epinephrine differ from norepinephrine in that its cardiac effects are greater, constriction of blood vessels in skeletal muscle is less, and metabolic effects are greater. Circulating norepinephrine and epinephrine released by the adrenal medulla and acting as hormones can substitute for SNS innervation of an organ. Another important role of the adrenal medulla is the ability of circulating norepinephrine and epinephrine to stimulate areas of the body that are not directly innervated by the SNS. For example, the metabolic rate of all cells can be influenced by hormones released from the adrenal medulla even though these cells are not directly innervated by the SNS.

REFERENCES

Ahlquist RP. A study of adrenotropic receptors. Am J Physiol 1948;53:586–606.

Burns JH, Rand MJ. Sympathetic postganglionic mechanism. Nature 1959;184:163–5.

Guyton AC. Textbook of Medical Physiology. 7th ed. Philadelphia: WB Saunders, 1986:686.

Kirshner N. Function and organization of chromaffin vesicles. Life Sci 1974;14:1153–67.

Kunos G. Adrenoceptors. Annu Rev Pharmacol Toxicol 1978;18:291–311.

Lands AM, Arnold A, McAuliff JP, Luduena FP, Brown RG. Differentiation of receptor systems activated by sympathomimetic amines. Nature 1967;214:597–8.

Langer SZ, Hicks PE. Physiology of the sympathetic nerve ending. Br J Anaesth 1984;56:689–700.

Lester HA. The response to acetylcholine. Sci Am 1977;236:106–18.

Maze M. Clinical implications of membrane receptor function in anesthesia. Anesthesiology 1981;55:160–71.

Steer ML, Wood A. Regulation of human platelet adenylate cyclase by epinephrine, prostaglandin E and guanine nucleotides. J Biol Chem 1979;254:1791–7.

Weiner N, Taylor P. Drugs acting at synaptic and neuroeffector junctional sites. In Gilman AG, Goodman LS, Rall TW, Murad F. The Pharmacological Basis of Therapeutics. New York, 7th edition. Macmillan Publishing Company. 1985;66.

Westfall TC. Local regulation of adrenergic neurotransmission. Physiol Rev 1977;57:659–728.

Wurtman RJ, Pohorecky LA, Baliga BS. Adrenocortical control of the biosynthesis of epinephrine and proteins in the adrenal medulla. Pharmacol Rev 1972;24:411–26.

Pain

INTRODUCTION

Pain (nociception) is a protective mechanism that occurs only when tissues are being damaged and causes the individual to react to remove the painful stimulus (Abram, 1985; Liebeskind *et al*, 1985). For example, pressure on a certain part of the body during sitting results in painful ischemia which causes the person to unconsciously shift the weight.

TYPES OF PAIN

Pain has been described as (1) stabbing, (2) burning, and (3) aching. Stabbing pain is perceived when a needle penetrates the skin or the skin is cut with a knife. Burning pain is the type of pain felt when the skin is exposed to high temperatures. Aching pain is not felt on the surface of the body but instead is a deep sensation that is often poorly localized. Stabbing pain results from stimulation of myelinated A-delta fibers with conduction velocities of 6 to 25 m sec^{-1} (Wilson, 1974). Burning and aching pain results from stimulation of more primitive unmyelinated C fibers with conduction velocities of 0.5 to 2 m sec^{-1}. Therefore, a painful stimulus creates a double perception of pain (*i.e.,* double innervation) consisting of a fast stabbing sensation followed by a slow burning sensation. It is the immediate stabbing pain that instantly tells the person that tissue damage is occurring while

burning pain becomes the source of continued discomfort.

Fibers for temperature follow the same pathways as fibers for pain. Indeed, artificially applied pain in the form of a heat stimulus causes pain in almost all subjects when skin temperature exceeds 43 Celsius (*i.e.,* pain threshold). This is the temperature that, if maintained, can produce tissue damage. Although pain threshold is fairly constant among individuals, different people, nevertheless, react quite differently to the same intensity of painful stimulation emphasizing the importance of personality and ethnic origin on pain tolerance and description.

PAIN RECEPTORS

Pain receptors (nociceptors) in the skin and other tissues are free afferent nerve endings of A-delta fibers and C fibers (Yaksh and Hammond, 1982). These nerve endings are widespread in superficial layers of the skin and also in certain internal tissues such as the periosteum, joint surfaces, skeletal muscle, and tooth pulp. Most of the other deep tissues are not richly supplied with pain receptors although widespread tissue damage can summate to cause aching pain in these areas.

Three categories of pain receptors are described in skin (Abram, 1985). Pain receptors that are activated by intense mechanical stimulation and conduct impulses by way of A-delta fibers are termed mechanosensitive pain receptors. Mechanothermal pain receptors are activated by mechanical and thermal (greater than 43 Celsius) stimulation and also conduct impulses by way of A-delta fibers. Polymodal pain receptors respond to mechanical, thermal, and chemical stimuli and conduct impulses by way of C fibers. Chemicals capable of activating these receptors include acetylcholine, bradykinin, histamine, lactic acid, potassium ions, prostaglandins, and proteolytic enzymes.

In contrast to other sensory receptors, pain receptors do not adapt. Indeed, under some conditions, the threshold for excitation of pain receptors becomes progressively lower as the pain stimulus continues allowing more and more receptors to become activated with time. This increase in sensitivity of pain receptors is termed *hyperalgesia*. Failure of pain receptors to adapt is protective for it allows the person to remain aware of continued tissue damage. After damage has occurred, pain is usually minimal.

The onset of pain in a tissue rendered acutely ischemic is related to its rate of metabolism. For example, pain occurs in exercising ischemic muscle in 15 to 20 seconds but not for 20 to 30 minutes in ischemic skin.

Skeletal muscle spasm is a common cause of pain and may become the basis for myofascial pain syndromes. This pain most likely reflects direct effects of skeletal muscle spasm in stimulating mechanosensitive pain receptors as well as an indirect effect of muscle spasm causing ischemia and thereby stimulating polymodal pain receptors. Skeletal muscle spasm compresses blood vessels and diminishes blood flow but also simultaneously increases the rate of metabolism in the muscle tissue, thus making the relative ischemia even greater and creating ideal conditions for release of pain-inducing chemicals.

Painful stimulation may evoke reflex increases in sympathetic nervous system efferent activity. It is possible that associated vasoconstriction leads to acidosis, tissue ischemia, and release of chemicals that further activate pain receptors. Resulting sustained painful stimulation produces further increases in sympathetic nervous system activity and the vicious cycle termed *reflex sympathetic dystrophy* may develop (Abram, 1985).

Following certain types of nerve injury, pain may arise without activation of pain receptors. Spontaneous firing that occurs from injured peripheral nerves, especially in response to sympathetic nervous system stimulation, may reflect a proliferation of alpha-adrenergic receptors on the increased number of neuroma sprouts (Devor, 1983). Spontaneous firing may also occur from dorsal root ganglia whose peripheral projections have been interrupted as follows nerve transection or limb amputation.

TRANSMISSION OF PAIN SIGNALS

Pain signals are transmitted from peripheral pain receptors to the dorsal horns of the spinal cord by A-delta fibers at rapid conduction velocities and by C fibers at slow conduction velocities (see the section entitled Types of Pain). The A-delta and C fibers enter the spinal cord through the dorsal roots and terminate on cells in the dorsal horns (see the section entitled Conceptual Model). Specifically, A-delta fibers synapse with cells in laminae I and V (wide dynamic range neurons) of the spinal cord while C fibers synapse with cells in laminae II and III which is also known as the substantia gelatinosa (see Fig. 41-7).

The spinothalamic tract, as well as other ascending pathways, is responsible for cephalad transmission of pain impulses after they have been processed in the dorsal horns of the spinal cord. Cells in laminae I and V are spinothalamic cells and about 75% of fibers originating from these cells cross to the contralateral spinothalamic tract. The phylogenetically newer portion of the spinothalamic tract projects to posterior portions of the thalamus and is considered to be involved with the spatial and temporal aspects of pain perception. The older paleospinothalamic tract projects to the medial thalamus and is responsible for initiation of unpleasant aspects of pain as well as autonomic nervous system responses to pain. Other pathways involved in cephalad transmission of pain impulses include the spinocervical tract, spinoreticular tract and spinomesencephalic tract. Pain impulses travel from the thalamus to the somatosensory cortex. Complete removal of the somatic areas of the cerebral cortex does not destroy the person's ability to perceive pain suggesting that the thalamus participates in the conscious perception of pain. It is speculated that the cerebral cortex is important in interpreting the intensity of pain even though perception of pain seems predominantly to be a function of lower brain centers.

Fibers conducting burning and aching pain

terminate in the reticular area of the brain stem. This area transmits activating signals into essentially all parts of the brain especially upward through the thalamus to the cerebral cortex and to the hypothalamus. Activation of the reticular activating system by burning and aching pain serves to arouse the person from sleep and produce generalized activation of the entire nervous system. These signals are poorly localized and serve only the purpose of alerting the person to continuing tissue damage. Even weak pain signals via this pathway may summate with time converting initially tolerable discomfort into intolerable pain.

Localization of pain probably results from simultaneous activation of tactile receptors along with pain stimulation. Nevertheless, burning and aching types of pain transmitted by C fibers are poorly localized, which is consistent with the fact that these fibers terminate diffusely in the hindbrain and thalamus.

Conceptual Model

A conceptual model of pain transmission includes ascending excitatory pain pathways, descending inhibitory pain pathways, and a variety of neurotransmitters (Fig. 43-1) (Cousins and Mather, 1984). Pain impulses traveling via afferent nerves from pain receptors enter the dorsal horns of the spinal cord. At this site, substance P and possibly other peptides (prostaglandins, vasoactive intestinal peptide, somatostatin, cholecystokinin) act as the neurotransmitter for stimulation of second order neurons necessary for further cephalad transmission of the pain impulse (Hokfelt *et al,* 1977; Yaksh and Hammond, 1982). Indeed, release of substance P into the cerebrospinal fluid is inhibited by concurrent administration of intrathecal morphine (Yaksh and Hammond, 1982). Furthermore, depletion of substance P renders animals insensitive to noxious thermal stimuli (Yaksh *et al,* 1980).

Transmission of pain impulses may be modified by activation of descending inhibitory pain pathways that pass from the brain to the spinal cord. Activation of these inhibitory pathways blocks the release of substance P, or other excitatory neurotransmitters, and thus prevents the cephalad transmission of nociceptive signals (Fig. 43-1) (Cousins and Mather, 1984; Yaksh and Elde, 1981). It seems likely that a central nervous system substrate, presumably endorphins, is responsible

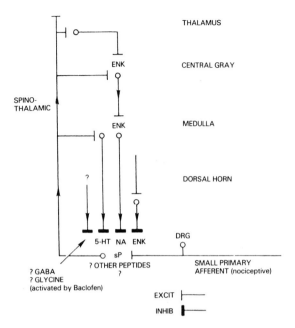

FIGURE 43- 1. A conceptual model of pain transmission includes ascending excitatory and descending inhibitory pain pathways and a variety of neurotransmitters. Primary afferent pain (nociceptive) signals travel by the dorsal root ganglion (DRG) to cells in the dorsal horns of the spinal cord where substance P acts as the neurotransmitter. The endogenous endorphin (ENK) system is activated by pain signals that reach the thalamus. Activation of descending inhibitory pain pathways by ENK results in inhibition of dorsal horn neurons in the spinal cord by virtue of the release of inhibitory neurotransmitters which may include serotonin (5-HT), norepinephrine (NA), endorphins (ENK), gammaaminobutyric acid (GABA), and glycine. (From Cousins MJ, Mather LE. Intrathecal and epidural administration of opioids. Anesthesiology 1984;61:276–310. Reproduced by permission of the authors and publisher.)

for activating descending inhibitory pathways. Electrical stimulation of the periaqueductal gray area of the midbrain also activates these pathways and produces profound analgesia in humans (Hosobuchi *et al,* 1977; Richardson and Akil, 1977). Opioid binding sites and endorphins are present in brain regions where electrical stimulation-produced analgesia can be evoked. Thus endorphins and their receptors are well situated to function in an endogenous pain suppression system. Indeed, electrical stimulation-produced analgesia may evoke the release of endorphins as suggested by the ability of naloxone to partially block this form of analgesia (Akil *et al,* 1976).

In addition to endorphins, other inhibitory neurotransmitters released by descending pathway fibers may include serotonin, norepinephrine, and possibly glycine and gamma-aminobutyric acid (Fig. 43-1) (Cousins and Mather, 1984; Reddy and Yaksh, 1980; Yaksh, 1981). Evidence for a role of norepinephrine as an inhibitory neurotransmitter is production of spinal analgesia by the alpha-1 adrenergic agonist, clonidine. This clonidine-induced analgesia is antagonized by an alpha-1 antagonist, prazosin. Likewise, serotonin-induced spinal analgesia is reversed by a known serotonin antagonist, methysergide (Yaksh and Wilson, 1979). The net effect of activation of these descending inhibitory pathways and release of inhibitory neurotransmitters is inhibition of transmission of pain impulses from pain receptors by way of afferent fibers.

The physiology of primary afferent transmission of pain impulses is of major importance in understanding the management of clinical pain. Utilizing the conceptual model of pain, it appears that the various inhibitory systems do not act through a final common pathway but instead appear to be independent (Fig. 43-1) (Cousins and Mather, 1984). Furthermore, these inhibitory systems appear to produce additive effects and pain seems to be blocked selectively, leaving sensory, motor, and sympathetic nervous system function intact.

Cordotomy

Surgical section through the anterolateral quadrant of the spinal cord (cordotomy) at the thoracic level interrupts the anterolateral spinothalamic tracts and relieves pain from the limb on the side opposite the cord transection (Lipton, 1968). Cordotomy may be unsuccessful in some patients because pain fibers from the upper part of the body do not cross to the opposite side of the spinal cord until they have reached the brain. Furthermore, pain which is often more intense than the original pain, may develop several months after the cordotomy. An alternative to cordotomy may be selective surgical destruction of certain areas of the thalamus.

Tactile Inhibition

Stimulation of large sensory fibers from peripheral tactile receptors depresses transmission of pain impulses either from the same area of the body or even from areas located many segments away. This explains why rubbing an injured area or application of irritant ointments produces varying degrees of pain relief. Stimulating electrodes (*e.g,* transcutaneous electrical nerve stimulation) also take advantage of this tactile inhibition of pain.

Gate Control Theory

The dorsal horns of the spinal column may function as gates for controlling entry of pain signals into pain pathways (Melzack and Wall, 1965). Furthermore, pain signals may be balanced against tactile signals, each capable of inhibiting the other. Despite its deficiencies, this theory has been important in stimulating physiologic and psychologic investigation in pain mechanisms and therapy (Bonica, 1985).

REACTION TO PAIN

Although pain threshold is similar, people's reaction to pain varies greatly. Pain causes both reflex motor reactions and psychic reactions. Involuntary reflex withdrawal actions occur in the spinal cord before pain signals reach the brain. Psychic reactions to pain vary greatly and include anxiety, depression, crying, and excess skeletal muscle excitability. Pain and anxiety are interrelated such that increased anxiety makes pain less tolerable while increased pain enhances anxiety. Indeed, the preoperative level of anxiety is a useful predictor of the intensity of postoperative pain (Scott *et al,* 1983). Intensity of pain signals transmitted through the spinal cord to the brain also varies greatly at different times and under different conditions even in the same person. This variation may reflect activity of endorphins and the endogenous pain suppression system (see the section entitled Conceptual Model).

REFERRED PAIN

Referred pain is perception of pain at a site considerably removed from the tissue causing the pain.

Typically, this type of pain is initiated in one of the visceral organs and referred to an area of the body surface. The mechanism of referred pain is most likely the conduction of pain signals from the viscera through common neurons for conduction of pain signals from the skin. As a result, the person has the false impression that pain is originating in the skin. Skeletal muscle spasm caused by damage in adjacent tissues may also be a cause of referred pain. For example, pain from the ureter can cause reflex spasm of the lumbar muscles.

VISCERAL PAIN

Viscera have sensory receptors for perception of pain. Nevertheless, highly localized damage to a viscus, as associated with a surgical incision, is not associated with severe pain. Conversely, a stimulus that causes diffuse stimulation of nerve endings throughout a viscus causes pain that can be severe. For example, ischemia to a portion of the gastrointestinal tract causes intense pain presumably due to the formation of acidic metabolic products or tissue degenerative products such as bradykinin. Other causes of visceral pain include (1) distention of a hollow viscus such as the gallbladder, common bile duct, or ureter, (2) stretching of ligament attachments, and (3) spasm of visceral smooth muscle. Often, visceral pain occurs as rhythmic cramps reflecting rhythmic contractions of smooth muscle. A cramping type of pain frequently accompanies gastroenteritis, menstruation, parturition, gallbladder disease, or ureteral obstruction. Distention of a hollow viscus results in pain due to stretch of the tissues and possibly ischemia due to compression of blood vessels by the overdistention.

Visceral pain originating in the thoracic and abdominal cavities is transmitted through sensory nerve fibers that travel in sympathetic nervous system nerves. These are type C fibers such that visceral pain is characteristically burning, aching, diffuse, and poorly localized. Indeed, visceral pain may be referred to surface areas of the body far removed from the painful viscus.

Parenchyma of the brain, liver, and alveoli of the lungs are devoid of pain receptors. Nevertheless, the liver capsule is highly sensitive to both direct trauma and stretch. Furthermore, bile ducts are sensitive to pain. In the lungs, even though the alveoli are insensitive, the bronchi and parietal pleura are very sensitive to pain (see the section entitled Parietal Pain).

Cardiac Visceral Pain

Pain impulses from the heart are conducted through sympathetic nervous system nerves to the middle cervical ganglia, stellate ganglion, and the first four or five thoracic ganglia of the sympathetic chain. These impulses enter the spinal cord through the second, third, fourth, and fifth thoracic nerves. The cause of pain impulses from the heart is almost always myocardial ischemia.

Pain that localizes under the sternum most likely reflects stimulation of sensory nerve endings passing from the heart through the pericardial reflections. In addition, the oppressive sensation beneath the sternum associated with profound myocardial ischemia is possibly due to reflex spasm of blood vessels, bronchioles, or skeletal muscles in the chest region.

PARIETAL PAIN

In addition to true visceral pain, some pain signals are also transmitted from the viscera through nerve fibers that innervate the parietal peritoneum, parietal pleura, or parietal pericardium. The parietal surfaces of visceral cavities are supplied mainly by spinal nerve fibers that penetrate from the surface of the body inward.

Disease of a viscus that spreads to the parietal wall elicits stabbing pain that is transmitted by spinal nerves. In this respect, the parietal wall resembles the skin in being extensively innervated by spinal nerves. Indeed, a surgical incision through parietal peritoneum is exquisitely painful while incision of visceral peritoneum is not painful. In contrast to poorly localized visceral pain, parietal pain is usually localized directly over the damaged area.

EMBRYOLOGIC ORIGIN AND LOCALIZATION OF PAIN

The position in the spinal cord to which visceral afferent fibers pass from each organ depends on the segment of the body from which the organ developed embryologically. For example, the heart originates in the neck and upper thorax such that visceral afferents from the heart enter the spinal cord at C3 to T5 (see the section entitled Cardiac Visceral Pain). The gallbladder originates from the ninth thoracic segment so visceral afferents from the gallbladder enter the spinal cord at T9. As such, the dermatome of the segment from which the visceral organ was originally developed in the embryo is the site of referred pain on the surface of the body.

A second set of pain fibers penetrates inward from spinal nerves to innervate the parietal peritoneum, parietal pleura, and parietal pericardium. Retroperitoneal visceral organs are also innervated by parietal pain fibers. For example, the kidneys are supplied by both visceral and parietal fibers.

The presence of both visceral and parietal pain pathways can result in localization of pain from viscera to two surface areas of the body at the same time. For example, pain impulses from an inflamed appendix pass through the sympathetic nervous system visceral pain fibers into the sympathetic chain and then into the spinal cord at T10–11. This pain is referred to an area around the umbilicus and is aching or cramping in quality. In addition, pain impulses originate in the parietal peritoneum where the inflamed appendix touches the abdominal wall, and these impulses pass through the spinal nerves into the spinal cord at L1–2. This stabbing pain is localized directly over the irritated peritoneal surface in the right lower quadrant.

REFERENCES

Abram SE. Pain pathways and mechanisms. Semin Anes 1985;4:267–74.

Akil H, Mayer DJ, Liebeskind JC. Antagonism of stimulation-produced analgesia by naloxone, a narcotic antagonist. Science 1976;191:961–2.

Bonica JJ. History of pain concepts and pain therapy. Semin Anes 1985;4:189–208.

Cousins MJ, Mather LE. Intrathecal and epidural administration of opioids. Anesthesiology 1984;61:276–310.

Devor M. Nerve pathophysiology and mechanisms of pain in causalgia. J Auton Nerv Syst 1983;7:371–85.

Hokfelt T, Ljungdahl A, Elde R, Nilsson G, Terenius L. Immunohistochemical analysis of peptide pathways possibly related to pain and analgesia: Enkephalin and substance P. Proc Natl Acad Sci 1977;74:3081–5.

Hosobuchi Y, Adams JE, Linchitz R. Pain relief by electrical stimulation of the central gray matter in humans and its reversal by naloxone. Science 1977;197:183–6.

Liebeskind JC, Sherman JE, Cannon JT, Terman GW. Neural and neurochemical mechanisms of pain inhibition. Semin Anes 1985;4:218–22.

Lipton S. Percutaneous electrical cordotomy in relief of intractable pain. Br Med J 1968;2:210–2.

Melzack R, Wall PD. Pain mechanisms: A new theory. Science 1965;150:971–9.

Reddy SVR, Yaksh TL. Spinal noradrenergic terminal system mediates antinociception. Brain Res 1980;189:391–401.

Richardson DE, Akil H. Pain reduction by electrical brain stimulation in man. Part I: Acute administration in periaqueductal and periventricular sites. J Neurosurg 1977;178–83.

Scott LE, Clum GA, Peoples JB. Preoperative predictors of postoperative pain. Pain 1983;15:283–93.

Wilson ME. The neurological mechanisms of pain. A review. Anaesthesia 1974;29:407–24.

Yaksh TL. Spinal opiate analgesia: characteristics and principles of action. Pain 1981;11:293–346.

Yaksh TL, Elde RP. Factors governing the release of methionine-enkephalin-like immunoreactivity from the mesencephalon and spinal cord of the cat in vivo. J Neurophysiol 1981;46:1056–75.

Yaksh TL, Hammond DL. Peripheral and central substances involved in the rostrad transmission of nociceptive information. Pain 1982;13:1–86.

Yaksh TL, Jessell TM, Gamse R, Mudge AW, Leeman SE. Intrathecal morphine inhibits substance P release from mammalian spinal cord in vivo. Nature 1980;286:155–6.

Yaksh TL, Wilson PR. Spinal serotonin terminal system mediates antinociception. J Pharmacol Exp Ther 1979;208:446–53.

CHAPTER 44

Systemic Circulation

INTRODUCTION

The systemic circulation supplies blood to all the tissues of the body except the lungs. Important considerations in understanding the physiology of the systemic circulation include (1) components of the systemic circulation, (2) physical characteristics of the systemic circulation, (3) physical characteristics of blood, (4) determinants and control of tissue blood flow, (5) regulation of arterial blood pressure, and (6) regulation of cardiac output and venous return. In addition, the fetal circulation possesses many unique features which distinguish it from the systemic circulation after birth.

COMPONENTS OF THE SYSTEMIC CIRCULATION

Components of the systemic circulation are the arteries, arterioles, capillaries, venules, and veins (Mellander, 1970) (see Chapter 45).

Arteries

The function of arteries is to transport blood under high pressure to tissues. For this reason, arteries have strong vascular walls and blood flows rapidly to tissues.

Arterioles

Arterioles have diameters less than 200 μ and are the last small branches of the arterial system. These vessels act as control valves through which blood is released into the capillaries. Arterioles have strong muscular walls that are capable of closing the lumen completely or dilating several fold, thereby greatly altering blood flow to the capillaries. Indeed, blood flow to each tissue is controlled almost entirely by the degree of contraction or dilatation of the arterioles. Metarterioles arise at right angles from arterioles and branch several times forming 10 to 100 capillaries.

Capillaries

Capillaries serve as the site for exchange of nutrients and metabolic by-products between tissues and the circulation.

Venules and Veins

Venules collect blood from capillaries for delivery to veins which act as conduits for transmitting blood to the right atrium. Since the pressure in the venous system is low, venous walls are thin. Nevertheless, walls of veins are muscular which allows these vessels to contract or expand and thus store a small or large volume of blood depending on physiologic needs. As a result, veins serve an important function beyond being conduits to return blood to the right atrium. A venous pump mechanism is important for propelling blood forward to the heart.

PHYSICAL CHARACTERISTICS OF THE SYSTEMIC CIRCULATION

The systemic circulation contains about 80% of the entire blood volume with the remainder present in the pulmonary circulation and heart (Fig. 44-1) (Guyton, 1986a). Of the blood volume in the systemic circulation, about 64% is in veins, 13% in arteries, and 5% in capillaries. The heart contains about 7% of the systemic blood volume. The heart ejects blood intermittently into the aorta such that arterial pressure in the aorta fluctuates between a systolic level of about 120 mmHg and diastolic level of about 80 mmHg (see the section entitled Regulation of Systemic Blood Pressure).

Velocity of Blood Flow

Velocity of blood flow in each portion of the systemic circulation is inversely proportional to the cross-sectional area of the blood vessel. Thus, blood flow velocity averages 330 mm sec^{-1} in the aorta and only 0.3 mm sec^{-1} in capillaries (Good-

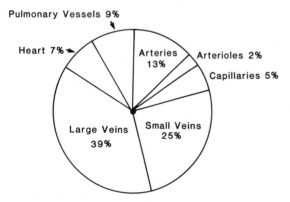

FIGURE 44-1. Distribution of blood volume in each portion of the systemic and pulmonary circulation. (From Guyton AC. Textbook of Medical Physiology. 7th ed. Philadelphia: WB Saunders, 1986:218. Reproduced by permission of the author and publisher.)

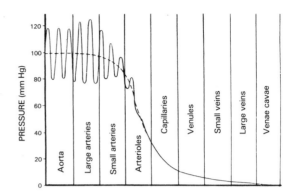

FIGURE 44-2. Blood pressure declines as the blood travels from the aorta to large veins. (From Guyton AC. Textbook of Medical Physiology. 7th ed. Philadelphia: WB Saunders, 1986:218. Reproduced by permission of the author and publisher.)

man *et al*, 1974). Despite this slow velocity of blood flow in capillaries, the short length of these vessels (0.3 – 1 mm) results in blood remaining in the capillaries for only 1 to 3 seconds. All diffusion that is going to take place through the capillary walls must occur in this short period of time.

Progressive Declines in Blood Pressure

As blood flows through the systemic circulation, its pressure falls progressively to nearly zero mmHg by the time it reaches the right atrium (Fig. 44-2) (Guyton, 1986a). The decrease in arterial pressure in each portion of the systemic circulation is directly proportional to the resistance to flow in the vessel. Resistance to blood flow in the aorta and other large arteries is minimal, and mean arterial pressure decreases only 3 to 5 mmHg as blood travels into arteries as small as 3 mm in diameter. Resistance to blood flow begins to increase rapidly in very small arteries causing the mean arterial pressure to decrease to about 85 mmHg at the beginning of the arterioles. Resistance to blood flow in arterioles is the greatest of any part of the systemic circulation, accounting for about one-half the resistance in the entire systemic circulation. As a result, blood pressure decreases to about 30 mmHg at the point where blood enters the capillaries. At the venous end of capillaries, the intravascular pressure has decreased to about 10 mmHg. The decline in blood pressure from 10 mmHg to nearly zero mmHg as blood traverses veins indicates that these vessels have far more resistance than one would expect for vessels of their large sizes. This resistance is caused by compression of the veins from the outside, which keeps many of them, especially the vena cavae, collapsed for a large portion of time.

Pulse Pressure in Arteries

The heart is a pulsatile pump that ejects blood into the aorta intermittently causing pressure pulses (Table 44-1). In the normal young adult, the pressure at the height of a pulse (*i.e.*, systolic pressure) is about 120 mmHg and at its lowest point (*i.e.*, diastolic pressure) is about 80 mmHg. The difference between systolic and diastolic pressures is the pulse pressure.

The typical pressure pulse curve recorded from a large artery is characterized by a rapid rise in pressure during ventricular systole, followed by a maintained high level of pressure for 0.2 to 0.3 second (Fig. 44-3). This plateau is followed by a sharp incisura at the end of systole and a subsequent more gradual decline of pressure back to the diastolic level. The incisura reflects a decline in the intraventricular pressure and a backflow of blood in the aorta that closes the aortic valve. In the presence of aortic regurgitation, the incisura is

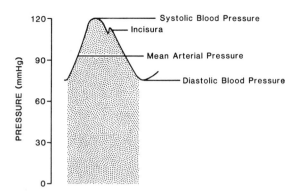

FIGURE 44-3. Schematic depiction of blood pressure recorded from a large systemic artery. Mean arterial pressure is equal to the area under the blood pressure curve divided by the duration of cardiac systole.

located lower on the downslope of the pressure curve. After systole is over, the pressure in the central aorta decreases rapidly initially and then more slowly.

Factors that Alter Arterial Pulse Pressure

The most important factors that alter pulse pressure in arteries are the (1) left ventricular stroke volume, and (2) compliance of the arterial tree (Remington and O'Brien, 1970). Pulse pressure is largely determined by the ratio of stroke volume to compliance of the arterial vessels. A third less important determinant of pulse pressure is the character of ejection from the left ventricle during systole.

LEFT VENTRICULAR STROKE VOLUME. The greater the stroke volume, the greater is the volume of blood that must be accommodated in the arterial vessels with each cardiac contraction. The end result of this increased stroke volume is a greater pulse pressure. Pulse pressure also increases when peripheral vascular resistance declines and flow of blood from arteries to veins is accelerated. Pulse pressure is increased in the presence of patent ductus arteriosus and aortic regurgitation reflecting rapid runoff of blood into the pulmonary circulation or left ventricle respectively. Sudden ejection of blood from the left ventricle causes a greater pulse pressure than a more prolonged ejection. An increase in heart rate

Table 44-1
Normal Pressures in the Systemic Circulation

	Mean Value (mmHg)	Range (mmHg)
Systolic blood pressure*	120	90–140
Diastolic blood pressure*	80	70–90
Mean arterial pressure	92	77–97
Left ventricular end-diastolic pressure	6	0–12
Left atrium	8	2–12
a wave	10	4–16
v wave	13	6–20
Right atrium	5	3–8
a wave	6	2–10
c wave	5	2–10
v wave	3	0–8

* Measured in radial artery

while the cardiac output remains constant causes the stroke volume and pulse pressure to decrease.

COMPLIANCE OF THE ARTERIAL TREE. The greater the compliance of the arterial system, the less will be the rise in pressure for a given stroke volume. Arterial compliance is altered by (1) changes in mean arterial pressure, and (2) pathological changes that affect the distensibility of the arterial walls. For example, with aging, the elastic and muscular tissues of the arterial walls are often replaced by fibrous tissue and sometimes calcified plaques, which cannot stretch. These changes decrease the compliance of the arterial system which in turn causes the arterial pressure to rise substantially during systole and to fall greatly during diastole as blood passes from arteries to veins.

Transmission of the Arterial Pulse Pressure

There is often enhancement of the pulse pressure as the pressure wave is transmitted peripherally (Fig. 44-4) (Guyton, 1986a). At least three factors contribute to this pulse pressure augmentation effect. Part of the augmentation results from a progressive decrease in compliance of the more distal portions of the large arteries. Secondly, pressure waves are reflected to some extent by the peripheral arteries. Specifically, when a pressure pulse enters the peripheral arteries and distends them,

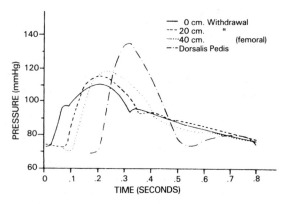

FIGURE 44-4. There is enhancement of the pulse pressure as the arterial blood pressure is transmitted peripherally. (From Guyton AC. Textbook of Medical Physiology. 7th ed. Philadelphia: WB Saunders, 1986:218. Reproduced by permission of the author and publisher.)

the pressure in these peripheral arteries causes the pulse wave to begin traveling backward. If the returning pulse wave strikes an oncoming wave, the two summate, causing a much higher wave than would otherwise occur. Finally, the pulse pressure is also augmented by transmission of certain parts of the pulse wave at more rapid rates than other parts. Augmentation of the peripheral pulse pressure must be remembered whenever blood pressure measurements are made in peripheral arteries as systolic pressure is sometimes as much as 20% to 30% above that in the central aorta and diastolic pressure is often reduced as much as 10% to 15%.

The pulse pressure becomes less and less as it passes through small arteries and arterioles until it becomes almost absent in capillaries (Fig. 44-2) (Guyton, 1986a). This dampening of the pulse pressure is primarily due to a combined effect of vascular distensibility and vascular resistance. Resistance in these small vessels is great enough that the flow of blood and consequently the transmission of pressure are greatly impeded. At the same time, distensibility of small vessels is great so that the small amount of blood that is caused to flow during a pressure pulse produces progressively less and less pressure rise in the more distal vessels.

Pulsus Paradoxus

Pulsus paradoxus is characterized by a series of weak followed by strong peripheral arterial pulsations that are related to the phase of ventilation (see the section entitled Respiratory Variations in Blood Pressure).

Pulsus Alternans

Pulsus alternans is alternating weak and strong cardiac contractions causing a similar alternation in the strength of the peripheral pulse. Digitalis intoxication and varying degrees of atrioventricular heart block are commonly associated with pulsus alternans.

Pulse Deficit

In the presence of atrial fibrillation or ectopic beats, two beats of the heart may occur so close together that the ventricle does not fill adequately and the second cardiac contraction pumps insufficient blood to create a peripheral pulse. In this circumstance, a second heart beat is audible with a stethoscope applied directly over the heart but one cannot palpate a corresponding pulsation in the radial artery. This phenomenon is called a pulse deficit.

Right Atrial Pressure

Blood from all the systemic veins flows into the right atrium. Pressure in the right atrium is commonly designated the central venous pressure. Right atrial pressure is regulated by a balance between venous return and the ability of the right ventricle to eject blood (Guyton and Jones, 1973). If the right ventricle is contracting strongly, right atrial pressure tends to decrease. Conversely, poor right ventricular contractility tends to elevate right atrial pressure. Likewise, any event that increases flow of blood into the right atrium, such as hypervolemia or venoconstriction, will tend to elevate right atrial pressure.

Normal right atrial pressure is about 5 mmHg (Table 44-1). The lower limit of right atrial pressure is about minus 5 mmHg corresponding to the pressure in the pericardial and intrapleural spaces that surround the heart. Right atrial pressure approaches these low values when right ventricular contractility is increased or venous return to the heart is greatly reduced as in the presence of severe hemorrhage.

Peripheral Venous Pressure

Large veins offer almost no resistance to blood flow when they are distended. Most large veins, however, are compressed at multiple extrathoracic sites. For example, pressure in the neck veins often is so low that the atmospheric pressure on the outside of the neck causes them to collapse. Veins coursing through the abdomen are compressed by different organs and by intra-abdominal pressure so they often are almost totally collapsed. Normal pressure in the peritoneal cavity averages about 2 mmHg but may increase to as high as 15 to 20 mmHg as a result of pregnancy or ascites. When this occurs, pressure in the veins of the legs must increase above abdominal pressure before the abdominal veins will open. For these reasons, large veins usually provide considerable resistance to blood flow manifesting as a venous pressure in these veins that is 6 to 10 mmHg

higher than the right atrial pressure. It is important to recognize that veins inside the thorax are not collapsed because of the distending effect of negative intrathoracic pressure.

Effect of Right Atrial Pressure on Peripheral Venous Pressure

Peripheral venous pressure does not begin to rise until right atrial pressure increases sufficiently to cause blood to pool in the large veins. This usually occurs when the right atrial pressure rises to about 4 to 6 mmHg.

Effect of Hydrostatic Pressure

In a standing person, pressure in the right atrium remains near zero mmHg because the heart pumps into arteries any excess blood that accumulates. Pressure in the veins of the feet. however, is about 90 mmHg because of the distance from the heart to the feet (Fig. 44-5) (Guyton, 1986a). Pressure increases about 0.7 mmHg for each centimeter below the level of the heart. Conversely, neck veins collapse almost completely due to atmospheric pressure on the outside of the neck. Veins inside the skull cannot collapse as they are held open by bone. As a result, negative pressure can exist in the dural sinuses. Indeed, venous pressure in the sagittal sinus is about minus 10 mmHg because of the hydrostatic suction between the top of the skull and the base of the skull. Thus, if the sagittal sinus is entered during surgery, air can be entrained immediately producing a potentially fatal venous air embolism.

Hydrostatic pressure affects peripheral pressures in arteries and capillaries as well as veins. For example, a standing person who has an arterial pressure of 100 mmHg at the level of the heart has an arterial pressure of about 190 mmHg in the feet.

Venous Valves and the Pump Mechanism

Valves in veins are arranged so that the direction of blood flow can be only toward the heart. In a standing person, movement of the legs compresses skeletal muscles against the fascia and the fascia against the skin so that the veins of the leg are compressed and blood is directed toward the

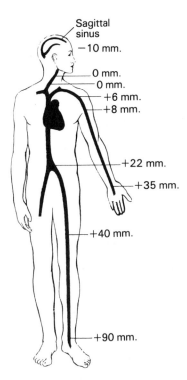

FIGURE 44-5. Effect of hydrostatic pressure on venous pressures throughout the body. (From Guyton AC. Textbook of Medical Physiology. 7th ed. Philadelphia: WB Saunders, 1986:218. Reproduced by permission of the author and publisher.)

heart. This venous pump or skeletal muscle pump is usually sufficient to maintain venous pressure in the feet of a walking adult below 25 mmHg.

If a person stands immobile, the venous pump does not function and venous pressures in the lower part of the leg can rise to the full hydrostatic value of 90 mmHg in about 30 seconds. Under these conditions, elevated pressures in capillaries can increase greatly the amount of fluid that leaks from the intravascular space into the tissue spaces. As a result, the legs swell and the blood volume diminishes. Indeed, as much as 15% of the blood volume can be lost from the intravascular space in the first 15 minutes of quiet standing.

Varicose Veins

Valves of the venous system can be destroyed when the veins are chronically distended by in-

creased venous pressure as occurs during pregnancy or in a person who stands most of the time. The end-result is varicose veins characterized by bulbous protrusions of the veins beneath the skin of the leg. Venous and capillary pressures remain elevated because of the incompetent venous pump and this causes constant edema in the legs of these individuals. Edema prevents adequate diffusion of nutrients from capillaries to tissues so that skeletal muscles become painful and weak while the skin frequently atrophies and finally ulcerates.

Reference Level for Measuring Venous Pressures

Hydrostatic pressure factors do not affect venous or arterial pressure that is measured at the level of the tricuspid valve. As a result, the reference point for pressure measurement is considered to be the level of the tricuspid valve. The reason for lack of hydrostatic effects at the tricuspid valve is the ability of the right ventricle to act as a regulator of pressure at this point. For example, if the pressure at the tricuspid valve rises, the right ventricle fills to a greater extent thereby decreasing the pressure at the tricuspid valve toward normal. Conversely, if the pressure declines at the tricuspid valve, the right ventricle fails to fill adequately, its pumping decreases, and blood pools in the veins until pressure at the tricuspid level again rises to a normal value.

External reference points for the level of the tricuspid valve are one-third the distance from the anterior chest and about one-fourth the distance above the lower end of the sternum. Regardless of body position, the right atrial pressure when referenced to the level of the tricuspid valve will not change. This does not mean that right atrial pressure at this point is zero mmHg but, rather, regardless of the value, changing body position will not significantly alter the pressure.

A precise hydrostatic point (*e.g.*, level of the tricuspid valve) in the chest to which pressures are referred is essential for accurate interpretation of venous filling pressure measurements. For example, each centimeter below the hydrostatic point adds 0.7 mmHg to the measured pressure while 0.7 mmHg is subtracted for each centimeter above this point. When venous pressures are normally low, an error introduced by 5 cm of hydrostatic pressure (*i.e.*, plus or minus 3.5 mmHg) can be substantial. Conversely, a precise hydrostatic point is less important for measurement of arterial pressures, since the error introduced by hydrostatic pressure is a small percentage of the total pressure.

Measurement of right atrial pressure is accomplished using a water-filled manometer or transducer referenced to the level of the tricuspid valve. A venous pressure measurement in cm H_2O can be converted to mmHg by dividing this value by 1.36. Venous pressure can also be estimated by observing distention of the neck veins. For example, neck veins become visibly distended in the sitting position only when venous pressure exceeds 10 to 15 mmHg.

Pressure Waves in Veins

Pressure pulses from the arteries are greatly dampened before they pass through the capillaries into the systemic veins. Right atrial pulsations (a, c, and v waves) can be transmitted retrograde to cause pressure pulses in the veins (Table 44-1) (see Chapter 47).

Centrifugal Acceleratory Forces

The most important effect of centrifugal acceleration is on the circulatory system (Burton *et al,* 1974). Positive gravitational forces displace blood toward the lower portions of the body causing vessels to passively dilate. As a result, venous return decreases, cardiac output declines, and cerebral blood flow becomes inadequate to maintain consciousness. Activation of baroreceptors offsets these effects up to about 3.3 times normal gravity. Compression bags applied to the legs and lower abdomen also reduce pooling of blood in these areas.

Negative gravity displaces excess blood into the head which elicits an intense baroreceptor reflex characterized by profound bradycardia. Hyperemia in the eyes during negative gravity causes temporary blindness ("redout").

Acceleration and deceleration forces in space travel are examples of linear acceleration (Burton *et al,* 1974). Forces equal to nine times normal gravity occur during acceleration or deceleration but in a semi-reclining position are distributed transverse to the axis of acceleration. This amount of gravitational force can be tolerated for several

minutes and is the reason reclining seats are used by the astronauts.

Physiology of Weightlessness

In the absence of resistance to movement that occurs in space, the effect of gravity is equal on all objects with the net effect being weightlessness (Adey, 1974). Important physiologic effects of weightlessness are (1) translocation of fluids within the body because of failure of gravity to cause hydrostatic pressure, and (2) diminishment of skeletal muscle tone because no strength of muscle contraction is required to oppose the force of gravity. Prolonged stay in space is associated with (1) reductions in plasma volume and erythrocyte mass, (2) reduction in cardiac output, and (3) loss of calcium from bones. Indeed, orthostatic hypotension may be marked on return to sea level reflecting translocation of a diminished blood volume to the legs and abdomen. All these changes resemble alterations that occur with inactivity at sea level and can be offset by a planned exercise program.

PHYSICAL CHARACTERISTICS OF BLOOD

Blood is a viscous fluid composed of cells and plasma. More than 99% of the cells in plasma are erythrocytes. As a result, leukocytes exert a minimal influence on the physical characteristics of blood. Plasma is considered extracellular fluid, and fluid inside cells is intracellular fluid. The percent of blood that is erythrocytes is the hematocrit.

Viscosity of Blood

Friction between successive layers of blood determines viscosity of blood. Therefore, viscosity of blood is greatly influenced by hematocrit (Fig. 44-6) (Guyton, 1986b). Assuming water has a viscosity of 1, viscosity of blood is about three times greater. This means that three times as much pressure is required to force blood through a given blood vessel than to force water through the same vessel. When hematocrit increases to 60% or 70%, viscosity of blood is increased about tenfold compared to water and flow through blood vessels is greatly reduced. The concentrations and types of protein in the plasma influence viscosity of blood only minimally.

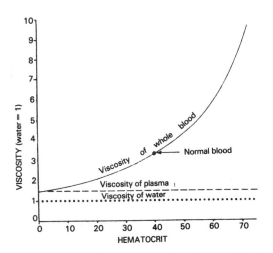

FIGURE 44-6. Hematocrit greatly influences the viscosity of blood. (From Guyton AC. Textbook of Medical Physiology. 7th ed. Philadelphia: WB Saunders, 1986:206. Reproduced by permission of the author and publisher.)

In addition to hematocrit and plasma proteins, three additional factors affect blood viscosity in small blood vessels of the circulatory system. For example, viscosity exerts far less effect on blood flow in small than in large blood vessels. Indeed, in blood vessels as small as capillaries, the impact of viscosity on blood flow is reduced about 50%. This reduced impact of viscosity most likely reflects alignment of erythrocytes as they pass through small blood vessels rather than the random arrangement characteristic of flow through larger vessels (Schmid-Schonbein, 1976). This alignment of erythrocytes, which greatly reduces the viscous resistance that occurs normally between cells, is largely offset by a reduced velocity of flow that greatly increases viscosity. For example, blood viscosity in capillaries with low flow can be increased as much as tenfold presumably reflecting adherence of erythrocytes to each other and to the walls of the blood vessel. The net effect may be that viscous effects in small blood vessels are similar to those that occur in large blood vessels.

Plasma

Plasma is part of the extracellular fluid. It is almost identical to interstitial fluid except that plasma contains more proteins. This difference reflects the inability of plasma proteins to easily pass through capillary channels into the interstitial spaces. As a result, most of the plasma proteins are held in the circulatory system giving it a protein concentration three to four times greater than that of fluid outside the capillaries. Plasma proteins consist of albumin (4.5 g dl^{-1}), globulins (2.5 g dl^{-1}), and fibrinogen (0.3 g dl^{-1}).

Albumin

The primary function of albumin is to create colloid osmotic pressure at the capillary membrane. This colloid osmotic pressure prevents fluid from leaking out of capillaries into interstitial spaces.

Globulins

Globulins are divided into alpha, beta, and gamma globulins. Alpha and beta globulins participate in transport of other substances by combining with them. The gamma globulins, and to a lesser extent beta globulins, are important in their function as antibodies that resist infection and provide the body with immunity.

Fibrinogen

Fibrinogen plays an important role in coagulation of blood (see Chapter 57).

DETERMINANTS OF TISSUE BLOOD FLOW

Blood flow is determined entirely by the pressure difference tending to push blood through the blood vessel and the resistance (*i.e.*, impediment) to blood flow through the vessel. It is important to appreciate that the difference in pressure between two points, and not the absolute pressure, is the determinant of blood flow. The relationship between flow, pressure, and resistance can be expressed mathematically as a variant of Ohms' law in which blood flow (*i.e.*, amperes) is directly proportional to the pressure drop across two points (*i.e.*, voltage) and inversely proportional to resistance (Fig. 44-7*A*). Rearrangement of this formula emphasizes that pressure is directly proportional to flow times resistance (Fig. 44-7*B*). Likewise, resistance is directly proportional to pressure and inversely proportional to flow (Fig. 44-7*C*). Furthermore, resistance is directly pro-

A   Blood Flow (Q)= $\dfrac{\text{Pressure Difference Between Two Points } (\Delta P)}{\text{Resistance To Flow (R)}}$

B $\Delta P \quad = Q \times R$

C $R \quad = \Delta P / Q$

FIGURE 44-7. The relationship between blood flow, pressure, and resistance to flow can be expressed as a variant of Ohm's law.

portional to viscosity of blood and the length of the vessel and inversely proportional to the fourth power of the radius of the vessel (*i.e.*, doubling the radius of the vessel decreases resistance to flow 16-fold) (Poiseuille's law). These observations emphasize that increasing tissue blood flow by hemodilution or vasodilation is more energy efficient than similar increases in flow produced by elevations in pressure. Indeed, tissue blood flow is normally the result of local variations in resistance to blood flow through vessels at a relatively constant blood pressure.

Blood flow is the quantity of blood that passes a given point in the circulation in a given period of time. Total blood flow is the cardiac output which is the amount of blood pumped by each ventricle of the heart in a given period of time. Obviously, the cardiac output into the systemic and pulmonary circulations must be the same.

Measurement of Blood Pressure

Blood pressure measured in mmHg is that force exerted by the blood against any unit area of the vessel wall. Occasionally, pressure is measured in centimeters of water. One mmHg equals 1.36 cm H_2O because the density of mercury is 13.6 times that of water.

Measurement of blood pressure using a mercury manometer is commonly employed. Mercury has so much inertia, however, that it cannot respond to pressure changes that occur more rapidly than about one cycle every 2 to 3 seconds. Accu-

rate recording of rapidly changing pressures requires utilization of pressure transducers that convert pressure into electrical signals that can be displayed and recorded. Recorders capable of monitoring pressure changes with frequencies of 20 to 100 cycles sec^{-1} are in common use.

Measurement of blood pressure by auscultation utilizes the principle that blood flow in large arteries is laminar and not audible. If blood flow is arrested by an inflated cuff and the pressure in the cuff is released slowly, audible tapping sounds (Korotkoff sounds) can be heard when the pressure of the cuff falls just below systolic blood pressure and blood starts flowing in the brachial artery. These tapping sounds occur because flow velocity through the constricted portion of the blood vessel is increased, resulting in turbulence and vibrations that are heard through the stethoscope. Diastolic blood pressure correlates with the onset of muffled auscultatory sounds. The auscultatory method for determining systolic and diastolic blood pressure usually gives values within 10% of those determined by direct measurement from the arteries.

Resistance to Blood Flow

Resistance to blood flow through a vessel is directly proportional to the viscosity of blood and length of the vessel and inversely proportional to the fourth power of the radius of the vessel. Resistance to blood flow cannot be measured directly. Instead, resistance is calculated as the difference between mean arterial and right atrial pressure divided by cardiac output (Fig. 44-7C). Total pulmonary vascular resistance is calculated as the difference between mean pulmonary artery and left atrial pressure divided by cardiac output. Resistance is expressed in units or dynes sec^{-1} cm^{-5} if the calculated value is multiplied by 80.

Conductance

Conductance is the reciprocal of resistance and is a measure of the amount of blood flow that can pass through a blood vessel in a given time for a given pressure gradient. Slight changes in diameter of a blood vessel cause large changes in conductance. Indeed, the conductance (*i.e.*, blood flow) of the vessel increases in proportion to the fourth power of the radius.

Vascular Distensibility

Blood vessels are distensible such that increases in blood pressure cause the vascular diameter to increase which in turn reduces resistance to blood flow (Dorbin, 1978). Conversely, reductions in intravascular pressure increase the resistance to blood flow. Blood pressure can eventually decline to the level that the intravascular pressure is no longer capable of keeping the vessel open. This pressure is defined as the critical closing pressure. Laplace's law, which states that the distending force to keep the blood vessel open is directly proportional to the diameter of the vessel times the pressure, helps explain why critical closing occurs more suddenly than would be predicted by the decline in blood pressure alone. The average critical closing pressure is 20 mmHg.

The level of activity of the sympathetic nervous system influences the critical closing pressure. For example, inhibition of sympathetic nervous system activity can reduce critical closing pressure to as low as 5 mmHg while stimulation of the sympathetic nervous system can increase critical closing pressure to as high as 100 mmHg. When the heart is abruptly stopped, the pressure in the entire circulatory system equilibrates (i.e., mean circulatory pressure) at about 7 mmHg (Manning et al, 1979).

The ability of blood vessels to distend as intravascular pressure increases varies greatly in different parts of the circulation. Anatomically, walls of arteries are stronger than those of veins. As a result, veins are six to ten times as distensible as the arteries.

Vascular Compliance

Compliance or capacitance of a blood vessel is defined as the increase in volume of the vessel produced by an increase in intravascular pressure. The compliance of the entire circulatory system is estimated to be 100 ml for each 1 mmHg increase in intravascular pressure (Guyton, 1986b). Distensibility and compliance are very different. For example, a distensible vessel which has a small volume may have far less compliance (i.e., distensibility times volume) than a much less distensible vessel which has a large volume. Compliance of a vein is about twenty-four times that of the corresponding artery because it is about eight times as distensible and has a volume about three times as great. This difference in compliance is important because it means that large amounts of blood can be stored in veins compared with arteries. For example, the volume of blood normally present in all veins is about 2500 ml while the arterial system contains only about 750 ml of blood when the mean arterial pressure is 100 mmHg.

Sympathetic nervous system activity can greatly alter the distribution of blood volume. Enhancement of sympathetic nervous system tone to the blood vessels, especially the veins, reduces the dimensions of the circulatory system, and the circulation continues to operate almost normally even when as much as 25% of the total blood volume has been lost.

Laminar Flow of Blood

The velocity of flow in the center of a blood vessel is greater than that toward the walls of the vessel. This phenomenon is called *laminar flow* or *streamline flow*. The cause of laminar flow is the adherence of molecules to the vessel wall while molecules towards the center of the lumen slip past one another easily. In small vessels, essentially all the blood is near the vessel wall so that a rapidly flowing central stream of blood does not exist. As the diameter of the blood vessel wall increases, there are progressive increases in the velocities of blood flow near the center of the lumen.

Turbulent Flow of Blood

Blood flow may become turbulent rather than laminar when the (1) rate of flow is excessive, (2) flow passes by an obstruction or rough surface in the blood vessel, or (3) blood vessel makes an abrupt turn. Turbulent blood flow causes eddy currents to form and greatly increases resistance to blood flow. The Reynolds number is the measure of the tendency for turbulence to occur.

CONTROL OF TISSUE BLOOD FLOW

Control of blood flow to different tissues includes (1) local mechanisms, (2) autonomic nervous system responses, and (3) release of hormones

(Lundgren and Jodal, 1975) (see Chapter 52). Total blood flow to tissues (*i.e.*, cardiac output) is about 5 L min^{-1} with large amounts being delivered to the heart, brain liver, and kidneys (Table 44-2) (Guyton, 1986c). Excessive accumulation of carbon dioxide and hydrogen ions in the brain is prevented by a high cerebral blood flow. A high hepatic blood flow is necessary to support the high level of metabolic activity of this organ. Skeletal muscle represents 35% to 40% of total body mass but receives only about 15% of the total cardiac output reflecting the low metabolic rate of inactive skeletal muscle.

Local Control of Blood Flow

Local control of blood flow is most often based on the need for delivery of oxygen or other nutrients such as glucose or fatty acids to the tissues. In some tissues, however, local blood flow may be determined by factors other than delivery of nutrients. For example, cutaneous blood flow is determined by the need to transfer heat from the body to the surrounding air. In the kidneys, the need to deliver substances for excretion is a major determinant of renal blood flow. The carbon dioxide and hydrogen ion concentrations in brain fluids are important determinants of cerebral blood flow.

Tissue Oxygen Needs

Local tissue blood flow increases whenever the availability of oxygen to the tissue decreases. This response to decreased oxygen delivery may reflect the local release of vasodilatory substances (adenosine, carbon dioxide, lactic acid, potassium ions) in response to tissue hypoxia. Alternatively, local lack of oxygen may interfere with the ability of the vessels that supply these tissues to maintain vascular contraction. Regardless of the mechanism, the net effect is local vasodilation in response to tissue oxygen lack. Local vasodilation increases tissue blood flow and the subsequent delivery of oxygen to tissues.

Vasomotion

Vasomotion is the cyclic opening and closure of precapillary sphincters. The number of precapillary sphincters that are open at any given time is approximately proportional to the nutrient (*i.e.*, oxygen) requirements of tissues.

Autoregulation of Blood Flow

Autoregulation is a local mechanism of control of blood flow in which a specific tissue is able to maintain a relatively constant blood flow over a wide range of mean arterial pressure. Concep-

Table 44-2
Tissue Blood Flow

| | Approximate Blood Flow | | Cardiac Output |
	(ml min^{-1})	(ml 100g^{-1} min^{-1})	(% of total)
Brain	750	50	15
Liver	1450	100	29
Portal vein	1100		
Hepatic artery	350		
Kidneys	1000	320	20
Heart	225	75	5
Skeletal muscle (at rest)	750	4	15
Skin	400	3	8
Other tissues	425	2	8
TOTAL	5000		100

(Adapted from Guyton AC. Textbook of Medical Physiology. 7th ed. Philadelphia; WB Saunders, 1986:230; by permission of the author and publisher.)

tually, when the mean arterial pressure becomes elevated, the resulting excess flow will provide too many nutrients to the tissues or will flush out all vasodilator substances, either of which will cause the blood vessels to constrict. As a result, increased perfusion pressure will not increase blood flow because of the modifying effect of vasoconstriction. Conversely, reductions in mean arterial pressure result in decreased delivery of nutrients to tissues such that vasodilation occurs to maintain an unchanged tissue blood flow despite a decreased perfusion pressure.

Autoregulation of renal and cerebral blood flow is determined by factors in addition to the requirements for nutrients. For example, autoregulation of renal blood flow is greatly influenced by the serum concentration of sodium and end-products of protein metabolism. An increase in either will increase renal blood flow. In the brain, a powerful mechanism for local regulation of blood flow is the concentration of carbon dioxide and hydrogen ions. When the concentration of these substances increases, blood vessels dilate, allowing more rapid blood flow to remove excess carbon dioxide. In addition, the hydrogen ion concentration declines because removal of carbon dioxide also removes carbonic acid. Conversely, a decrease in carbon dioxide and hydrogen ion concentration causes vasoconstriction, which allows these substances to accumulate in the tissues until their levels increase back toward normal values.

Autoregulatory responses to sudden changes in mean arterial pressure occur within 60 to 120 seconds. The ability of autoregulation to return local tissue blood flow to normal, however, is incomplete. Long-term changes over several days are necessary to return blood flow completely to normal values (see the section entitled Long-Term Local Control of Blood Flow).

Reactive hyperemia is a manifestation of local control of blood flow in which the temporary occlusion of blood flow to a tissue is followed by an instant increase in blood flow to that tissue when the occlusion is removed. Active hyperemia is local vasodilation that occurs whenever a previously resting tissue such as skeletal muscle or a gastrointestinal secretory gland becomes active.

Long-Term Local Control of Blood Flow

Long-term regulatory mechanisms are necessary to return local tissue blood flow completely to normal values following an initial rapid adjustment provided by autoregulation in response to changes in blood pressure. Chronic alterations in tissue metabolic requirements also produce long-term changes in blood flow.

The mechanism of long-term local control of blood flow is a change in the vascularity of tissues. For example, sustained elevation of mean arterial pressure to specific tissues, as occurs with coarctation of the aorta, is accompanied by a decrease in the size and number of blood vessels. Likewise, if the metabolism in a given tissue becomes chronically elevated, vascularity increases; or if metabolism is reduced, vascularity decreases. Indeed, there seems to be a built-in mechanism in most tissues to keep the degree of vascularity of the tissue almost exactly that required to supply the nutrient needs of the tissue.

This long-term change in vascularity occurs more promptly in young compared with older tissues. Therefore, the time required for long-term regulation to take place may be only a few days in the neonate or as long as several months in elderly people. Furthermore, the adequacy of response is more complete in the young than elderly.

A likely stimulus for increased or decreased tissue vascularity is the local tissue need for oxygen. Indeed, increased tissue vascularity occurs in animals that live in the low oxygen environment of high altitudes. Newborn infants exposed to excessive concentrations of oxygen may manifest cessation of new vascular growth in the retina of the eye. Subsequent removal of the neonate from a high oxygen environment causes an overgrowth of new vessels to offset the abrupt decrease in availability of oxygen. There may be so much overgrowth that the new vessels grow into the vitreous humor and cause blindness (*i.e.*, retrolental fibroplasia).

COLLATERAL CIRCULATION. Development of collateral circulation when blood flow to a tissue is blocked is a manifestation of long-term local blood flow regulation. Inadequate delivery of essential nutrients seems to be the stimulus for the development of collateral vessels.

Autonomic Nervous System Control of Blood Flow

Autonomic nervous system regulation of blood flow is characterized by a rapid response time (within 1 second) and an ability to control blood flow to certain tissues at the expense of other tissues (Folkow, 1960). For example, autonomic nervous system responses can transiently reduce blood flow to certain tissues despite the fact that local blood flow control mechanisms oppose this response. The sympathetic nervous system is the important component of the autonomic nervous system in the regulation of blood flow. Indeed, all blood vessels, with the exception of metarterioles and capillaries, are innervated by the sympathetic nervous system. Release of norepinephrine stimulates alpha-adrenergic receptors to produce peripheral vasoconstriction characteristic of sympathetic nervous system stimulation. The role of the parasympathetic nervous system in regulation of tissue blood flow is minimal being manifest primarily by changes in heart rate.

Innervation of small arteries and arterioles allows sympathetic nervous system stimulation to increase the resistance and thus to change the rate of blood flow through tissues. Innervation of large vessels, particularly veins, makes it possible for sympathetic nervous system stimulation to change the capacity of these vessels, resulting in alterations in the volume of blood present in the peripheral circulatory system.

Although sympathetic nervous system fibers are distributed essentially to all parts of the circulation, this distribution is greater in some tissues than others. For example, sympathetic nervous system innervation is prominent in the kidneys, gastrointestinal tract, spleen, and the skin. Conversely, effects of sympathetic nervous system stimulation on the cerebral circulation are minimal.

Vasomotor Center

The vasomotor center is located bilaterally in the reticular substance of the lower one third of the pons and upper two thirds of the medulla. This center transmits sympathetic nervous system impulses through the spinal cord and vasoconstrictor fibers to all blood vessels. The upper and lateral portions of the vasomotor center are continuously active, accounting for a sustained partial state of vasoconstriction (*e.g.*, vasomotor tone) in blood vessels. Evidence for this background vasomotor tone is the abrupt decline in blood pressure that occurs when sympathetic nervous system innervation of the vasculature is suddenly interrupted as by traumatic spinal cord transection or regional anesthesia.

The medial and lower portions of the vasomotor center do not participate in transmission of vasoconstrictor impulses but rather function as an inhibitor of sympathetic vasoconstrictor tone which allows blood vessels to dilate. Conceptually, this portion of the vasomotor center is functioning as the parasympathetic nervous system.

In addition to controlling peripheral vascular tone, the vasomotor center also influences cardiac activity (see Chapter 47). The lateral portions of the vasomotor center transmit excitatory impulses through sympathetic nervous system fibers that act to increase heart rate and myocardial contractility. The medial portion of the vasomotor center is near the dorsal motor nucleus of the vagus nerve and transmits impulses via the vagus nerve to reduce heart rate. The effects of the vasomotor center on cardiac function complement the peripheral vascular effects evoked by activity of this center.

Activity of the vasomotor center can be influenced by impulses from a number of sites including diffuse areas of the reticular activating system, hypothalamus, and cerebral cortex. Thus, widespread areas of the central nervous system can exert profound effects on the vasomotor center and, in turn, influence sympathetic nervous system-mediated vasoconstriction, either enhancing or inhibiting this response.

Sympathetic nervous system impulses are transmitted to the adrenal medulla at the same time they are transmitted to the peripheral vasculature (see Chapter 42). These impulses stimulate the adrenal medulla to secrete both epinephrine and norepinephrine into the circulation where they act directly on adrenergic receptors in the walls of vascular smooth muscle.

Vasodilator System

Sympathetic nervous system fibers to skeletal muscles include both constrictor and vasodilator fibers. It is likely that the vasodilator substance in humans is epinephrine, and not acetylcholine, as is the case in lower animals such as cats. The anterior hypothalamus is the principal central nervous system control site for the vasodilator system. It seems unlikely that sympathetic nervous system vasodilator fibers are important in the control of blood flow to skeletal muscles because blockade of these nerves minimally influences the ability of skeletal muscles to control their blood flow according to local needs. Prior to exercise, however, this vasodilator system is likely to be responsible for an initial vasodilatation to allow an anticipatory increase in blood flow even before the skeletal muscles require increased nutrients.

SYNCOPE. Emotional fainting (vasovagal syncope) may be due to intense stimulation of the anterior hypothalamus resulting in such profound skeletal muscle vasodilatation that blood pressure declines abruptly and syncope occurs. Associated vagal stimulation results in bradycardia. This phenomenon may occur in patients who have an intense fear of needles resulting in syncope during placement of an intravenous catheter.

MASS REFLEX. The mass reflex is characterized by stimulation of all portions of the vasomotor center resulting in generalized vasoconstriction and an increase in cardiac activity. In addition, the adrenal medulla is stimulated to release epinephrine and norepinephrine into the circulation. The net effect of these responses is (1) increased peripheral vascular resistance to increase arterial blood pressure, (2) venoconstriction to improve venous return, and (3) cardiac stimulation to evoke an increased cardiac output. All these changes result in increased delivery of tissue nutrients via increased tissue blood flow.

ALARM REACTION. The alarm reaction resembles the mass reflex. In addition, there is skeletal muscle vasodilatation and psychic excitement due to diffuse stimulation of the hypothalamus. This alarm pattern prepares an individual for extreme stress.

Hormone Control of Blood Flow

Vasoconstrictor hormones that control tissue blood flow are epinephrine, norepinephrine, angiotensin, and antidiuretic hormone. Bradykinin, serotonin, histamine, and prostaglandins are vasodilating substances (see Chapters 21 and 22). Chemical factors, including plasma concentrations of various ions, may also influence local tissue blood flow.

Epinephrine and Norepinephrine

Epinephrine and norepinephrine are secreted by the adrenal medulla in response to sympathetic nervous system stimulation (see Chapter 42). Norepinephrine activates alpha-adrenergic receptors

causing vasoconstriction in almost all vascular sites. Epinephrine also produces vasoconstriction by a similar mechanism. Conversely, low circulating concentrations of epinephrine stimulate beta-adrenergic receptors in skeletal muscle and coronary arteries to produce vasodilation.

Angiotensin

Angiotensin is an intensely potent vasoconstrictor substance that is formed from renin. Renin is released from the kidneys in response to (1) a reduction in renal blood flow due to hypotension or (2) decreased serum concentration of sodium. Effects of angiotensin on control of arterial blood pressure are related to (1) vasoconstriction of arterioles, (2) moderate venoconstriction, and (3) vasoconstriction of renal arterioles causing the kidneys to retain both water and sodium.

Antidiuretic Hormone

Antidiuretic hormone is more potent than angiotensin as a vasoconstrictor. Nevertheless, only small amounts of this hormone are secreted, and it seems probable that antidiuretic hormone has little effect in control of circulation. During severe hemorrhage, however, plasma concentrations of antidiuretic hormone may increase sufficiently to raise arterial blood pressure.

Bradykinin

Bradykinin is a polypeptide that causes intense vascular vasodilation and increased capillary permeability. The potential for bradykinin to be formed anywhere in the body suggests this substance plays an important role in the regulation of circulation.

Serotonin

Serotonin is present in high concentrations in chromaffin tissue and platelets. Depending on the characteristics of the local circulation, serotonin can produce vasodilatation or vasoconstriction.

Histamine

Histamine is released from virtually all tissues when they are damaged. Like bradykinin, histamine has an intense vasodilator effect on arterioles and can increase capillary permeability resulting in marked tissue edema.

Prostaglandins

Prostaglandins are capable of producing vasoconstriction or vasodilatation. The widespread distribution of prostaglandins in tissues for release into the circulation suggests a possible role for these substances particularly in the local regulation of tissue blood flow.

Chemical Factors

An increase in the plasma concentration of calcium causes vasoconstriction. Vasodilatation produced by increased plasma concentrations of potassium or magnesium reflects the ability of these ions to cause relaxation of vascular smooth muscle. Increased plasma concentrations of sodium cause arteriolar vasodilation as a result of an increase is osmolarity produced by this ion. An increase in carbon dioxide concentration or hydrogen ion concentration causes vasodilatation in most tissues. Carbon dioxide, however, has an indirect vasoconstrictor effect by virtue of stimulating the outflow of sympathetic nervous system impulses from the vasomotor center.

REGULATION OF ARTERIAL BLOOD PRESSURE

The ability of each tissue to control its own blood flow by local vasodilation or vasoconstriction of arterioles requires that mean arterial pressure be maintained reasonably constant. Indeed, the circulation has an intricate system for regulation of arterial blood pressure and maintenance of mean arterial pressure between 90 and 110 mmHg (Mancia *et al*, 1976). Nervous system and hormonal mechanisms act rapidly to regulate blood pressure. Conversely, long-term regulation of blood pressure includes slow responding mechanisms related to kidney function and blood volume regulation.

Normal Arterial Blood Pressures

Systolic, diastolic, and mean arterial pressure tend to increase progressively with age (Fig. 44-8) (Guyton, 1986d). Mean arterial pressure is the average pressure throughout each cardiac cycle. Since a greater portion of the cardiac cycle is nearer the diastolic blood pressure, it follows that

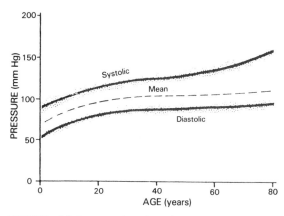

FIGURE 44-8. Systolic, diastolic, and mean arterial pressure tend to increase progressively with age. The shaded areas reflect range of changes. (From Guyton AC. Textbook of Medical Physiology. 7th ed. Philadelphia: WB Saunders, 1986:244. Reproduced by permission of the author and publisher.)

mean arterial pressure is not an arithmetic average of the systolic and diastolic blood pressure.

Mean arterial pressure is the average pressure tending to drive blood through the systemic circulation. For this reason, the mean arterial pressure is the important determinant of tissue blood flow. Mean arterial pressure, like systolic and diastolic blood pressure is lowest immediately after birth increasing from 70 mmHg to 100 mmHg at adolescence where it remains until middle age.

Arterial pressure is equal to the cardiac output times peripheral vascular resistance (Fig. 44-7*B*). Both these factors are often manipulated for the regulation of blood pressure.

Rapidly Acting Mechanisms for Regulation of Arterial Blood Pressure

Rapidly acting mechanisms for regulation of blood pressure involve nervous system responses as reflected by the (1) baroreceptor reflexes, (2) chemoreceptor reflexes, (3) atrial reflexes, and (4) central nervous system ischemic reflex. These reflex mechanisms respond almost immediately to changes in blood pressure. Furthermore, within about 30 minutes, these nervous system reflex responses are further supplemented by activation of hormonal mechanisms and shift of fluid into the circulation to readjust the blood volume. These short-term mechanisms can return arterial blood pressure toward, but never entirely back to normal. Indeed, the impact of many of the rapidly acting regulatory mechanisms, such as the baroreceptor reflex, diminish with time as these mechanisms adapt to the new level of arterial blood pressure.

Baroreceptor Reflexes

Baroreceptors are spray-type nerve endings in the walls of large arteries in the neck and thorax especially in the internal carotid arteries slightly above the carotid bifurcations and arch of the aorta (Fig. 44-9) (Guyton, 1986d). Impulses from baroreceptors are transmitted to the vasomotor center in the medullary area of the brain stem. An increase in intravascular blood pressure produces stretch

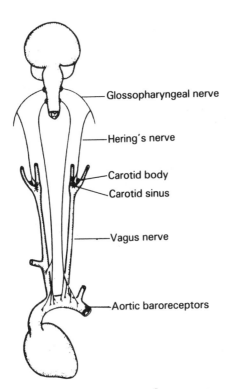

- Glossopharyngeal nerve
- Hering's nerve
- Carotid body
- Carotid sinus
- Vagus nerve
- Aortic baroreceptors

FIGURE 44-9. Baroreceptor reflex responses originate from sensors in the internal carotid arteries and arch of the aorta. (From Guyton AC. Textbook of Medical Physiology. 7th ed. Philadelphia: WB Saunders, 1986:244. Reproduced by permission of the author and publisher.)

of these baroreceptors, and increased numbers of nerve impulses are transmitted to the depressor portion of the medullary vasomotor center leading to a relative decline in the central nervous system outflow of sympathetic nervous system (e.g., vasoconstrictor) impulses. The net effects are vasodilatation throughout the peripheral circulatory system, decreased heart rate, and reduced myocardial contractility. Therefore, excitation of the baroreceptors by blood pressure elevations causes reflex changes that tend to reduce the blood pressure back toward normal levels. Conversely, declines in blood pressure reflexly produce changes likely to elevate the blood pressure.

The greatest increase in the number of impulses for each unit change in arterial blood pressure occurs near the normal mean arterial pressure (Fig. 44-10) (Guyton, 1986d). This emphasizes that the increase in baroreceptor activity occurs maximally at the level of mean arterial pressure where the response needs to be most prominent. Thus, in the normal range of mean arterial pressure, even a slight decline in blood pressure causes strong baroreceptor-mediated sympathetic nervous system reflexes to return the arterial pressure back toward normal. Baroreceptors respond extremely rapidly to changes in arterial blood pressure. For example, the number of impulses even increases during systole and decreases again during diastole. The ability of baroreceptors to reflexly regulate blood pressure is crucial for maintaining normal arterial pressures when individuals change from the supine to standing position.

Baroreceptors adapt in 1 to 3 days to whatever blood pressure level they are exposed to, emphasizing that these reflexes are probably of no importance in long-term regulation of arterial blood pressure (Krieger, 1970). Volatile anesthetics, particularly halothane and to a lesser extent isoflurane inhibit the heart rate response portion of the baroreceptor reflex that occurs in response to changes in blood pressure (see Chapter 2).

Chemoreceptor Reflexes

Chemoreceptors are chemosensitive cells located in carotid bodies that lie in the bifurcations of the common carotid arteries, and in aortic bodies adjacent to the aorta (Fig. 44-9) (Guyton, 1986d). Each carotid or aortic body is supplied with an abundant blood flow through a nutrient artery so that the chemoreceptors are always exposed to oxygenated blood. Whenever the blood pressure

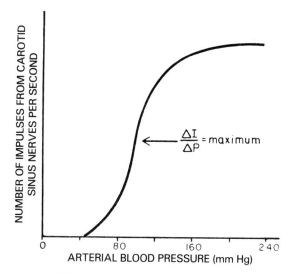

FIGURE 44-10. The greatest activity of baroreceptors occurs over a narrow range corresponding to normal mean arterial pressure. (From Guyton AC. Textbook of Medical Physiology. 7th ed. Philadelphia: WB Saunders, 1986:244. Reproduced by permission of the author and publisher.)

and thus blood flow falls below a critical level, chemoreceptors are stimulated by decreased availability of oxygen and also because of excess carbon dioxide and hydrogen ions that are not removed by the slow flow of blood. Impulses from the chemoreceptors are transmitted to the vasomotor center which results in reflex changes that tend to elevate blood pressure back toward the normal level. Nevertheless, chemoreceptors do not respond strongly until blood pressure declines below 80 mmHg. Instead, chemoreceptors are more important in elevating minute ventilation when the PaO_2 declines below 60 mmHg (*e.g.*, ventilatory response to hypoxemia) (see Chapter 49). The ventilatory response to arterial hypoxemia is inhibited by subanesthetic concentrations of volatile anesthetics (0.1 MAC) as well as injected drugs such as barbiturates and opioids (see Chapter 2).

Atrial Reflexes

Atria contain low pressure stretch receptors similar to baroreceptor stretch receptors in large systemic arteries (Goetz *et al*, 1975). Stretching of the atria evokes reflex vasodilatation and de-

creases the blood pressure back toward the normal level. Reflex vasodilatation also occurs in afferent arterioles in the kidneys leading to increased glomerular capillary pressure with resultant increases in filtration of fluid into the renal tubules. Furthermore, signals transmitted simultaneously to the hypothalamus to decrease the secretion of antidiuretic hormone also contribute to fluid loss into the urine and return of the blood volume to normal.

An increase in atrial pressure causes an acceleration in heart rate due to a direct effect of the increased atrial volume on stretch of the sinoatrial node as well as by the Bainbridge reflex. Stretch receptors in the atria that elicit the Bainbridge reflex transmit afferent signals through the vagus nerves to the medullary vasomotor center. The increase in heart rate evoked by stretching of the atria prevents accumulation of blood in the atria, veins, or pulmonary circulation.

Central Nervous System Ischemic Reflex

Most of the regulation of blood pressure achieved by nervous system reflexes originates in the baroreceptors, chemoreceptors, and low pressure atrial receptors, all of which are located in the peripheral circulation outside the brain. The central nervous system ischemic reflex response occurs when blood flow to the medullary vasomotor center is reduced to the extent that ischemia of this vital center occurs (Sagawa *et al*, 1961). As a result, there is an intense outpouring of sympathetic nervous system activity resulting in profound elevations in the mean arterial pressure. Peripheral sympathetic nervous system-induced vasoconstriction is so extreme that urine production ceases as a reflection of intense constriction of the renal arterioles.

The central nervous system ischemic reflex response is believed to be caused by failure of slowly flowing blood to remove carbon dioxide from the vasomotor center. As a result, the local concentration of carbon dioxide increases greatly and evokes an intense activation of sympathetic nervous system outflow from the central nervous system. Accumulation of lactic acid may also contribute to the marked stimulation of the vasomotor center.

The central nervous system ischemic reflex response does not become highly active until mean arterial pressure decreases below 50 mmHg and reaches its greatest degree of stimulation at pressures of 15 to 20 mmHg. This reflex response is not useful for regulation of normal blood pressure but rather acts as an emergency control system to prevent further reductions in blood pressure when cerebral blood flow is dangerously reduced.

CUSHING REFLEX. The Cushing reflex is a special type of central nervous system ischemic reflex response that results from increased intracranial pressure. Specifically, when intracranial pressure rises to equal the arterial pressure and thus compresses and occludes the arteries, the resulting cerebral ischemia evokes an intense central nervous system ischemic reflex response. This Cushing reflex response helps to protect vital central nervous system centers by elevating arterial pressure above intracranial pressure.

Role of Veins in Regulation of Blood Pressure

Much of the regulatory effect of the central nervous system on blood pressure is carried out by sympathetic nervous system-evoked venoconstriction. Indeed, veins constrict in response to weaker sympathetic nervous system stimulation than do arterioles and arteries. Constriction of veins does not greatly change resistance to flow but rather decreases their capacity to hold blood. This reduced capacitance causes translocation of blood out of veins into the heart, lungs, and arteries. Increased venous return leads to an improvement in cardiac output and a subsequent increase in blood pressure.

Role of Skeletal Muscles in Regulation of Arterial Blood Pressure

Any reflex response that increases central nervous system outflow of sympathetic nervous system impulses is associated with a concomitant increase in neural traffic to skeletal muscle, particularly the abdominal muscles. The resulting contraction of abdominal skeletal muscles compresses venous reservoirs of the abdomen serving to translocate blood toward the heart. This abdominal compression reflex is obviously absent in the presence of drug-induced skeletal muscle paralysis. Contraction of skeletal muscles accompanies exercise and contributes to increased venous return and the five- to sixfold increase in cardiac output that may accompany strenuous exercise.

Respiratory Variations in Arterial Blood Pressure

Arterial blood pressure usually rises and falls 4 to 6 mmHg in a wavelike manner during quiet spontaneous breathing. A contributing mechanism to this phenomenon is decreased return of blood to the heart during inspiration. This occurs because inspiration causes the intrathoracic pressure to become more negative and the thoracic blood vessels to expand. Typically, arterial blood pressure is increased during late inspiration and early exhalation and reduced during the remainder of the respiratory cycle. Positive pressure ventilation of the lungs produces a different sequence because the initial positive pressure pushes more blood toward the left ventricle followed by impaired venous return. As a result, blood pressure becomes maximal during the early phases of the mechanically provided inspiration.

Arterial Pressure Vasomotor Waves

Cyclical rises and falls in blood pressure lasting 7 to 10 seconds are referred to as *vasomotor waves* or *Traube-Hering* waves (Guyton and Satterfield, 1952). The presumed cause of vasomotor waves is oscillation in the reflex activity of baroreceptors. For example, increased blood pressure stimulates baroreceptors which then inhibit the sympathetic nervous system resulting in a reduction in blood pressure. Decreased blood pressure reduces baroreceptor activity and allows the vasomotor center to become active once again, elevating the blood pressure to a higher value.

Hormonal Mechanisms for the Moderately Rapid Regulation of Arterial Blood Pressure

In addition to the rapidly acting central nervous system reflex mechanisms for the prompt regulation of blood pressure, there are at least three hormonal mechanisms that also provide either rapid or moderately rapid control of blood pressure. These hormonal mechanisms are (1) catecholamine-induced vasoconstriction, (2) renin-angiotensin-induced vasoconstriction, and (3) antidiuretic hormone-induced vasoconstriction.

Catecholamine-Induced Vasoconstriction

Epinephrine and norepinephrine released from the adrenal medulla circulate to all portions of the body and are capable of indirectly evoking circulatory responses similar to those occurring as a result of direct stimulation from the sympathetic nervous system (see Chapter 42). Circulating catecholamines may even reach parts of the circulation that are devoid of sympathetic nervous system innervation such as the metarterioles. Furthermore, circulating catecholamines produce uniquely intense actions on some vascular beds, especially the cutaneous blood vessels.

Renin-Angiotensin-Induced Vasoconstriction

Low blood pressure and decreased renal blood flow evoke the release of renin from the kidney leading to the formation of angiotensin II, one of the most potent vasoconstrictors known. Blood pressure is increased by the intense angiotensin-induced peripheral vasoconstriction that occurs to a greater degree in arterioles than in veins. The renin-angiotensin vasoconstrictor mechanism requires about 20 minutes to become fully active, distinguishing it from the more rapidly acting central nervous system reflex responses for regulating blood pressure (Brough *et al,* 1975).

Antidiuretic Hormone-Induced Vasoconstriction

When blood pressure declines, the hypothalamus causes large amounts of antidiuretic hormone to be released from the posterior pituitary. Antidiuretic homone is even a more potent vasoconstrictor than angiotensin II. The resulting vasoconstriction elevates peripheral vascular resistance and blood pressure.

Intrinsic Mechanisms for Regulation of Arterial Blood Pressure

In addition to central nervous system and hormonal mechanisms, there are two intrinsic mechanisms which begin to act within minutes of changes in blood pressure. These two mechanisms manifest as capillary fluid shift and stress-relaxation of blood vessels.

Capillary Fluid Shift

Changes in blood pressure produce corresponding changes in capillary pressure with a resulting appropriate directional movement of fluid between capillaries and interstitial fluid. This shift in fluid produces a beneficial effect in the control of blood pressure by virtue of adjustment in blood volume.

Stress-Relaxation

Stress-relaxation is the gradual change in vessel size to adapt to changes in intravascular pressure and the amount of blood that is available. For example, excess infusion of fluid or blood initially elevates blood pressure, but within 60 minutes blood pressure returns toward normal. Conversely, acute hemorrhage causes blood vessels to gradually adapt their size to the blood volume that is present. The stress-relaxation mechanism has definite limitations such that increases in blood volume greater than about 30% or reductions of more than about 15% cannot be corrected by this mechanism.

Long-Term Mechanisms for Control of Arterial Blood Pressure

Long-term mechanisms for control of blood pressure, unlike the short-term regulatory mechanisms, have a delayed onset but do not adapt, providing a prolonged effect on blood pressure. The renal-body fluid system plays a predominant role in long-term control of blood pressure. This crucial role is supplemented by accessory mechanisms including the renin-angiotensin system, aldosterone, and antidiuretic hormone.

Renal-Body Fluid System

Increased arterial blood pressure evokes sodium (pressure natriuresis) and water (pressure diuresis) excretion by the kidneys. The resultant decrease in circulating blood volume leads to reductions in cardiac output and arterial blood pressure. After several weeks, the cardiac output returns toward normal and peripheral vascular resistance declines to maintain the lower but more acceptable blood pressure. Conversely, a decline in blood pressure stimulates the kidneys to retain fluid. A special feature of this regulatory mechanism is its ability to return blood pressure completely back to normal values. This contrasts with short-term mechanisms which cannot return blood pressure entirely back to normal. Overall, the renal-body fluid system is the major long-term determinant of arterial blood pressure as it controls both the cardiac output and peripheral vascular resistance.

Small, but persistent, changes in circulating blood volume may cause marked changes in blood pressure. For example, a 2% chronic increase in blood volume can increase the venous return and cardiac output by as much as 5%. An increase in cardiac output of 5% can increase peripheral vascular resistance 25% to 50% with a corresponding increase in blood pressure. Thus, a chronic increase of only a few hundred milliliters of extracellular fluid can lead to sustained hypertension. Indeed, patients with hypertension can often be rendered nearly normotensive by treatment with a diuretic which does nothing more than reduce the extracellular fluid volume by about 500 ml.

Pressure natriuresis and diuresis are supplemented by decreased secretion of renin and aldosterone as well as reduced sympathetic nervous system stimulation of the kidneys. These events further increase fluid loss as evidenced by urine output above that which occurs with the renal-body fluid regulatory system alone. Acute administration of fluids that greatly increase extracellular fluid volume fail to produce sustained elevations of arterial blood pressure because of the impact of short-term regulatory mechanisms.

Renin-Angiotensin System

Aldosterone secretion that results from the action of angiotensin II on the adrenal cortex exerts a long-term effect on blood pressure by virtue of stimulating the kidneys to retain sodium and water. The resulting increase in extracellular fluid volume causes cardiac output and subsequently arterial blood pressure to increase. Furthermore, a direct effect of angiotensin II on the kidneys is to decrease urine output by increasing sodium and water retention.

REGULATION OF CARDIAC OUTPUT AND VENOUS RETURN

Cardiac output is the amount of blood pumped by the left ventricle into the aorta each minute (*i.e.*,

heart rate times stroke volume), and venous return is the quantity of blood flowing from the veins into the right arium each minute. Over a prolonged period, cardiac output must equal venous return. For a few heartbeats, however, cardiac output and venous return may not be the same because blood volume can temporarily increase or decrease in the heart and lungs.

Normal Values for Cardiac Output

Cardiac output for the average 70-kg adult male with a body surface area of 1.7 m² is about 5 L min⁻¹ or 3 L min⁻¹ m⁻². This value is about 10% less in females. Cardiac output usually remains proportional to overall metabolism. In a well-traind athlete, cardiac output may increase five- to sevenfold during strenuous exercise.

Determinants of Cardiac Output

Venous return is more important than myocardial contractility in determining cardiac output (Guyton, 1967). The magnitude of venous return is directly related to blood pressure and inversely proportional to the peripheral vascular resistance. In essence, the metabolic requirements of tissues control cardiac output by virtue of alterations in resistance to tissue blood flow. For example, increased local metabolic needs lead to regional vasodilation with a resulting increase in tissue blood flow and thus venous return. Cardiac output is increased an amount equivalent to the venous return (Coleman *et al,* 1974).

Sympathetic nervous system stimulation increases myocardial contractility and heart rate to increase cardiac output beyond that possible from venous return alone. Maximal stimulation by the sympathetic nervous system can double cardiac output. Nevertheless, this nervous system-induced elevation of cardiac output is only transient despite sustained elevations in sympathetic nervous system activity. A reason for this transient effect is the automatic autoregulatory responses of tissues to increases in blood flow that manifest as vasoconstriction which reduces venous return and cardiac output back toward normal. In addition, the slightly increased blood pressure that results from nervous system-induced increases in cardiac output raises capillary pressure, and fluid filters out of the capillaries into interstitial fluid thereby decreasing the blood volume and also venous return back toward normal. Furthermore, increased blood pressure causes the kidneys to increase the excretion of sodium and water until blood pressure and cardiac output return to normal. These responses to sympathetic nervous system stimulation of the heart emphasize that conditions which cause chronic elevations of the cardiac output result from decreased peripheral vascular resistance and not increased cardiac activity.

Decreases in Cardiac Output

Any factor that interferes with venous return can lead to decreased cardiac output. Decreased blood volume, most often due to acute hemorrhage, is the likely peripheral event leading to decreased cardiac output. Hemorrhage reduces blood volume such that there is insufficient volume in the peripheral vessels to create the pressure necessary to drive blood back to the heart. Acute venodilatation, as caused by inadequate sympathetic nervous system activity, can so increase the capacitance of peripheral vessels that venous return is reduced and cardiac output declines. For example, total blockade of the sympathetic nervous system as produced by spinal anesthesia can substantially decrease cardiac output. Positive pressure ventilation of the lungs, particularly in the presence of a reduced circulating blood volume, causes a decrease in venous return and cardiac output.

Increases in Cardiac Output

Factors that increase cardiac output are all associated with reductions in peripheral vascular resistance. For example, anemia reduces the viscosity of blood leading to a decrease in peripheral vascular resistance. As a consequence. venous return and cardiac output increase.

An acute increase in blood volume of about 20% increases cardiac output to about 2.5 to 3 times normal. Increased blood volume acts to increase cardiac output by increasing the mean systemic filling pressure (*e.g.*, gradient for flow to the right atrium) and by distending blood vessels which reduces their resistance to blood flow. Increased cardiac output caused by the increased blood volume lasts only a few minutes because of compensatory effects that are immediately initiated. For example, increased cardiac output elevates capillary pressure which causes fluid to leave capillaries and enter tissues, thereby returning the blood volume to normal. Increased pressure in veins caused by the increased blood volume causes the veins to gradually distend (*i.e.*, stress-relaxation). Finally, excess blood flow through peripheral tissues causes an autoregulatory increase in the peripheral vascular resistance. These factors cause the mean systemic filling pressure to return to normal and also cause the resistance vessels of the systemic circulation to constrict. Therefore, over a period of 20 to 40 minutes, the cardiac output returns almost to normal.

The most important factor that increases cardiac output during exercise is vasodilatation that occurs in all exercising skeletal muscle. The large reduction in peripheral vascular resistance allows increased amounts of blood to flow through skeletal muscles and thus into the veins to be returned to the heart. When cardiac output must increase above about 15 L min^{-1}, however, venous return alone is not sufficient, and sympathetic nervous system stimulation becomes essential. This nervous system stimulation manifests as vasoconstriction throughout the body which delivers blood from peripheral veins for return to the heart. Sympathetic nervous system stimulation also increases cardiac output during exercise.

In hyperthyroidism, the metabolism of all tissues is greatly increased resulting in increased oxygen usage and often the local release of vasodilator products if oxygen availability to tissues is inadequate. Therefore, peripheral vascular resistance declines and cardiac output often increases 40% to 80% above normal.

An arteriovenous shunt, as present in patients on hemodialysis, allows large amounts of blood to flow directly from arteries to veins which lowers peripheral vascular resistance and increases venous return and cardiac output.

Lack of thiamine in the diet (*e.g.*, beriberi) diminishes the ability of tissues to utilize cellular nutrients including oxygen (see Chapter 34). The resulting vasodilatation leads to an increase in cardiac output.

Ventricular Function Curves

Ventricular function curves depict the cardiac output at different atrial filling pressures (Fig. 44-11). The basic factors that determine the precise char-

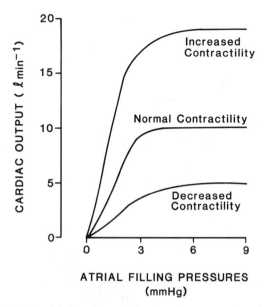

FIGURE 44-11. Ventricular function curves (Frank-Starling curves) depict the volume of forward ventricular ejection (*i.e.*, cardiac output) at different atrial filling pressures and varying degrees of myocardial contractility.

acteristics of the cardiac output curve are the (1) effectiveness of the heart as a pump and (2) extracardiac pressure. Improved cardiac function is characterized by a shift of the cardiac output curve to the left of the normal curve while a shift of the curve to the right of normal reflects decreased cardiac function. Clinically, ventricular function curves are used to estimate myocardial contractility.

Effectiveness of the Heart as a Pump

Factors that increase the cardiac output at a given atrial filling pressure (*i.e.*, curve shifted to the left) include (1) sympathetic nervous system stimulation of the heart, (2) hypertrophy of the heart, and (3) inhibition of the parasympathetic nervous system innervation to the heart. A reduced ability to achieve a given cardiac output at a given atrial filling pressure (*i.e.*, curve shifted to the right) is associated with (1) myocardial infarction, (2) myocardial ischemia, (3) valvular heart disease, (4) increased blood pressure, and (5) inhibition of the sympathetic nervous system inner-

vation to the heart or a predominance of parasympathetic nervous system activity.

Extracardiac Pressure

Normal extracardiac pressure is equal to the intrapleural pressure of about minus 4 mm Hg. An increase in intrapleural pressure means the right atrial pressure must increase by the same amount to overcome the increased pressure on the outside of the heart. The impact of increased extracardiac pressure is to shift the cardiac output curve to the right. Events that increase intrapleural pressure and thereby shift the cardiac output curve to the right include (1) positive pressure ventilation of the lungs, (2) opening the chest to atmospheric pressure, (3) pneumothorax, and (4) cardiac tamponade.

Balance of Output Between the Ventricles

An acute reduction in left ventricular contractility and stroke volume leads to increased pulmonary filling pressures which increase venous return to the left heart and restore left ventricular output. Simultaneously, the reduction in systemic filling pressure decreases right heart venous return and right ventricular output. This process continues until the output of the left ventricle rises to equal the falling output of the right ventricle. Thus, the outputs of the two ventricles become rebalanced within a few heart beats. Similar events occur in the opposite direction when the contractility of the right ventricle diminishes. Problems of balance between the two ventricles are of particular importance when selective ventricular failure occurs as when myocardial infarction or valvular disease causes poor function of only one ventricle.

Measurement of Cardiac Output

Indirect methods of cardiac output measurement are the (1) oxygen Fick method, (2) indicator dilution method, and (3) thermodilution method.

Oxygen Fick Method

Cardiac output is calculated as oxygen consumption divided by the arteriovenous difference for oxygen (Fig. 44-12) (Guyton, 1986e). Oxygen consumption is usually measured by a respiro-

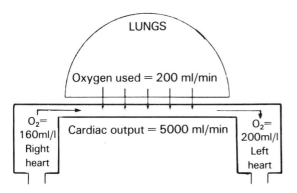

FIGURE 44-12. The Fick method calculates cardiac output as oxygen consumption divided by the arteriovenous difference for oxygen. (From Guyton AC. Textbook of Medical Physiology. 7th ed. Philadelphia: WB Saunders, 1986:272. Reproduced by permission of the author and publisher.)

meter containing a known oxygen mixture. The patient's exhaled gases are collected in a Douglas bag. The volume and oxygen concentration of the expired gas allow calculation of oxygen consumption. Venous blood for calculation of oxygen content must be obtained from the right ventricle or ideally the pulmonary artery to ensure adequate mixing. Blood from the right atrium may not yet be adequately mixed to provide a true mixed venous sample. Blood used for determining the oxygen saturation in arterial blood can be obtained from any artery because all arterial blood is thoroughly mixed before it leaves the heart and, therefore, has the same concentration of oxygen.

Indicator Dilution Method

In measuring the cardiac output by the indicator dilution method, a nondiffusible dye (indocyanine green) is injected into the right atrium (or central venous circulation), and the concentration of dye is subsequently measured continuously in the arterial circulation by a spectrophotometer. The area under the resulting time-concentration curve before recirculation of the dye occurs combined with knowing the amount of dye injected allows calculation of the pulmonary blood flow (*i.e.*, cardiac output). It is necessary to extrapolate the dye curve to zero because recirculation of the dye occurs before the downslope of the curve reaches zero. Early recirculation of dye may indi-

cate a patent foramen ovale or other similar intracardiac septal defects permitting direct passage of a portion of the dye to the left heart without passing through the lungs.

Thermodilution

Thermodilution cardiac outputs are determined by measuring the change in blood temperature between two points (right atrium and pulmonary artery) following injection of a known volume of cold saline at the proximal site (*i.e.*, right atrium) (Ganz and Swan, 1972). The change in blood temperature as measured at the distal site (*i.e.*, pulmonary artery) is proportional to pulmonary blood flow (*i.e.,* cardiac output). Recirculation is not a problem, and thermodilution cardiac outputs can be determined frequently. A pulmonary artery catheter with ports in the right atrium and pulmonary artery and a temperature sensor at the distal port is used to measure thermodilution cardiac output. A computer converts the area under the temperature–time curve to its equivalent in cardiac output.

FETAL CIRCULATION

Fetal circulation is considerably different than circulation after birth. For example, *in utero* blood flow through the lungs and liver is minimal. Oxygenated blood (oxygen saturation 80%) returning from the placenta through a single umbilical vein passes predominately through the ductus venosus, and into the inferior vena cava thus bypassing the liver (Fig. 44-13) (Guyton, 1986f). Most of this blood entering the right atrium from the inferior vena cava preferentially passes through the foramen ovale into the left atrium thus bypassing the lungs. Passage of this oxygenated blood directly to the left atrium allows perfusion of the fetal brain with optimal concentrations of oxygen.

Blood entering the right atrium from the superior vena cava is mainly deoxygenated blood from the fetal head regions. This blood enters the right ventricle for delivery into the pulmonary artery and then to the descending thoracic aorta by the ductus arteriosus. As a result, this deoxygenated flow is delivered distal to the blood vessels that supply the fetal brain. Blood is returned to the placenta for oxygenation by two umbilical arteries.

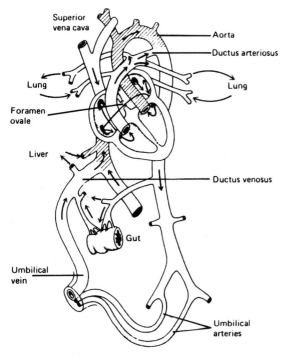

FIGURE 44-13. Anatomy of the fetal circulation. (From Guyton AC. Textbook of Medical Physiology. 7th ed. Philadelphia: WB Saunders, 1986:993. Reproduced by permission of the author and publisher.)

The primary changes in circulation at birth are increased peripheral vascular resistance and blood pressure due to cessation of blood flow through the placenta. In addition, pulmonary vascular resistance declines dramatically with expansion of the lungs leading to a marked increase in pulmonary blood flow. During fetal life, only an estimated 12% of the cardiac output passes through the lungs. These alterations in pulmonary and peripheral vascular resistance also change the pressure gradient across the foramen ovale. As a result of the higher pressure in the left atrium after birth, the right-to-left direction of blood flow through the foramen ovale present before birth is reversed. This reversal of pressure gradients serves to close the flaplike valve that is present on the left atrial septum thus occluding the foramen ovale. In about two thirds of individuals, this valve becomes adherent over the foramen ovale in a few months. In the absence of permanent closure of the flap over the foramen ovale, events that in-

crease right atrial pressure above left atrial pressure may introduce a right-to-left intracardiac shunt at this site (see Chapter 47). Indeed, unexplained arterial hypoxemia may be the initial manifestation of this intracardiac shunt when right atrial pressure is acutely and selectively increased. Events that may increase right atrial pressure more than left atrial pressure include (1) positive pressure ventilation of the lungs especially utilizing positive end-expiratory pressure, (2) right ventricular failure, and (3) pulmonary embolism.

Flow through the ductus arteriosus diminishes after birth due to constriction of the muscular wall of this vessel on exposure to higher concentrations of oxygen. Failure of the ductus arteriosus to close after birth results in a reversal of flow compared with that present before birth. This reversal of flow occurs because pressure in the aorta exceeds pressure in the pulmonary artery following birth. The muscular wall of the ductus venosus also contracts following birth diverting portal venous blood through the liver.

REFERENCES

Adey WR. The physiology of weightlessness. Physiologist 1974;16:179-83.

Brough RB, Cowley AW, Guyton AC. Quantitative analysis of the acute response to hemorrhage of the renin-angiotensin-vasoconstrictor feedback loop in areflexic dogs. Cardiovas Res 1975;9:722-33.

Burton RR, Leverett SD, Michaelson ED. Man at high sustained +Gz acceleration: A review. Aerospace Med 1974;45:1115-36.

Coleman TG, Manning RD, Normal RA, Guyton AC. Control of cardiac output by regional blood flow distribution. Ann Biomed Eng 1974;2:149-63.

Dorbin PB. Mechanical properties of arteries. Physiol Rev 1978;58:397-460.

Folkow B. Role of the nervous system in the control of vascular tone. Circulation 1960;21:760-8.

Ganz W, Swan HJC. Measurement of blood flow by thermodilution. Am J Cardiol 1972;29:241-6.

Goetz KL, Bond GC, Bloxham DD. Atrial receptors and renal function. Physiol Rev 1975;55:157-205.

Goodman AH, Guyton AC, Drake R, Loflin JH. A television method for measuring capillary red cell velocities. J Appl Physiol 1974;37:126-30.

Guyton AC. Regulation of cardiac output. N Engl J Med 1967;277:805-12.

Guyton AC. Textbook of Medical Physiology. 7th ed. Philadelphia: WB Saunders, 1986a:218.

Guyton AC. Textbook of Medical Physiology. 7th ed. Philadelphia: WB Saunders, 1986b:206.

Guyton AC. Textbook of Medical Physiology. 7th ed. Philadelphia: WB Saunders, 1986c:230.

Guyton AC. Textbook of Medical Physiology. 7th ed. Philadelphia: WB Saunders, 1986d:244.

Guyton AC. Textbook of Medical Physiology. 7th ed. Philadelphia: WB Saunders, 1986e:272.

Guyton AC. Textbook of Medical Physiology. 7th ed. Philadelphia: WB Saunders, 1986f:993.

Guyton AC, Jones CE. Central venous pressure: Physiologic significance and clinical implications. Am Heart J 1973;86:431-7.

Guyton AC, Satterfield JH. Vasomotor waves possibly resulting from CNS ischemic reflex oscillation. Am J Physiol 1952;170:601-5.

Krieger EM. Time course of baroreceptor resetting in acute hypertension. Am J Physiol 1970;218:486-90.

Lundgren O, Jodal M. Regional blood flow. Annu Rev Physiol 1975;37:395-414.

Mancia G, Lorenz RR, Shepherd JT. Reflex control of circulation by heart and lungs. Int Rev Physiol 1976;9:111-44.

Manning RD, Coleman TG, Guyton AC, Norman RA, McCaa RE. Essential role of mean circulatory filling pressure in salt-induced hypertension. Am J Physiol 1979;236:R40-7.

Mellander S. Systematic circulation: Local control. Annu Rev Physiol 1970;32:313-44.

Remington JW, O'Brian LJ. Construction of aortic flow pulse from pressure pulse. Am J Physiol 1970; 218:437-47.

Sagawa K, Ross JM, Guyton AC. Quantitation of cerebral ischemic pressor response in dogs. Am J Physiol 1961;200;1164-8.

Schmid-Schonbein H. Microrheology of erythrocytes, blood viscosity, and the distribution of blood flow in the microcirculation. Int Rev Physiol 1976;9:1-62.

C H A P T E R 45

Capillaries
and Lymph Vessels

CAPILLARIES

Capillaries serve as the site for exchange of nutrients and metabolic by-products between tissues and the circulation (Baez, 1977). About 10 billion capillaries, having a total surface area of about 100 m², provide this function. It is unlikely that any functional cell is more than 50 μ away from a capillary.

Anatomy of the Microcirculation

Blood from the arterioles passes into the metarterioles, which have a structure midway between arterioles and capillaries (Fig. 45-1). After leaving the metarterioles, blood enters capillaries, some of which are large and are called *preferential channels* and others that are small and designated *true capillaries*. At the origin of true capillaries from metarterioles, a smooth muscle fiber usually encircles the capillary serving as a precapillary sphincter. After passing through capillaries, the blood enters venules.

Capillaries

The thickness of capillary walls is about 0.5 μ consisting of a single layer of endothelial cells surrounded by a thin basement membrane on the outside (Fig. 45-2). Thin slits 6 to 7 nm wide exist between endothelial cells and function as channels (*e.g.*, pores or intracellular clefts) through which fluid and ions move inward or outward across capillary membranes (Fig. 45-2) (see the section entitled Fluid Movement Across Capillary Membranes). The width of these capillary channels is about 25 times the diameter of the water molecule (0.3 nm) which is the smallest molecule that normally passes through capillary channels (see Chapter 39). Plasma protein molecules have diameters that exceed the width of capillary pores. Other substances, such as sodium ions, potassium ions, chloride ions, and glucose have intermediate diameters (0.39 – 0.86 nm) such that permeability of capillary channels for different substances varies according to their molecular weights (Table 45-1) (Guyton, 1986) (see the section entitled Exchange of Nutrients).

In addition to channels, there are also present in the endothelial cells structures known as *pinocytic vesicles* (Fig. 45-2). Pinocytic vesicles form at one surface of the endothelial cell where they ingest plasma or interstitial fluid and then move to the opposite surface where they discharge their contents (*i.e.*, pinocytosis) (see the section entitled Exchange of Nutrients).

The diameter of capillaries is 7 to 9 μ which is barely sufficient to permit passage of erythrocytes (Guyton, 1986). The thin walls of the capillaries are able to withstand the intraluminal pressure because their small diameter prevents excessive wall tension (Laplace's law).

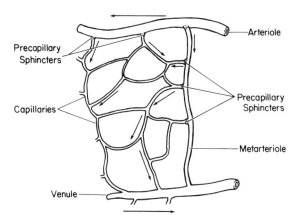

FIGURE 45-1. Schematic diagram of the microcirculation.

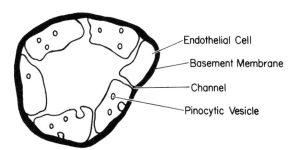

FIGURE 45-2. The capillary wall consists of a single layer of endothelial cells surrounded by a thin basement membrane on the outside. Channels are intracellular slits between endothelial cells. Pinocytic vesicles ingest plasma or interstitial fluid and migrate to the opposite surface to discharge their contents.

Table 45-1
Permeability of Capillary Membranes

	Molecular Weight	Relative Permeability
Water	18	1.0
Sodium chloride	58.5	0.96
Glucose	180	0.6
Hemoglobin	66,700	0.01
Albumin	69,000	0.0001

Blood Flow in Capillaries

Blood flow in capillaries is intermittent rather than continuous. This intermittent blood flow reflects contraction and relaxation of metarterioles and precapillary sphincters in alternating cycles 6 to 12 times min^{-1}. The phenomenon of alternating contraction and relaxation is known as *vasomotion*.

Oxygen is the most important determinant of the degree of opening and closing of metarterioles and precapillary sphincters. Low oxygen partial pressure allows more blood to flow through capillaries to supply tissues. In this regard, the impact of oxygen on capillary blood flow provides a form of autoregulation of tissue blood flow.

In addition to nutritive blood flow through tissues that is regulated by oxygen, there is also nonnutritive blood flow regulated by autonomic nervous system activity. This nonnutritive blood flow is characterized by direct vascular connections between arterioles and venules. Some of these arteriovenous connections have strong muscular coverings so that blood flow can be altered over a wide range. In some parts of the skin, these arteriovenous anastomoses provide a mechanism to permit rapid inflow of arterial blood to warm the skin (see Chapter 44).

Fluid Movement Across Capillary Membranes

The four pressures that determine whether fluid will move outward across capillary membranes (filtration) or inward across capillary membranes (reabsorption) are (1) capillary pressure, (2) interstitial fluid pressure, (3) plasma colloid osmotic pressure, and (4) interstitial fluid colloid osmotic pressure (Guyton, 1986). The net effect of these four pressures is a positive filtration pressure at the arterial end of capillaries causing fluid to move outward across cell membranes into the interstitial fluid spaces (Table 45-2). At the venous end of capillaries, the net effect of these four pressures is a positive reabsorption pressure causing fluid to move inward across capillary membranes into capillaries (Table 45-3). Overall, the mean values of the four pressures acting across capillary membranes are nearly identical such that the amount of fluid filtered nearly equals the amount reabsorbed (Table 45-4). Any fluid that is not

Table 45-2

Filtration of Fluid at the Arterial Ends of Capillaries

Pressures favoring outward movement	
Capillary pressure	25 mmHg
Interstitial fluid pressure	−6.3 mmHg
Interstitial fluid colloid osmotic pressure	5 mmHg
Total	36.3 mmHg
Pressure favoring inward movement	
Plasma colloid osmotic pressure	28 mmHg
Net filtration pressure	8.3 mmHg

Table 45-3

Reabsorption of Fluid at the Venous Ends of Capillaries

Pressures favoring outward movement	
Capillary pressure	10 mmHg
Interstitial fluid pressure	−6.3 mmHg
Interstitial fluid colloid osmotic pressure	5 mmHg
Total	21.3 mmHg
Pressure favoring inward movement	
Plasma colloid osmotic pressure	28 mmHg
Net Reabsorption pressure	6.7 mmHg

Table 45-4

Mean Values of Pressures Acting Across Capillary Membranes

Pressures favoring outward movement	
Capillary pressure	17 mmHg
Interstitial fluid pressure	−6.3 mmHg
Interstitial fluid colloid osmotic pressure	5 mmHg
Total	28.3 mmHg
Pressure favoring inward movement	
Plasma colloid osmotic pressure	28 mmHg
Net overall filtration pressure	0.3 mmHg

reabsorbed enters the lymph vessels (see the section entitled Lymph Vessels).

It is important to distinguish between filtration and diffusion through capillary membranes. Filtration is the net outward movement of fluid at the arterial end of capillaries. Diffusion of fluid occurs in both directions across capillary membranes.

Capillary Pressure

Capillary pressure tends to move fluid outward across the arterial ends of capillary membranes. It is estimated that capillary pressure at the arterial end of capillaries is 25 mmHg while pressure at the venous end of capillaries is 10 mmHg corresponding to that pressure present in venules. The mean pressure in capillaries is about 17 mmHg (Intaglietta, 1973).

Interstitial Fluid Pressure

Interstitial fluid pressure tends to move fluid inward across the capillary membrane. This pressure is difficult to measure precisely because the width of interstitial spaces is only about 1 μ. By indirect measurements, it is estimated that average interstitial fluid pressure is -6.3 mmHg (Guyton *et al*, 1971). Indeed, this negative pressure acts as a vacuum in some areas to hold tissues together. When tissues lose their negative interstitial fluid pressure, fluid accumulates in the spaces manifesting as edema (see the section entitled Edema).

The normal tendency for capillaries to absorb fluid from interstitial spaces and thus create a negative interstitial fluid pressure causes the structures of the interstitial spaces to be compacted together. This maintenance of a minimal distance between cells is important for rapid diffusion of nutrients to tissues. Indeed, rate of diffusion of nutrients between two points is inversely proportional to the distance between the cells and capillaries.

It is estimated that about 17% of the average tissue is composed of interstitial fluid, but almost none of this is in the mobile state. An exception is the brain which lacks collagen fibers between cells such that interstitial fluid represents only 12% of total weight.

Under normal conditions, almost all of the interstitial fluid is held in a gel that fills the spaces between cells. This gel contains large quantities of mucopolysaccharides, the most abundant of which is hyaluronic acid. The gel structure acts to hold the interstitial fluid in place and provide interstitial fluid spaces between cells to facilitate optimal diffusion of nutrients (Comper and Laurent, 1978).

Plasma Colloid Osmotic Pressure

The plasma colloid osmotic (oncotic) pressure tends to cause movement of fluid inward through capillary membranes. Dissolved proteins of the plasma and interstitial fluids are primarily responsible for the osmotic pressure that develops at capillary membranes. The concentration of protein in the plasma averages four times that in the interstitial fluid. The interstitial fluid concentration of

proteins remains low because proteins cannot diffuse readily across capillary membranes. Furthermore, protein is rapidly removed from interstitial fluid spaces by lymph vessels (see the section entitled Lymph Vessels).

Each gram of albumin exerts twice the colloid osmotic pressure of a gram of globulins. Since there is about twice as much albumin as globulin in the plasma, about 70% of the total colloid osmotic pressure results from albumin and only about 30% from the globulins and fibrinogens.

A special phenomenon known as *Donnan equilibrium* causes the colloid osmotic pressure to be about 50% greater than that caused by proteins alone. This reflects the negative charge characteristic of proteins that necessitates the presence of an equal number of positively charged ions, mainly sodium ions, on the same side of the membrane as the proteins. These extra positive ions increase the number of osmotically active substances and thus increase the colloid osmotic pressure.

Normal plasma colloid osmotic pressure is about 28 mmHg. About 19 mmHg of this pressure is caused by dissolved proteins, and the remainder is due to the positively charged ions held in the plasma by proteins.

Interstitial Fluid Colloid Osmotic Pressure

Interstitial fluid colloid osmotic pressure tends to cause movement of fluid outward through capillary membranes. The average interstitial fluid colloid osmotic pressure is about 5.5 mmHg. This pressure reflects the presence of proteins, predominately albumin, in interstitial fluids. Albumin molecules, because they are smaller than most globulin molecules, normally leak 1.6 times as readily as globulins through capillaries causing the proteins in interstitial fluids to have a disproportionately high albumin to globulin ratio.

The total amount of protein in the entire 12 liters of interstitial fluid is similar to the total quantity of protein in plasma, but because this volume is four times the volume of plasma, the average protein concentration of the interstitial fluid is only one-fourth that in plasma or about 1.8 g dl^{-1}.

Exchange of Nutrients

Diffusion is the most important mechanism for transfer of nutrients between the plasma and interstitial fluids. Substances such as sodium ions, chloride ions, and glucose are insoluble in lipid capillary membranes and, therefore, must pass through channels to gain access to interstitial fluids. The ease with which these substances pass through capillary channels is inversely related to their molecular weight (Table 45-1). As a result, the capillary membrane is almost impermeable to albumin, accounting for the substantial colloid osmotic pressure difference that exists between plasma and surrounding interstitial fluids (Table 45-2).

Oxygen and carbon dioxide are lipid-soluble molecules that can diffuse directly through capillary membranes independent of the channels. Anesthetic gases are also examples of highly lipid-soluble molecules that rapidly traverse capillary membranes at all sites in the body. The rate of diffusion of lipid-soluble molecules across capillary membranes in either direction is proportional to the concentration difference between the two sides of the membrane. For this reason, large amounts of oxygen move from blood toward the tissues while carbon dioxide moves in the opposite direction. Typically, only slight concentration differences suffice to maintain adequate transport between the plasma and interstitial fluid. For example, the concentration of oxygen in the interstitial fluid immediately outside the capillary is normally no more than 1% less than the concentration in the blood (see Chapter 50). Nevertheless, this 1% difference causes sufficient movement of oxygen to sustain tissue metabolism.

Pinocytosis is another mechanism by which molecules are transported through capillary membranes. This process is characterized by endothelial cells of the capillary wall ingesting small amounts of plasma or interstitial fluid followed by migration to the opposite surface where the fluid is released. This is a minor mechanism for transport of low molecular weight substances. Conversely, transport of high molecular substances such as plasma proteins, glycoproteins, and polysaccharides (*e.g.,* dextran) most likely occur principally by pinocytosis.

LYMPH VESSELS

Lymph vessels represent an alternate route by which excess fluids can flow from interstitial fluid spaces into the blood (Nicoll and Taylor, 1977). The most important function, however, of the lymphatic system is return of protein to the circulation and maintenance of a low protein concentration in the interstitial fluid. The small amount of protein that escapes from the arterial end of the capillary cannot undergo reabsorption at the venous end of the capillary. If lymph vessels were not available, this protein would become progressively concentrated in the interstitial fluid resulting in increases in interstitial fluid colloid osmotic pressure that, within a few hours, would be incompatible with life.

Anatomy

Essentially, all the lymph flows into the thoracic duct which empties into the venous system at the juncture of the left internal jugular vein and subclavian vein. Lymph vessels contain flaplike valves between endothelial cells that open toward the interior allowing the unimpeded entrance of interstitial fluid and proteins into the vessel (Leak and Burke, 1968). Backflow out of the lymph vessel is not possible because any flow in this direction causes the flaplike valve to close. Lymph vessels, like veins, also contain one-way valves that direct lymph toward the thoracic duct and ultimately the venous circulation.

Formation

Lymph is interstitial fluid that flows into lymphatic vessels. As such, the protein concentration of lymph is about 1.8 g dl^{-1} with the exception of lymph from the gastrointestinal tract and liver which contains two to three times this concentration of protein. Because about one half of the lymph is derived from the gastrointestinal tract and liver, the thoracic lymph, which is a mixture of lymph from all areas of the body, usually has a protein concentration of 3 to 5 g dl^{-1}. The lymphatic system is also one of the major channels for absorption of nutrients, especially fat, from the gastrointestinal tract. Bacteria that enter lymph vessels are removed and destroyed by lymph nodes.

Flow

Flow of lymph through the thoracic duct is about 100 ml hr^{-1}. A decrease in the negative value of interstitial fluid pressure increases the flow of interstitial fluid into the terminal lymph vessels and consequently also increases the rate of lymph flow. For example, at zero interstitial fluid pressure the rate of lymph flow is increased 10 to 50 times compared with flow at a normal interstitial fluid pressure of -7 mmHg. When interstitial fluid pressure increases above zero mmHg, lymph flow does not increase further because the interstitial fluid begins to compress the outsides of the lymphatics and thus increases the resistance to flow. Skeletal muscle contraction and passive movements of the extremities facilitate flow of lymph. For example, during exercise lymph flow is increased up to 14 times that present at rest.

EDEMA

Edema is the presence of excess interstitial fluid in peripheral tissues. As long as interstitial fluid pressure remains negative, edema does not occur. As soon as interstitial fluid pressure exceeds atmospheric pressure, the volume of interstitial fluid increases precipitously. Therefore, the mechanism of edema is positive pressure in the interstitial fluid spaces. Edema usually is not detectable in tissues until the interstitial fluid volume has risen to 20% to 30% above normal. When this occurs external pressure in one area will displace fluid to another area resulting in pitting edema. Also, fluid flows downward in tissues because of gravity resulting in dependent edema. Coagulation of edema fluid as may occur with infection or severe trauma may result in nonpitting or brawny edema.

Edema may also be accompanied by the presence of fluid in potential spaces such as the pleural cavity, pericardial space, peritoneal cavity, and synovial spaces. Fluid that collects in these spaces is usually called *transudate* if it is sterile and *exudate* if it contains bacteria. Excessive fluid in the peritoneal space, one of the spaces most prone to develop extra fluid, is called *ascites*. The peritoneal cavity is highly susceptible to the development of excess fluid because any increased pressure in the liver, as due to cirrhosis or cardiac failure, causes transudation of protein-containing fluids from the liver into the peritoneal cavity. Increased lymph flow that accompanies increases in interstitial fluid pressure prevents the formation of edema.

Causes of increased interstitial fluid volume that manifests as edema include (1) increased capillary pressure, (2) decreased plasma proteins, (3) obstruction of lymph vessels, and (4) increased permeability of capillaries. Renal dysfunction leading to excessive retention of fluid is another cause of edema.

Increased Capillary Pressure

Increased capillary pressure results in filtration of fluid in excess of reabsorption. Most often, capillary pressure is increased by impaired venous return as due to cardiac failure. Likewise, when arteriolar dilatation occurs in localized areas of the body, blood flows rapidly through the locally dilated arterioles, and the capillary pressure increases, resulting in local edema. Local edema associated with allergic reactions reflects histamine-induced smooth muscle relaxation of the arterioles and constriction of the veins. The localized areas of edema are referred to as *hives* or *urticaria*. Angioneurotic edema is most likely caused by localized decreases in arteriolar tone due to abnormal vascular control by the autonomic nervous system.

Decreased plasma concentrations of protein lower the colloid osmotic pressure such that capillary pressure predominates and excess fluid leaves the circulation. It is estimated that edema begins to appear when the plasma colloid osmotic pressure declines below 11 mmHg.

Albumin may be lost from the plasma in large quantities when the skin is burned. Renal disease may be associated with urinary loss of albumin sufficient to lower the plasma colloid osmotic pressure. Nutritional edema ocurs when dietary intake is not adequate to support formation of sufficient amounts of protein.

Obstruction of Lymph Vessels

Obstruction of lymph vessels results in accumulation of protein in interstitial fluid. The subsequent rise in interstitial fluid colloid osmotic pressure causes excess fluid to collect in the interstitial fluid space. Obstruction of lymph vessels with associated edema may follow operations such as radical mastectomy when it is necessary to remove lymph nodes as part of the operation. Edema due to this cause typically regresses over 2 to 3 months as new lymph vessels develop.

REFERENCES

Baez S. Microcirculation. Annu Rev Physiol 1977;39: 391–95.

Comper WD, Laurent TC. Physiological function of connective tissue polysaccharides. Physiol Rev 1978; 58:255–315.

Guyton AC. Textbook of Medical Physiology. 7th ed. Philadelphia: WB Saunders, 1986:348.

Guyton AC, Granger HJ, Taylor AE. Interstitial fluid pressure. Physiol Rev 1971;51:527–63.

Intaglietta M. The measurement of pressure and flow in the microcirculation. Microvasc Res 1973;5:357–61.

Leak LV, Burke JF. Ultrastructural studies on the lymphatic anchoring of filaments. J Cell Biol 1968; 36:129–49.

Nicoll PA, Taylor AE. Lymph formation and flow. Annu Rev Physiol 1977;39:73–95.

CHAPTER 46

Pulmonary Circulation

INTRODUCTION

The pulmonary circulation is a low-pressure and low-resistance system in series with the systemic circulation. The volume of blood flowing through the lungs and systemic circulation is essentially identical. Blood passes through pulmonary capillaries in about 1 second during which time it is oxygenated and excess carbon dioxide is removed. Increasing the cardiac output may shorten capillary transit time to less than 0.5 second.

ANATOMY

Anatomically, the right ventricle is wrapped halfway around the left ventricle. The semilunar shape of the right ventricle allows it to pump with minimal shortening of its muscle fibers. The thickness of the right ventricle is one-third that of the left ventricle reflecting the difference in pressures between the two ventricles. The wall of the right ventricle is only about three times as thick as the atrial walls.

The pulmonary artery extends only 4 cm beyond the apex of the right ventricle and then divides into the right and left main pulmonary arteries. The pulmonary artery is also a thin structure with a wall thickness about twice that of the vena cavae and one-third that of the aorta. The large diameter and distensibility of the pulmonary arteries allows the pulmonary circulation to easily accommodate the stroke volume output of the right ventricle. Pulmonary veins, like pulmonary arteries, are large in diameter and highly distensible. Pulmonary capillaries supply the estimated 300 million alveoli providing a gas-exchange surface of about 70 m².

The sympathetic nervous system supplies vasoconstrictor and vasodilator fibers to pulmonary vessels. For example, alpha-adrenergic stimulation from norepinephrine produces vasoconstriction while beta-adrenergic stimulation, as produced by isoproterenol results in vasodilation (Porcelli and Bergofsky, 1973). The vagus nerve supplies cholinergic parasympathetic fibers which produce vasodilation. Despite the presence of innervation from the autonomic nervous system, the resting vasomotor tone is minimal and pulmonary vessels are almost maximally dilated in the normal resting state.

The diameter of pulmonary vessels, because of their thin walls, is more likely to change from variations in intraluminal pressures than from changes in tone of vascular smooth muscle. Therefore, the caliber of these vessels depends mainly on differences between intraluminal pressures and alveolar pressures. For example, if alveolar pressure exceeds intravascular pressure, as during positive pressure ventilation of the lungs, pulmonary capillaries collapse and flow ceases. The size of larger vessels embedded in the lung parenchyma is largely dependent on lung volume. Therefore, resistance to flow through these vessels decreases at large lung volumes. The largest pulmonary vessels in the hilum of the lung vary in size with changes in intrapleural pressure.

Bronchial Circulation

Bronchial arteries from the thoracic aorta supply oxygenated blood to the supporting tissues of the lungs, including connective tissue, septa, and bronchi. After this bronchial arterial blood has passed through supporting tissues, it empties into pulmonary veins and enters the left atrium rather than passing back to the right atrium. This entrance of deoxygenated blood into the left atrium dilutes oxygenated blood and accounts for an inherent anatomic shunt. Indeed, an average of 1% to 2% of the total cardiac output passes through bronchial arteries creating the effect of an anatomic shunt and making the left ventricular output slightly greater than the right ventricular output.

Pulmonary Lymph Vessels

Lymph vessels extend from all the supportive tissues of the lung to the hilum of the lung and then to the thoracic duct. Particulate matter entering the alveoli is usually removed rapidly by lymph vessels. In addition, protein is also removed from lung tissues to prevent formation of interstitial pulmonary edema.

INTRAVASCULAR PRESSURES

Pressures in the pulmonary circulation are about one-fifth those present in the systemic circulation (Fig. 46-1) (Guyton, 1986). The normal systolic pressure in the pulmonary artery averages 22 mmHg with a diastolic pressure of 8 mmHg. The mean pulmonary artery pressure averages 13 mmHg. The mean pulmonary capillary pressure is about 10 mmHg, and the mean pressure in the pulmonary veins is about 4 mmHg such that the pressure gradient across the pulmonary circulation is 9 mmHg.

Approximately 0.16 second prior to ventricular contraction, the atria contract, delivering blood into the ventricles. Immediately following this priming by the right atrium, the right ventricle contracts and the right ventricular pressure rises rapidly until it equals the pressure in the pulmonary artery. At this time, the pulmonary valve

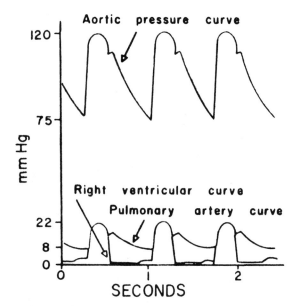

FIGURE 46-1. Comparison of intravascular pressures in the systemic and pulmonary circulations. (From Guyton AC. Textbook of Medical Physiology. 7th ed. Philadelphia: WB Saunders, 1986:287. Reproduced by permission of the author and publisher.)

opens and blood flows from the right ventricle into the pulmonary artery. When the right ventricular pressure begins to decline, the pulmonary valve closes and the right ventricular pressure continues to fall to a diastolic pressure near zero mmHg (Harlan *et al*, 1967).

At low pulmonary artery pressures, pulmonary resistance is high due to compression of vessels by extravascular structures. Once pressure in the vessels is high enough to overcome this compression, pulmonary vessels distend and resistance falls to low values. The greatest resistance to flow from the right ventricle is in precapillary vessels. Overall, the resistance offered by the pulmonary circulation to ejection of blood from the right ventricle is about one-tenth the resistance in the systemic circulation.

Pulmonary artery pressure is not influenced by left atrial pressures below 7 mmHg. When left atrial pressure exceeds 7 mmHg previously collapsed pulmonary veins have all been reexpanded and pulmonary artery pressure rises in parallel with increases in left atrial pressure. In the absence of left ventricular failure, even marked increases in peripheral vascular resistance do not cause the left atrial pressure to rise above this level. Consequently, the right ventricle continues to eject its stroke volume against a normal pulmonary artery pressure despite the increased work load imposed on the left ventricle. This means, also, that the right ventricular stroke volume is not measurably altered by changes in peripheral vascular resistance unless the left ventricle fails.

When the left ventricle fails, left atrial pressure can increase above 15 mmHg. Mean pulmonary artery pressures also increase, placing an increased work load on the right ventricle. Up to a mean pulmonary artery pressure of 30 to 40 mmHg, however, the right ventricle continues to eject its normal stroke volume with only a slight elevation in right atrial pressure. Above this pulmonary artery pressure, the right ventricle begins to fail, so that further increases in pulmonary artery pressure cause exaggerated increases in right atrial pressure with associated reductions in stroke volume.

Measurement of Left Atrial Pressure

The left atrial pressure can be estimated by inserting a catheter into a small pulmonary artery and inflating a balloon on its distal end such that flow does not occur around the catheter. As a result, pressure equilibrates with that in the pulmonary veins. This pulmonary artery occlusion pressure is usually only 2 to 3 mmHg greater than in the left atrium. In the absence of pulmonary hypertension, the pulmonary artery end-diastolic pressure correlates with the pulmonary artery occlusion pressure.

INTERSTITIAL FLUID SPACE

The interstitial fluid space in the lung is minimal and a continual negative pulmonary interstitial pressure of about −8 mmHg acts to dehydrate interstitial fluid spaces of the lungs and pull alveolar epithelial membranes towards capillary membranes (Parker *et al,* 1978). As a result, the distance between gas in the alveoli and the blood is minimal averaging about 0.4 μ in distance. Another consequence of negative pressure in pulmonary interstitial spaces is that it pulls fluid from alveoli through alveolar membranes and into interstitial fluid spaces thus keeping the alveoli dry. Furthermore, mean pulmonary capillary pressure

is about 10 mmHg, whereas, plasma colloid osmotic pressure is 28 mmHg. This net pressure gradient of 15 mmHg encourages movement of fluids into capillaries (see the section entitled Pulmonary Edema).

PULMONARY BLOOD VOLUME

Blood volume in the lungs is about 450 ml. Of this amount, about 70 ml is in capillaries, and the remainder is divided equally between pulmonary arteries and veins. Cardiac failure or increased resistance to flow through the mitral valve causes pulmonary blood volume to increase.

Cardiac output can increase nearly four times before pulmonary arterial pressure becomes elevated (Fig. 46-2) (Guyton, 1986). This reflects the distensibility of the pulmonary arteries and opening of previously collapsed pulmonary capillaries. The ability of the lungs to accept greatly increased amounts of pulmonary blood flow, as during exercise, without excessive elevations in pulmonary artery pressures is important to prevent development of pulmonary edema or right heart failure.

Pulmonary blood volume can increase up to 40% when an individual changes from the standing to supine position. This sudden shift of blood from systemic to pulmonary circulation is respon-

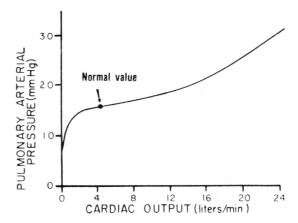

FIGURE 46-2. Cardiac output can increase nearly fourfold without greatly increasing the pulmonary arterial pressure. (From Guyton AC. Textbook of Medical Physiology. 7th ed. Philadelphia: WB Saunders, 1986:287. Reproduced by permission of the author and publisher.)

sible for the decrease in vital capacity in the supine position and the occurrence of orthopnea in the presence of left ventricular failure.

PULMONARY BLOOD FLOW AND DISTRIBUTION

Optimal oxygenation is dependent on matching pulmonary blood flow to ventilation (Racz, 1974). Although the lungs are richly innervated, it is doubtful that the autonomic nervous system has a major function in the normal control of pulmonary blood flow. Sympathetic nervous system stimulation, however, causes exaggerated vasoconstriction in the presence of alveolar hypoxia. Clinically, segmental pulmonary blood flow can be studied by intravenous injection of radioactive xenon while monitoring externally over the chest with radiation detectors. Xenon, because of its low solubility, rapidly diffuses into the alveoli and in well perfused regions of the lung radioactivity is detected early.

Hypoxic Pulmonary Vasoconstriction

Alveolar hypoxia (PAO_2 below 70 mmHg) causes vasoconstriction of pulmonary arterioles supplying these alveoli (Domino *et al*, 1984). The net effect is to divert blood flow away from poorly ventilated alveoli and thus optimize matching of pulmonary blood flow to ventilation and minimize any adverse effect on arterial oxygenation. The mechanism for this hypoxic pulmonary vasoconstriction is presumed to be locally mediated. Indeed, this response occurs in isolated and denervated lungs as well as intact lungs. It is possible that release of a vasoconstrictor substance by the periarterial mast cells acts on alpha-adrenergic receptors causing vasoconstriction (Bergofsky, 1974). Many drugs, including inhaled and injected anesthetics and potent vasodilating drugs have been reported to inhibit hypoxic pulmonary vasoconstriction leading to reductions in arterial oxygenation (Benumof and Wahrenbrock, 1975). Nevertheless, halothane and isoflurane do not further impair arterial oxygenation during one-lung ventilation in patients previously anesthetized with diazepam and fentanyl suggesting these volatile anesthetics do not inhibit hypoxic pulmonary

vasoconstriction (Fig. 46-3) (Rogers and Benumof, 1985).

In addition to the effects of low oxygen concentrations in the alveoli on regional pulmonary vasculature, arterial hypoxemia causes increased pulmonary artery and right ventricular pressures. For example, pulmonary hypertension may occur in those who reside at high altitudes.

Effect of Respiration

Inspiration increases venous return to the heart due to contraction of the diaphragm and abdominal muscles which increases the gradient from the intra-abdominal portion of the inferior vena cava to its intrathoracic portion. In addition, decreases in intrapleural pressure associated with inspiration serve to distend the intrathoracic portion of the vena cavae further facilitating venous return. The resulting augmented blood flow to the right atrium increases right ventricular stroke volume. In contrast to spontaneous breathing, a mechanically delivered inspiration impedes venous return to the heart and reduces right ventricular stroke volume.

Hydrostatic Pressure Gradients

In standing humans, the uppermost part of the lung is about 30 cm above the lowest point. As a result, pulmonary artery pressure at the top of the lung in the standing position is about 15 mmHg less than mean pulmonary artery pressure, while pressure in the lowest portion of the lung is about 8 mmHg greater (Reed and Wood, 1970). These differences in pulmonary artery pressure allow gravity to exert profound effects on blood flow through the different areas of the lung. Indeed, in the standing position, there is little pulmonary blood flow to the apex of the lung while the lower lung receives excess perfusion. This effect of gravity on distribution of pulmonary blood flow is minimized when an individual changes from the standing to supine positon. In patients with mitral stenosis or acute pulmonary edema, as may accompany a myocardial infarction, blood flow to the lung apex is increased while flow to bases is reduced (Kazemi *et al*, 1970). Presumably, a rise in pulmonary venous pressure leads to perivascular interstitial edema which subsequently in-

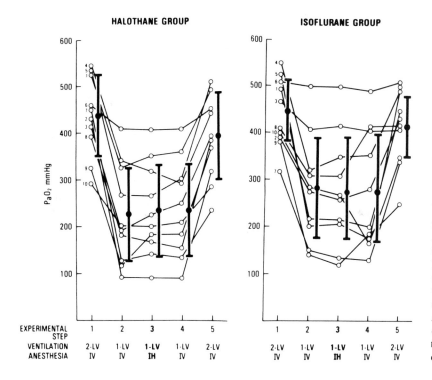

HALOTHANE GROUP

ISOFLURANE GROUP

EXPERIMENTAL STEP	1	2	3	4	5
VENTILATION	2-LV	1-LV	1-LV	1-LV	2-LV
ANESTHESIA	IV	IV	IH	IV	IV

FIGURE 46-3. PaO_2 was measured during two-lung ventilation (2-LV) and then during one-lung ventilation (1-LV) in patients anesthetized with fentanyl and diazepam without (experimental steps 2 and 4) and with halothane or isoflurane (experimental step 3). Addition of halothane or isoflurane (about 1.2 MAC) does not alter the PaO_2, suggesting these drugs do not inhibit hypoxic pulmonary vasoconstriction. Clear circles are individual patient data and closed circles are mean ± SD for each group. (From Rogers SN, Benumof JL. Halothane and isoflurane do not decrease PaO_2 during one-lung ventilation in intravenously anesthetized patients. Anesth Analg 1985;64:946. Reproduced by permission of the authors and the International Anesthesia Research Society.)

creases resistance to blood flow through the bases of the lungs.

Blood Flow Zones

The lung is often divided into three different blood flow zones (Fig. 46-4) (Guyton, 1986; West, 1974). These three zones reflect the impact on the caliber of pulmonary blood vessels produced by pulmonary artery pressure, alveolar pressure, and pulmonary venous pressure.

Zone 1

Zone 1 is an area of no pulmonary blood flow as the pressure in the alveoli exceeds pulmonary capillary pressure. This compression effect on pulmonary capillaries occurs at the apices of the lungs in the standing position when the pulmonary artery pressure is low. The extent of zone 1 is increased by hemorrhage which lowers pulmonary artery pressure. Likewise, positive pressure ventilation of the lungs can create an area of zone 1. Under normal circumstances, pulmonary artery pressure is just sufficient to deliver blood flow to

the apex of the lung and a zone 1 pattern of no blood flow does not occur.

Zone 2

Zone 2 is an area of intermittent pulmonary blood flow in which the hydrostatic pressure effect is such that pulmonary artery pressure exceeds alveolar pressure during systole but not diastole. In a standing patient, zone 2 begins 7 to 10 cm above the level of the heart and extends to the uppermost portion of the lungs.

Zone 3

Zone 3 is an area of continuous pulmonary blood flow as pulmonary artery pressure always exceeds alveolar pressure. This zone extends from about 7 to 10 cm above the heart to the lowermost portions of the lung. In the supine position, all portions of the lung become zone 3 with pulmonary blood flow being more evenly distributed. Exercise and associated increases in pulmonary artery pressures also tend to convert most of the lung to a zone 3 pattern of blood flow.

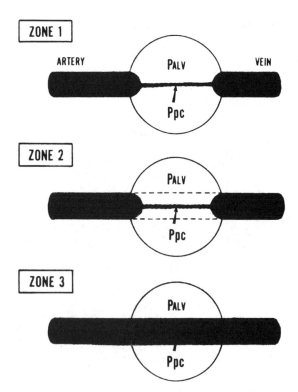

FIGURE 46-4. The lung is divided into three different blood flow zones based on the relationship between alveolar pressure (PALV) and capillary pressure (Ppc). (From Guyton AC. Textbook of Medical Physiology. 7th ed. Philadelphia: WB Saunders, 1986:287. Reproduced by permission of the author and publisher.)

PULMONARY EDEMA

Pulmonary edema is present when there are excessive quantities of fluid either in pulmonary interstitial spaces or in alveoli (Staub, 1974). Dehydrating forces of the colloid osmotic pressure of the blood in the lungs provide a large safety factor against development of pulmonary edema (see the section entitled Intravascular Fluid Space). In humans, plasma colloid osmotic pressure is about 28 mmHg so that pulmonary edema will rarely develop below a pulmonary capillary pressure of 30 mmHg. The most common cause of acute pulmonary edema is a greatly elevated pulmonary capillary pressure resulting from left ventricular failure and pooling of blood in the lungs.

During chronic elevations of left atrial pressure, pulmonary edema may not occur despite pulmonary capillary pressures as high as 45 mmHg. Enlargement of the pulmonary lymph vessels allowing lymph flow to increase up to 20 times is the most likely reason pulmonary edema does not occur in the presence of chronically elevated left atrial pressures.

Pulmonary edema can also result from local capillary damage as occurs with inhalation of acidic gastric fluid or irritant gases such as smoke. The result is rapid transudation of fluid and protein into the alveoli and interstitial spaces.

Mild degrees of pulmonary edema may be limited to only an increase in the interstitial fluid volume. The alveolar epithelium is not able to withstand more than a modest increase in interstitial fluid pressure, however, before fluid spills into alveoli.

EVENTS THAT OBSTRUCT PULMONARY BLOOD FLOW

Common causes of obstruction to pulmonary blood flow include pulmonary embolism, pulmonary emphysema, anthracosis, and atelectasis.

Pulmonary Embolism

Total blockage of one of the major branches of the pulmonary artery by an embolus is usually not immediately fatal because the opposite lung can accommodate all the pulmonary blood flow. As the blood clot extends, however, death ensues because of right ventricular failure due to excessive elevations in pulmonary artery pressure (McIntyre and Sasahara, 1974). Tachypnea and dyspnea are characteristic responses in awake patients experiencing pulmonary embolism. Tachypnea may reflect stimulation of pulmonary deflation receptors that are innervated by the vagus. Anticoagulation is recommended to prevent extension of the clot and in occasional patients, surgical removal of the embolus may be life-saving.

Diffuse pulmonary emboli, as occur with fat or air, produce increased pulmonary artery pressure similar to that which occurs with an isolated embolus. In addition, reflex-mediated pulmonary vasospasm initiated by pulmonary emboli further increases resistance to blood flow (Stein and Levy, 1974). This vasospasm may reflect reflex sympathetic nervous system stimulation or release of chemical mediators such as histamine or serotonin.

Pulmonary Emphysema

Destruction of alveoli that characterizes pulmonary emphysema is accompanied by a concomitant loss of pulmonary vasculature and elevation in pulmonary artery pressures. Pulmonary hypertension is further exaggerated by arterial hypoxemia which increases the cardiac output and thus enhances blood flow into the pulmonary circulation. Modest increases in the inhaled concentration of oxygen may be sufficient to lower pulmonary artery pressures in these patients.

Anthracosis

Anthracosis is an example of a condition in which there is fibrosis of the supportive tissues in the lungs. Pulmonary artery pressures may remain normal at rest. Conversely, even modest activity may evoke severe increases in pulmonary artery pressures because vessels surrounded by fibrous tissue cannot expand with increases in pulmonary blood flow (Bergofsky, 1974). In chronic situations, pulmonary artery pressure remains elevated and right ventricular failure eventually occurs.

Atelectasis

Atelectasis most commonly occurs when pulmonary blood flow absorbs air from unventilated alveoli as occurs when secretions plug bronchi. Subsequent collapse of these alveoli increases resistance to pulmonary blood flow and thus diverts blood flow to better perfused alveoli. In addition, the hypoxic pulmonary vasoconstriction reflex response diverts pulmonary blood flow to better ventilated alveoli (see the section entitled Hypoxic Pulmonary Vasoconstriction).

REFERENCES

Benumof JL, Wahrenbrock E. Local effects of anesthetics or regional hypoxic pulmonary vasoconstriction. Anesthesiology 1975;43:525–32.

Bergofsky EH. Mechanisms underlying vasomotor regulation of regional pulmonary blood flow in normal and disease states. Am J Med 1974;57:378–94.

Domino KB, Chen L, Alexander CM, Williams JJ, Marshall C, Marshall BE. Time course and responses of sustained hypoxic pulmonary vasoconstriction in the dog. Anesthesiology 1984;60:562–6.

Guyton AC. Textbook of Medical Physiology. 7th ed. Philadelphia: WB Saunders, 1986:287.

Harlan JC, Smith EE, Richardson TQ. Pressure-volume curves of systemic and pulmonary circuits. Am J Physiol 1967;213:1499–503.

Kazemi H, Parsons EF, Valenca LM, Stieder DJ. Distribution of pulmonary blood flow after myocardial ischemia and infarction. Circulation 1970;41:1025–30.

McIntyre KM, Sasahara AA. Hemodynamic and ventricular responses to pulmonary embolism. Prog Cardiovasc Dis 1974;17:175–90.

Parker JC, Guyton AC, Taylor AE. Pulmonary interstitial and capillary pressures estimated from intra-alveolar fluid pressures. J Appl Physiol 1978;44:267–76.

Porcelli RJ, Bergofsky EH. Adrenergic receptors in pulmonary vasoconstrictor responses to gaseous and humoral agents. J Appl Physiol 1973;34:488–94.

Racz GB. Pulmonary blood flow in normal and abnormal states. Surg Clin North Am 1974;54:967–77.

Reed JH, Wood EH. Effect of body position on vertical distribution of pulmonary blood flow. J Appl Physiol 1970;28:303–11.

Rogers SN, Benumof JL. Halothane and isoflurane do not decrease PaO$_2$ during one-lung ventilation in intravenously anesthetized patients. Anesth Analg 1985;64:946–54.

Staub NC. Pulmonary edema. Physiol Rev 1974;54:678–811.

Stein M, Levy SE. Reflex and humoral responses to pulmonary embolism. Prog Cardiovas Dis 1974;17:167–74.

West JB. Blood flow to the lung and gas exchange. Anesthesiology 1974;41:124–38.

Heart

CARDIAC PHYSIOLOGY

The heart can be characterized as a pulsatile four-chamber pump composed of two atria and two ventricles (Alpert *et al,* 1979). The atria function primarily as conduits (primer pumps) to the ventricles, but they also contract weakly to facilitate movement of blood into the ventricles. The ventricles serve as power pumps to supply the main force that propels blood through the systemic and pulmonary circulation. Special mechanisms in the heart maintain cardiac rhythm and transmit action potentials through cardiac muscle to initiate contraction.

Systole means contraction and is the time interval between closure of the tricuspid and mitral valves and closure of the pulmonary and aortic valves. Diastole is a period of relaxation corresponding to the interval between closure of the pulmonary and aortic valves and closure of the tricuspid and mitral valves.

Cardiac Muscle

Cardiac muscle consists of atrial muscle, ventricular muscle, and specialized excitatory and conductive muscle fibers. Atrial and ventricular cardiac muscle fibers contract similar to skeletal muscle (see Chapter 55). In contrast, excitatory and conductive fibers contain few contractile fibers but instead provide a rapid pathway for conduction of the cardiac action potential.

Cardiac muscle is striated in the same manner as skeletal muscle. Furthermore, cardiac muscle, like skeletal muscle has myofibrils that contain actin and myosin filaments. These filaments interdigitate and slide along each other during contraction in the same manner as occurs in skeletal muscle.

Cardiac muscle is a syncytium in which cardiac muscle cells are so tightly bound together that when one of these cells becomes excited, the action potential spreads to all of them. As a result, stimulation of a single atrial or ventricular cell causes the action potential to travel over the entire muscle mass such that the atria or ventricles contract as a single unit. The atrial syncytium is separated from the ventricular syncytium by the fibrous tissue surrounding the valvular rings. The cardiac action potential is conducted from the atrial syncytium into the ventricular syncytium by a specialized conduction pathway known as the *atrioventricular bundle.*

Cardiac Action Potential

The resting transmembrane potential of the normal cardiac muscle cell membrane is about −90 mv. For purposes of discussion, the cardiac action potential is divided into phases 0 through 4 (Fig. 47-1). The phase of depolarization and reversal of the transmembrane potential is designated phase 0. The three phases of repolarization are labeled 1, 2, and 3, and the resting transmembrane

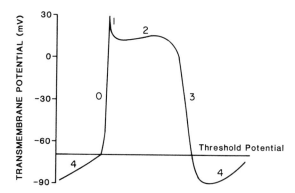

FIGURE 47-1. The action potential of a pacemaker cardiac cell is divided into phase 0, 1, 2, 3, and 4. The action potential of a nonpacemaker cardiac cell differs only in that phase 4 is constant in contrast to spontaneous phase 4 depolarization characteristic of pacemaker cells.

brief phase 1 followed by a plateau lasting 150 to 300 msec known as phase 2 (Trautwein, 1973). Phase 2 is due to closure of sodium channels and inward flux of calcium ions through specific slow calcium channels. Both these events maintain the positive charge inside the cell membrane necessary for sustaining phase 2. A third event contributing to the plateau of phase 2 is a decrease in permeability of the potassium channels that prevents rapid outflow of potassium ions further prolonging depolarization. The sustained plateau of phase 2 distinguishes the cardiac cell action potential from that developed by skeletal muscle cells.

Termination of phase 2 and further return of the transmembrane potential towards -90 mv occurs during phase 3. Phase 3 is due principally to a return to normal of cardiac cell membrane permeability to sodium ions and a sudden increase in permeability to potassium ions allowing a rapid loss of this ion so as to restore the transmembrane potential to -90 mv.

The velocity of conduction of the cardiac action potential in atrial and ventricular muscle averages 0.3 to 0.5 m sec^{-1}, which is about 10 times slower than in skeletal muscle and 250 times slower than in large nerve fibers. Cardiac muscle, like other excitable tissue, is refractory to restimulation during the action potential. The absolute refractory period extends through phases 1, 2, and part of phase 3 of the cardiac action potential. During the remainder of phase 3, the cardiac cells respond to a stimulus of greater than normal intensity (e.g., relative refractory period). The absolute refractory period of atrial muscle is much shorter than that for the ventricular muscle such that the rhythmical rate of contraction of the atria can be much faster than that of the ventricles.

potential is designated phase 4. These phases are clearly evident in recording of action potentials from Purkinje fibers. Many cardiac cells, however, develop action potentials that differ substantially from those of the Purkinje fibers. For example, sinoatrial and atrioventricular nodal cells have slowly rising phase 0, and phases 1, 2, and 3 cannot be clearly distinguished. Also, in nonpacemaker contractile atrial and ventricular cardiac muscle cells, phase 4 is constant during diastole, and these cells remain at rest until activated by a propagated cardiac impulse or an external stimulus. In contrast, pacemaker cardiac cells exhibit spontaneous phase 4 depolarization resulting in self-excitation and propagation of an action potential when threshold potential is reached (about -70 mv) (Fig. 47-1) (see the section entitled Cardiac Pacemakers).

Phase 0 of the cardiac action potential is generated by the inward movement of sodium ions through specific channels that are activated when spontaneous phase 4 depolarization reaches the threshold potential of about -70 mv. The influx of sodium ions is intense but brief. The rate of depolarization during phase 0 is referred to as V_{max}. During this phase, the resting transmembrane potential across cardiac cell membranes relative to extracellular fluid changes from about -90 mv to a peak spike potential of about 30 mv (Fig. 47-1).

Repolarization that follows phase 0 includes a

Contraction of Cardiac Muscle

Contraction of cardiac muscle is under the regulatory control of the sympathetic nervous system. At the cellular level, combination of catecholamines with membrane-bound beta-adrenergic receptors activates the enzyme adenylate cyclase. The subsequent increase in cyclic AMP then promotes myocardial contraction presumably by facilitating transmembrane flux of calcium ions. Release of calcium ions into the muscle sarcoplasm during phase 2 of the cardiac action potential is followed by diffusion into the myofibrils where this ion catalyzes chemical reactions that promote sliding of the actin and myosin filaments along each other (Fabiato and Fabiato, 1979). The sustained plateau characteristic of phase 2 of the cardiac action potential provides the prolonged period of contraction necessary for the ventricles to eject blood. Extra calcium ions stored in T tubules distinguish cardiac muscle from skeletal muscle. The T tubules are filled with extracellular fluid such that availability of calcium ions to cause cardiac muscle contraction depends on the extracellular fluid concentration of calcium. In contrast, the concentration of calcium ions in the extracellular fluid does not greatly influence the contractility of skeletal muscle. At the end of the plateau of phase 2 depolarization, the supply of new calcium ions to the interior of the cardiac muscle fiber suddenly ceases. At this point, calcium ions in the sarcoplasmic reticulum are rapidly pumped back into T tubules for reuse during the next cardiac action potential.

Cardiac Cycle

The cardiac cycle consists of a period of relaxation called *diastole* followed by a period of contraction called *systole* (Fig. 47-2) (Guyton, 1986a). The period from the end of one heart contraction to the end of the next is defined as the cardiac cycle. Each cycle is initiated by spontaneous generation

of an action potential in the sinoatrial node. This node is located in the posterior wall of the right atrium near the opening of the superior vena cava. Delay of transmission of this action potential for 0.1 second in the atrioventricular node allows the atria to contract before the ventricles, thereby pumping blood into the ventricles prior to forceful ventricular contraction. As such, the atria act as primer pumps for the ventricles, and the ventricles then provide the major source of power for moving blood through the systemic and pulmonary circulations.

When the heart rate increases, the duration of each total cycle of the heart must decrease. The duration of contraction (systole) decreases but not as much as the relaxation (diastole) phase. Excessive increases in heart rate may so shorten diastole that insufficient time is available for complete filling of the cardiac chambers prior to the next contraction.

Atrial Pressure Curves

Atrial pressure curves consists of a, c, and v waves (see Table 44-1). The a wave is caused by atrial contraction (Fig. 47-2) (Guyton, 1986a). Ordinarily, right atrial pressure rises 4 to 6 mmHg, and left atrial pressure rises 6 to 8 mmHg during contraction. The c wave occurs when the ventricles begin to contract and is caused by bulging of the tricus-

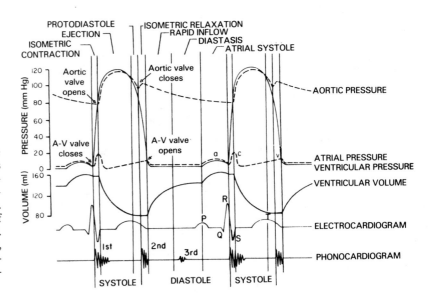

FIGURE 47-2. Events of the cardiac cycle including changes in intravascular pressures, ventricular volume, electrocardiogram, and phonocardiogram. (From Guyton AC. Textbook of Medical Physiology. 7th ed. Philadelphia: WB Saunders, 1986:150. Reproduced by permission of the author and publisher.)

pid and mitral valves backward toward the atria because of increasing pressure in the ventricles. In addition, pulling on atrial muscle by the contracting ventricles contributes to the c wave. The v wave occurs toward the end of ventricular contraction and is due to accumulation of blood in the atria. A large v wave occurs when blood flows retrograde into the atria through an incompetent tricuspid or mitral valve.

Atria as Pumps

During ventricular systole, large amounts of blood accumulate in the atria because of the closed tricuspid and mitral valves. At the conclusion of ventricular systole and when ventricular pressures fall rapidly, the higher pressures in the atria force the valves open and allow blood to flow rapidly into the ventricles. This period of rapid filling of the ventricles lasts for the first one third of diastole and accounts for about 70% of the blood that enters the ventricles. During the latter portion of diastole, the atria contract to deliver about 30% of the blood that normally enters the ventricles during each cardiac cycle.

Ventricles as Pumps

The start of ventricular contraction causes an abrupt increase in intraventricular pressure resulting in closure of the tricuspid and mitral valves (Fig. 47-2) (Guyton, 1986a). An additional 0.02 to 0.03 second is required for each ventricle to develop sufficient pressure to open the pulmonary and aortic valves which are kept closed by the back pressure of blood in the pulmonary artery and aorta. During this brief period of isovolemic contraction, there is no blood ejection from the ventricles. When intraventricular pressures are sufficient, the pulmonary and aortic valves open and about 60% of the total ventricular ejection of blood occurs during the first one fourth of systole. At the end of systole, intraventricular pressure declines rapidly allowing high pressures in the large arteries to close the pulmonary and aortic valves.

During diastole, filling of the ventricles with blood from the atria normally increases the volume of blood in each ventricle to about 130 ml. This volume is known as the *end-diastolic volume.* Subsequent ventricular ejection creates a stroke volume of about 70 ml. The remaining volume in the ventricle is called the *end-systolic volume.* When the heart contracts strongly, the end-systolic volume can decrease to as little as 10 ml.

Function of the Heart Valves

Heart valves open passively along a pressure gradient and close when a backward pressure gradient develops due to a high pressure in the pulmonary artery and aorta. Papillary muscles are attached to the vanes of the tricuspid and mitral valves by the chorda tendineae. These papillary muscles prevent the valves from bulging too far backward into the atria during ventricular contraction. Rupture of a chorda tendinea or dysfunction of a papillary muscle results in an incompetent valve during contraction of the ventricle.

High pressures in arteries at the conclusion of systole cause the pulmonary and aortic valves to snap to a closed position in comparison with a much softer closure of the tricuspid and mitral valves. Because of the rapid closure and rapid velocity of blood ejection, the edges of the pulmonary and aortic valves are subjected to much greater mechanical trauma than the tricuspid and mitral valves.

When listening to the heart with a stethoscope, one does not normally hear the opening of the valves because this is a relatively slow developing process that makes no noise. When the valves close, however, blood vibrates under the influence of the sudden pressure differentials that develop, creating a sound that travels in all directions through the chest (see the section entitled Dynamics of Heart Sounds).

Work of the Heart

The work of the heart is the amount of energy that the heart converts to work while pumping blood into the arteries. Work required to raise the pressure for ejection of blood is calculated as stroke volume times ejection pressure. Right ventricular work output is usually about one-seventh the work output of the left ventricle because of the difference in systolic pressure against which the two ventricles must pump. The energy required for the work of the heart is derived mainly from metabolism of fatty acids and to a lesser extent from metabolism of other nutrients, especially lactate and glucose.

Intrinsic Autoregulation of Cardiac Function

Intrinsic ability of the heart to adapt itself to changing loads of inflowing blood is called the Frank-Starling law of the heart. This law states that the greater the heart is filled with blood during diastole, the greater will be the quantity of blood ejected into the aorta. Within physiologic limits, the heart pumps all the blood that comes to it without allowing excessive accumulation of blood in the veins. In other words, the heart automatically adapts to the venous return as long as the total amount does not exceed the physiologic limit the heart can pump.

The mechanism by which the heart adapts to changing venous return reflects the increased stretch of cardiac muscle produced by increased filling of the ventricles from the atria. When the cardiac muscle becomes stretched, it contracts with greater force (analogous to increased stretch of a rubber band) thereby pumping additional blood into the arteries. The ability of stretched cardiac muscle to contract with increased force is characteristic of all striated muscle, not just cardiac muscle. The increased force of contraction is probably caused by the fact that actin and myosin filaments are brought to a more nearly optimal degree of interdigitation for achieving contraction. A plot of cardiac output with changes in atrial filling pressures (*i.e.,* ventricular function curves) reflects the degree of stretch applied to cardiac muscle (see Chapter 44).

In addition to the Frank-Starling mechanism, another less important mechanism for increasing cardiac output is a 10 to 30 beat min^{-1} increase in heart rate evoked by increased stretch of the right atrium. Changes in blood pressure within a physiologic limit have almost no effect on cardiac output. This emphasizes that the most important factor determining cardiac output is the atrial pressure created by venous return.

Neural Control of the Heart

The atria are abundantly innervated by the sympathetic and parasympathetic nervous system, but the ventricles are supplied principally by the sympathetic nervous system (Fig. 47-3) (Guyton, 1986a) (see the section entitled Cardiac Rhythm and Autonomic Nervous System Stimulation). These nerves affect cardiac output by changing the

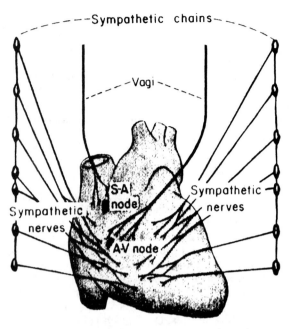

FIGURE 47-3. Innervation of the atria is from the sympathetic and parasympathetic (vagi) nervous systems while the ventricles are supplied principally by the sympathetic nervous system. (From Guyton AC. Textbook of Medical Physiology. 7th ed. Philadelphia: WB Saunders, 1986:150. Reproduced by permission of the author and publisher.)

heart rate and strength of myocardial contraction. Sympathetic nervous system fibers to the heart continually discharge at a slow rate that maintains a strength of ventricular contraction about 20% to 25% above its strength in the absence of sympathetic nervous system stimulation. Maximal sympathetic nervous system stimulation can increase cardiac output by about 100% above normal. Conversely, maximal parasympathetic nervous system stimulation decreases ventricular contractile strength and subsequent cardiac output only about 30%, emphasizing that parasympathetic nervous system stimulation of the heart is small compared with the effect of sympathetic nervous system stimulation. Increased myocardial contractility associated with sympathetic nervous system stimulation of the heart is most likely due to norepinephrine-induced increases in the permeability of cardiac muscle cell membranes to calcium ions.

Evaluation of Myocardial Contractility

The rate of change of ventricular pressure with time (dp/dt) is a useful method for evaluation of myocardial contractility. Nevertheless, dp/dt is affected by factors other than myocardial contractility including pressure in the aorta into which the ventricle is ejecting blood. The rate of shortening of ventricular muscle (V_{max}) is also a reflection of myocardial contractility.

CORONARY BLOOD FLOW

Unique features of coronary blood flow include absence of anastomosis between the left and right coronary arteries and interruption of blood flow during systole due to mechanical compression of vessels by myocardial contraction. In other organs, blood flow is continuous being uninfluenced by the phase of the cardiac cycle. The prevalence of atherosclerotic changes in the coronary arteries emphasizes the potential serious aspect of lack of anastomosis between the two major coronary arteries. Another characteristic of the coronary circulation is the maximal oxygen extraction (*e.g.,* up to two-thirds the oxygen content) that occurs, resulting in a coronary venous oxygen saturation of 25% or less. For this reason, the most reliable way to increase myocardial oxygen delivery is by vasodilation of the coronary arteries.

Anatomy of the Coronary Circulation

The left and right coronary arteries arise from the sinuses of Valsalva located behind the cusps of the aortic valve at the root of the aorta (Fig. 47-4). These main coronary arteries lie on the epicardial surface of the heart, and small perforating branches are primarily responsible for delivery of nutrients to cardiac muscle. Indeed, only the inner 75 to 1000 μ of the endocardial surface obtain nutrients directly from blood in the cardiac chambers. Even in the presence of cardiac hypertrophy, the ratio of capillaries to myocardial fibers is 1:1 (Guyton, 1986b). As a result, in the presence of cardiac hypertrophy each capillary must supply a greater bulk of muscle, and the distance that the nutrients have to travel to reach the center of the muscle is increased. This limits the amount of cardiac hypertrophy that can occur without the development of myocardial ischemia.

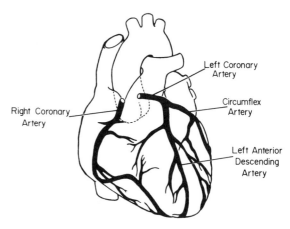

FIGURE 47-4. Anatomy of the coronary circulation.

The left coronary artery supplies the anterior part of the left ventricle while the right coronary artery supplies the right ventricle and the posterior portion of the left ventricle. In about 50% of individuals, more blood flows through the right coronary artery than the left, in about 30% the flow in both arteries is similar and in about 20% the left coronary artery is predominant (Guyton, 1986b).

Most of the venous blood that has perfused the left ventricle enters the right atrium via the coronary sinus. This accounts for about 75% of the total coronary blood flow. The majority of coronary blood flow to the right ventricle enters anterior cardiac veins that empty into the right atrium independent of the coronary sinus. A small amount of coronary blood flows back into the heart through Thebesian veins which can empty into any cardiac chamber. Thebesian veins that empty into the left heart contribute to the inherent anatomic shunt.

The resting coronary blood flow is about 225 ml min^{-1} or 4% to 5% of the cardiac output. Assuming the usual heart weighs about 280 g, this is equivalent to a flow of 75 ml^{-1} 100 g^{-1} min^{-1}. During strenuous exercise, coronary blood flow may increase fivefold. Resting myocardial oxygen consumption is about 40 ml min^{-1} or 15% of the total body consumption of oxygen.

Coronary blood flow occurs predominantly during diastole when cardiac muscle relaxes and no longer obstructs blood flow through ventricular capillaries. Coronary blood flow, especially to the left ventricle, is greatly reduced during systole reflecting contraction of left ventricular muscle around blood vessels. Intramyocardial pressure that develops during ventricular contraction compresses left ventricular subendocardial vessels far more than outer endocardial coronary arteries. During systole, blood flow through subendocardial arteries of the left ventricle falls almost to zero. Indeed, it is estimated that at least 75% of total coronary blood flow occurs during diastole. To compensate for minimal subendocardial blood flow during systole, subendocardial arteries are much larger than the perforating endocardial arteries. Therefore, during diastole, blood flow through subendocardial arteries is considerably greater than is blood flow in other arteries. Nevertheless, the subendocardial region of the left ventricle is the most common site for myocardial infarction. Tachycardia with an associated decrease in the time for coronary blood flow to occur during diastole further jeopardizes the adequacy of myocardial oxygen delivery particularly if coronary arteries are narrowed by atherosclerosis. The impact of systole on coronary blood flow through the right ventricle is minimal. This reflects the fact that pressure in the coronary arteries is greater than the pressure developed in the right ventricle.

Determinants of Coronary Blood Flow

Coronary blood flow is determined almost entirely by vascular responses to the local needs of the cardiac muscle for nutrients, especially oxygen (Klocke and Ellis, 1980). Indeed, coronary blood flow is regulated almost exactly in proportion to the need of cardiac muscle for oxygen. This regulatory role of oxygen is independent of nervous system innervation of the heart. Presumably, low oxygen concentrations evoke the local release of vasodilator substances that dilate coronary arterioles and thus increase oxygen delivery by virtue of increased coronary blood flow. Increased extraction of oxygen is not likely to offset local increases in oxygen needs since even in the normal resting state oxygen extraction by cardiac cells is nearly maximal. Therefore, little additional oxygen can be made available in the absence of increased coronary blood flow.

Arterial blood pressure acts as the perfusion pressure to drive blood through coronary arteries. For example, an increase in perfusion pressure will increase coronary blood flow. This increased flow, however, is transient as autoregulation of coronary blood vessel tone acts to return blood

flow toward normal. Perfusion pressure is particularly important in maintaining coronary blood flow through atherosclerotic arteries that cannot dilate in response to autoregulatory mechanisms (e.g., pressure-dependent perfusion).

Local Vasodilators

The most potent local vasodilator substance released by cardiac cells is adenosine (Berne and Rubio, 1974). Other vasodilators may include potassium ions, hydrogen ions, carbon dioxide, bradykinin, and possibly prostaglandins. An alternative explanation to release of a vasodilator substance is local vasodilation due to relaxation of vascular smooth muscle in the presence of low concentrations of oxygen.

Myocardial Oxygen Consumption

Myocardial oxygen consumption, which is the major determinant of coronary blood flow, is influenced by the pressure against which the heart is pumping blood times the cardiac output. When blood pressure increases, myocardial oxygen consumption increases almost directly in proportion. Conversely, when cardiac output increases without an increase in blood pressure, oxygen consumption increases only a modest amount. Sympathetic nervous system stimulation (tachycardia, increased myocardial contractility) also increases myocardial oxygen consumption. In contrast, parasympathetic nervous system stimulation slows heart rate and modestly reduces myocardial contractility, both of which reduce myocardial oxygen consumption and thus lead to constriction of the coronary arteries.

Myocardial oxygen consumption parallels peak myocardial muscle tension. Thus, when arterial pressure increases, myocardial muscle tension rises and oxygen consumption also increases. Likewise, when the heart dilates, heart muscle must generate increased tension to pump against even a normal arterial pressure. This results from Laplace's law, which states that tension required to generate a given pressure increase is proportional to the diameter of the heart.

Increasing venous return (i.e., volume work) is the least costly means of increasing cardiac output in terms of myocardial oxygen consumption. This emphasizes that the most important aspect of hemodynamic management is to first optimize venous return by appropriate adjustments in the intravascular fluid volume. Clinically, venous return is equivalent to preload and is estimated by measurement of the right atrial pressure or pulmonary artery occlusion pressure.

RATE–PRESSURE PRODUCT. The rate–pressure product (product of heart rate and systolic blood pressure) is the simplest clinical method for estimating myocardial oxygen consumption. Maintenance of the rate–pressure product below 12,000 in awake patients is considered unlikely to result in myocardial oxygen consumption exceeding myocardial oxygen delivery and the subsequent development of myocardial ischemia (Kaplan, 1979). It is important to appreciate that the magnitude of the rate–pressure product is less important than the absolute value of the individual components, with elevations in heart rate increasing myocardial oxygen consumption more than increases in systolic blood pressure. Furthermore, the validity of maintaining the rate–pressure product below a certain value has not been documented in anesthetized patients.

TRIPLE INDEX. The triple index (product of heart rate, systolic blood pressure, and pulmonary artery occlusion pressure), like the rate–pressure product, is a clinical indicator of myocardial oxygen consumption. Maintenance of the triple index below 150,000 is considered desirable particularly in patients with coronary artery disease (Kaplan, 1979).

Nervous System Innervations

Alpha- and beta-adrenergic receptors as well as histamine receptors are present in coronary arteries. In general, epicardial coronary arteries have a preponderance of alpha receptors while the intramuscular arteries have a preponderance of beta receptors. In some persons, alpha vasoconstrictor effects seem to be excessive resulting in vasospastic myocardial ischemia (*e.g.,* Prinzmetal's angina). The distribution of parasympathetic nervous system fibers to the coronary arteries in the ventricles is sparse, and any direct effect on coronary blood flow is unlikely.

DYNAMICS OF HEART SOUNDS

Closure of the heart valves is responsible for the audible sounds designated as the first and second heart sounds (Guyton, 1986c). Audible sounds are not normally produced by opening of heart valves.

First and Second Heart Sounds

Closure of the mitral and tricuspid valves produces the first heart sound while the second heart sound is due to closure of the aortic and pulmonary valves. An audible sound is produced by vibration of the taut valves immediately after closure as well as vibration of the adjacent blood, walls of the heart, and major vessels around the heart. These vibrations then travel to the chest wall where they can be heard as sound by a stethoscope.

The duration of the first heart sound is about 0.14 second, and the second heart sound lasts about 0.11 second (Guyton, 1986c). The reason the second heart sound is shorter in duration than the first heart sound is probably that the second heart sound is damped out by the vascular walls much more rapidly than is the first heart sound by the ventricular walls.

The loudness of the first heart sound is almost directly proportional to the rate of development of pressure differences across the mitral and tricuspid valves. For example, when the force of ventricular contraction is enhanced, the first heart sound is greatly accentuated. Conversely, in a weakened heart, in which the onset of contraction is sluggish, the intensity of the first heart sound is diminished.

The loudness of the second heart sound is determined by the rate of decrease in ventricular pressure at the end of systole. For this reason, the intensity of the second heart sound is accentuated in the presence of systemic or pulmonary hypertension. Conversely, when arterial pressure is low as in shock or cardiac failure, the second heart sound, as heard through a stethoscope, is diminished in intensity.

Third Heart Sound

Occasionally, a third heart sound is heard at the beginning of the middle third of diastole. The third heart sound is of such low frequency that it usually cannot be detected with a stethoscope but can be recorded on the phonocardiogram. This sound presumably results from the flaccid and inelastic condition of the heart during diastole.

Fourth Heart Sound

The fourth heart sound is caused by rapid inflow of blood into the ventricles due to atrial contraction. The frequency of this heart sound is so low that it rarely can be heard using a stethoscope.

Auscultation of Heart Sounds

The optimal areas for auscultation of heart sounds on the chest are not directly over the specific valve (Fig. 47-5) (Guyton, 1986c). The optimal area for auscultation of the aortic or pulmonary valve is upward along the aorta and pulmonary artery respectively. The tricuspid heart sound is best heard over the right ventricle. Closure of the mitral valve is best heard over the apex of the heart. This is true because the cardiac apex is the only portion of the left ventricle near the surface of the chest as the heart is rotated such that most of the left ventricle lies behind the right ventricle. For this reason, the sounds caused by closure of the mitral and tricuspid valves are transmitted to the chest wall through each respective ventricle and sounds from the aortic and pulmonary valves are transmitted along the courses of the respective vessels leading from the heart. This emphasizes that vibrations of the ventricles or large arteries are the cause of heart sounds.

Abnormal Heart Sounds

Abnormal heart sounds known as murmurs occur in the presence of abnormalities of the cardiac valves.

Murmur of Aortic Stenosis

Resistance to ejection of blood through a stenotic aortic valve causes pressure in the left ventricle to increase to values as great as 350 mmHg while pressure in the aorta remains normal. Thus, a nozzle effect is created during systole with blood jetting at a high velocity through the small opening of the aortic valve. This turbulent flow causes vibrations, and a systolic murmur is transmitted throughout the upper aorta and even into the carotid arteries. Vibrations in the form of a thrill can often be felt by placing the hand on the upper chest.

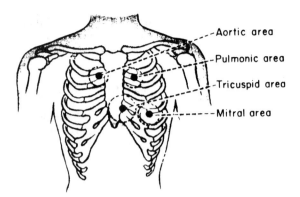

FIGURE 47-5. Optimal sites for auscultation of heart sounds due to opening or closing of specific cardiac valves. (From Guyton AC. Textbook of Medical Physiology. 7th ed. Philadelphia: WB Saunders, 1986:316. Reproduced by permission of the author and publisher.)

Murmur of Aortic Regurgitation

In aortic regurgitation, a murmur occurs during diastole as a result of vibrations from turbulence created by blood jetting backward into blood already in the left ventricle. The murmur of aortic regurgitation is not as loud as that of aortic stenosis because the pressure differential between the aorta and left ventricle is not nearly as great as it is in aortic stenosis.

Murmur of Mitral Stenosis

In the presence of mitral stenosis, a low intensity murmur occurs in diastole. The abnormal sounds present in mitral stenosis are of low intensity because, except for brief periods, the pressure differential forcing blood from the left atrium into the left ventricle rarely exceeds 35 mmHg.

Murmur of Mitral Regurgitation

Backward flow of blood through an incompetent mitral valve during left ventricular contraction produces a loud swishing systolic murmur. The left atrium is located so deeply in the chest that it is difficult to hear this murmur directly over the atrium. As a result, the sound of mitral regurgitation is transmitted to the chest wall mainly through the left ventricle and typically is heard best at the apex of the heart. Presumably, the murmur of mitral regurgitation is caused by vibrations from turbulence of blood ejected backward through the mitral valve against the atrial wall or into blood already in the left atrium. The quality of the murmur of mitral regurgitation is similar to that of aortic regurgitation, but it occurs during systole rather than diastole.

CONDUCTION OF THE CARDIAC IMPULSE

The adult heart contracts at a rate of 70 to 80 beats min^{-1} (Guyton, 1986d). A special excitatory and conductive system controls these rhythmic cardiac contractions (Fig. 47-6). The self-excitatory impulse is initially generated in the sinoatrial node and conducted to the atrioventricular node where it is delayed before passing into the ventricles. In the ventricles, the cardiac impulse travels via the atrioventricular bundle (bundle of His) to the left and right bundles of Purkinje fibers which are distributed over the surfaces of both ventricles.

Sinoatrial Node

The sinoatrial node is a strip of specialized cardiac muscle about 3 mm wide and 10 mm long located in the posterior wall of the right atrium immediately beneath and medial to the opening of the superior vena cava. The fibers of the sinoatrial node are continuous with the atrial fibers such that an action potential that begins in the sinoatrial node spreads immediately into the atria.

Sinoatrial fibers exhibit a resting transmembrane potential of only about -60 mv in comparison with -90 mv in most other cardiac fibers (Vasselle, 1979). This low resting transmembrane potential is caused by increased leakiness of the membrane of sinoatrial fibers to sodium ions. This leakage of sodium ions is responsible for the self-excitation and rhythmical repetitiveness of the action potentials in the sinoatrial node. Immediately after the action potential is over, the transmembrane potential reaches its greatest degree of negativity (*i.e.,* hyperpolarization) reflecting maximum permeability of the membrane to potassium ions. Potassium ions diffusing out of the cell carry positive charges away from the interior of the cell. This phenomenon does not persist because the high degree of negativity inside the membrane causes the membrane to become progressively less permeable to potassium ions and the natural leakiness of the membrane to sodium ions returns. As a result, the transmembrane potential slowly drifts back toward a less negative value until it reaches again the threshold for self-excitation of the fiber.

Internodal Pathways

Action potentials originating in the sinoatrial node spread through the entire atrial muscle mass on their way to the atrioventricular node. There are, however, internodal pathways that conduct the

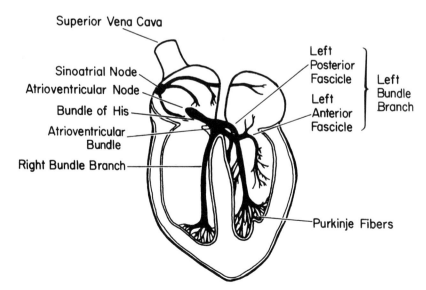

FIGURE 47-6. Anatomy of the conduction system for transmission of the cardiac impulse.

cardiac impulse from the sinoatrial to atrioventric-ular node more rapidly (0.45 – 0.6 m sec^{-1}) than in the general mass of the atrial muscle (0.3 m sec^{-1}) (Guyton, 1986d).

Atrioventricular Node

There is a delay of transmission of the cardiac im-pulse in the atrioventricular node which allows the atria to empty blood into the ventricles before ventricular systole is initiated. The cardiac im-pulse originating in the sinoatrial node typically reaches the atrioventricular node in about 0.04 second. Between this time and the time the im-pulse emerges from the atrioventricular node, an-other 0.11 second elapses. The cause of slow con-duction in the atrioventricular node is related to the small size of the fibers and the presence of fewer points of tight fusion between the cardiac muscle cells in this node. Both of these character-istics slow conduction of the cardiac impulse through the atrioventricular node.

Purkinje System

Purkinje fibers originating in the atrioventricular node form the atrioventricular bundle (bundle of His) which passes between the valves of the heart into ventricular muscle (Fig. 47-6). The atrioven-tricular bundle divides almost immediately into left and right bundle branches that lie beneath the endocardium on each side of the septum. The left bundle divides into the left anterior and left poste-rior fascicle. These branches descend towards the apex of each ventricle dividing into smaller branches that spread around each ventricle.

Purkinje fibers that lead from the atrioventric-ular node through the atrioventricular bundle and into the ventricles are large fibers that transmit cardiac impulses at a velocity of 1.5 to 4 m sec^{-1}. This rapid velocity permits nearly immediate transmission of cardiac impulses through the en-tire ventricular system. Indeed, only 0.03 second elapses from when the cardiac impulse first enters the atrioventricular bundle and when it reaches the terminations of Purkinje fibers. This rapid spread of excitation throughout the entire ventric-ular muscle mass causes ventricular muscle in both ventricles to contract at almost exactly the same time. Effective pumping by the two ventricu-lar chambers requires this synchronous type of

contraction. Any delay in transmission of cardiac impulses through the ventricle can make it possi-ble for impulses from the last excited ventricular muscle fiber to re-enter the first muscle fiber and produce ventricular fibrillation. Ordinarily, rapid transmission of cardiac impulses means the first stimulated fibers are still refractory at the time the last fibers are stimulated.

Cardiac Pacemakers

A cardiac pacemaker cell is one that undergoes spontaneous phase 4 depolarization to reach threshold potential and thus undergo self-excita-tion and propagation of the cardiac potential. The rate at which cardiac pacemaker cells discharge is determined by the (1) slope of phase 4 depolari-zation, (2) resting transmembrane potential, and (3) threshold potential (see the section entitled Cardiac Action Potential). The normal rate of dis-charge is accelerated by (1) increasing the slope of phase 4 depolarization, (2) raising the resting transmembrane potential (*i.e.,* less negative), and (3) lowering the threshold potential (*i.e.,* more negative).

Although many cardiac cells can undergo spontaneous phase 4 depolarization, propagation of the cardiac impulse from the sinoatrial node will interrupt this process in other cells (*e.g.,* la-tent cardiac pacemakers) before they reach threshold potential. The role of the sinoatrial node as the normal cardiac pacemaker reflects the higher intrinsic rate of discharge of this node rela-tive to other portions of the specialized cardiac conduction system (Irisawa, 1978). For example, atrioventricular nodal fibers discharge at an intrin-sic rate of 40 to 60 times min^{-1} and Purkinje fibers discharge at rates of 15 to 40 times min^{-1} com-pared with an intrinsic sinoatrial node rate of 70 to 80 times min^{-1}. As a result, the sinoatrial node excites these other potentially self-excitatory tis-sues before they can discharge independently. For this reason, the sinoatrial node functions as the normal pacemaker of the heart. A cardiac pace-maker other than the sinoatrial node is called an *ectopic pacemaker.*

Cardiac Rhythm and Autonomic Nervous System Innervation

Parasympathetic nervous system fibers (vagal) are distributed mainly to the sinoatrial node and atrioventricular node with less distribution to atrial muscle and even less to ventricular muscle. Sympathetic nervous system fibers are distributed to these same areas but have a greater presence in ventricular muscle than do parasympathetic nervous system fibers.

Parasympathetic Nervous System

Stimulation of parasympathetic nervous system fibers to the heart causes the release of acetylcholine which depresses the intrinsic rate of discharge of the sinoatrial node and slows the rate of transmission of the cardiac impulse through atrial internodal pathways to the atrioventricular node. Acetylcholine also depresses activity of the atrioventricular node. The mechanism of these effects is the ability of acetylcholine to increase permeability of cardiac muscle cell membranes to potassium ions allowing the rapid leakage of these ions to the exterior. This loss of potassium ions results in hyperpolarization of cell membranes and renders excitable tissue less excitable. Strong stimulation by the parasympathetic nervous system can completely stop activity of the sinoatrial node and block transmission of the cardiac impulse to the ventricles. In this instance, an ectopic cardiac pacemaker, usually in the atrioventricular bundle, causes ventricular contraction at a rate of 15 to 40 beats min^{-1}. This phenomenon is known as *ventricular escape.*

Sympathetic Nervous System

Stimulation of sympathetic nervous system fibers to the heart causes the release of norepinephrine which is presumed to act by increasing permeability of cardiac muscle cell membranes to sodium and calcium ions. In the sinoatrial node, an increase in permeability to sodium ions facilitates the decay of the resting transmembrane potential toward the threshold potential. As a result, the intrinsic rate of discharge of the sinoatrial node is increased and the heart rate is elevated. A similar increase in permeability to sodium ions in the atrioventricular node decreases conduction time for cardiac impulses to travel to the ventricles.

CIRCULATORY EFFECTS OF HEART DISEASE

Valvular heart disease produces circulatory effects related to volume overload (regurgitant lesions) or pressure overload (stenotic lesions) of the atria or ventricles. Congenital heart disease produces circulatory effects predominantly due to the presence of a left-to-right or right-to-left intracardiac shunt.

Aortic Valve Disease

Aortic stenosis or aortic regurgitation results in a decrease in forward left ventricular stroke volume. Compensatory responses to offset this decreased cardiac output include hypertrophy of left ventricular muscle and an increase in circulating blood volume. Hypertrophy of left ventricular muscle allows the ventricle to develop high pressures to eject blood across a stenotic valve or to accommodate the large volume of blood associated with aortic regurgitation. The left ventricle may hypertrophy to four or five times normal such that the heart may weigh 1000 g compared to a normal weight of about 280 g. In severe aortic regurgitation, the hypertrophied cardiac muscle allows the left ventricle to eject a stroke volume as high as 300 ml although most of this returns to the ventricle during diastole. Diminished renal blood flow associated with these valvular lesions stimulates fluid retention and a subsequent increase in circulating blood volume that facilitates venous return. In addition, hematocrit increases because of a modest degree of tissue hypoxia. These compensatory responses often prevent symptoms. Indeed, severe degrees of aortic stenosis or aortic regurgitation may be present before the patient becomes symptomatic. This emphasizes the importance of seeking the presence of cardiac murmurs during the preoperative physical examination in an otherwise asymptomatic patient.

Myocardial ischemia commonly occurs in patients with aortic valve disease. In aortic stenosis, high intraventricular pressures reduce coronary blood flow to almost zero during systole. If intraventricular pressures remain elevated during diastole, coronary blood flow is also impaired. The subendocardium is particularly vulnerable to myocardial ischemia in the presence of elevated intracavitary pressures. In aortic regurgitation, the problem is further compounded because the diastolic aortic pressure frequently falls to very low values as blood regurgitates back into the left ventricle. Because most of the coronary blood flow to the left ventricle occurs during diastole, this low diastolic blood pressure can be particularly detrimental to myocardial oxygenation. Furthermore, development of collateral coronary vasculature may not occur to the same extent as the mass of cardiac muscle resulting in myocardial ischemia.

Mitral Valve Disease

Net movement of blood from the left atrium into the left ventricle is reduced by mitral stenosis or mitral regurgitation. Accumulation of blood in the left atrium causes progressive increases in left atrial pressure which eventually lead to pulmonary edema. Pulmonary edema usually does not occur, however, until the mean left atrial pressure rises above 30 mmHg. Often, the mean left atrial pressure must rise to as high as 45 mmHg before pulmonary edema occurs, reflecting enlargement of the pulmonary lymph vessels which can carry excess fluid away from the lung tissues (see Chapter 46).

High left atrial pressure also causes progressive enlargement of the left atrium which increases the distance that the cardiac impulse must travel in the atrial wall. Eventually, this pathway becomes so long that it predisposes to the development of circus movements manifesting as atrial fibrillation. The onset of atrial fibrillation further compromises the cardiac output.

As the left atrial and pulmonary capillary pressures increase, blood also begins to pool in the pulmonary artery. This, combined with incipient pulmonary edema, evokes intense constriction of the pulmonary arterioles with elevations in the pulmonary artery pressure to as high as 60 mmHg. Right ventricular hypertrophy and pulmonary hypertension are end-results of these changes.

Compensatory responses to mitral valve disease include increased circulating blood volume to maintain venous return. Left ventricular hypertrophy does not occur in mitral stenosis. Moderate left and right ventricular hypertrophy may accompany chronic mitral regurgitation.

Exercise and Valvular Heart Disease

During exercise, large quantities of venous blood are returned to the heart from the peripheral circulation resulting in exacerbation of all the circulatory abnormalities associated with valvular heart disease. In patients who are asymptomatic at rest, exercise may result in dyspnea and pulmonary edema within a few minutes reflecting an inability to increase cardiac output in the presence of increased tissue oxygen demands. For this reason, exercise tolerance is a valuable clinical indicator of both the presence and severity of valvular heart disease.

Congenital Heart Disease

Three major types of congenital heart disease are (1) stenosis of a cardiac valve or major blood vessel, (2) left-to-right intracardiac shunt, and (3) right-to-left intracardiac shunt. The three most common types of stenotic lesions are coarctation of the aorta, congenital pulmonary stenosis, and congenital aortic stenosis. Examples of left-to-right intracardiac shunts in which pulmonary blood flow is greatly increased include patent ductus arteriosus, atrial septal defect, and ventricular septal defect. In these patients, the cardiac output is increased to offset the increased pulmonary blood flow and thus maintain a relatively normal systemic blood flow. This creates an extra work load on the heart such that cardiac failure often occurs at an early age. Right-to-left intracardiac shunts are characterized by decreased pulmonary blood flow and direct return of venous blood to the arterial circulation. As a result, arterial hypoxemia is chronically present in these patients. The most common type of right-to-left intracardiac shunt is tetralogy of Fallot. Congenital defects of the heart are often associated with other congenital defects elsewhere in the body.

Patent Ductus Arteriosus

At birth, the lungs expand allowing pulmonary arterial pressures to fall, and at the same time systemic pressures increase because of cessation of blood flow through the low-resistance placenta. As a result, forward blood flow through the ductus arteriosus ceases abruptly at birth and within a few hours the ductus arteriosus becomes occluded in most newborns. It is likely that the high arterial oxygen concentration of the aortic blood that perfuses the ductus arteriosus after birth causes vasoconstriction of the ductus muscle. Nevertheless, in about 1 out of every 5500 newborns the ductus arteriosus does not close spontaneously and the phenomenon known as patent ductus arteriosus occurs.

In the presence of a patent ductus arteriosus,

blood flows backward from the aorta into the lungs. The magnitude of blood flow through the ductus arteriosus increases as the child grows older and systemic pressures become greater. Pulmonary blood flow may be two to three times systemic blood flow. Because cardiac output is elevated at rest, these patients exhibit reduced exercise tolerance. Left ventricular hypertrophy reflects the increased work load of the heart to maintain a normal cardiac output. Increased pulmonary blood flow results in elevated pulmonary artery pressures and right ventricular hypertrophy. Furthermore, sustained exposure of pulmonary vessels to excessive blood flow leads to progressive sclerosis of the vessels and increased resistance to blood flow. Cyanosis does not occur unless severe cardiac failure develops.

At birth, the amount of reversed blood flow may be inadequate to cause a murmur. As the child grows, a continuous murmur becomes audible in the pulmonic area being most intense during systole when pressure in the aorta is elevated and less intense during the low pressure phase of diastole. This accounts for a murmur that waxes and wanes with each heart beat creating the so-called machinery murmur. Treatment of patent ductus arteriosus is surgical ligation.

Atrial Septal Defect

An atrial septal defect produces a left-to-right intracardiac shunt. This defect may occur at the foramen ovale or another site in the atrial septa leading to increasing pulmonary blood flow, pulmonary hypertension, and right ventricular hypertrophy.

FORAMEN OVALE. Normally, the foramen ovale closes at birth when pulmonary artery pressures decline and systemic blood pressures increase leading to corresponding changes in the right and left atrial pressures (see Chapter 44). In about one third of patients, however, the flap-like opening covering the foramen ovale does not adhere to the atrial septum. Nevertheless, the left atrial pressure which is 1 to 3 mmHg greater than the right atrial pressure keeps the flap closed over the foramen ovale. Clearly, events that abruptly and selectively increase right atrial pressure over left atrial pressure could produce an unexpected right-to-left intracardiac shunt and arterial hypoxemia in patients with a "probe" patent foramen ovale. Positive pressure ventilation of the lungs

with or without positive end-expiratory pressure can selectively increase right arterial pressure and open a "probe" patent foramen ovale (Moorthy and LoSasso, 1974).

Ventricular Septal Defect

A ventricular septal defect produces a left-to-right intracardiac shunt reflecting the fact that pressure in the left ventricle is about six times that in the right ventricle. Blood flow through the intracardiac shunt elevates right ventricular pressure and pulmonary blood flow leading to right ventricular hypertrophy and ultimately pulmonary hypertension. The presence of a ventricular septal defect is indicated by a systolic blowing murmur and the presence of oxygenated blood in the right ventricle. The presence of the murmur only during systole rather than continuously, as occurs with a patent ductus arteriosus, emphasizes that blood flow from the systemic circulation to the pulmonary circulation occurs only during systole and not continuously as through a patent ductus arteriosus.

Tetralogy of Fallot

Tetralogy of Fallot is the classic cause of right-to-left intracardiac shunt. Abnormalities associated with tetralogy of Fallot include an aorta that overrides the interventricular septum, pulmonary artery narrowing, a ventricular septal defect, and right ventricular hypertrophy. The major physiologic derangement caused by tetralogy of Fallot is shunting of as much as 75% of returning venous blood through the ventricular septal defect directly to the aorta resulting in poor pulmonary blood flow and profound arterial hypoxemia even at birth. The left ventricle may be smaller than the hypertrophied right ventricle.

MYOCARDIAL INFARCTION

Relatively few communications exist among the larger coronary arteries while many anastomoses exist among smaller arteries up to 250 μ in diameter (Cosby *et al*, 1974). When a sudden occlusion occurs in a larger coronary artery, these small vessels dilate maximally in a few seconds. Blood flow through these small vessels, however, is inadequate to maintain viability of all the supplied cardiac muscle. True collaterals do not enlarge further for the next 8 to 24 hours. Coronary blood flow via collaterals may be returned to normal within 1 month. When atherosclerosis constricts the coronary arteries slowly over many years rather than suddenly, collaterals can develop simultaneously and prevent overt evidence of coronary artery disease.

Causes of Mortality

The four major causes of mortality following a myocardial infarction are (1) decreased cardiac output, (2) pulmonary edema, (3) ventricular fibrillation, and (4) rarely rupture of the heart (Guyton and Daggett, 1976).

Decreased Cardiac Output

Low cardiac output usually occurs immediately after a myocardial infarction. The overall pumping ability of the ventricle is impaired when some cardiac muscle fibers are infarcted or ischemic and thus too weak to contract vigorously. In some instances, when normal portions of the ventricle contract, the damaged muscle is forced outward (*i.e.,* aneurysmal) by the intracavitary pressure (Fig. 47-7) (Guyton, 1986b). As a result, much of the pumping force is dissipated into the area of the ventricular aneurysm. An inadequate cardiac output leading to cardiogenic shock almost always occurs when more than 40% of the left ventricular muscle is infarcted. Mortality is greater than 80% when cardiogenic shock follows myocardial infarction.

Pulmonary Edema

Diminished cardiac output invariably leads to pooling of blood in pulmonary capillaries with associated increases in capillary pressure. Furthermore, decreased cardiac output causes reduced renal blood flow with subsequent retention of large volumes of fluid. Often, pulmonary edema develops suddenly, several days following myocardial infarction in patients who previously had been recovering without complications (see the section entitled Selective Left Ventricular Failure).

Ventricular Fibrillation

Ventricular fibrillation is a common cause of sudden death related to myocardial infarction. At least

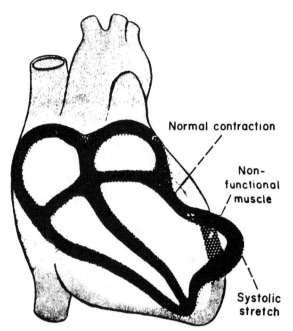

FIGURE 47-7. Aneurysmal dilatation of ischemic left ventricular muscle may follow a myocardial infarction leading to reductions in cardiac output. (From Guyton AC. Textbook of Medical Physiology. 7th ed. Philadelphia: WB Saunders, 1986:295. Reproduced by permission of the author and publisher.)

four different factors contribute to the likelihood of ventricular fibrillation. First, acute ischemia or infarction causes depletion of potassium ions from the damaged cardiac muscle. The subsequent elevation in the extracellular concentration of potassium ions increases the irritability of cardiac muscle. Second, ischemic cardiac musculature cannot repolarize (*i.e.,* current of injury) such that electrical current flows to the normal myocardium where it can evoke abnormal impulses. Third, sympathetic nervous system reflexes accompany myocardial infarction and can contribute to myocardial irritability. Fourth, dilatation of the ventricle associated with myocardial infarction lengthens the pathway for conduction of the cardiac impulse and may result in abnormal conduction pathways around the infarcted area.

Rupture of the Infarcted Area

Rupture of an area of acute myocardial infarction is unlikely in the first day. Several days later, however, the infarcted cardiac muscle may degenerate and increase the likelihood of cardiac rupture with subsequent acute cardiac tamponade.

Stages of Recovery from Acute Myocardial Infarction

Within 1 hour after myocardial infarction, the muscle fibers in the center of the ischemic area die. During the next few days, collateral channels growing into the outer rim of the infarcted area cause the nonfunctional area of cardiac muscle to become smaller. At the same time, fibrous tissue begins developing among the infarcted fibers because ischemia stimulates growth of fibroblasts and promotes development of greater than normal amounts of fibrous tissue. Fibrous tissue subsequently contracts such that the scar becomes smaller over a period of several months. This scarring process usually reverses any aneurysmal effect associated with an infarcted area. Furthermore, normal areas of the heart gradually hypertrophy to compensate for the damaged cardiac musculature. Nevertheless, the ability of the heart to increase its cardiac output following recovery from a myocardial infarction is commonly less than in otherwise normal hearts.

The magnitude of cardiac cell death is determined by the degree of ischemia times the metabolism of the heart muscle. This emphasizes the need to rest and avoid sympathetic nervous system stimulation following an acute myocardial infarction.

ANGINA PECTORIS

The likely cause of angina pectoris is stimulation of nerve endings in cardiac muscle by the release of lactic acid, histamine, or kinins from ischemic muscle. Distribution of pain into the arms and neck reflects the embryonic origin of the heart and arm in the neck (see Chapter 43). Therefore, both these structures receive pain fibers from the same spinal cord segments (*e.g.,* T2 – T5). Angina pectoris occurs when metabolic requirements for oxygen exceed oxygen delivery via coronary blood flow as may occur during exercise or events associated with stimulation of the sympathetic nervous system. Nitroglycerin most likely relieves angina pectoris by reducing venous return to the heart resulting in decreased cardiac output, blood pressure, and thus myocardial oxygen requirements (see Chapter 16). Associated dilation of large epi-cardial arteries may provide additional benefit. Nitroglycerin, however, does not dilate coronary arterioles. Blockade of beta receptors is also useful in relieving angina pectoris presumably by decreasing heart rate and myocardial contractility and thus reducing myocardial oxygen requirements.

CARDIAC FAILURE

The principal defect in cardiac failure (*e.g.,* congestive heart failure) is an inability of the myocardium to optimally utilize energy available for contraction. This results in a decreased force of contraction of the ventricles manifesting as a decreased maximal velocity of shortening (V_{max}). The weakened ventricle is unable to pump the blood delivered to it such that venous pressure is elevated and ventricular end-diastolic pressure rises. As the heart becomes weaker, the ventricles begin dilating and their residual volume increases thus stretching the myocardial muscles and, according to the Frank-Starling law, raises the cardiac output. As the intraventricular diameter increases even further, tension that has to be developed by the myocardial muscle to achieve that same intraventricular pressure increases (Laplace's law). Finally, a point is reached where further increases in myocardial fiber length do not produce additional improvement in cardiac output and the force of myocardial contraction decreases.

Cardiac failure leads to an increase in atrial pressures because the ventricles are unable to pump the blood they receive. This increased atrial pressure is reflected in the pulmonary and peripheral venous systems. The increase in peripheral venous pressure will raise intracapillary pressure leading to tissue edema. If the increase in atrial pressure is predominantly in the left atrium, increased venous pressure will be reflected primarily in the lungs and the principal complaint is dyspnea. Pulmonary edema is present when fluid enters the alveoli. Selective elevations in right atrial pressure manifest as distention of the neck veins, hepatomegaly, ascites, and peripheral edema.

Cardiac failure manifests as decreased cardiac output or pulmonary edema due to accumulation of blood in the lungs. Selective left ventricular failure occurs 30 times more often than selective right ventricular failure (Guyton, 1986e). Myocardial infarction and chronic hypertension are common causes of left ventricular cardiac failure. Valvular heart disease may produce left or right ventricular failure depending on the location of the diseased valve. Inhaled anesthetics produce exaggerated reductions in myocardial contractility when administered in the presence of cardiac failure (Kemmotsu et al, 1973).

Sympathetic nervous system stimulation plays an important role in the acute compensatory responses to cardiac failure. These reflex responses increase the tone of the vasculature, especially the veins, resulting in increased venous return and filling pressures, which helps the heart pump larger quantities of blood. Elevated plasma concentrations of catecholamines or increased urinary excretion of catecholamines is invariably present in patients with cardiac failure. Density of beta-adrenergic receptors is also decreased in cardiac cell membranes of failing left ventricles (Bristow et al, 1982).

Renal Effects of Cardiac Failure

Chronic reductions in cardiac output associated with cardiac failure result in renal-induced retention of fluid in an effort to raise the circulating blood volume and thus improve venous return to the heart (Barger, 1960). For example, decreased cardiac output reduces glomerular filtration rate due to reduced blood pressure and intense sympathetic nervous system-induced constriction of the renal arterioles. Reduced renal blood flow also stimulates renin release with subsequent production of angiotensin and resulting stimulation of aldosterone secretion by the adrenal cortex (see Chapter 52). Increased plasma concentrations of potassium associated with decreased renal function also act as a powerful independent stimulus for the secretion of aldosterone. Decreased hepatic blood flow associated with cardiac failure further prolongs the duration of action of aldosterone by reducing its rate of metabolism. Therefore, the net loss of water and salt into the urine is greatly reduced, and extracellular fluid volume increases. Finally, increased secretion of antidiuretic hormone stimulates water reabsorption by the renal tubules.

Modest fluid retention is helpful as a compensatory mechanism for decreased cardiac output. Indeed, increased blood volume distends veins which reduces resistance to flow and thus permits increased ease of venous return of blood to the heart. Excess fluid accumulation, however, can evoke detrimental effects as characterized by overstretching of an already weakened heart and pulmonary edema with associated reductions in arterial oxygenation.

Compensated Cardiac Failure

Compensated cardiac failure is characterized by chronically elevated right atrial pressures that help maintain cardiac output at near normal despite a reduced cardiac reserve. Slight elevations of right atrial pressure have little harmful effect except perhaps a modest degree of hepatomegaly and a tendency to develop ankle edema. However, any increased stress, such as exercise, sepsis, anesthesia, and surgery, may unmask the reduced cardiac reserve in these patients. Dyspnea and excessive activity of the sympathetic nervous system are likely to manifest when increased cardiac output is required.

Decompensated Cardiac Failure

When cardiac failure is severe, compensation via fluid retention and activation of the sympathetic nervous system cannot return the cardiac output to normal even at rest. As a result, cardiac output cannot increase sufficiently to restore normal renal function. Indeed, the main basis for decompensated cardiac failure is an inability of the heart to pump sufficient blood to restore renal blood flow and normal kidney function. Right atrial pressures also continue to increase, and eventually cardiac output begins to decline. When cardiac output declines, fluid retention is accelerated. Clinically, pulmonary edema and peripheral edema are prominent.

In addition to progressive fluid retention, there is also progressive deterioration of myocardial contractility and depression of the calcium mechanism responsible for causing excitation–contraction coupling. Furthermore, the amount of norepinephrine stored in cardiac sympathetic nerve endings is depleted in the chronically failing heart. For this reason, the failing myocardium may respond poorly to sympathetic nervous system stimulation or inotropic drugs.

Treatment of decompensated cardiac failure is administration of inotropic drugs to strengthen myocardial contractility and thus restore cardiac output and renal blood flow (see Chapter 13). In addition, limitation of sodium intake and administration of diuretics facilitate excretion of excess fluid.

Selective Left Ventricular Failure

Selective left ventricular failure leads to accumulation of blood in the lungs and pulmonary edema if mean pulmonary capillary pressure rises above 30 mmHg. In moderate acute left ventricular failure, pulmonary capillary pressures may not rise sufficiently to cause pulmonary edema initially, but progressive retention of fluid by the kidneys eventually causes further increases in capillary pressures and the sudden onset of pulmonary edema several days after the initial insult.

Selective Right Ventricular Failure

Selective right ventricular failure is characterized by a shift of blood from the pulmonary to systemic circulations. The compliance of the systemic circulation fails to sufficiently increase venous return to maintain an acceptable right ventricular stroke volume. As a result, acute right ventricular failure can cause greater depression of cardiac output than the same degree of left ventricular failure.

Systemic congestion alone can occur in selective chronic right ventricular failure. In this condition, there is no pulmonary congestion and, if sufficient fluids have been retained, the cardiac output is maintained near normal.

High Output Cardiac Failure

High output cardiac failure is due to excessive venous return of blood to the heart rather than decreased myocardial contractility. Decreased peripheral vascular resistance and increased venous return to the heart, as associated with arteriovenous fistulae or thyrotoxicosis, may lead to high output cardiac failure.

Cardiac Reserve

Cardiac reserve is the maximum amount cardiac output can increase above normal in response to stress. In the normal young adult, cardiac output can increase 3 to 4 times. Coronary artery disease or valvular heart disease reduces cardiac reserve. At rest, patients with reduced cardiac reserve are often asymptomatic but with any stress, such as increased exercise activity, the heart is unable to increase its cardiac output. As a result, tissue blood flow and oxygen delivery are inadequate leading to dyspnea and skeletal muscle weakness.

Ventricular Function Curves

Ventricular function curves (also known as Frank-Starling curves) describe the interrelationship between the ventricular end-diastolic pressure and the cardiac output (see Fig. 44-11). Under normal conditions, cardiac ventricular muscle operates on the ascending limb of the curve such that an increase in end-diastolic pressure results in an increase in stroke volume. Further stretching of the cardiac muscle beyond a certain point, however, results in a reduction in stroke volume. In a failing heart, a decrease in myocardial contractility is depicted as a downward shift of the ventricular function curve.

CIRCULATORY SHOCK

Circulatory shock is characterized by inadequate tissue blood flow and oxygen delivery to cells resulting in generalized deterioration of organ function. The usual cause of inadequate tissue perfusion in circulatory shock is inadequate cardiac output due either to direct myocardial depression as follows a myocardial infarction or decreased venous return as associated with a diminished blood volume.

Shock Due to Hypovolemia

Hemorrhage is the most common cause of shock due to hypovolemia. Venous return is reduced by hemorrhage leading to a reduction in cardiac output. About 10% of the blood volume can be lost with no significant effect on blood pressure or cardiac output. Additional blood loss, however, usually diminishes cardiac output first and later the blood pressure. Any decrease in blood pressure initiates powerful baroreceptor-mediated increases in sympathetic nervous system activity manifesting as arterial constriction, venoconstriction, and direct myocardial stimulation. Venoconstriction is particularly important in maintaining venous return to the heart and cardiac output. Sympathetic nervous system-mediated arterial constriction is responsible for initially maintaining blood pressure despite reductions in cardiac output (Chien, 1967). This maintenance of blood pressure sustains cerebral and coronary blood flow because significant vasoconstriction does not occur in these organs (Kovach and Sandor, 1976). In other organs, such as the kidneys, intense sympathetic nervous system-mediated vasoconstriction may reduce blood flow dramatically.

Decreased cardiac output associated with shock reduces tissue oxygen delivery which in turn reduces the level of metabolism that can be maintained by different cells of the body. Skeletal muscle weakness is prominent reflecting inadequate delivery of oxygen to this tissue. Metabolism is depressed, and the amount of heat liberated is reduced. As a result, body temperature tends to decrease especially in the presence of a cold environment. In the early stages of shock, consciousness is usually maintained although mental clarity may be impaired. Consciousness is likely to be lost as shock progresses. Low cardiac output greatly diminishes urine output or even causes anuria because glomerular pressure falls below the critical value required for filtration of fluid into Bowman's capsule. Furthermore, the kidney has such a high rate of metabolism and requires such large amounts of nutrients that reduced renal blood flow often causes tubular necrosis and renal failure.

Persistent Shock

An important feature of persistent shock is eventual progressive deterioration of the heart. Thrombosis may occur in minute vessels of the circulation reflecting agglutination of cells. After many hours of capillary hypoxia, permeability of the capillaries gradually increases and large amounts of fluid begin to transudate into the tissues further reducing cardiac output (Zweifach, 1974). In addition to myocardial depression caused by decreased coronary blood flow, the myocardium can also be depressed by toxic factors transported to the heart from other parts of the body. Examples of toxic factors are (1) lactic acid, (2) myocardial

depressant factor, and (3) bacterial toxins absorbed from the gastrointestinal tract.

MYOCARDIAL DEPRESSANT FACTOR. Myocardial depressant factor is a peptide with a molecular weight of 500 to 1000 that is released from the pancreas which has been rendered ischemic by vasoconstriction of the splanchnic circulation during shock (Lefer and Martin, 1970). The most prominent effect of myocardial depressant factor is depression of myocardial contractility by as much as 50%. This toxin may act by interfering with the function of calcium ions in the excitation–contraction coupling process. Indeed, administration of calcium or a cardiac glycoside that causes increased concentrations of calcium in cardiac muscle nullifies the negative inotropic effect of myocardial depressant factor. Regardless of the mechanism of action, release of myocardial depressant factor exacerbates the shock syndrome and is part of the positive feedback deteriorative process that causes progression of shock.

BACTERIAL TOXINS. Another toxic factor that probably contributes to progression of shock is endotoxin released from gram-negative bacteria in the gastrointestinal tract. Diminished blood flow to the gastrointestinal tract causes enhanced absorption of endotoxin which then causes systemic vasodilatation and direct myocardial depression. The release of endotoxin is of obvious importance in septic shock and may be less important during hemorrhagic shock.

Progressive Shock

As shock becomes more severe, there may be signs of generalized cellular deterioration throughout the body. The liver is particularly vulnerable reflecting lack of sufficient nutrients to support the normally high rate of metabolism in hepatic cells. Furthermore, hepatic cells manifest an extreme response to any toxic or abnormal metabolic factors present in shock. For example, active transport of sodium and potassium ions through cell membranes of hepatic cells is greatly diminished leading to loss of potassium ions from the cell. In addition, swelling of hepatic cells occurs. Mitochondrial activity in hepatic cells as well as other tissues including the heart becomes severely depressed.

In the absence of adequate tissue oxygen delivery, cells obtain their energy by the anaerobic process of glycolysis that results in production of excess lactic acid and the appearance of metabolic acidosis that is characteristic of shock. In addition, tissue blood flow may be inadequate to remove carbon dioxide, contributing further to intracellular acidosis.

Irreversible Shock

Irreversible shock is present when so much tissue damage has occurred, so many destructive enzymes have been released into the body fluids, and so much acidosis has developed that even a normal cardiac output cannot reverse the continuing deterioration. High energy phosphate reserves, especially in the liver and in the heart, are greatly diminished in severe degrees of shock. New adenosine triphosphate can be synthesized at the rate of only about 2% an hour. Ultimately, cardiac failure despite aggressive therapy seems to be the cause of irreversible shock. It seems clear that the most important nutrient necessary to prevent cellular deterioration and death during shock is oxygen.

Shock Caused by Plasma Loss

Loss of plasma from the circulatory system in the absence of whole blood loss can result in shock similar to that produced by hemorrhage. Intestinal obstruction results in extreme loss of plasma volume into the gastrointestinal tract. This loss of fluid into the intestine may reflect elevated capillary pressures caused by increased resistance in the stretched veins over the surface of the intestine, or it may be caused by direct damage to capillaries. Severe burns may also be associated with sufficient plasma loss to result in shock. Hypovolemic shock that results from plasma loss has almost the same characteristics as hemorrhagic shock except that selective loss of plasma greatly increases viscosity of blood and exacerbates sluggishness of blood flow.

Neurogenic Shock

Neurogenic shock occurs in the absence of blood loss when vascular capacity increases so greatly that even a normal blood volume is not capable of maintaining venous return and cardiac output. A classic cause of loss of vasomotor tone and subsequent neurogenic shock is acute blockade of the peripheral sympathetic nervous system by spinal or epidural anesthesia.

Septic Shock

Septic shock is characterized by (1) marked peripheral vasodilation throughout the body but particularly in infected tissues, (2) high cardiac output caused by the peripheral vasodilation and high metabolic rate if body temperature is elevated, and (3) the development of disseminated intravascular coagulation. The end-stages of septic shock are not greatly different from the end-stages of hemorrhagic shock, even though the initiating factors are markedly different.

Septic shock due to release of endotoxin occurs frequently when a portion of the gastrointestinal tract loses its blood supply and gram-negative bacteria in the area multiply rapidly. Extension of a urinary tract infection can also result in septic shock. Upon entering the circulation, endotoxin produces direct myocardial depression, peripheral vasodilation, and possibly an anaphylactic reaction.

REFERENCES

Alpert NR, Hemrell BB, Mulieri LA. Heart muscle mechanics. Annu Rev Physiol 1979;41:521–37.

Barger AC. The kidney in congestive heart failure. Circulation 1960;21:124–8.

Berne RM, Rubio R. Adenine nucleotide metabolism in the heart. Circ Res 1974;35:262–71.

Bristow MR, Ginsburg R, Minobe W et al. Decreased catecholamine sensitivity and β-adrenergic-receptor density in failing human hearts. N Engl J Med 1982;307:205–11.

Chien S. Role of the sympathetic nervous system in hemorrhage. Physiol Rev 1967;47:214–88.

Cosby RS, Giddings JA, See JR. Coronary collateral circulation. Chest 1974;66:27–31.

Fabiato A, Fabiato F. Calcium and cardiac excitation–contraction coupling. Annu Rev Physiol 1979;41:473–84.

Guyton AC. Textbook of Medical Physiology. 7th ed. Philadelphia: WB Saunders, 1986a:150.

Guyton AC. Textbook of Medical Physiology. 7th ed. Philadelphia: WB Saunders, 1986b:295.

Guyton AC. Textbook of Medical Physiology. 7th ed. Philadelphia: WB Saunders, 1986c:316.

Guyton AC. Textbook of Medical Physiology. 7th ed. Philadelphia: WB Saunders, 1986d:165.

Guyton AC. Textbook of Medical Physiology. 7th ed. Philadelphia: WB Saunders, 1986e:305.

Guyton RA, Daggett WM. The evolution of myocardial infarction: Physiological basis for clinical intervention. Int Rev Physiol 1976;9:305 – 39.

Irisawa H. Comparative physiology of the cardiac pacemaker mechanism. Physiol Rev 1978;58:461 – 98.

Kaplan JA. Hemodynamic monitoring. In: Kaplan JA, ed. Cardiac Anesthesia. New York, Grune & Stratton. 1979:71 – 115.

Kemmotsu O, Hashimoto Y, Shimosato S. Inotropic effects of isoflurane on mechanics of contraction in isolated cat papillary muscles from normal and failing hearts. Anesthesiology 1973;39:470 – 7.

Klocke FJ, Ellis AK. Control of coronary blood flow. Annu Rev Med 1980;31:489 – 508.

Kovach AGB, Sandor P. Cerebral blood flow and brain function during hypotension. Annu Rev Physiol 1976;38:571 – 96.

Lefer AM, Martin J. Relationship of plasma peptides to the myocardial depressant factor in hemorrhagic shock in cats. Circ Res 1970;26:59 – 69.

Moorthy SS, LoSasso AM. Patency of the foramen ovale in the critically ill patient. Anesthesiology 1974; 41:405 – 7.

Trautwein W. Membrane currents in cardiac muscle fibers. Physiol Rev 1973;53:793 – 835.

Vasselle M. Electrogenesis of the plateau and pacemaker potential. Annu Rev Physiol 1979;41:425 – 40.

Zweifach BW. Mechanisms of blood flow and fluid exchange in microvessels: Hemorrhagic hypotension model. Anesthesiology 1974;41:157 – 68.

The Electrocardiogram
and Analysis of
Cardiac Dysrhythmias

ELECTROCARDIOGRAM

Transmission of the cardiac impulse, which is actually a depolarization and repolarization wave, creates electrical currents which can be recorded as the electrocardiogram. The normal electrocardiogram consists of a (1) P wave, (2) QRS complex which is actually the combination of the Q, R, and S waves, and (3) T wave (Fig. 48-1). The P wave is caused by electrical currents generated as the atria depolarize prior to atrial contraction. The QRS complex is caused by electrical currents generated when the ventricles depolarize prior to ventricular contraction. Therefore, both the P wave and the components of the QRS complex are depolarization waves that occur immediately before actual contraction of the atria or ventricles. The T wave is caused by electrical currents generated as the ventricles recover (*i.e.,* undergo repolarization) from depolarization. This process occurs in ventricular muscle 0.25 to 0.3 second after depolarization, and the resulting T wave is that of repolarization. Ventricular repolarization is prolonged explaining the low voltage of the T wave compared with the QRS complex. The atrial T wave, which reflects repolarization of the atria, is obscured on the electrocardiogram by the larger QRS complex.

Recording of the Electrocardiogram

Paper used for recording of the electrocardiogram is designed so that when calibration of the record-

ing system is appropriate each horizontal line on the paper corresponds to 0.1 mv and each vertical line corresponds to 0.04 second. The voltage of the waves recorded on the normal electrocardiogram depends on the site of the electrode placement. When an electrode is placed directly over the heart, the voltage of the QRS complex will be 3 to 4 mv compared with about 1 mv when the electrodes are placed on the extremities. These voltages are quite small considering the action potential of 120 mv that can be recorded directly from the cardiac muscle membrane.

Electrical currents generated by cardiac muscle during each cardiac cycle can change potentials and polarity in less than 0.01 second. Therefore, any device for recording the electrocardiogram must be capable of responding rapidly to these changes in electrical potentials. An oscilloscope to display the electrocardiogram is commonly utilized for clinical monitoring. Recording of the electrocardiogram on paper utilizes a pen recorder system often with special heat-sensitive paper which turns black when it is exposed to the heated stylus.

The duration of time from the beginning of the P wave and the beginning of the Q wave is the interval between the beginning of contraction of the atria and the beginning of contraction of the ventricles. The normal P–Q interval (often called the P–R interval because the Q wave is frequently absent) is 0.12 to 0.2 second (Fig. 48-1). The QRS complex reflects the time of depolarization corresponding to ventricular excitation and normally lasts 0.05 to 0.1 second. The T wave is in the same

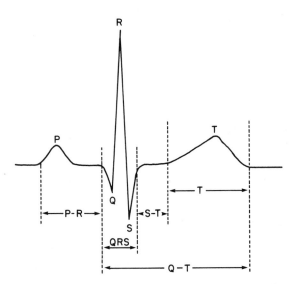

FIGURE 48-1. The normal waves and intervals on the electrocardiogram.

direction as the major deflection of the QRS complex. The Q – T interval represents the time necessary for complete depolarization and repolarization of the ventricle. Depending on the heart rate, the Q – T interval is normally 0.26 to 0.45 second.

Electrocardiogram Leads

In recording the electrocardiogram, various standard positions for placement of electrodes are used. The polarity of the recording on the electrocardiogram during each cardiac cycle is positive or negative depending on the orientation of electrodes with respect to electrical current flow in the heart. Electrical current flow is normally from the base of the heart toward the apex during most of the depolarization phase with the exception being at the very end of the wave. Therefore, an electrode nearer the base of the heart will record a negative potential with respect to an electrode placed nearer the apex of the heart. The usual 12-lead electrocardiogram consists of three standard limb leads, six chest leads, and three augmented unipolar leads.

Standard Limb Leads

Standard limb leads are placed on the left and right arms and the left leg (Fig. 48-2). These leads

record the potential difference between two points on the body. In recording lead I, the positive terminal of the electrocardiograph is connected to the left arm and the negative terminal to the right arm. Lead I, therefore, is the potential difference between the left arm and right arm. In recording lead II, the positive electrode is on the left leg and the negative electrode is on the right arm. Lead III is on the left leg as the positive electrode and the left arm as the negative electrode. Polarity is positive for electrocardiograms recorded from these standard limb leads. The sum of the voltages in leads I and III equals the voltage in lead II. Mathematically, this principle is called Einthoven's law. The axes of the three standard limb leads form the arms of an equilateral triangle known as Einthoven's triangle (Fig. 48-2).

The direction of depolarization of the atria parallels lead II. For this reason, P waves are prominent in this lead. In right atrial hypertrophy, the amplitude and duration of the right atrial component of the P wave overshadows those of the left atrial component and a tall peaked P wave results. This contrasts with left atrial hypertrophy in which the peak of the wave from the left atrium results in a notched P wave.

Chest Leads

Usually six different chest (precordial) leads (V_1 to V_6) are recorded by placing an electrode on the anterior surface of the chest over one of six separate points (Table 48-1). The anterior chest wall electrode is connected to the positive terminal of the electrocardiograph, and the negative or indifferent electrode is normally connected simultaneously through electrical resistances to the right arm, left arm, and left leg.

Each chest lead records mainly the electrical potential of the cardiac muscle immediately beneath the electrode. The nearness of the heart sur-

---

Table 48–1
Placement of Precordial Leads

V_1	Fourth intercostal space at the right sternal border
V_2	Fourth intercostal space at the left sternal border
V_3	Equidistant between V_2 and V_4
V_4	Fifth intercostal space in the left midclavicular line
V_5	Fifth intercostal space in the left anterior axillary line
V_6	Fifth intercostal space in the left midaxillary line

face to the electrode means that relatively minute abnormalities in the ventricles, particularly in the anterior ventricular wall, can produce marked changes in the corresponding electrocardiogram. In leads V_1 and V_2, the normal QRS recordings are mainly negative because the chest electrode in these leads is nearer the base of the heart than the apex. Conversely, the QRS complexes in V_4, V_5, and V_6 are mainly positive because the chest electrode in these leads is nearer the apex of the heart which is the direction of electropositivity during depolarization.

Augmented Unipolar Limb Leads

Augmented unipolar limb leads are recorded when two limbs are connected to the negative terminal of the electrocardiograph while the third limb is connected to the positive terminal. When the positive terminal is on the right arm, the lead is aVR; when on the left arm, the lead is aVL; and when on the left leg, the lead is aVF. The three augmented leads are similar to the standard limb lead recordings except that the recording from the aVR lead is inverted.

Interpretation of the Electrocardiogram

Abnormalities of the heart can be detected by analyzing the contours of the different waves in the various leads of the electrocardiogram. The electrical axis of the heart can be determined from the standard limb leads of Einthoven's triangle. The direction of the vector is denoted in degrees with the zero reference being horizontal towards the subject's left side (Fig. 48-3). From this zero reference point, the scale of vectors rotates clockwise. In a normal heart, the average direction of the vector during spread of the depolarization wave is about 59 degrees. When one ventricle of the heart hypertrophies, the axis of the heart shifts toward the enlarged ventricle. For example, left axis deviation (counterclockwise displacement of the electrical axis to less than 0 degrees) occurs in the presence of left ventricular hypertrophy or left bundle branch block. Right axis deviation (clockwise displacement of the electrical axis to greater than 100 degrees) occurs in the presence of right ventricular hypertrophy or right bundle branch block (Fig. 48-3).

The predominant direction of the vector through the heart during repolarization of the ven-

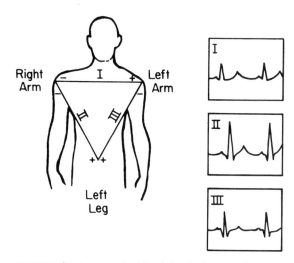

FIGURE 48-2. Standard limb leads (I, II, III) of the electrocardiogram and typical recordings.

tricles is from base to apex, which is also the predominant direction of the vector during depolarization. As a result, the T wave in the normal electrocardiogram is positive, which is also the polarity of most of the normal QRS complex. The vector of current flow during depolarization in the atria is similar to that in the ventricles. As a result, the P waves recorded from standard leads I, II, and III are positive.

Abnormalities of the QRS Complex

Normally, the voltage of the QRS complex in the standard limb leads of the electrocardiogram varies between 0.5 and 2 mv with lead III usually recording the lowest voltage and lead II the highest. High voltage QRS complexes are considered to be present when the sum of the voltages of all the QRS complexes of the three standard limb leads is greater than 4 mv. The most frequent cause of high voltage QRS complexes is ventricular hypertrophy.

The normal QRS complex lasts about 0.06 second and is considered to be prolonged when it lasts more than 0.1 second. Hypertrophy of the ventricles prolongs the duration of the QRS complex to as much as 0.1 second reflecting the longer pathway the ventricular depolarization wave must travel. Blockade of the Purkinje system for conduction of the cardiac impulse greatly slows conduction and prolongs the duration of the QRS

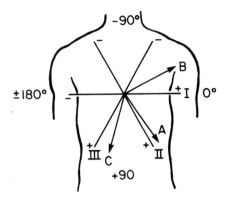

FIGURE 48-3. Electrical axis of the heart as determined from the standard limb leads of the electrocardiogram. In the normal heart, the electrical axis is about 59 degrees (*A*). Left axis deviation shifts the electrical axis to less than 0 degrees (*B*) while right axis deviation is associated with an electrical axis greater than 100 degrees.

complex to 0.12 second or longer. Multiple peaks in an abnormally prolonged QRS complex most often reflect multiple local blocks in conduction of the cardiac impulse in the Purkinje system as may occur from scar tissue formed at sites of myocardial infarction.

Decreased Voltage in the Standard Limb Leads

Causes of decreased voltage on the electrocardiogram recorded from standard limb leads are (1) multiple small myocardial infarctions that prevent generation of large quantities of electrical currents, (2) rotation of the apex of the heart toward the anterior chest wall, and (3) abnormal conditions around the heart so electrical currents cannot be easily conducted from the heart to the surface of the body. For example, pericardial fluid diminishes voltage recorded from standard limb leads due to the ability of this fluid to rapidly conduct electrical currents to multiple sites. Pulmonary emphysema is associated with reduced conduction of electrical current through the lungs because of insulating effects of excessive amounts of air in the lungs.

Current of Injury

A current of injury is due to the inability of damaged areas of the heart to undergo repolarization (*i.e.,* membranes are persistently depolarized) during diastole. The current of injury results when current flows between the pathologically depolarized (negative) and normally polarized (positive) areas. The most common cause of a current of injury is myocardial ischemia or infarction. Mechanical trauma to the heart and infectious processes that damage cardiac muscle membranes (*e.g.,* pericarditis, myocarditis) may also be responsible for a current of injury. In these conditions, a current of injury occurs when the period of depolarization of some cardiac muscle is so long that the muscle fails to repolarize completely before the next cardiac cycle begins.

Specific leads of the electrocardiogram are more likely than other leads to reflect myocardial ischemia that develops in areas of the myocardium supplied by an individual coronary artery (Table 48-2) (McCammon, 1983). Complete interruption of a coronary artery with infarction of the cardiac muscle results in a deep Q wave in the electrocardiogram leads recording from the infarcted area. The Q wave occurs because there is no electrical activity in the infarcted area. A Q wave whose amplitude is more than one-third that of the corresponding R wave and whose duration is more than 0.04 second is diagnostic of a myocardial infarction. In the presence of an old anterior myocardial infarction, a Q wave develops in lead I because of loss of muscle mass in the anterior left wall of the left ventricle. Conversely, in posterior infarction, a Q wave develops in lead III because of loss of cardiac muscle in the posterior apical part of the ventricle.

Abnormalities of the T Wave

The T wave is normally positive in all the standard limb leads reflecting occurrence of repolarization of the apex of the heart before the endocardial surfaces of the ventricles. The direction that repolarization spreads over the heart is backward to the direction in which depolarization takes place. The T wave becomes abnormal when the normal sequence of repolarization does not occur. For example, delay of conduction of the cardiac impulse through the ventricles (*i.e.,* prolonged depolarization), as occurs with left or right bundle branch block or ventricular premature contractions, results in a T wave with a polarity opposite the QRS complex.

Myocardial ischemia is the most common cause of prolonged depolarization of cardiac mus-

Table 48–2

Relationship of Electrocardiogram Lead Reflecting Myocardial Ischemia to Area of Myocardium Involved

Electrocardiogram Lead	Coronary Artery Responsible for Ischemia	Area of Myocardium Supplied by Coronary Artery
II, III, aVF	Right coronary artery	Right atrium Interatrial septum Right ventricle Sinoatrial node Atrioventricular node
V_3–V_5	Left anterior descending coronary artery	Anterior laterial left ventricle
I, aVL	Circumflex coronary artery	Lateral aspects of left ventricle Sinoatrial node Atrioventricular node

(By permission, McCammon RL. Coronary artery disease. In: Stoelting RK, Dierdorf SF, eds. Anesthesia and Co-Existing Disease. Churchill Livingstone Inc., New York, 1983.)

cle. When myocardial ischemia occurs in only one area of the heart, the duration of depolarization of this area increases out of proportion to that in other portions resulting in abnormalities (inversion, biphasic) of the T wave. Myocardial ischemia also leads to elevation of the ST segment on the electrocardiogram. To be clinically significant, the ST segment elevation should be at least 1 mm above the base line (Mason *et al,* 1967). During exercise, the development of any change in T waves or ST segments is evidence that some portion of ventricular muscle has become ischemic and is manifesting an increased period of depolarization out of proportion to the rest of the heart.

CARDIAC DYSRHYTHMIAS

Mechanisms

Cardiac dysrhythmias may be caused by (1) altered automaticity of pacemaker cardiac cells, (2) altered excitability of myocardial cells, and (3) altered conduction of the cardiac impulse through the specialized conduction system of the heart (Cranefield and Wit, 1979). Manifestations of these alterations may be the (1) appearance of an

ectopic cardiac pacemaker, (2) development of heart block, or (3) appearance of a reentry circuit.

Automaticity

Automaticity depicts the ability of a cardiac cell to undergo spontaneous depolarization (see Chapter 47). Under normal circumstances, automaticity is exhibited by cells in the sinoatrial node, atrioventricular node, and the specialized conducting fibers of the atria and ventricles.

Enhanced automaticity is due to an increase in the rate of spontaneous phase 4 depolarization manifesting as an increase in heart rate. Activation of the sympathetic nervous system by events such as arterial hypoxemia, acidosis, or release of catecholamines is the most common cause of enhanced automaticity. In addition, enhanced automaticity occurs when the threshold potential becomes more negative such that the difference between the threshold potential and resting transmembrane potential is less. In these abnormal states, any cardiac cell may exhibit automaticity and initiate an ectopic beat.

Depressed automaticity is produced by increased vagal activity which reduces responsiveness of sinoatrial and atrioventricular node cells by increasing outward potassium flux. This increased outward movement of potassium ions evoked by acetylcholine hyperpolarizes cardiac cell membranes and prevents them from depolarizing. Halothane slows heart rate by reducing the rate of spontaneous phase 4 depolarization and by increasing the threshold potential (Reynolds *et al,* 1970).

Vagal stimulation may decrease the vulnerability of the heart to develop ventricular fibrillation especially in the presence of sympathetic nervous system stimulation (Lown and Verrier, 1976). Carotid sinus stimulation decreases the frequency of premature ventricular contractions and can abolish ventricular tachycardia (Weiss *et al,* 1975).

ECTOPIC PACEMAKER. An ectopic cardiac pacemaker (focus) manifests as a premature contraction of the heart that occurs between normal cardiac beats (Irisawa, 1978). A depolarization wave spreads outward from the ectopic pacemaker and initiates the premature contraction. The usual cause of an ectopic pacemaker is an irritable area of cardiac muscle resulting from a local area of myocardial ischemia or excessive use of stimulants such as caffeine or nicotine. Sometimes, an ectopic pacemaker becomes persistent and assumes the role of pacemaker in place of the sinoatrial node. The most common point for development of an ectopic pacemaker is the atrioventricular node or atrioventricular bundle.

Excitability

Excitability is the ability of a cardiac cell to respond to a stimulus by depolarizing. A measure of excitability is the difference between the resting transmembrane potential and threshold potential of the cardiac cell membrane. The smaller the difference between these potentials, the more excitable, or irritable, is the cell. Although epinephrine enhances automaticity, this is somewhat offset by a concomitant small increase in the negativity of the resting transmembrane potential. Once a cell depolarizes, it is no longer excitable, being refractory to all stimuli. After this absolute refractory period, cardiac cells enter a relative refractory period during which greater than normal stimuli can cause cardiac cell membranes to depolarize.

Conduction

Conduction of the cardiac impulse proceeds through the specialized conduction system of the heart such that a coordinated contraction occurs. Abnormalities of conduction of the cardiac impulse manifest as the development of heart block or reentry circuits.

HEART BLOCK. Occasionally, transmission of the cardiac impulse is blocked at a critical point in the specialized conduction system of the heart (see Chapter 47). The most frequent sites of heart block are the atrioventricular bundle or one of the bundle branches. Causes of heart block at these sites include (1) excessive parasympathetic nervous system stimulation, (2) drug-induced depression of impulse conduction, (3) myocardial infarction, (4) pressure on the conduction system by artherosclerotic plaques, and (5) age-related degenerative processes of the conduction system.

REENTRY. Reentry (circus movements) implies re-excitation of cardiac tissue by return of the same cardiac impulse utilizing a circuitous pathway (Fig. 48-4) (Akhtar, 1982). This contrasts with automaticity in which a new cardiac impulse is generated each time to excite the heart. Reentry circuits can develop anywhere in the heart where there is an imbalance between conduction and refractoriness. Causes of this imbalance include (1) elongation of the conduction pathway as occurs in dilated hearts (especially a dilated left atrium associated with mitral stenosis), (2) decreased velocity of conduction of the cardiac impulse as occurs with myocardial ischemia or hyperkalemia, and (3) a shortened refractory period of cardiac muscle as produced by epinephrine or electrical shock from an alternating current. Each of these conditions creates a situation in which the cardiac impulse conducted by a normal Purkinje fiber can return retrograde through the abnormal Purkinje fiber which is not in a refractory state (*e.g.,* a reentry circuit). Furthermore, myocardial ischemia and resulting tissue hypoxia prevent cardiac muscle fibers from maintaining normal ionic differentials across their cell membranes. Therefore, polarization of cell membranes is reduced and excitability may be so altered that automatic rhythmicity disappears.

Maintenance of a reentry circuit is favored by (1) slow conduction of the cardiac impulse by nor-

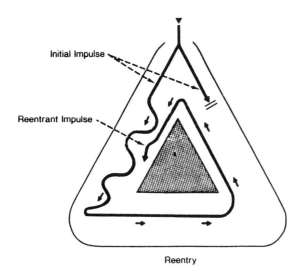

Reentry

FIGURE 48-4. The essential requirement for initiation of a reentry circuit is a unilateral block that prevents uniform anterograde propagation of the initial cardiac impulse. This same cardiac impulse can, under appropriate conditions, transverse the area of block in a retrograde direction and become a reentrant cardiac impulse. (By permission, Akhtar M. Management of ventricular tachyarrhythmias. JAMA 1982;247:671–4. Copyright 1982, American Medical Association.)

mal tissue around the nonconductive area, and (2) a short refractory period in normal cardiac cells. Reentry circuits can be eliminated by (1) speeding conduction through normal tissue so the cardiac impulse reaches its initial site of origin when the fiber is still refractory or (2) prolonging the refractory period of normal cells so the returning impulse cannot reenter.

The presence of a reentry circuit manifests as a premature cardiac contraction or a tachydysrhythmia. When multiple anatomic pathways contribute to reentry, the results are a random type of impulse propagation. Indeed, a reentry circuit is the most likely mechanism for supraventricular tachycardia, atrial flutter, atrial fibrillation, premature ventricular contractions, ventricular tachycardia, and ventricular fibrillation.

Types of Cardiac Dysrhythmias

Sinus Tachycardia

Sinus tachycardia is usually defined as a heart rate above 100 beats min^{-1}. A common cause of sinus tachycardia is sympathetic nervous system stimulation as may occur during a noxious stimulus in the presence of low concentrations of anesthetic. Increased body temperature elevates heart rate about 18 beats min^{-1} for every degree Celsius elevation. Fever causes tachycardia because increased temperature elevates the rate of metabolism in the sinoatrial node. Reflex stimulation of the heart rate accompanies reductions in blood pressure as produced by vasodilator drugs or acute hemorrhage.

Sinus Bradycardia

Sinus bradycardia is usually defined as a heart rate less than 60 beats min^{-1}. Heart rate slowing accompanies parasympathetic nervous system stimulation of the heart. Bradycardia in athletes reflects the fact that the heart is able to eject a greater stroke volume with each heart beat compared with the less conditioned heart.

Sinus Arrhythmia

Sinus arrhythmia is present during normal breathing with heart rate varying about 5% during various phases of the quiet respiratory cycle. This variation may increase to 30% during deep breathing. These variations in heart rate with breathing most likely reflect baroreceptor reflex activity and changes in the negative intrapleural pressure that elicits a waxing and waning Bainbridge reflex.

Atrioventricular Heart Block

First degree atrioventricular heart block is considered to be present when the P–R interval exceeds 0.2 second at a normal heart rate. Second degree atrioventricular heart block is classified as the Wenckebach phenomenon (Type I) or Mobitz (Type II) heart block. Wenckebach phenomenon is characterized by a progressive prolongation of the P–R interval until conduction of the cardiac impulse is completely interrupted and a P wave is recorded without a subsequent QRS complex. After this dropped beat, the cycle is repeated. Mobitz heart block is the occurrence of a nonconducted atrial beat without a prior change in the P–R interval.

Third degree (complete) atrioventricular heart block occurs when there is complete block of the transmission of the cardiac impulse from the atrium to the ventricles. In this instance, P waves are completely dissociated from QRS – T complexes. The atria may have a rate of 100 beats min^{-1} while the ventricles are contracting independently at an inherent rate of 30 to 40 beats min^{-1}. In this situation, the ventricles have escaped from control of the atrial pacemakers and are beating at their own natural rate under the influence of an ectopic pacemaker in the ventricles. In some patients, third degree heart block may be intermittent. The shape of the QRS complex depends on the site of the ectopic ventricular pacemaker. If the pacemaker is near the atrioventricular node, the QRS complexes of the resulting beats appear normal. If, however, the site of the ectopic ventricular pacemaker is in a bundle branch, the QRS complex is wide resembling a bundle branch block or premature ventricular contraction. Patients may experience syncope (Stokes-Adams syndrome) at the onset of third degree heart block reflecting the 5- to 10-second period of asystole that may precede ventricular escape and appearance of an ectopic ventricular pacemaker. Occasionally, the interval of ventricular standstill at the onset of third degree heart block is so long that death occurs. Treatment of patients with third degree heart block is insertion of a permanent artificial cardiac pacemaker.

Premature Atrial Contractions

Premature atrial contractions are recognized by an abnormal P wave and a shortened P – R interval. The QRS complex of the premature atrial contraction has a normal configuration. Also, the interval between the premature atrial contraction and the next succeeding contraction is usually not prolonged. Premature atrial contractions are usually benign and often occur in persons without heart disease.

Premature Nodal Contractions

Premature nodal contractions are characterized by the absence of a P wave preceding the QRS complex. The P wave is obscured by the QRS complex of the premature contraction because the cardiac impulse travels retrograde into the atria at the same time it travels forward into the ventricles.

Premature Ventricular Contractions

Premature ventricular contractions result from an ectopic pacemaker in the ventricles. The QRS complex on the electrocardiogram is typically

prolonged as the cardiac impulse is conducted mainly through the slowly conducting muscle of the ventricle rather than the Purkinje system. The voltage of the QRS complex of the premature ventricular contraction is increased reflecting the absence of the usual neutralization phenomenon that occurs when a normal cardiac impulse passes through both ventricles simultaneously. In this normal situation, depolarization waves on the two sides of the heart partially neutralize each other. When a ventricular premature contraction occurs, the cardiac impulse travels in only one direction so there is no neutralization effect. Premature ventricular contractions often reflect significant cardiac disease. For example, myocardial ischemia may be responsible for initiation of a premature contraction from an irritable site in poorly oxygenated ventricular muscle.

Following almost all premature ventricular contractions, the T wave has an electrical potential opposite to that of the QRS complex. This occurs because the slow conduction of the impulse through the cardiac muscle causes the area first depolarized also to repolarize first. As a result, the direction of current flow in the heart during repolarization is opposite to that during depolarization and the polarity of the T wave is reversed to that of the QRS complex.

A compensatory pause is often present following a premature ventricular contraction. This occurs because the first impulse from the sinoatrial node reaches the ventricle during the refractory period of the ventricle. The second impulse from the atria, however, reaches the ventricle during the excitable period and conduction is normal. As a result, the sum of the intervals after the normal beat and the one following the premature ventricular contraction is equal to two normal cardiac cycles.

When a premature ventricular contraction occurs, the ventricle may not have filled adequately with blood and the stroke volume resulting from this contraction fails to produce a detectable pulse. The succeeding stroke volume, however, may be increased due to added ventricular filling that occurs during the compensatory pause that typically follows a premature ventricular contraction.

Atrial Paroxysmal Tachycardia

Atrial paroxysmal tachycardia is caused by rapid rhythmic discharges of impulses from an ectopic atrial pacemaker. The rhythm on the electrocardiogram is perfectly regular and the P waves are abnormal, often inverted, indicating a site of origin other than the sinoatrial node. The rapid discharge rate causes this ectopic focus to become the pacemaker. Typically, the onset of atrial paroxysmal tachycardia is abrupt (a single beat) and may end just as suddenly with the pacemaker shifting back to the sinoatrial node. Atrial paroxysmal tachycardia can often be terminated by producing parasympathetic nervous system stimulation at the heart with drugs or unilateral external pressure applied to the carotid sinus. This cardiac dysrhythmia often occurs in otherwise healthy young persons.

Nodal Paroxysmal Tachycardia

Nodal paroxysmal tachycardia resembles atrial paroxysmal tachycardia except P waves are not distinguishable on the electrocardiogram. The P waves are obscured by the QRS complexes because the atrial impulse travels backward from the atrioventricular node at the same time the ventricular impulse travels through the ventricles.

Ventricular Tachycardia

Ventricular tachycardia on the electrocardiogram resembles a series of ventricular premature contractions that occur at a rapid and regular rate (70 – 180 beats min⁻¹) without any normal beats interspersed. This cardiac dysrhythmia predisposes to ventricular fibrillation because it creates a situation in which reentry can occur. Stroke volume is often severely depressed during ventricular tachycardia because the ventricles have insufficient time for cardiac filling.

Sustained ventricular tachycardia is when drugs or electrical cardioversion is required to terminate the dysrhythmia. Nonsustained ventricular tachycardia is when the dysrhythmia undergoes spontaneous termination.

Atrial Flutter

Atrial flutter on the electrocardiogram is characterized by 2:1, 3:1, or 4:1 conduction of atrial impulses to the ventricle. This occurs because the functional refractory period of Purkinje fibers and ventricular muscle is such that not over 200 impulses min⁻¹ can be transmitted into the ventricles. As a result, when the atrium contracts as rapidly as 300 beats min⁻¹, only one of every two (2:1), three (3:1), or four (4:1) atrial impulses reaches the ventricles.

An important distinguishing feature of atrial flutter is the high voltage (0.2 – 0.3 mv) of the P waves in lead II. This reflects the circus movement pathway of the impulse around the atria from top to bottom. As a result, the electrical current flow in the atria parallels the axis of lead II which causes high voltages in this lead, but low voltages in lead I. In addition, P waves have a characteristic sawtooth appearance.

Atrial Fibrillation

During atrial fibrillation, numerous small depolarization waves spread in all directions through the atria. These waves usually neutralize each other because they are weak and many are of an opposite polarity at any given time. Therefore, on the electrocardiogram, there are no visible P waves but rather a high-frequency and low-voltage wavy record. QRS complexes, however, are normal but completely irregular in their occurrence reflecting arrival of atrial impulses at the atrioventricular node at times that may, or may not, correspond to the refractory period of the node from a previous discharge.

Stroke volume is reduced during atrial fibrillation because the ventricles do not have sufficient time to fill optimally between cardiac cycles. Treatment of atrial fibrillation is classically with digitalis which prolongs the refractory period of the atrioventricular node, probably by enhancement of parasympathetic nervous system activity at the atrioventricular node (see Chapter 13). This prolongation of the atrioventricular node refractory period decreases the rate of ventricular response and improves stroke volume by permitting additional time for filling of the ventricles between cardiac cycles.

A pulse deficit in atrial fibrillation reflects the inability of each ventricular contraction to eject a sufficient stroke volume to produce a detectable peripheral pulse (see Chapter 44). For this reason, the heart rate, as counted by listening with a stethoscope placed over the heart or from the electrocardiogram may be greater than that determined by palpating a peripheral pulse.

Ventricular Fibrillation

Ventricular fibrillation on the electrocardiogram is characterized by an irregular wavy line with maximum initial voltages of about 0.5 mv. Within 30 seconds, voltage decreases to about 0.25 mv.

Fibrillation, whether atrial or ventricular, results in total incoordination of contraction and cessation of any pumping activity. Therefore, blood pressure is not obtainable when ventricular fibrillation occurs. Flutter or fibrillation is usually confined to either the atria or ventricles alone because the two masses of muscle are electrically insulated from each other by the rings of fibrous tissue around the heart valves.

The only effective treatment of ventricular fibrillation is the delivery of a direct electrical current through the ventricles (*i.e.,* defibrillation) for a brief period, which simultaneously depolarizes all ventricular muscle. This depolarization allows the reestablishment of a cardiac pacemaker at a site other than the irritable focus that was responsible for ventricular fibrillation. Mechanisms of atrial or ventricular fibrillation include the development of a rapidly discharging ectopic pacemaker or the establishment of a reentry circuit.

Most instances of flutter or fibrillation are due to a reentry mechanism.

REFERENCES

Akhtar M. Management of ventricular tachyarrhythmias. JAMA 1982;247:671–4.

Cranefield PF, Wit AL. Cardiac arrhythmias. Annu Rev Physiol 1979;41:459–72.

Irisawa H. Comparative physiology of the cardiac pacemaker mechanism. Physiol Rev 1978;58:461–98.

Lown B, Verrier RL. Neural activity and ventricular fibrillation. N Engl J Med 1976;294:1165–70.

Mason RE, Likar I, Bierm RO, Ross RS. Multiple lead exercise electrocardiography. Circulation 1967;36:517–25.

McCammon RL. Coronary artery disease. In: Stoelting RK, Dierdorf SF, eds. Anesthesia and Co-Existing Disease. New York, Churchill Livingstone, 1983;1.

Reynolds AK, Chiz JF, Pasquat AF. Halothane and methoxyflurane: A comparison of their effects on cardiac pacemaker fibers. Anesthesiology 1970;33:602–10.

Weiss T, Lattin GM, Engelman K. Vagally mediated suppression of premature ventricular contractions in man. Am Heart J 1975;89:700–7.

CHAPTER 49

Lungs

ANATOMY OF THE LUNGS

The trachea begins at the lower border of the cricoid cartilage opposite the level of the sixth cervical vertebra and extends downward until it bifurcates at the carina opposite the fifth thoracic vertebra. In an adult, the overall length of the trachea is about 11 cm and the inside diameter is about 12 mm. The capacity of the trachea is about 30 ml constituting 20% of the anatomic dead space. The mucosal lining of the trachea consists of ciliated columnar epithelium and mucus-secreting cells.

The bifurcation of the trachea at the carina gives rise to the left and right mainstem bronchi. The right mainstem bronchus is wider and more in line with the trachea. As a result, foreign bodies, suction catheters, and endotracheal tubes are more likely to pass into the right then left mainstem bronchus. Continued division of the right and left mainstem bronchi gives rise to bronchioles characterized by absence of cartilage and ultimately respiratory bronchioles which are the transitional zones between the bronchioles and alveolar ducts. Alveoli which are about 0.25 mm in diameter arise from these alveolar ducts as well as alveolar sacs. The branching of the bronchopulmonary segments is completed *in utero,* and the growth of the airways after birth is entirely by increase in size. Alveoli, however, continue to proliferate for about the first 10 years of life (Mead, 1973).

At birth, the walls of alveoli are kept collapsed by surface tension. For this reason, the first inspirations of the newborn infant must be capable of creating as much as 60 mmHg negative pressure in the intrapleural space.

PULMONARY VENTILATION

The lungs are responsible for accepting gases from the atmosphere and the subsequent distribution of these gases to the alveoli (see Chapter 50). Pulmonary ventilation is accomplished almost entirely by the muscles of inspiration. The inherent elastic properties of the lungs and chest cause the lungs to passively contract following relaxation of the muscles of inspiration.

Mechanics of Breathing

The lungs can be expanded and contracted by downward and upward movement of the diaphragm to lengthen or shorten the chest cavity and by elevation and depression of the ribs to increase and decrease the anteroposterior diameter of the chest cavity (Macklem, 1978). Normal quiet breathing is accomplished almost entirely by inspiratory movement of the diaphragm. During inspiration, contraction of the diaphragm moves abdominal contents downward and forward, creating a potential space which is filled by expansion of the lungs. It is estimated that the diaphragm moves 10 to 12 cm vertically during each inspiration. During exhalation, the diaphragm relaxes and the elastic recoil of the lungs, chest wall, and abdominal structures compresses the lungs. The nerve supply of the diaphragm is the phrenic nerve which arises from the third, fourth, and fifth cervical nerves.

In addition to movement of the diaphragm, the lungs can also be expanded by raising the rib cage. Elevation of the ribs expands the lungs because, in the natural resting position, the ribs slant downward, thus allowing the sternum to fall backward toward the vertebrae (Thurlbeck, 1977). Therefore, when the ribs are elevated, the ribs project forward so the sternum moves forward away from the vertebrae increasing the anteroposterior thickness of the chest. Skeletal muscles that elevate the ribs are muscles of inspiration (sternocleidomastoid muscles, anterior serrati, external intercostals), and those that depress the ribs are muscles of exhalation (abdominal recti, internal intercostals).

During inspiration, expansion of the lungs causes the pressure within alveoli to become slightly negative with respect to atmospheric pressure. As a result of this pressure differential, gas flows inward through the respiratory passages.

In contrast to inspiration, exhalation is passive. During inspiration, potential energy is stored in the elastic tissues of the lung and thoracic cage. The recoil of these stretched tissues leads to a rise in the alveolar pressure to above atmospheric pressure and gas is forced outward. Muscles of exhalation are active only during forced breathing or obstruction to the flow of gas. The most important muscles of exhalation are the abdominal recti and the internal intercostal muscles.

The inherent tendency for the lungs to collapse (*i.e.,* recoil away from the chest wall) is due to elastic fibers that are stretched by lung inflation and, therefore, attempt to shorten. Even more important, surface tension of the fluid lining the alveoli causes a continual elastic tendency for alveoli to collapse (see the section entitled Pulmonary Surfactant). Elastic fibers in the lungs normally account for about one third of the recoil tendency, and surface tension accounts for the remainder. Elastic recoil of the lungs is responsible for the negative intrapleural pressure of about -4 mmHg. This negative intrapleural pressure keeps the lungs expanded to normal size. Expansion of the lungs during maximum inspiration creates an intrapleural pressure of -12 to 18 mmHg.

PULMONARY SURFACTANT

Pulmonary surfactant is a lipoprotein secreted by Type II alveolar epithelial cells lining the alveoli (Clements, 1970). The phospholipid component of pulmonary surfactant, dipalmitoyl lecithin, decreases surface tension of fluids lining the alveoli. Surface tension results from the attraction of atoms in a liquid. Pulmonary surfactant lowers surface tension thus reducing the muscular effort required for expansion of alveoli. Furthermore, because surface tension changes with the size of the alveoli, surfactant stabilizes alveoli thus preventing their collapse. In the absence of surfactant, lung expansion is difficult requiring intrapleural pressures often approaching -30 mmHg to overcome the collapse tendency of the alveoli.

Pulmonary surfactant acts by forming a monomolecular layer at the interface between the fluid lining alveoli and the gas in alveoli. This prevents the development of a water–gas interface, which has up to 14 times as much surface tension as the surfactant–gas interface. Absence or inadequate amounts of pulmonary surfactant is called *hyaline membrane disease* or *respiratory distress syndrome of the newborn*. Formation of pulmonary surfactant may be hastened by administration of corticosteroids during pregnancy. Pulmonary surfactant may also be diminished after cardiopulmonary bypass, pulmonary embolism, and prolonged inhalation of 100% oxygen.

The effect of surface tension for causing alveolar collapse is exaggerated as the diameter of the alveolus decreases (Laplace's law). According to Laplace's law, the pressure inside a bubble necessary to keep it expanded is directly proportional to twice the tension in the wall of the bubble tending to collapse it divided by the radius of the bubble. If the tension is maintained constant and the radius of the bubble is diminished, then the pressure in the bubble will rise, thus emptying its content to a bigger bubble. In the absence of pulmonary surfactant, all smaller alveoli would empty into larger alveoli.

The transalveolar pressure required to keep an alveolus expanded is directly proportional to the surface tension of the lining fluid divided by diameter of the alveolus. As an alveolus decreases in size, the pulmonary surfactant becomes more concentrated at the surface of the alveolar lining fluid and the surface tension is reduced. This prevents the development of high transalveolar pres-

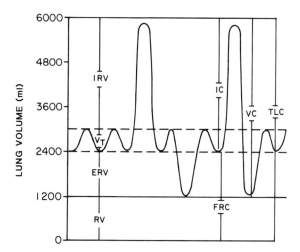

FIGURE 49-1. Schematic diagram of breathing excursions at rest and during maximum inhalation or exhalation. The amount of gas in the lungs is categorized as inspiratory reserve volume (IRV), tidal volume (V_T), expiratory reserve volume (ERV), residual volume (RV), inspiratory capacity (IC), functional residual capacity (FRC), vital capacity (VC), and total lung capacity (TLC).

sure which would collapse alveoli as they become smaller. Conversely, as alveoli become larger and the surfactant is spread more thinly on the fluid surface, the surface tension becomes greater. Thus, pulmonary surfactant helps to stabilize the sizes of alveoli, causing larger alveoli to contract more and smaller ones to contract less. The net effect is the maintenance of alveoli in any area of the lung at about the same size.

Surface tension, in addition to causing collapse of alveoli, acts to pull fluid into the alveoli. In the absence of pulmonary surfactant, this surface tension may cause the alveoli to fill with fluid causing pulmonary edema. Indeed, in respiratory distress syndrome of the newborn, the amount of pulmonary surfactant is greatly decreased and a large number of alveoli are filled with fluid.

COMPLIANCE

Compliance is expressed as the increase in the volume of the lungs for each unit increase of alveolar pressure. The combined compliance of

normal lungs and the thorax is 0.13 L cmH_2O^{-1}. This means that the lungs expand 130 ml for every 1 cm water pressure increase in the alveoli. Any condition that destroys lung tissue or blocks bronchioles causes decreased pulmonary compliance. Deformities of the thoracic cage such as kyphosis or scoliosis reduce thoracic compliance.

In the normal resting adult, the work of breathing is 1% to 2% of the total oxygen consumption. More than two thirds of the work of quiet breathing is spent in overcoming the elastic recoil of the lungs and thorax. When the respiratory rate increases or airways are narrowed, a large proportion of work is spent in overcoming the resistance to gas flow.

LUNG VOLUMES AND CAPACITIES

The amount of gas in the lungs has been subdivided into four different volumes and four capacities (Fig. 49-1). A lung capacity is the sum of two or more lung volumes. Data related to pulmonary ventilation and lung volumes are often designated by abbreviations to simplify their presentation and use in mathematical formulas (Table 49-1).

In normal persons, the volume of gas in the lungs depends primarily on body size and build. For example, large and athletic persons have greater lung volumes than small and asthenic indi-

Table 49-1
Lung Volumes and Capacities

Lung Volume	Abbreviation	Normal Adult Value
Tidal volume	V_T	500 ml
Inspiratory reserve volume	IRV	3000 ml
Expiratory reserve volume	ERV	1200 ml
Residual volume	RV	1200 ml
Inspiratory capacity	IC	3500 ml
Functional residual capacity	FRC	2400 ml
Vital capacity	VC	4500 ml
Forced exhaled vital capacity in 1 second	FEV_1	80%
Total lung capacity	TLC	5900 ml

viduals. All pulmonary volumes and capacities are about 25% less in females than in males. Lung volumes and capacities also change with body position, most of them decreasing when the patient is supine and increasing when the patient is standing. Decreases in lung volumes in the recumbent position reflect the tendency for abdominal contents to press upward against the diaphragm plus an increase in pulmonary blood volume, both of which decrease space available in the lungs for gas.

Lung Volumes

The four lung volumes are tidal volume (V_T), inspiratory reserve volume (IRV), expiratory reserve volume (ERV), and residual volume (RV).

Tidal Volume (V_T)

V_T is the volume of gas inhaled and exhaled with each normal breath. A typical V_T is 6 to 8 ml kg^{-1} or about 500 ml in an average adult.

Inspiratory Reserve Volume (IRV)

IRV is the additional volume of gas that can be inhaled beyond the normal V_T. A typical IRV is about 3000 ml.

Expiratory Reserve Volume (ERV)

ERV is the additional volume of gas that can be forceably exhaled at the end of a normal V_T. A typical ERV is about 1200 ml.

Residual Volume (RV)

RV is the volume of gas remaining in the lungs at the conclusion of a maximum forced exhalation. A typical RV is about 1200 ml. The RV is important because it provides gas in the alveoli to oxygenate the blood between breaths. In the absence of an RV, the concentrations of oxygen and carbon dioxide in the blood would vary widely with each breath.

Lung Capacities

The four lung capacities are inspiratory capacity (IC), functional residual capacity (FRC), vital capacity (VC), and total lung capacity (TLC).

Inspiratory Capacity (IC)

IC is the maximum volume of gas that a person can inhale beginning at the end of a normal V_T. A normal IC is about 3500 ml being equal to the sum of the V_T and IRV.

Functional Residual Capacity (FRC)

FRC is the amount of gas remaining in the lungs at the conclusion of a normal exhalation. A normal FRC is about 2400 ml being equal to the sum of the ERV and RV. The FRC is measured by asking the patient to inhale from a spirometer containing a known concentration of helium starting at end-exhalation. As a result, the helium becomes diluted by the FRC gas. The volume of the FRC can be calculated from the degree of dilution of the helium. Once the FRC is determined, the RV can be calculated by subtracting the ERV from the FRC. Also, the TLC can be determined by adding the IC to the FRC.

The FRC buffers changes in the inhaled concentration of gases such that abrupt alterations in gaseous concentrations in the blood do not occur. For example, at a normal V_T of 500 ml only about 350 ml of new gas enters the alveoli for each breath. This new gas represents only about one seventh of the residual gases (e.g., FRC) such that several breaths are required to exchange most of the alveolar gas (Engel and Macklem, 1977). This slow replacement of alveolar gas provides stability to the ventilatory control mechanism and helps to prevent excessive increases and decreases in (1) tissue oxygenation, (2) tissue carbon dioxide concentration, and (3) tissue pH when ventilation of the lungs is transiently interrupted as during direct laryngoscopy for intubation of the trachea.

Vital Capacity (VC)

VC is the maximum amount of gas that can be exhaled following a maximum inhalation. A normal VC is 60 to 70 ml kg^{-1} or about 4500 ml in an adult. The VC is the sum of three volumes, the IRV, V_T, and ERV.

Other than the anatomical build of an individual, the major factors that determine VC are the strength of the muscles of ventilation and the compliance of the lungs and chest. A tall thin person usually has a larger vital capacity than an obese person. A well-conditioned athlete may have a VC 30% to 40% above normal. Fibrotic changes in the lungs produced by chronic bronchial asthma or chronic bronchitis reduce pulmonary compliance and thus decrease VC. Any excess fluid in the lungs, as may occur with cardiac failure, decreases pulmonary compliance and thus the VC. Indeed, an improvement in VC may reflect a decrease in pulmonary edema associated with left ventricular dysfunction.

FORCED EXHALED VITAL CAPACITY. The forced exhaled vital capacity is the total volume of gas that can be rapidly and completely exhaled starting from a maximal inhalation (Fig. 49-2). The rate at which gas can be exhaled varies among patients and is greatly slowed in the presence of obstructive airways disease.

The greatest impact of obstructive airways disease on the expiratory flow rate is in the first second during determination of the forced exhaled vital capacity. Therefore, it is customary to record the forced exhaled volume during the first second (FEV_1). In the normal person, the percentage of the forced exhaled vital capacity that is exhaled in the first second is above 80%. In the presence of obstructive airways disease, this value is less than 50%.

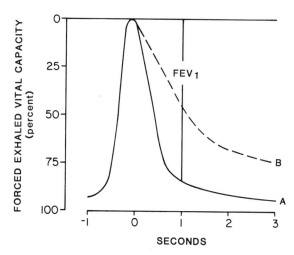

FIGURE 49-2. Schematic diagram of forced exhaled vital capacity in normal patients (*A*) and in individuals with obstructive airways disease (*B*). The normal patient can exhale about 80% of the vital capacity in 1 second (FEV_1) compared with 50% in 1 second in patients with obstructive airways disease.

Total Lung Capacity (TLC)

TLC is the volume to which the lungs can be expanded with maximum inspiration. A normal TLC is about 5900 ml being equal to the sum of all four individual lung volumes or IC plus FRC.

MINUTE VENTILATION

Minute ventilation is the total amount of gas moved into the lungs each minute and is thus equal to the V_T (500 ml) times the rate of breathing (12 breaths min^{-1}) (Table 49-1). Therefore, the average minute ventilation is about 6 L min^{-1}.

In diseases associated with airway obstruction, such as asthma and emphysema, it is usually much more difficult to exhale than to inhale because the expiratory closing tendency of the airways is greatly increased, while the negative intrapleural pressure of inspiration actually pulls the airways open. As a result, gas tends to enter the lungs easily and become trapped in the lungs leading to an increased RV and TLC.

Alveolar Ventilation (VA)

VA is the volume of gas each minute that enters areas of the lungs capable of participating in gas exchange with pulmonary capillary blood. The VA is less than minute ventilation because a portion of inhaled gases fill respiratory passageways that do not participate in gaseous exchange with the pulmonary capillary blood (*e.g.,* dead space gas). The VA is equal to the frequency of breathing times the V_T from which dead space gas volume is subtracted. Assuming a normal V_T of 500 ml, a dead space gas volume of 150 ml, and breathing rate of 12 breaths min^{-1}, the normal VA is about 4200 ml min^{-1}. The concentration and partial pressure of carbon dioxide, and to a lesser extent oxygen, in the blood are determined by VA. The rate of breathing, V_T, and minute ventilation are important only insofar as they influence VA.

During inspiration, only a small portion of the inhaled gas flows beyond the terminal bronchioles into the alveoli. Instead, diffusion of gas caused by kinetic motion of molecules is responsible for gas flow into the alveoli. All gases in the alveoli become completely mixed within a fraction of a second.

Dead Space

Dead space is that volume of the lungs containing gases that do not participate in gas exchange with pulmonary capillary blood (see Chapter 50). Anatomic dead space includes those areas of the respiratory tract (nasal passageways, pharynx, trachea, and bronchi) that do not normally participate in gas exchange with pulmonary capillary blood. Physiologic dead space is the gas volume of alveoli that are not functional or only partially functional because of absent or poor blood flow through corresponding pulmonary capillaries (*e.g.,* wasted ventilation) (see Chapter 50).

During exhalation, gas in dead space is exhaled before gas coming from the alveoli. This is the reason anesthetic breathing systems are designed to preferentially conserve dead space gas (no oxygen or anesthetic removed and no carbon dioxide added) and eliminate alveolar gas (depleted of oxygen and anesthetic and carbon dioxide added). Conceptually, rebreathing of dead space gas is similar to delivering fresh gases from the anesthesia machine.

The volume of dead space is determined by measuring the exhaled concentration of nitrogen following a single breath of pure oxygen. Gas being exhaled from dead space contains no nitrogen. The normal dead space volume is about 2 ml kg^{-1} or 150 ml in most adults, and this increases slightly with age. Normally, the contribution of anatomic and physiologic dead space to total dead space is nearly equal. Chronic lung disease, however, tends to selectively increase physiologic dead space volume.

CONTROL OF VENTILATION

Control of ventilation is designed to make adjustments in the VA so as to maintain an optimal and unchanging concentration of hydrogen ions and partial pressures of oxygen and carbon dioxide in the arterial blood. This fine control of ventilation is provided by the respiratory center under the influence of chemical stimuli and a peripheral chemoreceptor system (Cohen, 1979; Guz, 1975; Mitchell and Berger, 1975).

Respiratory Center

The respiratory center is a widely dispersed group of neurons located bilaterally in the reticular sub-

stance of the medulla oblongata and pons (Fig. 49-3) (Guyton, 1986). This center is divided into (1) an inspiratory area, (2) an area in the pons which influences the rate of breathing called the pneumotaxic area, and (3) an expiratory area.

Inspiratory Area

The inspiratory area is located bilaterally in the dorsal portion of the medulla. Vagal and glossopharyngeal nerves transmit signals from peripheral chemoreceptors to the inspiratory area. In addition, vagal nerves transmit sensory signals from the lungs that help to control lung inflation and the rate of breathing.

Rhythmic inspiratory cycles are generated in the inspiratory area (Cohen, 1979). This rhythmicity seems to result from intrinsic excitability of inspiratory area neurons that subsequently initiate neuronal signals to the diaphragm and intercostal muscles. Following forceful contraction of the diaphragm and intercostal muscles, the inspiratory area becomes dormant until intrinsic rhythmic activity again occurs.

Pneumotaxic Area

The pneumotaxic area transmits signals continuously to the inspiratory area. The purpose of

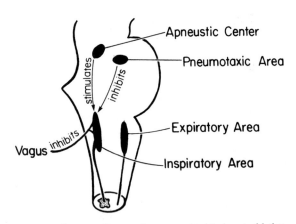

FIGURE 49-3. The respiratory center is located bilaterally in the reticular substance of the medulla oblongata and pons. (Redrawn from Guyton AC. Textbook of Medical Physiology. 7th ed. Philadelphia: WB Saunders, 1986:504; by permission of the author and publisher.)

these impulses is to inhibit the inspiratory signal before the lungs become overinflated. As such, the function of the pneumotaxic area is to limit the duration of inspiration which indirectly influences the rate of breathing. For example, a strong pneumotaxic signal limits the duration of inspiration but the cycle may begin sooner so the net effect is a more rapid rate of breathing. A weak pneumotaxic signal results in a slow rate of breathing.

Apneustic Center

The apneustic center is also located in the pons (Fig. 49-3) (Guyton, 1986). This center transmits signals to the inspiratory area that, in the absence of pneumotaxic area activity, prevents cessation of inspiration. As long as the pneumotaxic area is active, the apneustic center is suppressed. When apneustic center activity is unmasked because of damage to the pneumotaxic area, the pattern of breathing is maximal lung inflation with occasional expiratory gasps.

INFLATION REFLEX. Stretch receptors in the walls of bronchi transmit signals over the vagal nerves to the inspiratory area when overinflation of the lungs occurs. These signals limit the duration of inspiration in the same way as signals from the pneumotaxic area. This mechanism to limit inspiration is designated the *inflation reflex* or *Hering-Breuer reflex.* It is unlikely, however, that the inflation reflex is important in controlling normal lung inflation as it becomes activated only when the V_T is greater than about 1.5 liters (Guyton, 1986). Rapid shallow breathing during inhalation of volatile anesthetics is not likely to be related to the inflation reflex (Paskin *et al,* 1968). Conversely, in situations of decreased pulmonary compliance such as pulmonary fibrosis the pattern of breathing becomes shallow and rapid to minimize elastic work presumably by virtue of stimulation of these inflation receptors.

DEFLATION REFLEX. Deflation receptors are believed to be involved in tachypnea associated with pulmonary edema and pulmonary embolism. Tachypnea associated with inhalation of halothane may reflect stimulation of deflation receptors (Paintal, 1973). These deflation receptors are occasionally referred to as J receptors because of their juxtacapillary position.

Expiratory Area

The expiratory area in the ventral portion of the medulla is normally dormant as exhalation results from passive recoil of the elastic structures of the lung and surrounding chest wall. When the need for increased VA is great, however, the expiratory area becomes active providing signals that evoke forceful contraction of the muscles of expiration.

Chemical Control

Excess carbon dioxide or hydrogen ions affect ventilation mainly by direct excitatory effects on the respiratory center causing increased strength of both the inspiratory and expiratory signals to the respiratory muscles (Cohen, 1968). Conversely, oxygen seems to act almost exclusively on peripheral chemoreceptors located in the carotid and aortic bodies which in turn transmit neuronal signals to the respiratory center (Biscoe, 1971).

Chemosensitive Area of the Respiratory Center

An area independent of the inspiratory area, pneumotaxic area, and expiratory area is located a few microns below the ventral surface of the medulla near the site of entry of the glossopharyngeal and vagal nerves (Fig. 49-4) (Guyton, 1986; Mitchell and Berger, 1975). This chemosensitive area (also known as the medullary chemoreceptor) is highly responsive to changes in the concentration of carbon dioxide and hydrogen ions in the cerebrospinal fluid. Increases in activity of the chemosensitive area result in transmission of signals to the inspiratory area that increase the rate of breathing.

Hydrogen ions are the most important stimulus of the chemosensitive area, but these ions do not easily cross the blood–brain barrier to enter the cerebrospinal fluid. For this reason, changes in the hydrogen ion concentration of the blood have less effect in stimulating the chemosensitive area neurons than does carbon dioxide which readily crosses the blood–brain barrier. Carbon dioxide stimulates the chemosensitive area by virtue of its reaction with water in the cerebrospinal fluid to form carbonic acid which subsequently dissociates to provide the hydrogen ions necessary for stimulation (Fig. 49-4) (Guyton, 1986; Mitchell and Berger, 1975).

It seems that changes in the hydrogen ion

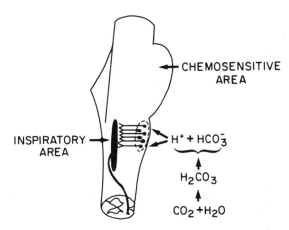

CHEMOSENSITIVE AREA

INSPIRATORY AREA

$H^+ + HCO_3^-$

H_2CO_3

$CO_2 + H_2O$

FIGURE 49-4. The chemosensitive area, located a few microns below the ventral surface of the medulla, transmits stimulatory impulses to the inspiratory area. This chemosensitive area is highly responsive to hydrogen ions in the cerebrospinal fluid that result from hydration of carbon dioxide. (From Guyton AC. Textbook of Medical Physiology. 7th ed. Philadelphia: WB Saunders, 1986:504. Reproduced by permission of the author and publisher.)

concentration of the cerebrospinal fluid are more important than changes in the pH of interstitial fluid for stimulating the chemosensitive area (Lausen, 1972). This is probably due to the limited buffering capacity of cerebrospinal fluid in contrast to the protein-rich interstitial fluid. As a result, a given change in the carbon dioxide concentration of cerebrospinal fluid results in a greater change in the hydrogen ion concentration than occurs in the buffered interstitial fluid. An advantage of a cerebrospinal fluid system in the control of ventilation is the rapidity with which changes in the blood carbon dioxide concentration are reflected in the cerebrospinal fluid. This change occurs within seconds compared with at least 1 minute that is required for changes in the $PaCO_2$ to be reflected in interstitial fluid. Hydrogen ions formed in the cerebrospinal fluid diffuse rapidly to the chemosensitive area neurons located a few microns below the surface of the medulla.

The effect of an increased $PaCO_2$ on ventilation peaks within 1 minute. After several hours, however, the stimulant effect wanes reflecting active transport (*i.e.,* an ion pump) of bicarbonate ions into the cerebrospinal fluid from the blood to return the cerebrospinal fluid pH to a normal

value of 7.32 (Heinemann and Goldring, 1974; Mitchell and Berger, 1975). These bicarbonate ions combine with excess hydrogen ions in the cerebrospinal fluid and thus stimulation of the chemosensitive area decreases with time. Therefore, a change in the $PaCO_2$ has an intense initial effect on the control of ventilation but only a weak effect after several hours during which time adaptation occurs (*i.e.,* return of cerebrospinal fluid pH to 7.32) by active transport of bicarbonate ions.

Chemoreceptors

The carotid and aortic bodies are chemoreceptors located outside the central nervous system which are responsive to changes in the concentration of hydrogen ions and the partial pressures of oxygen and carbon dioxide (Biscoe, 1971). These chemoreceptors transmit signals via the glossopharyngeal nerves (carotid bodies) and vagal nerves (aortic bodies) to the respiratory center in the medulla. Blood flow to peripheral chemoreceptors far exceeds their metabolic needs such that these tissues are exposed to blood gas values and pH values similar to arterial blood.

The carotid body consists of Type I or glomus cells as well as Type II cells. Glomus cells contain vesicles in which dopamine is stored. Dopamine functions as an inhibitory neurotransmitter acting to reduce the activity of the carotid body (see Chapter 12).

The carotid bodies are more involved with ventilatory responses than are the aortic bodies. Conversely, aortic bodies are much more prominent than the carotid bodies in influencing cardiovascular responses. The contribution of chemoreceptor drive to ventilation at a PaO_2 up to 170 mmHg is estimated to be about 10% (Downes and Lambertsen, 1966). Removal or denervation of the carotid bodies as may occur during carotid endarterectomy results in loss of the ventilatory response to hypoxemia and about a 30% reduction in the ventilatory response to carbon dioxide. The resting level of ventilation, however, remains unchanged. In the absence of carotid body function, the duration for which an individual can voluntarily breath-hold may be prolonged.

Changes in the partial pressure of oxygen in the arterial blood have no direct stimulatory effect on the respiratory center. Peripheral chemoreceptors, however, become strongly stimulated when the PaO_2 decreases below about 60 mmHg (Guz, 1975). This is important because saturation of hemoglobin with oxygen decreases rapidly when the PaO_2 decreases below 60 mmHg. Conversely, the stimulating effect of increased arterial concentrations of carbon dioxide and hydrogen ions on the peripheral chemoreceptors is much less than the direct effects of these ions on the respiratory center via changes in the cerebrospinal fluid pH. The mechanism by which a low PaO_2 activates nerve endings in peripheral chemoreceptors is not known.

Blood flow through the peripheral chemoreceptors is the highest of any tissue in the body, which means that the chemoreceptor tissue and venous PO_2 are nearly equal to the PaO_2. Therefore, it is the PaO_2 and not the arterial concentration of oxygen that determines the level of stimulation of the peripheral chemoreceptors. Nevertheless, when mean arterial pressure declines below 60 mmHg, blood flow through peripheral chemoreceptors becomes sluggish and tissue PO_2 declines below the PaO_2. As a result, peripheral chemoreceptors are stimulated by the low tissue PO_2 despite a normal PaO_2. This stimulation manifests as increased VA and peripheral vasoconstriction that increase mean arterial pressure back toward normal.

Even the 1.5-fold increase in VA evoked by a PaO_2 of 40 mmHg is modest compared with the tenfold increase in VA caused by a 50% increase in $PaCO_2$. This limited stimulating effect of oxygen on VA is due to the simultaneous effect of increased VA on the blood concentration of carbon dioxide and hydrogen ions. For example, increased VA due to arterial hypoxemia also lowers the $PaCO_2$ and increases the pH which act to depress ventilation thus offsetting the stimulant effect of a low PaO_2 on ventilation. Conversely, when intrinsic lung disease, such as pneumonia or emphysema, prevents a decrease in $PaCO_2$ when VA increases, the ventilatory response to arterial hypoxemia is no longer offset and VA may increase as much as fivefold in response to reductions in the PaO_2. Furthermore, with time, the respiratory center adapts to a lower $PaCO_2$ such that the stimulating effect of arterial hypoxemia on VA again manifests. This form of acclimatization is important for adapting to the decreased atmospheric concentration of oxygen encountered when ascending above sea level.

The ventilatory response of peripheral chemoreceptors to arterial hypoxemia is abolished by injected and inhaled anesthetics including even subanesthetic concentrations (0.1 MAC) of volatile anesthetics (Knill *et al,* 1979). For this reason, arterial hypoxemia that might occur in the early postanesthetic period is unlikely to increase alveolar ventilation.

A sensitive response of VA to changes in PaO_2 is not necessary because alveolar PO_2 is usually much higher than needed to saturate almost completely the hemoglobin. Even a 50% reduction in VA is unlikely to reduce hemoglobin saturation of oxygen much below 90%. Conversely, changes in VA have substantial effects on tissue concentrations of carbon dioxide which influence vital metabolic reactions. Therefore, it is mandatory that carbon dioxide, and not oxygen, be the major factor in the regulation of ventilation under normal conditions.

Effect of Exercise on Ventilation

An increase in ventilation occurs simultaneously with the onset of exercise due to direct stimulation of the respiratory center by the cerebral cortex (*i.e.,* anticipatory stimulation) and indirect stimulation of the respiratory center by proprioceptors that are activated by joint movement. These neurogenic factors usually stimulate the respiratory center almost exactly the proper amount to maintain an unchanged PaO_2, $PaCO_2$, and pH during even strenuous exercise.

Other Factors that Regulate Ventilation

Voluntary control of VA is mediated through the cerebral cortex rather than the respiratory center. Stimulation of the medullary vasomotor center is associated with spillover of impulses to the nearby respiratory center. As a result, decreases in blood pressure that evoke increases in sympathetic nervous system activity from the vasomotor center also evoke increases in VA due to increased activity of the respiratory center. Increased body temperature directly stimulates the respiratory center in addition to the indirect stimulation provided by increased carbon dioxide production.

The respiratory center is depressed by inhaled anesthetics and other centrally acting depressant drugs such as barbiturates and opioids. Acute cerebral edema may lead to increases in intracranial pressure that compress blood vessels supplying the respiratory center leading to ischemia and even infarction of the respiratory center.

Cerebral vascular accidents may damage the respiratory center leading to abnormalities of the breathing pattern.

Periodic Breathing

Cheyne-Stokes breathing, which is characterized by a waxing and waning pattern of ventilation, is the most common form of periodic breathing (Milhorn and Guyton, 1965). Cyclic increases and decreases in the $PaCO_2$ are the presumed mechanism for this form of periodic breathing. The normal absence of Cheyne-Stokes breathing reflects the damping effect provided by large tissue stores of carbon dioxide. When there is a delay in blood flow, however, from the lungs to the brain as in cardiac failure, the respiratory center may lag behind the $PaCO_2$ causing cyclic variations in the VA (Cherniack and Longobardo, 1973). Brain stem damage may increase the feedback gain control of the respiratory center such that a small change in the $PaCO_2$ causes a large change in VA.

RESPIRATORY PASSAGEWAYS

Inhaled gases are warmed, filtered, and humidified by the extensive vascular surfaces of the nasal turbinates and septum. Bypassing of the nasal passageways, as in the presence of a translaryngeal tracheal tube or tracheostomy, can lead to an undesirable drying effect in the lower lung.

The filtering function of the nose is due to the mucous covering of the main respiratory passages. This function is so efficient that almost no particles larger than 4 to 6 μ in diameter (*i.e.,* smaller than an erythrocyte) enter the lungs through the nose (Stuart, 1973). Foreign particles such as dust and bacteria are filtered out of the inhaled gases by adhering to the mucous blanket. Cilia move this mucus toward the pharynx where it is swallowed. Anesthetic drugs depress the velocity of mucous flow by diminishing ciliary activity. For example, mucous flow decreases from a normal 20 mm min^{-1} to 7 mm min^{-1} during halothane anesthesia (Lichtiger *et al,* 1975).

Inhaled particles that can reach the airways often accumulate in smaller bronchioles as a result of gravitational precipitation. For example, bronchiolar disease is common in coal miners reflecting the presence of settled dust particles. Even smaller particles (less than 0.5 μ) as present in cigarette smoke are exhaled or precipitated in

the alveoli. Particles that are trapped in alveoli eventually cause fibrous tissue growth in the alveolar septa, leading to irreversible damage.

Cough Reflex

Cough is the mechanism by which passageways of the lungs are maintained free of foreign particles. The larynx and carina are particularly sensitive to stimulation which results in the transmission of afferent impulses via the vagal nerves to the medulla. The medulla initiates a series of effects characterized by an inhalation followed by closure of the glottis and contraction of abdominal muscles. The result is an increase in pressure in the lungs such that air is forced outwards when the glottis suddenly opens. This rapidly moving air usually carries with it any foreign matter that is present in the larger passageways below the glottis. Depressant drugs such as opioids and volatile anesthetics as well as increasing age are associated with depression of the cough reflex (Fig. 49-5) (Pontoppidan and Beecher, 1960).

Sneeze Reflex

The sneeze reflex is similar to the cough reflex except that it applies to the nasal passageways instead of passageways below the nose. The initiating stimulus for the sneeze reflex is stimulation in the nasal passageways. Subsequent afferent impulses travel in the trigeminal nerve to the medulla where the sequence of events leading to a sneeze are initiated. The uvula is depressed so large amounts of air pass rapidly through the nose as well as through the mouth, thus helping to clear the nasal passageways of secretions.

Speech

Speech is composed of phonation, which is achieved by the larynx, and articulation, which is determined by structures in the mouth. The larynx is specially adapted to act as a vibrator. The vibrating elements are the vocal cords which are folds along the lateral walls of the larynx. The vocal cords are stretched between the thyroid cartilage and arytenoid cartilages. Specific skeletal muscles control the position and degree of stretch of the vocal cords. The vocal cords vibrate laterally in

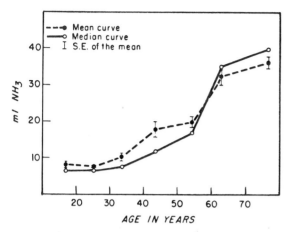

FIGURE 49-5. Volume of inhaled ammonia necessary to cause breath holding increases noticeably after 60 years of age suggesting a decline in the sensitivity of protective airway reflexes with increasing age. (By permission, Pontoppidan H, Beecher HK. Progressive loss of protective reflexes in the airway with the advance of age. JAMA 1960;174:2209–13. Copyright 1960, American Medical Association.)

response to air flow. The pitch of the sound emitted by the larynx is dependent on the degree of stretch of the vocal cords and the shape and mass of the vocal cord edges. The three organs of articulation are the lips, tongue, and soft palate. Resonators include the mouth, nose, nasal sinuses, and the pharynx.

Innervation of the Larynx

A knowledge of the innervation of the larynx is important when performing topical laryngeal anesthesia. The sensory innervation of the larynx is derived from the branches of the glossopharyngeal nerve (posterior tongue, pharynx, and tonsils) and the superior laryngeal nerve branch of the vagus nerve (epiglottis and mucous membranes of the larynx to the level of the false vocal cords). The vocal cords and upper trachea receive sensory innervation from the recurrent laryngeal nerve branch of the vagus nerve. Motor innervation of the laryngeal muscles is from the recurrent laryngeal nerve with the exception of the cricothyroid muscle, a vocal cord tensor, which is innervated by the superior laryngeal nerve.

NONVENTILATORY FUNCTIONS OF THE LUNGS

Because all blood must flow through the lungs, the function of the pulmonary capillaries as a filter for foreign particles and air is predictable. This filter effect is lost in the presence of a right-to-left intracardiac shunt or during cardiopulmonary bypass. Metabolic functions of the lung include removal of vasoactive substances such as norepinephrine, histamine, and prostaglandins as they pass through the lungs (Marshall, 1973). Inhaled anesthetics may interfere with the normal removal of norepinephrine from the blood by the lungs (Naito and Gillis, 1973).

REFERENCES

Biscoe TJ. Carotid body: Structure and function. Physiol Rev 1971;51:427–95.

Cherniack NS, Longobardo GS. Cheyne-Stokes breathing. An instability in physiologic control. N Engl J Med 1973;288:952–7.

Clements JA. Pulmonary surfactant (editorial). Am Rev Resp Dis 1970;101:984–90.

Cohen MI. Discharge patterns of brain-stem respiratory neurons in relation to carbon dioxide tension. J Neurophysiol 1968;31:142–65.

Cohen MI. Neurogenesis of respiratory rhythm in the mammal. Physiol Rev 1979;59:1105–73.

Downes JJ, Lambertsen CJ. Dynamic characteristics of ventilatory depression in man on abrupt administration of oxygen. J Appl Physiol 1966;21:447–53.

Engel LA, Macklem PT. Gas mixing and distribution in the lung. Int Rev Physiol 1977;14:37–82.

Guyton AC. Textbook of Medical Physiology. 7th ed. Philadelphia: WB Saunders, 1986:504.

Guz A. Regulation of respiration in man. Annu Rev Physiol 1975;37:303–23.

Heinemann HO, Goldring RM. Bicarbonate and the regulation of ventilation. Am J Med 1974;57:361–70.

Knill RL, Manninen PH, Clement JL. Ventilation and chemoreflexes during enflurane sedation and anesthesia in man. Can Anaesth Soc J 1979;26:353–60.

Lausen I. Regulation of cerebrospinal fluid composition with reference to breathing. Physiol Rev 1972;52:1–56.

Lichtiger M, Landa JF, Hirsch MA. Velocity of tracheal mucous in anesthetized women undergoing gynecologic surgery. Anesthesiology 1975;42:753–6.

Macklem PT. Respiratory mechanics. Annu Rev Physiol 1978;40:157–84.

Marshall BE. Non-respiratory functions of the lung. Anesthesiology 1973;39:573–4.

Mead J. Respiration: Pulmonary mechanics. Ann Rev Physiol 1973;35:169–92.

Milhorn HT, Guyton AC. An analog computer analysis of

Cheyne-Stokes breathing. J Appl Physiol 1965; 20:328–33.

Mitchell RA, Berger AJ. Neural regulation of respiration. Am Rev Resp Dis 1975;111:206–24.

Naito H, Gillis CN. Effects of halothane and nitrous oxide on removal of norepinephrine from the pulmonary circulation. Anesthesiology 1973;39:575–80.

Paintal AS. Vagal sensory receptors and their reflex effects. Physiol Rev 1973;53:159–227.

Paskin S, Skovsted P, Smith TC. Failure of the Hering-Breuer reflex to account for tachypnea in anesthetized man: A survey of halothane, fluroxene, methoxyflurane, and cyclopropane. Anesthesiology 1968;29:550–8.

Pontoppidan H, Beecher HK. Progressive loss of protective reflexes in the airway with the advance of age. JAMA 1960;174:2209–13.

Stuart BO. Deposition of inhaled aerosols. Arch Intern Med 1973;131:60–73.

Thurlbeck WM. Structure of the lungs. Int Rev Physiol 1977;14:1–36.

Pulmonary Gas Exchange and Blood Transport of Gases

PULMONARY GAS EXCHANGE

Oxygen leaves alveoli to enter pulmonary capillary blood, and carbon dioxide enters alveoli from pulmonary capillary blood by the process of diffusion (West, 1977). There is always a net diffusion of molecules from areas of high pressure to areas of low pressure which is directly proportional to the pressure difference divided by the distance for diffusion (*i.e.,* diffusion gradient). When the pressures of gas molecules in each phase are identical, net transfer of molecules ceases (*i.e.,* the number of molecules entering a phase is equal to the number leaving). In addition to the diffusion gradient, the rate of gas diffusion is influenced by the (1) solubility of gas in the fluid, (2) cross-sectional area of the membrane, (3) molecular weight of the gas, and (4) temperature of the fluid in the body.

Partial Pressure

The partial pressure that a gas exerts is due to the constant impaction of the kinetically moving molecules against a surface. The greater the concentration of gas, the greater also will be the sum of the forces of impaction of all the molecules striking the surface at any instant. As a result, the partial pressure of a gas is directly proportional to its concentration. In addition, temperature influences the kinetic energy of the molecules.

In a mixture of gases, the partial pressure that each gas contributes to the total pressure is directly proportional to its relative concentration (Table 50-1). For example, at sea level, 79% of the total atmospheric pressure of 760 mmHg is due to nitrogen (*i.e.,* PN_2 597 mmHg) and 21% is due to oxygen (*i.e.,* PO_2 159 mmHg). The total atmospheric pressure is equal to the sum of all the individual partial pressures.

When a gas–liquid or gas–tissue interface exists, gas molecules dissolve in the liquid or tissue until equilibrium is achieved. Equilibrium is present when the number of molecules leaving the gas phase equals the number returning to the gas phase. At equilibrium, the partial pressure of the dissolved gas is equal to the pressure of gas in the gas phase, each pushing against each other at the interface with equal force.

The concentration of a gas in liquid is determined not only by the partial pressure the gas exerts but also by the solubility coefficient of the gas. For example, some molecules are physically or chemically attracted to water (*e.g.,* carbon dioxide) while others are repelled. Molecules that are attracted to water dissolve in water without building up excess partial pressure in the solution. Conversely, molecules that are repelled will develop high partial pressures for minimal solubility in a solution. Henry's law states that the concentration of a dissolved gas is equal to the partial pressure of that gas times its solubility coefficient.

Table 50-1
Partial Pressures of Respiratory Gases at Sea Level (760 mmHg)

	Inhaled Air (mmHg)	Alveolar Gases (mmHg)	Exhaled Gases (mmHg)
Oxygen	159	104	120
Carbon dioxide	0.3	40	27
Nitrogen	597	569	566
Water	3.7	47	47

Vapor Pressure of Water

Water in tissues has a tendency to escape into an adjoining gas phase just as molecules in the gas phase pass into the water. The pressure that water molecules exert to escape to the surface is the vapor pressure of water (PH_2O). At normal body temperature of 37 Celsius, the PH_2O is 47 mmHg. The PH_2O depends entirely on the temperature of water. The greater the temperature, the greater is the kinetic activity of the molecules and thus the greater is the likelihood that water molecules will escape from the surface into the gas phase.

Composition of Alveolar Gases

Composition of alveolar gases is different than the composition of inhaled (atmospheric) gases because (1) oxygen is constantly being absorbed from the alveoli, (2) carbon dioxide is constantly being added to the alveoli, and (3) dry inhaled gases are humidified by the addition of water vapor (Table 50-1). Because the total partial pressure of gases in the alveoli remains unchanged, the addition of water vapor and carbon dioxide to the inhaled gases dilutes the delivered partial pressure of oxygen from 159 to 104 mmHg and the partial pressure of nitrogen from 597 to 569 mmHg.

Alveolar Partial Pressure of Oxygen (PAO₂)

The PAO_2 is determined by the rate of delivery of new oxygen by alveolar ventilation and the rate of absorption of oxygen into pulmonary capillary blood. The normal rate of absorption of oxygen is

250 ml min^{-1}. Exercise increases oxygen absorption into blood and the PAO_2 declines unless alveolar ventilation increases oxygen input sufficiently to offset the increased absorption. Regardless of the level of alveolar ventilation, the PAO_2 can never exceed 149 mmHg breathing air (*i.e.*, 21% oxygen).

The inhaled partial pressure of oxygen is diluted by the alveolar partial pressure of carbon dioxide (40 mmHg) and water vapor (47 mmHg) both of which remain nearly constant regardless of barometric pressure. The impact of this dilution on the PAO_2 is greater when the inhaled partial pressure of oxygen is already reduced by decreased barometric pressure. Breathing pure oxygen offsets the dilutional effect of carbon dioxide and water vapor.

Alveolar Partial Pressure of Carbon Dioxide (PACO₂)

The $PACO_2$ is determined by the rate of delivery of carbon dioxide to the alveoli from pulmonary capillary blood and the rate of removal of this carbon dioxide from the alveoli by alveolar ventilation. The normal rate of delivery of carbon dioxide to alveoli by blood is 200 ml min^{-1}. In the presence of a constant delivery of carbon dioxide to alveoli, the $PACO_2$ is directly proportional to the alveolar ventilation.

Composition of Exhaled Gases

The composition of exhaled gases is determined by the proportion that is alveolar gas and the proportion that is dead space gas (Table 50-1) (see Chapter 49). The first portion of exhaled gas is dead space gas. The composition of this dead space gas resembles the composition of inhaled gas. Progressively, more and more alveolar gas becomes mixed with dead space gas until all the dead space gas has been exhaled and only alveolar gas remains. For this reason, collection of the last portion of exhaled gas (*i.e.*, end-tidal sample) is a method for analyzing the composition of alveolar gas.

Gas Diffusion from Alveoli to Blood

There are an estimated 150 million alveoli in each lung with each alveolus having a diameter of about

0.25 mm (Weibel, 1973). Alveolar walls are extremely thin and within these walls, there is almost a solid network of interconnecting capillaries. The average thickness of the respiratory membrane is estimated to be 0.5 μ. The total surface area of the respiratory membrane is about 70 m², and the 60 to 140 ml of blood in the pulmonary capillaries at any time is spread as a thin sheet over this surface ensuring rapid diffusion of gases.

The average diameter of the pulmonary capillaries is only 8 μ, which means that erythrocytes must actually squeeze through these vessels. As a result, the surface of the erythrocyte usually touches the capillary wall so that the distance for diffusion of oxygen and carbon dioxide is minimal. This anatomic arrangement increases the rapidity of diffusion.

Rate of Gas Diffusion

Factors that determine how rapidly a gas molecule will pass through the respiratory membrane include the (1) thickness of the membrane, (2) the surface area of the membrane, (3) the diffusion coefficient of the gas in the substance of the membrane, and (4) the partial pressure difference between the two sides of the membrane.

THICKNESS OF MEMBRANE. The thickness of the respiratory membrane may be increased as a result of edema fluid in alveoli or interstitial space of the membrane resulting in an increase in the diffusion distance for molecules. The rate of diffusion through the membrane is inversely proportional to the thickness of the membrane. Any factor that increases the thickness of the membrane by two to three times can significantly interfere with exchange of gases across the respiratory membrane.

SURFACE AREA. The surface area of the respiratory membrane is decreased by emphysema in which many of the alveoli coalesce into large sacs but with less surface area because of loss of alveolar walls. When the total surface area is reduced to about one-fourth normal, exchange of gases through the respiratory membrane is inadequate even under resting conditions.

DIFFUSION COEFFICIENT. The diffusion coefficient for the transfer of each gas through the respiratory membrane depends on its solubility in the constituents of the membrane and inversely on the square root of the molecular weight of the gas. The rate of diffusion of gases through constituents of the respiratory membrane is about the same as through water. Therefore, carbon dioxide (molecular weight 44) diffuses through the respiratory membrane about 20 times as rapidly as oxygen, while oxygen diffuses about twice as rapidly as nitrogen.

PARTIAL PRESSURE DIFFERENCE. The partial pressure difference for gases in blood and alveoli determines the direction of diffusion. PAO_2 exceeds that in blood such that oxygen molecules diffuse from alveoli into pulmonary capillary blood. The partial pressure gradient for carbon dioxide is reversed and carbon dioxide readily diffuses from pulmonary capillary blood into alveoli.

Diffusing Capacity

The diffusing capacity is the volume of gas that can diffuse through the respiratory membrane for each 1 mmHg of partial pressure difference. At rest, the diffusing capacity for oxygen is about 21 ml min^{-1} mmHg^{-1}, and the partial pressure difference across the respiratory membrane is about 11 mmHg. This results in a net transfer of about 230 (21×11) ml min^{-1} of oxygen into pulmonary capillary blood from alveoli. This rate of oxygen transfer parallels the minute oxygen consumption by the body. During exercise, there is dilatation of pulmonary capillaries as well as opening of previously closed capillaries resulting in an increased surface area for diffusion to occur. Indeed, diffusing capacity may approach 65 ml min^{-1} mmHg^{-1} during strenuous exercise.

Carbon dioxide diffuses through the capillary endothelium so rapidly that the partial pressure difference between pulmonary capillary blood and alveolar gas for carbon dioxide is less than 1 mmHg. Based on the fact that the diffusion coefficient of carbon dioxide is 20 times that of oxygen, the estimated diffusing capacity for carbon dioxide is 400 to 450 ml min^{-1} mmHg^{-1}. This high diffusing capacity is the reason damage to the alveolar-capillary membrane jeopardizes diffusion of oxygen more than carbon dioxide.

Ventilation to Perfusion Ratio

The ratio of alveolar ventilation to pulmonary capillary blood flow (V/Q) determines ultimately the composition of the alveolar gas. In the presence of an optimal V/Q ratio, the PaO$_2$ is about 104 mmHg, and the PaCO$_2$ is 40 mmHg. The V/Q ratio is also important in determining the effectiveness of gas exchange across the respiratory membrane, particularly oxygen exchange.

A V/Q ratio of zero is present when there is no ventilation to an alveolus that continues to be perfused by pulmonary capillary blood. The remaining gas in such an alveolus equilibrates with the partial pressures of oxygen (40 mmHg) and carbon dioxide (45 mmHg) in the blood that continues to perfuse the alveolus.

A V/Q ratio equal to infinity means that there is alveolar ventilation but no pulmonary capillary blood flow to that alveolus. The alveolar gas content of these unperfused alveoli approaches and ultimately equals inhaled gas concentrations (*i.e.*, PO$_2$ 159 mmHg, PCO$_2$ zero). These alveoli, like those alveoli that receive no ventilation (V/Q ratio zero), do not participate in gas exchange.

The V/Q ratio is higher at the apex than at the base of the lung. The higher V/Q ratio at the apex of the lung manifests as a higher PAO$_2$ in this area of the lung. Similarly, PACO$_2$ differs from the top to lower portions of the lung with venous blood from the apex having a lower partial pressure of carbon dioxide than blood from the base. The effect of this uneven V/Q ratio, however, in total gas exchange is practically insignificant.

Physiologic Shunt

Physiologic shunt occurs when the V/Q ratio is below normal such that there is inadequate ventilation to optimally oxygenate the pulmonary capillary blood perfusing the alveolus. The fraction of pulmonary capillary blood that does not become oxygenated is referred to as *shunted blood*. This shunted blood plus the approximately 2% of the cardiac output which normally bypasses the lungs by flowing through the bronchial veins into pulmonary veins and Thebesian and anterior cardiac veins draining into the left side of the heart is designated the *physiologic shunt*. In the standing position, ventilation to the lower portions of the lung is decreased relative to pulmonary blood flow. As a result, a small fraction of blood flowing through the lower portions of the lungs is inadequately oxygenated representing physiologic shunt. Obstructive airways disease most often associated with cigarette smoking interferes with ventilation of perfused alveoli and is a common cause of phys-

iologic shunt. Physiologic shunt is calculated from measurements of the oxygen concentration of mixed venous and arterial blood (Table 50-2).

Physiologic Dead Space

When ventilation to an alveolus exceeds the pulmonary capillary blood flow to that alveolus, the excess ventilation is wasted. This wasted ventilation combined with that inhaled gas that fills the respiratory dead space is designated the *physiologic dead space*. In the standing position, blood flow to upper portions of the lung is decreased more than ventilation, which causes a modest degree of physiologic dead space in this area of the lung. The ratio of physiologic dead space to tidal volume is calculated by measuring the tidal volume, PaCO$_2$, and the average partial pressure of carbon dioxide in the exhaled air (P$_E$CO$_2$) (Table 50-3).

Table 50-2
Calculation of Physiologic Shunt Fraction

$$Q_s/Q_T = \frac{CcO_2 - CaO_2}{CcO_2 - CvO_2}$$

Q$_s$ = fraction of pulmonary blood flow not exposed to ventilated alveoli
Q$_T$ = total pulmonary blood flow
CcO$_2$ = oxygen content of pulmonary capillary blood, ml dl^{-1}
CaO$_2$ = oxygen content of arterial blood, ml dl^{-1}
CvO$_2$ = oxygen content of mixed venous blood, ml dl^{-1}

Table 50-3
Calculation of the Physiologic Dead Space to Tidal Volume Ratio

$$V_D/V_T = \frac{PaCO_2 - P_ECO_2}{PaCO_2}$$

V$_D$/V$_T$ = ratio of physiologic dead space to tidal volume
PaCO$_2$ = arterial partial pressure of carbon dioxide, mmHg
P$_E$CO$_2$ = mixed exhaled partial pressure of carbon dioxide, mmHg

BLOOD TRANSPORT OF OXYGEN AND CARBON DIOXIDE

After diffusion from alveoli into pulmonary capillary blood, oxygen is transported principally in combination with hemoglobin to tissue capillaries where it is released along a partial pressure gradient for use by cells (Wagner, 1977). Carbon dioxide, formed in the cells from oxygen-dependent metabolic pathways, enters tissue capillaries along a partial pressure gradient for transport back to alveoli.

Oxygen Uptake in the Blood

The partial pressure of oxygen in the mixed venous blood (PvO_2) returning to the lungs is about 40 mmHg, reflecting the large amount of oxygen that has been removed from the blood as it flows through various tissues (Fig. 50-1) (Guyton, 1986). This mixed venous blood is exposed to a PAO_2 of about 104 mmHg leading to a rapid diffusion of oxygen along a partial pressure gradient (*e.g.,* 64 mmHg) into pulmonary capillary blood. Indeed, the PO_2 of pulmonary capillary blood is essentially equal to the PAO_2 after passing through

only the first third of the capillary (Fig. 50-1) (Guyton, 1986). This rapid equilibration of pulmonary capillary blood with the PAO_2 provides an important safety factor for transfer of oxygen when blood flow through the lungs is accelerated as during exercise.

Blood leaving the pulmonary capillaries has a PO_2 of about 104 mmHg while the arterial blood, which contains bronchial blood flow that has bypassed the lungs, has a PaO_2 of about 95 mmHg (Fig. 50-2) (Guyton, 1986). This is due to the dilutional effect produced by the low PO_2 in the bronchial blood.

Diffusion of Oxygen from the Capillaries

The PO_2 in interstitial fluid averages about 40 mmHg providing a large initial partial pressure gradient for diffusion of oxygen from tissue capillaries where the PaO_2 is about 95 mmHg (Fig. 50-3) (Guyton, 1986). At the end of the capillary, the PO_2 in blood and the interstitial fluid have nearly equilibrated such that the PvO_2 is also about 40 mmHg.

Interstitial fluid PO_2 is increased when tissue blood flow increases, reflecting greater oxygen delivery to the tissues. Associated increases in tissue oxygen requirements, if present, will offset the effect of increased oxygen delivery and interstitial fluid PO_2 is unchanged or even decreased if tissue oxygen utilization exceeds delivery. Since about 97% of the oxygen transported in the blood is carried by hemoglobin, a decrease in the concentration of hemoglobin has the same effect on interstitial fluid PO_2 as does a decrease in tissue blood flow (Bruley, 1973).

Diffusion of Carbon Dioxide from the Cells

Continuous formation of carbon dioxide in cells maintains a partial pressure gradient for diffusion of this gas into the capillary blood (Fig. 50-4) (Guyton, 1986). Diffusion of carbon dioxide from cells into interstitial fluid and then into capillaries is rapid despite a partial pressure gradient of only 1 to 6 mmHg compared with about 64 mmHg for oxygen. Indeed, carbon dioxide diffuses about 20 times as easily as oxygen.

The lower limit to which interstitial PCO_2 can decline from its normal value of 45 mmHg is to that of the $PaCO_2$, which is about 40 mmHg. For

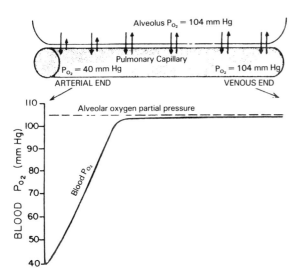

FIGURE 50-1. Schematic depiction of the uptake of oxygen by the pulmonary capillary blood. (From Guyton AC. Textbook of Medical Physiology. 7th ed. Philadelphia: WB Saunders, 1986:493. Reproduced by permission of the author and publisher.)

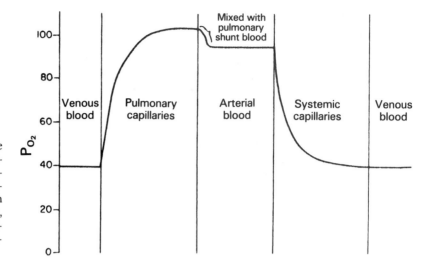

FIGURE 50-2. Changes in the PO_2 as blood traverses the systemic and pulmonary circulations. (From Guyton AC. Textbook of Medical Physiology. 7th ed. Philadelphia: WB Saunders, 1986:493. Reproduced by permission of the author and publisher.)

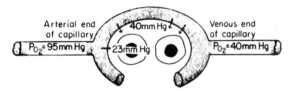

FIGURE 50-3. Schematic depiction of the diffusion of oxygen from tissue capillaries into the interstitial fluid. (From Guyton AC. Textbook of Medical Physiology. 7th ed. Philadelphia: WB Saunders, 1986;493. Reproduced by permission of the author and publisher.)

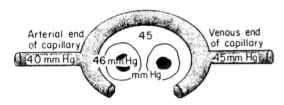

FIGURE 50-4. Schematic depiction of uptake of carbon dioxide by capillary blood. (From Guyton AC. Textbook of Medical Physiology. 7th ed. Philadelphia: WB Saunders, 1986:493. Reproduced by permission of the author and publisher.)

example, an increase in tissue blood flow to six times normal reduces the tissue PCO_2 only to 41 mmHg. Conversely, reductions in tissue blood flow or increases in metabolic rate can substantially increase the tissue PCO_2.

On arrival at alveoli the venous PCO_2 is only 5 to 6 mmHg greater than the $PACO_2$, a diffusion gradient some 10 to 12 times less than that for oxygen. As for passage into the capillaries, however, the fact that the diffusion coefficient for carbon dioxide is 20 times that for oxygen facilitates the rapid passage of carbon dioxide from blood to alveoli.

Blood Transport Oxygen

About 97% of oxygen transported from alveoli to the tissues is carried to tissues in chemical combination with hemoglobin (Bruley, 1973; Perutz, 1978). Indeed, the most important feature of the hemoglobin molecule is its ability to combine loosely with molecular oxygen. A single molecule of hemoglobin can combine with four molecules of oxygen. About 3% of oxygen is transported to tissues in the dissolved state in plasma.

When the PO_2 in pulmonary capillaries is elevated, oxygen binds with hemoglobin, but when the PO_2 is low, as in tissue capillaries, oxygen is released from hemoglobin (Perutz, 1978). This is the basis of transport of oxygen from alveoli to tissues and emphasizes that the combination of oxygen with hemoglobin is very loose varying with the partial pressure of oxygen in the blood. This reaction occurs independent of any enzyme action or change in the ferrous state of iron in the hemoglobin molecule. Therefore, this uptake of oxygen by hemoglobin is termed oxygenation rather than oxidation.

Each gram of hemoglobin can combine with about 1.34 ml of oxygen (1.39 ml when hemoglobin is chemically pure) (Perutz, 1978). Therefore, in the presence of a normal hemoglobin concentration of 15 g dl^{-1}, blood will carry about 20 ml of oxygen when the hemoglobin is 100% saturated. About 5 ml of these 20 ml of oxygen carried in each 100 ml of blood pass from capillaries into tissues. The loss of 5 ml of oxygen from each 100 ml of blood reduces the hemoglobin saturation with oxygen to about 75% corresponding to a mixed venous PO$_2$ of about 40 mmHg.

About 0.29 ml of oxygen is dissolved in every 100 ml of blood when the PO$_2$ is 95 mmHg (Bruley, 1973). When the PO$_2$ of blood declines to 40 mmHg in tissue capillaries, about 0.12 ml of oxygen remains dissolved. This means that about 0.17 ml of oxygen is delivered to the tissues in the dissolved state in every 100 ml of blood compared with about 5 ml of oxygen attached to hemoglobin in the same amount of blood. Breathing enriched concentrations of oxygen increases the amount of dissolved oxygen in every ml of blood by 0.003 ml for every mmHg rise in the partial pressure of oxygen (*i.e.,* 0.3 ml of oxygen is dissolved for every 100 mmHg of partial pressure of oxygen).

Under resting conditions, about 5 ml of oxygen is released to the tissues from every 100 ml of blood resulting in a total delivery of 250 ml of oxygen to tissues each minute when the cardiac output is 5 L min^{-1} (West, 1977). This tissue oxygen delivery can be increased by increasing the cardiac output. In cells, the partial pressure of oxygen required to maintain chemical reactions is only 3 to 5 mmHg (Whalen, 1971). Under normal conditions, the rate of intracellular utilization of oxygen is dependent on the concentration of adenosine triphosphate and not the availability of oxygen to the cells. Cells are rarely more than 50 μ from a capillary, and oxygen can readily diffuse this short distance. Ultimately, the total amount of oxygen available each minute for use in any given tissue is determined by the content of oxygen in the blood and the tissue blood flow.

Hemoglobin

Hemoglobin is a conjugated protein with a molecular weight of 66,700 (Perutz, 1978). Synthesis of hemoglobin begins in the erythroblasts and continues through formation of reticulocytes (see Chapter 56). The four heme molecules with a central iron atom combine with globin, a globulin protein synthesized in the ribosomes of the endoplasmic reticulum to form hemoglobin. The globin portion of the hemoglobin molecule is composed of four polypeptide chains of more than 700 amino acids. The sequence of these amino acids, which is determined genetically, influences the binding affinity of hemoglobin for oxygen.

TYPES OF HEMOGLOBIN. Types of hemoglobin are designated as A through S depending on the sequence of amino acids in the polypeptide chains. Normal adult hemoglobin A consists of two identical alpha polypeptide chains and two identical beta polypeptide chains. Fetal erythrocytes contain fetal hemoglobin (hemoglobin F) which has a low concentration of 2,3-diphosphoglycerate and a resulting high affinity for oxygen. The oxyhemoglobin dissociation curve of hemoglobin F is shifted to the left, which facilitates transfer of oxygen from the placenta to the fetus. Indeed, at a normal umbilical vein PO$_2$ of 28 mmHg, fetal hemoglobin is 80% saturated with oxygen while adult hemoglobin (*i.e.,* hemoglobin A) would only be about 50% saturated with oxygen at this same PO$_2$ (Fig. 50-5). After birth,

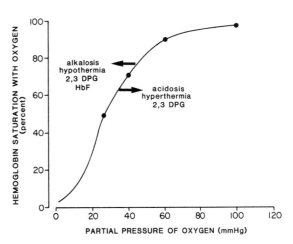

FIGURE 50-5. Oxyhemoglobin dissociation curve for adult hemoglobin (HbA) at pH 7.4 and 37 Celsius. Changes in arterial pH, body temperature, concentration of 2,3-disphosphoglycerate (2,3-DPG), and presence of different types of hemoglobin (fetal hemoglobin, HbF) shift the oxyhemoglobin dissociation curve to the left or right of its normal position.

the presence of hemoglobin F impairs release of oxygen to tissues accounting for the disappearance of fetal hemoglobin by 4 to 6 months of age.

With the exception of hemoglobin A and hemoglobin F, all other forms of hemoglobin are considered abnormal. The oxyhemoglobin dissociation curves for these abnormal hemoglobins are shifted to the right of hemoglobin A. This rightward shift of the oxyhemoglobin dissociation curve interferes with the transfer of oxygen from the alveoli to hemoglobin (see the section entitled Oxyhemoglobin Dissociation Curve). Abnormal types of hemoglobin result from changes in the amino acid sequences of the polypeptide chains of globin. For example, substitution of valine for glutamic acid in two of the four polypeptide chains of hemoglobin A results in hemoglobin S. Erythrocytes containing hemoglobin S become elongated when exposed to low concentrations of oxygen and are known as *sickle cells.*

MYOGLOBIN. Myoglobin has a structural formula similar to hemoglobin. Unlike hemoglobin, however, myoglobin binds only one molecule rather than four molecules of oxygen. As a result, its dissociation curve is a hyperbola rather than S-shaped. The main function of myoglobin is to provide a source of oxygen to skeletal muscle (Wittenberg, 1970). Oxygen cannot be released from myoglobin until the PaO_2 has decreased to very low values.

Oxyhemoglobin Dissociation Curve

The percent saturation of hemoglobin with oxygen at different partial pressures of oxygen in the blood is described by the oxyhemoglobin dissociation curve (Fig. 50-5). The S-shape of the oxyhemoglobin dissociation curve explains several important properties of hemoglobin. For example, increasing PaO_2 above 100 mmHg increases the concentration of oxygen in the blood only slightly. This reflects the fact that hemoglobin is already at least 97% saturated with oxygen when the PaO_2 is 100 mmHg. Likewise, reducing the PaO_2 to 60 mmHg maintains at least 90% saturation of hemoglobin with oxygen reflecting the flat aspect of the oxyhemoglobin dissociation curve over this range. At tissue capillaries where the PO_2 is 20 to 40 mmHg, the oxyhemoglobin curve is steep such that small changes in PaO_2 result in transfer of large amounts of oxygen from hemoglobin to tissues.

Shift of the Oxyhemoglobin Dissociation Curve

A number of different factors can displace the oxyhemoglobin dissociation curve to the left or to the right (Wagner, 1974). Acidosis, increased body temperature, and increased concentrations of 2,3-diphosphoglycerate (2,3-DPG) shift the curve to the right while alkalosis, decreased body temperature, decreased concentrations of 2,3-DPG, and the presence of fetal hemoglobin have an opposite effect (Fig. 50-5).

For unknown reasons, inhaled anesthetics produce a modest rightward shift of the oxyhemoglobin dissociation curve (Gillies *et al,* 1970; Kambam, 1982). A convenient indicator of the position of the oxyhemoglobin dissociation curve is the partial pressure of oxygen when only 50% of the hemoglobin is saturated with oxygen (*i.e.,* P_{50}). In the normal adult at a pH of 7.4 and body temperature of 37 Celsius, the P_{50} is about 26 mmHg (Fig. 50-5). A shift of the oxyhemoglobin dissociation curve to the right is reflected by an increase of the P_{50} above 26 mmHg, while P_{50} is less than 26 mmHg when the oxyhemoglobin curve is shifted to the left. For example, inhaled anesthetics increase the P_{50} by 2 to 3.5 mmHg. A shift of the oxyhemoglobin curve to the left means the PO_2 must decline further before oxygen is released from hemoglobin to tissues.

BOHR EFFECT. The Bohr effect is the shift in the oxyhemoglobin dissociation caused by changes in the blood concentration of carbon dioxide. In the lungs, diffusion of carbon dioxide into alveoli increases the pH of the blood (alkalosis) which shifts the oxyhemoglobin dissociation curve to the left thus enhancing the affinity of hemoglobin for oxygen. At tissues, carbon dioxide enters blood causing the pH to decrease and the oxyhemoglobin dissociation curve to shift to the right facilitating the release of oxygen from hemoglobin.

DIPHOSPHOGLYCERATE (2,3-DPG). The effect of 2,3-DPG is to shift the oxyhemoglobin dissociation curve to the right (*i.e.,* decrease the affinity of hemoglobin for oxygen) causing oxygen to be released to the tissues at a higher PaO_2 than in the absence of this substance. The increase in the concentration of 2,3-DPG evoked by arterial hypoxemia, as occurs with ascent to altitude, could thus serve as a compensatory response to improve the unloading of oxygen from hemoglobin to tissues. This beneficial effect, however, may be offset by impaired loading of oxygen to hemoglobin at the lungs. Other events associated with increased concentrations of 2,3-DPG in the erythrocyte include anemia and hormones such as thyroid and growth hormone. Storage of whole blood is associated with a progressive decline in the erythrocyte concentration of 2,3-DPG. This decline is less in blood preserved in citrate-phosphate-dextrose than in acid-citrate-dextrose.

During exercise, the oxyhemoglobin dissociation curve for skeletal muscle is shifted to the right reflecting release of carbon dioxide by exercising muscle so as to increase the hydrogen ion concentration of muscle capillary blood. In addition, phosphate compounds are released and the temperature of the exercising skeletal muscle may increase 3 to 4 degrees Celsius. These changes allow hemoglobin to continue to release oxygen to the skeletal muscle (*i.e.,* oxyhemoglobin dissociation curve shifted to the right) even when the PO_2 in the blood has decreased to as low as 40 mm Hg.

Carbon Monoxide

Carbon monoxide combines with hemoglobin at the same point on the hemoglobin molecule as does oxygen. Furthermore, the strength of this bonding is about 230 times greater than that exhibited by oxygen. Therefore, a carbon monoxide partial pressure of 0.4 mmHg is equivalent to an oxygen partial pressure of 92 mmHg. At this partial pressure of carbon monoxide about half the hemoglobin is bound with this gas rather than oxygen. A carbon monoxide partial pressure of 0.7 mmHg can bind nearly all the hemoglobin sites normally occupied by oxygen. High inhaled concentrations of oxygen that greatly increase the partial pressure of oxygen in the blood effectively displace carbon monoxide from hemoglobin. This is the reason for considering the use of a hyperbaric oxygen chamber in the treatment of severe carbon monoxide poisoning.

Cyanosis

Cyanosis is the term used to describe blueness of the skin caused by the presence of excessive amounts of deoxygenated hemoglobin in the cutaneous blood vessels. More than 5 g of deoxygenated hemoglobin causes cyanosis regardless of the overall concentration of oxyhemoglobin. Therefore, patients with polycythemia may appear cyanotic despite adequate arterial concentrations of oxygen while the anemic patient may lack sufficient hemoglobin to produce enough deoxygenated hemoglobin to cause cyanosis even in the presence of profound tissue hypoxia. The degree of cyanosis is influenced by the rate of blood flow through the skin. If cutaneous blood flow is sluggish, even low skin metabolism may result in production of sufficient deoxygenated hemoglobin to cause cyanosis. This is the explanation for the occurrence of peripheral cyanosis in cold weather particularly when thin skin permits transmission of the color of deoxygenated hemoglobin from the deeper vascular structures.

Blood Transport of Carbon Dioxide

Carbon dioxide formed as a result of metabolic processes in cells readily diffuses across cell membranes into capillary blood. Despite the fact that the partial pressure difference of carbon dioxide between tissues and blood is only 1 to 6 mmHg, the high solubility of this gas permits rapid transfer. An average of 4 ml of carbon dioxide in each 100 ml of blood is transported to the lungs as (1) dissolved carbon dioxide, (2) bicarbonate ions, and (3) carbaminohemoglobin (Fig. 50-6) (Guyton, 1986).

Dissolved Carbon Dioxide

About 0.3 ml of the 4 ml of carbon dioxide in every 100 ml of blood (*i.e.,* about 7% of the total) is transported to the lungs in the dissolved state. The partial pressure of carbon dioxide in the mixed venous blood is increased from 40 mmHg to about 45 mmHg by the addition of this dissolved carbon dioxide to that already present in the blood. This increase in the $PACO_2$ lowers the pH of the venous blood to 7.36 compared with a pH of 7.4 in arterial blood and a $PaCO_2$ of 40 mmHg. The ratio of dissolved carbon dioxide to bicarbonate ions is normally 20:1.

Bicarbonate Ions

The vast majority of carbon dioxide (about 2.8 ml of the 4 ml) that enters the tissue capillaries for transport to the lungs reacts with water in the erythrocytes to form carbonic acid. This reaction in the erythrocytes is almost instantaneous due to

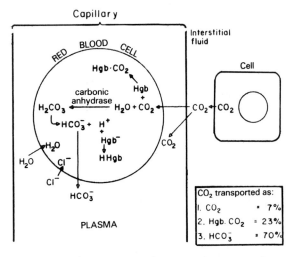

FIGURE 50-6. Schematic depiction of transport of carbon dioxide in blood. (From Guyton AC. Textbook of Medical Physiology. 7th ed. Philadelphia: WB Saunders, 1986:493. Reproduced by permission of the author and publisher.)

the accelerating effects of the enzyme, carbonic anhydrase, on the reaction (Maren, 1967). Administration of a carbonic anhydrase inhibitor such as acetazolamide, interferes with this transport mechanism, and resulting accumulation of carbon dioxide leads to tissue acidosis. Carbonic anhydrase is essentially absent in the plasma. Immediately following the formation of carbonic acid, there is dissociation of this weak acid into hydrogen ions and bicarbonate ions. Most of the hydrogen ions then combine with hemoglobin which acts as a powerful acid–base buffer. Bicarbonate ions diffuse from erythrocytes into plasma while chloride ions enter the erythrocytes to take their place (*i.e.,* chloride shift). As a result of this chloride shift, the chloride content of venous erythrocytes is greater than that of arterial erythrocytes. The increase in osmotically active ions such as chloride and bicarbonate ions in the erythrocytes of venous blood leads to water retention by the cell leading to an increase in its size. Indeed, this is the reason the venous hematocrit is about 3% greater than the arterial hematocrit.

Carbaminohemoglobin

A third transport mechanism for the transport of carbon dioxide to the lungs is the formation of carbaminohemoglobin due to the combination of carbon dioxide with hemoglobin (Kilmartin and Ross-Bernardi, 1973). A small amount of carbon dioxide interacts in a similar way with plasma proteins. It is estimated that 0.9 ml of the 4 ml of carbon dioxide in each 100 ml of blood is transported to the lungs by this mechanism.

HALDANE EFFECT. At the lungs, the combination of oxygen with hemoglobin causes hemoglobin to become a stronger acid. As a result, carbaminohemoglobin dissociates, and the increased acidity provides hydrogen ions to combine with bicarbonate ions to form carbonic acid. Carbonic acid rapidly dissociates into water and carbon dioxide, with the carbon dioxide instantly diffusing from pulmonary capillary blood into alveoli. The phenomenon of displacement of carbon dioxide from hemoglobin by oxygen that occurs at the lungs is known as the *Haldane effect.* Conversely, the Haldane effect at the tissues facilitates the passage of carbon dioxide into capillary blood.

Body Stores of Carbon Dioxide

In contrast to total body oxygen stores of about 1500 ml (about 1000 ml in arterial blood), there are an estimated 120 liters of carbon dioxide dissolved in the body. In the presence of apnea, but provision of oxygen (*i.e.,* apneic oxygenation) the rate of rise of the PCO_2 during the first minute of apnea is about 5 to 10 mmHg (Eger and Severinghaus, 1961). This initial rapid rise in the $PaCO_2$ represents equilibration of the alveolar gas with the mixed venous PCO_2. Following this first minute of apnea, the $PaCO_2$ increases about 3 mmHg min^{-1} reflecting metabolic production of carbon dioxide.

Respiratory Quotient

The ratio of carbon dioxide output to oxygen uptake is the respiratory quotient. During resting conditions, the amount of oxygen added to blood (*i.e.,* 5 ml dl^{-1}) exceeds the amount of carbon dioxide that is removed from the blood (*i.e.,* 4 ml dl^{-1}) resulting in a respiratory quotient of 0.8. The respiratory quotient varies with different metabolic conditions increasing to 1 when carbohydrates are being used exclusively for metabolism and declining to 0.7 when fat is the primary source of metabolic energy. The reason for this difference is the formation of one molecule of carbon dioxide for every molecule of oxygen consumed when carbohydrates are metabolized. When oxygen reacts with fats a substantial amount of oxygen combines with hydrogen atoms to form water instead of carbon dioxide thus reducing the respiratory quotient to near 0.7. Consumption of a normal diet consisting of carbohydrates, fats, and proteins results in a respiratory quotient of about 0.83.

CHANGES ASSOCIATED WITH HIGH ALTITUDE

Barometric pressure, which is the total pressure of all the gases in the atmosphere, decreases progressively as distance above sea level increases (Table 50-4). For example, barometric pressure is 760 mmHg at sea level and 523 mmHg at 3300 m (10,000 ft) above sea level. Since the concentration of oxygen remains constant at about 21%, the decrease in barometric pressure above sea level is associated with a progressive decrease in the partial pressure of oxygen. For example, the partial pressure of oxygen at sea level is 159 mmHg (21% times 760 mmHg) and 110 mmHg at 3300 m (21% times 523 mmHg).

The pharmacologic effect of inhaled anesthetics is reduced by decreased barometric pressure. For example, 60% inhaled nitrous oxide produces a partial pressure of 456 mmHg at sea level compared with 314 mmHg at 3300 m. The inhaled concentration of nitrous oxide at 3300 m would have to be 87% to produce a partial pressure similar to that produced by breathing 60% nitrous

oxide at sea level. Likewise, 1% inhaled isoflurane producing 7.6 mmHg partial pressure at sea level would have to be increased to nearly 1.5% to produce the same partial pressure at 3300 m.

Mental function remains intact up to 2700 to 3300 m above sea level. The rate of breathing ordinarily does not increase until one ascends above 2400 m at which point the peripheral chemoreceptors are stimulated (Pace, 1974).

Acclimatization to Altitude

Acclimatization to altitude occurs because of increased (1) alveolar ventilation, (2) production of hemoglobin, (3) production of 2,3-DPG, (4) diffusing capacity of the lungs, (5) vascularity of the tissues, and (6) ability of the cells to utilize oxygen despite the low PaO_2 (Frisancho, 1975).

Alveolar Ventilation

The initial increase in alveolar ventilation lowers $PaCO_2$ which blunts the magnitude of this compensatory response. Within a few days, however, active transport of bicarbonate ions returns the cerebrospinal fluid pH to normal and alveolar ventilation again increases despite a low $PaCO_2$ (see Chapter 49).

Hemoglobin

Increased production of hemoglobin requires several months to reach its maximal effect during which time the hemoglobin concentration may increase to over 20 g dl^{-1} (Dill *et al*, 1969). In addi-

Table 50-4
Effects of Altitude on Respiratory Gases While Breathing Air

Altitude (m/feet)	Barometric Pressure (mmHg)	Inhaled PO_2 (mmHg)	Alveolar PO_2 (mmHg)	Alveolar PCO_2 (mmHg)	Arterial O_2 Saturation (%)
Sea level	760	159	104	40	97
3300/10,000	523	110 (436)*	67	36	90
6600/20,000	349	73	40	24	70
9900/30,000	226	47	21	24	20

* Breathing pure O_2

tion, the plasma volume may increase as much as 30%.

Diphosphoglycerate (2,3-DPG)

Within a few hours of ascending to altitude, there are increased quantities of 2,3-DPG formed in the erythrocytes. This phosphate compound decreases the affinity of hemoglobin for oxygen resulting in facilitation of oxygen delivery to tissues. This beneficial effect, however, is offset by reduced affinity of hemoglobin for oxygen at the lungs.

Diffusing Capacity

Increased diffusing capacity during acclimatization reflects increased pulmonary artery pressures and blood volume which serve to open more pulmonary capillaries and thus increase the alveolar surface area for diffusion of oxygen.

Vascularity of Tissues

Cardiac output often increases as much as 30% immediately after ascending to altitude, but this increase is transient, returning to normal in a few days (Korner, 1959). Concomitant with this change, blood flow through the skin and kidneys decreases while blood flow through skeletal muscles, heart, and brain increases. There is also greatly increased vascularity in tissues that are ischemic accounting for the accommodation of an increased blood volume without a change in blood pressure.

Utilization of Oxygen

Chronic exposure to altitude is associated with increased numbers of mitochondria and certain cellular oxidative enzyme systems presumably reflecting improved ability to utilize available oxygen.

Chronic Mountain Sickness

An occasional sea level native who remains for prolonged periods at altitude may develop chronic mountain sickness characterized by extreme polycythemia, pulmonary hypertension, and right ventricular failure (Stickney, 1972). Presumably, the increased hemoglobin concentra-

tion so increases the viscosity of the blood that tissue blood flow becomes inadequate while at the same time chronic arterial hypoxemia causes vasospasm of pulmonary arterial vessels. Recovery is usually prompt when these individuals return to sea level.

CHANGES ASSOCIATED WITH EXCESSIVE BAROMETRIC PRESSURE

Barometric pressure increases the equivalent of 1 atmosphere for every 10 m below the surface of water. For example, a person 10 m beneath the water surface is exposed to 2 atmospheres reflecting the 1 atmosphere of pressure caused by the weight of the air above the water and the second atmosphere by the weight of the water. At 20 m below the water surface, barometric pressure is equivalent to 3 atmospheres. Another important effect of increased barometric pressure below the surface of the water is compression of gases in the lungs to smaller volumes (Lanphier, 1972).

High atmospheric pressure produces nitrogen narcosis when the inhaled gases are air. Presumably, high partial pressures of nitrogen at elevated atmospheric pressure cause sufficient absorption and deposition of nitrogen molecules in lipid membranes to produce an anesthetic effect. Helium can be substituted for nitrogen to avoid narcosis associated with absorption of nitrogen. In addition to a lesser sedative effect, helium is less soluble, thus reducing the quantity of bubbles that result with return to atmospheric pressure.

Nitrogen that is absorbed at high atmospheric pressure remains dissolved in the tissues until the partial pressure of nitrogen in the lungs decreases. Decompression sickness (caisson disease) occurs when sudden decreases in atmospheric pressure allow nitrogen bubbles to develop in body tissues and fluid. Nitrogen bubbles develop because pressure on the outside of the body is no longer able to keep the excess gas absorbed during high atmospheric pressure in solution. As a result, nitrogen can escape from the dissolved state and form bubbles in the tissues. The most frequent sign of nitrogen bubble formation is pain in the extremities while the most serious sequelae are seizures and cerebral ischemia that occur as a result of bubble formation in the central nervous system. Nitrogen bubbles that form in the blood block pulmonary blood flow manifesting as dyspnea ("chokes"). The onset of symptoms of decompression sickness usually appear within minutes but may also be delayed for as long as 6 hours or more after decompression. The period of time a diver must be decompressed depends upon the depth of submersion and duration of exposure. For example, submersion at 60 m for 1 hour requires about 3 hours for decompression.

Breathing pure oxygen at excessive barometric pressures can cause acute oxygen toxicity characterized by seizures followed by coma. It is likely that excess oxygen concentrations (PO_2 greater than 1500 mmHg) inactivate oxidative enzymes and cause tissue toxicity by reducing the ability of cells to form high energy phosphate bonds.

REFERENCES

Bruley DF. Mathematical considerations for oxygen transport to tissue. Adv Exp Med Biol 1973;37: 749–59.

Dill DB, Horvath SM, Dahms TE, Parker RE, Lynch JR. Hemoconcentration at altitude. J Appl Physiol 1969;27:514–8.

Eger EI, Severinghaus JW. The rate of rise of $PaCO_2$ in the apneic anesthetized patient. Anesthesiology 1961;22:419–25.

Frisancho AR. Functional adaptation to high altitude hypoxia. Science 1975;187:313–9.

Gillies IDS, Bird BD, Norman J, Gordon-Smith EC, Whitwam JG. The effect of anaesthesia on the oxy-haemoglobin dissociation curve. Br J Anaesth 1970; 42:561.

Guyton AC. Textbook of Medical Physiology. 7th ed. Philadelphia: WB Saunders, 1986:493.

Kambam JR. Isoflurane and oxy-hemoglobin dissociation. Anesthesiology 1982;57:A496.

Kilmartin JV, Ross-Bernardi L. Interaction of hemoglobin with hydrogen ions, carbon dioxide, and organic phosphates. Physiol Rev 1973;53:836–90.

Korner PI. Circulatory adaptations in hypoxia. Physiol Rev 1959;39:687–730.

Lanphier EH. Human respiration under increased pressures. Symp Soc Exp Biol 1972;26:379–94.

Maren TH. Carbonic anhydrase: Chemistry, physiology, and inhibition. Physiol Rev 1967;47:595–781.

Pace N. Respiration at high altitude. Fed Proc 1974;33: 2126–32.

Perutz MF. Hemoglobin structure and respiratory transport. Sci Am 1978;239:92–125.

Stickney JC. Some problems in homeostasis in high-altitude exposure. Physiologist 1972;15:349–59.

Wagner PD. Diffusion and chemical reaction in pulmonary gas exchange. Physiol Rev 1977;57:257–312.

Wagner PD. The oxyhemoglobin dissociation curve and pulmonary gas exchange. Sem Hematol 1974;11: 405–21.

Weibel ER. Morphological basis of alveolar capillary gas exchange. Physiol Rev 1973;53:419–95.

West JB. Pulmonary gas exchange. Int Rev Physiol 1977;14:83–106.

Whalen WJ. Intracellular PO_2 in heart and skeletal muscle. Physiologist 1971;14:69–82.

Wittenberg JB. Myoglobin-facilitated oxygen diffusion role of myoglobin in oxygen entry into muscle. Physiol Rev 1970;50:559–636.

C H A P T E R 51

Acid – Base Balance

INTRODUCTION

Regulation of hydrogen ion concentration in cells and blood is the determinant of acid–base balance (Kintner, 1972; Malnic and Giebisch, 1972). Slight changes in the hydrogen ion concentration from the normal value can cause marked alterations in enzyme activity and the rates of chemical reactions in the cells, some being depressed and others accelerated. The hydrogen ion concentration is regulated to maintain the arterial blood pH (pHa) between 7.35 and 7.45. The pH is equivalent to the negative logarithm of the hydrogen ion concentration which is most often expressed in nmol L^{-1}. A normal pHa of 7.4 is equivalent to a hydrogen ion concentration of 40 nmol L^{-1}. At a pH of 7, the hydrogen ion concentration is 100 nmol L^{-1}, and at a pH of 7.7 is 20 nmol L^{-1}. A pH range of 7 to 7.7, which is equivalent to a fivefold change in the hydrogen ion concentration, is compatible with life. This large variation is conceptually masked by expression of hydrogen ion concentration as pH.

The hydrogen ion concentration in blood is minimal compared with other ions. For example, the normal plasma concentration of sodium ions is 140,000,000 nmol L^{-1} which is 1 million times greater than the normal hydrogen ion concentration. For this reason, the osmotic effect of hydrogen ions in blood is considered to be negligible.

Venous blood and interstitial fluids have a pH of about 7.35 because of extra quantities of carbon dioxide that form carbonic acid in these fluids.

The intracellular pH ranges between 6.0 and 7.4 in different cells, averaging about 7.0 (Waddell and Bates, 1969). A rapid rate of metabolism in cells increases the rate of carbon dioxide formation and consequently decreases intracellular pH. Poor blood flow to any tissue also causes accumulation of carbon dioxide and a decrease in intracellular pH.

MECHANISMS FOR REGULATION OF HYDROGEN ION CONCENTRATION

Mechanisms for regulation of the hydrogen ion concentration over a narrow range include (1) buffer systems, (2) ventilatory responses, and (3) renal responses. The buffer system mechanism is rapid but incomplete. Ventilatory and renal responses develop less rapidly but often produce nearly complete correction of the pH.

Buffer Systems

All body fluids contain acid–base buffer systems that instantly combine with any acid or alkali so as to prevent excessive changes in the hydrogen ion concentration thus maintaining the pHa near 7.4. By convention, an acid is any substance that increases the hydrogen ion concentration (*i.e.,* a proton donor) in solution while an alkali decreases the hydrogen ion concentration (*i.e.,* a proton acceptor). A strong acid, such as hydrochloric acid, is fully dissociated to hydrogen ions and chloride ions, whereas carbonic acid, which is a weaker acid, dissociates less completely to hydrogen ions and bicarbonate ions.

Buffer systems include the (1) bicarbonate buffer system, (2) phosphate buffer system, and (3) protein buffer system.

Bicarbonate Buffer System

The bicarbonate buffer system consists of carbonic acid (H_2CO_3) and sodium bicarbonate ($NaHCO_3$). Carbonic acid is a weak acid because of its limited degree of dissociation (estimated to be less than 5%) into hydrogen ions and bicarbonate ions compared with that of other acids (Fig. 51-1). Furthermore, 99% of carbonic acid in solution almost immediately dissociates into carbon dioxide and water with the net result being a high concentration of dissolved carbon dioxide but only a weak concentration of acid. Ordinarily, the amount of dissolved carbon dioxide is about 1000 times the concentration of the undissociated acid. In intracellular fluid, bicarbonate ions are present mainly as potassium bicarbonate and magnesium bicarbonate, while in extracellular fluid sodium bicarbonate predominates.

Bicarbonate buffer is the most available buffer in blood accounting for greater than 50% of the total buffering capacity of blood. Bicarbonate ions diffuse relatively easily into erythrocytes such that about one third of the bicarbonate-buffering capacity of blood occurs in erythrocytes. In contrast, the electrical charge of bicarbonate ions limits diffusion of these ions into cells other than erythrocytes.

The addition of a strong acid such as hydrochloric acid to the bicarbonate buffer system results in conversion of this strong acid to weak carbonic acid (Fig. 51-2). Therefore, a strong acid lowers the pH of a body fluid only slightly. The addition of a strong base, such as potassium hydroxide, to the bicarbonate buffer system, results in the formation of a weak base and water (Fig. 51-3).

It is not possible to measure the concentration of undissociated carbonic acid in solution because it is continually in reversible equilibrium with dissolved carbon dioxide in solution. The amount of undissociated carbonic acid, however, is proportional to the amount of dissolved carbon dioxide, which can be measured. The Henderson-Hasselbach equation can be used to calculate the pH of a solution if the concentrations of bicarbonate ion and dissolved carbon dioxide are known (Fig. 51-4). The ratio of bicarbonate ions to carbonic acid is 20:1.

The bicarbonate system is not a powerful buffer because its pK of 6.1 differs greatly from normal pH of 7.4. Furthermore, the concentrations of the two elements of the bicarbonate buffer system, carbon dioxide and bicarbonate ions, are not great. The difference in pK and pH means that about 20 times as much of the bicarbonate buffer is in the form of bicarbonate ion as in the form of dissolved carbon dioxide. The importance of the bicarbonate buffer system, however, is enhanced by the fact that the concentration of its two elements can be regulated by the lungs and kidneys.

Phosphate Buffer System

The phosphate buffer system acts in a manner similar to the bicarbonate buffer system being composed of two elements (Fig. 51-5). The pK of the

$$H_2CO_3 \rightleftharpoons H^+ + HCO_3^-$$

FIGURE 51-1. Dissociation of carbonic acid (H_2CO_3) into hydrogen ions and bicarbonate ions.

$$HCL + NaHCO_3 \longrightarrow H_2CO_3 + NaCl$$

FIGURE 51-2. The addition of a strong acid (HCl) to the bicarbonate buffer system results in the formation of weak carbonic (H_2CO_3) acid.

$$KOH + H_2CO_3 \longrightarrow KHCO_3 + H_2O$$

FIGURE 51-3. The addition of a strong base (KOH) in the presence of carbonic acid (H_2CO_3) results in the formation of a weak base.

$$pH = 6.1 + \log \frac{HCO_3^-}{CO_2}$$

FIGURE 51-4. The Henderson-Hasselbach equation can be used to calculate the pH of a solution.

$$H_2PO_4 \rightleftharpoons H^+ + HPO_4^{--}$$

FIGURE 51-5. The phosphate buffer system acts in a manner similar to the bicarbonate buffer system.

phosphate buffer system is 6.8, which is near the normal pH of 7.4. This allows the phosphate buffer system to operate near its maximum buffering power. Nevertheless, the buffering power of this buffer system in the extracellular fluid is far less than that of the bicarbonate buffer system. This occurs because the concentration of the two phosphate buffer elements is only about one-twelfth that of the two buffer elements of the bicarbonate buffer system (bicarbonate ions and carbonic acid).

The phosphate buffer system is especially important in the renal tubules where phosphate is greatly concentrated because of its poor reabsorption and concomitant reabsorption of water. Furthermore, renal tubular fluid is more acidic than extracellular fluid, bringing the pH of tubular fluid closer to the pK of the buffer system. The phosphate buffer system is also important in intracellular fluids because the concentration of phosphate in these fluids is much greater than the concentration in extracellular fluids. Furthermore, like the renal tubular fluid, the pH of intracellular fluid is closer to the pK of the phosphate buffer system than is the pH of extracellular fluid.

Protein Buffer System

The protein buffer system, because of the high intracellular concentration of proteins, is the most potent buffering system in the body. Furthermore, the pK of some of the protein buffers is near 7.4. It is estimated that about 75% of all the buffering of body fluids occurs intracellularly and most of this results from intracellular proteins. For example, hydrogen ions produced in the mitochondria are buffered by local proteins. Ultimately, however, excess hydrogen ions diffuse into the extracellular fluid.

The method by which the protein buffer system operates within the cells is identical to the bicarbonate buffer system. For example, a protein is composed of amino acids bound together by peptide linkages, and some of these amino acids have free acidic radicals that can dissociate into base plus hydrogen ions. In the plasma, proteins act as weak acids. The low concentration of plasma proteins, however, limits their role as buffers in the extracellular fluid.

Hemoglobin, because of its greater concentration, is a more effective buffer than plasma proteins. Furthermore, the buffering capacity of hemoglobin varies with oxygenation with reduced hemoglobin being a weaker acid than oxyhemoglobin. As a result, at the capillaries, dissociation of oxyhemoglobin makes more base available to combine with carbonic acid produced in the tissues. The buffering capacity of hemoglobin is due to the imidazole group of the histidine molecules in the protein, globin.

Ventilatory Responses

Ventilatory responses for regulation of pH manifest as alterations in activity of the respiratory center within 1 to 5 minutes of the change in hydrogen ion concentration. As a result, alveolar ventilation increases or decreases to produce appropriate changes in the concentration of carbon dioxide in tissues and body fluids. In the presence of a constant rate of metabolic formation of carbon dioxide, the dissolved concentration of carbon dioxide is inversely proportional to alveolar ventilation. Doubling alveolar ventilation eliminates sufficient carbon dioxide to increase the pHa to about 7.63. Conversely, reducing alveolar ventilation to one fourth of normal results in retention of carbon dioxide sufficient to reduce the pHa to about 7.0.

Degree of Ventilatory Response

Ventilatory responses cannot return the pHa to 7.4 when a nonrespiratory abnormality is responsible for the acid–base disturbance. This occurs because the intensity of the stimulus that has been causing either increased or decreased alveolar ventilation will begin to diminish as the pHa returns toward 7.4. As a buffer, ventilatory responses are able to buffer one to two times as much acid or base as all the chemical buffers combined.

Renal Responses

Renal responses that regulate the hydrogen ion concentration are accomplished by increasing or decreasing bicarbonate ion concentration in the body. This regulation manifests as acidification or alkalization of the urine. Regulation of bicarbonate ion concentration is achieved by complex reactions that occur in the renal tubules (see Chapter 53).

The basic mechanism by which the kidney corrects either acidosis or alkalosis is by incomplete titration of hydrogen ions against bicarbonate ions, leaving one or the other of these ions to enter the urine and, therefore, to be removed from the extracellular fluid (Arruda and Kurtzman, 1978). The majority of this titration process occurs in the proximal renal tubules. In the presence of acidosis, the rate of hydrogen ion secretion exceeds the rate of bicarbonate ion filtration into the renal tubules. As a result, an excess of hydrogen ions are excreted into the urine. In the presence of alkalosis, the effect of the titration process in the renal tubules is to increase the number of bicarbonate ions filtered into the renal tubules relative to hydrogen ions secreted. Because bicarbonate ions cannot be reabsorbed without first reacting with hydrogen ions, all the excess bicarbonate ions pass into the urine and carry with them sodium ions or other positive ions. The net effect is removal of sodium bicarbonate from the extracellular fluid.

Renal Tubular Secretion of Hydrogen Ions

Hydrogen ions are secreted into the renal tubular fluid by epithelial cells lining proximal renal tubules, distal renal tubules, and collecting ducts (Fig. 51-6). Presumably, carbon dioxide either diffuses into or is formed by metabolism in the renal tubular epithelial cells. This carbon dioxide combines with water under the influence of carbonic anhydrase to form carbonic acid. Carbonic acid then dissociates into bicarbonate ions and hydrogen ions. Hydrogen ions are subsequently secreted by active transport from the epithelial cells into the lumens of the renal tubules. Sodium ions are actively reabsorbed in place of the secreted hydrogen ions. At the same time, bicarbonate ions formed in the renal tubular epithelial cells pass into peritubular capillaries to combine with sodium ions. As a result, the amount of sodium bicarbonate in the plasma is increased during the secretion of hydrogen ions into the lumen of the renal tubule (Fig. 51-6).

The greater the concentration of carbon dioxide in the extracellular fluid, the more rapidly are hydrogen ions formed for secretion into the renal tubules. Conversely, any event that decreases the concentration of carbon dioxide, such as hyperventilation of the lungs or decreased metabolism, also decreases the rate of hydrogen ion secretion. In the presence of normal concentrations of carbon dioxide, the rate of hydrogen ion secretion from the lining epithelial cells into the renal tubules is about 3.5 mM min^{-1}.

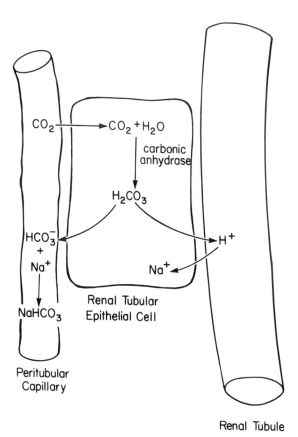

FIGURE 51-6. Schematic depiction of the renal tubular secretion of hydrogen ions.

Over 80% of hydrogen ion secretion occurs in the proximal renal tubule, but the tubular fluid pH can be reduced to only about 6.9. Below this pH, epithelial cells lining the proximal renal tubules are unable to secrete hydrogen ions into the lumen of the renal tubule. Conversely, in collecting ducts, hydrogen ion secretion can continue until the concentration of hydrogen ions in the tubules decreases to about 4.5, which is equivalent to a hydrogen ion concentration nearly 900 times that present in the extracellular fluid (Steinmetz, 1974).

Renal Tubular Transport of Excess Hydrogen Ions

Hydrogen ions must combine with buffers in the lumens of the renal tubules to prevent the tubular fluid pH from declining below the maximum limit that allows continued secretion of hydrogen ions by the lining epithelial cells. Buffer systems in the renal tubular fluid for transport of excess hydrogen ions into the urine utilize phosphate buffer and ammonia buffer (Tannen, 1980).

PHOSPHATE BUFFER. Excess hydrogen ions in the renal tubules combine with HPO_4 to form H_2PO_4 which passes into the urine (Fig. 51-5).

AMMONIA BUFFER. The other important buffer mechanism for hydrogen ions in renal tubular fluid is provided by ammonia which is synthesized in the lumens of the renal tubules (Fig. 51-7). In the renal tubule, ammonia combines

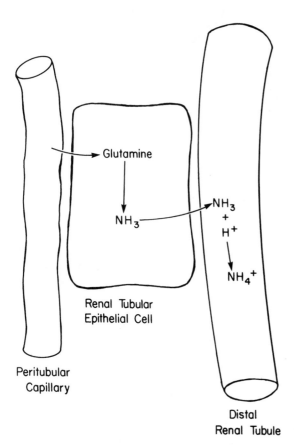

FIGURE 51-7. Ammonia (NH_3) formed in the renal tubular lining epithelial cells combines with hydrogen ions in the renal tubules to form ammonium (NH_4^+) ions.

with hydrogen ions to form ammonium. Ammonium ions are excreted in the urine in combination with chloride as the weak acid, ammonium chloride. Again, the net effect of these reactions is to increase the concentration of bicarbonate ions in plasma. For example, each time an ammonia molecule combines with a hydrogen ion to form an ammonium ion, the concentration of ammonia in the renal tubular fluid decreases, which allows additional ammonia to diffuse from the lining epithelial cells into the renal tubular fluid. Therefore, the rate of ammonia secretion into the renal tubular fluid is actually controlled by the amount of excess hydrogen ions to be transported.

About two thirds of the ammonia secreted by the renal tubular epithelial cells is derived from the amino acid, glutamine. The remaining ammonia is derived from other amino acids, especially glycine and alanine. The formation of ammonia can increase as much as tenfold over several days if excess hydrogen ions persist in the renal tubular fluid.

Regulation of Chloride Ion

The kidneys have the ability to conserve bicarbonate ions in the plasma when acidosis develops, or to remove bicarbonate ions when alkalosis is present. As such, bicarbonate ions are transported back and forth as one of the principal means of adjusting the acid–base balance of the plasma. In the process of altering the plasma concentration of bicarbonate ions, it is mandatory to remove some other anion each time the concentration of bicarbonate ions is increased, or to increase some other anion when the bicarbonate ion concentration is decreased. Typically, the anion that follows changes in the concentration of bicarbonate ion is chloride ion. Thus, in controlling the pH of the body fluids, the renal acid–base regulating system also regulates the ratio of chloride ions to bicarbonate ions in the extracellular fluid.

Degree of Renal Response Compensation

Renal responses for regulation of acid–base balance are slow to act (hours to days) but continue until the pH returns almost exactly to normal rather than a certain percentage of the way as occurs with respiratory responses. Thus, the value of renal regulation of hydrogen ion concentration is not rapidity of action but instead its ability to nearly completely neutralize any excess acid or alkali that enters the body fluids. Ordinarily, the kidneys can remove up to 500 mM of acid or alkali each day. If greater quantities than this enter the body fluids, the kidneys are unable to maintain normal acid–base balance, and acidosis or alkalosis occurs.

In the process of adjusting the hydrogen ion concentration of plasma, the kidneys often excrete urine at pHs as low as 4.5 or as high as 8.0. Even when the pH of plasma is 7.4, a small amount of acid is still lost each minute. This reflects the daily production of 50 to 80 mM more of acid than alkali. Indeed, the normal urine pH of about 6.4, rather than 7.4, is due to the presence of this excess acid in the urine.

ACID – BASE DISTURBANCES

Acid–base disturbances are categorized as respiratory or metabolic acidosis (pHa below 7.35) or alkalosis (pHa above 7.45) (Relman, 1972). An acid–base disturbance that results primarily from changes in alveolar ventilation is described as *respiratory acidosis or alkalosis*. An acid–base disturbance due to changes in the metabolic component of blood is designated as *metabolic acidosis or alkalosis. Compensation* is used to describe the secondary physiologic changes that occur in response to the primary acid–base disturbance. These compensatory changes tend to return the pHa towards a normal value.

The major effect of respiratory or metabolic acidosis is depression of the central nervous system. For example, patients with severe diabetic acidosis or uremic acidosis usually become comatose. The major effect of alkalosis is increased excitability of the central and peripheral nervous system. Nerves are so excitable that they automatically and repetitively fire causing skeletal muscles to go into a state of continuous contraction known as *tetany*. Tetany of muscles of respiration may interfere with adequate ventilation of the lungs. Central nervous system excitability may manifest as seizures, especially in patients with epilepsy.

Respiratory Acidosis

Any factor that decreases alveolar ventilation results in an increased concentration of dissolved carbon dioxide in the plasma (*e.g.,* increased $PaCO_2$), which in turn leads to formation of car-

bonic acid and hydrogen ions. By convention, carbonic acid resulting from dissolved carbon dioxide is called a *respiratory acid,* and respiratory acidosis is present when the pHa declines below 7.35. Any disease or drug (*e.g.,* anesthetics) that depresses the respiratory center in the medulla as well as intrinsic disease of the lungs can lead to respiratory acidosis.

Respiratory Alkalosis

Respiratory alkalosis is present when increased alveolar ventilation removes sufficient carbon dioxide from the body to reduce hydrogen ion concentration and thus increase the pHa above 7.45. A physiologic cause of respiratory alkalosis occurs when a person ascends to altitude and the low inspired concentration of oxygen leads to a reduction of PaO_2. The low PaO_2 stimulates chemoreceptors to increase alveolar ventilation which leads to excess loss of carbon dioxide (*e.g.,* decreased $PaCO_2$). The kidney can compensate for this alkalosis by excreting bicarbonate ions in association with sodium ions and potassium ions. This renal compensation is evident in people residing at altitude who have nearly normal pHa values despite a low $PaCO_2$. Tetany that accompanies alkalosis reflects hypocalcemia due to the greater affinity of plasma proteins for calcium in an alkaline compared with an acidic solution.

Metabolic Acidosis

Any acid formed in the body other than carbon dioxide is called a *metabolic acid,* and its accumulation results in metabolic acidosis. Causes of metabolic acidosis include failure of the kidneys to excrete acids formed each day by normal metabolic processes. Severe diarrhea and associated loss of sodium bicarbonate also rapidly lead to metabolic acidosis especially in the pediatric age-group. Lack of insulin secretion prevents normal use of glucose for metabolism, forcing tissues to utilize fat for energy requirements. As a result, the concentration of acetoacetic acid in the plasma often increases sufficiently to cause metabolic acidosis. Excess potassium ions compete with hydrogen ions for secretion by the distal renal tubules and collecting ducts. For this reason, fewer hydrogen ions are eliminated in the urine and metabolic acidosis occurs. Inhibition of carbonic anhydrase enzyme by acetazolamide results in metabolic acidosis due to interference with the reabsorption of bicarbonate ions from the renal tubular fluid. As a result, excess bicarbonate ions are lost in the urine, and the plasma concentration of bicarbonate ions is decreased.

Metabolic Alkalosis

Causes of metabolic alkalosis include vomiting with excess loss of hydrochloric acid and chronic administration of thiazide diuretics (see Chapter 25). Excess secretion of aldosterone is also associated with the development of metabolic alkalosis.

Respiratory compensation in metabolic alkalosis is unpredictable. This may be due to divergence between the intracellular and extracellular changes in the concentration of hydrogen ions. Renal compensation is by increased reabsorption of hydrogen ions. This metabolic compensation, however, is limited by the amount of sodium, potassium, and chloride ions present in the body. For example, during protracted vomiting, there is excessive loss of chloride ions along with sodium or potassium ions. When this occurs, the kidneys preferentially conserve sodium and potassium ions, and the urine becomes paradoxically acid. Indeed, the presence of paradoxical aciduria indicates electrolyte depletion.

Compensation for Acid – Base Disturbances

Metabolic acidosis stimulates alveolar ventilation and thus causes rapid removal of carbon dioxide from the body fluids which reduces the hydrogen ion concentration toward normal. This respiratory compensation for metabolic acidosis, however, is only partial because the pHa is not returned completely to normal.

Metabolic alkalosis diminishes alveolar ventilation which in turn causes accumulation of carbon dioxide and a subsequent increase in the concentration of hydrogen ions. As with metabolic acidosis, this respiratory compensation for metabolic alkalosis is only partial.

Respiratory acidosis is compensated for within 6 to 12 hours by increased secretion of hydrogen ions by the kidneys resulting in an increased plasma concentration of bicarbonate ions. After a few days, the pHa will be normal despite persistence of an increased $PaCO_2$.

In the presence of respiratory alkalosis, the kidneys respond by decreasing the reabsorption of bicarbonate ions from the renal tubules. As a result, bicarbonate ions are lost in the urine thus decreasing the plasma concentration of bicarbonate ions and returning pHa toward normal despite persistence of a reduced $PaCO_2$.

REFERENCES

Arruda JAL, Kurtzman NA. Relationship of renal sodium and water transport to hydrogen ion secretion. Annu Rev Physiol 1978;40:43 – 66.

Kintner EP. Acid – base, blood gas, and electrolyte balances. Prog Clin Pathol 1972;4:143 – 80.

Malnic G, Giebisch G. Symposium on acid – base homeostasis, mechanism of renal hydrogen ion secretion. Kidney Int 1972;1:280 – 96.

Relman AS. Metabolic consequences of acid – base disorders. Kidney Int 1972;1:347 – 59.

Steinmetz PR. Cellular mechanisms of urinary acidification. Physiol Rev 1974;54:890 – 956.

Tannen RL. Control of acid excretion by the kidney. Annu Rev Med 1980;31:35 – 49.

Waddell WJ, Bates RG. Intracellular pH. Physiol Rev 1969;49:285 – 329.

C H A P T E R   52

Endocrine System

INTRODUCTION

Functions of the body are regulated by the nervous system and the endocrine system (Guyton, 1986a). Glands of the endocrine system are primarily concerned with regulation of different metabolic functions of the body. The product of secretion of endocrine glands is known as a *hormone* (Table 52-1). A hormone is a chemical substance that is secreted directly by the endocrine gland into the blood for delivery to a distant target site where it exerts an effect. Hormones can only affect the rate of cellular reactions and do not act as substrates during metabolic reactions.

Chemically, hormones are steroids or derivatives of amino acids. For example, hormones from the pancreas (insulin, glucagon) and anterior pituitary are proteins, hormones from the posterior pituitary are peptides, and those from the thyroid gland are derivatives of amino acids.

Hormone output from most endocrine glands is controlled physiologically by negative feedback systems in which increased circulating plasma concentrations of the hormone act to reduce its subsequent release from the gland. Tumors that secrete hormones, however, usually escape from this negative feedback control, and excess plasma concentrations of the hormone occur. Unrecognized endocrine dysfunction is unlikely if it can be established preoperatively that (1) body weight is unchanged, (2) heart rate and blood pressure are normal, (3) glycosuria is absent, (4) sexual function is normal, and (5) there is no history of recent medication.

MECHANISM OF ACTION OF HORMONES

Hormones may activate cyclic AMP systems of cells or stimulate genes in the cells to form specific intracellular proteins that initiate cellular functions. Examples of hormones that activate cyclic AMP include anterior pituitary hormones, antidiuretic hormone, glucagon, catecholamines (see Chapter 12) and hypothalamic-releasing factors. It is believed that the hormone combines with a receptor on the cell membrane of the target cell (Catt and Dufau, 1977). The combination of hormone and receptor activates adenylate cyclase enzyme in the cell membrane, and the portion of adenylate cyclase that is exposed to the cytoplasm (*e.g.*, interior of the cell) causes conversion of cytoplasmic adenosine triphosphate (ATP) into cyclic AMP. This intracellular cyclic AMP then initiates any number of cellular functions. An alternate mechanism of action for hormones is illustrated by steroids that cause synthesis of proteins in target cells. These proteins then function as enzymes or carrier proteins, which, in turn, activate other functions of cells.

PITUITARY GLAND

The pituitary gland lies in the sella turcica at the base of the brain and is connected with the hypothalamus by the pituitary stalk. Physiologically, the pituitary gland is divided into the anterior pituitary (adenohypophysis) and posterior pituitary (neurohypophysis). Hormones secreted by the an-

Table 52-1
Hormones

Anterior Pituitary
Growth hormone
Prolactin
Luteinizing hormone
Follicle-stimulating hormone
Adrenocorticotrophic hormone (ACTH)
Thyroid-stimulating hormone (TSH)
Posterior Pituitary
Antidiuretic hormone (ADH, vasopressin)
Oxytocin
Adrenal Cortex
Mineralocorticoids
Aldosterone
Desoxycorticosterone
Glucocorticoids
Cortisol
Corticosterone
Cortisone
Thyroid Gland
Thyroxine (T_4)
Triiodothyronine (T_3)
Calcitonin
Parathyroid Glands
Parathyroid hormone (parathormone)
Pancreas
Insulin
Glucagon
Testes
Testosterone
Ovaries
Estrogens
Progesterone
Placenta
Chorionic gonadotropin
Estrogens
Progesterone
Somatomammotropin

fibers originating in the hypothalamus and terminating in the posterior pituitary (Brodish and Lymangrover, 1977). Hormones designated as hypothalamic-releasing factors and hypothalamic-inhibitory factors originating in the hypothalamus control secretions from the anterior pituitary (Labrie *et al*, 1979; Reichlin *et al*, 1976).

Synthesis and release of hypothalamic-releasing factors and hypothalamic-inhibitory factors may be controlled by adrenergic and dopaminergic mechanisms (Weiner and Ganong, 1978). Indeed, drugs that alter central adrenergic mechanisms exert a significant influence on the secretion of hormones by the anterior pituitary. In addition, the hypothalamus receives signals, including pain signals, emotions, olfactory sensations, and impulses related to concentrations of water and electrolytes, from numerous sites in the nervous system. As such, the hypothalamus is a collecting center for information that is often used to control secretions of pituitary hormones (see Chapter 41).

Anterior Pituitary

Cells of the anterior pituitary are categorized as acidophils, basophils, and chromophobes, based on their staining characteristics with dyes. Acidophils are the source of growth hormone and prolactin; the basophils produce gonadotropins (*i.e.,* luteinizing hormone and follicle-stimulating hormone), ACTH, and TSH; and chromophobes are believed to be nonsecreting developing cells.

The anterior pituitary is a highly vascular gland connected to the hypothalamus by the hypothalamic-hypophyseal portal vessels. Special neurons in the hypothalamus secrete hypothalamic-releasing factor and, in some instances, a corresponding hypothalamic-inhibitory factor.

Growth Hormone

Growth hormone is a polypeptide hormone containing 191 amino acids that is synthesized and stored in acidophils of the anterior pituitary referred to as *somatotrophs*.

PHYSIOLOGIC EFFECTS. Growth hormone stimulates growth of all tissues of the body and evokes intense metabolic effects (Kostyo and Isaksson, 1977). For example, growth hormone stimulates growth of cartilage and bone by causing

terior pituitary include growth hormone, prolactin, luteinizing hormone, follicle-stimulating hormone, adrenocorticotrophic hormone (ACTH), and thyroid stimulating hormone (TSH). The two hormones secreted by the posterior pituitary are antidiuretic hormone (ADH) and oxytocin.

The function of the pituitary is under the control of the hypothalamus by virtue or direct neural and vascular connections (hypothalamic-hypophyseal portal vessels). For example, secretion from the posterior pituitary is controlled by nerve the formation of proteins called *somatomedins.* Somatomedins in turn act directly on cartilage and bone to promote their growth. An excess of growth hormone results in gigantism. Acromegaly occurs when the epiphyses of long bones have closed and the bones can no longer increase in length but can increase in thickness. A deficiency of growth hormone in childhood results in short stature.

Generalized metabolic effects of growth hormone include (1) increased rate of protein synthesis, (2) increased mobilization of fatty acids, and (3) decreased rate of glucose utilization. Increased protein synthesis may reflect the ability of growth hormone to enhance transport of amino acids through cell membranes to the interior of cells. This control of amino acid transport is similar to the effect of insulin in controlling glucose transport through cell membranes. Growth hormone also stimulates protein synthesis by causing formation of increased amounts of ribonucleic acid (RNA). At the same time that growth hormone is stimulating synthesis of proteins, the increased mobilization of fatty acids for energy use acts to spare protein breakdown.

The major effects of growth hormone on cellular metabolism of glucose are (1) decreased utilization of glucose for energy, (2) increased deposition of glycogen in cells, and (3) reduced uptake of glucose by the cells. A diabetogenic effect of growth hormone reflects stimulation of insulin output from the pancreas in response to an elevated blood–glucose concentration. Sustained stimulation of pancreatic beta cells may lead to their eventual exhaustion (see the section entitled Diabetes Mellitus). Diabetes mellitus owing to elevated blood–glucose concentrations secondary to excess secretion of growth hormone (also ACTH, TSH, and prolactin) is known as pituitary diabetes. In pituitary diabetes, the levels of circulating insulin are normal, and additional exogenous insulin has little beneficial effect.

REGULATION OF SECRETION. Secretion of growth hormone is regulated by growth hormone–releasing factor and growth hormone–releasing inhibitory factor (somatostatin), which are secreted by the hypothalamus and transported to the anterior pituitary by the hypothalamic-hypophyseal portal vessels. Somatostatin is also secreted by delta cells of the islets of Langerhans in the pancreas and can inhibit secretion of insulin and glucagon by beta and alpha cells of the pan-

creas in the same way that it inhibits secretion of growth hormone. As such, somatostatin may have a widespread role in regulating the functions of multiple hormonal systems. Placed in the epidural space, somatostatin produces postoperative analgesia that is not altered by naloxone (Chrubasik *et al,* 1985).

Growth hormone secretion may increase within minutes in response to hypoglycemia, physical exertion, anxiety, and stress as produced by anesthesia. Obesity causes a reduction in the release of growth hormone in response to hypoglycemia and other stimuli. Likewise, free fatty acids inhibit the release of growth hormone. Plasma concentrations of growth hormone characteristically increase during the first 2 hours of sleep, independent of circadian rhythm.

Drugs can influence the secretion of growth hormone, presumably by interfering with the release of regulatory hypothalamic factors. For example, large doses of glucocorticoids suppress secretion of growth hormone, which may be responsible for the inhibitory effects on growth observed in children receiving high doses of these drugs for prolonged periods. Conversely, dopaminergic agonists acutely increase the secretion of growth hormone.

Prolactin

Prolactin is synthesized in specific acidophils of the anterior pituitary as well as the placenta (Golander *et al,* 1978). The elimination half-time of prolactin is 15 to 20 minutes.

PHYSIOLOGIC EFFECTS. Secretion of prolactin by the anterior pituitary is responsible for growth and development of the breast in preparation for breast feeding. The mammotrophic actions of prolactin suggest a possible role of prolactin in the development of mammary tumors. Nevertheless, there is no evidence that disorders of prolactin metabolism have etiologic significance in human mammary carcinogenesis.

REGULATION OF SECRETION. The hypothalamus plays an essential role in regulating the secretion of prolactin. A difference, however, is that the hypothalamus inhibits prolactin production, whereas for other hormones, the effect is stimulatory. The inhibitory factor from the hypothalamus is probably dopamine (MacLeod, 1976). Conversely, suckling seems to evoke a signal from the hypothalamus that increases secretion of prolactin. Therefore, it is postulated that there is a prolactin-releasing factor as well as an inhibitory factor produced by the hypothalamus.

Prolactin secretion in response to suckling is a potent inhibitor of ovarian function, explaining the usual lack of ovulation and infertility during breast feeding. Indeed, prolactin-secreting tumors are often accompanied by galactorrhea and, in females, amenorrhea. Prolactin concentrations in the plasma typically increase during anesthesia and surgery, which may reflect stimulation of the release of this hormone from the anterior pituitary by exogenous opioids or endogenous endorphins (Bovill *et al,* 1983; Sebel *et al,* 1981).

Gonadotrophins

The two gonadotrophins, luteinizing hormone and follicle-stimulating hormone, are synthesized and stored by specific basophils in the anterior pituitary. Gonadotropins of placental origin include chorionic gonadotropin, which is absorbed into the maternal circulation in quantities sufficient to inhibit menstruation. The detection of this placental gonadotropin in the urine is the basis of pregnancy tests. Assays of chorionic gonadotropin are also used to diagnose and evaluate the treatment of trophoblastic tumors (*e.g.,* choriocarcinoma, hydatidiform moles).

PHYSIOLOGIC EFFECTS. Gonadotropins bind to specific receptors on cell membranes and presumably act by stimulating the synthesis of cyclic AMP. At puberty, secretion of these hormones increases as a result of diminished feedback inhibition of secretion by sex steroids. Both hormones are involved in the secretion of hormones by the ovary, whereas in the testes, luteinizing hormone plays a predominant role stimulating the production of gonadotropin.

Adrenocorticotrophic Hormone

ACTH is a polypeptide hormone containing 39 amino acids synthesized and stored in specific basophils of the anterior pituitary. The first 24 amino acids are common to all species, whereas amino acids 25 to 33 confer species specificity.

PHYSIOLOGIC EFFECTS. ACTH stimulates the adrenal cortex, particularly the zona reticularis and zona fasiculata, leading to the formation and release of various corticosteroids, especially cortisol and, to a much lesser extent, aldosterone. In the absence of ACTH, the adrenal cortex undergoes atrophy, but the zona glomerulosa, which secretes aldosterone, is least affected. Indeed, hypophysectomy has minimal effects on electrolyte balance, reflecting the continued release of aldosterone from the adrenal cortex. Excess presence of ACTH induces hyperplasia of the adrenal cortex with sustained high output of corticosteroids from the adrenal cortex.

ACTH stimulates synthesis of corticosteroids by interacting with specific receptors on cell membranes of the adrenal gland, leading to an increased intracellular concentration of cyclic AMP. In addition, ACTH stimulates the formation of cholesterol in the adrenal cortex by activating the enzyme cholesterol esterase. Cholesterol is the initial building block for synthesis of corticosteroids.

REGULATION OF SECRETION. Secretion of ACTH from the anterior pituitary is under the control of corticotropin-releasing factor from the hypothalamus as well as a negative feedback mechanism dependent on the circulating concentration of cortisol.

Administration of certain corticosteroids suppresses secretion of ACTH, reduces the amount of ACTH stored in the anterior pituitary, and leads to atrophy of the adrenal cortex. In the patient with inadequate or absent adrenocortical function, the concentration of ACTH in the blood is increased.

Secretory rates of corticotropin-releasing factor and ACTH are high in the morning and low in the evening. This diurnal variation results in high plasma cortisol concentrations in the morning (about 20 μg dl^{-1}) and low levels (about 5 μg dl^{-1}) around midnight. For this reason, plasma concentrations of cortisol must be interpreted in terms of the time of day when they are measured. Diurnal variations in ACTH and thus plasma cortisol concentrations are not observed in patients with excessive adrenal cortex activity (*i.e.,* Cushing's disease).

Thyroid Stimulating Hormone

TSH is a glycoprotein that is synthesized and stored by specific basophils of the anterior pituitary.

PHYSIOLOGIC EFFECTS. TSH accelerates all the steps involved in the formation of thyroid hormone, including initial uptake of iodide into the thyroid gland. In addition, TSH causes proteolysis of thyroglobulin in the follicles of thyroid cells, with the resultant release of thyroid hormones into the circulation. These effects of TSH are due to attachment to specific receptors on cell membranes, leading to activation of adenylate cyclase and increased intracellular formation of cyclic AMP.

REGULATION OF SECRETION. Secretion of TSH from the anterior pituitary is under the control of thyrotropin-releasing factor from the hypothalamus as well as a negative feedback mechanism, depending on the circulating concentration of thyroid hormones. For example, when the rate of thyroid hormone secretion rises to about 1.75 times normal, the rate of TSH secretion declines almost to zero. Likewise, sympathetic nervous system stimulation and corticosteroids also suppress the secretion of TSH and thus diminish activity of the thyroid gland.

Hypothyroidism with elevated plasma concentrations of TSH indicates a primary defect at the thyroid gland. A defect at the hypothalamus or anterior pituitary is indicated by low circulating concentrations of both TSH and thyroid hormones. The only clinical use of TSH is in the evaluation of thyroid gland function to differentiate hypopituitarism from primary myxedema.

Long-acting thyroid stimulator is an immunoglobulin G protein that can bind to receptor sites on thyroid cells. Presumably, the binding of these thyroid-stimulating antibodies can mimic the effects of TSH and account for hyperthyroidism (Volpe, 1978). Indeed, patients with hyperthyroidism often have detectable circulating concentrations of these proteins.

Thyrotropin-releasing factor is widely distributed in the central nervous system. Indeed, this tripeptide hormone exerts a variety of physiologic actions in addition to regulation of the secretion of TSH. For example, thyrotropin-releasing factor is a potent analeptic. Furthermore, it is effective in reversing experimental hypovolemic and septic shock (Faden, 1984).

Posterior Pituitary

The posterior pituitary (neurohypophysis) is composed of cells that act as supporting structures for terminal nerve endings of fibers from the supraoptic and paraventricular nuclei of the hypothalamus. These nerve fibers pass to the posterior pituitary through the pituitary stalk. The nerve endings are bulbous knobs that lie on the surfaces of capillaries into which they secrete the two posterior pituitary hormones, ADH and oxytocin (Seif and Robinson, 1978).

Antidiuretic Hormone

ADH is secreted by nerve fibers originating in the supraoptic nuclei of the hypothalamus. Granules containing ADH and its carrier protein, neurophysin, are transported down axons that terminate in the posterior pituitary. The formed hormone is stored in the posterior pituitary for release in response to appropriate stimuli. The primary functions of ADH are regulation of the osmotic pressure of extracellular fluid and regulation of blood volume.

MECHANISM OF ACTION. ADH is transported by way of the blood to the kidneys, where it acts to increase the permeability of the renal collecting ducts to water (see Chapter 53). It is believed that ADH attaches to receptors on the surface of epithelial cells that line the renal collecting ducts, causing them to form large amounts of cyclic AMP. This, in turn, opens pores on the epithelial cell membranes and allows free permeability (*i.e.,* diffusion) of water (Strewler and Orloff, 1977). Circulating ADH has an elimination half-time of 5 to 10 minutes. Enzymatic cleavage, principally in the kidney, is responsible for removal of ADH from the circulation.

REGULATION OF SECRETION. Osmoreceptors in the hypothalamus most likely regulate activity of hypothalamic neurons that provide signals for release of ADH. When the osmolarity of plasma increases above about 280 mOsm L^{-1} (*i.e.,* threshold), the supraoptic nuclei are stimulated and impulses are transmitted to the posterior pituitary and ADH is secreted (Robertson *et al*, 1973). The secreted ADH passes to the kidneys where it causes the reabsorption of water and a return of plasma osmolarity to normal.

Hemorrhage or sodium depletion that decreases extracellular fluid volume evokes the release of ADH, regardless of the osmolarity of plasma. Receptors that mediate release of ADH in response to decreased extracellular fluid volume are different from those that mediate the response to changes in plasma osmolarity. Volume receptors are present in the left atrium, pulmonary veins, carotid sinus and aorta. Secretion of ADH is believed to be under tonic inhibitory control by the baroreceptors, such that hormone is released when blood pressure declines and release is inhibited when the blood pressure rises. In addition to baroreceptors, the carotid body may contain chemoreceptors sensitive to arterial hypoxemia that stimulate secretion of ADH (Schrier *et al*, 1979). Increased concentrations of ADH in the plasma in response to acute reductions of extracellular fluid volume may be sufficient to exert direct pressor effects on arterioles and thus contribute to maintenance of blood pressure (Cowley *et al*, 1974).

FACTORS THAT ALTER SECRETION. In the absence of painful stimulation, secretion of ADH is not altered by opioids or inhaled anesthetics (Fig. 52-1) (Philbin and Coggins, 1978). Painful stimulation, however, in association with the onset of surgery results in significant increases in circulat-

ing concentrations of ADH (Fig. 52-1) (Philbin and Coggins, 1978). This release of ADH in response to surgical stimulation is blocked by high doses of morphine (2 mg kg^{-1}), fentanyl (60 μg kg^{-1}), or sufentanil (15 μg kg^{-1}) (Bovill *et al*, 1983; Sebel *et al*, 1981). Prolonged mechanical ventilation of the lungs, particularly if combined with positive end–expiratory pressure may be associated with increased circulating concentrations of ADH and subsequent water retention (Kumar *et al*, 1974; Sladen *et al*, 1968).

Elevated plasma concentrations of fluoride ions resulting from the metabolism of fluorinated inhaled anesthetics (methoxyflurane and, to a lesser extent, enflurane) may result in impaired ability to concentrate urine in the postoperative period (see Chapter 2). Presumably, fluoride interferes with the normal response of renal tubules to ADH. Calcium nephropathy, hypokalemia, amyloidosis, and sarcoidosis also interfere with responsiveness of the kidneys to ADH and are associated with an inability to adequately concentrate the urine.

Ethanol and phenytoin inhibit the secretion of ADH. Occasionally, excess ADH is secreted by certain types of tumors, especially oat cell carcinoma of the lung (*i.e.*, syndrome of inappropriate ADH secretion). Ethanol does not inhibit release of ADH from hormone-secreting tumors.

Diabetes insipidus results when there is destruction of neurons in or near the supraoptic and paraventricular nuclei of the hypothalamus. It will not occur when the posterior pituitary alone is damaged, because the cut fibers of the pituitary stalk can still continue to secrete ADH. Diabetes insipidus, which develops in association with pituitary surgery, typically is due to trauma to the posterior pituitary and is usually transient.

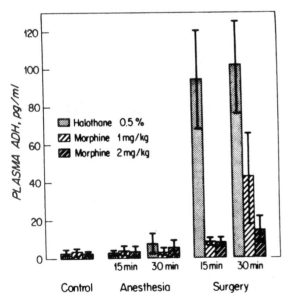

FIGURE 52-1. Plasma antidiuretic hormone (ADH) levels in adult patients are not altered by anesthesia in the absence of surgical stimulation. (From Philbin DM, Coggins CH. Plasma antidiuretic hormone levels in cardiac surgical patients during morphine and halothane anesthesia. Anesthesiology 1978;49:95–8. Reproduced by permission of the authors and publisher.)

CARDIOVASCULAR EFFECTS. Normal circulating concentrations of ADH are responsible for about 5 to 10 mmHg of the normal blood pressure (Smith *et al*, 1979). Moderate to high circulating concentrations of ADH cause intense vasoconstriction of the arterioles and thus increase blood pressure. A powerful stimulus for the secretion of ADH is acute loss of intravascular fluid volume. This increased secretion is believed to result mainly from the low pressure in the atria of the heart caused by low blood volume. The subsequent relaxation of atrial stretch receptors is believed to stimulate the release of ADH.

Oxytocin

Oxytocin is a cyclic octapeptide hormone synthesized in nerve cell bodies in the paraventricular nuclei of the hypothalamus. This hormone travels in secretory granules along axons of the hypothalamic neurons to the posterior pituitary, where it is stored. Oxytocin can be released abruptly and independently of ADH.

Oxytocin is a potent hormone for causing contraction of the pregnant uterus, especially toward the end of gestation. The effect of ADH on the uterus is 1/100 that of oxytocin (Guyton, 1986a). In addition, oxytocin causes milk to be expressed from the alveoli into the ducts so that it can be obtained by suckling. This reflects contraction of the myoepithelial cells that surround the alveoli of the mammary glands.

ADRENAL CORTEX

The two major classes of corticosteroids are mineralocorticoids and glucocorticoids. Mineralocorticoids affect the plasma concentrations of sodium and potassium ions, whereas glucocorticoids influence glucose, fat, and protein metabolism as well as exhibiting anti-inflammatory effects. More than 30 different corticosteroids have been isolated from the adrenal cortex, but only two are of major importance: aldosterone, a mineralocorticoid, and cortisol, the principal glucocorticoid. These corticosteroids are not stored in the adrenal cortex, emphasizing that the rate of synthesis determines the secretion and plasma concentrations (Table 52-2).

Anatomically, the adrenal cortex is divided into three zones: The zona glomerulosa secretes mineralocorticoids; the zona fasiculata secretes glucocorticoids; and the zona reticularis produces androgens and estrogens.

Mineralocorticoids

Aldosterone accounts for about 95% of the mineralocorticoid activity produced by corticosteroids (Table 52-2). Desoxycorticosterone is the other naturally occurring mineralocorticoid, but it has only 3% of the sodium ion – retaining potency of aldosterone. Cortisol induces sodium retention and potassium ion secretion, but much less effectively than does aldosterone.

Physiologic Effects

Aldosterone causes absorption of sodium ions and simultaneous secretion of potassium ions by the lining renal tubular epithelial cells of the distal renal tubules and collecting ducts (Raisz et al, 1977). As a result, aldosterone causes sodium ions to be conserved in the extracellular fluid while potassium ions are excreted in the urine. Water follows sodium ions such that the extracellular fluid volume tends to change in proportion to the rate of aldosterone secretion. Indeed, in the presence of excess secretion of aldosterone, the extracellular fluid volume, blood volume, cardiac output, and blood pressure are increased (McCaa et al, 1979).

Aldosterone has effects on sweat glands and

Table 52-2
Physiologic Effects of Endogenous Corticosteroids

	Daily Secretion (mg)	Sodium Retention*	Gluconeogenesis*	Anti-Inflammatory Effect*
Aldosterone	0.125	3000	0.3	Insignificant
Desoxycorticosterone		100	0	0
Cortisol	20	1	1	1
Corticosterone	minimal	15	0.35	0.3
Cortisone	minimal	0.8	0.8	0.8

* Relative to cortisol

salivary glands that are similar to its effects on the renal tubules. For example, aldosterone increases the reabsorption of sodium ions and secretion of potassium ions by sweat glands. This effect is important to conserve sodium ions in hot environments or when excess salivation occurs. Aldosterone also enhances sodium ion reabsorption by the gastrointestinal tract. When the plasma concentration of potassium is reduced about 50% owing to excess secretion of aldosterone, skeletal muscle weakness or even paralysis occurs, reflecting hyperpolarization of nerve and muscle membranes, which prevents transmission of action potentials.

Mechanism of Action

Aldosterone is able to diffuse to the interior of the lining renal tubular epithelial cells where it combines with a highly specific cytoplasmic receptor protein. This complex diffuses into the nucleus, where it induces deoxyribonucleic acid (DNA) to form a type of messenger RNA necessary for the transport of sodium ions and potassium ions. It is speculated that this RNA is a specific ATPase that catalyzes energy transfer from cytoplasmic ATP to the sodium transport mechanism of the cell membrane. It takes up to 30 minutes before the new RNA appears and about 45 minutes before the rate of sodium ion transport begins to increase.

Regulation of Secretion

Aldosterone is secreted by the zona glomerulosa, a thin layer of cells on the surface of the adrenal cortex immediately beneath the capsule. These cells function almost entirely independently of the deeper cells in the zona fasiculata and zona reticularis, which secrete cortisol and androgens. The most important factors in regulation of aldosterone secretion are the (1) extracellular fluid concentrations of potassium ions, (2) total body sodium content, and (3) renin–angiotensin system (see Chapter 22). Mineralocorticoid secretion is not under the primary control of ACTH. For this reason, hypoaldosteronism does not accompany loss of ACTH secretion from the anterior pituitary.

POTASSIUM ION CONCENTRATION. An increase in the extracellular fluid concentration of potassium ions of less than 1 mEq L^{-1} will triple the rate of aldosterone secretion. This establishes a powerful negative feedback system that acts to main-

tain the plasma concentration of potassium in a normal range. This negative feedback mechanism is the most potent of all the factors controlling secretion of aldosterone. The effect of potassium ions on aldosterone secretion is a direct effect of these ions on cells of the zona glomerulosa.

Glucocorticoids

At least 95% of the glucocorticoid activity results from the secretion of cortisol (Table 52-2). In addition, a small amount of glucocorticoid activity is provided by corticosterone and an even smaller amount by cortisone.

Physiologic Effects

The most important physiologic effects of cortisol are (1) increased gluconeogenesis, (2) protein catabolism, (3) fatty acid mobilization, and (4) antiinflammatory effects.

GLUCONEOGENESIS. Cortisol has the ability to stimulate gluconeogenesis by the liver by as much as tenfold (Guyton, 1986b). Increased gluconeogenesis reflects several effects of cortisol, including (1) enhanced transport of amino acids into liver cells for conversion to glucose, (2) stimulation of formation of enzymes necessary to convert amino acids to glucose, and (3) mobilization of amino acids from extrahepatic tissues. A manifestation of increased gluconeogenesis is a marked increase in the glycogen content of hepatic cells. Cortisol also causes a decrease in the rate of glucose utilization by cells.

The increased rate of gluconeogenesis and the moderate reduction in the rate of glucose utilization produced by cortisol causes the blood–glucose concentration to rise, producing adrenal diabetes. Administration of insulin lowers the blood–glucose concentration more than with pituitary diabetes and less than with pancreatic diabetes.

PROTEIN CATABOLISM. Cortisol decreases protein stores in essentially all cells except those in the liver. This is caused by decreased protein synthesis and increased catabolism of protein already in cells. Decreased protein synthesis reflects increased transport of amino acids to the liver such that less is available to extrahepatic cells for synthesis. At the same time, catabolism of proteins in extrahepatic cells continues to release amino acids from the already existing proteins, and these diffuse from the cells to increase the plasma amino acid concentration. In this regard, cortisol mobilizes amino acids from tissues for delivery to the liver and gluconeogenesis. In the presence of sustained excesses of cortisol concentrations, skeletal muscle weakness may become profound.

FATTY ACID MOBILIZATION. Cortisol promotes mobilization of fatty acids from adipose tissue. In addition, cortisol enhances oxidation of fatty acids in cells. Despite these effects on fat metabolism, excess amounts of cortisol cause deposition of fat in the head and chest regions, giving rise to a buffalo-like torso. This peculiar distribution of fat reflects deposition of fat at these sites at a rate that exceeds its mobilization.

ANTI-INFLAMMATORY EFFECTS. Cortisol in large amounts has anti-inflammatory effects, reflecting its ability to cause stabilization of the lysosomal membranes (Parrillo and Fauci, 1979). Since substances that cause inflammation are formed in the lysosomes, the effect of cortisol is to greatly reduce the amount of these substances that are released. Other anti-inflammatory effects of cortisol reflect decreased capillary permeability, which prevents loss of plasma into tissues and also reduces the migration of leukocytes into the inflamed area. Finally, cortisol decreases tissue reactions in that reduced amounts of antibodies and sensitized leukocytes enter the inflamed area.

Even after inflammation has become well established, administration of cortisol can reduce its manifestations. This effect of cortisol is important in attenuating inflammation associated with disease states such as rheumatoid arthritis and acute glomerulonephritis.

Cortisol decreases the number of eosinophils and lymphocytes in the blood within a few minutes of its injection. In addition, there is atrophy of lymphoid tissue throughout the body, which results in decreased production of antibodies. As a result, the level of immunity against bacterial or viral infection is decreased, and fulminating infection can occur. Conversely, this ability of cortisol to suppress immunity is useful in preventing immunologic rejection of transplanted tissues.

The beneficial effect of cortisol in the treatment of allergic reactions reflects prevention of inflammatory responses that are responsible for many of the serious effects (*e.g.,* laryngeal edema) of an allergic reaction. Cortisol does not, however, alter the antigen–antibody interaction or histamine release associated with allergic reactions.

Mechanism of Action

Cortisol reacts with receptor proteins in the cytoplasm of responsive cells (Ballard *et al,* 1974). As a result, there is stimulation of the synthesis of RNA that codes for enzymes whose production is stimulated by these hormones (Iynedjian and Hanson, 1977).

Regulation of Secretion

Cortisol is the most important hormone secreted by the adrenal cortex, being released at the rate of about 20 mg daily. Secretion of cortisol is regulated by ACTH from the anterior pituitary (see the section entitled Adrenocorticotrophic Hormone). In addition, circulating cortisol exerts a direct negative feedback effect on the (1) hypothalamus to decrease the formation of corticotropin-releasing factor and (2) anterior pituitary to reduce the formation of ACTH. In the circulation, about 90% of cortisol is bound to a specific globulin, designated transcortin. Degradation of cortisol occurs mainly in the liver with the formation of glucuronides. These inactive glucuronides appear in the urine.

The normal 8 A.M. plasma concentration of cortisol is 8 to 25 μg dl^{-1}. Secretion of cortisol and growth hormone is stimulated by stress as associated with surgery, infection, and hypothermia (Traymor and Hall, 1981). These stress stimuli can override the normal negative feedback control mechanisms, and plasma concentrations of cortisol are elevated. The beneficial effect of increased plasma concentrations of cortisol and growth hormone is not known but may reflect the acute mobilization of cellular stores of proteins and fats for energy and synthesis of other compounds, including glucose. Large doses of opioids, including morphine, fentanyl, and sulfentanil abolish the cortisol and growth hormone response to surgical stimulation (Bovill *et al,* 1983; Sebel *et al,* 1981). Volatile anesthetics provide less suppression to this stress-induced endocrine response.

THYROID GLAND

The thyroid gland secretes two principal hormones, thyroxine (T4) and triiodothyronine (T3). These hormones have profound effects on the metabolic rate of the body. For example, absence of thyroid gland hormones causes the basal metabolic rate to decrease to about 40% below normal, whereas excesses of these hormones can elevate the basal metabolic rate as much as 100% above normal. The thyroid gland also secretes calcitonin, which is an important hormone for calcium metabolism (see the section entitled Calcitonin).

Formation and Secretion

About one third of orally ingested iodides that are absorbed from the gastrointestinal tract are selectively absorbed by the thyroid gland (*i.e.,* iodide trapping). In a normal gland, iodide can be concentrated to about 40 times its concentration in blood. Iodide ions are oxidized to iodine, which is then capable of combining directly with the amino acid tyrosine. Successive stages of iodination of tyrosine to monoiodotyrosine and diiodotyrosine lead ultimately to the formation of the thyroid hormones. Diiodotyrosine molecules become coupled to form T4, whereas T3 is the result of coupling of one molecule of monoiodotyrosine and one molecule of diiodotyrosine.

Anatomically, the thyroid gland is composed of follicles that are filled with a secretory substance called *colloid.* The major constituent of colloid is the glycoprotein thyroglobulin. Thyroid hormones are stored in combination with thyroglobulin. Under the influence of TSH, T4 and T3 are first cleaved by proteinases from thyroglobulin for subsequent release into the circulation. When thyroglobulin is cleaved, monoiodotyrosine and diiodotyrosine are also liberated but usually do not leave the thyroid gland. Instead, these substances are metabolized, and the resulting iodide is reused. In the circulation, most of the thyroid hormones are combined with an acidic glycoprotein, thyroxine-binding globulin. Binding of T3 is less avid than that of T4. Thyroid hormones are also bound to albumin and thyroxine-binding prealbumin. Protein binding of thyroid hormones protects them from metabolism and excretion, resulting in a long elimination half-time. For example, T4 has an elimination half-time of 6 to 7 days, whereas less avidly protein bound T3 has an elimi-

nation half-time approaching 2 days. It is estimated that only about 0.03% of circulating T4 and 0.2% to 0.5% of T3 is available to act on receptors (Utiger, 1974). Pregnancy or administration of estrogens results in increased circulating concentrations of thyroxine-binding globulin, which could reduce the available free fraction of thyroid hormones. This effect, however, is offset by increased secretion of thyroid hormones. Thyroid hormones are conjugated in the liver with glucuronic acid and sulfuric acids and are excreted in the bile.

The normal daily secretion of T4 is 70 to 90 μg, whereas that of T3 is 15 to 30 μg. About 35% of T4, however, is converted to T3 in the peripheral tissues (Schimmel and Utiger, 1977). The function of both hormones is qualitatively the same, but they differ in rapidity and intensity of action. For example, T3 is about four times as potent as T4 but is also present in the blood in smaller amounts and for a shorter period of time.

Physiologic Effects

Important physiologic effects of thyroid hormones include (1) stimulation of growth in children, presumably as a result of protein synthesis, (2) maintenance of body temperature, and (3) generalized increase in metabolic rate except in the brain. Failure of thyroid hormones to greatly alter the metabolic rate of the brain is consistent with the minimal changes in anesthetic requirements that accompany hyperthyroidism or hypothyroidism (Fig. 52-2) (Babad and Eger, 1968). Uncoupling of oxidative-phosphorylation in mitochondria may be produced by thyroid hormones. The enzyme sodium-potassium-ATPase, necessary for the transport of sodium and potassium ions through cell membranes, is also stimulated by thyroid hormones.

Thyroid hormones stimulate all aspects of carbohydrate metabolism, including glycolysis, gluconeogenesis, and insulin secretion. Mobilization of free fatty acids and their subsequent oxidation are accelerated by thyroid hormones. Despite increased mobilization of fatty acids, the amount of cholesterol, phospholipids, and triglycerides in the blood is actually decreased by increased concentrations of thyroid hormones. Conversely, the large increase in circulating blood lipids in hypothyroidism is often associated with the development of atherosclerosis. Thyroid hormones increase the utilization of vitamins, and vitamin

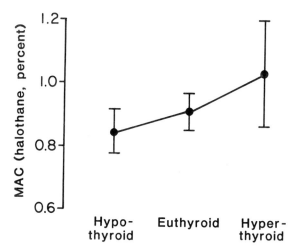

FIGURE 52-2. Anesthetic requirements (MAC, mean ± SD) are not significantly altered by changes in activity of the thyroid gland. (Data from Babad AA, Eger EI. The effects of hyperthyroidism and hypothyroidism on halothane and oxygen requirements in dogs. Anesthesiology 1968;29:1087–93.)

deficiency can develop if dietary intake does not match thyroid activity.

Increased metabolism produced by thyroid hormones causes vasodilation in tissues to provide the required blood flow to deliver necessary oxygen and carry away metabolites and heat. As a result of this increased tissue blood flow, the cardiac output increases as much as 50%. Heart rate often increases out of proportion to the increase in cardiac output. Mean arterial pressure is not altered, as the impact of increased cardiac output is offset by peripheral vasodilation.

The rate and depth of breathing are increased by thyroid hormones. Gastrointestinal tract motility is enhanced, and diarrhea is likely to accompany excess secretion of thyroid hormones. Excess protein catabolism associated with increased secretion of thyroid hormones is the presumed mechanism of skeletal muscle weakness characteristic of hyperthyroidism. The fine muscle tremor that accompanies hyperthyroidism is probably due to increased sensitivity of neuronal synapses in the area of the spinal cord that control skeletal muscle tone.

Increased secretion of thyroid hormones causes corresponding elevations in other endocrine gland secretions, including insulin and cortisol. Increased cortisol secretion is evoked in part by increased hepatic breakdown of glucocorticoids in the presence of thyroid hormones.

Injection of exogenous T4 is followed by a latent period of 48 to 72 hours before effects on metabolic rate manifest (see Chapter 23). Once activity begins, it increases progressively and reaches a maximum in 10 to 12 days. The latent period following injection of T3 is 6 to 12 hours, with maximal cellular effects occurring in 48 to 72 hours. A large part of the latent period and prolonged duration of action is due to binding to proteins in the plasma and cells.

Mechanism of Action

It is generally believed that thyroid hormones exert most, if not all, of their effects through control of protein synthesis. This most likely reflects the ability of thyroid hormones to activate the DNA transcription process in the cell nucleus, with resulting formation of new cell proteins, including enzymes. These effects could also manifest as an increased number and activity of mitochondria, which, in turn, enhance the rate of formation of ATP to fuel cellular function.

Regulation of Secretion

Optimal secretion of thyroid gland hormones is dependent on a negative feedback mechanism that operates through the hypothalamus and anterior pituitary (see the section entitled Thyroid-Stimulating Hormone).

Calcitonin

Calcitonin is a polypeptide hormone consisting of 32 amino acids that is secreted by the thyroid gland. In contrast to parathyroid hormone, calcitonin causes a reduction in the plasma concentration of calcium. Calcitonin reduces the plasma concentration of calcium by (1) decreasing the activity of osteoclasts, (2) increasing osteoblastic activity, and (3) preventing the formation of new osteoclasts. In the adult, calcitonin has only a weak effect on the plasma concentration of calcium, since any reduction in calcium serves as an intense stimulus for secretion of parathyroid hormone. Calcitonin is more important in children for regulating the plasma calcium concentration, because osteoclastic activity in this age group is much greater than that in adults. Also, in certain diseases of the bone, such as Paget's disease, in which osteoclastic activity is greatly accelerated, calcitonin has a potent effect in reducing calcium absorption. In hypercalcemic patients, the administration of calcitonin lowers the plasma concentration of calcium and phosphate for 6 to 10 hours. Other approaches, however, are more practical than calcitonin for reducing the serum calcium concentration (see Chapter 35). Furthermore, the development of antibodies is common with chronic therapy.

A 10% increase in the plasma concentration of calcium evokes an immediate twofold increase in the rate of secretion of calcitonin. This provides a second hormonal negative feedback mechanism for controlling the plasma calcium ion concentration. This negative feedback mechanism, however, works exactly opposite to the parathyroid hormone system, which responds to increased plasma concentrations of calcium by reducing output of parathyroid hormone. The calcitonin system responds more rapidly, reaching peak activity in less than 1 hour, compared with several hours required for peak activity to be attained following secretion of parathyroid hormone. Ultimately, however, the role of calcitonin as a regulator of the calcium ion concentration is quickly overridden by the more powerful parathyroid control mechanism. Therefore, over a prolonged period of time, it is almost entirely the secretion of parathyroid hormone that regulates the level of calcium ions in the extracellular fluid. Calcitonin is most important in the early moments following ingestion of a high-calcium meal. Nevertheless, a total thyroidectomy and subsequent absence of calcitonin does not measurably influence regulation of the plasma concentration of calcium, again emphasizing the predominant role of the parathyroid hormone mechanism.

PARATHYROID GLANDS

The four parathyroid glands secrete an 84 amino acid polypeptide known as parathyroid hormone. Removal of three of the four parathyroid glands usually causes transient hypoparathyroidism. Nevertheless, even a small amount of remaining parathyroid tissue can undergo sufficient hypertrophy with time to prevent persistent hypoparathyroidism.

Physiologic Effects

The primary function of parathyroid hormone is to elicit adaptive changes that serve to maintain a constant plasma concentration of calcium ions (see Chapter 35). The most prominent effect of parathyroid hormone is to promote mobilization of calcium from bone. A part of this mobilization is due to activation of osteoclastic activity by parathyroid hormone. In addition, parathyroid hormone evokes the immediate urinary loss of phosphate ions. At this same time, parathyroid hormone increases the renal tubular reabsorption of calcium ions at the distal renal tubules and collecting ducts.

Hypoparathyroidism is a predictable cause of hypocalcemia. Hyperparathyroidism results in hypercalcemia owing to excessive secretion of parathyroid hormone from the parathyroid glands (adenoma, hyperplasia) or from tumors arising at other sites. There is decalcification of bone and the occurrence of spontaneous fractures.

Commercially available parathyroid hormone must be administered parenterally. Following subcutaneous injection, the maximal effect is obtained after about 18 hours. The peak effect following intravenous injection occurs much sooner. Metabolism seems to be extensive, as less than 1% is excreted unchanged in the urine. There are currently no therapeutic uses for parathyroid hormone.

Mechanism of Action

Parathyroid hormone is likely to exert its effect on target cells in bone, renal tubules, and the gastrointestinal tract by virtue of stimulating the formation of cyclic AMP. Indeed, a portion of the cyclic AMP synthesized in the kidney escapes into the urine, and its assay serves as a measure of parathyroid gland activity. It is likely that parathyroid hormone functions in bone in the same way that it works in the kidneys and gastrointestinal tract, by causing the conversion of vitamin D to its active form, 1,25-dihydroxycholecalciferol (see Chapter 34).

Regulation of Secretion

Slight decreases in the plasma concentration of calcium are potent stimulants for the release of parathyroid hormone. An acute reduction of 1 mg dl⁻¹ in the plasma calcium ion concentration approximately doubles the plasma concentration of parathyroid hormone. Conversely, any increase in the plasma concentration of calcium is accompanied by a decrease in the activity of the parathyroid gland.

PANCREAS

The pancreas secretes digestive substances into the duodenum, whereas the islets of Langerhans secrete insulin and glucagon directly into the blood. The islets of Langerhans contain alpha, beta, and delta cells. Beta cells secrete insulin, alpha cells secrete glucagon, and delta cells secrete somatostatin. Somatostatin is the same as growth hormone releasing-inhibitory factor that is secreted by the hypothalamus. Secretion of both insulin and glucagon is also inhibited by somatostatin produced by the delta cells of the pancreas (Unger *et al,* 1978).

Insulin

Preproinsulin is synthesized in the membrane-associated polyribosomes of the rough endoplasmic reticulum of the beta cells of the pancreas and converted at this site to proinsulin. Enzymatic conversion of proinsulin to insulin occurs in storage granules. Structurally, insulin is a protein composed of two amino acid side chains connected by disulfide linkages (see Fig. 24-1). The mechanism by which insulin exerts its effects on cells is largely unknown. Circulating insulin is removed from the blood within 10 minutes and degraded in the kidneys and liver.

Physiologic Effects

Insulin exerts important effects on carbohydrate, fat, and protein metabolism. Basically, insulin promotes the utilization of carbohydrates for energy while it depresses utilization of fats. Conversely, lack of insulin causes utilization of mainly fat to the exclusion of glucose except by brain cells. As such, insulin controls whether glucose or fat will be utilized by cells for energy. The effect of insulin is not uniform on every organ. For example, entrance of glucose into skeletal muscle but not the central nervous system is dependent on insulin.

CARBOHYDRATE METABOLISM. Glucose that is absorbed into the circulation causes prompt secretion of insulin by the pancreas. Insulin facilitates uptake and storage of glucose as glycogen, especially in the liver, skeletal muscles, and fat. Between meals, when the blood glucose concentration declines and insulin is not available, glycogen is converted back to glucose, which is released into the plasma to maintain a normal blood–glucose concentration.

Insulin facilitates glucose uptake and storage in the liver by inhibiting or stimulating specific enzymes. For example, insulin inhibits phosphorylase enzyme, which normally causes liver glycogen to split into glucose. Enhanced uptake of glucose into liver cells reflects insulin-induced increases in the activity of the glucokinase enzyme. Glucokinase is the enzyme that causes the initial phosphorylation of glucose after it diffuses into the liver cells. Once phosphorylated, glucose is trapped inside cells, being unable to diffuse back through cell membranes. Liver cells, however, remain highly permeable to the continued passage of glucose into the cells. Insulin also increases the activity of other enzymes, including phosphofructokinase, which promotes glycogen synthesis. The net effects of these actions of insulin on enzymes is to increase hepatic stores of glycogen up to a maximum of about 100 g. Ordinarily, about 60% of the glucose in a meal is stored in the liver as glycogen (Guyton, 1986c).

Normal resting skeletal muscle membrane is almost impermeable to glucose except in the presence of insulin. Between meals, the circulating level of insulin is too low to promote glucose entry into skeletal muscle. As a result, resting skeletal muscle depends on fatty acids for energy. Exercise increases the permeability of the skeletal muscle membrane to glucose, perhaps reflecting the release of insulin from within the skeletal muscle itself or its vasculature (Koivisto and Felig, 1978).

Glucose that enters resting skeletal muscle under the influence of insulin is stored as glycogen for subsequent use as energy. The amount of glycogen that can be stored in skeletal muscle, however, is much less than that which can be stored in the liver. Furthermore, glycogen in skeletal muscle, in contrast to that stored in the liver, cannot be reconverted to glucose and released into the circulation. This occurs because skeletal muscle lacks glucose phosphatase enzyme, which is necessary for splitting glycogen.

Insulin promotes glucose transport into skeletal muscle cells differently than in the liver, where phosphorylation traps the glucose intracellularly. In contrast, glucose entry into skeletal muscle is more dependent on a carrier transport system. This carrier transport system is activated in an unknown manner by insulin. Glucose movement occurs only in the direction of a lower concentration of glucose, emphasizing that the carrier transport system for glucose is an example of facilitated diffusion (see Chapter 39).

Brain cells are unique in that permeability of the cell membrane to glucose is not dependent on the presence of insulin. This is crucial because brain cells use only glucose for energy, and it emphasizes the importance of maintaining the blood concentration of glucose above a critical level of about 50 mg dl^{-1}.

FAT METABOLISM. Insulin promotes conversion of liver glucose into fatty acids, and these fatty acids are subsequently transported to adipose tissue and deposited as fat. Glucose that enters liver cells becomes available for synthesis of fat when maximal amounts of hepatic glycogen have been formed. Insulin facilitates storage of fat in adipose cells by inhibiting lipase enzyme, which normally causes hydrolysis of triglycerides in fat cells.

PROTEIN METABOLISM. Insulin, like growth hormone, promotes active transport of amino acids into cells. In addition, formation of new proteins is facilitated by insulin-induced stimulation of RNA formation. Catabolism of proteins is also diminished by insulin. In the liver, insulin inhibits enzymes necessary for formation of glucose from amino acids (*i.e.,* gluconeogenesis), thus conserving amino acid stores.

Regulation of Secretion

Regulation of insulin secretion seems to involve a coordinated interaction between the availability of food, autonomic mechanisms, and the effects of other hormones. In man, glucose is the only nutrient that stimulates both the synthesis and secretion of insulin at physiologic concentrations. Indeed, secretion of insulin parallels elevations in the blood–glucose concentration (Hedeskov, 1980). Nevertheless, amino acids, fatty acids, and ketone bodies also evoke the release of insulin, emphasizing the role of this hormone in stimulating storage of all fuels.

It has been speculated that glucose acts as a secretagogue by means of interactions with glucoreceptors on cell membranes of pancreatic beta cells. The fact that beta-2 agonists stimulate secretion of insulin suggests a role of cyclic AMP. The presence of extracellular calcium ions is also necessary for glucose-induced secretion of insulin. Inhaled anesthetics do not seem to exert a selective effect on secretion of insulin (Merin *et al,* 1971).

Insulin secretion is minimal in the presence of a normal fasting blood–glucose concentration. Abrupt elevations of the blood–glucose concentration stimulate the immediate release of preformed insulin from the pancreas as well as activation of the enzyme system for synthesis of insulin. When the blood–glucose concentration is 300 to 400 mg dl^{-1}, the rate of insulin secretion may be increased 20-fold, compared with the basal level. Hypertrophy of the beta cells occurs when increases in the blood concentration of glucose are sustained for a week or more. The decline in insulin secretion when the blood–glucose concentration falls is as rapid as the response to increased levels of blood glucose. These rapid responses in the rate of insulin secretion provide a sensitive negative feedback mechanism to regulate the blood concentration of glucose over a narrow range.

GASTROINTESTINAL MECHANISMS. Oral glucose is more effective than intravenous glucose in evoking the release of insulin, suggesting the presence of an anticipatory signal from the gastrointestinal tract to the pancreas. Indeed, gastrointestinal hormones, including secretin, gastrin, and glucagon, stimulate insulin release from the pancreas (Hedeskov, 1980). Consistent with this enteropancreatic axis is the observation that glycosuria is more likely to accompany intravenous than oral administration of glucose. This observation has obvious implications for the intravenous infusion of fluids containing glucose during the perioperative period.

ADRENERGIC MECHANISMS. The sympathetic and parasympathetic nervous systems richly innervate the beta cells of the pancreas. For example, alpha-adrenergic stimulation produced by norepinephrine and epinephrine inhibits secretion of insulin by the pancreas. Likewise, beta-adrenergic blockade or cholinergic blockade inhibits release of insulin into the circulation.

Events such as arterial hypoxemia, hypothermia, stress as produced by trauma, burns, or surgery all result in suppression of insulin secretion by means of activation of alpha-adrenergic receptors. Conversely, selective activation of beta-2 adrenergic receptors, cholinergic drugs, and vagal nerve stimulation enhance the secretion of insulin.

OTHER HORMONES. Glucagon, growth hormone, and glucocorticoids can potentiate glucose-induced stimulation of insulin secretion (Marks and Samols, 1970). Prolonged secretion of these hormones or their exogenous administration can lead to the exhaustion of pancreatic beta cells and development of diabetes mellitus. Indeed, diabetes mellitus often occurs in patients who develop acromegaly or in those persons with a diabetic tendency who are treated with glucocorticoids.

Diabetes Mellitus

Insulin-dependent diabetes mellitus (juvenile-onset) is characterized by the absence of insulin in the pancreas and circulation. Severe hyperglycemia and ketoacidosis are likely complications in these patients. Persons with noninsulin-dependent diabetes mellitus (maturity-onset) have functional pancreatic beta cells as evidenced by the presence of insulin in the plasma, but there are abnormalities in the initial secretion of insulin by these pancreatic cells when stimulated by glucose. In addition, less insulin is secreted at any given blood–glucose concentration in both diabetic patients and in those persons with latent disease. The defect in these patients is not known but may be associated with an alteration in the glucoreceptors on pancreatic beta cell membranes. Most patients with maturity-onset diabetes mellitus are obese. Indeed, weight reduction is important in the treatment of maturity-onset diabetes mellitus.

HYPERGLYCEMIA. In the absence of sufficient insulin, there is a marked reduction in the rate of transport of glucose across certain cell membranes. Because of the inability of glucose to gain entrance into cells, the oxidation of glucose to carbon dioxide and its conversion to glycogen and fat are slowed. Nevertheless, insulin does not influence the rate of transfer of glucose across all cell membranes. For example, glucose entrance into hepatic cells is not significantly reduced in the absence of insulin. Likewise, the rate of entry of glucose into the brain is unaffected by diabetes mellitus, and function of the central nervous system remains normal unless a state of ketoacidosis develops.

In the absence of insulin, there is a marked decrease in the activity of the enzyme system that catalyzes the conversion of glucose to glycogen. There is an accompanying high rate of conversion of protein to glucose. Furthermore, the protein catabolic actions of glucagon, corticosteroids, and thyroid hormones are unopposed in insulin deficiency. The formation of glucose from protein accounts for the observation that glucose lost in urine may exceed oral intake. Much of the protein for glucose formation comes from skeletal muscle. Protein wasting is a serious side effect of diabetes mellitus, leading to skeletal muscle weakness as well as deranged function of multiple organ systems.

HYPERLIPEMIA AND KETONEMIA. Increased free fatty acid concentrations in the plasma of diabetic patients reflects loss of insulin-induced inhibition of the lipase enzyme system such that mobilization of fatty acids proceeds unopposed. The liver takes up large quantities of these liberated free fatty acids and oxidizes them to acetyl coenzyme A. The reduced ability of the insulin-deficient liver, however, to synthesize fatty acids from acetyl coenzyme A results in diversion of this substrate to ketone bodies such as acetone, acetoacetate, and beta-hydroxybutyrate. These ketone bodies are subsequently used as a source of energy by skeletal muscle and cardiac muscle. In extreme circumstances, the liver can store 30% or more of its weight in the form of fat. Sustained elevations of the circulating concentrations of lipids are associated with the development of atherosclerosis in patients with diabetes mellitus.

DIABETIC KETOACIDOSIS. Diabetic ketoacidosis is caused by a marked deficiency of insulin relative to metabolic demands that may be abruptly increased by trauma or infection. Diabetic katoacidosis is a continuum ranging from slight ketonemia and ketonuria to the syndrome of diabetic coma, which is characterized by glycosuria, ketonemia, ketonuria, metabolic acidosis, diuresis-induced hypovolemia, and coma. Hyperventilation may be present. Abdominal pain accompanied by leukocytosis and elevated serum amylase concentrations may result in confusion of diabetic acidosis with a surgical disease.

Production of large amounts of acetoacetate and beta-hydroxybutyrate, which are relatively strong acids, causes the acidosis of insulin deficiency. Urinary excretion of these anions is in part responsible for the loss of fixed cation and contributes to the depletion of electrolytes characteristic of diabetic ketoacidosis. For example, the loss of potassium ions averages 5 mEq kg^{-1} in patients with ketoacidosis. Concentrations of potassium in the plasma, however, are usually not decreased, because intracellular potassium is exchanged for extracellular potassium to compensate for the acidosis. Increased urinary excretion of ammonia is a renal homeostatic mechanism that is stimulated by ketoacidosis.

The treatment of diabetic coma is with the continuous intravenous infusion of insulin, 2 to 10 units hr^{-1} and intravascular fluid and electrolyte replacement (Kreisberg, 1978). Normal saline is a useful replacement for intravascular fluid volume losses owing to glycosuria-induced diuresis. There is intracellular depletion of potassium despite an initial normal or moderately elevated plasma concentration, reflecting intracellular buffering of metabolic acids. During treatment, as the production of ketoacids diminishes and potassium ions move intracellularly under the influence of insulin, and as the patient is rehydrated, hypokalemia may manifest. For these reasons, intravenous administration, 10 to 20 mEq hr^{-1}, of potassium is recommended in the initial treatment regimen.

Deficiency of phosphorus accompanies ketoacidosis and may result in decreased concentrations of 2,3-diphosphoglycerate in erythrocytes, with consequent changes in the affinity of hemoglobin for oxygen. Skeletal muscle weakness may also be due to hypophosphatemia.

Low plasma concentrations of insulin, although inadequate to prevent hyperglycemia, may be quite effective in blocking lipolysis. This differential effect of insulin explains the common observation in patients with diabetes mellitus that hyperglycemia can exist without the presence of ketone bodies. Ketosis can be easily prevented by continuously providing all diabetic patients with small amounts of glucose and insulin. This is particularly appropriate in the perioperative period when nutritional intake is greatly altered.

HYPEROSMOLAR COMA. Hyperosmolar coma is a variant of diabetic ketoacidosis, but severe ketosis is usually absent (Podolsky, 1978; Wulfson and Dalton, 1974). Typically, the thirst mechanism is impaired. Patients are often obese, elderly, and diabetic with an infection that accentuates hyperglycemia, leading to diuresis and profound intravascular volume depletion. Plasma glucose concentration may exceed 1500 mg dl^{-1}, and the plasma osmolarity is usually greater than 350 mOsm L^{-1}. Seizures, coma, and death occur unless there is aggressive intravascular fluid replacement. Insulin infusion is the same as that used for treatment of diabetic coma.

Glucagon

Glucagon is a single-chain polypeptide hormone consisting of 29 amino acids secreted by the alpha cells of the pancreas (Sherwin and Felig, 1977). Human glucagon is identical in structure to the bovine and porcine hormone. The primary action of glucagon is to increase the blood concentration of glucose, accounting for the designation of this hormone as the hyperglycemic factor.

Physiologic Effects

Glucagon is able to abruptly increase the blood concentration of glucose by stimulation of glycogenolysis in the liver. This reflects activation of adenylate cyclase by glucagon and the subsequent formation of cyclic AMP. Enzyme systems necessary for degradation of glycogen are activated by the increased intracellular concentrations of cyclic AMP. Infusion of glucagon for about 4 hours can totally deplete liver glycogen stores. In this regard, the metabolic effects of glucagon at the liver mimic those produced by epinephrine. Indeed, the study of the mechanism of the hyperglycemic action of glucagon and epinephrine led to the discovery of cyclic AMP (Rall and Sutherland, 1958).

Glucagon also causes hyperglycemia by virtue of stimulation of gluconeogenesis in the liver cells. This process continues even when hepatic glycogen stores have been depleted. Other effects of glucagon such as enhanced myocardial contractility and increased secretion of bile probably occur only when exogenous administration elevates plasma concentrations of the hormone far above those that occur normally (see Chapter 13).

Regulation of Secretion

Reductions in the blood concentration of glucose are the principal stimulus for the secretion of glucagon by pancreatic alpha cells (Gerich *et al,* 1976). During exercise, release of glucagon is important in mobilizing glucose from the liver for use by skeletal muscles. Amino acids enhance the release of glucagon and thus prevent hypoglycemia that would occur from ingestion of a pure protein meal and associated stimulation of insulin secretion. Other events that enhance secretion of glucagon include infection and stress as produced by trauma, burns, and surgery.

Glucagon undergoes enzymatic destruction to an inactive compound in the liver, kidney, and plasma and at receptor sites in cell membranes (Pohl *et al,* 1972). The elimination half-time of glucagon is brief, being only 3 to 6 minutes (Alberti and Nattrass, 1977).

MALE SEX HORMONES

The testes secrete male sex hormones, which are collectively called *androgens.* Testosterone is the most potent and abundant of the androgens. This hormone is formed by the interstitial cells of Leydig, which are present in the interstices between seminiferous tubules and constitute about 20% of the mass of the adult testes. The adrenal cortex also secretes androgens, but the effects of these hormones are usually inconsequential unless a hormone-secreting tumor develops. For example, in males, about 10% of androgens are produced in the adrenal cortex. This is an insufficient amount to maintain spermatogenesis or secondary sexual features in an adult male. In abnormal conditions, such as the adrenogenital syndrome, the adrenal cortex can secrete large quantities of steroids and androgenic precursors. The Stein-Leventhal syndrome is characterized by virilization resulting from excessive ovarian secretion of androgens.

All androgens are steroid compounds that can be synthesized from cholesterol or acetyl coenzyme A. Circulating testosterone is loosely bound to proteins, becoming attached to tissues or degraded to inactive metabolites in the liver. In cells, testosterone is often converted to dihydrotestosterone.

Physiologic Effects

Testosterone is responsible for the development and maintenance of male sex characteristics (Wilson, 1978). Testosterone typically causes growth of hair but paradoxically decreases growth of hair on the top of the head. Many virile men, however, do not become bald; baldness is also determined genetically. Hypertrophy of the laryngeal mucosa accompanies secretion of testosterone, leading to the characteristic change in voice at puberty. Testosterone increases secretion of sebaceous glands, leading to acne. Beard growth is the last manifestation of puberty. Skeletal muscle growth is an anabolic effect of testosterone in the male.

Mechanism of Action

At most sites of action, testosterone is not the active form of the hormone being converted in target tissues to the more active dihydrotesterone by a reductase enzyme. Dihydrotesterone binds to a cytoplasmic protein receptor that results in increased synthesis of specific RNA and protein. In the absence of sufficient reductase enzyme, external genitalia fail to develop despite secretion of adequate amounts of testosterone (*i.e.,* pseudohermaphroditism) (Imperato-McGinley *et al,* 1979). Not all target tissues, however, require the conversion of testosterone to dihydrotestosterone for activity. For example, androgenic and anabolic effects in skeletal muscle and bone marrow are mediated by testosterone or a metabolite other than dihydrotestosterone (Givens, 1978).

Regulation of Secretion

Testosterone is produced in the testes only when stimulation occurs from luteinizing hormone secreted by the anterior pituitary. Follicle-stimulating hormone from the anterior pituitary is necessary to initiate spermatogenesis. Both of these anterior pituitary hormones are secreted by the anterior pituitary in response to releasing factors produced by the hypothalamus. Puberty occurs when the hypothalamus begins to secrete these releasing factors. At puberty (10 – 13 years of age), production of testosterone increases rapidly and continues throughout the remainder of life. The amount produced, however, decreases beyond the age of 40 years to become about one- fifth the peak value by 80 years of age.

FEMALE SEX HORMONES

The two types of ovarian hormones, estrogen and progesterone, are secreted in response to luteinizing hormone and follicle-stimulating hormone from the anterior pituitary (*i.e.,* gonadotropins) (Linder *et al,* 1977). These anterior pituitary hormones are secreted in response to a hypothalamic-releasing factor.

Ovarian changes during the female sexual cycle depend entirely on secretion of gonadotropins. Following ovulation, the secretory cells of the follicle develop into a corpus luteum that secretes progesterone and estrogen (Richards, 1980). The rise in body temperature (about 0.5°C) that accompanies ovulation is due to progesterone. After about 14 days, the corpus luteum degenerates and menstruation begins when the plasma concentration of progesterone has declined to a critical level. Pregnanediol in urine accounts for about 15% of the metabolized progesterone. This percentage increases up to 30% during the luteal phase of the menstrual cycle and during pregnancy (Fatherby and James, 1972). Measurement of urinary pregnanediol provides a valuable index of the secretion and metabolism of progesterone.

Physiologic Effects

Estrogens

Estrogens are responsible for the development of female sexual characteristics. In the nonpregnant female, significant amounts of estrogen are secreted by the ovaries, although minute amounts are also secreted by the adrenal cortex. During pregnancy, large amounts of estrogen are secreted by the placenta. The three most important estrogens are beta-estradiol, estrone, and estriol. The liver conjugates these estrogens into almost totally inactive metabolites, which appear in the urine.

Progesterone

Progesterone is necessary for preparation of the uterus for pregnancy and the breasts for lactation. Almost all the progesterone in the nonpregnant female is secreted by the corpus luteum during the latter half of each ovarian cycle. The adrenal cortex forms minute amounts of progesterone. During pregnancy, large amounts of progesterone are formed by the placenta. The liver is the site of metabolism of progesterone to pregnanediol.

Pregnancy

In pregnancy, the placenta forms large amounts of chorionic gonadotropin, estrogens, progesterone, and chorionic somatomammotropin (Thorburn and Challis, 1979). Secretion of chorionic gonadotropin prevents sloughing of the endometrium of the uterus that typically occurs 14 days after ovulation (*i.e.,* menstruation). Chorionic gonadotropin also prevents the usual involution of the corpus luteum and instead causes it to secrete large amounts of progesterone and estrogens, which stimulate the endometrium to continue growing. After about 12 weeks, the placenta secretes sufficient amounts of progesterone and estrogens to maintain pregnancy and the corpus luteum involutes.

Secretion of estrogen by the placenta is different from secretion by the ovaries. For example, about 90% of the estrogen secreted by the placenta is estriol, which is found in only small amounts in the nongravid female. Increased circulting concentrations of estrogen cause enlargement of the breasts and uterus. Estrogens also relax pelvic ligaments so that the sacroiliac joints become limber and the symphysis pubis becomes elastic.

Progesterone is essential for pregnancy. Initially, moderate amounts of progesterone are secreted by the corpus luteum, and, as pregnancy progresses, large amounts are secreted by the placenta until delivery. This hormone is necessary for the development of decidual cells in the uterine endometrium and suppression of uterine contractions that could result in abortion. Near term, the production of progesterone remains constant, whereas estrogen production increases. This change in the ratio of estrogen to progesterone may be at least partially responsible for the onset of uterine contractions.

Increased plasma concentrations of progesterone and associated sedative effects during pregnancy have been proposed as the explanations for a 25% to 40% decrease in anesthetic requirements (*i.e.,* MAC) for volatile drugs in gravid animals (Palahniuk *et al,* 1974). Nevertheless, anesthetic requirements in animals return to non-pregnant values within 5 days postpartum, while the plasma concentration of progesterone remains elevated, suggesting that the reduction in MAC cannot be attributed entirely to progesterone (Strout and Nahrwold, 1981). Increased plasma concentrations of progesterone are presumed to be the stimulus for elevations in minute ventilation during pregnancy.

Chorionic somatomammotropin begins to be produced by the placenta about the fifth week of gestation. This hormone has important metabolic effects, including decreased insulin activity, making more glucose available to the fetus.

The parturient with asthma may experience unpredictable changes in airway reactivity. Exacerbation of asthma may reflect bronchoconstriction evoked by prostaglandins of the F series, which are present in all trimesters of pregnancy, but especially during labor (see Chapter 20). Conversely, prostaglandins of the E series are bronchodilators and predominate during the third trimester. A role of glucocorticoids in altered airway responsiveness is questionable, because increased plasma concentrations of cortisol associated with pregnancy are offset by concomitant increases in the carrier protein transcortin, with the net effect being an unchanged level of available cortisol.

REFERENCES

Alberti KGMM, Nattrass M. The physiological function of glucagon. (Editorial). Eur J Clin Invest 1977;7:151–4.

Babad AA, Eger EI. The effects of hyperthyroidism and hypothyroidism on halothane and oxygen requirements in dogs. Anesthesiology 1968;29:1087–93.

Ballard PL, Baxter JD, Higgens SJ, Rousseau GC, Tomkins GM. General presence of glucocorticoid receptors in mammalian tissues. Endocrinology 1974;94:988–1002.

Bovill JG, Sebel PS, Fiolet JW, Touber JL, Kok K, Philbin DM. The influence of sufentanil on endocrine and metabolic responses to cardiac surgery. Anesth Analg 1983;62:391–7.

Brodish A, Lymangrover JR. The hypothalamic-pituitary adrenocortical system. Int Rev Physiol 1977;16:93–149.

Catt KJ, Dufau ML. Peptide hormone receptors. Annu Rev Physiol 1977;39:529–57.

Chrubasik J, Meynadier J, Scherpereel P, Wunsch E. The effect of epidural somatostatin on postoperative pain. Anesth Analg 1985;64:1085–8.

Cowley AW, Monos E, Guyton AC. Interaction of vasopressin and the baroreceptor reflex system in the regulation of arterial blood pressure in the dog. Cir Res 1974;34:505–14.

Faden AI. Opiate antagonists and thyrotropin-releasing hormone. 1. Potential role in the treatment of shock. JAMA 1984;252:1177–80.

Fatherby K, James F. Metabolism of synthetic steroids. Adv Steroid Biochem Pharmacol 1972;3:67–165.

Gerich JE, Charles MA, Grodsky GM. Regulation of pancreatic insulin and glucagon secretion. Annu Rev Physiol 1976;38:353–88.

Givens JR. Normal and abnormal androgen metabolism. Clin Obstet Gynecol 1978;21:115–23.

Golander A, Hurley T, Barrett J, Hizi A, Handivergen S. Prolactin synthesis by human choriondecidual tissue: a possible source of prolactin in the amniotic fluid. Science 1978;202:311–3.

Guyton AC. Textbook of Medical Physiology, 7th ed. Philadelphia: WB Saunders, 1986a:876.

Guyton AC. Textbook of Medical Physiology, 7th ed. Philadelphia: WB Saunders, 1986b:909.

Guyton AC. Textbook of Medical Physiology, 7th ed. Philadelphia: WB Saunders, 1986c:923.

Hedeskov CJ. Mechanism of glucose-induced insulin secretion. Physiol Rev 1980;60:442–509.

Imperato-McGinley J, Peterson RE, Gautier T, Sturla E. Androgens and the evaluation of male gender identify among male pseudohermaphrodites with 5 alpha-reductase deficiency. N Engl J Med 1979;300:1233–7.

Iynedjian PB, Hanson RW. Messenger RNA for renal phosphoenolpyruvate carboxykinase and its regulation by glucocorticoids and by changes in acid–base balance. J Biol Chem 1977;152:8398–403.

Koivisto VA, Felig P. Effects of leg exercise on insulin absorption in diabetic patients. N Engl J Med 1978;298:79–83.

Kostyo JL, Isaksson O. Growth hormone and the regulation of somatic growth. Int Rev Physiol 1977;13:255–74.

Kreisberg RA. Diabetic ketoacidosis:new concepts and trends in pathogenesis and treatment. Ann Intern Med 1978;88:681–95.

Kumar A, Pontoppidan H, Baratz RA, Laver MB. Inappropriate response to increased plasma ADH during mechanical ventilation in acute respiratory failure. Anesthesiology 1974;40:215–21.

Labrie F, Borgeat P, Drouin J et al. Mechanism of action of hypothalamic hormones in the adenohypophysis. Annu Rev Physiol 1979;41:555–69.

Linder HR, Amsterdam A, Solomon Y et al. Intraovarian factors in ovulation: determinants of follicular response to gonadotropins. J Repro Fertil 1977;51:215–35.

MacLeod RM. Regulation of prolactin secretion. In: Martini L, Ganong E, eds. Frontiers in Neuroendocrinology, New York, Raven Press, 1976:169.

Marks V, Samols E. Intestinal factors in the regulation of insulin secretion. Adv Metab Disord 1970;4:1–38.

McCaa RE, McCaa CS, Bengis RG, Guyton AC. Role of aldosterone in experimental hypertension. J Endocrinol 1979;81:69P–78P.

Merin RG, Samuelson PN, Schalch DS. Major inhalation anesthetics and carbohydrate metabolism. Anesth Analg 1971;50:625–32.

Palahniuk RJ, Shnider SM, Eger EI. Pregnancy decreases the requirement for inhaled anesthetic agents. Anesthesiology 1974;41:82–3.

Parrillo JE, Fauci AS. Mechanisms of glucocorticoid action on immune processes. Annu Rev Pharmacol Toxicol 1979;19:179–201.

Philbin DM, Coggins CH. Plasma antidiuretic hormone levels in cardiac surgical patients during morphine and halothane anesthesia. Anesthesiology 1978; 49:95–8.

Podolsky S. Hyperosmolar nonketotic coma in the elderly diabetic. Med Clin North Am 1978;62:815–28.

Pohl SL, Michiel H, Krans J, Bernbaumer L, Rodbell M. Inactivation of glucagon by plasma membranes of rat liver. J Biol Chem 1972;247:2295–2301.

Raisz LG, Mundy GR, Dietrich JW, Canalis EM. Hormonal regulation of mineral metabolism. Int Rev Physiol 1977;16:199–240.

Rall TW, Sutherland EW. Formation of a cyclic adenine ribonucleotide by tissue particles. J Biol Chem 1958;232:1065–76.

Reichlin S, Saperstein R, Jackson IMD, Boyd AE, Patel Y. Hypothalamic hormones. Annu Rev Physiol 1976;38:389–450.

Richards JS. Maturation of ovarian follicles: Actions and interactions of pituitary and ovarian hormones on follicular cell differentiation. Physiol Rev 1980; 60:51–89.

Robertson GL, Mahr EA, Athar S, Sinha T. Development and clinical application of a new method for the radioimmunoassay of arginine vasopressin in human plasma. J Clin Invest 1973;52:2340–52.

Schimmel M, Utiger RD. Thyroidal and peripheral production of thyroid hormones. Ann Intern Med 1977:87:760–8.

Schrier RW, Berl T, Anderson RJ. Osmotic and nonosmotic control of vasopressin release. Am J Physiol 1979;236:F321–32.

Sebel PS, Bovill JG, Schellekens APM, Hawker CD. Hormonal responses to high-dose fentanyl anesthesia. Br J Anaesth 1981;53:941–8.

Seif SM, Robinson AG. Localization and release of neurophysins. Annu Rev Physiol 1978;40:345–76.

Sherwin R, Felig P. Glucagon physiology in health and disease. Int Rev Physiol 1977;16:151–71.

Sladen A, Laver MB, Pontoppidan H. Pulmonary complications and water retention in prolonged mechanical ventilation. N Engl J Med 1968;279:448–53.

Smith MJ, Cowley AW, Guyton AC, Manning RP. Acute and chronic effects of vasopressin on blood pressure, electrolytes, and fluid volumes. Am J Physiol 1979;237:F232–40.

Strewler GJ, Orloff J. Role of cyclic nucleotides in the transport of water and electrolytes. Adv Cyclic Nucleotide Res 1977;8:311–61.

Strout CD, Nahrwold ML. Halothane requirement during pregnancy and lactation in rats. Anesthesiology 1981;55:322–3.

Thorburn GD, Challis JRG. Endocrine control of parturition. Physiol Rev 1979;59:863–918.

Traymor C, Hall GM. Endocrine and metabolic changes during surgery: anaesthesia implications. Br J Anaesth 1981;53:153–60.

Unger RH, Dobbs RE, Orci L. Insulin, glucagon, and somatostatin secretion in the regulation of metabolism. Annu Rev Physiol 1978;40:307–43.

Utiger RD. Serum triiodothyronine in man. Annu Rev Med 1974;29:289–302.

Volpe R. The pathogenesis of Graves' disease: an overview. Clin Endocrinol Metab 1978;7:3–29.

Weiner RI, Ganong WF. Role of brain monoamines and histamine in regulation of anterior pituitary secretion. Physiol Rev 1978;58:905–76.

Wilson JD. Sexual differentiation. Annu Rev Physiol 1978;40:279–306.

Wulfson HD, Dalton B. Hyperosmolar hyperglycemic nonketotic coma in a patient undergoing emergency cholecystectomy. Anesthesiology 1974; 41:286–90.

Kidneys

INTRODUCTION

The kidneys perform two essential physiologic functions (Lassiter, 1975). First, these organs excrete end products of metabolism such as urea while essential body nutrients, including amino acids and glucose, are retained. Second, kidneys control the electrolyte and hydrogen ion composition of body fluids, emphasizing the importance of renal function in maintaining a normal plasma osmolarity and pH. In addition to these two physiologic functions, the kidneys secrete hormones, including renin and erythropoietin.

NEPHRON

The nephron is the basic anatomic unit of the kidneys. Each kidney contains about 1.2 million nephrons, and this number does not change after birth. The nephron is composed of a glomerulus from which fluid is filtered and a long tubule in which the filtered fluid is converted into urine on its way to the renal pelvis (Fig. 53-1) (Pitts, 1974). Components of the renal tubule are the proximal convoluted tubule, loop of Henle, and distal convoluted tubule.

The glomerulus is formed selectively in the renal cortex by a tuft of capillaries that invaginate into the dilated blind end of the nephron known as *Bowman's capsule.* The capillaries that form the glomerulus are unique anatomically in being interposed between two sets of arterioles. Blood enters the glomerulus through afferent arterioles and leaves through efferent arterioles. Pressure in glomerular capillaries can be altered by changing the vascular activity of either the afferent or efferent arterioles. It is the pressure of the blood in glomerular capillaries that causes water and low–molecular weight substances to filter into Bowman's capsule, which is in direct continuity with the proximal renal tubule. This glomerular filtrate flows into the proximal renal tubule, which, along with the glomerulus, lies entirely in the renal cortex.

From the proximal renal tubule, glomerular filtrate passes into the loop of Henle. Those loops that extend into the renal medulla are termed *juxtamedullary nephrons,* while those that lie close to the surface of the kidneys are called *cortical nephrons.* From the loop of Henle, fluid flows back into the renal cortex by way of the distal renal tubule. Finally, the glomerular filtrate enters the collecting duct, which gathers fluid from several nephrons. The collecting duct passes from the renal cortex downward through the medulla, paralleling the loops of Henle, before it empties into the renal pelvis.

As the glomerular filtrate travels along the renal tubule, most of its water and varying amounts of its solutes are reabsorbed from the renal tubular lumen into peritubular capillaries. In addition, small amounts of other solutes are secreted into the lumen of the renal tubule. The resulting glomerular filtrate and solutes become urine.

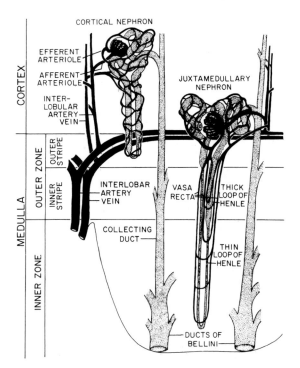

FIGURE 53-1. Schematic depiction of the nephron and accompanying blood supply. (Reproduced with permission from Pitts RF. Physiology of the Kidney and Body Fluids, 3rd edition. Copyright 1974 by Year Book Medical Publishers, Inc., Chicago.)

Nephrons clear the plasma of waste products by filtering a large proportion of plasma through the glomerular capillary membrane into the tubules of the nephron. The unwanted metabolic substances, unlike water and electrolytes, are not reabsorbed as the glomerular filtrate progresses through the renal tubule. A second mechanism by which the nephron clears the plasma of unwanted substances is by secretion. Specifically, substances are secreted from the plasma directly through the epithelial cells lining the renal tubules and into the tubular fluid. Thus, the urine that is eventually formed is composed mainly of substances filtered through the glomerular capillaries and small amounts of secreted substances.

RENAL BLOOD FLOW

Renal blood flow is about 1000 ml min^{-1} when the cardiac output is 5.0 L min^{-1}. This represents about 20% of the resting cardiac output passing through the kidneys. The renal cortex receives about 75% of the renal blood flow.

Blood Supply to the Nephron

The nephron is supplied by the glomerular capillary bed and peritubular capillaries (Fig. 53-1) (Pitts, 1974). The glomerular capillary bed receives its blood from the afferent arteriole, which is separated from the glomerulus by the efferent arteriole. The efferent arteriole offers significant resistance to blood flow, causing the glomerular capillaries to be a high-pressure system. Conversely, peritubular capillaries are a low-pressure system. High pressure in glomerular capillaries causes them to function in the same manner as arterial ends of tissue capillaries, with fluid filtering continuously out of the glomerular capillaries into Bowman's capsule. Conversely, low pressure in peritubular capillaries causes them to function in much the same way as the venous ends of the tissue capillaries, with fluid from the renal tubules being absorbed continually into these capillaries.

Vasa Recta

The vasa recta are a specialized portion of the peritubular capillary system. These specialized peritubular capillaries form a network that descend around the lower portions of the loops of Henle in the renal medulla before returning to the renal cortex to empty into the veins. Only 1% to 2% of the renal blood flow passes through the vasa recta, emphasizing that blood flow through the medulla of the kidney is sluggish compared with the rapid blood flow that occurs in the renal cortex. The vasa recta are particularly important in the formation of a concentrated urine, by virtue of controlling the rate of solute removal from the interstitium (*i.e.,* countercurrent mechanism).

Role of Peritubular Capillaries

About 180 L of fluid are filtered daily through the glomeruli, and all but about 1.5 L of this is reabsorbed from the renal tubules into renal interstitial spaces and subsequently into peritubular capillaries. This represents about four times as much fluid as that reabsorbed at the venous ends of all the other tissue capillaries. Peritubular capillaries are able to achieve this necessary reabsorption by virtue of being extremely porous in comparison with other tissue capillaries. As a result, colloid osmotic pressure provided by plasma proteins can provide for the rapid reabsorption of fluid from the renal interstitial space into peritubular capillaries.

Intravascular Pressures in the Renal Circulation

Blood enters the renal arteries at a mean pressure of about 100 mmHg and drains into veins with an intravascular pressure of about 8 mmHg (Fig. 53-2) (Guyton, 1986a). In the afferent arterioles, the pressure declines from 100 mmHg at its arterial end to an estimated 60 mmHg in the glomerulus. As the blood flows through the efferent arterioles from the glomerulus into the peritubular capillary system, the pressure again declines substantially from 60 mmHg to an average 13 mmHg.

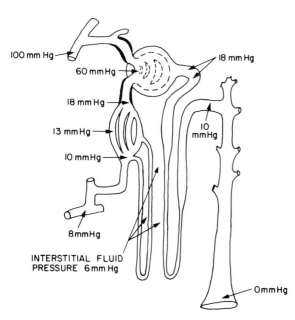

FIGURE 53-2. Intravascular pressures in the renal circulation. (From Guyton AC. Textbook of Medical Physiology, 7th ed. Philadelphia: WB Saunders, 1986:393. Reproduced by permission of the author and publisher.)

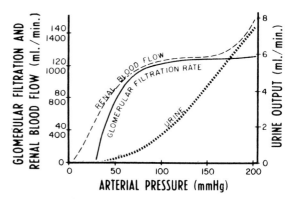

FIGURE 53-3. Renal blood flow and glomerular filtration rate, but not urine output, are autoregulated between a mean arterial pressure of about 70 to 160 mmHg. (From Guyton AC. Textbook of Medical Physiology, 7th ed. Philadelphia: WB Saunders, 1986:410. Reproduced by permission of the author and publisher.)

Autoregulation of Renal Blood Flow

Changes in arterial blood pressure between about 70 and 160 mmHg initially autoregulate both renal blood flow and glomerular filtration rate (Fig. 53-3) (Guyton, 1986b). Renal blood flow autoregulation is due to an intrinsic mechanism that results in appropriate vasodilatation or vasoconstriction of afferent renal arterioles. For example, reductions in arterial blood pressure and renal blood flow cause a decrease in glomerular capillary pressure and glomerular filtration rate. As a consequence, a negative feedback mechanism is activated, and signals from the macula densa cells cause vasodilation of the afferent renal arterioles. This vasodilation allows renal blood flow to increase despite a persisting reduction in arterial blood pressure. The same mechanism operates in the opposite direction, causing afferent arteriole vasoconstriction when arterial blood pressure and renal blood flow become excessive. The fact that autoregulation occurs, even in a denervated kidney, confirms the intrinsic nature of the mechanism responsible for this response. Autoregulation of renal blood flow has been demonstrated to remain intact during administration of halothane (Fig. 53-4) (Bastron *et al,* 1977).

Autoregulation of renal blood flow is not sustained in the presence of persistent changes in arterial blood pressure, which contrasts with sus-

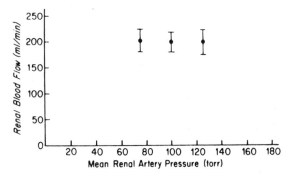

FIGURE 53-4. Autoregulation of renal blood flow seems to remain intact during halothane anesthesia. (From Bastron RD, Perkins FM, Pyne JL. Autoregulation of renal blood flow during halothane anesthesia. Anesthesiology 1977;46:142–4. Reproduced by permission of the authors and publisher.)

tained effects of autoregulation on glomerular filtration rate. This is due to the fact that initial autoregulation of both renal blood flow and glomerular filtration rate is due almost entirely to changes in resistance to blood flow in afferent renal arterioles. After about 5 to 10 minutes, however, angiotensin II is formed, and vasoconstriction of efferent renal arterioles becomes the predominant mechanism. This vasoconstrictor mechanism causes decreased, rather than increased, renal blood flow. As a result, when arterial blood pressure remains low for more than about 10 minutes, autoregulation of renal blood flow wanes. This allows the glomerular filtration rate to remain near normal despite marked reductions in renal blood flow, which can be redistributed to other vital organs during prolonged periods of hypotension.

Plasma Clearance

Plasma clearance is the amount of plasma that can be cleared of a substance by the kidneys each minute. Plasma clearance of urea is 70 ml min^{-1}, which means that 70 ml of plasma is cleared of urea each minute. As such, plasma clearance is a reflection of the ability of the kidneys to remove substances from extracellular fluid.

Free Water Clearance

Free water clearance is the total volume of plasma that is cleared of excess water each minute. This value reflects how rapidly the kidneys are changing the balance between water and osmotic substances in tissue fluids. Early renal ischemia may be detected by measuring free water clearance (Baek *et al,* 1973).

GLOMERULAR FILTRATE

Fluid that filters across glomerular capillaries into Bowman's capsule is designated glomerular filtrate (Renkin and Robinson, 1974). The permeability of the membrane of the glomerular capillary is 100 to 1000 times as great as that of the usual tissue capillary. This increased capillary permeability is due to the presence of numerous pores in the endothelial cells of the glomerular capillary membrane. In addition, fluid must pass through slit-pores of the epithelial cells and the meshwork of the basement membrane of the glomerular capillary membrane. The size of these various openings is sufficient to allow rapid filtration of fluid and small molecular weight substances (less than 30,000 molecular weight) but prevent loss of plasma proteins, which have high molecular weights (albumin is the smallest plasma protein, with a molecular weight of 69,000). Furthermore, plasma proteins are somewhat larger than the 7-micron size of the slit-pores. Therefore, the glomerular capillary membrane is almost impermeable to plasma proteins but is highly permeable to all other smaller dissolved substances in plasma.

Glomerular filtrate has almost the same electrolyte composition as the fluid that filters from the arterial ends of other tissue capillaries into the interstitial fluid. For all practical purposes, glomerular filtrate is the same as plasma except that it lacks proteins.

Glomerular Filtration Rate

Glomerular filtration rate is the amount of glomerular filtrate formed each minute by all the nephrons. In normal persons, glomerular filtration rate averages 125 ml min^{-1} (Brenner *et al,* 1976). Filtration fraction is that fraction of the renal blood flow that becomes glomerular filtrate. The normal filtration fraction is about 20%.

Mechanism of Glomerular Filtration

Glomerular filtration occurs by the same mechanisms by which fluid filters out of any tissue capillary (Wright, 1974). Specifically, pressure inside glomerular capillaries causes filtration of fluid through the capillary membrane into Bowman's capsule. The filtration pressure in glomerular capillaries is estimated to be about 60 mmHg. Colloid osmotic pressure of the blood in the glomerular capillaries and pressure in Bowman's capsule (estimated to be 18 mmHg) oppose this filtration pressure. Colloid osmotic pressure increases from about 28 to 36 mmHg (average 32 mmHg) as blood passes through glomerular capillaries, reflecting a progressive increase in the concentration of protein owing to loss of plasma into Bowman's capsule. The net filtration pressure is the difference between these two sets of opposing pressures. Normal filtration pressure is about 10 mmHg (*i.e.,* 60 mmHg minus pressure in Bowman's capsule and colloid osmotic pressure). The normal glomerular filtration rate is 12.5 ml min^{-1} mmHg^{-1} of filtration pressure, resulting in a glomerular filtration rate of 125 ml min^{-1} when the net filtration pressure is 10 mmHg.

Factors that Influence Glomerular Filtration Rate

Arterial blood pressure, cardiac output, and sympathetic nervous system activity play important roles in determining glomerular filtration rate (Wright and Briggs, 1979). It should be understood that changes in these factors as produced by anesthetic drugs can exert profound effects on glomerular filtration rate and urine formation.

Arterial Blood Pressure

The impact of arterial blood pressure changes on glomerular filtration rate is blunted by autoregulation. Tubuloglomerular feedback, which probably occurs primarily at the juxtaglomerular apparatus, is responsible for autoregulation of glomerular filtration rate. Specifically, signals from the macula densa cells in the distal renal tubule cause efferent or afferent renal arterioles to vasodilate or vasoconstrict and thus adjust the capillary pressure in the glomerulus so as to maintain an almost constant glomerular filtration rate, regardless of changes in the mean arterial pressure between about 70 and 160 mmHg (see Fig. 53-3) (Guyton, 1986b). For example, when blood pressure rises, afferent arteriolar constriction occurs automatically. This intrinsic response prevents a

significant rise in glomerular capillary pressure despite the rise in blood pressure. Nevertheless, even a 5% increase in glomerular filtration rate can result in a large increase in urine output. For this reason, an increase in blood pressure can greatly increase urine output, even though it affects glomerular filtration rate only slightly. Likewise, even small reductions in blood pressure can produce dramatic reductions in urine output despite minimal changes in glomerular filtration rate.

JUXTAGLOMERULAR APPARATUS. The juxtaglomerular apparatus is the site where the distal renal tubule passes in the angle between renal afferent and efferent arterioles. Those epithelial cells of the distal renal tubule that actually contact arterioles are more dense than the other distal renal tubular epithelial cells and are collectively designated the *macula densa.* Smooth muscle cells (*i.e.,* juxtaglomerular cells) of afferent and efferent arterioles that contact these macula densa cells contain granules that are composed mainly of inactive renin. Renin is released into the circulation during hypotension, renal ischemia, or sympathetic nervous system stimulation in an effort by the kidney to maintain a normal renal blood flow.

The anatomic structure of the juxtaglomerular apparatus suggests that glomerular filtrate in distal renal tubules in some way provides feedback signals to both afferent and efferent renal arterioles so as to maintain an optimal and unchanging glomerular filtration rate. For example, a low glomerular filtration rate results in excessive reabsorption of chloride ions and a decline of the chloride ion concentration in macula densa cells. As a result, these cells release renin, and the subsequent formation of angiotensin II causes greater vasoconstrictor effects on the efferent than on the afferent renal arterioles. Efferent arteriole vasoconstriction raises the glomerular capillary pressure so as to increase the glomerular filtration rate back toward normal.

Cardiac Output

The rate of renal blood flow greatly influences glomerular filtration rate. Renal blood flow parallels cardiac output, emphasizing the important impact of changes in cardiac output on glomerular filtration rate. For example, the greater the renal blood flow and thus the flow of plasma into the glomerulus, the greater the glomerular filtration rate.

Sympathetic Nervous System Activity

Sympathetic nervous system stimulation of the kidneys results in preferential constriction of afferent renal arterioles, decreased pressure in glomerular capillaries, and a reduction in glomerular filtration rate. Excessive sympathetic nervous system stimulation can reduce glomerular capillary blood flow such that urine output decreases to almost zero. Decreased sympathetic nervous system stimulation allows a modest degree of dilatation of renal afferent arterioles, and urine output increases.

Small doses of catecholamines have more vasoconstrictor effects on the efferent than on the afferent arterioles, thus maintaining the glomerular filtration rate. Large doses, however, decrease both renal blood flow and glomerular filtration rate.

RENAL TUBULAR FUNCTION

Glomerular filtrate flows through renal tubules and collecting ducts into the pelvis of the kidney. As the glomerular filtrate passes through renal tubules, substances are selectively reabsorbed from tubules into peritubular capillaries or secreted into tubules by tubular epithelial cells. The resulting glomerular filtrate entering the pelvis is urine.

About 80% of the sodium, chloride, and water filtered through the glomeruli is reabsorbed from proximal renal tubules into peritubular capillaries. The transfer of sodium ions from inside renal tubular epithelial cells through cell membranes and into peritubular capillaries is against a concentration gradient. The only way to move sodium ions against this gradient is through a pump mechanism (sodium pump), which requires energy (Glynn and Karlish, 1976). Reabsorption of sodium ions accounts for the greatest energy expenditure of the kidney. The transfer of chloride ions and water is passive. These ions follow sodium ions in an effort to maintain electroneutrality and isotonicity of the ultrafiltrate. As a result, the glomerular filtrate fluid leaving proximal renal tubules is still isotonic with plasma. Reabsorption is more important than secretion in the overall formation of urine. Secretion, however, is particularly important in determining the amounts of potassium ions and hydrogen ions that appear in the urine (Giebisch and Stanton, 1979).

Greater than 99% of the water in the glomerular filtrate is normally reabsorbed into peritubular capillaries as it passes through renal tubules. Therefore, for any dissolved constituent of the glomerular filtrate that is not reabsorbed, the reabsorption of water will concentrate this substance more than 99 times. Conversely, substances such as glucose and amino acids are almost completely reabsorbed, so their concentrations decrease almost to zero before the glomerular filtrate becomes urine (Ullrich, 1979).

Active Transport of Ions from the Renal Tubules

Active transport is responsible for the movement of sodium ions from the lumens of proximal renal tubules into the epithelial cells lining renal tubules and then into peritubular capillaries. The continual active transport of sodium ions out of renal tubular epithelial cells causes an electrical potential inside these cells of about -70 mv as well as a concentration gradient for sodium ions between lumens of the renal tubules and the interior of the cells. This negative intracellular voltage as well as the low concentration of sodium ions inside the renal tubular epithelial cells sustains the electrochemical gradient, which is important in maintaining diffusion of sodium ions from the lumens of the renal tubules into lining epithelial cells.

Substances other than sodium ions that are actively absorbed through the renal tubular epithelial cells include glucose, amino acids, calcium ions, potassium ions, chloride ions, and phosphate ions. Glucose and amino acids are transported from the lumens of renal tubules into the lining epithelial cells by sodium cotransport (see Chapter 39). Specifically, glucose or amino acids and sodium combine with a common carrier, which enters the epithelial cell. Inside the epithelial cell, glucose or amino acids split from the carrier and then diffuse through the cell membrane to enter peritubular capillaries.

Active Secretion of Ions into the Renal Tubules

Hydrogen ions and potassium ions are examples of substances that are actively secreted into all or some portions of renal tubules. Active secretion occurs in the same way as active absorption except that renal tubular epithelial cells transport the secreted substance into lumens of the renal tubules rather than into peritubular capillaries.

Passive Reabsorption of Water

Transport of solutes through the renal tubular epithelial cells creates a concentration difference that causes osmosis of water in the same direction that the solutes have been transported. Nevertheless, lining epithelial cells in some portions of the renal tubule system are more permeable to water than others, regardless of the concentration gradient for osmosis. For example, osmosis of water through proximal renal tubules is so rapid that the osmolar concentration of solutes on the peritubular capillary side of cell membranes is almost never more than a few milliosmoles greater than in the lumen of the tubules. Conversely, distal renal tubules are almost completely impermeable to water, which is important in the mechanism for controlling the specific gravity of urine.

Passive Reabsorption of Solutes

Passive reabsorption of water concentrates solutes such as urea in renal tubules. The resulting concentration gradient leads to the passive diffusion of urea or other diffusible solutes from lumens of renal tubules into peritubular capillaries. The rate of passive reabsorption of a solute is determined by (1) the amount of water that is reabsorbed, because this determines the concentration gradient, and (2) permeability of renal tubule cell membranes for the solute. Permeability of cell membranes for urea in most parts of the renal tubule is less than that for water, such that far less urea is reabsorbed than water. As a result, about 50% of the urea that enters the glomerular filtrate is lost in the urine. Permeability of renal tubule cell membranes for creatinine, insulin, and mannitol is zero, which means that all that enters the glomerular filtrate appears in the urine.

Diffusion Due to Electrical Differences

Active reabsorption of sodium ions from renal tubules produces negativity inside the tubule lumens with respect to the peritubular capillary fluid. This negative electrical potential inside

renal tubules repels negative ions such as chloride ions and phosphate ions, causing them to diffuse into peritubular capillaries from the renal tubules. Conversely, positive ions such as sodium ions and potassium ions will be attracted from peritubular capillaries into renal tubules. In distal renal tubules where the electrical potential is positive, ions with a positive charge move toward peritubular capillaries, and negative ions migrate toward renal tubule lumens.

Differences in Reabsorptive Capabilities

The reabsorptive capabilities of various portions of renal tubules are different (Lameire *et al,* 1977).

Proximal Renal Tubule

Proximal renal tubule lining epithelial cells have large numbers of mitochondria to support the metabolic activity associated with the active transport processes that occur in these cells. Indeed, about two thirds of all reabsorptive and secretory processes that occur in renal tubules take place in proximal renal tubules. As a result, only about one third of the original glomerular filtrate normally passes the entire distance through proximal renal tubules to reach the loops of Henle.

Loop of Henle

Epithelial cells lining the lumens of the loops of Henle contain few mitochondria, indicating a minimal level of metabolic activity. Descending portions of the loops of Henle are highly permeable to water and moderately permeable to urea and sodium ions. Conversely, ascending limbs of the loops of Henle are far less permeable to water and urea than are the descending portions. This is vital for the optimal function of the countercurrent mechanism for concentrating urine (see the section entitled Countercurrent Mechanism).

Distal Renal Tubule

Distal renal tubules begin at the ascending limbs of the loops of Henle where the lining epithelial cells become grossly thickened. This segment ascends all the way back to the same glomerulus from which the renal tubule originated and passes through the angle between the afferent and efferent arterioles forming the juxtaglomerular apparatus (see the section entitled Juxtaglomerular Apparatus). Beyond the juxtaglomerular apparatus, distal renal tubules become convoluted and at the end of the convolutions become collecting ducts.

Distal renal tubules are divided into two functional segments, the diluting segment and the late distal tubule.

DILUTING SEGMENT. The function of the diluting segment of the distal renal tubule is to dilute the glomerular filtrate in the renal tubule. Lining epithelial cells of this portion of the distal renal tubule are uniquely adapted for active transport of chloride ions from the tubule into peritubular capillaries. Transport of negatively charged chloride ions out of the renal tubule creates a positive electrical potential in the tubule lumen. This positive electrical potential facilitates the diffusion of sodium ions from the lumen of the tubule into peritubular capillaries. This segment of the distal tubule is almost impermeable to water such that those substances that remain in the tubule fluid are very dilute (*i.e.*, diluting segment).

LATE DISTAL TUBULE. The late distal tubule portion of the distal renal tubule has lining epithelial cells that are adapted for active transport of positively charged ions such as sodium. The late distal tubule is essentially impermeable to urea.

Collecting Ducts

Distal ends of several distal renal tubules join together to form collecting ducts. Epithelial cells that line collecting ducts have the ability to pump ions, including sodium, potassium, hydrogen, and calcium ions against large electrochemical gradients. In the collecting ducts, urine becomes either highly concentrated or dilute and highly acidic or basic. The permeability of the epithelial cells lining the collecting ducts is determined primarily by the circulating concentration of antidiuretic hormone (ADH). When ADH is present in large amounts, collecting duct epithelial cells become highly permeable to water. As a result, most of the water is reabsorbed from the collecting ducts and returned to peritubular capillaries, resulting in the excretion of minimal amounts of highly concentrated urine. In the absence of large amounts of ADH, little water is reabsorbed and large volumes of dilute urine are excreted.

Reabsorption and Secretion of Specific Substances

Water

Water transport out of renal tubules occurs mainly by osmotic diffusion as a result of reabsorption or diffusion of substances into peritubular capillaries. Of the 125 ml min^{-1} of water that becomes glomerular filtrate, only 45 ml reaches the loops of Henle and 1 ml becomes urine. This emphasizes that two thirds of the glomerular filtrate water is reabsorbed in proximal renal tubules.

Glucose, Proteins, Amino Acids, and Vitamins

Glucose, proteins, amino acids, and vitamins are examples of substances that are reabsorbed by active processes in proximal renal tubules (Ullrich, 1979). As much as 30 g of protein filter into the glomerular filtrate daily. This filtered protein is reabsorbed by the process known as *pinocytosis*. Pinocytosis is when the membrane of the epithelial cell lining the proximal renal tubule invaginates to incorporate the protein into the interior of the cell (Mainsbach, 1976). Once inside the lining epithelial cell, the protein is digested into its constituent amino acids, which are then absorbed into peritubular capillaries.

Metabolic End Products

Urea and creatinine are examples of metabolic end products that undergo modest (urea) or no (creatinine) reabsorption during their passage through the renal tubules. In fact, small quantities of creatinine are actually secreted into the tubular fluid by epithelial cells lining the proximal renal tubules such that the total quantity of creatinine increases about 20% above the amount originally entering the glomerular filtrate.

Inulin and Para-Aminohippuric Acid

Inulin is a large polysaccharide that is not reabsorbed or secreted in any segment of the renal tubules. These characteristics combined with the fact that the small molecular weight of inulin (5200) allows it to pass through the glomerular capillary membrane as freely as water is the reason that the plasma clearance of inulin can be used to calculate the glomerular filtration rate. For example, if the plasma concentration of inulin is

100 mg dl^{-1}, and 125 mg min^{-1} of inulin enters the urine, it is calculated that 125 ml of glomerular filtrate must be formed each minute in order to deliver that amount of inulin to the urine.

Mannitol is another substance that is totally diffusible through glomerular capillary membranes and is neither reabsorbed nor secreted. As a result, the plasma clearance of mannitol is also equal to the glomerular filtration rate.

Para-aminohippuric acid (PAH), like inulin, is freely diffusible through glomerular capillary membranes. In addition, PAH is secreted into the tubular fluid by epithelial cells lining the proximal renal tubule. PAH is not reabsorbed in any segment of the renal tubule.

Various Ions

In most segments of renal tubules, positively charged ions are transported through the lining epithelial cells by active transport mechanisms. Negatively charged ions are usually transported passively as a result of electrical potential differences developed across the membranes while the positively charged ions are actively transported. For example, when sodium ions are actively transported out of the proximal tubular fluid, the resulting electronegativity that develops in the remaining tubular fluid causes chloride ions to follow.

Potassium ions and hydrogen ions are secreted into the proximal renal tubules, distal renal tubules, and collecting ducts.

Bicarbonate ions are probably reabsorbed in the form of carbon dioxide rather than as bicarbonate ions. Bicarbonate ions in the renal tubular fluid first combine with hydrogen ions that are secreted into the fluid by the lining epithelial cells. This combination forms carbonic acid, which then dissociates into water and carbon dioxide (see Fig. 51-1). Carbon dioxide, being highly lipid soluble, diffuses rapidly through renal tubule lining epithelial cells into peritubular capillaries. When more bicarbonate ions than hydrogen ions are present in renal tubules, the excess bicarbonate ions enter the urine because the tubules are only slightly permeable to this ion.

Concentrations of Different Substances at Various Sites in the Renal Tubules

Reabsorption of a substance relative to the reabsorption of water determines how concentrated the substance becomes as it travels through renal tubules. For example, greater reabsorption of a substance relative to water results in its dilution in renal tubules. Conversely, limited reabsorption of a substance relative to water results in that material becoming concentrated in renal tubules.

Nutritionally important materials such as glucose and amino acids are reabsorbed so much more rapidly than water in proximal renal tubules that their concentrations in the glomerular filtrate decline to almost zero. Metabolic end products become progressively more concentrated as they travel through renal tubules. Sodium and chloride ions are normally reabsorbed from renal tubules to the same extent as water.

The presence or absence of circulating ADH greatly influences the concentration or dilution of substances that occurs in collecting tubules. For example, in the absence of ADH, reabsorption of water by collecting ducts is greatly reduced, and the subsequent presence of extra water in the urine greatly dilutes all substances. Conversely, release of ADH, as in response to painful surgical stimulation, can result in greater concentration of substances in the collecting ducts.

Countercurrent Mechanism

The countercurrent mechanism is responsible for the kidneys being able to eliminate solutes with minimal excretion of water (Stephenson, 1978). The special anatomic arrangement of peritubular capillaries known as vasa recta to those loops of Henle that extend into the renal medulla make the countercurrent mechanism possible. Countercurrent refers to an anatomic arrangement in which blood inflow is parallel and in the opposite direction to outflow.

The first step in the excretion of excess solutes in the urine is the formation of a high osmolarity renal medullary interstitial fluid. Indeed, this osmolarity increases from about 300 mOsm L^{-1} in the renal cortex to nearly 1200 mOsm L^{-1} in the pelvic tip of the renal medulla. At least four different factors contribute to the accumulation of solutes and the subsequent marked increase in the osmolarity of the renal medullary interstitial fluid. The primary cause is the active transport of chloride ions plus the associated passive transfer of sodium ions out of the ascending limbs of the loops of Henle into medullary peritubular capillaries. In collecting ducts, there is active transport of sodium ions and passive absorption of chloride ions along with the sodium ions. Furthermore, there is passive diffusion of large amounts of urea from collecting ducts into the renal medulla in the presence of large amounts of circulating ADH. Finally there is further transport of sodium ions and chloride ions into medullary peritubular capillaries from the thin segments of the loops of Henle.

In the absence of special characteristics of the renal medullary vascular system, excess solutes in the medullary interstitial fluid would be rapidly removed in peritubular capillaries. To prevent this, renal medullary blood flow is minimal, amounting to only 1% to 2% of the total renal blood flow. This sluggish medullary blood flow minimizes removal of solutes from the interstitial fluid of the renal medulla. Furthermore, the U-shaped arrangement of the vasa recta allows the solutes to function as a countercurrent exchanger, which prevents washout of solutes from the interstitial fluid of the renal medulla by flow through peritubular capillaries.

In the presence of the hyperosmolarity characteristic of the medullary interstitial fluid, water freely leaves collecting ducts by osmosis when lining epithelial cells of this portion of the renal tubules are rendered permeable to water by the presence of high circulating concentrations of ADH. As a result, it is possible to excrete a concentrated urine that results in loss of excess solutes from the body fluids while at the same time conserving as much water as possible.

TUBULAR TRANSPORT MAXIMUM

Tubular transport maximum (Tm) is the maximal amount of a substance that can be actively reabsorbed from the lumens of renal tubules each minute. The Tm is dependent on the amounts of carrier substance and enzyme available to the specific active transport system in the lining epithelial cells of renal tubules.

The Tm for glucose is about 320 mg min^{-1}. When the amount of glucose that filters through the glomerular capillary membrane exceeds this amount (i.e., hyperglycemia), the excess glucose cannot be reabsorbed but instead passes into the urine. The usual amount of glucose in the glomerular filtrate entering proximal renal tubules is 125 mg min^{-1}, and there is no detectable loss into the urine. When the tubular load, however, ex-

ceeds about 220 mg min^{-1} (i.e., threshold concentration), glucose first begins to appear in the urine. A blood–glucose concentration of 180 mg dl^{-1} in the presence of a normal glomerular filtration results in delivery of 220 mg min^{-1} of glucose into the renal tubular fluid. Maximal loss of glucose occurs at concentrations above the Tm for glucose.

REGULATION OF THE CHARACTERISTICS OF BODY FLUIDS

The kidneys are the most important organs for regulating the characteristics of body fluids (Anderson, 1977). This regulation is apparent in the control of (1) blood volume, (2) extracellular fluid volume, (3) osmolarity of body fluids, and (4) concentrations of various ions, including hydrogen ion concentrations and resulting pH of body fluids. Often, the thirst mechanism also plays a vital role in controlling some of the characteristics of body fluids.

Control of Blood Volume

Blood volume is maintained almost constant despite marked daily variations in fluid and solute intake or loss. The basic mechanism for the control of blood volume is the same feedback loop that also influences extracellular fluid volume, cardiac output, blood pressure, and urine output. Specifically, an increase in blood volume increases cardiac output, which elevates blood pressure. Increased blood pressure subsequently leads to renal changes that cause an increased urine output and a return of blood volume to normal. The reverse sequence of events occurs when the blood volume is decreased. Blood pressure is likely to be the most important factor in determining the long-term level of fluid volume excretion. The effect of elevated blood pressure on urine output seems to be sustained indefinitely. Elevated blood pressure increases pressure in the glomerular capillaries, which causes an increase in glomerular filtration rate, which leads to diuresis. An increase in blood pressure also increases pressure in peritubular capillaries, which decreases reabsorption of solutes and water from the renal tubules, also leading to an increased urine output. A reduction in blood pressure produces opposite effects on glomerular filtration rate and reabsorption, leading to a reduction in fluid volume excretion by way of the urine.

The effects of changes in blood volume on cardiac output, blood pressure, and urine output are slow to develop, requiring several hours to produce a full effect. This process, however, can be greatly accelerated by (1) volume receptor reflexes, (2) ADH, (3) aldosterone, and (4) inherent vascular capacity of the circulation (Gauer and Henry, 1976).

Volume Receptor Reflexes

Volume receptors are stretch receptors located in the walls of the right and left atrium (Goetz *et al,* 1975). Increased blood volume causes increased pressure in the atria, and the resultant stretch of the volume receptors initiates reflex responses that accelerate the return of blood volume toward normal. Specific reflex responses initiated by increased stretch of the volume receptors include inhibition of (1) sympathetic nervous system activity to the kidneys and peripheral arterioles and (2) decreased release of ADH. These responses facilitate increased renal excretion of fluid. Changes in arterial blood pressure produced by alterations in blood volume also activate baroreceptors in the carotid arteries and aorta. Resulting responses evoked by baroreceptors complement the reflex responses initiated by activation of the volume stretch receptors in the atria.

In most instances, these volume receptors can cause the blood volume to return almost to normal within 1 hour, but the final precise adjustment in blood volume is still dependent on the sequence of events that involve cardiac output changes. The reason for this is adaptation of volume receptors that occurs over 1 to 3 days such that they no longer transmit corrective signals.

Antidiuretic Hormone

ADH exerts a minimal impact on control of blood volume. For example, absence of ADH in diabetes insipidus results in minimal alterations in blood volume since the thirst mechanism compensates for increased fluid losses. Blood volume, however, will decrease dramatically if fluid intake is not maintained to match losses. Failure of the blood volume to increase more than 5% in the presence of a tremendous excess of ADH (*i.e.,* syndrome of inappropriate ADH secretion) reflects the ability of increased blood pressure to

offset the fluid-retaining effects of this hormone (Zerbe *et al,* 1980).

Increased circulating concentrations of ADH cause an abrupt reduction in excretion of fluid volume by way of the urine. This is due to the ability of ADH to increase reabsorption of water from the lumens of collecting ducts and, to a lesser extent, from the late distal renal tubules. As a result, a small volume of highly concentrated urine is excreted. When large amounts of ADH persist in the circulation for prolonged periods of time, the acute effect to reduce urine output is not sustained. This reflects the ability of blood pressure, tubular osmolar balance, and plasma colloid osmotic pressure to eventually offset the effects of ADH.

ADH works by activating adenylate cyclase in the lining epithelial cells of the collecting tubules (see Chapter 52). The subsequent formation of cyclic AMP increases permeability of lining epithelial cell membranes to water, leading to an increase in water reabsorption from the lumens of the collecting ducts.

Aldosterone

Aldosterone causes reabsorption of sodium ions from the late distal renal tubules, which in turn leads to the osmotic reabsorption of water (see Chapter 52). As a result, urine output decreases and extracellular fluid volume and blood volume increase. Aldosterone is also necessary for secretion of potassium ions into distal renal tubules.

Inherent Vascular Capacity of the Circulation

Blood volume is automatically regulated in response to changes in the inherent vascular capacity of the circulation. For example, persistent stimulation of the sympathetic nervous system and associated vasoconstriction as may occur in the presence of a pheochromocytoma lead to a reduction in blood volume. Conversely, blood volume may be increased by chronic drug-induced vasodilatation or the effects of severe varicose veins.

Control of Extracellular Fluid Volume

Control of extracellular fluid volume by the kidneys occurs by the same mechanisms and at the same time as control of blood volume. It is not possible, for example, to alter blood volume without also simultaneously changing extracellular fluid volume (Guyton, 1986c). Indeed, extracellular fluid becomes a reservoir for excess fluid that may be administered intravenously during the perioperative period.

Control of Osmolarity of Body Fluids

Osmolarity of body fluids is determined almost entirely by the concentration of sodium ions in the extracellular fluid. Control of sodium ion concentration and, thus, osmolarity of body fluids is under the influence of the osmoreceptor–ADH mechanism and the thirst reflex. The aldosterone feedback system plays a minor role in controlling the extracellular fluid concentration of sodium ions. Sodium intake is regulated by a conscious desire for salt in the presence of depletion of this ion.

The kidneys excrete excessive amounts of water as urine when osmolarity of body fluids is too low. Conversely, the kidneys excrete increased amounts of solutes when osmolarity of body fluids is too high. A shift of the kidneys from excreting excess water to excreting excess solutes is controlled by ADH (Andreoli and Schaefer, 1976). In the absence of ADH, the kidneys excrete a dilute urine containing excessive amounts of water. When the circulating concentration of ADH is elevated, the kidneys excrete a concentrated urine containing excessive amounts of solutes.

Osmoreceptor–ADH

The osmoreceptor–ADH control system for regulation of sodium ion concentration in the extracellular fluid is a typical negative feedback control circuit. An increase in osmolarity of the extracellular fluid owing to excess sodium ions activates specialized neuronal cells called *osmoreceptors* in the supraoptic nuclei of the hypothalamus. Increased osmolarity of the extracellular fluid pulls fluid out of the osmoreceptors, causing them to shrink and thereby increase their rate of discharge of impulses through the pituitary stalk to the posterior pituitary gland where they promote the release of ADH (Cross and Wakerley, 1977). ADH increases the permeability of renal collecting ducts for water. The resulting retention of water dilutes the concentration of sodium ions in body fluids and returns osmolarity downward toward

normal. Conversely, when extracellular fluid becomes too dilute, the osmoreceptors swell, and the discharge of impulses is decreased. As a result, less ADH is formed, and more water than solutes is excreted by the kidneys, thus concentrating sodium ions and returning osmolarity upward toward a normal value. In essence, the release of ADH is directly proportional to changes in the osmolarity (*i.e.,* sodium ion concentration) of the extracellular fluid. Changes in osmolarity of only 1% to 5% evoke substantial increases in the circulating concentration of ADH. Conversely, decreases in blood volume have minimal effects on release of ADH, with a 10% loss in blood volume required before a significant release of ADH occurs.

Osmoreceptors respond to changes in the extracellular fluid concentration of sodium ions but not to changes in the concentration of potassium ions. Likewise, these receptors respond minimally to changes in the fluid concentrations of urea and glucose. Therefore, for practical purposes, the osmoreceptors may be considered as sodium ion concentration receptors.

Thirst Reflex

Thirst is as important for regulating body water and sodium ion concentration as is the osmoreceptor–ADH mechanism. Indeed, this reflex is the primary regulator for the intake of water (Fitzsimons, 1972).

Neurons in the thirst center located in the lateral preoptic area of the hypothalamus regulate the conscious desire for water. The most common cause for thirst is an increased sodium ion concentration in the extracellular fluid, which causes osmosis of fluid from the neuronal cells of the thirst center. Another important cause for shrinkage of thirst center neuronal cells is excessive loss of potassium ions from the body. Any change in the circulation that leads to increased production of angiotensin II, such as acute hemorrhage or cardiac failure, also leads to thirst. It is likely that the major site of action of angiotensin II is not directly on the thirst center but, instead, on a specialized area on the surface of the third cerebral ventricle, stimulation of which transmits signals to the thirst center to increase water intake. Although the sensation of a dry mouth is often associated with the thirst reflex, the blockade of salivary secretion, as by anticholinergic drugs, does not cause animals or humans to drink excessively.

Relief from thirst occurs almost immediately after drinking water, even before water has been absorbed from the gastrointestinal tract. This temporary but rapid relief of thirst is necessary to prevent people from ingesting more water than necessary to return plasma osmolarity to normal. A delayed relief of thirst would result in the ingestion of excess water, which would adversely dilute the plasma concentration of sodium ions.

The thirst mechanism is activated when the plasma concentration of sodium increases about 2 mEq L^{-1} above normal or when the plasma osmolarity rises about 4 mOsm L^{-1}. People typically drink the correct amount of water, allowing precise maintenance of the osmolarity of the extracellular fluid.

Aldosterone

Compared with the osmoreceptor–ADH hormone mechanism and the thirst reflex, the effect of aldosterone on plasma osmolarity is insignificant (Knox and Diaz-Buxo, 1977). Indeed, in the complete absence of aldosterone, the serum sodium concentration varies less than 2% over a sixfold range of sodium intake (Fig. 53-5) (Guyton, 1986c; Young *et al*, 1976). The minimal effect of aldosterone seems paradoxical, considering the

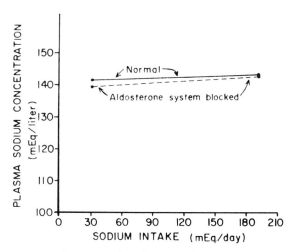

FIGURE 53-5. In the absence of aldosterone, the serum sodium concentration varies less than 2% over a sixfold range of sodium intake. (From Guyton AC. Textbook of Medical Physiology. 7th ed. Philadelphia: WB Saunders, 1986:425. Reproduced by permission of the author and publisher.)

ability of this hormone to greatly increase the reabsorption of sodium ions from renal tubules. Nevertheless, this sodium ion reabsorption is accompanied by a simultaneous reabsorption of water and increase in extracellular fluid volume. An increase of only a few percent in the volume of extracellular fluid leads to an increase in blood pressure and glomerular filtration rate that offsets the effect of aldosterone on extracellular fluid concentration of sodium ions.

Patients with primary aldosteronism manifest only 2 to 3 mEq L^{-1} increases in the serum sodium concentration. This minimal response to even large excesses of aldosterone again emphasizes the more prominent role of ADH and thirst in controlling the serum sodium concentration.

Control of Extracellular Concentrations of Ions

Potassium Ions

Aldosterone is extremely important in the control of the excellular fluid concentration of potassium ions. In the presence of aldosterone, there is increased secretion of potassium ions into renal tubules, leading to increased loss of this ion in the urine. When aldosterone activity is blocked, as may be produced by certain diuretics, the serum potassium concentration parallels intake of potassium, making hypokalemia or hyperkalemia possible (Fig. 53-6) (Guyton, 1986c; Young *et al*, 1976). The absence of aldosterone associated with Addison's disease may result in dangerous hyperkalemia. Excessive amounts of aldosterone in patients with primary aldosteronism produces profound hypokalemia with associated skeletal muscle weakness owing to failure of nerve transmission because of hyperpolarization of the nerve membrane.

ADH and thirst reflex can override aldosterone control of the extracellular fluid concentration of sodium ions but not potassium ions. Indeed, the rate of aldosterone secretion is controlled closely by the extracellular fluid concentration of potassium ions (Fig. 53-7) (Guyton, 1986c; McCaa *et al*, 1972). This is characteristic of a properly functioning negative feedback system in which the factor that is controlled (*i.e.*, potassium ion concentration) has a feedback effect to control the controller (*i.e.*, aldosterone).

In addition to aldosterone, the concentration

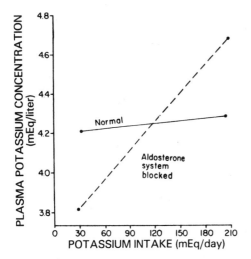

FIGURE 53-6. Plasma potassium concentration parallels intake when aldosterone activity is impaired. (From Guyton AC. Textbook of Medical Physiology. 7th ed. Philadelphia: WB Saunders, 1986:425. Reproduced by permission of the author and publisher.)

of hydrogen ions and sodium intake may exert modest effects on the extracellular fluid concentration of potassium ions. For example, hydrogen ions compete with potassium ions for secretion into renal tubules. The level of sodium intake may influence extracellular fluid concentrations of potassium ions, because sodium is reciprocally transported through the late distal renal tubule and collecting duct lining epithelial cells in exchange for potassium ions.

Potassium ions are unique among the normal constituents of blood in that this ion is both reabsorbed and secreted by renal tubules. Most of the filtered potassium ions are reabsorbed in the proximal renal tubule. Potassium ions are transported through the lining epithelial cells of proximal renal tubules and the diluting segment of distal tubules in almost parallel fashion to sodium ions (Giebisch and Stanton, 1979). As for the sodium ions, less than 10% of the potassium ions that originally enter the glomerular filtrate reach the late distal renal tubules.

Considerable amounts of potassium ions are secreted into the late distal renal tubules and collecting ducts. It is likely that the negative electrical potential created in the lining epithelial cells as a result of outward transport of sodium ions attracts the positively charged potassium ions into the cells. Once potassium ions have entered the epithelial cells, they diffuse passively from these cells into the lumens of renal tubules.

The secretory transport of potassium ions into distal renal tubules is vital to eliminating excess potassium ions from the body and maintaining a normal plasma concentration of potassium. Aldosterone is necessary for the secretion of potassium ions into distal renal tubules. In the absence of aldosterone, secretion of potassium ions ceases and reabsorption of potassium ions from distal renal tubules predominates.

Potassium ions are secreted in exchange for sodium ions. Sodium ions can also be exchanged for hydrogen ions. For example, when the concentration of hydrogen ions is excessive, these ions are excreted in preference to potassium ions. Conversely, alkalosis facilitates secretion of potassium ions. The amount of potassium ions secreted depends on the intracellular content of this ion, particularly in renal tubule epithelial cells. The extracellular concentration of potassium ions has minimal effect on potassium ion excretion, because this ion is principally intracellular.

Sodium Ions

Active transport of sodium ions through the lining epithelial cells of the proximal renal tubules

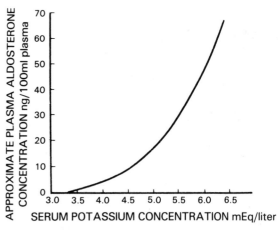

FIGURE 53-7. Small changes in the plasma concentration of potassium evoke large changes in the plasma concentration of aldosterone. (From Guyton AC. Textbook of Medical Physiology. 7th ed. Philadelphia: WB Sanders, 1986:425. Reproduced by permission of the author and publisher.)

causes diffusion of negative chloride ions through the cell membranes as well (Glynn and Karlish, 1976). Furthermore, the reabsorption of sodium ions and chloride ions creates an osmotic gradient that causes water to move across proximal renal tubule membranes. The lining epithelial cells of proximal renal tubules are so permeable to water that almost identical proportions of water and ions are reabsorbed from the lumens of renal tubules. Overall, about two thirds of the sodium ions are reabsorbed from proximal renal tubules.

In the diluting segment of distal renal tubules, the active transport of chloride ions causes sodium ions and other positively charged ions to be reabsorbed along with the chloride ions. As a result of these efficient reabsorption mechanisms, less than 10% of sodium ions that initially enter the glomerular filtrate reach the late distal renal tubules and collecting ducts.

Aldosterone also influences reabsorption of sodium ions from the late distal renal tubules and collecting ducts. In the presence of large amounts of aldosterone, almost all the remaining sodium ions are reabsorbed, and urinary excretion of sodium ions approaches zero. Conversely, in the absence of aldosterone, the remaining sodium ions are not reabsorbed from the late distal renal tubules and collecting ducts, and urinary excretion of sodium ions is increased. Aldosterone acts by entering the lining epithelial cells of the renal tubules where it combines with a receptor protein. The receptor protein activates DNA molecules to form messenger RNA, which subsequently causes the formation of carrier proteins or protein enzymes, which are necessary for the sodium and potassium ion transport process. The formation of these substances requires about 45 minutes following the release of aldosterone.

Hydrogen Ions

The kidneys excrete excess hydrogen ions by (1) exchanging a hydrogen ion for a sodium ion, thus acidifying the urine, and (2) by the synthesis and excretion of ammonia (see Chapter 51).

Calcium Ions

Calcium ion concentration is controlled principally by the effect of parathyroid hormone on bone reabsorption (Dennis *et al,* 1979) (see Chapter 52). For example, a decrease in the extra-cellular fluid concentration of calcium ions causes the release of parathyroid hormone, which acts on bone to cause reabsorption of calcium ions from bone. When the calcium ion concentration is too high, the secretion of parathyroid hormone is reduced to the point at which almost no bone reabsorption occurs. The osteoblastic system, however, continues to form new bone such that calcium ions are removed from the extracellular fluid and the extracellular concentration of calcium ions declines toward normal. In addition to effects on bone, parathyroid hormone increases reabsorption of calcium ions from the late distal renal tubules, collecting ducts, and gastrointestinal tract.

Magnesium Ions

Magnesium ions are reabsorbed by all portions of the renal tubules. Urinary excretion of magnesium ions parallels the extracellular fluid concentration of this ion.

Phosphate Ions

Phosphate ion concentration in the extracellular fluid is regulated primarily by a renal overflow mechanism that occurs when the normal Tm is exceeded (Dennis *et al,* 1979) (see the section entitled Tubular Transport Maximum). When the phosphate ion concentration in the glomerular filtrate exceeds this Tm, excess ions are excreted in the urine. When the glomerular filtrate is below the Tm, all phosphate ions are reabsorbed from the renal tubules. As a result, the extracellular fluid concentration of phosphate ions is regulated over a narrow range, despite large daily variations in intake.

Parathyroid hormone decreases the Tm for phosphate ions. This effect combined with the increased concentrations of phosphate ions in the glomerular filtrate because of parathyroid hormone – induced reabsorption of bone leads to increased urinary excretion of phosphate ions and depletion of the extracellular fluid concentration of this ion.

Other important negatively charged ions in the body, including sulfates, nitrates, urates, lactates, and amino acids have a Tm similar to that of phosphate ions. The Tm acts to maintain precise control of the extracellular fluid concentrations of these ions in the same way as for phosphate ions.

Urea

Urea is the most abundant of the metabolic waste products. It must be excreted in the urine to prevent excess accumulation in body fluids. High lipid solubility of urea results in its rapid diffusion through all cell membranes except for the blood–brain barrier.

The normal plasma concentration of urea is about 25 mg dl^{-1}. The major factors that determine the rate of urea excretion are the (1) plasma concentration of urea and (2) glomerular filtration rate. The amount of urea that enters proximal renal tubules is equal to the product of the plasma urea concentration and the glomerular filtration rate. Typically, about 50% of the urea that initially enters the proximal renal tubules appears in the urine.

When the glomerular filtration rate is low, the filtrate remains in the renal tubules for prolonged periods of time before it finally becomes urine. The longer the period of time that the filtrate remains in the renal tubules, the greater is the reabsorption of urea. As a result, the amount of urea that reaches the urine is reduced, and the plasma concentration of urea (*i.e.,* blood urea nitrogen, BUN) is increased. Conversely, when the glomerular filtration rate is high, filtrate passes through renal tubules so rapidly that very little urea is reabsorbed into peritubular capillaries.

ACUTE RENAL FAILURE

Acute renal failure is most often a result of acute glomerulonephritis or acute damage or obstruction of the renal tubules.

Acute Glomerulonephritis

In approximately 95% of patients, the abnormal immune reaction that causes acute glomerulonephritis occurs 1 to 3 weeks following an infection with group A beta streptococci at a site other than the kidney. Antibodies that develop against the streptococcal antigen become entrapped in the basement membrane of the glomerulus. Once the immune complex has deposited in the glomeruli, the cells begin to proliferate and large numbers of leukocytes become entrapped in the glomeruli. Many of the glomeruli become blocked entirely by this inflammatory reaction, and those that are not blocked often become excessively permeable, allowing both protein and erythrocytes to leak into the glomerular filtrate. In severe cases, acute renal failure may occur, but, in most cases, the acute inflammation of the glomeruli subsides in 10 to 14 days and renal function recovers. Sometimes, many of the glomeruli are irreversibly damaged, and, in a few patients, progressive renal deterioration continues.

Acute Tubular Necrosis

Acute tubular necrosis, which is due to the destruction of epithelial cells lining the renal tubules, is most often due to nephrotoxins such as carbon tetrachloride or severe renal ischemia caused by circulatory shock and associated reductions in renal blood flow. A transfusion reaction results in precipitation of excess hemoglobin from hemolysis of erythrocytes in the renal tubules, causing blockage of the nephron.

CHRONIC RENAL FAILURE

Chronic renal failure (uremia or urine in the blood) results when so many nephrons are damaged that the remaining nephrons cannot perform the normal functions of the kidney.

Chronic Glomerulonephritis

Chronic glomerulonephritis begins with the accumulation of precipitated antigen–antibody complex in the glomerular membrane, although this is rarely caused by streptococcal infection. Inflammation of the glomeruli results in progressive thickening of the glomerular membrane, which is eventually invaded by fibrous tissue. In the final stages of chronic glomerulonephritis, many of the glomeruli are replaced by fibrous tissue, and the function of the nephron is lost.

Pyelonephritis

Pyelonephritis is an infectious and inflammatory process that usually begins in the renal pelvis but extends progressively into the renal parenchyma, destroying glomeruli and renal tubules. Infection can result from many different types of bacteria but is often due to colon bacilli that originate from fecal contamination of the urinary tract. Infection usually affects the structures in the medulla of the kidney more than the renal cortex. As a result, the countercurrent mechanism may be impaired. Indeed, patients with pyelonephritis may have almost normal renal function but lack ability to concentrate urine.

Manifestations of Chronic Renal Failure

Chronic renal failure is characterized by inability of the kidneys to handle large loads of electrolytes or substances that must be excreted. Under normal circumstances, one third of the usual numbers of nephrons can eliminate sufficient amounts of waste products to prevent any significant accumulation in the body fluids. Any further reduction, however, leads to retention of waste products and potassium ions. As progressively more nephrons are destroyed, the specific gravity of the urine approaches that of the glomerular filtrate, about 1.008.

Chronic renal failure is almost always associated with severe anemia. Presumably, damaged kidneys are less able to secrete the enzyme that splits erythropoietin from a plasma protein. Erythropoietin normally stimulates bone marrow to produce erythrocytes.

Osteomalacia is a frequent accompaniment of chronic renal failure. This occurs because kidney damage interferes with the conversion of vitamin D to its active form, 1,25-dihydroxycholecalciferol, in the kidneys. This active form of vitamin D is necessary to promote calcium ion absorption from the gastrointestinal tract. In the absence of 1,25-dihydroxycholecalciferol, the availability of calcium ions to bones is greatly reduced and osteomalacia is likely to occur.

Chronic renal failure leading to a decreased glomerular filtration rate and subsequent retention of water and sodium ions is often associated with hypertension. Hypertension is likely to develop in patients in whom one part of the kidney is ischemic, as occurs when one renal artery is severely constricted. The ischemic kidney tissue secretes large quantities of renin, which leads to the formation of angiotensin II, subsequent vasoconstriction, and hypertension.

Generalized edema results from water and sodium retention, and acidosis reflects failure to excrete acidic waste products. Each day, the metabolic processes of the body produce 50 to 100 mM more metabolic acid than metabolic alkali. Normally, buffers of tissue fluids can buffer up to 1000 mM of acid without a decrease in the pH (see Chapter 51). Uremic coma is most likely due to reductions in pH. Rapid and deep breathing during uremic coma is an attempt to compensate for metabolic acidosis.

Hemodialysis

The basic principle of hemodialysis is to pass the patient's blood through channels bounded by a thin membrane such as cellophane. On the other side of the membrane is dialyzing fluid into which unwanted substances in the blood pass by diffusion. Cellophane is porous enough to allow all constituents of the plasma except proteins to diffuse freely in both directions. If the concentration of a substance is greater in the plasma than in the dialyzing fluid, there will be net transfer of the substance from the plasma into the dialyzing fluid. The amount of substance that transfers depends on the concentration difference between the two sides of the membrane, molecular size, and the length of time that the blood and dialyzing fluid remain in contact with the membrane.

During hemodialysis, blood flows continually from an artery, through the artificial kidney, and back into a vein. The total amount of blood in the artificial kidney is usually less than 500 ml. Heparin is added to the blood as it enters the artificial kidney, and protamine is added before the blood is returned to the patient. Danger from excess heparin, hemolysis of blood, and infection limit the use of hemodialysis to no more often than every 3 to 4 days.

NEPHROTIC SYNDROME

Nephrotic syndrome is characterized by the loss of large amounts of plasma proteins (up to 30 g daily) into the urine, reflecting increased permeability of the glomerular capillary membrane. The extreme loss of protein causes a reduction of colloid osmotic pressure that manifests as edema, including ascites and accumulation of fluid in the joints, pleural cavity, and pericardium.

Causes of the nephrotic syndrome include chronic glomerulonephritis, amyloidosis, and lipoid nephrosis. Glucocorticoids will usually cause complete remission of lipoid nephrosis but not the other causes of nephrotic syndrome.

TRANSPORT OF URINE TO THE BLADDER

Urine is transported to the bladder through the ureters, which originate in the pelvis of each kidney. Each ureter is innervated by both sympathetic and parasympathetic nervous systems. As urine collects in the renal pelvis, the pressure in the pelvis increases and initiates a peristaltic contraction that travels downward along the ureter to force urine toward the bladder. Parasympathetic nervous system stimulation increases the frequency of this peristalsis, whereas sympathetic nervous system stimulation decreases it. At its distal end, the ureter penetrates the bladder obliquely such that pressure in the bladder compresses the ureter, thereby preventing backflow of urine when pressure in the bladder increases during micturition.

Ureters are well supplied with nerve fibers such that blockade of a ureter by a stone causes intense reflex constriction and severe pain. In addition, pain impulses are likely to elicit a sympathetic nervous system reflex that causes constriction of the renal arterioles and a concomitant reduction in urine output from that kidney. This ureterorenal reflex is important to prevent excessive flow of urine into the pelvis of a kidney with a blocked ureter.

As the bladder fills with urine, stretch receptors in the bladder wall initiate micturition contractions. Sensory signals are conducted to the sacral segments of the spinal cord through the pelvic nerves and then back again to the bladder through parasympathetic nervous system fibers. The micturition reflex is a completely automatic spinal cord reflex that can be inhibited or facilitated by centers in the brain. These higher centers in the brain can prevent micturition by continual tonic contraction of the external urinary sphincter. Spinal cord damage above the sacral region leaves the micturition reflex intact, but it is no longer controllable by the brain.

REFERENCES

Anderson B. Regulation of body fluids. Annu Rev Physiol 1977;39:185–200.

Andreoli TE, Schaefer JA. Mass transport across cell membranes: The effects of antidiuretic hormone on water and solute flows in epithelia. Annu Rev Physiol 1976;38:451–500.

Baek SM, Brown RS, Shoemaker WC. Early prediction of acute renal failure and recovery: 1. Sequential measurements of free water clearance. Ann Surg 1973;177:253–8.

Bastron RD, Perkins FM, Pyne JL. Autoregulation of renal blood flow during halothane anesthesia. Anesthesiology 1977;46:142–4.

Brenner BM, Deen WM, Robertson CR. Determinations of glomerular filtration rate. Annu Rev Physiol 1976;38:9–19.

Cross BA, Wakerley JB. The neurohypophysis. Int Rev Physiol 1977;16:1–34.

Dennis VW, Stead WW, Myers JL. Renal handling of phosphate and calcium. Annu Rev Physiol 1979;41:257–71.

Fitzsimons JT. Thirst. Physiol Rev 1972;52:468–562.

Gauer OH, Henry JP. Neurohormonal control of plasma volume. Int Rev Physiol 1976;9:145–90.

Giebisch G, Stanton B. Potassium transport in the nephron. Annu Rev Physiol 1979;41:241–56.

Glynn IM, Karlish SJD. The sodium pump. Annu Rev Physiol 1976;37:13–36.

Goetz KL, Bond GC, Bloxham DD. Atrial receptors and renal function. Physiol Rev 1975;55:157–205.

Guyton AC. Textbook of Medical Physiology, 7th ed. Philadelphia: WB Saunders, 1986a:393.

Guyton AC. Textbook of Medical Physiology, 7th ed. Philadelphia: WB Saunders, 1986b:410.

Guyton AC. Textbook of Medical Physiology, 7th ed. Philadelphia: WB Saunders, 1986c:425.

Knox FG, Diaz-Buxo JA. The hormonal control of sodium excretion. Int Rev Physiol 1977;16:173–98.

Lameire NH, Lifschitz MD, Stein JH. Heterogeneity of nephron function. Annu Rev Physiol 1977;39:159–84.

Lassiter WE. Kidney. Annu Rev Physiol 1975;37:371–93.

Mainsbach AB. Cellular mechanisms of tubular protein transport. Int Rev Physiol 1976;11:145–67.

McCaa RE, McCaa CS, Read DG, Bower JD, Guyton AC.

Increased plasma aldosterone concentrations in response to hemodialysis in nephrectomized man. Cir Res 1972;31:473–86.

Pitts RF. Physiology of the Kidney and Body Fluids, 3rd ed. Chicago, Year Book Medical Publishers, 1974.

Renkin EM, Robinson RR. Glomerular filtration. N Engl J Med 1974;290:785–92.

Stephenson JL. Countercurrent transport in the kidney. Annu Rev Biophys Bioeng 1978;7:315–39.

Ullrich KL. Sugar, amino acids, and Na$^+$ cotransport in the proximal tubule. Annu Rev Physiol 1979; 41:181–95.

Wright FS. Intrarenal regulation of glomerular filtration rate. N Engl J Med 1974;291:135–41.

Wright FS, Briggs JP. Feedback control of glomerular blood flow, pressure, and filtrate rate. Physiol Rev 1979;59:958–1006.

Young DB, McCaa RE, Pan Y-J, Guyton AC. Effectiveness of the aldosterone-sodium and -potassium feedback control system. Am J Physiol 1976;231:945–53.

Zerbe R, Stopes L, Robertson G. Vasopressin function in the syndrome of inappropriate antidiuresis. Annu Rev Med 1980;31:315–27.

Liver and Gastrointestinal Tract

LIVER

The basic roles of the liver can be divided into (1) vascular functions for storage and filtration of blood, (2) secretory functions for delivering bile into the gastrointestinal tract, and (3) metabolic functions (Guyton, 1986a).

The liver of the newborn is not optimally developed, as reflected by decreased ability to conjugate bilirubin with glucuronic acid and deficient formation of plasma proteins, including coagulation factors. The role of the newborn liver in gluconeogenesis is particularly deficient, rendering the newborn susceptible to hypoglycemia.

Anatomy

The basic functional unit of the liver is the hepatic lobule (Fig. 54-1) (Guyton, 1986a), which is a cylindrical structure constructed around a central vein that subsequently empties into hepatic veins and then into the vena cava. The liver contains 50,000 to 100,000 individual hepatic lobules. Each hepatic lobule is composed of hepatic cells (*i.e.,* hepatocytes) that radiate centrifugally from the central vein. Between hepatic cells are located bile canaliculi, which empty into terminal bile ducts. Blood from portal venules flows into hepatic sinuses on its way to the central vein. As a result, hepatic cells are constantly exposed to portal venous blood. Hepatic arterioles may also empty into hepatic sinuses.

Hepatic sinuses are lined by Kupffer's cells, which are capable of phagocytizing bacteria and other foreign material in the blood (Fig. 54-1) (Guyton, 1986a). These cells can remove 99% or more of bacteria in the portal venous blood (Kappas and Alvares, 1975). This is crucial, since the portal venous blood drains the gastrointestinal tract and almost always contains colon bacilli.

Endothelial cells that line the hepatic sinuses contain large pores, permitting easy diffusion of large substances, including plasma proteins, into extravascular spaces of the liver that connect with terminal lymphatics. The extreme permeability of the lining endothelial cells allows large quantities of lymph to form, which contain protein concentrations that are only slightly less than the protein concentration of plasma. Indeed, about one third to one half of all the lymph is formed in the liver (see Chapter 45).

Blood Flow

The liver receives a dual afferent blood supply from the hepatic artery and portal vein (Fig. 54-2). Total hepatic blood flow is about 1450 ml min^{-1} (*i.e.,* about 29% of the cardiac output), with 1100 ml provided by the portal vein (*i.e.,* about 75% of the total) and the remainder supplied by the hepatic artery. On a weight basis, hepatic blood flow is about 100 ml 100 g^{-1} min^{-1} (Greenway and Stark, 1971). Clearly, the majority of hepatic blood flow is with deoxygenated venous

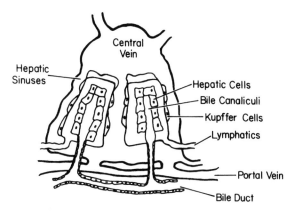

FIGURE 54-1. Schematic depiction of the hepatic lobule, which serves as the basic functional unit of the liver. (Redrawn from Guyton AC. Textbook of Medical Physiology. 7th ed. Philadelphia: WB Saunders, 1986:835. Reproduced by permission of the author and publisher.)

blood delivered by the portal vein. Nevertheless, about 50% of the liver's oxygen requirements are provided by portal venous blood. The extreme permeability of hepatic sinuses brings the hepatic blood flow into close contact with hepatic cells and facilitates the rapid exchange of nutrient materials.

The portal vein is formed by the junction of the superior mesenteric vein and splenic veins. As a result, this vein drains most of the abdominal viscera. Portal venous blood flows through the hepatic sinuses and then enters central veins of the liver for delivery to the inferior vena cava (Fig. 54-1) (Guyton, 1986a).

Fibrotic constriction involving hepatic sinuses, characteristic of hepatic cirrhosis, can increase resistance to blood inflow, as evidenced by portal venous pressures of 20 to 30 mmHg. Conversely, cardiac failure impairs outflow of blood from the liver by virtue of increased central venous pressure, which is transmitted to hepatic veins. The resulting continual stretching of hepatic sinuses caused by hepatic congestion can lead to necrosis of hepatic cells. An increase of 3 to 7 mmHg in hepatic venous pressure causes transudation of fluid through the outer surface of the liver capsule directly into the abdominal cavity (*i.e.,* ascites) (see the section entitled Portal Venous Pressure).

Blockage of portal venous flow into or through the liver causes high capillary pressures

in the entire gastrointestinal tract, resulting in edema of the gastrointestinal wall and transudation of fluid into the abdominal cavity. This, too, can cause ascites but is less likely than hepatic congestion, because collateral vascular channels develop rapidly from splenic veins to the esophageal veins (see the section entitled Portal Venous Pressure). These collateral venous channels decrease capillary pressure in the gastrointestinal wall back to normal.

Hepatic artery blood flow maintains nutrition of connective tissues and walls of bile ducts. For this reason, loss of hepatic artery blood flow can be fatal because of ensuing necrosis of vital liver structures. Blood from the hepatic artery, after it has supplied the structural elements of the liver, empties into hepatic sinuses to mix with the portal vein blood.

Control of Hepatic Blood Flow

Portal vein blood flow is determined by the various factors that determine flow through the gastrointestinal tract and spleen (see the section entitled Control of Gastrointestinal Blood Flow). Hepatic artery blood flow is influenced by local metabolic factors in the liver, including the concentration of oxygen, the lack of which causes vasodilation.

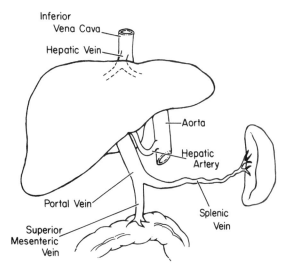

FIGURE 54-2. Schematic depiction of the dual afferent blood supply to the liver provided by the portal vein and hepatic artery.

Autoregulation of hepatic blood flow is present by means of the hepatic artery only, because portal vasculature does not exhibit this response (Richardson, 1982). Hypotension or splanchnic vasoconstriction from arterial hypoxemia or hypercapnia reduces hepatic blood flow (Strunin, 1975). Vasoconstriction reflects innervation of the hepatic vasculature by sympathetic nervous system fibers derived from T3–T11. Positive pressure ventilation of the lungs increases venous pressure, which is transmitted to hepatic veins with a subsequent reduction in hepatic blood flow. Similar effects on venous pressure and hepatic blood flow accompany cardiac failure.

Inhaled anesthetics, as well as regional anesthesia, reduce hepatic blood flow 20% to 30% in the absence of surgical stimulation (see Chapter 2). These changes reflect drug or technique-induced effects on perfusion pressure or splanchnic vascular resistance or both. Surgical stimulation may further decrease hepatic blood flow, with the greatest reductions occurring during intra-abdominal operations (Fig. 54-3) (Gelman, 1976).

Reservoir Function

The liver normally contains about 500 ml of blood, or 10% of the total blood volume. Elevations of the right atrial pressure cause back pressure, and the liver, being a distensible organ, may accommodate as much as 1 L of extra blood. As

such, the liver acts as a storage site when blood volume is excessive, as in cardiac failure, and is capable of supplying extra blood when hypovolemia occurs. Indeed, the large hepatic veins and sinuses are constricted by stimulation from the sympathetic nervous system, discharging up to 350 ml of blood into the circulation. Therefore, the liver is the single most important source of additional blood during strenuous exercise or acute hemorrhage.

Bile Secretion

Hepatic cells continually form bile (600–1000 ml daily), which is secreted into bile canaliculi, which empty into progressively larger ducts, ultimately reaching the hepatic duct and common bile duct (Fig. 54-1) (Boyer, 1980; Guyton, 1986a). From these ducts, bile either empties directly into the duodenum or is diverted into the gallbladder (Gerolami and Sartes, 1977).

Bile secreted by hepatic cells is normally stored in the gallbladder until it is needed in the duodenum (Jones and Myers, 1979). Fat in food entering the small intestine causes release of cholecystokinin from the intestinal mucosa. This hormone enters the circulation and passes to the gallbladder, where it causes selective contraction of the gallbladder smooth muscle. This provides the pressure that forces bile toward the duodenum. Vagal stimulation causes an additional weak contraction of the gallbladder smooth muscle. Contraction of the gallbladder smooth muscle also causes relaxation of the sphincter of Oddi, allowing bile to flow by way of the common bile duct into the duodenum. Furthermore, peristalsis in the duodenum momentarily relaxes the sphincter of Oddi. This relaxation is a reflection of the receptive relaxation that travels ahead of the peristaltic contraction wave. When adequate amounts of fat are present, the gallbladder empties in about 1 hour.

Bile salts, bilirubin, cholesterol, and lecithin are secreted in large amounts in the bile. Water and electrolytes are reabsorbed by the gallbladder mucosa, resulting in concentration of the remaining substances in the gallbladder (Table 54-1). Bile contains no digestive enzymes and is important for digestion only because of the presence of bile salts, which help to emulsify fat globules so that they can be digested by the intestinal lipases (Jones and Myers, 1979). In addition, bile facili-

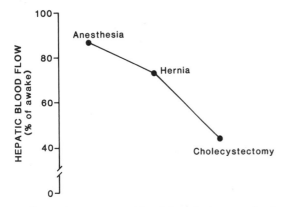

FIGURE 54-3. Hepatic blood flow during anesthesia in the absence of surgical stimulus and during operations removed from or near the liver. (Data from Gelman, SI. Disturbances in hepatic blood flow during anesthesia and surgery. Arch Surg 1976;111:881–4.)

Table 54-1
Composition of Bile

	Bile Formed in the Liver	Bile Present in the Gallbladder
Water	97.5 g dl⁻¹	92 g dl⁻¹
Bile Salts	1.1 g dl⁻¹	6 g dl⁻¹
Bilirubin	0.04 g dl⁻¹	0.3 g dl⁻¹
Cholesterol	0.1 g dl⁻¹	0.3 – 0.9 g dl⁻¹
Fatty Acids	0.12 g dl⁻¹	0.3 – 1.2 g dl⁻¹
Lecithin	0.04 g dl⁻¹	0.3 g dl⁻¹
Sodium	145 mEq L⁻¹	130 mEq L⁻¹
Potassium	5 mEq L⁻¹	9 mEq L⁻¹
Chloride	100 mEq L⁻¹	75 mEq L⁻¹
Bicarbonate	28 mEq L⁻¹	10 mEq L⁻¹

tates the transport of the end products of fat digestion to the intestinal villi so that they can be absorbed into lymphatics.

Bile Salts

The precursor of bile salts is cholesterol. Bile salts are essential for the gastrointestinal absorption of fats and accompanying fat-soluble vitamins. For example, within a few days after bile secretion ceases, one usually develops steatorrhea and a deficiency of vitamin K (see Chapter 34).

About 95% of bile salts are reabsorbed through the mucosa of the distal ileum by an active transport process. On reaching the liver, these bile salts are again secreted into the bile (*i.e.,* enterohepatic circulation). The amount of bile secreted by the liver each day is dependent on the availability of bile salts.

Bilirubin

Bilirubin, which is an end product of hemoglobin decomposition, is secreted in the bile (Fig. 54-4) (Guyton, 1986a). Specifically, after about 120 days, the cell membranes of erythrocytes rupture, and the released hemoglobin is phagocytized by reticuloendothelial cells throughout the body. The resulting bilirubin is released into the circulation where it binds with plasma albumin. Protein bound bilirubin is absorbed through hepatic cell membranes, becoming dissociated in the process from albumin. In hepatic cells, bilirubin is conju-

gated, predominantly with glucuronide and to a lesser extent with sulfate. In the gastrointestinal tract, bilirubin is converted by bacterial action mainly into urobilinogen.

JAUNDICE. Jaundice is the yellowish tint of body tissues that accompanies accumulation of bilirubin in extracellular fluid. Skin color usually begins to change when the plasma concentration of bilirubin increases to about three times normal (*i.e.,* above 1.5 mg dl⁻¹).

The most common types of jaundice are (1) hemolytic jaundice owing to increased destruction of erythrocytes, with rapid release of bilirubin into the blood and (2) obstructive jaundice owing to obstruction of bile ducts.

In hemolytic jaundice, the excretory function of the liver is not impaired, but the excess load of bilirubin exceeds the excretory capacity. Therefore, the plasma concentration of protein bound albumin increases.

In obstructive jaundice, bilirubin continues to

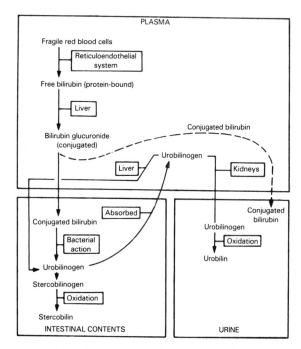

FIGURE 54-4. Schematic depiction of bilirubin formation and excretion. (From Guyton AC. Textbook of Medical Physiology. 7th ed. Philadelphia: WB Saunders, 1986:835. Reproduced by permission of the author and publisher.)

enter the liver and become conjugated. This conjugated bilirubin is then returned to the blood by rupture of the congested biled canaliculi and direct emptying of the bile into the lymph leaving the liver. As a result, the plasma concentration of conjugated bilirubin is increased in people with obstructive jaundice. Large amounts of conjugated bilirubin appear in the urine in contrast to the absence of protein bound bilirubin associated with hemolytic jaundice (Fig. 54-4) (Guyton, 1986a).

Cholesterol

No specific function is known for cholesterol secreted into bile. Under abnormal conditions (*e.g.,* excess absorption of water, excess dietary cholesterol, inflammation of the gallbladder epithelium), this cholesterol may precipitate, resulting in the formation of gallstones. Cholesterol gallstones can often be dissolved over 1 to 2 years by the daily oral administration of chenodeoxycholic acid (Boucheir, 1980). This substance, which is also one of the naturally occurring bile salts, adds greatly to the enterohepatic pool of bile salts. The increased quantity of bile salts increases the volume of bile formed, which reduces the concentration of cholesterol in the bile and renders that cholesterol more soluble.

Metabolic Functions

Metabolism of carbohydrates, lipids, and proteins is dependent on normal hepatic function (see Chapter 58). Furthermore, the liver is an important storage site for vitamins (see Chapter 34).

Carbohydrates

The liver is especially important for maintaining a normal blood – glucose concentration. This is accomplished by the formation of glycogen in the liver when the blood – glucose concentration is excessive. Amino acids can be converted to glucose by the process of gluconeogenesis when the blood – glucose concentration is reduced.

Lipids

Certain aspects of lipid metabolism occur more rapidly in hepatic cells than in other tissue cells. For example, beta-oxidation of fatty acids into two carbon acetyl radicals that form acetyl coenzyme A

occurs more rapidly in hepatic cells than in other sites. Lipoproteins, cholesterol, and phospholipids, such as lecithin, are formed in the liver. Furthermore, most of the synthesis of fats from carbohydrates and proteins also occurs in the liver.

Proteins

The most important functions of the liver in protein metabolism include (1) deamination of amino acids, (2) formation of urea for removal of ammonia from the body fluids, and (3) formation of plasma proteins.

Deamination of amino acids is required before these substances can be used for energy or converted into carbohydrates or fats. Reduction of portal blood flow through the liver, as may occur with a shunt between the portal vein and vena cava, can result in fatal hepatic coma owing to ammonia caused by activity of gastrointestinal tract bacteria. The liver can form 30 to 60 g of plasma proteins daily, and depletion of plasma proteins causes enlargement of hepatic cells.

Vitamins

The liver is important for storing vitamins, including vitamins A, D, and B_{12}. Sufficient amounts of vitamin A can be stored in the liver so as to prevent vitamin A deficiency for as long as 2 years.

Iron

Except for iron in hemoglobin, the liver is the most important storage site of iron. Iron combines with the protein apoferritin in the liver to form ferritin. When circulating concentrations of iron decline, ferritin releases iron into the blood.

GASTROINTESTINAL TRACT

The primary function of the gastrointestinal tract is to provide the body with a continual supply of water, electrolytes, and nutrients (Guyton, 1986b). To achieve this goal, the contents of the gastrointestinal tract must move through the entire system at an appropriate rate for digestive and absorptive functions to occur (Atanassova and Papasova, 1977). Each part of the gastrointestinal tract is adapted for specific functions such as (1) conduit for passage of food in the esophagus, (2) storage of food in the stomach or fecal matter in the colon, (3) digestion of food in the stomach, duodenum, jejunum, and ileum, and (4) absorption of the digestive end products and fluids in the entire small intestine and proximal portions of the colon.

Anatomy

The layers of a section of gastrointestinal wall from the outermost layer toward the interior are serosa, longitudinal muscle layer, circular muscle layer, submucosa, and mucosa. The motor functions of the gastrointestinal tract are performed by the different layers of smooth muscle. The smooth muscle of the gastrointestinal tract is a syncytium, which means that electrical signals originating in one smooth muscle fiber are easily propagated from fiber to fiber.

Smooth muscles of the gastrointestinal tract undergo almost continuous electrical activity. When the smooth muscle is stimulated by stretch, acetylcholine, or stimulation of the parasympathetic nervous system (PNS), the fibers undergo depolarization. Conversely, stimulation of the gastrointestinal tract smooth muscles by release of epinephrine or activation of the sympathetic nervous system (SNS) will decrease the resting membrane potential, causing hyperpolarization and a reduction of mechanical activity of the gastrointestinal tract to almost zero.

Tonic contraction of gastrointestinal smooth muscle at the pylorus, ileocecal valve, and anal sphincter helps regulate the rate of movement of materials through the gastrointestinal tract. In other parts of the gastrointestinal tract, rhythmic movements occur 3 to 12 times per minute (*i.e.,* peristalsis) to facilitate mixing and movement of food.

Blood Flow

About 80% (*i.e.,* about 850 ml) of the portal vein blood flow originates from the stomach and gastrointestinal tract, with the remainder coming from the spleen and pancreas (Jacobson, 1968). Over 60% of the blood flow to the gastrointestinal tract is to the mucosa to supply energy needed for production of intestinal secretions and for absorbing digested food.

Local regulatory mechanisms are primarily responsible for control of blood flow to the musculature of the gastrointestinal tract. Blood flow to the gastrointestinal mucosa and submucosa, where the glands are located and where absorption occurs, is controlled separately from blood flow to the musculature. Increases in activity of the gastrointestinal glands produces corresponding elevations in gastrointestinal blood flow. The mechanism by which alterations in gastrointestinal activity influence blood flow probably include the vasodilating effect of low concentrations of oxygen and peptide hormones (gastrin, secretin, cholecystokinin) released from the mucosa of the gastrointestinal tract during the digesting process.

Stimulation of PNS fibers to the stomach and lower colon increases local blood flow at the same time that it increases glandular secretions. Conversely, stimulation of SNS fibers causes vasoconstriction of the arterial blood supply to the gastrointestinal tract. After a few minutes, however, the blood flow returns to almost normal. This occurs because of local metabolic vasodilator mechanisms (*i.e.,* autoregulatory escape) elicited by ischemia as a result of the reduced blood flow induced by the intense vasoconstriction. The importance of this transient SNS-induced vasoconstriction is that it permits shunting of blood from the gastrointestinal tract for brief periods during exercise or when increased blood flow is needed by skeletal muscles and the heart.

Vasoconstriction of gastrointestinal veins, unlike the arteries, does not escape from the effects of SNS stimulation. As a result, large volumes of blood are displaced from these persistently constricted veins so as to sustain the circulating blood volume during periods of acute hemorrhage.

Portal Venous Pressure

The liver offers modest resistance to blood flow from the portal venous system. As a result, the pressure in the portal vein averages 8 to 10 mmHg, which is considerably higher than the almost zero pressure in the inferior vena cava. Cirrhosis of the liver, most frequently caused by alcoholism, is characterized by increased resistance to portal vein blood flow owing to replacement of hepatic cells with fibrous tissue that contracts around the blood vessels. The gradual increase in resistance to portal vein blood flow produced by cirrhosis of the liver causes large collateral vessels to develop between the portal veins and the systemic veins. The most important of these collaterals are from the splenic veins to the esophageal veins. These collaterals may become so large that they protrude into the lumen of the esophagus, producing esophageal varicosities. The esophageal mucosa overlying these varicosities eventually becomes eroded, leading to life-threatening hemorrhage.

In the absence of the development of adequate collaterals, sustained elevations of portal vein pressure may cause protein-containing fluid to escape from the surface of the mesentery, gastrointestinal tract, and liver into the peritoneal cavity. This fluid, known as *ascites,* is similar to plasma, and the high protein content causes an elevated colloid osmotic pressure in the abdominal fluid. This high colloid osmotic pressure draws additional fluid from the surfaces of the gastrointestinal tract and mesentery into the peritoneal cavity.

Splenic Circulation

The splenic capsule in humans, in contrast to that in many lower animals, is nonmuscular, which limits the ability of the spleen to release stored blood in response to SNS stimulation. A small amount (150–200 ml) of blood is stored in the splenic venous sinuses and can be released by SNS-induced vasoconstriction of the splenic vessels. Release of this amount of blood into the systemic circulation is sufficient to increase the hematocrit 1% to 2%.

The spleen functions to remove erythrocytes from the circulation. This occurs when erythrocytes re-enter the venous sinuses from the splenic pulp by passing through pores that may be smaller than the erythrocyte. Fragile cells do not withstand this trauma, and the released hemoglobin that results from their rupture is ingested by the reticuloendothelial cells of the spleen. These same reticuloendothelial cells also function, much like lymph nodes, to remove bacteria and parasites from the circulation. Indeed, asplenic patients may be more prone to bacterial infections (Likhite, 1976).

During fetal life, the splenic pulp produces erythrocytes in the same manner as does the bone marrow in the adult. As the fetus reaches maturity, however, this function of the spleen is lost.

Innervation

The gastrointestinal tract has an intrinsic nervous system that extends from the esophagus to the anus (Grossman, 1979). This intrinsic nervous system controls gastrointestinal tract movements and secretions. Signals from the autonomic nervous system influence the activity of this intrinsic system; for example, impulses from the PNS increase intrinsic activity, whereas signals from the SNS cause a decrease in intrinsic activity.

Intrinsic Nervous System

The intrinsic nervous system is composed of two layers of neurons and connecting fibers. The neuronal outer layer lies between the longitudinal and circular muscle layers and is designated the myenteric plexus, or Auerbach's plexus (Wood, 1975). The second neuronal layer is in the submucosa and is known as the submucosal plexus, or Meissner's plexus. The myenteric plexus controls mainly gastrointestinal tract activity, whereas the submucosal plexus is important in controlling secretions and responding to sensory signals principally from stretch receptors in the wall of the gastrointestinal tract. The excitatory fibers of the myenteric plexus are cholinergic and secrete acetylcholine.

PARASYMPATHETIC NERVOUS SYSTEM INNERVATION. The cranial component of PNS innervation to the gastrointestinal tract is by way of the vagus nerve. These fibers provide extensive innervation of the esophagus, stomach, pancreas, and proximal portion of the small intestine. The distal portion of the colon is richly supplied by the sacral parasympathetics. These fibers function particularly in the defecation reflex. Overall, stimulation of the PNS causes an increase in the activity of the intrinsic nervous system.

SYMPATHETIC NERVOUS SYSTEM INNERVATION. The fibers of the SNS destined for the gastrointestinal tract pass through outlying ganglia such as the celiac ganglion and various mesenteric ganglia. Postganglionic fibers leave these ganglia to innervate equally all portions of the gastrointestinal tract. This contrasts with the predominance of cephalad and caudad innervation of the gastrointestinal tract by the PNS. Overall, stimulation of the SNS causes a decrease in the activity of the intrinsic nervous system.

Afferent Nerve Fibers

Afferent nerve fibers arise from the gastrointestinal tract and pass with SNS and PNS fibers to the central nervous system. An estimated 80% of the nerve fibers are afferent rather than efferent (Guyton, 1986b). These fibers transmit signals to the medulla to initiate vagal impulses, which, in turn, control important functions of the gastrointestinal tract.

Hormonal Control

Gastrointestinal tract activity, in addition to control by nervous system impulses, is influenced by several hormones (Dickray, 1979). For example, gastrin is secreted by the mucosa of the stomach antrum when food enters. This hormone acts to increase motility of the stomach. Lower esophageal sphincter tone is also increased by gastrin, so as to reduce the likelihood of esophageal reflux.

Secretin is secreted by the mucosa of the duodenum in response to the movement of acidic gastric contents through the pylorus. This hormone has a mild inhibitory effect on motility of the gastrointestinal tract. In addition, gastric inhibitory peptide, secreted by the mucosa of the proximal small intestine, acts to slow activity of the gastrointestinal tract.

Cholecystokinin is secreted mainly by the mucosa of the jejunum in response to the presence of fatty substances in the gastrointestinal tract. This hormone increases contractility of the gallbladder, thus causing expulsion of bile into the small intestine, where it helps to emulsify fatty substances. Furthermore, cholecystokinin is present as a neurotransmitter in the central nervous system, where it may act as an endogenous opioid antagonist (see Chapter 3).

Types of Motility

The two types of gastrointestinal tract motility are mixing contractions and propulsive movements. The basic propulsive movement of the gastrointestinal tract is peristalsis, in which a contractile ring appears around the gut and then moves forward. Peristalsis is an inherent property of any syncytical smooth muscle tube, and stimulation at any point causes a contractile ring to spread in both directions, although cephalad movement is not sustained. The usual stimulus for peristalsis is distention.

Even though peristalsis is a basic feature of tubular smooth muscle structures, it occurs only weakly in portions of the gastrointestinal tract that have congenital absence of the myenteric plexus. Peristalsis is also greatly depressed by anticholinergic drugs that inhibit the cholinergic nerve endings of the myenteric plexus. Furthermore, the intensity of peristalsis can be greatly influenced by the level of PNS activity.

Motor Functions of the Upper Gastrointestinal Tract

The majority of the muscles of chewing are innervated by the motor portion of cranial nerve V, and the chewing process is controlled by nuclei in the brain. Chewing is important because digestive enzymes act only on the surfaces of food particles. As such, the rate of digestion is highly dependent on the total surface area exposed to the intestinal secretions. Furthermore, fruits and raw vegetables have undigestible cellulose membranes around their nutrient portions, which must be broken before the food can be utilized.

Swallowing

Swallowing is a complicated reflex mechanism that is almost always initiated by voluntary movement of food into the back of the mouth. For example, stimulation of swallowing receptor areas located all around the opening of the pharynx, but particularly in the tonsillar pillars, sends impulses primarily over the sensory portions of cranial nerves V and X to the brain stem, which initiates a series of automatic pharyngeal muscular contractions. The areas in the medulla and lower pons that control swallowing are collectively called the *swallowing,* or *deglutition center.* The motor impulses from the swallowing center travel to the pharynx by way of cranial nerves V, IX, X, and XII.

The entire pharyngeal stage of swallowing occurs in less than 1 to 2 seconds, thereby interrupting only briefly the usual breathing cycle. The swallowing center inhibits the respiratory center of the medulla, halting breathing at any point in the cycle to allow swallowing to proceed.

The esophagus serves as a conduit for passage of food from the pharynx to the stomach. The act of swallowing initiates a peristaltic wave in the esophagus, which propels food to the stomach. Peristaltic waves also occur in the esophagus as a result of distention by food. Vagal afferent and efferent fibers are responsible for peristaltic waves of the esophagus. In the absence of vagal innervation, the myenteric nerve plexus becomes sufficiently active after a few days to independently initiate peristaltic waves.

Lower Esophageal Sphincter

The lower 2 to 5 cm of the esophagus functions as the lower esophageal sphincter. Anatomically, this sphincter is not different from the rest of the esophagus, but, in contrast to the rest of the esophagus, this area remains tonically constricted except when a peristaltic wave arrives. Failure of the sphincter to relax appropriately results in achalasia.

A principal function of the lower esophageal sphincter is to prevent reflux of acidic stomach contents into the upper esophagus. Indeed, the esophageal mucosa is not capable of resisting the digestive action of gastric secretions. A valve-like mechanism of that portion of the esophagus that lies immediately beneath the diaphragm also acts to prevent esophageal reflux.

The difference between gastric pressure and lower esophageal sphincter pressure is termed *barrier pressure* (see Chapter 26). Barrier pressure, which normally exceeds 15 cm H_2O, is influenced by drug-induced alterations in lower esophageal sphincter tone. For example, anticholinergic drugs have been shown to decrease lower esophageal sphincter tone, whereas metoclopramide produces an opposite effect (Brocke-Utne *et al,* 1976). The influence, if any, of these drug-induced effects on barrier pressure and subsequent inhalation of gastric fluid during anesthesia remains undocumented.

Motor Functions of the Stomach

Motor functions of the stomach include (1) storage of food until it can be accommodated elsewhere, (2) mixing of food with gastric secretions until it forms a semiliquid mixture known as *chyme,* and (3) gradual release of food from the stomach into the small intestine at an optimal rate for digestion and absorption (Guyton, 1986b).

The stomach is divided into the fundus, corpus, or body and the antrum (Fig. 54-5).

Storage of Food

Normally, the body of the stomach has little muscular wall tone so that it can bulge passively outward, thereby accommodating more and more volume, up to about 1 L. The intragastric pressure remains low until this limit is approached.

Mixing of Food

Digestive juices are secreted by gastric glands, and these juices then mix with food. This mixing is facilitated by waves that pass through the stomach, propelling food toward the antrum. Chyme is present when food has been thoroughly mixed with gastric fluid.

Emptying of the Stomach

Emptying of the stomach is opposed by resistance of the pylorus to the passage of food and is promoted by peristaltic waves in the antrum of the stomach. Tone of the pylorus is great enough to prevent movement of chyme into the duodenum except when a strong antral peristaltic wave occurs. The degree of constriction of the pyloric sphincter can increase or decrease in response to signals from the stomach and the duodenum (*i.e.,* enterogastric reflex). Likewise, signals from these same sites can influence the intensity of the antral peristaltic waves. These feedback signals allow

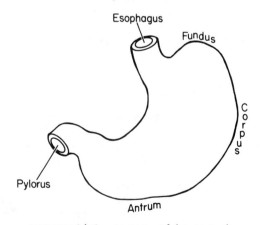

FIGURE 54-5. Anatomy of the stomach.

chyme to enter the duodenum only as rapidly as it can be processed by the small intestine.

Gastrin enhances the activity of the pyloric pump while at the same time relaxing the pylorus. This hormone also enhances tone of the lower esophageal sphincter to prevent reflux of gastric contents into the esophagus during this period of enhanced gastric activity.

Movements of the Small Intestine

As in the stomach, movements of the small intestine can be divided into mixing contractions and propulsive movements. Distention of the small intestine with chyme causes peristaltic contractions that promote mixing of food with the secretions of the small intestine. These mixing movements mainly depend on the reflex signals generated in the myenteric plexus in response to intestinal distention.

Chyme moves through the small intestine at an average of 1 cm min^{-1} (Guyton, 1986b). As a result, it takes 3 to 5 hours for chyme to pass from the pylorus to the ileocecal valve. On reaching the ileocecal valve, chyme is sometimes blocked for several hours until one eats another meal.

Functions of the Ileocecal Valve

A principal function of the ileocecal valve is to prevent backflow of fecal contents from the colon into the small intestine. The lips of the ileocecal valve protrude into the lumen of the cecum and can resist reverse pressure as great as 60 cm H$_2$O. The resistance to emptying at the ileocecal valve prolongs the stay of chyme in the ileum and, therefore, facilitates absorption. On the average, about 750 ml of chyme empty into the cecum daily.

The degree of contraction of the ileocecal valve is also influenced by reflexes from the cecum. For example, when the ileum is distended, reflexes mediated by the myenteric plexus intensify the tone of the ileocecal valve. An inflamed appendix can increase the tone of the ileocecal valve to the extent that emptying of the ileum ceases. Conversely, gastrin causes relaxation of the ileocecal valve.

Movements of the Colon

The functions of the colon are absorption of water and electrolytes from the chyme and storage of

fecal matter until it can be expelled (Guyton, 1986b). The proximal half of the colon is involved principally with absorption, and the distal portion of the colon is involved with storage. Since intense movements are not required for these functions, the movements of the colon are sluggish, although they still may be divided into mixing contractions and propulsive movements.

Mixing Contractions

Circular muscle of the colon contracts and, at the same time, strips of longitudinal muscle known as *tineae coli* contract, causing the unstimulated portion of the colon to bulge outward into baglike sacs or haustrations. This combination of circular and longitudinal muscle contraction causes maximal amounts of the fecal material to be exposed to the surface of the large intestine, resulting in absorption of all but about 100 ml of the original 750 ml of chyme that enters the colon daily.

Propulsive Movements

Propulsive movements characterized as peristalsis, as occur in the small intestine, rarely develop in the colon. Instead, most propulsive movement occurs by haustral contractions involved with mixing movements and mass movements. Most of the propulsion in the cecum and ascending colon results from the slow but persistent haustral contractions requiring as long as 8 to 15 hours to move the chyme the short distance from the ileocecal valve to the transverse colon. During this transit, the chyme becomes fecal in quality and also becomes semisolid.

Mass Movements

Mass movements predominate from the transverse to the sigmoid colon. When mass movement forces feces into the rectum, the desire for defecation is perceived. The appearance of mass movements after meals is caused at least in part by reflexes that result from distention of the stomach (gastrocolic reflex) and duodenum (duodenocolic reflex). These reflexes are transmitted through the myenteric plexus. Gastrin also plays a role by virtue of its ability to inhibit the ileocecal valve and stimulate the colon. Irritation of the colon, as associated with ulcerative colitis, can be responsible for almost continuous mass movements in the colon. Mass movements are also initiated by intense stimulation of the PNS or by mechanical overdistention of a segment of the colon.

Defecation

Movement of feces into a previously empty rectum initiates the urge for defecation. Distention of the rectum initiates afferent signals that spread through the myenteric plexus to initiate peristaltic waves in the descending colon, sigmoid colon, and rectum, forcing feces toward the anus. In addition, signals are transmitted from the rectum to the sacral portion of the spinal cord and then reflexively back to the descending colon, sigmoid colon, rectum, and anus by fibers of the PNS. These signals from the PNS are necessary to fortify the otherwise weak defecation reflexes. Signals from the PNS also initiate the characteristic deep breath, closure of the glottis, and contraction of the abdominal muscles that accompany the defecation reflex. Ultimately, it is conscious control, however, over the tone of the external anal sphincter that determines when defecation occurs. When conscious maintenance of external sphincter tone is present, the defecation reflex wanes after a few minutes and usually will not return until an additional amount of feces enters the rectum, sometimes several hours later.

Secretory Functions

The gastrointestinal tract secretes digestive enzymes, usually in response to the presence of food and in amounts necessary for proper digestion (Table 54-2) (Guyton, 1986c). In addition, glands secrete mucus to provide lubrication and protection of all parts of the gastrointestinal tract. Mucus is also necessary to allow easy passage of food particles through the lumen of the gastrointestinal tract. Stimulation of PNS fibers to the gastrointestinal tract almost invariably increases the rates of glandular secretion. Conversely, stimulation of the SNS reduces blood flow to the glands and, by this mechanism, tends to inhibit glandular secretion.

Gastrointestinal tract secretions are regulated by polypeptide hormones (Bloom, 1977). For example, hormones liberated from the gastrointestinal tract mucosa in response to the presence of food in the lumen are absorbed into the blood and are carried to glands, where they stimulate secretion of digestive enzymes. This type of stimulation is particularly valuable in increasing the output of gastric fluid and pancreatic fluid when food enters the stomach or duodenum. In addition, hormonal stimulation of the gallbladder wall causes it to eject bile into the duodenum.

Salivary Gland Secretions

The principal salivary glands are the parotid, submaxillary, and sublingual glands. The daily secretion of saliva averages 1200 ml (0.5 – 1 ml min^{-1}). This saliva acts to wash away pathogenic bacteria in the oral cavity as well as food particles that provide nutrition for the bacteria. Saliva also contains thiocyanate ions and proteolytic enzymes, which have antibacterial effects. Indeed, in the absence of saliva, oral tissues become ulcerated and infected. Saliva also contains an alpha-amylase enzyme that is important for digesting starches and mucin for lubricating purposes.

The PNS is responsible for the regulation of salivation. These fibers are stimulated by taste and tactile stimuli from the tongue. In addition, salivation may be influenced by the appetite area of the brain.

Saliva has a pH of 6 to 7 and contains large amounts of potassium and bicarbonate ions. Conversely, concentrations of sodium and chloride ions are much less in saliva than in plasma. This reflects active reabsorption of sodium ions from the salivary ducts and active secretion of potassium ions in exchange for the sodium ions. The net result of these active transport processes is a concentration of sodium and chloride ions in saliva equivalent to about 15 mEq L^{-1}, whereas potassium ions are concentrated to about

Table 54-2
Daily Secretions of the Gastrointestinal Tract

	Volume (ml in 24 hr)	pH
Saliva	1000	6.0 – 7.0
Gastric Fluid	1500	1.0 – 3.5
Pancreatic Fluid	1000	8.0 – 8.3
Bile	1000	7.8
Small Intestine	1800	6.5 – 7.5
Large Intestine	200	7.5 – 8.0

(Guyton, AC. Textbook of Medical Physiology, 7th ed. Philadelphia: WB Saunders, 1986: 770; by permission of the author and publisher.)

30 mEq L^{-1}. The bicarbonate ion concentration in saliva of 50 to 90 mEq L^{-1} is two to four times that in plasma. The high potassium concentration of saliva can result in hypokalemia and skeletal muscle weakness if excess salivation persists.

Esophageal Secretions

Esophageal secretions are entirely mucoid and provide lubrication for swallowing. Mucus secreted by the mucous glands prevents mucosal excoriation by food and protects the esophageal wall from irritation by acidic gastric fluid that may reflux into the lower esophagus. Despite this protection, a peptic ulcer may still develop at the gastric end of the esophagus.

Gastric Secretions

The mucosa of the stomach contains glands that secrete mucus, hydrochloric acid, pepsinogen, gastrin, and mucus (Bloom, 1977). Parietal cells secrete hydrochloric acid, whereas peptic or chief cells are responsible for the secretion of pepsinogen. Total daily gastric secretion is about 2000 ml, with a pH of 1 to 3.5.

PARIETAL CELLS. Parietal cells secrete a hydrogen ion–containing solution with a pH of about 0.8. At this pH, the hydrogen ion concentration is about three million times that present in the arterial blood. The importance of carbon dioxide in the chemical reactions for formation of hydrochloric acid is emphasized by the fact that carbonic anhydrase inhibition by acetazolamide almost completely blocks the formation of hydrochloric acid.

Intrinsic factor, which is essential for absorption of vitamin B$_{12}$ from the ileum, is secreted by the same cells in the gastric mucosa that secrete hydrochloric acid. For this reason, destruction of acid-producing cells in the stomach in association with chronic gastritis produces achlorhydria and, often, pernicious anemia.

PEPTIC CELLS. When pepsinogens are first secreted, they have no digestive activity. Activated pepsin is formed, however, whenever pepsinogen comes into contact with hydrochloric acid. Pepsin is a proteolytic enzyme that is most active in fluid with a pH of about 2. Above a pH of 5, pepsin possesses little proteolytic activity.

PYLORIC GLANDS. Pyloric glands in the gastric mucosa are responsible for secreting mucus, which protects the stomach wall from digestion by the gastric enzymes. In addition, the surface of the gastric mucosa between glands has a continuous layer of mucous cells that secrete a viscid and alkaline mucus that coats and protects.

REGULATION OF GASTRIC SECRETIONS. Gastric secretions are regulated by neural and hormonal mechanisms. Neural regulation involves intrinsic nerve plexus reflexes as well as impulses from the PNS that travel with the vagus nerves. Hormonal regulation of gastric secretions is by gastrin. The stimulant effect of gastrin on gastric secretion requires the presence of histamine. Indeed, blockade of H$_2$ receptors prevents the stimulant effects of gastrin on gastric secretion (Hirschowitz, 1979).

When food enters the stomach, it distends the antral portion of the gastric mucosa and causes the secretion of gastrin. Gastrin maintains the secretion of gastric fluid that continues throughout the several hours that the food remains in the stomach. Certain substances known as *secretagogues* (*e.g.,* alcohol, caffeine) are particularly likely to evoke the release of gastrin. Distention of the stomach, as well as the chemical action of secretagogues, elicits release of gastrin by means of a local nerve reflex. Specifically, these changes stimulate sensory nerve fibers in the gastric epithelium, which, in turn, synapse with the intrinsic nerve plexus. These nerves transmit efferent signals to gastrin-secreting cells. Gastrin is absorbed into the blood and is carried to the gastric glands, where it stimulates the production of hydrochloric acid. Blockade of the vagus nerves or administration of atropine, which prevents the action of acetylcholine on the intrinsic nerve cells, will prevent the release of gastrin.

The rate of gastric fluid secretion is greater in response to vagal stimulation than in response to gastrin. The two mechanisms together, however, produce a greater than additive effect. The stomach secretes only a few milliliters of gastric fluid each hour during the periods between digestion. The secretion that does occur at this time is mainly mucus containing very little pepsinogen or hydrogen ions. Strong emotional stimulation, however, as occurs preoperatively can increase interdigestive secretion of highly acidic gastric fluid to 50 ml hr^{-1} or more. This increased rate of gastric fluid secretion resembles the cephalic phase of gastric fluid secretion that occurs in anticipation of a meal. Attempts to regulate the volume and hydrogen ion concentration of gastric fluid with drugs may be particularly important in the period prior to the induction of anesthesia (see Chapter 21).

Pancreatic Secretions

The pancreas lies parallel and beneath the stomach and has a structure similar to the salivary glands. Digestive enzymes and large volumes of sodium bicarbonate ions (up to 145 mEq L^{-1}) are secreted by way of the pancreatic duct into the duodenum, mainly in response to the presence of chyme in the upper portions of the small intestine (Rothman, 1977). Digestive enzymes necessary for the breakdown of proteins, carbohydrates, and fats are secreted by the pancreas. Bicarbonate ions are important for neutralizing the acid chyme that empties from the stomach into the duodenum. The total volume of pancreatic secretions averages 1200 ml daily, and the pH is near 8.

The most important pancreatic enzyme for the digestion of protein is trypsin. Trypsin splits proteins into small peptides or amino acids. The digestive enzyme for carbohydrates is pancreatic amylase, which hydrolyzes carbohydrates to disaccharides The main enzymes for fat digestion are pancreatic lipase, which is capable of hydrolyzing fat into glycerol and fatty acids, and cholesterol esterase, which causes hydrolysis of cholesterol esters.

TRYPSIN. Trypsin synthesized in the pancreatic cells exists in an enzymatically inactive form known as *trypsinogen*. Trypsinogen is activated in the gastrointestinal tract by the enzyme enterokinase, which is secreted by the gastrointestinal mucosa when chyme comes in contact with the mucosa. Activation of trypsinogen before it reaches the gastrointestinal tract could cause autodigestion of the pancreas. Indeed, the same pancreatic cells that synthesize proteolytic enzymes also simultaneously secrete a trypsin inhibitor. Damage to the pancreas or blockage of a pancreatic duct can cause pooling of proteolytic enzymes, with the effect of the trypsin inhibitor being overwhelmed. When this occurs, acute pancreatitis rapidly ensues, reflecting digestion of the pancreas by the proteolytic enzymes it forms. Acute pancreatitis is often fatal because of the profound accompanying shock.

REGULATION OF PANCREATIC SECRETIONS.
Pancreatic secretion is regulated more by hormonal than by neural mechanisms. For example, the entrance of chyme into the duodenum causes the release and activation of secretin, which is subsequently absorbed into the circulation. Hydrochloric acid is the most important constituent of chyme that evokes the release of secretin in the duodenum. Secretin causes the pancreas to produce large amounts of fluid containing high concentrations of bicarbonate ions but almost no digestive enzymes. Neutralization of the acidic pH is important because the mucosa of the small intestine cannot withstand the intense digestive action of gastric fluid. Furthermore, pancreatic enzymes function optimally in a slightly alkaline or neutral solution.

In addition to the release of secretin, the presence of food in the duodenum causes the release of a second polypeptide hormone, cholecystokinin. Cholecystokinin also enters the circulation, but instead of causing pancreatic secretion of a fluid high in bicarbonate ions, this hormone evokes secretion of digestive enzymes. The response evoked by cholecystokinin resembles the response to stimulation of the PNS.

Impulses from the PNS are transmitted to the pancreas by way of the vagus nerves, resulting in release of acetylcholine and secretion of moderate amounts of enzymes into the pancreatic acini. Little fluid, however, flows through the pancreatic ducts to the duodenum because only small amounts of water and electrolytes are secreted along with the enzymes. As a result, most of the enzymes formed in response to stimulation of the PNS are temporarily stored.

Secretions of the Small Intestine

There are extensive numbers of mucous glands (Brunner's glands) located in the first few centimeters of the duodenum between the pylorus and the ampulla of Vater where pancreatic secretions and bile enter the duodenum. These glands secrete mucus to protect the duodenal wall from damage by the acidic gastric fluid. Stimulation of the SNS inhibits the mucus-producing function of these glands, leaving the duodenal bulb unprotected. Indeed, this may be one of the factors that causes this area of the gastrointestinal tract to be the most frequent site of peptic ulcer disease.

Crypts of Lieberkühn are located over the entire surface of the small intestine except for the area of the duodenum containing Brunner's glands. Intestinal secretions are formed by the epithelial cells in these crypts at a rate of about 2000 ml daily. These secretions lack digestive enzymes and mimic extracellular fluid, having a *p*H in the range of 6.5 to 7.5. This fluid is reabsorbed by the intestinal villi and provides a watery vehicle for absorption of substances from the chyme as it comes in contact with the villi. Indeed, this absorption of substances from chyme is one of the primary functions of the small intestine.

The epithelial cells in the crypts of Lieberkühn continually undergo mitosis, with an average life cycle of only about 5 days. This rapid growth of new cells allows rapid repair of any excoriation that occurs in the mucosa. This rapid turnover of cells also explains the vulnerability of the gastrointestinal epithelium to chemotherapeutic drugs (see Chapter 29).

The epithelial cells of the mucosa of the small intestine contain digestive enzymes that are thought to digest food substances while they are being absorbed through the epithelium. These enzymes include peptidases for splitting small peptides into amino acids, enzymes for splitting disaccharides into monosaccharides, and intestinal lipases.

REGULATION OF SMALL INTESTINE SECRETIONS. The most important mechanism for regulation of small intestine secretions is local neural reflexes, especially those initiated by tactile or irritative stimuli. For this reason, the volume of secretions is directly proportional to the volume of chyme in the small intestine. Hormones, such as secretin and cholecystokinin, play a minor role in the stimulation of secretions in the small intestine.

Secretions of the Large Intestine

The mucosa of the large intestine is lined by crypts of Lieberkühn, but, unlike the small intestine, the epithelial cells of these crypts do not contain significant amounts of digestive enzymes. Instead, these cells almost exclusively secrete mucus. The rate of secretion of this mucus is regulated principally by direct tactile stimulation of the mucus-secreting cells and by local myenteric reflexes. In addition, impulses from the PNS that increase motility of the distal portion of the large intestine also greatly increase mucous production in this portion of the colon. Therefore, during extreme stimulation of the PNS, there may be production of mucous bowel movements in the presence of little or no fecal material.

Mucus in the large intestine protects the mucosa against trauma and provides an adherent medium to hold fecal material together. Furthermore, this mucus protects the gastrointestinal mucosa from bacterial activity occurring inside the feces. The alkalinity of this mucus (*p*H about 8) owing to the presence of large amounts of bicarbonate also provides a barrier to keep acids that are formed deep in the feces from attacking the intestinal wall.

Irritation of a segment of the large intestine, as occurs with bacterial infection, causes the mucosa to secrete large quantities of water and electrolytes in addition to the normal viscid solution of mucus. This acts to dilute the irritating factors and to cause rapid movement of feces toward the anus (*i.e.,* diarrhea). As a result, there is the loss of large amounts of water and electrolytes.

Principles of Gastrointestinal Absorption

The total quantity of fluid that must be absorbed daily from the gastrointestinal tract is equal to that ingested (about 1.5 L) plus that secreted by the gastrointestinal tract (about 7.5 L) (Guyton, 1986d). Approximately 8 to 8.5 L of this total of 9 L of fluid is absorbed in the small intestine, leaving only 0.5 to 1 L to enter the large intestine each day.

Absorption from the Stomach

The stomach is a poor absorptive area of the gastrointestinal tract, because it lacks the villus structure characteristic of absorptive membranes. Furthermore, the junctions between the epithelial cells of the stomach are tight. As a result, only highly lipid-soluble substances, such as alcohol, and some drugs, such as aspirin, can be significantly absorbed from the stomach.

Absorption from the Small Intestine

In the small intestine, the absorptive surface is greatly increased by folds of the mucosa (valvulae conniventes) that may protrude as much as 8 mm into the intestinal lumen. These folds are particularly well developed in the duodenum and jejunum. The presence of villi on these mucosal folds further increases the absorptive area. In addition, the intestinal epithelial cells are characterized by a brush border consisting of microvilli about 1 μm in length and 0.1 μm in diameter protruding from each cell (Guyton, 1986d). This further increases the absorptive area of the gastrointestinal tract. Together, the mucosal folds, villi, and microvilli provide an absorptive surface area of about 250 m² for the small intestine.

Normally, absorption from the small intestine each day consists of carbohydrates, fat, amino acids, and 8 to 9 L of water. This absorptive capacity may be greatly increased when necessary. Indeed, 20 L or more of water per day can be absorbed through the small intestine. Water is transported through the gastrointestinal membrane by diffusion. For example, when chyme is dilute, water is absorbed through the gastrointestinal mucosa into the blood. Conversely, water can be transported from the plasma into the chyme whenever hyperosmotic solutions pass from the stomach to the duodenum.

As dissolved substances are absorbed from the lumen of the gastrointestinal tract into the blood, water also diffuses into the circulation to prevent changes in the osmotic pressure of the chyme. In this way, not only are the ions and nutrients almost entirely absorbed before the chyme passes through the ileocecal valve, but so is about 95% of the water.

The daily absorption of sodium ions from the small intestine is 25 to 35 g. This emphasizes the rapidity with which total body sodium depletion can occur if excessive intestinal secretions are lost, as occurs with extreme diarrhea. Absorption of sodium ions from the gastrointestinal tract is by active transport (Turnberg, 1973). Chloride ions follow the electrical gradient created by the active transport of sodium ions.

Epithelial lining cells of the distal ileum and the large intestine have the capability of exchanging chloride ions for bicarbonate ions. This provides bicarbonate ions for neutralization of acidic products by bacteria, especially in the large intestine. Bacterial toxins, as from cholera and staphylococci, can intensely stimulate this chloride–bicarbonate exchange mechanism. The secreted bicarbonate ions carry with them sodium ions and an isosmotic equivalent of water, resulting in life-threatening diarrhea.

Calcium ions are actively absorbed, especially from the duodenum. This gastrointestinal absorption of calcium is enhanced by the action of vitamin D. Phosphate is easily absorbed from the gastrointestinal tract except when excess calcium forms poorly soluble calcium–phosphate compounds. Iron and monovalent ions, such as potassium, are also actively absorbed from the small intestine (Forth and Rummel, 1973).

Absorption of Nutrients

Nutrients, with the exception of vitamins and minerals, can be classified as carbohydrates, fats, and proteins. These nutrients, however, cannot be absorbed in their natural form; first they must undergo digestion. The basic process in the digestion of carbohydrates, fats, and proteins is hydrolysis.

CARBOHYDRATES. The three major sources of carbohydrates in the human diet are sucrose, lactose, and starches, which are large polysaccharides present in almost all foods, especially grains. Sucrose and lactose are disaccharides found in sugar and milk, respectively. Cellulose is carbohydrate, but no enzymes capable of hydrolyzing cellulose are secreted by the human gastrointestinal tract.

When food is chewed and mixed with saliva, the enzyme alpha-amylase, which is secreted mainly by parotid glands, hydrolyzes starches into disaccharides. Nevertheless, food remains in the mouth for only a short period of time, such that no more than 5% of all the starches are hydrolyzed before swallowing. The action of alpha-amylase, however, continues in the stomach. Furthermore, pancreatic secretions contain alpha-amylase similar to that in saliva, such that hydrolysis of starches continues as chyme empties from the stomach into the duodenum. As a result of these alpha-amylase enzymes, almost all ingested starches are converted into maltose and isomaltose before passing beyond the jejunum.

The epithelial cells lining the small intestine contain the four enzymes capable of splitting the disaccharides lactose, sucrose, maltose, and isomaltose into the corresponding monosaccharides, which include galactose, fructose, and glucose. These digested monosaccharides are immediately absorbed into the portal vein. In the ordinary diet, glucose represents about 80% of the final products of carbohydrate digestion.

Absorption of monosaccharides is by active transport systems in the brush borders of epithelial cells lining the gastrointestinal tract (Olsen, 1974). Active transport systems are specific for each monosaccharide, and there is a transport maximum. For example, galactose and glucose transport ceases whenever active transport of sodium is blocked, suggesting that energy for transport of these two monosaccharides is actually provided by the sodium transport system.

PROTEINS. Dietary proteins are derived almost entirely from meats and vegetables and are represented by long chains of amino acids bound together by peptide linkages (Matthews, 1975). Pepsin is the enzyme in the stomach that is capable of digesting essentially all the different proteins present in the diet, including collagen. Collagen is a major constituent of the intercellular connective tissue of meats and must be first digested to permit access of other digestive enzymes. Pepsin is optimally active at a pH of about 2, splitting proteins by the process of hydrolysis at the peptide linkages between the amino acids. Upon leaving the stomach, the protein products in the form of proteoses, peptones, and large polypeptides are attacked by pancreatic enzymes, especially trypsin. Pancreatic enzymes are capable of hydrolyzing all the partial breakdown products of proteins to peptides, and even to the final stage of amino acids. The epithelial cells lining the small intestine also contain several different enzymes for hydrolyzing the final peptide linkages. All the proteolytic enzymes, including those of the gastric fluid, pancreatic fluid, and lining intestinal epithelial cells, are specific for hydrolyzing individual types of peptide linkages. This accounts for the large number of proteolytic enzymes and the fact that rarely can a single enzyme digest protein all the way to its constituent amino acid.

Most proteins are absorbed from the gastrointestinal tract as amino acids using active transport mechanisms (Matthews, 1975). As with monosaccharides, active transport systems located in the brush borders of the lining epithelial cells are specific for certain amino acids and function only in the presence of simultaneous transport of sodium ions. The existence of common carrier systems is suggested by the ability of one amino acid to interfere with the absorption of another amino acid. Amino acid absorption is rapid and occurs predominantly in the duodenum and jejunum. When food has been properly chewed and ingested in appropriate amounts, about 98% of all proteins become either amino acids or small peptides, usually dipeptides.

FATS. Triglycerides or neutral fats are the most common fats present in the diet. Cholesterol is derived from fats and is metabolized in a manner similar to fats, accounting for its dietary classification as a fat. Essentially all digestion of fat occurs in the small intestine. The first step in fat digestion is to break the fat globules into small sizes, so that water-soluble digestive enzymes can act on the surfaces of the globules. This process is called *emulsification* of fat and is achieved under the influence of bile salts present in bile. Subsequently, lipases attack the surface of the fat globules.

The most important enzyme for the digestion of fats is pancreatic lipase, which is present in the pancreatic secretions. Lining epithelial cells of the small intestine also contain enteric lipase. Both of these lipase enzymes act in a similar manner to cause hydrolysis of fat. Eventually, most of the triglycerides of the diet are split into monoglycerides, free fatty acids, and glycerol. Bile salts form micelles, which dissolve in water and act as a transport medium to carry the monoglycerides and free fatty acids to the lining epithelial cells of the gastrointestinal tract for absorption.

Absorption of fat occurs by diffusion through the lining epithelial cells. First, however, the monoglycerides and fatty acids must be transported to these epithelial cells by the bile salt micelles. After releasing fat, the bile salt micelles diffuse back into the chyme to absorb still more monoglycerides and fats for transport to the epithelial cells. In the presence of adequate amounts of bile salts to provide this "ferrying mechanism," about 97% of all fat is absorbed. In the absence of bile salts, essentially no cholesterol and only 5% to 60% of dietary fat is absorbed (Guyton, 1986d). Undigested triglycerides are only minimally absorbed, because bile acid micelles will not dissolve them for transport to the epithelial cells.

Bile salts are actively absorbed from the distal ileum after serving their function of ferrying fats to the lining epithelial cells of the gastrointestinal tract for absorption. These reabsorbed bile salts are then available for secretion into the bile and return to the upper small intestine. This bile salt circulation limits fecal loss of bile salts to less than 15%. Surgical resection of the ileum leads to the passage of bile salts into the large intestine. This causes irritation of the epithelial lining and results in severe diarrhea. Indeed, a complication of small bowel bypass operations for the treatment of morbid obesity is persistent diarrhea.

In the lining epithelial cell, many of the absorbed monoglycerides are further digested into glycerol and fatty acids by an epithelial cell lipase. Free fatty acids are subsequently reconstituted into triglycerides. The resulting triglycerides aggregate with absorbed cholesterol onto protein-coated globules known as *chylomicrons*. Chylomicrons are extruded from the lining epithelial cell and enter the lymphatic channels present in the villi. Ultimately, the chylomicrons enter the circulation through the thoracic duct.

Certain short-chain fatty acids are absorbed directly into the portal vein blood rather than being converted into triglycerides and absorbed into the lymphatics. The reason for this difference between short- and long-chain fatty acid absorption is presumed to be the greater water solubility of short-chain fatty acids, which allows direct diffusion of substances from the lining epithelial cells into the capillary blood of the villus.

Absorption in the Large Intestine

On the average, about 750 ml of chyme passes through the ileocecal valve daily. Most of the water and electrolytes in this chyme are absorbed in the colon, usually leaving less than 100 ml of fluid to be excreted in the feces. Almost all ions are also absorbed, leaving less than 1 mEq of sodium or chloride ions to be lost in the feces. Most of this absorption occurs in the proximal half of the colon, whereas the distal colon functions principally as a storage area.

The mucosa of the large intestine, like that of the small intestine, can actively absorb sodium ions, which leads to simultaneous absorption of chloride ions along the resulting electrical gradient. In addition, the mucosa of the large intestine actively secretes bicarbonate ions in exchange for chloride ions. The bicarbonate ions help to neutralize the acidic end products of bacterial action in the colon.

Numerous bacteria, especially colon bacilli, are present in the proximal colon. Substances formed as a result of bacterial activity include vitamin K, vitamin B_{12}, thiamin, riboflavin, and various gases (see Chapter 34).

REFERENCES

Atanassova E, Papasova M. Gastrointestinal motility. Int Rev Physiol 1977;12:35–69.

Bloom SR. Gastrointestinal hormones. Int Rev Physiol 1977;12:71–103.

Boucheir IAD. The medical treatment of gallstones. Annu Rev Med 1980;31:59–77.

Boyer JL. New concepts of mechanisms of hepatocyte bile formation. Physiol Rev 1980;60:303–26.

Brocke-Utne JG, Rubin J, Downing JW, Dimopoulos GE, Moshal MG, Naicker M. The administration of metoclopramide with atropine. A drug interaction effect on the gastrointestinal sphincter in man. Anaesthesia 1976;31:186–90.

Dickray G. Comparative biochemistry and physiology of gut hormones. Annu Rev Physiol 1979;41:83–95.

Forth W, Rummel W. Iron absorption. Physiol Rev 1973;53:724–92.

Gelman SI. Disturbances in hepatic blood flow during anesthesia and surgery. Arch Surg 1976;111:881–4.

Gerolami A, Sartes JC. Biliary secretion and motility. Int Rev Physiol 1977;12:223–56.

Greenway CV, Stark RD. Hepatic vascular bed. Physiol Rev 1971;51:23–65.

Grossman MI. Neural and hormonal regulation of gastrointestinal function: an overview. Annu Rev Physiol 1979;41:27–33.

Guyton AC. Textbook of Medical Physiology, 7th ed. Philadelphia: WB Saunders, 1986a:835.

Guyton AC. Textbook of Medical Physiology, 7th ed. Philadelphia: WB Saunders, 1986b:754.

Guyton AC. Textbook of Medical Physiology, 7th ed. Philadelphia: WB Saunders, 1986c:770.

Guyton AC. Textbook of Medical Physiology, 7th ed. Philadelphia: WB Saunders, 1986d:787.

Hirschowitz BI. H-2 histamine receptors. Annu Rev Pharmacol Toxicol 1979;19:203–44.

Jacobson ED. The gastrointestinal circulation. Annu Rev Physiol 1968;30:133–46.

Jones RS, Myers WC. Regulation of hepatic biliary secretion. Annu Rev Physiol 1979;41:67–82.

Kappas A, Alvares AP. How the liver metabolizes foreign substances. Sci Am 1975;232:22–31.

Likhite VL. Immunological impairment and susceptibility to infection after splenectomy. JAMA 1976;236:1376–7.

Matthews DM. Intestinal absorption peptides. Physiol Rev 1975;55:537–608.

Olsen WA. Carbohydrate absorption. Med Clin North Am 1974;58:1387–95.

Richardson PDI. Physiologic regulation of the hepatic circulation. Fed Proc 1982;41:2111–6.

Rothman SS. The digestive enzymes of the pancreas: a mixture of inconstant proportions. Annu Rev Physiol 1977;39:373–89.

Strunin L. Organ perfusion during controlled hypotension. Br J Anaesth 1975;47:793–8.

Turnberg LA. Absorption and secretion of salt and water by the small intestine. Digestion 1973;9:357–81.

Wood JD. Neurophysiology of Auerbach's plexus and control of intestinal motility. Physiol Rev 1975;55:307–24.

CHAPTER 55

Skeletal
and Smooth Muscle

SKELETAL MUSCLE

An estimated 40% of the body is skeletal muscle, and another 5% to 10% is smooth and cardiac muscle (Guyton, 1986a). Sarcolemma is the cell membrane of the muscle fiber. At the ends of skeletal muscle fibers, surfaces of the sarcolemma fuse with tendon fibers, which form tendons that insert into bones. Each skeletal muscle fiber contains thousands of myofibrils, which, in turn, contain protein molecules known as *myosin filaments* and *actin filaments* (Lyman, 1979). Myofibrils are suspended inside skeletal muscle fibers in a matrix known as *sarcoplasm*. The sarcoplasm contains large amounts of potassium ions, protein enzymes, and mitochondria. Mitochondria provide adenosine triphosphate (ATP) needed by the myofibrils responsible for contraction of the muscle (Tregear and Marston, 1979). The sarcoplasm also contains an extensive endoplasmic reticulum known as the *sarcoplasmic reticulum*.

Action Potential

Contraction of skeletal muscle begins with generation of an action potential that elicits electrical currents that spread to the interior of the myofibril, where they cause the release of calcium ions from the sarcoplasmic reticulum. Indeed, a special feature of sarcoplasmic reticulum is its high content of calcium ions (Tada *et al,* 1978). Calcium ions initiate the chemical events of skeletal

muscle contraction (see the section entitled Mechanism of Action).

Characteristics of action potentials in myofibrils and nerve fibers are similar except that the velocity of conduction of 3 to 5 m sec^{-1} in myofibrils is slower than the velocity of conduction in large myelinated nerve fibers. Transmission of the action potential deep within the skeletal muscle to all myofibrils is by way of transverse (T) tubules. The T tubule action potentials in turn cause the sarcoplasmic reticulum to release calcium ions in the immediate vicinity of all myofibrils.

Mechanism of Action

Skeletal muscle contraction occurs by the sliding filament mechanism in which actin filaments slide inward among the myosin filaments (Caputo, 1978). At rest, the attractive forces between actin and myosin filaments are inhibited. Arrival of an action potential causes release of calcium ions into the sarcoplasm surrounding the myofibrils. These calcium ions bind to troponin and abolish its inhibitory effect on actin and myosin.

Skeletal muscle contraction will continue as long as calcium ions are present in high concentrations in the sarcoplasm. A calcium pump, however, located in the walls of the sarcoplasmic reticulum, pumps calcium ions out of the sarcoplasm back into the sarcoplasmic reticulum. This pump can concentrate calcium ions about 2000-fold inside the sarcoplasmic reticulum. As a result, the calcium ion concentration in the sarcoplasm around the myofibril remains low except after an action potential. Failure of the calcium pump results in sustained skeletal muscle contraction and marked increases in heat production leading to malignant hyperthermia.

Energy necessary for the contractile process and activity of the calcium pump that returns calcium ions back into the sarcoplasmic reticulum is derived from ATP. However, the amount of ATP present in a skeletal muscle fiber is sufficient to maintain full contraction for less than 1 second. This emphasizes the importance of rephosphorylation of adenosine diphosphate (ADP) to form ATP. The energy source for this rephosphorylation is derived from oxidation of carbohydrates, lipids, and proteins, principally in mitochondria (see Chapter 58).

Blood Flow

Skeletal muscle blood flow can increase more than 20 times (a greater increase than in any other tissue of the body) during strenuous exercise (Bevegard and Shepherd, 1967). At rest, only 20% to 25% of the capillaries are open, and skeletal muscle blood flow is 3 to 4 ml 100 g^{-1} min^{-1}. During strenuous exercise, almost all skeletal muscle capillaries become patent. Opening of previously collapsed capillaries diminishes the distance that oxygen and other nutrients must diffuse from capillaries to skeletal muscle fibers and contributes an increased surface area through which nutrients can diffuse from blood.

Regulation of Skeletal Muscle Blood Flow

Increased skeletal muscle blood flow that occurs during exercise is caused primarily by local effects in skeletal muscles acting directly on the arterioles to cause vasodilation (Heistad and Abboud, 1974). Presumably, skeletal muscle activity lowers the concentration of oxygen, which, in turn, causes vasodilation because the vessel walls cannot maintain contraction in the absence of adequate amounts of oxygen. Alternatively, oxygen deficiency may cause release of vasodilator substances. Adenosine is a likely vasodilator substance that is released by oxygen lack, but potassium ions, acetylcholine, lactic acid, and carbon dioxide may also be important (Guyton, 1986b).

In addition to local tissue regulatory mecha-

nisms, skeletal muscles are innervated by vasoconstrictor fibers from the sympathetic nervous system. Maximally stimulated, these fibers produce vasoconstriction that can reduce skeletal muscle blood flow 75%. This degree of vasoconstriction is less than that which occurs in other tissues where blood flow may be reduced to almost zero. In addition to norepinephrine released from postganglionic sympathetic nerve endings, exercise evokes release of norepinephrine from the adrenal medulla, which also causes vasoconstriction of skeletal muscle vessels, presumably by acting on alpha-adrenergic receptors. Conversely, epinephrine released from the adrenal medulla stimulates beta-adrenergic receptors in skeletal muscle, producing vasodilation. Epinephrine may subserve the same function as sympathetic vasodilator fibers that are present in certain animals that release acetylcholine (Guyton, 1986b).

Exercise is associated with a centrally mediated stimulation of the sympathetic nervous system manifesting as vasoconstriction in nonmuscular tissues and increases in blood pressure. Excessive increases in blood pressure, however, are prevented by vascular vasodilation that occurs in the large tissue mass represented by skeletal muscle. A reduction in blood flow through most nonmuscular areas of the body makes more blood available to perfuse skeletal muscle. Furthermore, increased blood pressure also dilates skeletal muscle blood vessels and increases blood flow. Exceptions to vasoconstriction induced by exercise are the coronary and cerebral circulation, which have poor vasoconstrictor innervation. This is teleologically understandable because the heart and brain are as essential to the response to exercise as are the skeletal muscles. The increase in cardiac output that occurs during exercise results principally from local vasodilation in active skeletal muscles and subsequent increased venous return of blood back to the heart.

Innervation

Skeletal muscles are innervated by large myelinated nerve fibers that originate in motor neurons of the anterior horns of the spinal cord. Each motor neuron that leaves the spinal cord usually innervates several different skeletal muscle fibers. Skeletal muscle fibers innervated by a single motor nerve fiber are called a *motor unit* (Buchthal and Schmalbruch, 1980).

Skeletal muscle tone is a residual degree of skeletal muscle contraction that persists even at rest. Presumably, skeletal muscle tone reflects nerve impulses that are emitted continuously from the spinal cord. Denervation of skeletal muscle results in atrophy of the muscle. Rigor mortis, which occurs after death, is believed to be caused by loss of all the ATP in the muscle fibers, which is required in order for separation of the actin and myosin filaments to occur. Skeletal muscles remain rigid until skeletal muscle proteins are destroyed. This occurs in 15 to 25 hours after death and is due to autolysis caused by enzymes released from lysosomes.

Neuromuscular Junction

The neuromuscular junction is the site at which presynaptic nerve endings meet postsynaptic membranes of skeletal muscle fibers (*i.e.,* motor end-plates), approximately at the fibers' midpoint. As a result, the action potential spreads from the middle of the skeletal muscle fiber toward its two ends, thus ensuring almost coincident contraction of all myofibrils. The majority of skeletal muscle fibers have only a single neuromuscular junction.

Anatomy

The nerve fiber branches at its end to form a complex of nerve terminals that invaginate into the skeletal muscle fiber but lie entirely outside the sarcolemma to form the neuromuscular junction (see Fig. 8-1). The invagination of the sarcolemma is called the *synaptic trough,* and the space between the nerve terminal and the sarcolemma is called the *synaptic cleft.* The synaptic cleft is 20 to 30 nm wide and is filled with extracellular fluid. Subneural clefts are folds in the sarcolemma that greatly increase the area on the motor end-plate where the neurotransmitter, acetylcholine, can act.

Acetylcholine

Mitochondria in the nerve terminal supply energy for the synthesis of acetylcholine. Acetylcholine is synthesized in the cytoplasm of the nerve terminal but is rapidly absorbed into synaptic vesicles. There are an estimated 300,000 synaptic vesicles normally present in the nerve terminals of a single

neuromuscular junction. A nerve impulse arriving at the neuromuscular junction causes the release of about 300 synaptic vesicles containing acetylcholine into the synaptic cleft (Ceccarelli and Hurlbut, 1980). Calcium ions cause the vesicles of acetylcholine to pass through cell membranes by the process of exocytosis. In the absence of calcium ions or in the presence of excess magnesium ions, this release of acetylcholine is greatly reduced.

Acetylcholine diffuses across the synaptic cleft to excite skeletal muscles, but within 1 msec, the neurotransmitter is hydrolyzed (*i.e.,* inactivated) by acetylcholinesterase enzyme (true cholinesterase) in the subneural clefts. This rapid inactivation of acetylcholine prevents re-excitation after skeletal muscle fibers have recovered from the first action potential.

MECHANISM OF ACETYLCHOLINE EFFECTS. The mechanism by which acetylcholine increases permeability of skeletal muscle fiber membranes is presumed to reflect its action on protein molecules in muscle membranes designated acetylcholine receptors. Attachment of acetylcholine to this receptor causes the receptor to undergo a conformational change that increases the permeability of the skeletal muscle membranes to sodium ions. This conformational change is perceived to be an enlargement of channels through which sodium ions pass to enter the interior of membranes. It is estimated that for each molecule of acetylcholine that combines with the receptor, there is a flow of 50,000 ions across skeletal muscle membranes (Katz and Miledi, 1972). As a result, the resting transmembrane potential rises in this local area of the motor end-plate, creating a local action potential known as the *end-plate potential.* This end-plate potential initiates an action potential that spreads in both directions along the skeletal muscle fiber. The threshold potential at which skeletal muscle fibers are stimulated is about -50 mv.

ALTERED RESPONSES TO ACETYLCHOLINE. Drugs such as methacholine, carbachol, and nicotine have the same effect on skeletal muscle fibers as does acetylcholine. Unlike acetylcholine, however, these drugs are not destroyed rapidly by acetylcholinesterase. The nondepolarizing neuromuscular blocking drugs compete with acetylcholine for receptors and thus prevent changes in permeability of skeletal muscle membranes (see

Chapter 8). As a result, an end-plate potential does not occur and neuromuscular transmission is effectively prevented. Neostigmine and physostigmine are drugs that inactivate acetylcholinesterase enzyme, allowing accumulation of acetylcholine at the neuromuscular junction with resulting sustained stimulation of skeletal muscle fibers (see Chapter 9).

Myasthenia gravis is characterized by a reduction in the number of synaptic clefts as well as widening of the synaptic cleft. Furthermore, antibodies against the acetylcholine receptors may be present. These changes result in end-plate potentials that are too weak to initiate a propagated action potential.

Electromyogram

An electromyogram is the recording from skin electrodes of the electrical current that spreads from skeletal muscles to skin during simultaneous contraction of numerous skeletal muscle fibers.

Fasciculation

Fasciculation occurs when an entire motor unit contracts because of an abnormal impulse in motor nerve fibers, as accompanies destruction of anterior motor neurons by polio virus or following traumatic interruption of a nerve. As the peripheral nerve fibers die, spontaneous impulses are generated during the first few days and fasciculations manifest in the skeletal muscle.

Fibrillation

Fibrillation is a spontaneous impulse that appears in denervated skeletal muscle fibers 3 to 5 days following destruction of nerves to skeletal muscles. This reflects an intrinsic rhythmicity that develops in skeletal muscles that are released from innervation. After several weeks, atrophy of skeletal muscle fibers is so severe that fibrillation impulses cease. Electrodes must be inserted directly into the belly of the skeletal muscle to record fibrillation impulses.

SMOOTH MUSCLE

Smooth muscle, in contrast to skeletal muscle, is composed of fewer and shorter fibers, and the physical arrangement of smooth muscle fibers is unique. For example, smooth muscle is categorized as multiunit smooth muscle and visceral smooth muscle. Multiunit smooth muscle contraction is controlled almost exclusively by nerve signals, and spontaneous contractions rarely occur. Examples of multiunit smooth muscles are the ciliary muscles of the eye, iris of the eye, and smooth muscles of many large blood vessels. Visceral smooth muscle is characterized by cell membranes that contact adjacent cell membranes forming a functional syncytium that often undergoes spontaneous contractions, usually as a single unit. Visceral smooth muscle is prominent in the walls of the gastrointestinal tract, bile ducts, ureters, and smooth muscle.

Action Potential

Smooth muscles exhibit membrane potentials and action potentials similar to those that occur in skeletal muscle fibers. The normal resting transmembrane potential is about −60 mv, which is about 30 mv less negative than that in skeletal muscles. Action potentials in smooth muscles are characterized as spike potentials and action potentials with plateaus. Plateaus in the action potentials of smooth muscles lasting up to 30 seconds may occur in the ureters and uterus.

Visceral smooth muscle is often self-excitatory, with action potentials (pacemaker waves) occurring spontaneously in the absence of an extrinsic stimulus. These action potentials are particularly prominent in tubular structures, accounting for peristaltic motion in organs such as the ureter and gastrointestinal tract. Indeed, distention of a hollow viscus often evokes contraction of visceral smooth muscle.

Uterine Smooth Muscle

Uterine smooth muscle is characterized by a high degree of spontaneous electrical and contractile activity. Unlike the heart, there is no pacemaker, and the contraction process spreads from one cell to another at a rate of 1 to 3 cm sec^{-1}. Contractions of labor result in peak intrauterine pressures of 60 to 80 mmHg in the second stage. Resting uterine pressure during labor is about 10 mmHg. Movement of sodium ions appears to be the primary determinant in depolarization, whereas calcium ions are necessary for excitation–contraction coupling. Availability of calcium ions greatly influences the response of uterine smooth muscle to physiologic and pharmacologic stimulation and inhibition. Alpha excitatory and beta inhibitory receptors are present in the myometrium.

Mechanism of Contraction

Smooth muscles contain both actin and myosin filaments, having chemical characteristics similar to, but not identical to, actin and myosin filaments in skeletal muscles. In skeletal muscles, calcium ions activate contraction by binding with troponin, which causes activation of the actin filaments. It is doubtful that this same sequence occurs in smooth muscle because troponin has not been documented to even be present in smooth muscle cells (Guyton, 1986c). Instead, in smooth muscles, calcium ions excite ATPase activity of myosin filaments, which is believed to initiate contraction of smooth muscles. Despite these differences, it is clear that the sliding filament mechanism operates in smooth muscles as well as in skeletal muscles.

The source of calcium ions differs in smooth muscles compared with that in skeletal muscles because the sarcoplasmic reticulum of smooth muscles is poorly developed. Most of the calcium ions that cause contraction of smooth muscles enter from extracellular fluid at the time of the action potential. The time required for this diffusion is 200 to 300 msec and is called the *latent period* before the contraction begins. This latent period is about 50 times greater than for skeletal muscles. Subsequent relaxation of smooth muscles is achieved by a calcium pump that pumps calcium ions back into extracellular fluid or into the sarcoplasmic reticulum. This calcium pump is very slow-acting in comparison with the fast-acting sarcoplasmic reticulum pump in skeletal muscles. As a result, the duration of smooth muscle contractions is often seconds rather than milliseconds as is characteristic of skeletal muscles.

Neuromuscular Junction

A neuromuscular junction similar to that of skeletal muscles does not occur in smooth muscles. Instead, nerve fibers branch diffusely on top of a sheet of smooth muscle fibers without making actual contact. These nerve fibers secrete their neurotransmitter into an interstitial fluid space a few microns from the smooth muscle cells. Two different neurotransmitters, acetylcholine and norepinephrine, are secreted by the autonomic nervous system nerves that innervate smooth muscles. Acetylcholine is an excitatory neurotransmitter for smooth muscles at some sites and functions as an inhibitory neurotransmitter at other sites. Norepinephrine exerts the reverse effect of acetylcholine. It is believed that the presence of specific excitatory or inhibitory receptors in the membranes of smooth muscle fibers determines the response to acetylcholine or norepinephrine (Bolton, 1979). When the neurotransmitter interacts with an inhibitory receptor instead of an excitatory receptor, the membrane potential of the muscle fiber becomes more negative (*i.e.,* hyperpolarized).

Non-Nervous Stimulation

It is estimated that at least one half of all smooth muscle contraction is initiated by stimulatory factors acting directly on smooth muscles and not by action potentials. Examples of non-nervous stimulating events are local tissue factors such as lack of oxygen, excess carbon dioxide, and increased concentrations of hydrogen ions, all of which cause local vasodilation by direct effects on smooth muscles. In addition, hormones may cause excitatory or inhibitory effects on smooth muscle. Indeed, smooth muscle spasm may persist for hours in response to norepinephrine, antidiuretic hormone, or angiotensin. It is believed that local factors and hormones cause smooth muscle contraction by activating the calcium ion mechanism.

REFERENCES

Bevegard BS, Shepherd JT. Regulation of the circulation during exercise in man. Physiol Rev 1967;47:178–213.

Bolton TB. Mechanisms of action of transmitters and other substances on smooth muscle. Physiol Rev 1979;59:606–718.

Buchthal F, Schmalbruch H. Motor unit of mammalian muscle. Physiol Rev 1980;60:90–142.

Caputo C. Excitation and contraction processes in muscle. Annu Rev Biophys Bioeng 1978;7:63–83.

Ceccarelli B, Hurlbut WP. Vesicle hypothesis of the release of quanta of acetylcholine. Physiol Rev 1980;60:396–442.

Guyton AC. Textbook of Medical Physiology, 7th ed. Philadelphia: WB Saunders, 1986a:120.

Guyton AC. Textbook of Medical Physiology, 7th ed. Philadelphia: WB Saunders, 1986b:336.

Guyton AC. Textbook of Medical Physiology, 7th ed. Philadelphia: WB Saunders, 1986c:136.

Heistad DD, Abboud FM. Factors that influence blood flow in skeletal muscle and skin. Anesthesiology 1974;41:139–56.

Katz B, Miledi R. The statistical nature of the acetylcholine potential and its molecular components. J Physiol 172;224:665–99.

Lyman RW. Kinetic analysis of myosin and actinomysin ATPase. Annu Rev Biophys Bioeng 1979;8:145–63.

Tada M, Yamamoto T, Tonomura Y. Molecular mechanism of active calcium transport by sarcoplasmic reticulum. Physiol Rev 1978;58:1–79.

Tregear RT, Marston SB. The crossbridge theory. Annu Rev Physiol 1979;41:723–36.

CHAPTER 56

Erythrocytes
and Leukocytes

ERYTHROCYTES

Erythrocytes (red blood cells) are the most abundant of all cells in the body (25 trillion of the estimated total 75 trillion cells), emphasizing their irreplaceable role in delivery of oxygen to tissues (Guyton, 1986a). Indeed, the major function of erythrocytes is to transport hemoglobin, which, in turn, carries oxygen from the lungs to tissues (see Chapter 50). In addition to their function of transporting hemoglobin, erythrocytes contain large amounts of carbonic anhydrase. This enzyme speeds the reaction between carbon dioxide and water, making it possible to transport carbon dioxide from tissues to the lungs for elimination. Also, hemoglobin in erythrocytes is an excellent acid–base buffer, providing about 70% of the buffering power of whole blood (see Chapter 51).

Anatomy

Erythrocytes are biconcave disks with a mean diameter of 8μ. The shape of these cells can change greatly, conforming to the capillaries that erythrocytes must pass through. The average number of erythrocytes in each milliliter of plasma varies with the person's sex and barometric pressure. When the hematocrit is 40% to 45% and the quantity of hemoglobin in each erythrocyte is normal, the whole blood of an adult male contains an average of 16 g of hemoglobin in every 100 ml of plasma (*i.e,* 16 g dl^{-1}). The hemoglobin concen-

tration in an average adult female is 14 g dl^{-1}. Each gram of pure hemoglobin is capable of combining with about 1.34 ml of oxygen.

Site of Production

The bone marrow of almost all bones produces erythrocytes until one is about 5 years of age. The marrow of long bones, except for the proximal portions of the humerus and tibia, becomes fatty and produces few or no erythrocytes after one is about 20 years of age. After age 20 years, most erythrocytes are produced in the marrow of the membranous bones, including the vertebrae, sternum, ribs, and pelvis.

Erythrocytes are derived from hemocytoblasts that are being continually formed in bone marrow. Formation of hemoglobin is initiated in the basophil erythroblast. Cells in the reticulocyte stage pass into capillaries by squeezing through pores of the capillary membrane. This process is known as *diapedesis.* The remaining endoplasmic reticulum in the reticulocyte continues to produce a small amount of hemoglobin for 1 to 2 days, after which the endoplasmic recticulum completely disappears. In normal blood, the total proportion of reticulocytes among all the cells is slightly less than 1%. Once the endoplasmic reticulum has been completely resorbed, the cell is considered a mature erythrocyte.

When bone marrow produces erythrocytes at a rapid rate, many of the cells are released into the blood before they are mature cells. For example, during rapid erythrocyte production, the percent of circulating reticulocytes may increase from less than 1% to as high as 30% to 50%.

Control of Production

The total mass of erythrocytes in the circulation is regulated within narrow limits so that the number of cells is optimal to provide tissue oxygenation without an excessive number that would adversely increase viscosity of the blood and reduce tissue blood flow. It is not the concentration of erythrocytes in the blood that controls the rate of their production but rather the ability of cells to transport oxygen to tissues in relation to tissue demand for oxygen. Any event that causes the amount of oxygen transported to the tissues to decrease, as in the presence of anemia, chronic pulmonary disease, or cardiac failure will stimulate production of erythrocytes by the bone marrow. Destruction of bone marrow by x-ray or drugs causes hyperplasia of remaining bone marrow.

Erythropoietin

Erythropoietin is a glycoprotein produced in response to arterial hypoxemia and transported to the bone marrow to produce erythrocytes. The only means by which arterial hypoxemia stimulates bone marrow to produce erythrocytes is through erythropoietin (Peschle, 1980). It is speculated that hypoxia in the kidney evokes release of renal erythropoietic factor into the circulation. This enzyme acts on a globulin to split away the erythropoietin molecule. Erythropoietin circulates in the blood for about 24 hours, and, during this time, acts on bone marrow to cause erythropoiesis. The absence of kidneys removes the source of renal erythropoietic factor, which is consistent with the chronic anemia that accompanies renal failure.

Arterial hypoxemia results in formation of erythropoietin within minutes, but almost no new erythrocytes appear in the blood before 2 days, and the maximal new rate of erythrocyte production (6–8 times normal) does not occur until 5 days (Guyton, 1986a). After this maximum is reached, erythrocytes continue to be produced at an increased rate as long as the hypoxic stimulus persists. It is presumed that erythropoietin exerts a predominant effect on increasing the rate of divi-

sion of hemocytoblasts. When arterial hypoxemia dissipates, erythropoietin production decreases to zero almost immediately, followed in a few days by a similar decline in erythrocyte production. Erythrocyte production remains at a low level until enough cells have lived out their life spans, thus reducing the number of circulating erythrocytes to a level consistent with normal tissue oxygenation (*i.e.,* a negative feedback mechanism).

Vitamins Necessary for Formation

Cyanocobalamin (vitamin B_{12}) is necessary for the synthesis of deoxyribonucleic acid (DNA) (see Chapter 34). As a result, lack of this vitamin causes failure of nuclear maturation and division, which is particularly evident in rapidly proliferating cells such as erythrocytes. In addition to failing to proliferate rapidly, maturation failure occurs, as reflected by erythroblast cells in bone marrow that become larger than normal, developing into megaloblasts and macrocytes. Macrocytes have a weak cell membrane, causing them to exhibit a shorter life span than nomal erythrocytes.

The amount of vitamin B_{12} required each day to maintain normal erythrocyte maturation is less than 1 μg and the normal store in the liver is about 1000 times this amount. As a result, many months of impaired vitamin B_{12} absorption are necessary before maturation failure anemia manifests.

Folic acid is also necessary for maturation of erythrocytes. This vitamin, like vitamin B_{12}, is required for the formation of DNA and synthesis of ribonucleic acid (RNA).

Destruction

Erythrocytes normally circulate an average of 120 days after leaving the bone marrow. Mature erythrocytes lack a nucleus, mitochondria, and endoplasmic reticulum but still possess cytoplasmic enzymes capable of metabolizing glucose to form adenosine triphosphate (ATP). This ATP acts to maintain the (1) erythrocyte cell membrane, (2) transport of ions across the cell membrane, and (3) iron in the ferrous rather than ferric form. Indeed, the ferric form of iron causes the formation of methemoglobin, which will not transport oxygen. With increasing cell age, the metabolic systems of erythrocytes decline and cell membranes become fragile. Many fragile erythrocytes rupture in the spleen. Hemoglobin released from ruptured erythrocytes is almost immediately phagocytized by recticuloendothelial cells. Iron is released from hemoglobin back into the blood to be carried by transferrin either to bone marrow for production of new erythrocytes or to the liver and other tissues for storage as ferritin. The heme portion of the hemoglobin molecule is converted by the reticuloendothelial cells into bilirubin.

BLOOD GROUPS

At least 30 antigens, including A, B, O, Rh, M, N, P, Kell, Duffy, and Lewis, have been found on cell membranes of erythrocytes. Some of these antigens are highly antigenic (*e.g.,* A, B, O, Rh), whereas others are more important for establishing parentage. Blood is divided into different groups and types on the basis of the antigens present on cell membranes.

ABO Antigen System

Type A and type B antigens can occur alone or in combination on cell membranes of erythrocytes. Furthermore, cell membranes of erythrocytes may lack both these antigens. The presence or absence of these antigens is determined genetically. Blood is grouped for transfusion as A, B, O, or AB on the basis of the ABO antigen systems (Table 56-1). Based on the prevalence of different blood types among White Americans, it is obvious that the O and A genes occur frequently, whereas the gene for the B antigen is rare (Table 56-1). There are six possible combinations of genes resulting in six different genotypes. In the absence of the A or B antigen, the opposite antibody is present in the circulation (Table 56-1). These antibodies are gamma globulins, most often being immunoglobulin M or G molecules.

It seems paradoxical that antibodies are produced in the absence of the respective antigen on cell membranes of erythrocytes. It is likely that small amounts of group A and B antigens enter the body by way of food or bacteria, thus initiating the development of corresponding antibodies. Indeed, immediately after birth, the circulating level of antibodies to group A or B antigens is almost zero. It is only at 2 to 8 months of age that one begins to produce antibodies to the antigen not present on erythrocyte cell membranes. A maximal titer of antibodies is usually reached by 8 to 10 years of age and then gradually declines with increasing age. (Guyton, 1986b).

Blood Typing

Blood typing is the *in vitro* mixing of a drop of the patient's blood with plasma containing antibodies against the A or B antigen. This mixture is observed under a microscope for the presence or absence of agglutination. Using this procedure, blood can be typed as O, A, B, or AB. Cross-matching is the procedure that determines compatibility of the patient's blood with the donor's erythrocytes and plasma. Failure of agglutination when the erythrocytes from the donor and plasma from the recipient are mixed and when the erythrocytes of the recipient are mixed with plasma from the donor confirms compatibility.

Rh Blood Types

There are six common types of Rh antigens, designated C, D, E, c, d, and e, which are collectively known as the *Rh factor*. Only the C, D, and E antigens are sufficiently antigenic to cause develop-

---

Table 56-1
ABO Antigen System

Blood Type	Incidence (%)	Genotype	Antigens (Agglutinogens)	Antibodies (Agglutinins)
O	47	OO		Anti-A, Anti-B
A	41	OA or AA	A	Anti-B
B	9	OB or BB	B	Anti-A
AB	3	AB	A and B	

ment of anti-Rh antibodies that are capable of causing transfusion reactions. A person with C, D, and E antigens on erythrocyte cell membranes is Rh positive. A person is Rh negative when erythrocyte cell membranes contain c, d, and e antigens. Genes for the Rh factor are dominant, such that to be Rh negative, a person must have no genes that code for Rh-positive factors. About 85% of white Americans are Rh positive. Typing for Rh factors is performed in a manner similar to that for typing for ABO antigens (see the section entitled Blood Typing). Antibodies to Rh antigens, however, are much less potent in evoking agglutination than are the antibodies to the A and B antigens.

A person who is Rh negative develops antibodies only when exposed to erythrocytes containing the C, D, and E antigens. The development of antibodies is slow, but with multiple exposures, an Rh-negative person becomes strongly sensitized.

If an Rh-negative person receives Rh-positive blood, no immediate reaction occurs. In some people, however, antibodies develop in sufficient amounts after 2 to 4 weeks to cause agglutination of transfused cells that are still circulating. These cells are then hemolyzed in the reticuloendothelial system, producing a delayed and usually mild transfusion reaction. On subsequent transfusion of Rh-positive blood to this same person, however, the severity of the transfusion reaction is greatly enhanced and can be similar to reactions resulting from ABO incompatibility.

An Rh-negative mother having her first Rh-positive child does not usually develop sufficient antibodies to cause a reaction in the fetus. During the second pregnancy, however, antibodies to the Rh factor develop more rapidly and can cause hemolysis in the Rh-positive fetus (*i.e.,* erythroblastosis fetalis).

The Rh-negative mother typically becomes sensitized to the Rh-positive factor in her child during the first few days following birth of the baby, when large amounts of degenerating products from the placenta release their Rh-positive antigens into the maternal circulation. If this Rh-positive antigen is destroyed at this time, before it can initiate an antibody response, the mother will not be sensitized to the Rh-positive factor for subsequent pregnancies. This is achieved by injecting serum containing antibodies against the antigen, which destroys the circulating Rh factor before it can evoke the formation of antibodies.

Transfusion Reactions

Transfusion of blood from an ABO group that is different than that of the recipient results in agglutination of the transfused erythrocytes by antibodies present in the plasma of the recipient. Agglutination of the recipient's erythrocytes is less likely because antibodies in the incompatible blood are rapidly diluted in the recipient's plasma. In addition to agglutination, this antigen–antibody interaction may result in immediate hemolysis of the transfused erythrocytes. Hemolysis reflects activation of the complement system, which releases proteolytic enzymes that rupture cell membranes of erythrocytes. Indeed, blockage of blood vessels by agglutinated erythrocytes and concomitant intravascular hemolysis are well-recognized hazards of transfusion of mismatched or incompatible blood. Nevertheless, immediate intravascular hemolysis is less common than agglutination, presumably reflecting the need for very high titers of antibody to evoke hemolysis. Furthermore, a different type of antibody known as *hemolysins* seem to be necessary for hemolysis to occur. Ultimately, however, even agglutination leads to hemolysis of agglutinated erythrocytes.

When the rate of hemolysis is rapid, the plasma concentration of hemoglobin may exceed the binding capacity of haptoglobin, and free hemoglobin continues to circulate. This free hemoglobin is converted to bilirubin, and jaundice may occur. Nevertheless, if liver function is normal, jaundice usually does not appear unless more than 300 to 500 ml of blood is hemolyzed in less than a day (Guyton, 1986b). Acute renal failure often accompanies a severe transfusion reaction.

Pyrogenic reactions manifesting as chills and fever result from proteins in the transfused plasma to which the recipient is allergic.

TISSUE TYPING

It is possible to type tissues in much the same way that blood is typed. For example, the most important antigens that cause rejection of transplanted tissue are the HLA antigens (Amos and Ward, 1975). There are at least 50 different antigens on tissue cell membranes that are determined by four separate genes (Cunningham, 1977). These same HLA antigens are present on cell membranes of leukocytes. As a result, tissue typing can be accomplished by determining the types of antigens on membranes of lymphocytes separated from blood of the recipient. Some HLA antigens are poorly antigenic, negating the need for precise tissue matching of all antigens.

LEUKOCYTES

Leukocytes are formed partially in bone marrow (granulocytes and monocytes) and partially in lymph tissues (lymphocytes and plasma cells). These cells are selectively transported to areas of inflammation, providing a rapid defense against invading organisms.

Classification

The six different types of leukocytes present in blood are classified as (1) polymorphonuclear neutrophils, (2) polymorphonuclear eosinophils, (3) polymorphonuclear basophils, (4) monocytes, (5) lymphocytes, and (6) plasma cells (Table 56-2). A seventh type of cell present in the circulation is platelets, derived from megakaryocytes in bone marrow. The three types of polymorphonuclear cells are termed *granulocytes* because of their granular appearance. Granulocytes and monocytes protect the body against invading organisms by the process of phagocytosis. Lymphocytes destroy invading organisms by attaching to them.

An adult has about 7000 leukocytes and 300,000 platelets in every milliliter of blood. Approximately 62% of leukocytes are neutrophils, 30% lymphocytes, 5% lymphocytes, and 2% eosinophils (Table 56-2).

Formation

Polymorphonuclear cells and monocytes are normally formed and stored in bone marrow for subsequent release. Typically, about three times as many granulocytes are stored in bone marrow as circulate in blood, representing about a 6-day supply of these cells. Lymphocytes and plasma cells are produced in various lymph organs. These lymph organs include the lymph glands, spleen, thymus, tonsils, and lymphoid tissue in the gastrointestinal tract. Megakaryocytes are formed in bone marrow and subsequently fragment into smaller portions known as *thrombocytes,* or *platelets.*

Life Span

The life span of leukocytes in the blood is short. For example, once granulocytes are released from bone marrow, the life span in blood is 6 to 8 hours, followed by another 2 to 3 days in tissues. In the presence of infection, the life span in the circulation and tissues is even less, as granulocytes proceed rapidly to the infected area, ingest the foreign organism and, in this process, are also destroyed.

Monocytes rapidly leave the circulation, passing through capillary membranes into tissues. Once in tissues, monocytes persist for months or even years unless destroyed in the process of performing phagocytosis. As such, these cells form the basis of the tissue macrophage system.

Lymphocytes enter the circulatory system continually, along with drainage of lymph from lymph nodes. These cells enter tissues and then re-enter lymph, thus continually circulating through tissues.

The 300,000 platelets in each milliliter of blood are replaced about every 10 days. Therefore, about 30,000 platelets are formed each day for every milliliter of blood.

Table 56-2
Classification of Leukocytes

	Total (ml of plasma) (range)	% of Total (range)
Granulocytes		
Neutrophils	3000–6000	55–65
Eosinophils	0–300	1–3
Basophils	0–100	0–1
Monocytes (macrophages)	300–500	3–6
Lymphocytes	1500–3500	25–35

Characteristics

Neutrophils are mature cells in the blood and can destroy bacteria and viruses. Conversely, monocytes are immature cells in the blood but, on entering tissues, swell to become macrophages, which are capable of phagocytosis.

Diapedesis

Neutrophils and monocytes can squeeze through the pores of blood vessels by diapedesis. Specifically, even though the pore is smaller than the leukocyte, a small portion of the cell slides through the pore at a time, the portion sliding through being momentarily constricted to the size of the pore.

Chemotaxis

Chemotaxis is the phenomenon by which different chemical substances in tissues cause neutrophils and monocytes to move either toward or away from the chemical. For example, inflamed tissue may contain several chemicals (*i.e.,* bacterial toxins, degenerative products of inflamed tissues, products of the complement complex, reaction products caused by plasma clotting in the inflamed area) that cause neutrophils and monocytes to move toward (*i.e.,* chemotaxis) the inflamed area (Guyton, 1986c). Chemotaxis is effective up to 100 μ away from an inflamed tissue. Since almost no tissue is more than 30 to 50 μ away from a capillary, the chemotactic signal can rapidly attract large numbers of leukocytes to the inflamed area. Chemotaxis may be impaired by inhaled anesthetics (see Chapter 2).

Phagocytosis

The most important function of neutrophils and macrophages is phagocytosis. Neutrophils and monocytes are known as phagocytes. On approaching a particle to be phagocytized, the neutrophil projects pseudopodia around the particle. These pseudopodia fuse, creating a chamber containing the ingested particle. Phagocytosis is likely to occur when the (1) surface of the particle is rough, (2) particle is electropositive, and (3) particle is recognized as foreign. Most natural substances of the body, including neutrophils and monocytes, have electronegative surfaces. Conversely, dead tissues and foreign particles are often electropositve and, thus, attracted to phagocytes. Foreign particles also evoke the production of antibodies that adhere to cell membranes of these particles and make them vulnerable to phagocytosis.

A neutrophil can phagocytize 5 to 20 bacteria before it becomes inactivated and dies (Guyton, 1986c). Monocytes that have become macrophages are more powerful than neutrophils, being capable of phagocytizing as many as 100 bacteria. Furthermore, these cells can phagocytize large particles, including whole erythrocytes, necrotic tissue, and dead neutrophils. In contrast, neutrophils are not capable of phagocytizing particles much larger than bacteria.

Neutrophils and macrophages contain lysosomes filled with proteolytic enzymes capable of digesting bacteria and other foreign particles. Lysosomes of macrophages also contain lipases, which digest thick lipid membranes of tubercle bacteria. Neutrophils can produce hydrogen peroxide, which exerts an antibacterial effect. Eventually, neutrophils are killed by toxic products released inside themselves from lysosomes.

Tissue Macrophage System

The majority of monocytes, on entering tissues and becoming macrophages, attach to tissues until they are needed for phagocytosis. The combination of mobile and fixed tissue macrophages is collectively called the *reticuloendothelial system.*

Macrophages in different tissues are designated by different names; for example, macrophages in the liver are known as Kupffer's cells; in lymph nodes, spleen, and bone marrow as reticulum cells; in alveoli of the lungs as alveolar macrophages; in subcutaneous tissues as histiocytes; and in the brain as microglia.

Kupffer's Cells

Kupffer's cells line hepatic sinuses and serve as a filtration system to remove bacteria that have entered the portal blood from the gastrointestinal tract. Indeed, these tissue macrophages are capable of removing almost all bacteria from the portal blood (see Chapter 54).

Reticulum Cells

Reticulum cells line sinuses of lymph nodes. These macrophages effectively phagocytize foreign particles as they pass through lymph nodes.

Invading organisms that manage to find their way into the general circulation are vulnerable to phagocytosis by reticulum cells in the spleen and bone marrow. The spleen is similar to lymph nodes except that blood rather than lymph flows through the substance of the spleen. The spleen is also important for the removal of abnormal platelets and erythrocytes.

Alveolar Macrophages

Alveolar macrophages are present in alveolar walls and can phagocytize invading organisms that are inhaled. If the phagocytized particles are digestible, the resulting products are released into the lymph. If the particles are not digestible (*e.g.,* carbon silica), the macrophages often form a giant cell capsule around the particle.

Histiocytes

Histiocytes are tissue macrophages that are present in subcutaneous tissues. These cells phagocytize invading organisms that gain access when the skin is broken. When local inflammation occurs in the subcutaneous tissues, histiocytes are stimulated to divide and form additional macrophages.

INFLAMMATION

Inflammation is a series of sequential changes that occur in tissues in response to injury. Tissue injury, whether it is due to bacteria or trauma, causes the local release of several substances, including histamine, bradykinin, and serotonin, into the surrounding fluids. These substances, particularly histamine, increase local blood flow as well as the local permeability of the capillaries, allowing large amounts of fluid and protein, including fibrinogen, to leak into tissues. Local extracellular edema results, and the extracellular fluid and lymphatic fluid coagulate because of the coagulating effects of fibrinogen present in extravasated fluid. As a result, brawny edema develops in the spaces surrounding damaged tissues.

Tissue spaces and lymphatics in the inflamed area are blocked by clots of fibrinogen; thus, fluid flow through this area is minimal. This effectively isolates the injured area from normal tissues and minimizes the dissemination of bacteria or toxic products. Staphylococci liberate potent cellular

toxins, causing the rapid onset of inflammation and walling off of the infected area. Conversely, streptococci cause less intense local tissue destruction, such that the walling off process develops slowly, allowing streptococci to spread extensively. As a result, streptococci have a greater tendency to produce disseminated and life-threatening infection than do staphylococci, even though staphylococci produce more intense local tissue damage.

Soon after inflammation begins, the inflamed area is invaded by neutrophils and macrophages. These cells immediately begin their function of phagocytosis. For example, this phagocytic function is provided by *in situ* tissue macrophages such as histiocytes in subcutaneous tissues, alveolar macrophages in the lungs, and microglia in the brain. In addition, the number of neutrophils in blood increases as much as fivefold (*i.e.,* leukocytosis) within a few hours following the onset of inflammation. Leukocytosis is stimulated by release of a chemical substance from the inflamed tissues known as *leukocytosis-inducing factor.* This factor is believed to dilate venous sinusoids of bone marrow, thus facilitating release of stored neutrophils. Products of inflamed tissues also stimulate movement of neutrophils into the inflamed area from the circulation (see the section entitled Chemotaxis). When neutrophils and macrophages engulf large numbers of bacteria and necrotic tissue, almost all the neutrophils and many of the macrophages die. The collection of dead leukocytes and necrotic tissue is known as *pus.* The pus cavity may digest its way to the exterior or into an internal cavity and thus discharge its contents. Alternatively, the pus cavity may remain closed, and, eventually, its contents will undergo autolysis and absorption into surrounding tissues.

LEUKOCYTOSIS DUE TO NONINFLAMMATORY CAUSES

Almost any factor that causes tissue damage, including operative trauma as well as acute hemorrhage and debilitating diseases, can cause leukocytosis. For example, an increased circulating concentration of neutrophils accompanies acute myocardial infarction, presumably reflecting release of leukocytosis-inducing factor from degenerating cardiac muscle. Even severe exercise lasting only 1 minute can cause the number of circulating neutrophils to increase threefold (*i.e.,* physiologic neutrophilia).

Eosinophils

Eosinophils normally constitute about 2% of circulating leukocytes. These cells are only weak phagocytes but enter the circulation in increased amounts following the ingestion of foreign proteins. It is speculated that eosinophils are important in detoxifying foreign proteins before they cause tissue damage. Eosinophils migrate into blood clots where they release profibrinolysin, which becomes activated to fibrinolysin, an enzyme that digests fibrin.

Eosinophils show a special propensity to collect at sites of antigen–antibody reactions in tissues. The total number of circulating eosinophils increases during allergic reactions, presumably because tissue reactions release products that selectively increase the production of eosinophils in the bone marrow. The most common cause of large increases in the circulating concentration of eosinophils is the presence of parasites in blood. This may reflect the role of eosinophils in detoxifying foreign proteins.

Basophils

Basophils in blood are similar to large mast cells located in tissues. Mast cells release heparin into blood, where it prevents coagulation and speeds removal of fat particles from blood after a meal. It is possible that basophils in blood perform a function similar to tissue mast cells.

Mast cells and basophils are important in allergic reactions, because immunoglobulin E antibodies attach selectively to the membranes of these cells (Capra and Edmundson, 1977). Subsequent attachment of antigen to these antibodies causes cell membranes to rupture, releasing chemical mediators, including histamine and bradykinin. These chemical mediators are responsible for many of the manifestations of allergic reactions.

AGRANULOCYTOSIS

Agranulocytosis is the acute cessation of production of leukocytes by bone marrow. Within 2 to 3 days, ulcers appear in the mouth and colon, reflecting the uninhibited growth of bacteria that normally populate these areas. Irradiation of the body by gamma rays associated with a nuclear explosion or exposure to drugs or chemicals containing benzene or anthracine nuclei (*e.g.,* sulfonamides, chloramphenicol, thiouracil) can cause acute bone marrow aplasia in which neither erythrocytes nor leukocytes are produced. Usually sufficient stem cells (*i.e.,* hemocystoblasts) remain after injury to allow recovery of bone marrow function if fatal infection is prevented by appropriate antibiotic therapy. This regeneration, however, may require several months.

IMMUNITY

Immunity is the capacity of the body to resist organisms or toxins that cause tissue damage. Acquired or adaptive immunity is due to (1) a special mechanism that forms antibodies (humoral immunity) and (2) sensitized lymphocytes (cellular immunity) that seek and destroy specific organisms and toxins. In addition, immunity may be innate, as reflected by phagocytosis, destruction of organisms by acidic digestive enzymes, and action of chemical compounds in the blood, such as lysozyme or properdin.

Antigens

Antigens are foreign proteins that initiate the process known as *acquired immunity*. Bacteria or toxins contain unique chemical compounds that differ from normal body proteins, resulting in their role as antigens. For a substance to be antigenic, it usually must have a molecular weight of greater than 8000 (Guyton, 1986d). Nevertheless, immunity against low–molecular-weight substances can occur if the material acts as a hapten and binds to a protein, the combination resulting in an antigenic response. Haptens that elicit such an immune response are usually drugs, chemical constituents in dust, or breakdown products of dandruff from animals.

Role of Lymphoid Tissue

Lymphoid tissue is present in lymph nodes and special lymph tissues such as submucosal areas of the gastrointestinal tract, spleen, bone marrow, tonsils, and adenoids. These locations are ideal for intercepting ingested or inhaled antigens as well as those that reach the circulation.

Lymphocytes in lymphoid tissue are categorized as either T- or B-lymphocytes. Cellular immunity is due to formation of sensitized lymphocytes by T cells. The T designation emphasizes the role of the thymus gland in the origin of these cells. Antibodies that provide humoral immunity are derived from B-lymphocytes. The designation as B-lymphocytes reflects their original discovery in birds in which the formation of these cells occurs in the bursa of Fabricius.

Most of the preprocessing of T-lymphocytes of the thymus occurs shortly before birth and for a few months after birth. Removal of the thymus gland after this time usually will not interfere with cellular immunity.

Most of the preprocessing of B-lymphocytes that prepares them to manufacture antibodies occurs before and shortly after birth. In humans, it is likely that this preprocessing occurs predominantly in the lymphoid tissue in the fetal liver and to a lesser extent in bone marrow and the gastrointestinal mucosa. After formation of processed T- and B-lymphocytes, these cells are delivered by the circulation to lymphoid tissue where they are trapped.

It is believed that during the processing of T- and B-lymphocytes, all those clones of lymphocytes capable of destroying the body's own tissues are self-destroyed because of their continual exposure to the body's antigens (Guyton, 1986d). This immune tolerance to the body's own tissues may diminish, resulting in autoimmune diseases such as thyroiditis, rheumatic fever, glomerulonephritis, myasthenia gravis, and lupus erythematosus.

Sensitized Lymphocytes

Sensitized lymphocytes are released from lymphoid tissue in response to the stimulus of a specific antigen in a manner that parallels antibody release. These cells subsequently pass from lymph into the circulation and are delivered to all tissues of the body. As with antibodies, lymphocyte memory cells are also formed, providing the mechanism for an exaggerated response when reexposure to the same antigen occurs. It is believed that T-lymphocytes become sensitized against

specific antigens by forming, on their cell surfaces, a type of antibody. Sensitized lymphocytes, on coming in contact with specific antigens, combine with the antigens, resulting ultimately in the destruction of antigens by direct and indirect mechanisms. Combination of sensitized lymphocytes with antigens also causes the release of transfer factor from lymphocytes. Transfer factor reacts with adjacent lymphocytes, causing them to also attack antigens (*i.e.,* amplifying effect). Another product of activated and sensitized lymphocytes is macrophage chemotactic factor, which attracts macrophages to the site of the reaction for phagocytosis of the resulting debris. Cellular immunity by sensitized lymphocytes is particularly important in protecting the body against certain viral diseases, in destroying early cancer cells, and in causing the rejection of transplanted tissues.

Antibodies

Prior to exposure to a specific antigen, clones of B-lymphocytes remain dormant in the lymphoid tissue. Entry of antigens into lymphoid tissues causes clones of B-lymphocytes specific for the antigens to undergo changes, eventually resulting in the formation of plasma cells capable of producing gamma globulin antibodies (*i.e.,* primary response) (Fig. 56-1) (Guyton, 1986d). Some B-lymphocytes, however, remain dormant in the

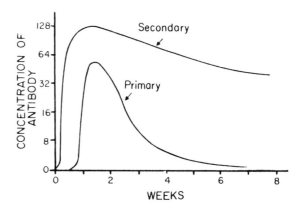

FIGURE 56-1. Time course of antibody response following primary and secondary injection of antigen. (From Guyton AC. Textbook of Medical Physiology. 7th ed. Philadelphia: WB Saunders, 1981:60. Reproduced by permission of the author and publisher.)

lymphoid tissue, functioning as memory cells. Subsequent exposure to the antigen causes these memory cells to participate in an exaggerated antibody response (*i.e.,* secondary response) compared with the primary response (Fig. 56-1) (Guyton, 1986d). The increased intensity and duration of the secondary response is the reason why vaccination is often achieved by injection of the antigen in multiple small doses several weeks apart.

Structure

Antibodies are gamma globulins grouped into five classes of immunoglobulins (*i.e.,* IgG, IgA, IgM, IgD, and IgE) (Table 56-3) (Roesch, 1983). About 75% of all antibodies are IgG. IgE antibodies constitute only a small percent of the total number of antibodies but are uniquely important in the mechanism of allergy. For example, an allergen is an antigen that reacts with a specific IgE antibody, leading to an allergic reaction. Urticaria results from antigen entering skin sites and evoking localized release of histamine. Hay fever results when the allergen–antibody reaction occurs in the nose in contrast to asthma, where the reaction occurs in the bronchioles of the lungs. Histamine seems to be primarily responsible for the symptoms of hay fever, whereas bronchospasm characteristic of asthma may be mainly due to leukotrienes (see Chapter 20). Indeed, antihistamines have beneficial effects in the treatment of hay fever; however, less effect is seen in their use for the prevention and treatment of asthma.

Immunoglobulins have molecular weights between 150,000 and 900,000. Each antibody that is specific for a particular antigen has a different organization of amino acids that lends steric shape. This steric shape fits the antigen and results in a rapid and tight chemical or physical bond between the antibody and the antigen (Capra and Edmundson, 1977).

Mechanism of Action

Antibodies act by direct effects on the antigen, activation of the complement system, or initiation of an anaphylactic reaction. Examples of direct effects of antibodies that destroy the antigens are (1) agglutination as occurs with transfusion of incompatible blood, (2) precipitation, (3) neutralization, and (4) lysis. More important, however, than these direct effects are the amplifying effects of the complement system or the anaphylactic response.

COMPLEMENT SYSTEM. Complement is a system of nine different enzyme precursors that are normally present in the plasma in an inactive form. These inactive complement enzymes are designated C1 through C9. Combination of an antibody with an antigen initiates a series of sequential (*i.e.,* cascade) reactions in the complement system. The resulting activated complement enzymes attack the antigen by a variety of mechanisms, including (1) lysis of the cell membrane, (2) facilitation of phagocytosis by the phenome-

---

Table 56-3
Properties of Immunoglobulins

	IgG	IgA	IgM	IgD	IgE
Location	Plasma, amniotic fluid	Plasma, saliva, tears	Plasma	Plasma	Plasma
Plasma Concentration (mg dl^{-1})	550–1900	60–333	45–145	0.3–30	Trace
Plasma Half-Time (days)	23	6	5	3	2.5
Function	Immunity and defense against infection	Topical defense against infection	Lysis of bacterial cells walls	?	Allergic reactions

(By permission, Roesch R. The Immune System. In: Stoelting RK, Dierdorf SF. Anesthesia and Co-Existing Disease. New York, Churchill Livingston, 1983:645.)

non of opsonization, (3) chemotaxis, (4) agglutination, (5) neutralization of viruses by alteration of their molecular structures, rendering them nonvirulent, and (6) inflammatory effects (Guyton, 1986d).

ANAPHYLACTIC REACTION. An anaphylactic reaction, although potentially harmful, can be protective in the sense of slowing the spread of infection by virtue of immobilizing the antigen. IgE antibodies are the class of immunoglobulins that are most likely to attach to cell membranes of circulating basophils or tissue mast cells. Subsequent attachment of antigens to these antibodies causes rupture of cell membranes and release of chemical mediators, including histamine, leukotrienes, and lysosomal enzymes. Chemotactic factors are also released, attracting neutrophils, macrophages, and eosinophils to the site of the antigen–antibody reaction. Eosinophils may be particularly important in phagocytizing the products of the antigen–antibody reactions (see the section entitled Eosinophils).

Interferons

Interferons are protein substances released by cells that are attacked by viruses (Burke, 1977)

(see Chapter 28). These substances prevent replication of either the RNA or DNA of the viruses, thus preventing any further damaging effects. Interferon is distributed by way of the circulation to all cells, providing protection beyond the affected cells.

REFERENCES

Amos DB, Ward FE. Immunogenetics of the HL-A system. Physiol Rev 1975;55:206–48.

Burke DC. The status of interferon. Sci Am 1977;236:42–50.

Capra JD, Edmundson AB. The antibody combining site. Sci Am 1977;236:50–9.

Cunningham BA. The structure and function of histocompatibility antigens. Sci Am 1977;237:96–107.

Guyton AC. Textbook of Medical Physiology, 7th ed. Philadelphia: WB Saunders, 1986a:42.

Guyton AC. Textbook of Medical Physiology, 7th ed. Philadelphia: WB Saunders, 1986b:70.

Guyton AC. Textbook of Medical Physiology, 7th ed. Philadelphia: WB Saunders, 1986c:51.

Guyton AC. Textbook of Medical Physiology, 7th ed. Philadelphia: WB Saunders, 1981d:60.

Peschle C. Erythropoiesis. Annu Rev Med 1980;31:303–14.

Roesch R. The Immune System. In: Stoelting RK, Dierdorf SF. Anesthesia and Co-Existing Disease. New York, Churchill Livingstone, 1983:645.

C H A P T E R   57

Hemostasis
and Blood Coagulation

HEMOSTASIS

Hemostasis in the presence of loss of integrity of a blood vessel is achieved by several mechanisms, including (1) vascular spasm, (2) formation of a platelet plug, (3) clot formation, and (4) growth of fibrous tissue into the blood clot to seal the break in the blood vessel (Guyton, 1986).

Vascular Spasm

The wall of a cut blood vessel immediately contracts, which serves to reduce flow of blood from the damaged vessel. This contraction results from neural reflexes initiated by pain impulses from the traumatized vessel as well as local myogenic initiated contraction. Vascular spasm is most intense in severely traumatized or crushed blood vessels. The sharply cut or transected blood vessel, as occurs during surgery, undergoes less vascular spasm, and blood loss is reduced less. Vascular spasm lasts 20 to 30 minutes, providing time for additional mechanisms of hemostasis to become active.

Platelet Plug

The second event in hemostasis is an attempt by platelets to form a plug in the opening of the blood vessel. Platelets are round or oval discs about $2\ \mu$ in diameter. When platelets come in contact with a damaged vascular surface, they begin to swell, become sticky, and secrete large amounts of adenosine diphosphate (ADP) as well as enzymes that cause formation of thromboxane A_2 in the plasma. The ADP and thromboxane A_2 activate adjacent platelets, causing them to adhere to the already activated platelets. These platelets accumulate to form a loose platelet plug. Subsequent attachment of fibrin threads to platelets results in a firm plug in the vessel opening. Prostacyclin, presumed to come primarily from the blood vessel wall, inhibits thrombosis.

The platelet plug mechanism is extremely important for closing minute breaks in small blood vessels that occur hundreds of times daily. When the number of platelets is reduced, small hemorrhagic areas appear under the skin and internally. Typically, the platelet plug does not occlude the lumen of the blood vessel.

Clot Formation

Formation of a blood clot in a severely traumatized blood vessel begins within 15 to 20 seconds (see the section entitled Blood Coagulation). Activator substances from the traumatized vascular wall and platelets initiate this process. After 3 to 6 minutes, the cut end of a blood vessel is filled with clot.

Growth of Fibrous Tissue

Invasion of a blood clot by fibroblasts causes formation of connective tissue throughout the clot.

Conversion of the clot to fibrous tissues is complete in 7 to 10 days.

BLOOD COAGULATION

More than 30 different substances that promote (procoagulants) or inhibit (anticoagulants) coagulation have been identified in blood and tissues (Ratnoff, 1974). Normally, anticoagulants predominate, and blood does not coagulate. When a blood vessel is transected or damaged, activity of the procoagulants in the area of damage becomes predominant and clot formation occurs. Continued clot formation occurs only where the blood is not flowing. This is true because the flow of blood dilutes thrombin and the other procoagulants released during the clotting process, thus preventing their concentration from rising high enough to sustain continued formation of clot (Goldsmith, 1974).

Within a few minutes after the clot is formed, it begins to contract and typically expresses most of the fluid from itself after 30 to 60 minutes. Platelets are necessary for this clot retraction to occur. Indeed, failure of clot retraction is an indication that the number of circulating platelets is inadequate. Normally, as the blood clot retracts, the edges of the broken blood vessel are pulled together, restoring the integrity of the vascular lumen.

Initiation of Coagulation

Initiation of coagulation requires activation of prothrombin by mechanisms that are stimulated by trauma to tissues, trauma to blood, or contact of blood with damaged epithelial cells or collagen. Regardless of the mechanism, the result is formation of prothrombin activator, which then facilitates the conversion of prothrombin to thrombin.

The two basic mechanisms by which prothrombin activator is formed are (1) the extrinsic pathway, which begins with trauma to tissues outside the vessel wall or with damage to the vascular wall, and (2) the intrinsic pathway, which begins in blood. In both the extrinsic and intrinsic pathways, a series of plasma proteins, often beta globulins, function as blood clotting factors (Table 57-1). Normally, these clotting factors exist as inactive forms of proteolytic enzymes, which, when activated, cause successive reactions of the clotting process. Blood coagulation culminates in formation of fibrin, following the interaction of more than a dozen proteins in a cascading series of proteolytic reactions (Fig. 57-1) (McNiece, 1983).

Extrinsic Pathway

The extrinsic pathway is stimulated to form prothrombin activator when blood comes into contact with traumatized vascular wall or extravascular tissues. Traumatized tissue releases a proteolytic en-

---

Table 57-1
Nomenclature of Blood Clotting Factors

Factor	Synonyms	Plasma Concentration ($\mu g\ ml^{-1}$)	Half-Time (hr)	Stability in Stored Whole Blood
I	Fibrinogen	2000 – 4000	95 – 120	No change
II	Prothrombin	150	65 – 90	No change
III	Thromboplastin			
IV	Calcium			
V	Proaccelerin	10	15 – 24	Half-time 7 days
VII	Proconvertin	0.5	4 – 6	No change
VIII	Antihemophilic factor	15	10 – 12	Half-time 7 days
IX	Christmas factor	3	18 – 30	No change
X	Stuart Prower factor	15	40 – 60	No change
XI	Plasma thromboplastin antecedent	5	45 – 60	Half-time 7 days
XII	Hageman factor	5	50 – 70	No change
XIII	Fibrin-stabilizing factor	20	72 – 120	No change

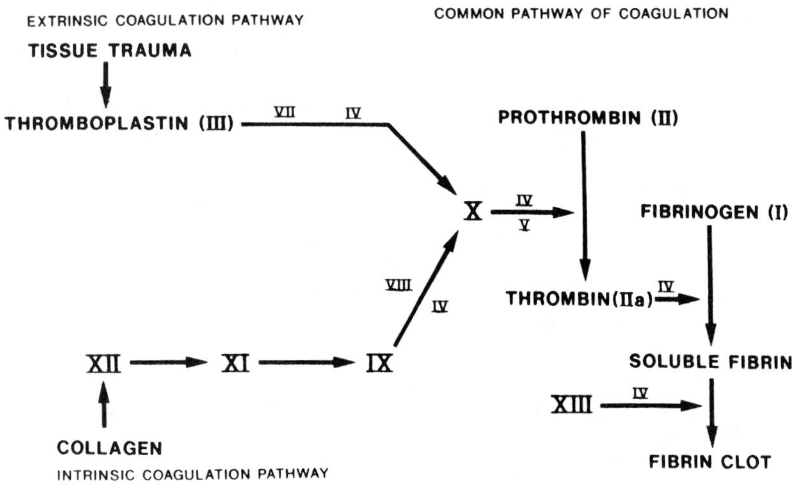

EXTRINSIC COAGULATION PATHWAY   COMMON PATHWAY OF COAGULATION

FIGURE 57-1. Schematic depiction of the extrinsic and intrinsic coagulation pathway culminating in the formation of a fibrin clot. (By permission, McNiece WL. Disorders of Coagulation. Stoelting RK, Dierdorf SF, eds: Anesthesia and Co-Existing Disease. New York, Churchill Livingstone Inc., 1983.)

zyme (tissue factor) and phospholipids from the tissue cell membranes, both of which initiate the clotting process (Fig. 57-1) (NcNiece, 1983). Calcium and factors V and VII are also necessary for the sequence of events that characterize the extrinsic pathway.

Intrinsic Pathway

The intrinsic pathway is stimulated to form prothrombin activator when there is trauma resulting in contact of factor XII and platelets in blood with collagen in the vascular wall (Fig. 57-1) (McNiece, 1983). Calcium and factors V and VIII are also necessary for the steps characteristic of the intrinsic pathway. The importance of calcium in the clotting process is emphasized by the ability of citrate or oxalate ions, which react with calcium, to prevent clotting of blood when it is removed from the body.

When blood is removed from the body and placed in a test tube, it is the intrinsic pathway alone that must initiate the coagulation process. Typically, this results from contact of factor VII and platelets with the wall of the container, leading to activation of the intrinsic pathway. If the surface of the container is very smooth, such as a siliconized surface, the clotting of blood is greatly slowed.

The extrinsic and intrinsic pathways differ with respect to the speed of their reactions. The intrinsic pathway proceeds slowly, usually requiring 2 to 6 minutes to cause clotting. Furthermore,

a variety of inhibitors act at different sites in the intrinsic pathway. Conversely, the formation of prothrombin activator by the extrinsic pathway is rapid, often resulting in the appearance of clot within 15 seconds.

Conversion of Prothrombin to Thrombin

Prothrombin activator is responsible for the conversion of prothrombin to thrombin. Prothrombin is an α_2-globulin present in the plasma in concentrations of about 15 mg dl^{-1} (Suttie and Jackson, 1977). It is an unstable protein and is easily split into smaller components, including thrombin.

Prothrombin is formed constantly in the liver. Failure of the liver to synthesize prothrombin leads to a decline in the plasma concentration below acceptable levels within 24 hours. Furthermore, vitamin K is required by the liver for normal formation of prothrombin. As a result, lack of vitamin K or severe liver disease may prevent normal prothrombin formation.

Conversion of Fibrinogen to Fibrin

Fibrinogen is a high–molecular-weight protein (340,000) present in the plasma in concentrations between 100 and 400 mg dl^{-1}. This clotting factor is formed in the liver, and severe liver dysfunction can cause an inadequate synthesis. Because of its large molecular weight, little fibrinogen normally leaks into interstitial fluids, accounting for the lack of coagulation that occurs in this fluid. When capillary permeability increases, however, as in the presence of inflammation, fibrinogen can enter interstitial fluids and initiate coagulation.

Thrombin is a proteolytic enzyme that acts on fibrinogen to remove two low–molecular weight peptides from each molecule of fibrinogen, resulting in a fibrin monomer that can polymerize with other fibrin monomers. A large number of fibrin monomers polymerize within seconds into long fibrin threads that form the reticulum of the clot. The strength of this fibrin clot is subsequently greatly enhanced by the action of fibrin-stabilizing factors, which is present in the plasma and is also released from adjacent platelets. Ultimately, the blood clot is composed of a meshwork of cross-linked fibrin threads that adhere to the damaged surfaces of blood vessels, entrapping platelets, erythrocytes, and plasma.

Prevention of Intravascular Clotting

The smoothness of the vascular endothelium, which prevents contact activation of the intrinsic clotting system, and a monomolecular layer of negatively charged protein on the inner layer of the vascular endothelium that repels clotting factors and platelets are the two factors that normally prevent intrinsic initiation of the clotting process (Wall and Harker, 1980). Damage to the endothelial wall disrupts its smoothness and destroys its negative charge, leading to activation of the intrinsic pathway. A further restraint to spontaneous intravascular coagulation is the ability of fibrin threads formed during clotting to remove excess thrombin and thus minimize extension of the clot. In addition, a circulating α_2-globulin known as antithrombin III prevents excessive activity of thrombin.

Heparin

Heparin is a powerful anticoagulant that is produced by many cells, but especially mast cells located in tissues around the capillaries. These cells continually secrete small amounts of heparin, which diffuses into the circulation. Basophils, present in the blood, resemble mast cells and also release small amounts of heparin into the plasma.

Mast cells are particularly abundant in tissues surrounding capillaries of the lungs and, to a lesser extent, those of the liver. This is important because capillaries of the lungs and liver receive many embolic clots formed in the slowly flowing venous blood. Heparin may prevent further growth of these clots. The concentration of heparin in normal blood has been estimated to be as much as 0.01 mg dl^{-1} (Guyton, 1986). Although this is 10 to 100 times less than that achieved clinically to prevent clotting, it is probably sufficient to be physiologically active (see Chapter 27). Conversely, platelet factor released from aggregated platelets during coagulation subsequently binds to and neutralizes endogenous heparin (Okuno and Crockatt, 1977). This neutralization of heparin may facilitate the local accumulation of thrombin and subsequent clot formation.

In addition to a possible effect on coagulation, heparin may bind histamine and serotonin, which are released endogenously. This binding is possible by virtue of the strong negative charge of heparin. It is of interest that heparin is released with histamine during allergic reactions.

Lysis of Blood Clots

Plasma proteins include a euglobulin known as *plasminogen*, which, when activated, becomes plasmin. Plasmin is a proteolytic enzyme that digests fibrin threads, causing lysis of clots. In addition, plasmin causes destruction of clotting factors such as factors I, II, V, VIII, and XII. As a result, lysis of clots may also be associated with hypocoagulability of the blood.

Tissues and blood contain substances, including (1) thrombin, (2) activated factor XII, (3) lysosomal enzymes from damaged tissues, and (4) factors from the vascular endothelium that can convert plasminogen to plasmin (Guyton, 1986). After 24 to 48 hours, blood that has leaked into tissues and clotted is dissolved by activation of plasminogen. Likewise, clots in blood vessels undergo lysis. This lysis, however, occurs more readily in small vessels than in large vessels. Indeed, the greatest importance of the fibrinolysin system is likely to be removal of minute clots from the millions of small peripheral vessels that otherwise would become occluded. Conversely, opening of large blood vessels by this process, rarely occurs.

Urokinase is an activator substance that is believed to be important in the lysis of clots that develop in the renal tubules. Streptokinase is released by streptococci, resulting in formation of plasmin from plasminogen and enhanced spread of the infection.

Thromboembolism

A thrombus is an abnormal clot that develops in a blood vessel, whereas an embolus is a fragment that breaks away from this clot. Typically, an embolus lodges at a site of vascular narrowing. For this reason, an embolus originating in an artery usually occludes a more distal and smaller artery. Conversely, an embolus originating in a vein commonly lodges in the lungs, causing pulmonary vascular obstruction.

Thromboembolism is likely to occur in the presence of (1) any condition that causes a roughened endothelial vessel wall, such as arteriosclerosis, infection, or trauma, and (2) a slowing of blood flow. Slow blood flow interferes with the normal dilution of procoagulants in the blood, resulting in an increased likelihood that localized clotting will occur. Indeed, vascular stasis in leg veins associated with postoperative immobility is a common precipitating event for formation of a venous thrombus and subsequent pulmonary embolism.

Disseminated Intravascular Coagulation

Disseminated intravascular coagulation is characterized by widespread activation of the coagulation process. A common cause of this activation is bacterial endotoxins. This generalized clotting consumes so many of the clotting factors that spontaneous hemorrhage often accompanies disseminated intravascular coagulation.

REFERENCES

Goldsmith HL. Blood flow and thrombosis. Thromb Diath Haemorrh 1974;32:35–48.

Guyton AC. Textbook of Medical Physiology, 7th ed. Philadelphia: WB Saunders, 1986:76.

McNiece WL. Disorders of coagulation. In: Stoelting RK, Dierdorf SF. Anesthesia and Co-Existing Disease. New York: Churchill Livingstone, 1983:541.

Okuno T, Crockatt D. Platelet factor 4 activity and thromboembolic episodes. Am J Clin Pathol 1977; 67:351–7.

Ratnoff OD. Some recent advances in the study of hemostasis. Circ Res 1974;35:1–14.

Suttie JW, Jackson CM. Prothrombin structure, activation and biosynthesis. Physiol Rev 1977;57:1–70.

Wall RT, Harker LA. The endothelium and thrombosis. Annu Rev Med 1980;31:361–71.

Metabolism of Nutrients

INTRODUCTION

Metabolism of carbohydrates, lipids, and proteins in cells is directed toward oxidation of these nutrients and the subsequent synthesis of adenosine triphosphate (ATP) (Fig. 58-1). ATP is present everywhere in the cytoplasm and nucleoplasm. Energy necessary for essentially all physiologic processes and chemical reactions is derived from the high phosphate bonds of ATP. Probably the most important intracellular process that requires energy from ATP is formation of peptide linkages between amino acids during the synthesis of proteins. Skeletal muscle contraction cannot occur without energy from ATP. ATP from metabolism of nutrients is necessary to provide energy for transport of ions across cell membranes and thus maintain the distribution of these ions, which is necessary for propagation of nerve impulses. In renal tubules, as much as 80% of ATP is used for membrane transport of ions.

METABOLISM OF CARBOHYDRATES

At least 99% of all the energy derived from carbohydrates is used to form ATP in the cells (Guyton, 1986a). The final products of carbohydrate digestion in the gastrointestinal tract are glucose, fructose, and galactose. After absorption into the circulation, fructose and galactose are rapidly converted to glucose. As a result, glucose becomes the predominant form of carbohydrate delivered to cells.

Transport of Glucose into Cells

Glucose must be transported through cell membranes into cellular cytoplasm before it can be used by cells (Lund-Andersen, 1979). The molecular weight of glucose is 180, which exceeds the maximal molecular weight of substances that can diffuse through channels (*i.e.,* pores) in cell membranes. Instead, glucose is actively transported to the interior of cells using protein carrier molecules by a process known as *carrier-mediated diffusion* (see Chapter 39). Carrier-mediated diffusion can transport glucose into or out of cells only in the direction from a higher concentration to a lower concentration. This diffusion mechanism differs from the transport of glucose through the gastrointestinal mucosa and renal tubules, where active transport of sodium provides the energy for absorbing glucose against a concentration gradient (*i.e.,* sodium cotransport) (see Chapter 39).

The rate of carrier-mediated diffusion of glucose is enhanced by insulin. Indeed, except for the liver and brain, the amount of glucose that can enter cells in the absence of insulin is too little to supply energy needs.

Immediately upon entering cells, glucose is converted to glucose-6-phosphate under the influence of the enzyme glucokinase. This phosphorylation of glucose prevents escape of glucose from cells back into the circulation.

The fetus derives almost all of its energy from glucose obtained by means of the maternal circu-

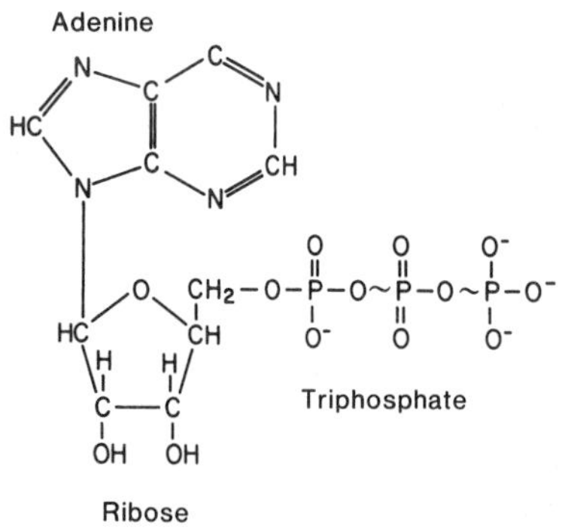

FIGURE 58-1. Metabolism of nutrients in cells is directed toward the ultimate synthesis of adenosine triphosphate (ATP). Energy necessary for physiologic processes and chemical reactions is derived from the high phosphate bonds of ATP.

lation. Immediately after birth, the infant's stores of glycogen are sufficient to supply adequate glucose for only a few hours. Furthermore, gluconeogenesis is limited in the newborn. As a result, the newborn infant may be vulnerable to hypoglycemia.

Storage of Glucose as Glycogen

After entering cells, glucose can be used immediately for release of energy to cells, or it can be stored as a polymer of glucose known as *glycogen* (Hems and Whitton, 1980). Although all cells can store at least some glucose as glycogen, the liver and skeletal muscles are particularly capable of storing large amounts of glycogen. The ability to form glycogen makes it possible to store substantial quantities of carbohydrates without significantly altering the osmotic pressure of intracellular fluids.

Gluconeogenesis

Gluconeogenesis is the formation of glucose from amino acids and the glycerol portion of fat. This process occurs when body stores of carbohydrates decrease below normal levels. An estimated 60% of the amino acids in the body's proteins can be converted easily to carbohydrates, whereas the remaining 40% have chemical configurations that make this difficult.

Gluconeogenesis is stimulated by hypoglycemia. In addition, simultaneous release of cortisol mobilizes proteins, making these available in the form of amino acids for gluconeogenesis, especially in the liver. Thyroxine is also capable of increasing the rate of gluconeogenesis.

Release of Energy from Glucose

Glucose is progressively broken down, and the resulting energy is used to form ATP. For each mole of glucose that is utilized by cells, a total of 38 moles of ATP is ultimately formed. The most important means by which energy is released from the glucose molecule is by glycolysis and the subsequent oxidation of the end products of glycolysis.

Glycolysis

Glycolysis is the splitting of the glucose molecule into two molecules of pyruvic acid. This occurs in 10 successive chemical steps, and each step is catalyzed by a specific protein enzyme. The net gain in ATP molecules by the entire glycolytic pathway is only 2 moles for each mole of glucose utilized.

Acetyl Coenzyme A

After the formation of pyruvic acid, the next step in the degradation of glucose is the conversion of pyruvic acid to acetyl coenzyme A. Coenzyme A is derived from the vitamin panothenic acid. No ATP is formed by the conversion of pyruvic acid to acetyl coenzyme A.

Citric Acid Cycle

The next step in the degradation of glucose after the formation of acetyl coenzyme A is a series of chemical reactions in which the acetyl portion of acetyl coenzyme A is converted to carbon dioxide and hydrogen ions in the citric acid cycle (same as the tricarboxylic acid cycle or Krebs cycle) (Fig. 58-2). These reactions all occur in the mitochondria. A total of 2 moles of ATP is formed by the citric acid cycle.

Oxidative Phosphorylation

Hydrogen ions released during glycolysis, during formation of acetyl coenzyme A, and in the citric

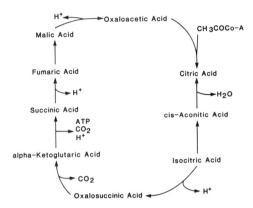

FIGURE 58-2. The acetyl portion of acetyl coenzyme A (CH_3COCo-A) is converted to ATP, carbon dioxide (CO_2), and hydrogen ions (H^+) in a sequence of chemical reactions known as the citric acid cycle.

acid cycle combine with nicotinamide adenine dinucleotide (NAD), which is a derivative of the vitamin niacin, to form NADH. This bound hydrogen can enter into oxidative chemical reactions to form large quantities of ATP (*i.e.,* oxidative phosphorylation) (Baltcheffsky and Baltcheffsky, 1974). During oxidative phosphorylation, electrons that are removed from hydrogen ions enter an electron transport chain that is an integral part of the inner membrane of the mitochondria. These electrons are transported through the electron transport chain until they reach cytochrome oxidase, where they are used to form water (Dickerson, 1980). During transport of these electrons through the electron transport chain, energy is released that is later used for the synthesis of ATP. The final step is the transfer of ATP from mitochondria back into the cytoplasm of cells. A total of 38 moles of ATP are formed for each mole of glucose that is completely degraded to carbon dioxide and water.

Anaerobic Glycolysis

In the absence of adequate amounts of oxygen, oxidative phosphorylation cannot occur. Under these circumstances, a small amount of energy can be released to cells by anaerobic glycolysis because conversion of glucose to pyruvic acid does not require oxygen. Indeed, carbohydrates are the only nutrient that can form ATP without oxygen.

Nevertheless, this is an extremely wasteful use of glucose, because only about 2% of the total energy in the glucose molecule is utilized. However, this release of glycolytic energy to the cells can be lifesaving for a few minutes when oxygen becomes unavailable.

During anaerobic glycolysis, most pyruvic acid is converted to lactic acid, which diffuses rapidly out of cells into extracellular fluid. When oxygen again becomes available, this lactic acid can be reconverted to glucose. This reconversion occurs predominantly in the liver. Indeed, severe liver disease may interfere with the ability of the liver to convert lactic acid to glucose, leading to metabolic acidosis.

The heart is particularly able to convert lactic acid to pyruvic acid for subsequent energy use. This occurs during strenuous exercise when large amounts of lactic acid are released into the circulation from skeletal muscles.

Phosphogluconate Pathway

The phosphogluconate pathway is an alternative pathway to glycolysis for the degradation and oxidation of glucose. This pathway is important because it can provide energy independently of all the enzymes in the citric acid cycle. This is uniquely important when there is an enzymatic abnormality of cells.

METABOLISM OF LIPIDS

Lipids include (1) neutral fat known as *phospholipids,* (2) cholesterol, and (3) triglycerides (Guyton, 1986b). Chemically, the basic lipid moiety of phospholipids and triglycerides is fatty acids. Fatty acids are long-chain hydrocarbon organic acids. The three fatty acids most commonly present in food and the body are (1) stearic acid, which has an 18 carbon chain and is fully saturated with hydrogen atoms, (2) oleic acid, which has an 18 carbon chain and a single double bond, and (3) palmitic acid, which has a 16 carbon chain and is fully saturated (Fig. 58-3). The basic structure of the triglyceride molecule is three long-chain fatty acids bound with one molcule of glycerol (Fig. 58-4). Cholesterol does not contain fatty acids, but its sterol nucleus is synthesized from degradation products of fatty acid molecules, thus giving it many of the physical and chemical properties characteristic of lipids (Fig. 58-5).

$$CH_3(CH_2)_{14} \overset{\overset{\text{O}}{\|}}{C}OH$$

FIGURE 58-3. Palmitic acid.

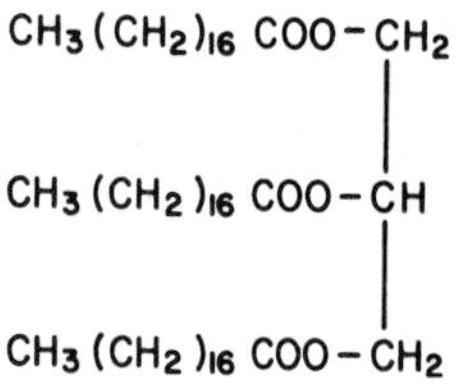

$$CH_3(CH_2)_{16} COO-CH_2$$
$$CH_3(CH_2)_{16} COO-CH$$
$$CH_3(CH_2)_{16} COO-CH_2$$

FIGURE 58-4. The basic structure of the triglyceride molecule is three long-chain fatty acids bound with one molecule of glycerol.

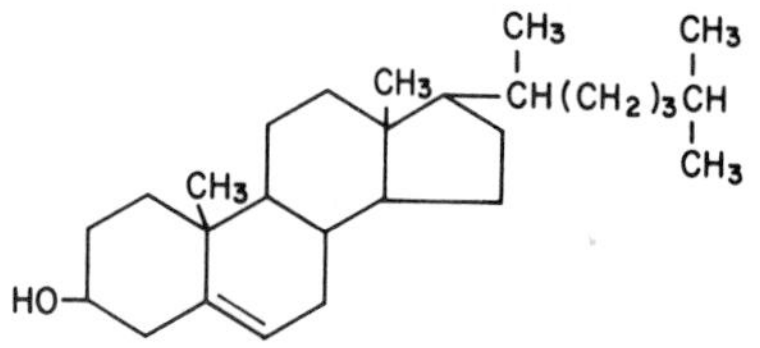

FIGURE 58-5. Cholesterol contains a sterol nucleus that is synthesized from degradation products of fatty acid molecules.

Triglycerides are used in the body mainly to provide energy for metabolic processes similar to carbohydrates. Other lipids, especially phospholipids and cholesterol, are used to provide other intracellular functions.

Transport of Lipids

Triglycerides, following absorption from the gastrointestinal tract, are transported in the lymph and then by way of the thoracic duct into the circulation in droplets known as *chylomicrons*. Most of the absorbed cholesterol and phospholipids is also transported in chylomicrons.

Following ingestion of large amounts of fat, plasma may appear turbid to yellow because of the large concentration of chylomicrons. Chylomicrons, however, are rapidly removed from the circulation and are stored as they pass through capillaries of adipose tissue and skeletal muscle. This stored fat is subsequently transported to other tissues as fatty acids combined with plasma albumin.

Fatty acids bound with albumin are called *free fatty acids,* or *nonesterified fatty acids* to distinguish them from other fatty acids in the plasma that exist in the form of esters of glycerol or cholesterol. The turnover of free fatty acids in blood is very rapid, with about one-half the plasma free fatty acids replaced by new fatty acids every 2 to 3 minutes.

Lipoprotein

In the postabsorptive state (*i.e.,* chylomicrons have been cleared from the blood), more than 95% of all lipids in plasma are lipoproteins (Jackson *et al,* 1976). Lipoproteins are synthesized principally in the liver and are mixtures of triglycerides, phospholipids, cholesterol, and proteins. Based on their densities, lipoproteins are classified as (1) very low-density, (2) low-density, (3) intermediate-density, (4) high-density, and (5) very high-density lipoproteins (see Chapter 32). The presumed function of lipoproteins is to provide a mechanism of transport for lipids throughout the body. For example, high-density lipoproteins are likely to be important for the transport of cholesterol from peripheral tissues to the liver, presumably playing a preventive role in the development of atherosclerosis. Low-density lipoproteins deliver cholesterol to the adrenal glands and skeletal muscles as well as to the liver.

Storage of Lipids

Large amounts of lipids can be stored in adipose tissue and in the liver. The major function of adipose tissue is to store triglycerides until they are needed to provide energy elsewhere in the body. A lesser function of adipose tissue is to provide heat insulation. The amount of triglycerides present in the liver is proportional to the rate at which lipids are being used for energy. Indeed, large amounts of triglycerides appear in the liver during starvation and in the presence of poorly controlled diabetes mellitus.

Phospholipids

The three major types of phospholipids in the body are (1) lecithins, (2) cephalins, and (3) sphingomyelins. About 90% of phospholipids are formed in hepatic cells. Functions of phospholipids include (1) constituents of lipoproteins, (2) formation of thromboplastin necessary for coagulation, (3) formation of sphingomyelin, which acts as an insulator in the myelin sheath around nerve fibers, and (4) formation of certain structural elements of cell membranes.

Triglycerides

The use of lipids by the body for energy is equally as important as the use of carbohydrates (Masoro, 1977). Furthermore, much of the carbohydrate ingested with each meal is converted to triglycerides for storage and subsequent use as an energy source. Nevertheless, when adequate amounts of carbohydrates are available, utilization of triglycerides for energy is greatly depressed.

The first step in the utilization of triglycerides for energy is hydrolysis into fatty acids and glycerol and subsequent transport of these products to tissues where they are oxidized. Almost all cells, except for brain cells, can use fatty acids interchangeably with glucose for energy.

Glycerol, on entering tissues, is converted by intracellular enzymes into glycerol-3-phosphate, which enters the glycolytic pathway. Degradation and oxidation of fatty acids occur only in mitochondria. The fatty acid molecule is degraded in mitochondria by progressive release of 2 carbon fragments (*i.e.,* beta-oxidation) in the form of acetyl coenzyme A. The acetyl coenzyme A molecules can enter the citric acid cycle in the same manner as acetyl coenzyme A formed from pyruvic acid during the metabolism of glucose, ultimately leading to the formation of ATP.

Formation of Acetoacetic Acid

In the liver, two molecules of acetyl coenzyme A formed from the degradation of fatty acids can combine to form acetoacetic acid (Robinson and Williamson, 1980). A substantial amount of acetoacetic acid is converted to beta-hydroxybutyric acid and minute quantities to acetone (Fig. 58-6). Acetoacetic acid and beta-hydroxybutyric acid freely diffuse from hepatic cells for transport to peripheral tissues. At peripheral tissues, these substances diffuse into cells where reverse reactions occur and acetyl coenzyme A is formed, which enters the citric acid cycle.

In the absence of adequate carbohydrate me-

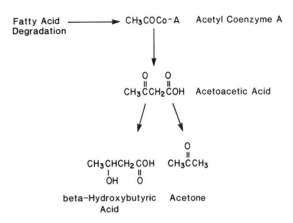

FIGURE 58-6. Fatty acid degradation in the liver leads to the formation of acetyl coenzyme A. Two molecules of acetyl coenzyme A combine to form acetoacetic acid, which, in large part, is converted to beta-hydroxybutyric acid and, in lesser amounts, to acetone.

tabolism, large quantities of acetoacetic acid, beta-hydroxybutyric acid, and acetone accumulate in the blood to produce ketosis (see Chapter 51). Indeed, when carbohydrates are not available for energy, as in starvation or uncontrolled diabetes mellitus, almost all the energy of the body must come from metabolism of lipids.

The ability of different cells of the body to store carbohydrates as glycogen is limited to only a few hundred grams. Conversely, many kilograms of lipids can be stored for subsequent energy use. Epinephrine and norepinephrine activate triglyceride lipase, which is present in cells, leading to the mobilization of fatty acids. A similar lipase enzyme is activated by cortisol and growth hormone.

Cholesterol

Cholesterol is absorbed from the gastrointestinal tract as well as being formed endogenously in the liver from acetyl coenzyme A. An intrinsic feedback control system decreases the endogenous production of cholesterol when exogenous intake is increased. As a result, the plasma concentration of cholesterol does not vary greatly.

The most important function of cholesterol is to form cholic acid in the liver. Indeed, as much as 80% of cholesterol is converted to cholic acid. A small amount of cholesterol is used by (1) the adrenal cortex to form steroids, (2) by the ovaries to form progesterone and estrogen, (3) and by the testes to form testosterone. These glands can also synthesize endogenous sterols for formation of these hormones.

METABOLISM OF PROTEINS

About 75% of the solid constituents of the body are proteins, including structural proteins, enzymes, genes, hemoglobin, and contractile elements of muscle. The principal constituents of proteins are amino acids, of which 20 are present in significant amounts and are considered essential, because they cannot be synthesized in adequate amounts endogenously (Table 58-1). Each amino acid has an acidic group (COOH) and a nitrogen radical, usually represented by an amino group (NH_2) (Fig. 58-7). In proteins, amino acids are connected into long chains by peptide linkages. Even the smallest proteins characteristically contain more than 20 amino acids combined by peptide linkages, whereas complex proteins have as many as 100,000 amino acids. In addition, more than one amino acid chain in a protein may be bound together by hydrogen bonds, hydrophobic bonds, and electrostatic forces.

Types of Proteins

Proteins exist as globular, fibrous and conjugated, or structural proteins.

Table 58-1
Amino Acids

Essential	Nonessential
Arginine	Alanine
Histidine	Asparagine
Isoleucine	Aspartic acid
Leucine	Cysteine
Lysine	Glutamic acid
Methionine	Glutamine
Phenylalanine	Glycine
Threonine	Proline
Tryptophan	Serine
Valine	Tyrosine

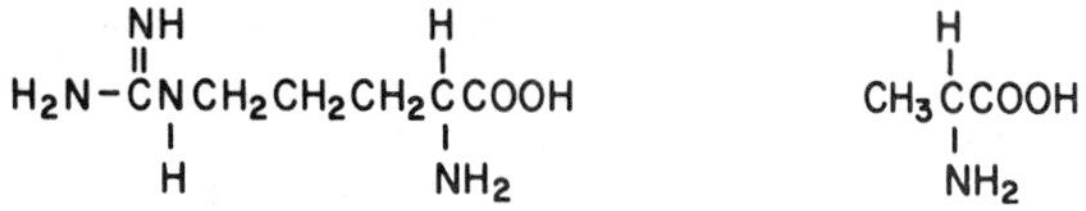

FIGURE 58-7. Examples of amino acids containing an acidic group (COOH) and an amino group (NH_2).

Globular Proteins

Most proteins of the body assume either a globular or an elliptical shape and are classified as globular proteins. Globular proteins include the proteins found in plasma, which are represented by albumin, globulin, fibrinogen, and hemoglobin. Furthermore, most of the cellular enzymes and nucleoproteins of the cell are globular proteins (see Chapter 39).

Fibrous Proteins

Fibrous proteins are characterized by elongated peptide chains that are often held together in parallel bundles by cross-linkages. Examples of fibrous proteins include collagen, which is the basic structural protein of connective tissue, tendons, cartilage, and bone. Other fibrous proteins include (1) elastic fibers of tendons and arteries, (2) keratins, which are the structural proteins of hair and nails, and (3) actin and myosin, the contractile proteins of muscle (Ross and Bornstein, 1971). In scar tissue, fibrous proteins tend to contract.

Conjugated Proteins

Examples of proteins that are conjugated with nonprotein substances (*i.e.,* conjugated proteins) include structural components of cells and mucoproteins, which are major components of all tissues and serve as a lubricant in joints (see Chapter 39). These proteins are responsible for the gel-like consistency of the vitreous humor of the eyes.

Transport of Amino Acids

Amino acids are relatively strong acids and exist in the blood principally in the ionized form. Even after a meal, the blood amino acid concentration increases only a few milligrams, reflecting rapid tissue uptake, especially by the liver. Passage of amino acids into cells requires active transport mechanisms, because these substances are too large to pass through channels in cell membranes (see Chapter 39).

In proximal renal tubules, amino acids that have entered the glomerular filtrate are actively transported back into the blood. These transport mechanisms have maximums above which amino acids appear in the urine. In the normal person, however, loss of amino acids in the urine each day is negligible.

Storage of Amino Acids

Immediately after entry into cells, amino acids are conjugated under the influence of intracellular enzymes into cellular proteins. As a result, concentrations of amino acids inside cells remain low. Indeed, storage of large amounts of amino acids does not occur, but rather, these substances are stored as actual proteins, especially in the liver, kidneys, and gastrointestinal mucosa. Nevertheless, these proteins can be rapidly decomposed again into amino acids under the influence of intracellular lysosomal digestive enzymes. The resulting amino acids can then be transported out of cells into blood to maintain optimal plasma amino acid concentrations. Tissues can synthesize new proteins from amino acids in blood. This response is especially apparent in relation to protein synthesis in cancer cells. Cancer cells are prolific users of amino acids, and, simultaneously, the proteins of the other tissues become markedly depleted.

Plasma Proteins

Plasma proteins are represented by (1) albumin, which provides colloid osmotic pressure, (2) globulins, necessary for natural and acquired immunity, and (3) fibrinogen, which polymerizes into long fibrin threads during coagulation of blood. Essentially all plasma albumin and fibrinogen and 60% to 80% of the globulins are formed in the liver. The remainder of the globulins are formed in lymphoid tissues and other cells of the reticuloendothelial system. The rate of plasma

protein formation by the liver can be greatly increased in situations such as severe burns where there is loss of large amounts of fluid and protein through denuded tissues. The rate of synthesis of plasma proteins by the liver depends on the blood concentration of amino acids. Even during starvation or severe debilitating diseases, the ratio of total tissue proteins to total plasma proteins in the body remains relatively constant at about 33 to 1 (Guyton, 1986c). Because of the reversible equilibrium between plasma proteins and other proteins of the body, one of the most effective of all therapies for severe acute protein deficiency is the intravenous administration of plasma protein. Within hours, amino acids of the administered protein become distributed throughout cells of the body to form proteins where they are needed.

Synthesis of Proteins

Proteins are synthesized in all cells, and the type formed depends on the genes of the cells (Wiessbach and Brot, 1974). The two basic steps are (1) the initial synthesis of amino acids, and (2) the subsequent appropriate conjugation of amino acids by peptide linkages to form individual proteins. Synthesis of amino acids depends first on the formation of appropriate alpha-keto acids (Truffa-Bachi and Cohen, 1973). For example, pyruvate formed during the glycolytic breakdown of glucose is the keto acid precursor of alanine. Necessary transamination of keto acids to form appropriate amino acids is regulated by transaminase enzymes, which are derivatives of the B vitamin pyridoxine. Cells of the body are able to synthesize 10 of the amino acids (nonessential amino acids), whereas the other 10 amino acids cannot be synthesized in adequate amounts and must, therefore, be supplied in the diet (essential amino acids) (Table 58-1).

Use of Proteins for Energy

After cells contain a maximal amount of protein, any additional amino acids are deaminated to keto acids that can enter the citric acid cycle to become energy or are stored as fat (Harper *et al,* 1970). Certain deaminated amino acids are similar to the breakdown products that result from glucose and fatty acid metabolism. For example, deaminated alanine is pyruvic acid, which can be converted to glucose or glycogen, or it can become acetyl coenzyme A, which is then polymerized to fatty acids. The conversion of amino acids to glucose or glycogen is gluconeogenesis, and the conversion of amino acids into fatty acids is ketogenesis.

In the absence of protein intake, about 20 to 30 g of endogenous protein are degraded into amino acids daily. In severe starvation, cellular functions deteriorate because of protein depletion. Carbohydrates and lipids spare protein stores because they are used in preference to proteins for energy.

Hormonal Regulation of Protein Metabolism

Growth hormone and insulin promote the rate of synthesis of cellular proteins, possibly by facilitating the transfer of amino acids into cells. Glucocorticoids increase the rate of breakdown of extrahepatic proteins, thereby making increased amino acids available to the liver. This allows the liver to synthesize increased amounts of cellular proteins and plasma proteins. Testosterone increases protein deposition in tissues, particularly the contractile proteins of skeletal muscles.

REFERENCES

Baltcheffsky H, Baltcheffsky M. Electron transport phosphorylation. Annu Rev Biochem 1974;43:871–97.

Dickerson RE. Cytochrome C and the evolution of energy metabolism. Sci Am 1980;242:136–53.

Guyton AC. Textbook of Medical Physiology, 7th ed. Philadelphia: WB Saunders, 1986a:808.

Guyton AC. Textbook of Medical Physiology, 7th ed. Philadelphia: WB Saunders, 1986b:818.

Guyton AC. Textbook of Medical Physiology, 7th ed. Philadelphia: WB Saunders, 1986c:829.

Harper AE, Benevenga NJ, Wohlhueter RM. Effects of ingestion of disproportionate amounts of amino acids. Physiol Rev 1970;50:428–558.

Hems DA, Whitton PD. Control of hepatic glycogenolysis. Physiol Rev 1980;60:1–50.

Jackson RL, Morrisett JD, Gotto AM. Lipoprotein structure and metabolism. Physiol Rev 1976;56:259–316.

Lund-Anderson H. Transport of glucose from blood to brain. Physiol Rev 1979;59:305–52.

Masoro EJ. Lipids and lipid metabolism. Annu Rev Physiol 1977;39:301–21.

Robinson AM, Williamson DH. Physiological roles of ketone bodies as substances and signals in mammalial tissues. Physiol Rev 1980;60:143–87.

Ross R, Bornstein P. Elastic fibers in the body. Sci Am 1971;224:44–52.

Truffa-Bachi P, Cohen GN. Amino acid metabolism. Annu Rev Biochem 1973;42:113–34.

Wiessbach H, Brot N. The role of protein factors in the biosynthesis of proteins. Cell 1974;2:137–44.

Drug Index

Drugs are listed by generic name
followed by trade name(s) in
parentheses.

Subject Index

Numbers followed by an *f* indicate a figure; *t* following a page number indicates tabular material. For listing of trade names corresponding to generic drug names, see Drug Index.